The Haemolytic Anaemias

VOLUME 2

The Hereditary Haemolytic Anaemias

PART 2

The Haemolytic Anaemias
VOLUME 2

The Hereditary Haemolytic Anaemias
PART 2

Sir John Dacie

MD (Lond) FRCP(Lond) FRCPath FRS
Emeritus Professor of Haematology,
University of London, Royal Postgraduate
Medical School, London

THIRD EDITION

CHURCHILL LIVINGSTONE
EDINBURGH LONDON MELBOURNE AND NEW YORK 1988

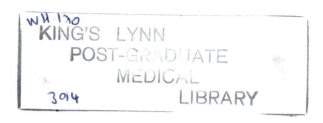
CHURCHILL LIVINGSTONE
Medical Division of Longman Group UK Limited

Distributed in the United States of America by Churchill
Livingstone Inc., 1560 Broadway, New York, N.Y. 10036,
and by associated companies, branches and representatives
throughout the world.

First edition 1954
Second edition 1960
Third edition 1988

ISBN 0-443-03242-4

British Library Cataloging in Publication Data
Dacie, *Sir* John V.
  The haemolytic anaemias. — 3rd ed.
  Vol. 2: The hereditary haemolytic anaemias.
  Part 2
  1. Hemolytic anaemia
  I. Title.
  616.1′52   RC641.7.H4

Library of Congress Cataloging in Publication Data
(Revised for volume 2)
Dacie, John V. (John Vivian)
  Haemolytic anaemias.
  Contents: v. 1-   .The hereditary haemolytic
anaemias.
  1. Hemolytic anemia — Collected works I. Title.
[DNLM: 1. Anemia, Hemolytic. WH 170 D118h]
RC641.7.H4D33 1985   616.1′52   84–5849

Printed and bound in Great Britain
at The Bath Press, Avon

Preface

The advances in understanding of the medical significance of the abnormal haemoglobins and thalassaemia that have taken place in recent years are at least as remarkable and exciting as any that have occurred in the whole field of medicine. The contrast between what is now known and what was known in the early 1950s when I wrote the chapters on 'sickle-cell disease and allied syndromes' and on 'Mediterranean anaemia and allied disorders' which were included in the first (1954) edition of *The Haemolytic Anaemias* could scarcely be greater. In the early 1950s only haemoglobins S, C and D had been discovered and almost nothing was known of the nature of thalassaemia.

In the present volume I have attempted to describe in chronological order what has been discovered and by whom in much the same way as I tried to do when writing the relevant chapters in the book's earlier editions. The amount of information now available and its complexity have made this task an almost superhuman one, but I hope I have done justice to those who have made the most important contributions. The interest of the subject and its importance in medical science and practice is such that I believe that a strong case could be made out for the writing of a fully comprehensive and definitive history of the subject. I wish I had had the time, knowledge and resources to have attempted to do this.

I am most grateful to friends and colleagues, and their publishers, who have generously allowed me to reproduce previously published illustrations which seem to me to have been of particular significance in the history of the development of knowledge of the subject. I am also grateful to colleagues who have allowed me to reproduce hitherto unpublished illustrations and to Dr Adrian Stephens and Dr Wanchai Wanachiwanawin who have provided me with blood films for photography. A list of the above-mentioned illustrations and my sincere acknowledgement to authors and publishers follow in a separate section. The photomicrographs new to this edition were taken for me by Mr W. F. Hinkes at the Royal Postgraduate Medical School and I am most grateful to him for his expertise.

The whole of the work has been typed and retyped by my wife whose skill and patience have been indispensable. I am indebted to Professor Lucio Luzzatto for helpful discussions and to the library staff at the Royal Postgraduate Medical School and the Royal Society of Medicine for their ready help, to Miss Eleanor Lloyd and Mrs Sylvia Barnes for help with photocopying, and to Mr John Hopwood of St Bartholomew's Hospital Medical College and Mr D. Simmonds of the Royal Postgraduate Medical School for the reproduction of certain illustrations. The staff of Churchill Livingstone have, too, been unfailingly helpful.

London, 1988   John Dacie

Acknowledgements

I am greatly indebted to the following authors and publishers of the journals cited for permission to reproduce the illustrations referred to below.

Chapter 11. Fig. 11.2: Professor L. Pauling and The American Association for the Advancement of Science (*Science*, **110**, 543, 1949). Fig. 11.3: Professor H. Lehmann and Blackwell Scientific Publications. Fig. 11.4: Dr Konotey-Ahulu. Fig. 11.5: Dr H. A. Pearson and the C. V. Mosby Company (*J. Pediat.*, **89**, 205, 1976). Fig. 11.6: Dr G. R. Serjeant and the British Medical Journal (*Brit. med. J.*, **285**, 633, 1982). Figs. 11.7, 11.8 and 11.9: Dr P. J. Milner and Grune & Stratton Inc. (*Blood*, **60**, 1411, 1982). Fig. 11.10: Dr J. E. Dacie. Fig. 11.11: Drs D. S. Gillett and R. S. Mibashan. Fig. 11.12: Dr G. R. Serjeant and Oxford University Press. Fig. 11.13: Dr J. F. Desforges and W. B. Saunders Co. (*Med. Clin. N. Amer.*, **50**, 1519, 1966). Fig. 11.14: Dr G. R. Serjeant and Churchill Livingstone. Fig. 11.15: Dr Konotey-Ahulu. Fig. 11.16: Dr J. E. Dacie. Fig. 11.17: Dr Konotey-Ahulu. Fig. 11.18: Dr J. E. Dacie. Fig. 11.19: Dr G. Honig and C. V. Mosby Company (*J. Pediat.*, **80**, 235, 1972).

Chapter 12. Figs. 12.1 and 12.2 and 12.6: Dr G. R. Serjeant and Blackwell Scientific Publications (*Brit. J. Haemat.*, **48**, 533, 1981). Figs. 12.3 and 12.4: Dr G. R. Serjeant and Oxford University Press. Fig. 12.5: Dr I. Schulman and Pediatrics (*Pediatrics*, **25**, 629, 1960). Fig. 12.7: Dr G. R. Serjeant and the New England Journal of Medicine (*New Engl. J. Med.*, **306**, 1441, 1982). Fig. 12.14: Dr E. Schwartz and Blackwell Scientific Publications (*Brit. J. Haemat.*, **44**, 547, 1980). Fig. 12.15: Dr G. R. Serjeant and Blackwell Scientific Publications (*Brit. J. Haemat.*, **52**,

455, 1982). Fig. 12.16: Dr H. Chaplin and the C. V. Mosby Company (*J. Lab. clin. Med.*, **88**, 546, 1976). Fig. 12.17: Dr O. Castro and the New England Journal of Medicine (*New Engl. J. Med.*, **308**, 527, 1983). Fig. 12.18: Dr A. Motulsky and the C. V. Mosby Company (*J. Lab. clin. Med.*, **35**, 721, 1950). Fig. 12.19: Dr U. M. Saarinen and Grune & Stratton Inc. (*Blood*, **67**, 1411, 1986). Figs. 12.20 and 12.21: Dr D. Hammond and the Annals of the New York Academy of Sciences (*Ann. N.Y. Acad. Sci.*, **149**, 516, 1968). Fig. 12.24: Professor M. Bessis and Springer Verlag.

Chapter 13. Figs. 13.1, 13.3, 13.6, 13.7 and 13.10: Dr G. R. Serjeant and Oxford University Press. Figs. 13.4, 13.12 and 13.13: Dr G. R. Serjeant and Blackwell Scientific Publications (*Brit. J. Haemat.*, **60**, 279, 1985). Fig. 13.5: Dr G. R. Serjeant and the New England Journal of Medicine (*New Engl. J. Med.*, **306**, 1441, 1982). Fig. 13.8: Dr C. T. Noguchi and the American Society for Clinical Investigation (*J. clin. Invest.*, **75**, 1632, 1985). Fig. 13.9: Dr S. H. Embury and the C. V. Mosby Company (*J. Lab. clin. Med.*, **106**, 75, 1985).

Chapter 14. Fig. 14.1: Dr T. Asakura and the C. V. Mosby Company (*J. Lab. clin. Med.*, **104**, 987, 1984). Figs. 14.2 and 14.3: Dr J. W. Harris and the Society of Experimental Biology and Medicine (*Proc. Soc. exp. Biol. Med.*, **75**, 197, 1950). Figs. 14.4 and 14.5: Dr M. Murayama and the American Association for Clinical Chemistry (*Clin. Chem.*, **14**, 578, 1967). Figs. 14.6 and 14.7: Professor S. Edelstein and Macmillan Magazines Limited [*Nature* (*Lond.*), **272**, 506, 1978]. Fig. 14.8: Dr J. G. White. Fig. 14.9: Dr S. B. Shohet and Grune & Stratton Inc. (*Blood*, **47**, 121,

1976). Fig. 14.10: Dr H. S. Jacob and Macmillan Magazines Limited [*Nature (Lond.)*, **246**, 105, 1973]. Fig. 14.11: Dr G. P. Rodgers and the New England Journal of Medicine (*New Engl. J. Med.*, **311**, 1534, 1984).

Chapter 15. Fig. 15.1: Dr D. L. Solanki and the British Medical Journal (*Brit. med. J.*, **287**, 725, 1983). Fig. 15.2: Dr W. C. Mentzer and Grune & Stratton Inc. (*Blood*, **64**, 161, 1984). Figs. 15.3 and 15.4: Dr F. L. Johnson and the New England Journal of Medicine (*New Engl. J. Med.*, **311**, 780, 1984).

Chapter 16. Figs. 16.1 and 16.8: Professor H. Lehmann and Blackwell Scientific Publications. Fig. 16.5: Dr C. L. Conley and Williams & Wilkins [*Medicine (Baltimore)*, **43**, 785, 1964]. Fig. 16.6: Dr R. E. Hirsch and Grune & Stratton Inc. (*Blood*, **66**, 775, 1985). Fig. 16.9: Dr P. Wasi and Baillière Tindall, W. B. Saunders Co. (*Clinics Haemat.*, **10**, 707, 1981).

Chapter 17. Figs. 17.2, 17.6, 17.7 and 17.13: Blackwell Scientific Publications (*Brit. J. Haemat.*, **10**, 388, 1964). Figs. 17.14, 17.15 and 17.16: Dr S. Shibata and the Kawasaki Medical Journal (*Kawasaki med. J.*, **9**, 205, 1983). Fig. 17.17: Professor J. M. White. Fig. 17.18: Dr H. Jacob (*Proc. natl. Acad. Sci. U.S.A.*, **65**, 697, 1970).

Chapter 18. Fig. 18.1: Dr E. Letsky. Fig. 18.4: Professor E. Kleihauer and Springer Verlag (*Blut*, **4**, 241, 1958). Figs. 18.6 and 18.7: Dr J. E. Dacie. Figs. 18.9, 18.10 and 18.11: Sir David Weatherall. Figs. 18.16 and 18.17: Professor S. N. Wickramasinghe and Blackwell Scientific Publications (*Clin. lab. Haemat.*, **7**, 353, 1985).

Chapter 19. Figs. 19.1 and 19.2: Blackwell Scientific Publications (*Brit. J. Haemat.*, **5**, 245, 1959). Fig. 19.3: Professor Ph. Fessas and Grune & Stratton Inc. (*Blood*, **21**, 21, 1963). Figs. 19.5 and 19.6: Professor S. N. Wickramasinghe and Akadémiai Kiadó (*Haematologia*, **17**, 35, 1984). Fig. 19.7: Sir David Weatherall.

Chapter 20. Fig. 20.1: Blackwell Scientific Publications (*Brit. J. Haemat.*, **12**, 44, 1966).

Contents of Volume 2

Contents of Volume 1

Forthcoming volumes:

Volume 3. **The Immune Haemolytic Anaemias**

Volume 4. **The Non-immune Acquired Haemolytic Anaemias**

Sickle-cell disease I: history, genetics and geographical distribution of haemoglobin S; clinical aspects of sickle-cell trait and homozygous sickle-cell disease

The present Chapter and the six that follow are concerned with the haemoglobinopathies in which there is evidence for a shortening of the life-span of the erythrocyte, with particular reference to the history of their discovery, the clinical consequences and the haematological and other laboratory findings, their pathogenesis and possible modes of treatment. The biochemical, molecular-biological, genetical and anthropological aspects of the subject are discussed more briefly. The sickle-cell disease syndromes are dealt with in this Chapter and in Chapters 12–15 and the haemoglobins other than Hb S associated with increased haemolysis in Chapters 16 and 17. The thalassaemia syndromes are dealt with in Chapters 18–20.

HISTORY

On the 5th of May 1910, Dr. James B. Herrick, a professor of medicine at the University of Michigan, gave a paper at the Annual Meeting of the Association of American Physicians entitled 'Peculiar elongated and sickle-shaped red blood corpuscles in a case of severe anemia' in which were described many of the more characteristic haematological and clinical findings of what became later to be known as sickle-cell anaemia (Herrick, 1910a,b). Although the sickle-shaped erythrocytes in the blood of his patient (a male black from the West Indies then aged 20) were well illustrated by photomicrographs (Fig. 11.1),

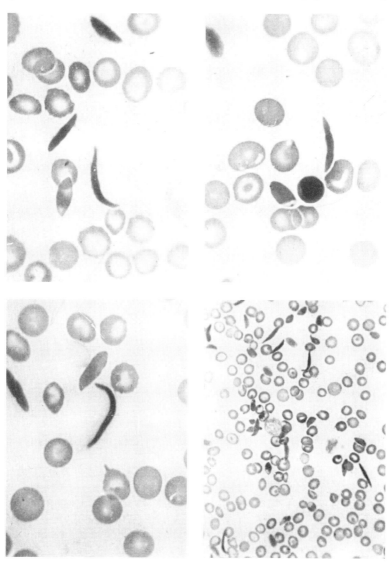

Fig. 11.1 Reproduction of the first published illustration of sickle cells.
[From Herrick (1910a,b).]

the development of sickling *in vitro* was not described until Emmel, studying the blood of a patient whose clinical history was described by Cook and Meyer (1915), noticed (as reported by Cook and Meyer) that the erythrocytes of the patient, and of his father and a sister, developed long, sharp projections when sealed preparations of blood were allowed to stand undisturbed at room temperature for several days. In 1917 Emmel published a full description of his observations on the development of sickle-shaped cells when the blood of these patients was 'cultured' *in vitro*.

In 1922 Mason introduced the term 'sickle-cell anemia' and suggested that the disease might be confined to the negro race. In 1923 Huck showed that the sickling phenomenon was unquestionably inherited, and an analysis of the data by Taliaferro and Huck (1923) indicated that the inheritance was probably controlled by a single dominant non-sex-linked abnormal gene. Out of 23 children in a single family, born of matings between presumed heterozygotes and normal subjects, 11 were normal, 11 showed sickling and one was untested.

Full clinical accounts soon followed. Sydenstricker's (1924) paper is particularly noteworthy: 'active' and 'latent' phases of the disease were recognized and the anaemia was attributed to excessive blood destruction resulting from the sickling phenomenon. The blood changes were described in detail. The previous year Sydenstricker, Mulherin and Houseal (1923) had reported on the post-mortem findings in two cases. They also tested the blood of a large number of white and black subjects for sickling and concluded that sickle-cell anaemia was a familial disease which only affected blacks.

Subsequent discoveries of seminal significance include those of Hahn and Gillespie (1927), who showed that sickling develops as the result of a fall in the partial pressure of oxygen, and Sherman (1940) who reported (without interpretation) that under the polarizing microscope sickled cells showed a definite birefringence which disappeared after the cells were aerated and had assumed the normal discoid form. Nine years later came the publication in November 1949 in the journal *Science* of a paper by Pauling, Itano, Singer and Wells, based on communications given in April 1949 to the National Academy of Sciences in Washington and to the American Society of Biological Chemists in Detroit, in which they presented evidence that sickling of erythrocytes in the sickle-cell trait (sicklemia) or sickle-cell anaemia is associated with the presence of molecules of a 'defective' haemoglobin which they referred to as 'sickle cell anemia hemoglobin' (Fig. 11.2). 'Sicklemia' erythrocytes were found to contain 40% of the defective haemoglobin and sickle-cell anaemia erythrocytes 100%. Later, Pauling and his co-workers (1950) reported that they had examined the haemoglobin of 25 individuals with the sickle-cell trait and found that the

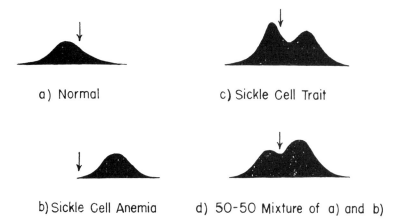

a) Normal

c) Sickle Cell Trait

b) Sickle Cell Anemia

d) 50-50 Mixture of a) and b)

Fig. 11.2 Scanning diagrams of carbonmonoxyhaemoglobins in phosphate buffer at 0.1 ionic strength and pH 6.9 after 20 hours' electrophoresis in a modified Tiselius apparatus.
[Reproduced by permission from Pauling, Itano, Singer and Wells (1949).]

amount of 'sickle cell anemia hemoglobin' present ranged from 25 to 44%. From these momentous discoveries has stemmed a new discipline, molecular genetics; more directly, they led to the recognition that sickle-cell anaemia is a disease of molecules, a 'molecular' disease, and provided an explanation for many of its puzzling laboratory features. They led, too, to the eventual recognition that a whole host of abnormal types of human haemoglobin exist and that some of the molecular variants are of major clinical importance.

The history of the gradual build-up of knowledge of sickle-cell anaemia and the abnormal haemoglobins has been dealt with in many reviews. An excellent recent one is that of Conley (1980).

The background of the discovery, referred to above, that the sickling phenomenon is associated with the presence of an abnormal haemoglobin makes a fascinating story. Credit for interesting Linus Pauling, a distinguished chemist, in the intriguing problems of sickle-cell anaemia and sickling belongs to W. B. Castle, then Professor of Medicine at Harvard, who called Pauling's attention to Sherman's discovery, published in 1940, that sickled erythrocytes exhibited birefringence in polarized light. Conley (1980) gives details of the relevant conversation, recalled by both Castle and Pauling, that took place between them whilst they were travelling in the overnight train between Denver and Chicago in 1945 [see also Strauss (1964)]. Brecher (1981) discusses who deserves the most credit for making what has turned out to be one of the most important and seminal discoveries of the present century in the field of medical science: Pauling or Itano, Singer and Wells (or Castle)?

The review of Bessis and Delpech (1982), described as a historical annotation, is remarkable and valuable because it comprises in the form of abstracts of papers and illustrations a chronological history of the evolution of knowledge of sickle-cell disease in man and of Hb S and the sickling phenomenon. Bessis and Delpech appended a minimal commentary of which the following is an extract: 'We have included many articles containing "firsts" in discovery, even if they have been quoted only rarely in historical reviews. We have sought out these previously neglected fore-runners who have been proven right in the course of time. We have also made reference to authors who were wrong or who did not fully appreciate the significance of their own observations.' Bessis and Delpech do not attempt to provide solutions to debatable questions of priority; in this connection they referred to a previous essay (Bessis and Delpech, 1981) which should be read in conjunction with their later review.

Sickle-cell anaemia before Herrick

In an interesting letter to the *Lancet*, Serjeant and Serjeant (1972) made some suggestions as to why sickle-cell anaemia had not been recognized previously. This was, in their view, because cardinal symptoms of the disease — the leg ulceration, rheumatism and jaundice — were features which were common in medical practice in the tropics and because the characteristic blood picture had remained unnoticed because blood films were not then commonly looked at. [This is understandable in Africa in the early 1900s but less readily so in North America.]

Serjeant and Serjeant were, however, able to unearth two 19th-century records in the American literature of blacks who, giving a history compatible with that of sickle-cell anaemia, were both found to lack a spleen at necropsy, a sign strongly suggesting that they had in fact had sickle-cell anaemia.

According to Konotey-Ahulu (1968) sickle-cell anaemia had been recognized in Ghana for centuries and had received a variety of tribal names. In the case of neighbouring Nigeria, however, this does not seem to be so. Onwubalili (1983) has suggested that the local (Nigerian) belief in reincarnation was based on the occurrence there of homozygous sickle-cell anaemia in certain families, with the 'reincarnate children' being born again into the same or a subsequent generation only to die young from sickle-cell anaemia, thus repeating the cycle.

THE ABNORMAL HAEMOGLOBINS

It was originally recommended that 'new' haemoglobins should be named alphabetically in the order of their discovery (Hematology Study Section, National Institutes of Health, 1953). However, haemoglobin S (Hb S) was retained to describe sickle-cell haemoglobin, rather than haemoglobin B, and haemoglobin F (Hb F) retained for fetal haemoglobin. Normal adult haemoglobin was referred to as haemoglobin A (Hb A).

Haemoglobin C (Hb C) was described by Itano and Neel in 1950 and haemoglobin D (Hb D) by Itano in 1951. Haemoglobin E (Hb E) was described independently in 1954 by Chernoff, Minnich and Chongchareonsuk and by Itano, Bergren and Sturgeon, and haemoglobin G (Hb G) by Edington and Lehmann (1954). Haemoglobins H, I, J, K, L, N, O, P and Q were subsequently discovered and named.

It soon became clear, however, that the alphabetical system of naming abnormal haemoglobins would have to be abandoned. One reason was that the same letter was being allotted to more than one type of haemoglobin as the result of discoveries being made more or less simultaneously in different parts of the world; another reason was that it seemed clear that all the available letters would soon be used up! These considerations led to 'new' haemoglobins being named after localities (*British Medical Journal*, 1960; *International Society of Haematology*, 1965), *e.g.*, after the town, city, county or hospital in which the bearer of the haemoglobin lived or was studied, *e.g.*, Hb Galveston (Schneider and Haggard, 1957), Hb Norfolk (Ager, Lehmann and Vella, 1958) and Hb Bart's (Ager and Lehmann, 1958).

The next 25 years or so have witnessed the recognition of more than 500 'new' haemoglobins, resulting from amino-acid substitutions in one or other of the globin chains or less commonly from deletions, chain elongations or chain fusions (Stamatoyannopoulos and Nute, 1974; Lehmann and Kynoch, 1976; International Hemoglobin Information Center, 1986). It has been the application of newly developed sophisticated biochemical techniques that has enabled the abnormality in each individual variant, *e.g.*, the amino-acid substitution, to be pin-pointed. Fortunately, only a small proportion of the variants that have been identified, with the exception of those which are unstable (dealt with separately in Ch. 17), are of clinical importance.

THE HAEMOGLOBIN MOLECULE

Some information on the chemical nature of the human haemoglobin molecule is necessary for an understanding of the abnormal haemoglobins. A short summary is given below. A more detailed account is beyond the scope of this book. Full details are given in several recent monographs, *e.g.*, those of Murayama and Nalbandian (1973), Lehmann and Huntsman (1974), Bunn, Forget and Ranney (1977), Winslow and Anderson (1978), Weatherall and Clegg (1981), Lehmann and Casey (1982) and Bunn and Forget (1986).

Human haemoglobin is formed of two pairs of globin chains to each of which is attached one molecule of haem. Six variants are normally formed: three are transient embryonic haemoglobins referred to as Hb Gower 1, Hb Gower 2 and Hb Portland (see Wood, Clegg and Weatherall, 1977); Hb F is the predominant haemoglobin of fetal life, and Hb A (more than 95%) and Hb A_2 (2.5–3.5%) are the characteristic haemoglobins of adults. Hb F, although present in large amounts at birth (65–95%), is normally formed subsequently only in traces.

The individual chains formed in post-natal life are designated α, β, γ and δ. Hb A is formed of two α chains and two β chains ($\alpha_2 \beta_2$); Hb F is formed of two α chains and two γ chains ($\alpha_2 \gamma_2$), and Hb A_2 of two α chains and two δ chains ($\alpha_2 \delta_2$). The α chain is thus common to all three types of haemoglobin molecule.

The realization that normal human adult haemoglobin is formed of two chemically different polypeptide chains (originally designated A and B), and that each molecule consists of four chains, stems from the pioneer work of Rhinesmith, Schroeder and Pauling (1957). That fetal haemoglobin is formed of two chains common to adult haemoglobin and two further chemically different chains was proposed by Schroeder and Matsuda in 1958.

The α chains are formed of 141 amino-acids and the β, γ and δ chains of 146; their exact sequence is known. They are arranged in a long right-handed spiral or α-helix folded to give rise to eight long helical segments joined by short non-helical segments or corners (Lehmann and Carrell, 1969). The long segments have been named A to H and the non-helical sequences between the long segments NA, AB, CD, EF and so on to GH. (BC and DE do not exist as non-helical sequences.) Each amino-acid is numbered according to its position in its chain or alternatively in its segment of chain, *e.g.*, β^6(A3).

The four chains are associated in the form of a tetramer: the $\alpha_1\beta_1$ contact is the strongest and involves many amino-acids with many interlocking side chains; the $\alpha_1\beta_2$ contact is less extensive, while the contacts between like chains are relatively weak. The binding of a molecule of haem into a 'haem pocket' in each chain is vital for the oxygen-carrying capacity of the molecule and stabilizes the whole molecule. If the haem attachment is weakened, the globin chains dissociate into dimers or monomers.

Much of the knowledge summarized above stems from the X-ray and crystallographic studies on sperm-whale myoglobin and horse haemoglobin carried out by Perutz, Kendrew and Watson and their co-workers in the early 1960s (Kendrew *et al.*, 1961; Watson and Kendrew, 1961). [White and Dacie (1971) and Bunn, Forget and Ranney (1977) give additional references to pioneer work on the structure and function of the haemoglobin molecule.]

The abnormal haemoglobin variants have arisen as the result of mutations in the genes controlling the globin chains; these have led usually to the substitution of one (normal) amino-acid by another. Such substitutions, occurring in either of the α or β chains of Hb A, but more commonly in the β chain, will have a clinical effect only if they affect the function or stability of the haemoglobin molecule. Fortunately, as already mentioned, the majority of the substitutions do no harm (and are unlikely to be detected unless they affect the electrophoretic mobility of the whole molecule). No attempt will be made in this book to list all the variants that have been described. For details, the reader is referred to reviews and monographs such as those of Huisman (1963), Lehmann and Huntsman (1974), Lehmann and Kynoch (1976), Bunn, Forget and Ranney (1977) and the International Hemoglobin Information Center's (1986) list.

Nature of haemoglobin S

Almost as soon as Hb S was recognized as a distinct form of haemoglobin it was realized that the difference between it and Hb A lay in the globin part of the molecule and not in the haem (Pauling *et al.*, 1950). It was the pioneer work of Ingram (1956, 1957) which established the nature of the difference, *i.e.*, the substitution of a valine residue for a glutamic acid residue in the β chain of each half-molecule (Ingram, 1957). Hb S is thus $\alpha_2\beta_2^{6Glu\rightarrow Val}$, the substitution affecting the sixth residue (A3) in the β chain. On deoxygenation, it is the alteration in the first part of the β chain which allows interaction with adjacent α chain receptor site(s) and consequent stacking of the molecules into filaments (see p. 190).

It is now realized that rarely a globin chain may be affected by two distinct amino-acid substitutions. Hb S Travis is an example of this remarkable event; Hb C Harlem is another example (see p. 297). Hb S Travis has the same substitution as Hb S, *i.e.* $\beta6$ Glu $\rightarrow$ Val, and in addition valine is substituted for alanine ($\beta142$) (Moo-Penn *et al.*, 1977). The 6 Glu $\rightarrow$ Val mutation in Hb S Travis confers on the haemoglobin similar properties to those of Hb S, *e.g.*, sickling of erythrocytes, insolubility when reduced, and a minimum gelling concentration identical to that of Hb S. The haemoglobin has, however, some additional properties, conferred on it presumably by the $\beta142$ substitution: these are, compared to Hb S, increased O_2 affinity, decreased affinity for 2,3-DPG, increased mechanical precipitability, an increased rate of heat denaturation at 65°C, and an increased rate of auto-oxidation (methaemoglobin formation) *in vitro* at 37°C.

Literature on the abnormal haemoglobins

This is now vast in extent. In 1951, at the start of the explosion of knowledge following the discovery by Pauling, Itano, Singer and Wells, (1949) of Hb S, Margolies listed 344 relevant references in a comprehensive review on sickle-cell anaemia. Early reviews dealing with the clinical, genetical and biochemical aspects of the new knowledge include those of White (1952–53), Pauling (1953–54), White and Beaven (1954), Chernoff (1955), Itano (1955, 1956, 1957), Singer (1955), Itano, Bergren and Sturgeon (1956), Watson (1956), Zuelzer, Neel and Robinson (1956), Neel (1957), Smith (1957), Huisman (1958), Beaven and Gratzer (1959), Ingram (1959), Lehmann (1959a) and Huehns and Shooter (1965). Since these reviews many hundreds, perhaps thousands, of papers and reviews have been published as well as monographs and numerous reports of symposia. Bunn and Forget's (1986) massive book is a mine of information.

Nomenclature. In 1957 the British Medical Colonial Research Committee described as a '*haemoglobinopathy*' a condition in which the production of Hb A is partly or wholly suppressed and partly or wholly replaced by one or more haemoglobin variants which might include Hb F. The term 'disease', *e.g.* sickle-cell disease, was used to refer to any morbid condition produced by one or more haemoglobin variants in the absence of Hb A. The combination of Hb A with an abnormal haemoglobin comprised a '*trait*'. These recommendations have generally been adhered to. The term 'trait' is still used to describe the presence of an abnormal haemoglobin, in addition to normal Hb A, a combination which normally (except when the abnormal haemoglobin is unstable) produces little or no clinical effect (see Lehmann, 1966). In this Chapter Hb-S trait or Hb AS will be used as a short synonym for (heterozygous) *sickle-cell trait* and Hb-SS disease or Hb SS as a short synonym for (homozygous) *sickle-cell anaemia*. Following the suggestion of Neel (1958), in designating the genotype of heterozygotes, the first haemoglobin named is the one present in the greater quantity.

The term *sickle-cell disease* will be used to describe an illness attributable to the presence of Hb S, which might be due to homozygosity for Hb S or result from the presence of Hb S and another abnormal haemoglobin or thalassaemia. The term *sickle-cell anaemia*, without the prefix homozygous, is best avoided. In the early literature it was used quite naturally to describe any haemolytic anaemia associated with sickling, long before it was realized that some of the cases might be due to compound heterozygosity for Hb S and another abnormal haemoglobin or thalassaemia rather than due to homozygosity for Hb S.

The short notation Hb-SC disease or Hb SC will be used to describe the combination of Hb S and Hb C and Hb-S/β-thalassaemia for the combination of Hb S and β-thalassaemia, etc.

GEOGRAPHICAL DISTRIBUTION OF HAEMOGLOBIN S

The early work in America suggested that the Hb-AS trait was entirely confined to the blood of blacks. Later, however, doubts arose and Mason (1938) accepted as authentic reports of sickling in white families 'without any reasonable suspicion of admixture with negro blood'. Wintrobe (1956) listed 13 instances, mostly in Greeks, Italians and Sicilians, but added that 'ancestral negro blood can be suspected'. Margolies (1951), who referred to 30 cases, and Plachta and Speer (1952) similarly concluded that ancestral admixture with negro blood was the most likely explanation.

The distribution of Hb S in the Old World is summarized in Figure 11.3. The Hb-S trait is found throughout all tropical Africa, although its frequency varies widely amongst the African races, the maximum incidence being about 40% (Lehmann, 1954, 1984). Hb S has, too, been found in scattered loci in the countries bordering on the Mediterranean, in the Middle East and in India (see Lehmann and Cutbush, 1952; Lehmann, 1954, 1956, 1956–57, 1959a; Neel, 1957). Lie-Injo (1957) reported finding two examples of Hb AS out of 4000 blood samples tested in Indonesia: one was from an individual of mixed Chinese, Indonesian and Javanese origin, the other from a pure Indonesian.

Figures for the percentage frequency of Hb S (and of Hb C and of β-thalassaemia) in populations throughout the continents of the world were published by WHO in 1966 [Report of a WHO Scientific Group (Lehmann, Chairman)].

Lehmann and Cutbush (1952) were the first to find Hb S in India [in certain primitive pre-

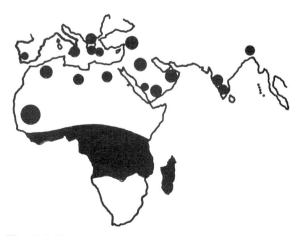

Fig. 11.3 Distribution of Hb S in the Old World.
[Redrawn from Lehmann (1959b).]

Dravidian tribes (Veddoids) living in the Nilgiri Hills in Southern India]. Subsequently, the Hb-S trait and Hb-SS disease were identified in other places in India, Assam and Ceylon (see Shukla and Solanki, 1958; Shukla, Solanki and Parande, 1958; de Silva *et al.*, 1962; Brittenham *et al.*, 1979; Kar *et al.*, 1986).

Foy, Kondi and Alexandrides (1951) described the occurrence of sickle-cell anaemia in a Greek girl living in Northern Greece. Choremis and co-workers (1951) found that the Hb-S trait was relatively frequent in certain localities in Greece (see also Veras, Démétriadès and Manios, 1953; Deliyannis and Tavlarakis, 1955a; Fessas, 1959). Dreyfus and Benyesch (1951) described its occurrence in Yemenite Jews.

Aksoy (1955, 1956) described a relatively high incidence of the trait (13.3%) in Turkey, and also Hb-SS disease in an isolated Eti-Turk community. Özsolu and Altinöz's (1977) report on Hb-SS disease in Turkey was based on 97 cases and is an indication of the relative frequency of Hb S in that country (see p. 10).

Aluoch and co-workers (1986) have more recently studied 71 Hb-SS Eti-Turk patients from South Turkey and compared their clinical, haematological and genetic findings with those of 25 black patients from Surinam, Nederlands Antilles and Kenya. The Turkish patients were found to be as severely affected as the others. Haplotyping (see p. 10), however, identified haplotype 19 as the common type in the Eti-Turks, a finding which suggests that their β^S chromosome originated from West Africa.

Recent reports of the Hb-S trait and Hb-SS disease in the Arabian peninsula include those of Gelpi and King (1976), Perrine *et al.* (1978), and Acquaye *et al.* (1985) (see also p. 49). According to El-Hazmi (1982), the trait is common in some areas although rare elsewhere, the incidence varying in five areas from <2% to 27%. White (1983) has recorded incidences of 1.3 to 5.8% in three ethnic groups. Lehmann, Maranjian and Mourant (1963) attributed the presence of Hb S in Saudi Arabia to spread from India.

Allison (1956), Walters and Lehmann (1956), Neel (1957) and Vandepitte (1959) reviewed the distribution of the trait in West Africa, and Edington (1959) stressed the frequency of Hb S

(and Hb C) in Ghana where he had found the combined incidence to be in the region of 30%. Cabannes *et al.* (1956) and Portier, Cabannes and Duzer (1959) provided data on the occurrence of Hb S (and other abnormal haemoglobins) in North Africa.

Whether the gene responsible for Hb S arose independently in the different ethnic groups referred to above or spread to each group from a common ancestor has been an intriguing problem (Neel, 1953). Lehmann (1953) suggested that Hb S was not an essentially negroid feature and that the trait had probably entered Africa from the north-east. According to Lehmann, (1956–57, 1959b), Veddoid races peopled Arabia in neolithic times, later spreading south into Africa and India, and perhaps carried the gene for Hb S with them. On the other hand, it seems highly probable that Hb S would have been imported into Southern Europe from Africa, and into the Middle East and India, too, via the slave trade (Gelpi, 1967, 1973; Gelpi and Perrine, 1973; Roth *et al.*, 1978) (see below).

The presence of Hb S in the New World is by contrast a relatively recent event; it was undoubtedly brought to the West Indies (Jelliffe, Stuart and Wills, 1954) and to North America, first in the 17th century, by the importation of slaves from West Africa. The incidence of the Hb-AS genotype in the black population in the United States was recorded as 8.3% by Diggs, Ahmann and Bibb (1933) and as 8–9% in the late 1950s, or almost 1% of the entire population (Schneider, 1956; Levin, 1958). More recent data indicate a slight lower incidence, 7–8% (Murphy, 1973), 6–14%, most likely 8% (Motulsky, 1973).

Serjeant (1981) recorded the incidence in Jamaica as 10.05%, a figure derived from screening 60 000 live births. (The incidence of the Hb-SS genotype in the same population was 0.317%).

Nature of the β^S gene and its origins

It has become apparent in recent years that the genetic change giving rise to the β^S gene has probably originated in at least three independent loci in Africa and possibly, too, independently in a locus or loci outside Africa. This new information has stemmed from the use of restriction enzymes to analyse the DNA of the β-globin gene cluster. These analyses have demonstrated not only a remarkable degree of DNA polymorphism but also the association of the β^S gene with certain haplotypes and differences between populations in these associations.

Kan and Dozy (1978, 1980) used the restriction enzyme *Hpa* 1 in the analysis of the β-globin gene region and found that while in most individuals the β-globin gene is contained in a chromosome that yields a 7.6 kb DNA fragment, in some individuals the gene is contained in a 7.0 kb fragment or a 13.0 kb fragment. Normally, in American blacks of genotype *AA* the gene is in the 7.6 kb fragment: in striking contrast, the gene bearing the Hb-S mutation was found in the great majority of those of genotype *AS* or *SS* to be in a chromosome that yields the 13.0 kb fragment. The β^C gene was found, too, to be usually carried in the 13.0 kb fragment. Since both the β^S and β^C were found to be linked to the 13.0 kb *Hpa* 1 variant, Kan and Dozy (1980) concluded that both arose separately in chromosomes containing the 13.0 kb site. In contrast to the findings in the American blacks (the great majority of whom had originated from West Africa), individuals of genotype *AS* or *SS* from Gabon, Kenya, Saudi Arabia and India were found to have their β^S genes almost without exception located in a chromosome yielding the 7.6 kb fragment. Kan and Dozy concluded that separate mutational events had produced the *same* abnormal haemoglobin in India and West Africa and that β^S genes might have arisen independently in Kenya and Saudi Arabia, too. In Africa, the high proportion of the 13.0 kb haplotype was thought to have been brought about by the β^S and β^C genes protecting against malaria (see p. 11), in contrast to the 13.0 kb haplotype containing the β^A gene which conferred no protection. Kan and Dozy suggested that the 13.0 kb mutation probably arose in Upper Volta or Ghana where the β^C gene is highly concentrated and that the β^S gene, associated with the 13.0 kb haplotype, spread from the Ghana-Nigeria area to North Africa and to Sicily and Cyprus.

Feldenzer and co-workers (1979) studied 70 Africans or Caucasians. They confirmed Kan and Dozy's (1978) observations on DNA polymorphism but found that the frequency with which the β^S gene was associated with the 13 kb fragment when the DNA was cleaved with the *Hpa* 1 enzyme (58%) was considerably less than in Kan and Dozy's series of β^S genes (87%). Twenty-nine of the individuals they studied had Hb-SS disease: 10 had the 13.0/13.0 kb genotype, 14 the 13.0/7.6 kb genotype and five the 7.6/7.6 kb genotype.

Data that supported Kan and Dozy's (1980) observations were provided by Mears *et al.* (1981b) who analysed DNA from Hb-AA, Hb-SS, Hb-SC, Hb-AS

and Hb-AC subjects from the Ivory Coast in the west and from Togo in the east of West Africa. In Togo strong linkage of the β^S gene to the 13 kb DNA fragment was demonstrated, using the *Hpa* 1 enzyme, and in the Ivory Coast almost as strong linkage to the 7.6 kb fragment. Their data were considered to be consistent with the selection and expansion of two different chromosomes bearing β^S genes in two physically close but ethnically different regions of West Africa.

Mears and co-workers (1981a) reported on a similar study carried out on 56 unrelated individuals from Algeria and Morocco, including 21 of *SS* and five of *AS* genotype. Their data indicated a very tight linkage of the β^S gene with the 13 kb *Hpa* 1 DNA fragment, strong evidence in their view that the gene had originated from West Africa rather than from Arab populations in the Middle East.

Further support for the concept of a multicentric origin of the β^S gene in Africa has been provided by Pagnier *et al.* (1983, 1984) who used eight different restriction enzymes capable of defining 11 different polymorphic sites in the β-globin gene cluster. They studied DNA obtained from 63 Hb-SS homozygotes from Senegal (in Atlantic West Africa), Benin (in central West Africa), Central African Republic and Algeria. In Benin all the chromosomes carrying the β^S gene were of identical haplotype and in the Bantu-speaking Central African Republic and in Senegal a large proportion of Hb-S-bearing chromosomes had a haplotype specific for each country, the three haplotypes differing from each other by at least three sites. The Hb-S chromosomes from Algeria were all of the Benin type (spread to Algeria probably via trans-Saharan caravan routes). Pagnier *et al.* concluded that the apparent multicentric origin of the β^S gene has important implications for the better understanding of the variable expression of Hb-SS disease and suggested that clinically relevant DNA sequences, such as those that perhaps control γ-chain expression, could be linked to specific haplotypes.

Wainscoat and co-workers (1983) studied polymorphism of the β-globin gene cluster in 244 β^S chromosomes derived from 122 Jamaican Hb-SS patients. Using five different restriction endonucleases, defining seven restriction enzyme polymorphic sites (five 5' to the β^S gene and two 3'), 12 different haplotypes were identified: 58% of the patients were homozygous for the 5' haplotype type 1. Wainscoat *et al.* concluded that their data indicated that the β^S mutation probably had multiple origins.

Antonarakis and co-workers (1984) analysed 170 β^S-bearing chromosomes derived from North-Americans of African origin: 16 different haplotypes were demonstrated. Three were particularly common (151 out of the 170 chromosomes); these three were, however, much less common in chromosomes bearing normal β^A genes (six out of 47). Antonarakis *et al.* concluded that the finding of 16 different haplotypes was best explained by (1) a number of simple recombination events 5' to the β-globin gene, and (2) by up to four independent mutations and/or interallelic gene conversions.

Further information on a possible link between haplotype and β^S gene and clinical and haematological expression has been provided by Nagel *et al.* (1984, 1985). They studied 69 patients with Hb-SS disease from Senegal, Benin and Bantu-speaking Equatorial, East and Southern Africa. Patients from Senegal were found to have relatively high Hb-F levels (with a predominance of $^G\gamma$ chains) and a low percentage of very dense cells and irreversibly sickled cells (ISCs) compared with those from Benin, who had lower Hb-F percentages (with a low percentage of $^G\gamma$ chains) and higher percentages of very dense cells and ISCs. Nagel and co-workers suggested that the low percentages of very dense cells and ISCs were probably secondary to the high levels of Hb F acting as an inhibitor of Hb-S polymerization; they pointed out that in the New World Hb S would be predominantly a mixture of the Senegal and Benin types.

Bakioglu and co-workers (1985) studied five adults with mild Hb-SS disease. They found that the patients, who came from Qatar, Turkey and South Africa, had a similar genotype, one haplotype being Type 31 and the other Type 19 (a common type in blacks and Turkish patients). All five patients had high Hb-F percentages (14.4–29.9), and it was suggested that this was the consequence of the presence of haplotype 31. One patient was also homozygous for α-thalassaemia ($-\alpha/-\alpha$); the others all had a normal α-globin genotype.

Additional observations linking haplotype 31 β^S chromosomes with high Hb-F levels were reported by Kutlar and co-workers (1985). They had studied seven Arabian patients suffering from relatively benign Hb-SS disease whose Hb-F levels fell between 21 and 34%: four were found to be homozygotes for haplotype 31 β^S chromosomes and three compound heterozygotes for haplotype 31 and haplotype 19 chromosomes. Kutlar *et al.*, emphasizing that Hb-AS heterozygotes with a haplotype 31 β^S chromosome did not have raised Hb-F levels, pointed out that the increased production of Hb F associated with haplotype 31 was likely to be a response to the presence of anaemia.

Pagnier and co-workers (1986) reported further observations on the expression of the Hb-S gene as it occurs in Bantu-speaking Africans resident in Central African Republic, Zaire and Congo. Thirty-six Hb-SS homozygotes were studied: the mean Hb-F percentage was 7.6, approximately the same as in similar patients in Benin but lower than those in Senegal; the mean $^G\gamma$ percentage was also low at 40.2. The incidence of the α-thalassaemia gene was high (40.2%).

Hattori and co-workers (1986) have reported further data on the incidence of haplotypes of β^S chromosomes in black Afro-Americans resident in Georgia. In all, 10 haplotypes were defined amongst Hb-SS patients. The most common haplotypes were those designated 19 (Benin) and 20 (Central African Republic) and the majority of the patients were genotypically 19/19 or 20/19: both groups, as well as seven 20/20 patients, were severely affected and had low Hb-F and $^G\gamma$ percentages. Haplotype 3 (Senegal) was present in 15% of chromosomes: three patients who were homozygotes (3/3) were mildly affected and had high Hb-F and $^G\gamma$ percentages. Seven patients had the A^T haplotype producing the variant $^{A}\gamma^T$ chain. This paper includes haematological and haemoglobin composition data from 83 patients (over 2 years of age), separated according to their haplotype combination (15 different genotypes in all).

INHERITANCE OF HAEMOGLOBIN S

The possibility that the sickle-cell phenomenon might be inherited was first hinted at by Emmel (1917), who observed that the blood of the father of a patient suffering from sickle-cell anaemia sickled *in vitro*. In 1923, as has already been mentioned, Taliaferro and Huck showed that sickling was inherited as a non-sex-linked dominant. It was realized by Sydenstricker (1924) that latent and active forms of sickle-cell anaemia occurred and that latent cases far outnumbered active cases. Later, the two forms became generally known as sickle-cell anaemia and (symptomless) sickle-cell trait (Cooley and Lee, 1926; Diggs, Ahmann and Bibb, 1933; Sherman, 1940).

The exact relationship between the anaemia and trait was not established until considerably later. In 1947, Neel stated: 'This [modification of Huck's original hypothesis] is that there is present in the colored population a certain factor which when heterozygous may have no discernible effects but usually results in sickling, and when homozygous tends to result in sickle cell anemia.' Proof of this hypothesis was provided by Neel (1949) when he reported that the erythrocytes of all of 42 parents of 29 patients with sickle-cell anaemia sickled. Further confirmatory data were published by Neel in 1951. Beet (1949) had independently come to the same conclusion as had Neel, based on the study of a single large family: he stated that 'sickle cell anemia occurs in homozygotes only, and that this may account for the occurrence of the anemia from time to time, for no apparent reason, in a drepanocytic population'. Large-scale family studies carried out in the Belgian Congo by the Lambotte-Legrands (1951, 1952, 1955a) and by Vandepitte (1954) provided further valuable evidence in support of the hypothesis of Neel and Beet. As will be described later, measurement of the proportion of Hb S present compared to that of Hb A in the two categories of case, sickle-cell trait and sickle-cell anaemia, when it was possible to determine this by electrophoresis of haemoglobin, also strongly favoured the hypothesis that the trait represents the heterozygous state and the anaemia the homozygous state of an inherited abnormality.

Homozygous sickle-cell anaemia is a serious disorder which even today may lead to death in childhood or prematurely in adults. Why, therefore, is the gene for Hb S so widespread, if homozygotes die abnormally frequently before reaching maturity? This was at one time the subject of much debate and speculation. It now seems clear, however, that the high incidence of the β^S gene in certain parts of the world is the consequence of a state of balanced polymorphism, with the heterozygotes having an advantage over normal and abnormal homozygotes. [The alternative possibility that the β^S gene could be maintained by fresh mutations implies a rate of mutation many times greater than other known mutation rates (Allison, 1954a, b, c; Vandepitte, 1954; J. and C. Lambotte-Legrand, 1955a; Vandepitte et al., 1955; Neel, 1957).]

As discussed below, a relative resistance to *Pl. falciparum* malaria seems to have been the most important mechanism in bringing about the persistence and high frequency of the β^S gene.

Resistance to malaria

Brain (1952) appears to have been the first to suggest in print that the erythrocytes of sicklers might offer a less favourable environment for malaria parasites than normal cells. He based this suggestion on the observation of Beet (1947), confirmed by himself, that the spleen, which he [Brain] presumed was enlarged due to malarial infection, was less frequently palpable in sicklers than in non-sicklers.

Beet (1946) had previously reported that the incidence of malaria parasites was lower in sicklers than in non-sicklers in the Balovale district of Northern Rhodesia. However, the difference in incidence between the two groups was found to be much less obvious when a similar study was carried out in another part of the country and the possible importance of his first observation seems not to have been appreciated (Beet, 1947). Unfortunately, too, Beet interpreted the finding of a reduced incidence of splenomegaly in sicklers as being due to infarction of the spleen rather than to a diminished incidence of malaria.

Raper (1949), too, had come near to suggesting that sickling might in some way protect against malaria. In discussing the higher percentage of positive sickling tests in adults (25.3%) compared with in children (16.4%), as reported from Dar es Salaam, he wrote an 'advocate might postulate that the sickling mutation established itself among negroes because at one time it was protective against parasites or other adverse conditions in the tropics'. He made, however, no direct reference to malaria.

At about the same time as the work referred to above was being carried out in East Africa, a relationship between the presence of sickling and malaria was also beginning to be appreciated in the Belgian Congo. J. and C. Lambotte-Legrand (1951) reported that the mortality rate was lower in infants who were sicklers than in non-sicklers and that, although the incidence of a variety of infections was about the same in the two groups, the mortality from malaria and the incidence of cerebral attacks were much lower in sicklers than in non-sicklers.

It was left to Allison (1954a,b,c) to provide the first definite evidence that the hypothesis that a person who was heterozygous for Hb S had an increased resistance to malaria was likely to be correct, and that the advantage applied apparently only to infection with *Pl. falciparum* (subtertian malaria).

The importance of malaria in protecting against malaria and ensuring the persistence of the β^S gene was quickly accepted (Deliyannis and Tavlarakis, 1955b; Raper, 1955, 1956; Edington and Lehmann, 1956; Lehmann and Raper, 1956; Allison 1957; Vandepitte and Delaisse, 1957; J. and C. Lambotte-Legrand, 1958; Lehmann, 1959a,c; Konotey-Ahulu, 1972a).

The sickle-cell trait occurs at its highest frequency in areas where malaria is or has been hyperendemic; this applies to its incidence in Greece (Deliyannis and Tavlarakis, 1955a) and India as well as in Africa. In North America, the incidence of the trait (about 9%)

is less than that of the trait in the areas of Africa from which the negro slaves were imported (15.4%; Allison, 1954c). This fall in incidence has, according to Allison, been brought about by the removal of the sicklers from a malarial environment. In Africa, in areas where malaria is hyperendemic, the parasite counts in children who are sicklers are lower than in non-sicklers (Allison, 1954a; Raper, 1955; Vandepitte and Delaisse, 1957). Similarly, serious complications such as cerebral malaria, blackwater fever or severe anaemia are much less frequently met with in sicklers than non-sicklers (J. and C. Lambotte-Legrand, 1952, 1958; Raper, 1956). It thus seems that the presence of Hb S, although it does not prevent malaria, limits the severity of *Pl. falciparum* infection.

It appears that the advantage conferred by the presence of Hb S is chiefly confined to young Hb-AS children before the development of immunity to malaria (Garlick, 1960). In adults exposed to experimental infections the difference in resistance is less clear cut (Beutler, Dern and Flanagan, 1955; Liachowitz *et al.*, 1958). Allison (1957) calculated that if the child mortality in Africa due to malaria was 10%, and if this was confined solely to non-sicklers, this could explain the high incidence of Hb S in Africa.

It is possible that, in addition to malaria, other factors contribute to the survival of the β^S gene (Foy *et al.*, 1955; Neel, 1957; J. and C. Lambotte-Legrand, 1958). The basis for this possibility is, however, less secure. Delbrouck (1958), nevertheless, concluded that in the Belgian Congo hyperfecundity might be more important than resistance to malaria.

Mechanism of resistance to *Pl. falciparum* infection. In an interesting letter Mackey and Vivarelli (1954) referred to the Annual Report of the Medical Laboratory for 1952 (in Tanganyika), in which they had suggested that heterozygosity for Hb S might confer advantage in respect of decreased susceptibility of a proportion of the erythrocytes to parasitization with *Pl. falciparum*. They found in an individual with the sickling trait and a severe infection that of the many cells that were parasitized very few sickled when the blood was sealed under a coverslip. They suggested that Hb S may be 'an unsuitable intracellular environment for the growth and metabolism of the trophozoite' or, alternatively, that 'parasitization of a cell containing a certain proportion of sickle-cell haemoglobin may lead to its *in vivo* sickling and phagocytosis, thus terminating the reproductive cycle in the case of the cells so invaded'.

Luzzatto, Nwachuku-Jarrett and Reddy's (1970) subsequent data supported the second expla-

nation. In Hb-AS children with acute malaria the rate at which parasitized erythrocytes sickled when their blood was incubated anaerobically was found to be 2–8 times faster than that of non-parasitized cells within the same sample. It was concluded that the presence of parasites increased the probability that a cell sickled and that, once sickled, the cell's quick removal from the circulation as the result of phagocytosis led to the life cycle of the parasite being terminated.

The recently acquired ability to grow *Pl. falciparum in vitro* in continuous culture has provided a means by which the effect of the presence of Hb S on the growth and multiplication of the parasites can be studied.

Roth and co-workers (1978a) infected Hb-AS erythrocytes with *Pl. falciparum* parasites *in vitro* and observed the rate at which the parasitized cells sickled under various degrees of deoxygenation. They compared this with the rate of sickling of uninfected Hb-AS cells. The cells that contained small ring forms sickled approximately 8 times faster than did uninfected cells. In contrast, cells containing large parasites (trophozoites or schizonts) appeared to sickle less readily — electron microscopy showed, however, that the Hb S they contained had, nevertheless, undergone polymerization.

Friedman (1978) compared the growth and multiplication of *Pl. falciparum* in AA, AS and SS erythrocytes under various oxygen tensions. At a high concentration of oxygen (18%) no sickling developed and growth was essentially the same in the three types of cells. At low concentrations of oxygen (1–5%) the SS cells sickled, the parasites were killed and most of them lysed. Under the low oxygen concentrations approximately 60% of AS cells sickled or became distorted; the parasites grew for a time but most subsequently died at the large ring stage. In contrast, the parasites in the AA cells continued to grow normally at the low oxygen tensions. Reduction in the sickling of AS erythrocytes as a result of prior exposure to sodium cyanate resulted in a reversal of protection against the growth of the parasites. Friedman concluded that resistance to parasite growth *in vivo* could be due solely to conditions within the erythrocytes engendered by the presence of Hb S. Friedman and Trager (1981) argued that it is loss of intracellular K^+ which takes place when AS erythrocytes sickle that leads to the intracellular death of the parasite. Experimentally, *in vitro*, when AS erythrocytes infected with *Pl. falciparum* were incubated in a medium containing an augmented concentration of K^+, sickling took place when the oxygen percentage was reduced to 3%; the parasites, nevertheless, survived. Friedman and Trager concluded that *in vivo* parasites develop normally in AS erythrocytes until the host cells became sequestered in the microcirculation when the low O_2 tension (and low intracellular pH associated with the presence of the parasite) together cause rapid sickling; the intracellular K^+ concentration then falls and the parasites die.

The possible role of Hb F in retarding the growth of malarial parasites is referred to later when the relative resistance of patients with β-thalassaemia to infection with *Pl. falciparum* malaria is considered.

SICKLE-CELL TRAIT (Hb AS)

Synonyms. Sickle-cell trait; Hb AS; sicklemia (Cooley and Lee, 1926); sicklemia trait (Committee for Clarification of Nomenclature, 1950).

CLINICAL FEATURES

It has generally been assumed that the presence of Hb AS is not associated with any clinical effects, and this is undoubtedly true in the great majority of instances (Sears, 1978). Nevertheless, symptoms and pathological changes have occasionally occurred that appear only to be explicable by the presence of the trait (Ende, Pizzolato and Ziskind, 1955; Singer, 1955; Levin, 1958). Haematuria is quite a common symptom and the spleen has become infarcted during flights in unpressurized aircraft, and there are a few reports of sudden collapse leading to death in which the presence of Hb AS may have played a contributory part and of intestinal or pulmonary infarction. Ulceration of the leg has also been described.

Haematuria. In 1950, Goodwin, Alston and Semans described a series of black Americans whose blood sickled and who had developed unexplained unilateral haematuria. Four of the patients were considered to have the sickle-cell trait. Similar cases were reported by Chapman *et al.* (1954) and Lund, Cordonnier and Forbes (1954). Goldman, Chapman and Cross (1955) investigated six patients with Hb AS who had had haematuria on several or 'innumerable' occasions. No urological cause could be found and in six of the patients it was noted at the time of investigation that the bleeding was confined to one kidney.

Mostofi, Vorder Bruegge and Diggs (1957) studied the pathology of kidneys removed from 22 young black patients thought to have Hb AS. Severe congestion with focal medullary and papillary haemorrhages and areas of necrosis, repair and regeneration (micro-infarcts) were demonstrated. In a review of the literature they referred to 58 patients; they stressed that the bleeding may be unilateral and that nephrectomy should be avoided. Further patients with Hb AS and gross haematuria were reported by Crone *et al.* (1957) and Lucas and Bullock (1960). Knochel (1969) observed improvement in two patients with long-standing haematuria following intravenous infusions of alkalis or distilled water. The effect of the latter was attributed to expansion of the erythrocyte volume and dilution of the Hb S.

The pathological lesions described above presumably follow sickling of the erythrocytes. This means that a major degree of oxygen unsaturation must occur somewhere in the renal circulation. Whether this can happen in a strictly normal kidney is uncertain; possibly ptosis of the kidney or other mechanism leading to partial obstruction to the blood supply is an important accessory factor. Another exacerbating factor is a concurrent coagulation defect. Brody, Levison and Jung (1977) referred to five unrelated patients with sickle-cell trait and haematuria, two of whom had become seriously anaemic. All four were shown to have the von Willebrand syndrome. The two who were seriously anaemic were treated with cryoprecipitate with the result that the bleeding soon ceased. Brody, Levison and Jung stressed that von Willebrand's syndrome should not be forgotten when investigating patients with the sickle-cell trait and haematuria.

Reeves, Lubin and Embury (1984) reported that haematuria is more frequent and impaired renal concentration is more pronounced in Hb-AS subjects with high rather than low concentrations of Hb S: thus in 11 patients with a history of gross haematuria the mean percentage of Hb S was 39.6 ± 3.6, whilst in 23 without such a history the mean percentage was 36.7 ± 3.7 ($P = 0.03$).

Hyposthenuria. Inability to concentrate urine to the normal degree is another symptomless accompaniment of the presence of Hb S. Schlitt and Keitel (1960a) studied 23 children with sickle-cell trait and 14 with sickle-cell disease. Ten of the former and all of the latter had a urine-concentrating ability less than the minimal normal level.

In both groups the impairment in concentrating power became worse as the children became older (see also p. 34, under homozygous sickle-cell anaemia.)

Splenic infarction. While splenic infarction is probably much more easily produced in patients with Hb-SC disease or Hb-S/β-thalassaemia, it seems clear that flying at a high altitude in a non-pressurized or an insufficiently pressurized aircraft can give rise to hypoxic sickling of the erythrocytes within the spleen and consequent congestion and infarction in subjects with Hb AS. Severe left-sided abdominal pain and nausea are the result.

Patients who probably had Hb AS only and who developed splenic infarction were first described by Conn (1954) and by Cooley, Peterson and Jernigan (1954). Smith and Conley (1955) reinvestigated 15 patients who had had splenic infarction during aeroplane flights and found that 12 of them had Hb AS; they concluded, nevertheless, that the incidence of infarction is low when the frequency of the trait is taken into account. Further examples of splenic congestion (? infarction) in Hb-AS patients, severe enough to produce symptoms, were reported by Rotter *et al.* (1956).

Experimentally, Levin and his colleagues (1957) obtained support for the idea that moderate degrees of hypoxia could lead to sickling of Hb-AS erythrocytes *in vivo* and their sequestration in the spleen. They found by in-vivo counting after labelling the erythrocytes of four subjects with ^{51}Cr that there was a significant increase in radioactivity over the spleen following exposure to hypoxia equivalent to an altitude of 7000–8000 ft (2100–2400 m).

Green, Huntsman and Serjeant (1971) described the histories of seven patients, with various types of sickle-cell disease, who developed serious symptoms during aeroplane flights. One of the patients had Hb AS: she had been a passenger in a local-service unpressurized aircraft at 10 000 ft (approximately 3050 m) and developed a local infarct in the small intestine. Green, Huntsman and Serjeant concluded that some Hb-AS patients are at risk in unpressurized aircraft flying at relatively high altitudes and that Hb-SC and Hb-S/β-thalassaemia patients are always at risk, even in pressurized aircraft. The risk for Hb-SS patients flying in pressurized aircraft they considered to be less, perhaps because of atrophy of the spleen. Konotey-Ahulu (1972b), commenting on the above report, emphasized the necessity of excluding Hb-S/β-thalassaemia before accepting an AS electrophoretic pattern as signifying a diagnosis of sickle-cell trait.

Another cause of splenic infarction in Hb-AS subjects is mountain climbing. O'Brien and co-workers (1972) referred to splenic infarcts developing at 2130–3050 m and gave details of a 26-year-old Caucasian male who, when climbing Mount Washington, developed acute left-sided upper abdominal pain at an unusually low altitude (760 m). Haemoglobin electrophoresis demonstrated a Hb-AS pattern and a [^{99m}Tc] sulphur colloid scan showed a large defect in the spleen image.

Ulceration of the leg. Intractable ulcers over or just above the malleoli have long been regarded as a frequent complication of sickle-cell disease (see p. 26): sickle-cell trait may be a predisposing factor, too. Serjeant and Gueri (1970) reported that of 250 patients with chronic leg ulcers attending a West-Indies hospital 49 had Hb AS (19.6%), whereas the expected incidence of the trait was only 10.8%.

Sudden death. The sickle-cell trait appears occasionally to have been a contributory factor in the collapse and death of patients who have been stressed by excessive exertion, infection, acidosis or dehydration, particularly if occurring in combination. Jones, Binder and Donowho (1970) described four such cases amongst 4000 black Americans undergoing combat training at 4060 ft (approximately 1240 m). All four had Hb AS but had apparently been healthy previously. At necropsy no clear cause for their death was found. The blood in grossly congested organs was, however, massively sickled, and it was suggested that this had been responsible for the men's death. The sickling was attributed to hypoxia, acidosis and dehydration, and the accumulation of endogenous reducing agents, in men exposed to moderate-to-severe exertion soon after arriving at a relatively high altitude. Cooper and Toole (1972), in a brief review of such cases, emphasized the importance of a normal haematocrit as a major contributory factor to the increased viscosity of blood containing sickled cells. They stressed, too, the role of vasoconstriction in precipitating ischaemia and infarction.

Miscellaneous conditions. Other conditions that have been attributed to the presence of Hb AS include occlusion of mesenteric vessels leading to acute abdominal symptoms (Ende,

Pizzolato and Ziskind, 1955; Ober *et al.*, 1960), avascular necrosis of bone (Ratcliff and Wolf, 1962), proliferative retinopathy (Nagpal *et al.*, 1977), pulmonary infarction (Israel and Salipante, 1979), and strokes, cerebral infarction and cerebral thrombosis (Handler and Perkin, 1982).

In connection with retinopathy the report of Nagpal *et al.* (1977) is of particular interest. Seven patients aged between 39 and 59 were described who undoubtedly had the Hb-AS trait. Retinal abnormalities were present which could not be distinguished from those occurring in Hb-SC disease, Hb-S/thalassaemia or Hb-SS disease. However, there was evidence in each patient of an associated systemic disease, *i.e.*, diabetes, syphilis, tuberculosis or sarcoidosis, that may have played a part in the pathogenesis of the retinal lesions.

Handler and Perkin (1982) stated that they had been able to trace in the English literature only seven patients in whom cerebrovascular thrombotic phenomena seemed possibly to be attributable to the Hb-AS trait. They described a patient of their own, a 22-year-old male West Indian, who gave a history of epilepsy and whose right leg was atrophic. A CAT scan revealed several low density areas consistent with cerebral infarcts.

Pregnancy

Margolies (1951) considered that the presence of the Hb-S trait did not affect conception or increase the likelihood of complications during pregnancy. Adams, Whitacre and Diggs (1953), however, concluded that pregnancy was in fact a hazard and that the incidence of toxaemia and the fetal death rate were both increased. These assertions were not, however, confirmed by Whalley, Pritchard and Richards (1963) who in a comparison of 500 black women with Hb AS and 500 with Hb AA found no difference in the incidences of abortion, toxaemia, prematurity or perinatal death. However, pyelonephritis occurred more frequently during pregnancy and the puerperium in the Hb-AS individuals.

Tuck, Studd and White (1983) came essentially to the same conclusions, namely, that pregnancy in a Hb-AS woman is not associated with an increased perinatal mortality and that the birthweight of the infant is not reduced. Urinary infections and haematuria were the only maternal complications the incidence of which was abnormally high.

Serjeant (1974a), who devoted a chapter of his monograph to a consideration of the possible pathogenicity of the sickle-cell trait, concluded that this was still a subject of controversy at the time of writing; he emphasized in particular the need for strict laboratory criteria in the diagnosis of the trait and that evidence pointing to the trait having clinical relevance must satisfy critical diagnostic and statistical criteria.

A further comprehensive review of the morbidity of the sickle-cell trait was published by Sears in 1978. He, too, stressed that some of the early records are unreliable because of the possibility that the patient was suffering from compound heterozygosity for Hb S and Hb C or β-thalassaemia, and also because of undue reliance on the post-mortem finding of sickling as an indicator of a pathogenetic role. He concluded that the presence of Hb AS does not impair life expectancy and that of the long list of morbid associations which have been attributed to its presence only six seemed to be very likely, namely, splenic infarction at the atmospheric pressure found at 10 000 ft (3050 m) or higher, reduced mortality from *Pl. falciparum* infection, an increased incidence of bacteriuria and of pyelonephritis in pregnancy, hyposthenuria and haematuria. Eleven other suggested associations were thought to be possible and 29 more considered unlikely and certainly unproved. It is certainly difficult to accept the presence of the simple Hb-AS trait as sufficient or sole explanation for the severe anaemia that affected three members of an African family described in an interesting report by Gelfand, Christie and Seymour (1962).

The percentage of Hb S in Hb-AS heterozygotes varies from less than 30 to more than 40 (see p. 107). Kennedy and co-workers (1986) investigated 355 hospitalized Hb-AS patients with the aim of determining whether there was any association between the Hb-S percentage and the occurrence of vascular events. They found that, although there was an inverse correlation between the Hb-S percentage and total haemoglobin and MCV, there appeared to be no relationship between Hb-S percentage and a history of pulmonary embolism, thrombophlebitis, myocardial infarct, cerebrovascular accident or idiopathic haematuria.

HOMOZYGOUS SICKLE-CELL DISEASE (Hb-SS DISEASE)

Synonyms. Sickle-cell anemia (Mason, 1922); drepanocytic anemia (Hahn, 1928); meniscocytic anemia (Graham and McCarty, 1930); sicklemia (Committee for Clarification of Nomenclature, 1950).

NATURAL HISTORY, PRESENTATION AND MORTALITY IN AFRICA

Prior to the early 1950s, sickle-cell anaemia was regarded as a rare disease in Africa. Raper, in a review published in 1950, stated that only about 33 reports on any aspect of sickle-cell disease had been published from African sources up to that time. However, it has transpired that the apparent rarity of sickle-cell anaemia in areas where the sickling trait was present in a relatively high proportion of the population was an artifact brought about by the very high death-rate in infancy and early childhood of homozygotes (Foy, Kondi and Brass, 1951; Foy and Kondi, 1951, 1952; J. and C. Lambotte-Legrand, 1951, 1955a,b; Edington, 1953; Vandepitte, 1954; Trowell, Raper and Wellbourn, 1957).

J. and C. Lambotte-Legrand (1952) reported that sickle-cell anaemia was in fact common in black Africa;

they had studied 130 cases in $2\frac{1}{2}$ years and found that only approximately one-quarter of the affected (homozygous) infants lived beyond 2 years. By 1955 the same authors were able to refer to 300 cases in the Belgian Congo, but almost one-half of the infants died before the age of 1 year; the number reaching adult life was thought to be minute. Vandepitte (1954) recorded 244 cases (at Leopoldville), almost all infants or small children; only 11 were more than 10 years of age and only two were adults. Trowell, Raper and Wellbourn (1957) were able to give a comprehensive account of sickle-cell anaemia as it then was occurring in Uganda, based on a study of 59 children. Their experience indicated that although homozygous sickle-cell disease may be suspected at the 3rd month, anaemia was not usually marked until the 5th or 6th month. By the 7th to 15th month severe anaemia was almost invariably present. Haemolytic crises, with involvement of the liver and increasing jaundice (serum bilirubin 5–15 mg/dl) were a potent cause of death of children between 6 and 24 months of age. After the age of 2 years the anaemia tended to become less severe. A characteristic early clinical sign in infancy was found to be recurrent swelling of the hands and feet, apparently due to periosteal thickening. The Lambotte-Legrands (1951) stated that this was often the first sign of the disease, appearing as a rule when the infant was 6–8 months old. According to Lambotte (1962), 80% of infants are affected (Fig. 11.4).

In recent years the death-rate of African infants and children due to Hb-SS disease has become far

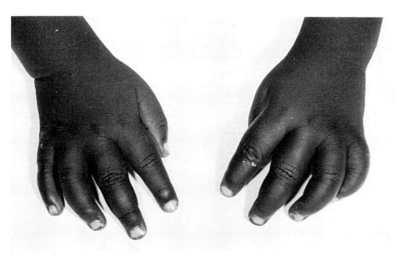

Fig. 11.4 Dactylitis in a 9-month-old infant.
(Reproduced by courtesy of Dr Konotey-Ahulu.)

less than that mentioned above, but it still remains a very serious problem. Data from Ghana, reported by Konotey-Ahulu (1971), illustrate this point. Of 256 children under the age of 5 years attending the sickle-cell (haemoglobinopathy) clinic at the Korle Bu Teaching Hospital in Accra, 204 (79.7%) had Hb-SS disease, compared with only 14% in the 25–35 age-group. (The reverse was true of patients with Hb-SC disease, who comprised the majority from the age of 15 years upwards.) Likewise, Attah and Ekere (1975), reporting from Ibadan on 28 deaths in Hb-SS and Hb-SC patients, found that half of these had occurred in children less than 5 years of age — all had Hb SS. Serious intercurrent infections were the most important cause.

Effiong (1982) has provided an excellent up-to-date account of sickle-cell disease as it now occurs in West Africa. Of 1877 children, patients at University College Hospital in Ibadan, Nigeria, none was less than 3 months of age when first diagnosed. Common complaints and symptoms in infancy and childhood were listed as fever, pain, swelling of the limbs, pain and swelling of the abdomen, poor appetite, vomiting and diarrhoea; other symptoms mentioned were bleeding from the nose or gums, darkening of the urine, polyuria and abnormal thirst. Most of the children are obviously pale on presentation and mildly to moderately jaundiced.

Effiong mentioned that while most affected children are below average in weight and height and have relatively long thin limbs, a protruberant abdomen and lumbar lordosis, some are well proportioned and robust. Most of the children, when in a steady state, are moderately anaemic and have a PCV of 18–30% (see also p. 78).

Painful (infarctive or vaso-occlusive) crises. Infections (which may be bacterial or viral or malaria), cold and wet weather, starvation, undue exertion and any cause of dehydration or acidosis were listed by Effiong as causes, in Nigeria, of painful crises. In infants and young children, the pain, which may be extremely severe, affects the hands and feet and digits, particularly, and the arms and legs in older children. The crises may last for a few hours only or persist for several days, or even weeks, and may be accompanied by an increase in haemolysis. 'Sequestration' crises, associated with a marked increase in the size of the spleen, are uncommon in children but quite frequently occur in pregnancy.

According to Effiong, dactylitis and the hand-foot syndrome are common complications, more than 90% of children aged 2 years or less presenting with one or other or both syndromes. The lesions usually clear up completely but may occasionally result in shortening or other deformity of the fingers or toes. Osteomyelitis, too, remains a common and serious complication. This usually presents combined with septicaemia: the affected child is seriously ill, has a high fever and is likely to become deeply jaundiced with greenish-yellow sclerae and bile in the urine. Species of Salmonella are the most common infecting organism: of 63 patients with Salmonella osteomyelitis diagnosed in Ibadan, 57 had Hb SS, one Hb SC, one Hb AS, two Hb-S/HPFH and only two Hb AA (Adeyokunnu and Hendrickse, 1980).

Liver and jaundice. The liver was recorded by Effiong to be palpable in approximately 50% of affected children on presentation. They are usually mildly to moderately jaundiced. Occasionally, however, mostly in children over 6 years of age, an obstructive type of jaundice develops associated with an enlarged firm liver and sometimes, too, with finger clubbing. Some, at least, of these children have developing cirrhosis.

Spleen. Effiong mentioned that approximately 70% of the children have a palpable spleen on presentation. Marked atrophy of the spleen ('autosplenectomy'), a characteristic feature of Hb-SS disease in the New World [so much so that the spleen is rarely palpable in children over 10 years of age (see p. 28)], occurs apparently less frequently in Nigeria. Massive enlargement of the spleen is quite common at that age, chronic infection with malaria being a likely cause.

Malaria. According to Effiong, infection with Pl. falciparum is less intense in Hb-SS than in Hb-AA individuals. The consequences, however, may be serious: infection may lead to crises — haemolytic, sequestration or infarctive — and is a common cause of death of both Hb-SS and Hb-SC patients. As an illustration of this, Adeloye, Luzzatto and Edington (1971) described how an 8-year-old Nigerian girl died following a heavy mixed infection with Pl. malariae and Pl. falciparum. Her haemoglobin fell to 3 g/dl and at necropsy her spleen was found to weigh only 3.0 g!

HOMOZYGOUS SICKLE-CELL DISEASE IN THE NEW WORLD

Age at diagnosis and presentation

In the United States the earliest descriptions of sickle-cell disease mostly dealt with its presentation in relatively old children and adolescents. Thus Wintrobe, in the fourth edition of his Textbook published in 1956, stated that only 12 cases in infants up to the age of 1 year had been recorded up to that time. Later reports emphasized the wide age-range at which patients present. Thus Scott and co-workers (1955) reported that although the mean age at first admission into hospital of 63 black children with Hb-SS disease was 4.7 years, their ages ranged from 4 months to 15 years.

Haggard and Schneider (1961) reported some interesting data on age and the onset of symptoms. Of 54 black infants with Hb-SS disease none had had symptoms attributable to this cause before the age of 3 months. However, half of them developed symptoms before the end of the second year. An early and frequent symptom was an osteopathy affecting metacarpals and proximal phalanges [as had been reported earlier from Africa by the Lambotte-Legrands (1951) (see above)].

O'Brien and co-workers (1976) have given an interesting account of the first 3 years of life of 12 infants in whom Hb-SS disease was identified at birth. Signs of haemolytic anaemia were evident by the time they were 12 weeks old and paralleled the post-natal decline in Hb F. Vaso-occlusive symptoms were recognized on at least 17 occasions in seven of the infants, in four before they were 1 year old, and the hand-foot

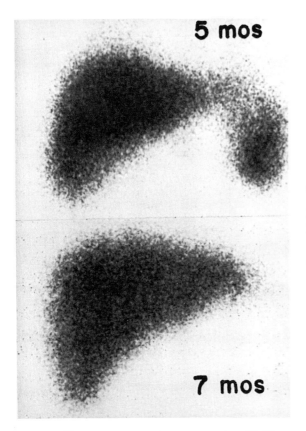

Fig. 11.5 [⁹⁹ᵐTc]sulphur colloid spleen scan in a Hb-SS infant.
Shows the presence of a spleen shadow at 5 months, and its disappearance by 7 months. [Reproduced by permission from O'Brien *et al.* (1976).]

syndrome was observed as early as 5 months. Aplastic crises developed in four of the infants on seven occasions; all were associated with febrile illnesses; most were not serious and resolved spontaneously and only one of the infants needed a transfusion. One of the infants developed pneumococcal sepsis.

Serial scans using [⁹⁹Tc]sulphur colloid were carried out on nine of the infants. In one, aged 5 months, impaired uptake by the spleen (functional asplenia) was already present; in eight, functional asplenia, for which there was no evidence during the first 6 months of life, developed subsequently (Fig. 11.5); in three, uptake by the spleen was still normal at 18, 20 and 29 months, respectively.

There are, however, a small number of reports of infants in whom sickle-cell anaemia has been diagnosed in the first few weeks of life (Cohen, Miller and Orris, 1947; Frazier and Rice, 1950; Heldrich, 1951; Leikin and McCoo, 1958; Russell, 1962; Porter and Thurman, 1963; Hegyi *et al.*, 1977). It is difficult in most cases to explain satisfactorily the infants' symptoms on the presence of the proportionately small amount of Hb S that must have been present in such young children. The infant described by Hegyi *et al.* was remarkable as she had many sickled cells in her blood film, although only 20% of her haemoglobin was Hb S; the remainder was Hb F. She died when 5 days old and the findings at necropsy were interpreted as being those of a sickle-cell crisis with multisystem involvement; severe multifocal necrotizing enterocolitis was the most striking finding. Blood cultures were negative. Anoxia and hyperviscosity were considered to be factors which led to the overt sickling and the infant's death.

Course

In older children, and in adolescents and adults, Hb-SS disease usually runs a fairly stable course: the main symptoms are those attributable to chronic anaemia, *i.e.* weakness and dyspnoea. From time to time, however, the patients have attacks of severe aching pain in the joints or elsewhere in the limbs and sometimes attacks of abdominal pain and nausea. These painful (infarctive or vaso-occlusive) crises are usually accompanied by mild to moderate pyrexia; they are caused by sickled cells blocking small blood vessels, and when leading to abdominal pain or respiratory symptoms such episodes often pose important problems of differential diagnosis. The crises are usually not associated with an increase in anaemia. Sudden increases in anaemia do, however, occur from time to time as the result of increased haemolysis, perhaps brought about by an intercurrent infection. Even more serious are the anaemic crises secondary to bone-marrow inhibition associated with viral infections (see p. 100) or to massive splenic sequestration of erythrocytes (see p. 28). Both these latter types of anaemic crises occur most frequently in young children.

Hb-SS patients are usually chronically mildly to moderately jaundiced due to an increase in unconjugated bilirubin.

Growth and development. Hb-SS disease patients are typically thin and of asthenic stature, and growth and puberty are often delayed (see p. 21). Whether the delay in growth and maturation is different from that found in other chronic anaemias of childhood and adolescence is uncertain. Probably it is not different. Chodorkoff and Whitten (1963) found that the intellectual and psychological function of 19 Hb-SS children (who gave no history of neurological disorder) was similar to that of siblings of similar age.

Mortality and longevity. The early mortality from Hb-SS disease in the United States has always been less than it was at one time in Africa, and the same is true of the Hb-SS population of the West Indies. Even so, the mortality in the 1940s and 1950s in the United States was disturbingly high. Thus Scott and co-workers (1951) reported that five out of 37 children with sickle-cell anaemia died, three of respiratory infections; and it was not unusual at that time for young children with Hb-SS disease to die in a severe anaemic crisis. Jenkins, Scott and Baird (1960) reported 10 such occurrences in children aged between 8 months and 9 years, seven of them being less than 3 years of age. These children had been admitted to hospital in a shock-like state (considered probably to have been brought on by an acute infection). In contrast to a generalized marked pallor, their spleens and livers were strikingly congested. One such patient had blood like 'pink water' (Hb < 1 g/dl): in contrast, the spleen was dark purplish in colour and weighed 274 g (estimated normal weight 30 g).

Porter and Thurman (1963), who reviewed the clinical progress of 64 children in whom Hb-SS disease had been diagnosed before the age of 1 year, reported that 10 died in the first year of life: in seven, acute infection had been the cause of death.

In 1975 Powars reviewed the outlook for patients in the western United States; 24 out of 422 patients, aged 1–7 years, died, 13 of infections. Based on this experience, the expected death-rate was calculated to be about 10% in the first decade and 5% or less in subsequent decades.

Rogers and co-workers (1978) provided relatively recent data from the West Indies. Of 109 Hb-SS infants diagnosed at birth, 13% died within the first 2 years [compared with 5% of 67 Hb-SC infants and 1% of normal (Hb AA) controls]. The infants that died were mostly between 6 and 12 months of age: the principal causes were acute splenic sequestration and pneumococcal infection. In a more recent report from Jamaica, Thomas, Pattison and Serjeant (1982) reported the age at death and its cause in 241 Hb-SS patients. Most deaths occurred in children who were less than 5 years of age (Fig. 11.6): the commonest causes were the acute chest syndrome (60 deaths, at all ages), acute splenic sequestration (23 deaths, small children only), renal failure (21 deaths, mostly adults), meningitis (18 deaths, mostly small children) and cardiovascular accident (18 deaths, mostly adults).

The proportion of patients who survive until late adult life has been gradually increasing as the years pass. In 1958, in the West Indies, Went and MacIver reported that only 19 out of 114 Hb-SS patients were over 26 years of age, and the clinical history of the female patient from Baltimore, who had been described by Charache and Richardson (1964) as living to the age of 66, was considered to be sufficiently unusual to warrant special notice (see p. 51). By 1968, however, Serjeant and co-workers were able to report on 60 patients in Jamaica who were over 30 years of age.

In 1970 was recounted at a Clinicopathologic Conference at the Washington University School of Medicine the clinical history and necropsy findings of a female who had survived for 48 years. This account is exceptionally interesting as the patient had suffered from many of the major complications of Hb-SS disease and had been followed closely for the last 25 years of her life, and had taken part in many therapeutic studies. She had received many blood transfusions and became eventually heavily iron-overloaded: her liver weighed 4360 g and contained 61.48 g of iron; the spleen weighed 10 g!

In the United States, Shurafa and co-workers (1982) reported on 10 patients aged between 40 and 76 years, all of whom attended a sickle-cell clinic in Detroit. The aim of the study, in which the clinical history and laboratory findings in these patients were compared with those of a group of 11 patients, attending the same clinic, who had died when aged between 20 and 31 years, was to ascertain whether there were any features in their history or in their laboratory findings that were associated with long survival. The long survivors had had in fact fewer painful crises, but they had experienced, perhaps because of their greater age, more long-term complications such as leg ulcer, congestive cardiac

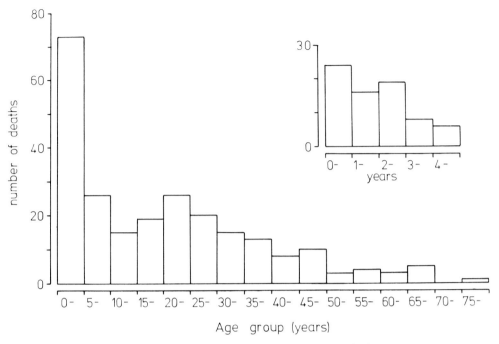

Fig. 11.6 Age at death of 241 Jamaican patients with Hb-SS disease.
[Reproduced by permission from Thomas, Pattison and Serjeant (1982).]

failure and aseptic hip necrosis. Cerebrovascular accidents were the cause of death in nine of the 11 short-term survivors but had not been experienced by any of the long survivors. No differences were established between the two groups in the severity of their anaemia, in the intensity of increased haemolysis or in Hb-A$_2$ levels. The long survivors had, however, higher Hb-F levels (mean 6.5 ± 3.5% compared with 3.6 ± 1.9%) and higher erythrocyte (but not plasma) zinc concentrations. α : β-chain synthesis ratios were normal in the long survivors and α-gene mapping, carried out on five of the long survivors, revealed αα/αα genotypes in four and a α−/αα genotype in one. The long survivors appeared to have better developed secondary sex characters, but the significance of this finding, and of the higher Hb-F and erythrocyte zinc levels, was considered to be uncertain. The concurrence of α-thalassaemia did not appear to be playing any part in long survival.

REVIEWS DEALING WITH THE CLINICAL ASPECTS OF SICKLE-CELL DISEASE

Many comprehensive accounts of the symptomatology of sickle-cell disease have been published. The early ones suffer from a lack of distinction between Hb-SS disease and compound heterozy-gous conditions such as Hb-SC disease and Hb-S/β-thalassaemia. Anderson and Ware's (1932) review was based on a study of 44 patients; Grover's (1947) paper dealt with the clinical manifestations in 48 patients; Henderson's (1950) review was based on a study of 54 cases. Margolies's (195i) review is a valuable source of information on the early literature. Serjeant's (1974a) monograph comprised a comprehensive review of the literature (about 1400 references) and of his own experience in Jamaica; his recent book (Serjeant, 1985b) is even more comprehensive and is based on his unique and valuable experience of approximately 2000 patients who are being monitored in sickle-cell clinics throughout the island and an additional cohort of 550 patients who were diagnosed at birth and who have been followed up subsequently as closely as possible. There are about 2000 references.

Other important recent reviews which deal with the clinical aspects of Hb-SS disease include those of Milner (1974), Powars (1975), Luzzatto (1981), Platt and Nathan (1981), Warth and Rucknagel (1983), Winslow and Anderson (1983) and Serjeant (1985a).

CLINICAL FEATURES OF HOMOZYGOUS SICKLE-CELL DISEASE IN MORE DETAIL

Habitus, growth and development

As already referred to (p. 19), patients with Hb-SS disease are typically thin and of asthenic stature and growth and puberty are often delayed.

Winsor and Burch (1944a), who studied 15 patients with sickle-cell anaemia, stressed the deep narrow chest, long extremities and enlarged abdomen in children and the linear build, emaciation, long legs, short trunk and increased dorsal kyphosis and lumbar lordosis in adults. Whitten (1961) compared 40 Hb-SS children with their unaffected siblings and with the accepted standards for normal children. As a group, the Hb-SS children weighed less and were shorter and thinner. Their spans were normal, but their upper-to-lower segment ratios, like those of their normal siblings, were smaller than those of normal white children. Skeletal maturation did not appear to be affected in childhood but was possibly affected in early adolescence.

Jimenez and co-workers (1966) contrasted the development of 20 girls with Hb-SS disease with that of 774 normal black girls. Their data indicated delay of the menarche, advancement of the age of the first pregnancy and decreased fertility. They, too, found that the Hb-SS children tended to be underweight and below normal stature and to have lower than normal upper-to-lower segment ratios; they concluded that it was uncertain whether the delay in growth and maturation they had observed was different from that found in other chronic anaemias of childhood and adolescence.

Similar observations were recorded by Ashcroft, Serjeant and Desai (1972), who studied 99 Jamaicans, aged 12–21 years, who had Hb-SS disease. Compared with controls (Hb AA or Hb AS), the patients' weight and skeletal age (based on hand radiographs) were less at all ages. The average height of the younger patients was less than normal but that of the older patients was at least as great as that of the controls.

Details of sexual function in 32 adult male Hb-SS disease patients were recorded by Abbasi et al. (1976). The secondary sex characters were delayed and under-developed in 29, and 31 of the men were considered to have a eunuchoid skeletal proportion. Androgen levels were subnormal, and erythrocyte and hair zinc concentrations were subnormal, too; and the question was raised as to the relationship, if any, between the zinc deficiency and apparent testicular failure. As the result of a seminal fluid investigation, carried out in Lagos, Osegbe, Akinyanju and Amaku (1981) reported finding evidence of lowered fertility potential in all of the 17 males, aged 17–30 years, they had studied.

Kramer and co-workers (1980) reported on the pre- and post-natal growth and development of a cohort of 14 Hb-SS children, whom they had followed from birth until 3–6 years of age, compared with that of 71 Hb-AA controls. None of the Hb-SS infants was premature and their birthweights were within the normal range. However, subsequently, there was unequivocal evidence of impaired height and weight, and of the laying down of body fat and of delayed skeletal maturation. The data of Stevens, Hayes and Serjeant (1981), who compared 64 Hb-SS children 4–6 years of age with 123 age-matched Hb-AA children, were similar: on the average, the weight, height, sitting height, limb length and skin-fold thickness of the Hb-SS children were less than those of the controls.

According to Alleyne, Rauseo and Serjeant (1981), the sexual maturation of female Hb-SS patients is retarded. They compared the development of 91 Jamaican patients with that of 51 controls of similar socio-economic class and found that there was a mean delay of 2–3 years in the onset of menstruation in the Hb-SS patients and a mean delay of 3.9 years in the age at first pregnancy. There was, however, no evidence of lesser fertility, although the number of infants born to the Hb-SS patients was less at all ages.

Daeschner and co-workers (1981) pursued the question of the possible relationship between zinc deficiency and delayed growth. Twenty-two Hb-SS and two Hb-SC disease patients were studied, aged between 1 year and 17 years. In 11 of them there was evidence of delayed growth; in 12 growth was considered to be normal. The plasma zinc concentration and the activity of the two zinc-dependent iso-enzymes, carbonic anhydrase B and C, were measured. The plasma zinc levels, although low, were not significantly different from those of the controls, but the activity of both carbonic anhydrase enzymes was significantly subnormal in the growth-retarded patients compared with the controls. Daeschner et al. concluded that measuring the enzyme activity was a more reliable way of demonstrating zinc deficiency than the estimation of its concentration in the plasma, and that their findings supported the contention that there is a relationship between delayed growth and puberty in sickle-cell disease patients and decreased availability or abnormal utilization of zinc.

The results of a more recent and much larger study of growth and sexual maturation were reported by Platt, Rosenstock and Espeland in 1984 on behalf of the Cooperative Study of Sickle Cell Disease Coordinating Center: 2115 patients who had Hb-SS disease, Hb-SC disease, Hb-S/β^+-thalassaemia or Hb-Sβ^0-thalassaemia were studied with respect to their height, weight and sexual maturation. The Hb-SS and Hb-S/β^0 patients were found to be consistently smaller and less well sexually developed than the Hb-SC and Hb-S/β⁺ patients. In all four groups, and in both sexes, subnormal weight was more pronounced than subnormal height, the differences becoming more apparent after the age of 7 years.

PAINFUL (VASO-OCCLUSIVE) CRISES

As already referred to, painful crises are a cause of much suffering. Detailed descriptions of their occurrence in American and African patients studied in Memphis and Ghana, respectively, were recorded by Diggs (1965) and Konotey-Ahulu (1974). The patients complain as a rule of the sudden onset of pain in the lumbo-sacral region or in one or more sites in the limbs, particularly in the vicinity of the knee, shoulder or hip joint, or in the thigh, or less commonly elsewhere, *e.g.*, in the orbit (Blank and Gill, 1981); or they may complain of pains in the abdomen or chest. The onset of pain is usually quickly followed by a rise in body temperature, which often reaches 101° F but may reach as high as 104° F. Not infrequently, in cases in which the pain is confined to the abdomen the physician may be presented with the difficult problem of excluding the possibility of an abdominal catastrophe requiring surgical intervention. The crises appear to be brought about by sickled erythrocytes blocking small blood vessels and leading to tissue ischaemia. Hence the qualification 'vaso-occlusive' or 'infarctive' used to describe this type of crisis. Increase in anaemia is not a characteristic accompaniment of the crisis (Diggs, 1956). The pain is often extremely severe: it persists as a rule for 4–6 days, but may last but a few hours or even as long as several weeks. According to Diggs (1965), it is typical for the pain to develop suddenly in the early hours or to affect the patient on waking in the morning. Painful crises affect patients of all ages, but they are particularly frequent in young people between the ages of 5 and 15 years; they tend to occur less frequently as the patient grows older and they are rare in patients over 30. Younger children seem particularly prone to develop the hand-foot syndrome (see p. 24) or to suffer from abdominal pain.

Most patients who suffer from crises have repeated attacks; some, however, have very few; others even escape them altogether (Karayalcin *et al.*, 1975). Factors that have been considered as likely to bring on a painful crisis include infections, cold, wet weather, exertion, dehydration and pregnancy. In some patients crises develop for no obvious reason.

Uncommonly, crises have followed pyrexial reactions to blood transfusions (Paterson and Sprague, 1959). Painful crises were also experienced by a 34-year-old female with Hb-SS disease and chronic renal failure of unknown origin following a successful cadaveric kidney transplant (Spector *et al.*, 1978). The re-emergence of crises, which had been absent for many years, was attributed to the rise in haematocrit and consequent increase in blood viscosity that followed the success of the transplant.

Effect of cold weather and rainfall. The possible influence of cold and wet weather has been the subject of considerable debate. In tropical Africa, the crises appear to be most frequent in the relatively cool, rainy season at a time when most infections occur (Konotey-Ahulu, 1972e; Effiong, 1982). Konotey-Ahulu (1965a) suggested that increases in atmospheric water pressure, associated with a fall in the partial pressure of oxygen, might be a factor. Addae (1971) stressed the possible importance, amongst other factors, of the redistribution of the circulation during exposure to a cool environment, resulting in a reduction of blood flow in certain regions such as the bones and joints.

In the United States, the effect of environmental temperature or rainfall seems to be less clear cut. As far back as 1927, Graham and McCarty described how a patient had repeatedly stated that he was liable to periods of illness after he had been exposed to cold or dampness; they added that the patient's 'fatal seizure began the day after a snowstorm during which he had become cold and wet.' Diggs (1965), too, mentioned that a common history is that of getting wet or chilled and developing pain immediately afterwards, several hours later or during the following night; he also described, however, how a patient, at Memphis, had been followed for 10 years from when he was 7 years old without there being any clear periodicity or seasonal relationship or tendency for the crises to alter in type or severity as the years passed. Diggs and Flowers (1971) later reported that they had closely observed over a 2-year period 35 children aged between 2 and 13 years who had Hb-SS disease. Careful record keeping revealed no periodicity and no relationship between the seasons and the occurrence of vaso-occlusive phenomena.

In Chicago, too, admission to hospital of children with sickle-cell anaemia was reported by Seeler (1973) to be fairly constant between 1969 and 1973 despite a large winter-to-summer temperature difference. In Buffalo, however, Amjad, Bannerman and Judisch (1974) found an apparent correlation between the admission to hospital of Hb-SS and Hb-SC patients for pain and the environmental humidity and temperature. A total of 134 admissions during the years 1967–71 were reviewed. The monthly totals varied considerably; most admissions were found to have been in December (when humidity was high and temperature very low) and fewest in June (when humidity was low and temperature high).

In the West Indies the relationship between admission to hospital and temperature seems to be similar to that observed in tropical Africa. Redwood and co-workers (1976), as the result of a 10-year study of patients with Hb-SS disease, were able to demonstrate a close correlation between the minimal environmental temperature (in November–February) and the highest admission rate to hospital. Admissions, however, were not positively correlated with the period of highest rainfall (July–November).

The possible role of serum cryoglobulins or cold auto-agglutinins was raised by Charmot, Reynaud and Bergot (1963). Of 15 children with sickle-cell anaemia observed in Brazzaville, Senegal, the seven in whom cryoglobulins were demonstrated appeared to have suffered from more painful crises than the children in whom cryoglobulins were absent. Diggs (1965), however, discounted the importance of cryoglobulins in the pathogenesis of crises. [Much would depend upon the highest temperature at which the plasma viscosity was increased by the presence of the cryoglobulins or at which auto-agglutination would take place, but clearly any mechanism which contributed to local slowing of the circulation would be likely to increase the possibility of a painful crisis developing.]

McSweeney, Mermann and Wagley, as long ago as 1947, had determined the cold-agglutinin titre in 30 patients with sickle-cell anaemia. In 60% of patients the titre was 40 or over and in 36% 80 or over. However, there appeared to be no clear correlation between the titre and the degree of sickling, haemoglobin or haematocrit levels, icterus index or clinical indications of disease severity or the occurrence of painful crises.

Accounts of patients with sickle-cell disease in whom the development of cold auto-antibodies of anti-I specificity resulted in acute exacerbations of their anaemia were recorded by Mann et al. (1975) and Maniatis, Bertles and Wethers (1977) (see also p. 54).

Bone pain: the causal lesion

Pain in the bones in sickle-cell disease is associated with local infarction of the bone marrow, and it may be possible to aspirate dead or dying marrow cells from the affected area. Radionuclides have been used with success in demonstrating the extent of the lesions.

Hammel and co-workers (1973) demonstrated abnormalities of the bone marrow, and of the mineral content of bone, in several patients with acute bone pain in whom X-rays revealed no evidence of infarction or infection. Using [^{99m}Tc]sulphur colloid, they were able to define discrete areas of decreased isotope concentration corresponding to where the pain was localized and using ^{85}Sr they obtained evidence of increased mineral turnover in the same areas. Scans with ^{18}F indicated a normal bone blood flow, in contrast to the diminished marrow blood flow.

Alavi and co-workers (1974) also used ^{99m}Tc. They studied 29 patients: in eight out of 17 patients who were free of symptoms areas of decreased uptake were present, suggestive of past infarcts and subsequent fibrosis, while six out of 10 patients, scanned during painful crises, were found to have areas of decreased activity corresponding with the localization of their pain. In four of these patients, re-scanned when no longer in crisis, the scan indicated healing and repopulation of the marrow.

Milner, Brown and Yoder (1982) investigated the possibility of a correlation between the occurrence of bone-marrow infarction and the haematological profile of the patients (Figs. 11.7–11.9). Forty-two Hb-SS patients had been studied using [^{99m}Tc]sulphur colloid over a 2-year period. Marrow defects were demonstrated in 28 of them and in 15 (aged between 19 and 52 years) they were matched with X-ray changes. Repeated imaging demonstrated in many cases resolution or decrease in size of the defects within a 3–6 months' period. In patients who were free from symptoms no defects were demonstrated. Milner, Brown and Yoder found that the patients who had suffered from marrow infarction tended to have relatively high levels of haemoglobin; however, a high Hb-F percentage or the presence of α-thalassaemia did not appear to be protective.

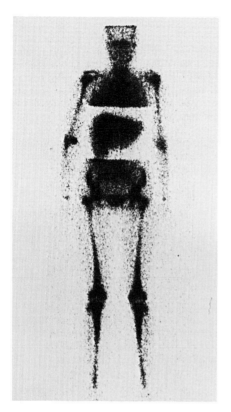

Fig. 11.7 [⁹⁹ᵐTc]sulphur colloid bone-marrow images in a 33-year-old Hb-SS female in an asymptomatic phase.
(Reproduced by courtesy of Drs Mark Brown and Paul S. Milner.)

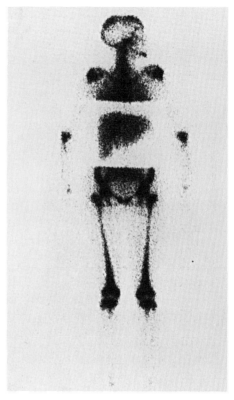

Fig. 11.8 [⁹⁹ᵐTc]sulphur colloid bone-marrow images in a 33-year-old Hb-SS female in a severe vaso-occlusive crisis (same patient as in Fig. 11.6).
Relative little colloid has been taken up by the arm bones and tibiae. (Reproduced by courtesy of Drs Mark Brown and Paul S. Milner.)

Hand-foot syndrome

Danford, Marr and Elsey (1941) described under the title 'Sickle cell anemia with unusual bone changes' how an 8-month-old black American infant became febrile, vomited and developed painful swollen hands. Fifteen days later an X-ray 'showed periosteal thickening and bone destruction of the metacarpals and phalanges'. A similar occurrence in a 1-year-old was reported by Ivy and Howard (1953). This account included good clinical photographs. The Lambotte-Legrands' (1951) description of the syndrome in the Belgian Congo has already been referred to (p. 16).

Watson and co-workers (1963) described the bone lesions in detail and reviewed the literature; they pointed out that the syndrome was often the first clinical manifestation. The child's hand and/or feet become swollen and painful (Fig. 11.4) and within 7–14 days X-rays show periosteal elevation and bone destruction of metatarsals, metacarpals and phalanges. The swelling usually subsides in 1–3 weeks and bony changes demonstrable by X-ray tend to heal in about 3 months. Diggs (1965), too, stressed the frequency of the 'hand-foot syndrome' or 'sickle-cell dactylitis' in children of 1–4 years of age, and attributed it to sickling of the erythrocytes leading to ischaemia of the marrow in the metacarpals, proximal phalanges and metatarsals.

That local cold might in some cases be a precipitating factor was demonstrated by Marsden and Shah (1964) who found that, although immersion of the hands in water at 0°C, with or without the application of a tourniquet for short periods of time, often had no ill effects, in a small number of individuals transient oedema and dactylitis developed.

Serjeant and Ashcroft (1971) stressed how shortening and other deformities of the small bones of the hands and feet may be late sequelae of the hand-foot syndrome

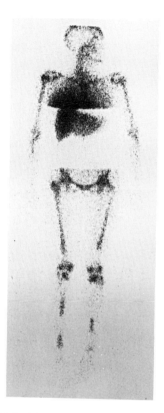

Fig. 11.9 [⁹⁹ᵐTc]sulphur colloid bone-marrow images in a 50-year-old Hb-SS female.

Shows an irregular distribution of colloid indicative of old infarcts in femora and tibiae. [Reproduced by permission from Milner, Brown and Yoder (1982).]

occurring in early childhood. They illustrated this with clinical and X-ray photographs of the hands and feet of five Hb-SS patients aged between 14 and 28 years.

Worrell and Butera (1976) emphasized the importance, from the orthopaedic surgeon's point of view, of not overlooking the possibility of sickle-cell dactylitis and the hand-foot syndrome in the differential diagnosis of acute osteomyelitis.

Acute infarction of long bones in children

Infarction of the diaphysis or metaphysis of the long bones occurs quite commonly in sickle-cell disease as an acute event. Clinically, it can simulate bacterial osteomyelitis quite closely. Infarction is, however, according to Keeley and Buchanan (1982), at least 50 times as common as osteomyelitis proved by bacterial culture.

Keeley and Buchanan (1982) reviewed the clinical histories of 192 children and adolescents with a major sickle haemoglobinopathy, aged from 9 months to 18 years, and found that 21 of them (17 Hb SS) had had 41 episodes of long-bone infarction. Nine of the children had had repeated episodes; 12 gave a history of dactylitis in infancy; six episodes involved two bones simultaneously. The humerus, tibia and femur were (in order of frequency) most commonly involved, particularly the distal parts. The onset of infarction was characterized by local tenderness, warmth and marked swelling. In contrast to bacterial infection (see p. 42), blood and/or bone cultures are negative, and the segmentation of the nuclei of the polymorphonuclears is not markedly shifted to the left. According to Keeley and Buchanan, plain X-rays or radionuclide scans of bone or bone marrow are not likely to help in differentiating infarction from infection.

Chronic avascular (aseptic) necrosis of bone

Localized obstruction of blood vessels by sickled cells is probably responsible for foci of avascular necrosis that lead to chronic destruction of bone. Infarction of the head of the femur is in fact a well-known and quite common complication of Hb-SS disease (Tanaka, Clifford and Axelrod, 1956; Rowe and Haggard, 1957; Carrington, Ferguson and Scott, 1958) (Fig. 11.10). Pain and obvious deformity may develop, but some patients

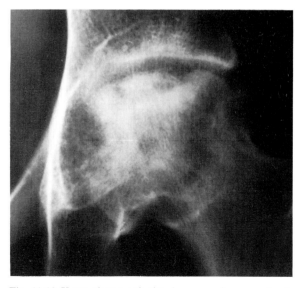

Fig. 11.10 X-ray photograph showing avascular necrosis of the head of the left femur.

Shows fragmentation of the bone and sclerosis. (Reproduced by courtesy of Dr Janet Dacie.)

have no symptoms although typical sclerosis and bony deformity may be visible on X-ray.

Hawker and co-workers (1982) compared the haematological indices of 50 West-Indian patients who had had avascular necrosis of the femoral head with those of 180 patients who had not suffered from this complication. When the results obtained from both sexes were combined, avascular necrosis appeared to be more frequent in patients with relatively high haemoglobin levels and low levels of Hb F, suggesting that both sickling and increased blood viscosity contribute to the necrosis.

Bone-marrow and fat embolism

A rare complication is bone-marrow and fat embolism secondary to bone-marrow infarction (Wade and Stevenson, 1941; Shelley and Curtis, 1958; Brown, 1972; Shapiro and Hayes (1984).

Wade and Stevenson's (1941) patient, a Greek female aged 49, in retrospect probably had Hb-S/thalassaemia. She died in coma. At necropsy, the bone marrow was necrotic in places and there were focal areas of necrosis in the brain. Fat emboli were demonstrated in small blood vessels in the brain, lung, kidney, liver and spleen (which weighed 350 g).

Shelley and Curtis (1958) described bone-marrow and fat embolism in two patients with Hb-SS disease and in a further patient with Hb-SC disease. Their initial complaint of bone pain was followed by mental depression, pyrexia and skin petechiae. Two of the patients were pregnant. Shelley and Curtis suggested that bone-marrow embolism may be the pathological basis of some of the instances of sudden death in sickle-cell disease.

More recently, Hutchinson, Merrick and White (1973) described a patient in whom bone-marrow infarction and fat embolism of the lungs were diagnosed in life. A 19-year-old West-Indian female had a flu-like illness. After 48 hours or so there were signs of consolidation in the lungs. The haemoglobin had dropped to 5.2 g/dl and the platelet count was $100 \times 10^9/l$. The total nucleated cell count was $45 \times 10^9/l$ of which $40 \times 10^9/l$ were normoblasts. The arterial pO_2 was markedly reduced at 66 mm Hg, and there was evidence of disseminated intravascular coagulation. Fat globules were identified in the sputum, and bone-marrow infarction with fat embolism was diagnosed. A [99mTc]sulphur colloid scan revealed multiple areas in which the expected radioactivity was absent; this was particularly so in the pelvis and in one femur, and biopsy of one of these areas revealed necrotic bone marrow. Two weeks later, a scan using ^{18}F showed that new bone was being formed in the infarcted areas.

Arthropathies

Arthralgia and effusions may develop acutely in Hb-SS disease independently of nearby overt infection. Schumacher, Andrews and McLaughlin (1973) reviewed the clinical presentation, and laboratory and X-ray findings, in seven such patients, all considered to have Hb-SS disease. Synovial fluid was obtained from six of the patients and synovial biopsies were carried out on five of them. The acute onset of the arthralgia, with or without obvious effusions, was stressed, with local warmth and tenderness simulating an inflammatory arthritis. In most cases one or two joints (especially the knees or elbows) were involved and usually the joint symptoms had occurred with other evidence of a painful crisis. The episodes were generally short lived and the effusions resolved within 2–14 days in six of the patients. The effusions were mostly clear and contained in addition to some sickled cells an exudate in which large mononuclear cells and lymphocytes predominated; 10% or less of the cells were polymorphonuclears. Synovial biopsy revealed microvascular thrombi and evidence of past vascular occlusion.

The results of a similar but larger study were reported by Espinoza, Spilberg and Osterland (1974). They had found that 32 (30 with Hb SS) out of 70 unselected patients with sickle-cell disorders gave a history of joint disease. The arthritis, which was usually of short duration, was usually polyarticular and had affected the larger rather than the smaller joints and those of the lower limb particularly. Joint aspiration produced a sterile exudate containing a variable number of cells: lymphocytes and mononuclears predominated except in cases where the count was high, when the majority of the cells might be polymorphonuclears.

Alavi and co-workers (1976) assessed the value of radionuclide bone scans in the investigation of arthropathies in patients with sickle-cell disorders. Eight patients (six with Hb SS) had joint symptoms at the time of study and in these patients the uptake of [99mTc]sulphur colloid in the vicinity of the affected joints was decreased, suggesting local obliteration of vessels. The scans appeared to be more sensitive than X-rays in demonstrating bony lesions in the vicinity of painful joints.

Chronic ulcers of the leg

Skin ulceration is a common finding in sickle-cell disease and was mentioned by Herrick (1910a, b) in his original descriptions of the disease. Diggs and Ching (1934) reported that ulcers or scars of ulcers are present 'in about three of four adults with the disease, but are infrequent in young children'. The leg is the commonest site (Fig. 11.11); the elbow has, however, been affected (Corrigan and Schiller, 1934) and, according to Konotey-Ahulu (1965b), no area of skin is exempt.

Chernoff, Shapleigh and Moore (1954) stated that 30–35% of Hb-SS disease patients are affected. The crural ulcers are more often than not bilateral and lie superficially to, or just above, the internal or external malleoli. Gueri and Serjeant (1970) reported that 190 out of 300 Jamaican patients had developed a leg ulcer at some time in their history and that they were most common in patients aged between 10 and 25 years. Serjeant (1974b) stated that the ulcers were bilateral in 49%, that the left leg alone was affected in 31% and the right leg alone in 20%. Vascular stasis, trauma, infection and thrombosis were held to be responsible. It is possible that zinc sulphate taken orally may help the ulcers to heal (Serjeant, Galloway and Gueri, 1970). According to Mont-gomery (1960), chronic leg ulceration is a relatively frequent source of tetanus in the tropics.

Priapism

Prolonged and painful penile erection lasting for many hours or even days is a well-recognized complication of sickle-cell disease (Diggs and Ching, 1934; Campbell and Cummins, 1951; Hasen and Raines, 1962; Karayalcin, Imran and Rosner, 1972; Emond et al., 1980, etc.). Campbell and Cummins (1951) stated that this had been the chief complaint in five out of 102 males admitted to hospital for sickle-cell anaemia. Sousa, Catoe and Scott (1962), in reporting priapism in boys aged 6 and 9 years, respectively, referred to 13 other instances in which children had been affected. Emond and co-workers (1980), stated that 42% of Jamaican males over 15 years of age had had short-lived attacks usually lasting less than 3 hours which in some instances heralded major attacks lasting 24 hours or more that frequently led to impotence. Vascular stasis leading to thrombosis appears to be the cause. In some cases alcohol has seemed to be the provoking factor, perhaps by causing dehydration (Conrad et al., 1980).

Duodenal ulceration

Duodenal ulcers (D.U.) appear to be unusually frequent in Hb-SS disease patients. Serjeant and co-workers (1973) reported that 27 out of 353 patients over 12 years of age were known to have had a D.U., and that as many as 30.5% of 72 male patients over 25 years of age were affected. They did not generally have the hyper-chlorhydria expected in D.U. patients, and it was suggested that ischaemic damage to the mucosa as the result of sickling was a factor in the causation of the ulcers.

Epistaxis

According to Hughes, Diggs and Gillespie (1940), epistaxis is a frequent symptom, although haemorrhage from other mucous membranes is rare; they mentioned that epistaxis often was followed by relief of headache (also mentioned by them as a frequent and bothersome symptom). Konotey-Ahulu (1965b) described how a 16-year-old Ghanaian girl suffered from torrential epistaxis which was associated with multiple ulcerated areas on her face.

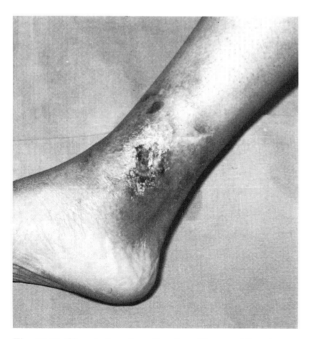

Fig. 11.11 Chronic leg ulceration in a 31-year-old patient with Hb-SS disease.
(Reproduced by courtesy of Drs D. S. Gillett and R. S. Mibashan.)

THE SPLEEN IN HOMOZYGOUS SICKLE-CELL DISEASE: HYPERSPLENISM AND ACUTE SPLENIC SEQUESTRATION

The spleen is probably always enlarged in young children with Hb-SS disease and it is often then palpable. Usually, however, it soon atrophies and it can seldom be palpated in adults.

Watson, Lichtman and Shapiro (1956) reported that the spleen was palpable in 18% of 115 patients: 33% of those in the first decade had a palpable spleen and 10% of those who were older. Haggard and Schneider (1961) recorded that the spleen was palpable in 15 out of 26 infants in the first 2 years of life. As will be referred to in Chapter 13, splenomegaly is more frequent, and persists into adult life, in Hb-SC disease and Hb-S/thalassaemia.

According to Serjeant (1974a, p. 98), the spleen can be felt in about 70% of young children at the age of 18 months, after which the incidence of splenomegaly gradually falls; in his series, however, it was still palpable in 6% of patients over the age of 30 years. Serjeant's (1970) West-Indian data suggest that the persistence of splenomegaly can be correlated with low levels of irreversibly sickled cells (ISCs): the mean ISC count of 42 patients with a palpable spleen was 6.36 ± 4.3% and in 271 patients with an impalpable spleen 13.0 ± 6.6%. The presence of splenomegaly was also associated with relatively high Hb-F percentages in all age-groups.

Hypersplenism

Rarely, the spleen becomes massively enlarged in children suffering apparently from genuine Hb-SS disease and this leads to increasingly severe anaemia and thrombocytopenia and the possibility of death in a shock-like state. Haggard and Schneider (1961) recorded four such cases out of a series of 54 infants who were less than 2 years of age. Their platelet count varied from 10 to 81 × 10^9/l. Splenectomy was carried out on one of the patients, after which the platelet count rose substantially. Similar striking examples of hypersplenism were described by Hilkovitz and Martin (1961), Egdahl, Martin and Hilkovitz (1963) and Rossi et al. (1964).

Hilkovitz and Martin's patients were two sisters, whose minimum haemoglobin was as low as 1.8 g/dl and 3.5 g/dl. They were splenectomized when aged 6 years and 13 years, respectively, and transfusions, which had had to be given repeatedly, were no longer required after the operation. Their spleens weighed 750 g and 1340 g.

Egdahl, Martin and Hilkovitz described five rather similar cases; three were children. Their minimum haemoglobin was recorded as between 1.6 and 3.8 g/dl and their minimum platelet count between 18 and 101 × 10^9/l. The total leucocyte count (including no doubt normoblasts, too) varied between 8.1 and 28.2 × 10^9/l; their reticulocyte count ranged between 32 and 52%. Splenectomy was carried out on all the patients with considerable benefit: their haemoglobin stabilized between 6 and 10 g/dl, the platelet count rose to normal levels and the reticulocyte count fell. The spleens weighed between 300 and 1235 g.

Rossi and co-workers' patient was a 6-year-old male child whose spleen eventually extended below the iliac crest. At this point, when his haemoglobin had fallen to 2.2–2.7 g/dl, and the platelet count to 44–66 × 10^9/l, splenectomy was carried out. Subsequently, the haemoglobin stabilized at 7–8 g/dl. The spleen weighed 808 g; microscopically, marked congestion, with closely packed sickled cells, and areas of fibrosis and siderosis were conspicuous. Before splenectomy, a ^{51}Cr erythrocyte auto-survival study gave a T_{50} of 20–24 hours; 45 days after splenectomy the T_{50} was 11 days.

Acute splenic sequestration. Seeler and Shwiaki (1972) described under the title 'acute splenic sequestration crisis' the occurrence in 14 young children, aged between 6 and 55 months, of episodes of severe anaemia and moderate thrombocytopenia associated with massive enlargement of the spleen and signs and symptoms of acute circulatory insufficiency. Four of the children died; four had one or more recurrences; in four the spleen involuted; two underwent splenectomy. In only four of the episodes was there evidence of an accompanying infection. The data were accumulated within a $4\frac{1}{2}$-year period during which time there had been 150–170 admissions to hospital annually of children with Hb-SS disease.

A further dramatic case was described by Schwartz (1972). The patient was a 6-year-old male who gave a history of 'sequestration crises'. Before splenectomy the platelet count had fallen to 60–100 × 10^9/l; it stabilized at 400–500 × 10^9/l subsequently.

More recent accounts of acute splenic sequestration and hypersplenism include an important paper by Topley et al. (1981) who had carried out a cohort study of 216 West-Indian Hb-SS children from the time of their birth: 52 of these children were recorded as

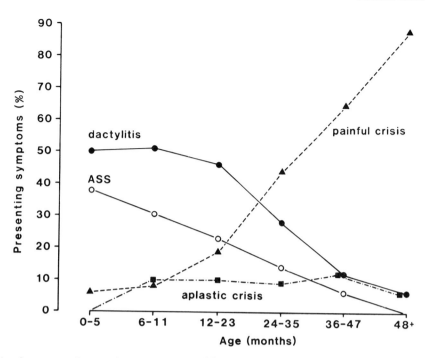

Fig. 11.12 Relative frequency of presenting symptoms at different ages in Hb-SS children: dactylitis, acute splenic sequestration (ASS), aplastic crisis and painful crisis.
[Reproduced by permission from Serjeant (1985b).]

suffering from 71 episodes of acute splenic sequestration (ASS); 10 of them died. Most of the episodes occurred in children less than 2 years of age (Fig. 11.12): eight of those who died were in this age-group, and their spleen at necropsy weighed between 60 and 445 g (2–10 times the normal weight for the child's age). Topley *et al.* stressed that, in addition to life-threatening 'classical' attacks of ASS, minor attacks also occurred, and that there was in fact a continuous spectrum of severity. As minimum criteria for diagnosing ASS, a fall in haemoglobin of at least 2 g, a sustained or increased reticulocyte count and an enlarging spleen were all required. The mean haemoglobin in all attacks was 4.8 g/dl (range 0.8–7.3 g) and the average fall was 3.2 g. Bacteriological examination failed to identify any specific infective agent. Topley *et al.* concluded that ASS was a major cause of morbidity and mortality in young children and that the minor attacks were predictive in some patients of later major episodes; they suggested that prevention of the latter by splenectomy should be considered for children who had developed minor episodes, particularly if they had been left with sustained hypersplenism.

In a subsequent report from Jamaica, Emond and co-workers (1985) recorded that 89 out of 308 Hb-SS children in the cohort had experienced 132 significant attacks of ASS within a 10-year period. The majority of the affected children were aged between 6 months and 2 years: 13 had died before transfusion could be organized, 11 during their first attack. Almost half of those who developed ASS had had a subsequent attack or attacks. Respiratory symptoms accompanied 52 of the 132 episodes, but there were relatively few significant bacterial isolates, and previous immunization with *Str. pneumoniae* vaccine or penicillin prophylaxis did not seem to be effective in preventing attacks. The presence of a high Hb-F percentage and possibly, too, of one or two genes for α-thalassaemia did, however, appear to be protective. Emond *et al.* stressed that ASS (and pneumococcal infection) were the most important causes of death in young Hb-SS children in Jamaica.

The cause and mechanism of these remarkable episodes has not really been established. The pathology of the spleen in Hb-SS disease is considered on page 181.

Estimation of spleen size using [99m]Technetium (Tc)

[99mTc]sulphur colloid has been used in several studies in an attempt to visualize the spleen in Hb-SS patients and to estimate its size. In the majority of cases no spleen shadow has been obtained (Pearson, Spencer and Cornelius, 1969; Samuels and Stewart, 1970; Casper *et al.*, 1976).

Pearson, Spencer and Cornelius studied 12 children aged 8 months to 14 years, five of whom had had severe bacterial infections. Howell-Jolly bodies, suggestive of splenic atrophy, were identified in the blood films of 11 of them. However, the spleen was palpable in nine of the children and there was X-ray evidence, too, of its enlargement. Despite this, it was successfully delineated by the [^{99m}Tc]sulphur colloid technique in only one of them. Pearson, Spencer and Cornelius suggested that the 'functional asplenia' which they had demonstrated, *i.e.*, the failure to clear the radioisotope-labelled sulphur colloid particles, was due either to masses of sickled cells obstructing the passage of blood through the spleen pulp, thus forcing much of the blood to traverse the spleen by intrasplenic shunts, or because the R.E. phagocytic cells were already overstuffed with particulate material. Later, Pearson and co-workers (1970) reported that the functional asplenia could be reversed by prior transfusion with normal blood. Eight children were studied: five were transfused with blood and ^{99m}Tc scans carried out on them subsequently were successful in demonstrating a spleen; in contrast, in the three given plasma only the scan failed to demonstrate a spleen. Pearson *et al.* suggested that an admixture of about 50% of normal erythrocytes was required to restore a sufficient flow of blood through the spleen pulp for the organ to be visualized.

Additional evidence of functional asplenia has been provided by studies using ^{51}Cr-labelled heat-damaged erythrocytes. Ringelhann and Konotey-Ahulu (1971) found that the uptake of the isotope by the spleen was very low in all of 13 patients with Hb SS, even if the spleen was palpably enlarged; it was variable with some low values in seven Hb-SC patients and similar to normal controls in patients with Hb CC, Hb-S/thalassaemia or Hb AS. The spleen:liver radioactivity ratio was 1.0 in the Hb-SS patients.

In an interesting recent study, Babiker and co-workers (1985) reported that they had carried out [^{99m}Tc]sulphur colloid scans in two different populations of Saudi-Arabian Hb-SS patients. In 21 out of 25 children originating from the South West of the country there was no uptake of colloid (indicating splenic dysfunction), whereas in eight out of 10 children from the Eastern Province the uptake in the spleen was equal to that in the liver. The South-Western children suffered from a severe form of the disease and had relatively low Hb-F levels (5.6–10%), while the Eastern-Province children were relatively mildly affected and had high Hb-F levels (see also p. 50).

JAUNDICE, GALLSTONES AND THE LIVER

Most Hb-SS patients are chronically mildly to moderately jaundiced. Margolies (1951) described

their conjunctivae as being typically greenish-yellow in colour. Some patients, particularly the older ones, suffer additionally from episodes of obstructive jaundice due to pigment gallstones and cholecystitis.

Gallstones. These were recorded by Weens (1945), Green, Conley and Berthrong (1953) and Jordan (1957) in about one-third of their patients. The stones are typically of the multiple pigment variety (as in other chronic haemolytic anaemias) but they seldom cause trouble (Barrett-Connor, 1968a). They have been reported in quite young children, *e.g.*, by Mintz, Church and Adams (1955) in a boy aged 10, by Mintz and Pugh (1970) in a 6½-year-old boy and by Lachman *et al.* (1979) in a 4-year-old boy. The incidence increases with age. Thus, Barrett-Connor (1968a), who reviewed the literature, described their presence in 16 out of 22 patients (73%) who were aged between 12 and 58 years.

More recently, McCall and co-workers (1977) reported that of 206 Jamaican Hb-SS patients 28% were found to have evidence of gallstones by means of a straight X-ray of the abdomen and 61% by oral cholecystography. The incidence of the stones was found to be directly related to the patient's age and to the apparent haemolytic rate, as judged by the height of the reticulocyte count. More females were affected than males. In only 17% of the patients with stones were the stones radio-translucent. In 10% of the patients oral cholecystography showed that the gall bladder was non-functional.

Lachman and co-workers (1979) described how they had detected gallstones in 29% of 31 Hb-SS patients who had no symptoms of gall-bladder disease. Ultrasonography was used as a screening procedure, supported by abdominal radiography and cholecystography.

Sarnaik and co-workers (1980) reported on the incidence of gallstones, as assessed by ultrasonography, in a large series of Hb-SS patients attending a clinic in Detroit. Of 226 patients aged between 2 and 18 years, 63 (27%) were shown to have developed stones and 14 (6.2%) were diagnosed as having 'sludge'. The patients who had stones had significantly higher mean serum bilirubin levels than those without stones, but their haemoglobin concentrations and reticulocyte counts were similar. The proportion of patients with stones who were female was higher in 15–18-year-olds than in the pre-adolescent children. Sarnaik *et al.* stressed the unexpectedly high incidence of stones in children less than 10 years old and also that the rather small proportion of patients (14% at all ages) who had complained of symptoms which could be attributed to the presence of stones raised doubts as to whether early surgical intervention was justified. Stephens and Scott (1980), who also reported on the incidence of gallstones in a large series of patients, recommended, however, that elective cholecystectomy should be carried out. Twenty-nine of their patients had undergone the operation without any major surgical complication. Stephens and Scott pointed out that urgent cholecystectomy in a Hb-SS patient with real or suspected cholecystitis was a risky procedure and that the removal of stones electively from a patient in a quiescent phase simplified the management of subsequent bouts of abdominal pain. Forty of their 100 Hb-SS patients were shown by means of cholecystography, ultrasonography or abdominal X-ray to have formed stones, and in approximately one-half of the patients the stones were sufficiently calcified to be visible on a straight X-ray. Their youngest patient was 3 years old.

The incidence of gallstones in Hb-SS patients is thus high in the Western World. According to Perrine (1973), stones are, however, far less common (only one-quarter to one-sixth as frequent) in Hb-SS oasis dwellers in Saudi Arabia.

Rarely, cholestasis had led to very intense jaundice (Muirhead, Halden and Wilson, 1956; Klion, Weiner and Schaffner, 1964). In Muirhead, Halden and Wilson's five patients cholescystectomy was followed by complete or almost complete disappearance of their jaundice. The gall bladders contained thick bile of almost 'putty-like' consistency, but no stones.

Very intense jaundice has, too, been recorded in patients who have developed hepatitis or have suffered from bile-duct obstruction due to stones. Hargrove (1970) gave details of six such patients whose serum bilirubin levels reached maxima of 43–103 mg/dl, of which 25–63.5 mg was conjugated bilirubin.

The liver

The liver is usually palpable in Hb-SS disease, particularly in children (Margolies, 1951; Green, Conley and Berthrong, 1953; Ferguson and Scott, 1959); its enlargement tends to become less frequent in the second and third decades, but becomes more common in patients surviving to 30 years or more (Green, Conley and Berthrong, 1953; Hilkovitz and Jacobson, 1961). The liver may enlarge further during painful crises. Brittain, de la Torre and Willey (1966) recorded the occurrence of an intrahepatic abscess which they attributed to secondary infection of an infarct with *E. coli*.

Hyperbilirubinaemic crises. Owen, Aldridge and Thompson (1965) described the occurrence in five patients of an unusual fatal liver disorder which they believed was peculiar to Hb-SS disease and not a form of hepatitis. The patients became deeply jaundiced; stasis of sickled cells in the hepatic sinuses and swelling of Kupffer cells were thought to have led to ischaemic necrosis of hepatocytes and biliary stasis. The patients' serum bilirubin levels were extremely high (maximum values 61–89 mg/dl) and there was marked biliuria. The leucocyte counts were also very high and reached $15.6–50.0 \times 10^9/l$, with a left shift of the neutrophils.

A similar occurrence was recorded by Desforges and Wang (1966) and referred to as 'hyperbilirubinemic crisis'. Their patient, a 12-year-old boy complained of abdominal pain and became deeply jaundiced, the total serum bilirubin reaching 50 mg/dl, of which 40 mg was conjugated. The liver enlarged and became tender, the urine contained bile pigment and the patient's temperature reached 103° F (Fig. 11.13). The serum glutamic oxaloacetic transaminase content was markedly increased. The jaundice subsided after 2 weeks, and a cholecystogram carried out later showed a normal gall bladder and no evidence of stones. Desforges and Wang suggested that the basis of the patient's crisis was sickling and sludging of blood in the liver leading to hepatic necrosis.

Further cases of extreme hyperbilirubinaemia were described by Buchanan and Glader (1977). Their patients were six children of whom one, aged 15, had had a cholecystectomy for stones when aged 6 years old and another, aged 11, had multiple stones in the gall bladder at the time of investigation. The other four children were aged between 5 and 11 years and had normal cholecystograms. Their serum bilirubin ranged between 28 and 58 mg/dl, of which 16–22 mg were conjugated: the serum transaminase levels were similarly markedly raised. Liver enlargement was apparently not a marked feature and the episodes resolved without treatment in 2–5 weeks. Buchanan and Glader concluded that intra-hepatic sickling was the cause of the deep jaundice and that in children such episodes were usually benign and self-limited.

Hepatic sequestration of sickled cells. Recently, further patients have been described as suffering from recurrent attacks of acute 'hepatic seques-

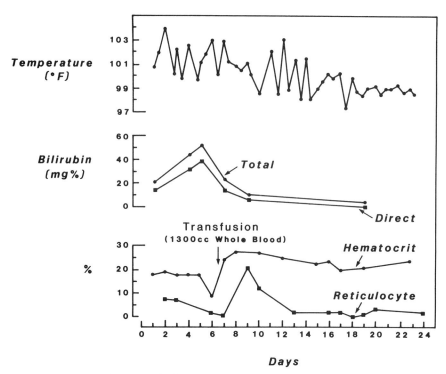

Fig. 11.13 Course of a hyperbilirubinaemic crisis in a 12-year-old male with Hb-SS disease.
[Reproduced by permission from Desforges and Wang (1966).]

tration'. Hatton, Bunch and Weatherall's (1985) two patients were Nigerian females aged 21 and 18 years, respectively, who presented with a rapidly enlarging liver, increasing jaundice and a sharp fall in haemoglobin accompanied by a rise in reticulocyte count. Sequestration of sickled cells in the liver was suggested as the causal mechanism. There were no appreciable disturbances of liver function and no signs of cardiac failure. Hatton, Bunch and Weatherall drew attention to the importance of assessing liver size in a patient experiencing a sudden fall in haemoglobin; they stressed that the hepatic enlargement could be associated with a painful bone crisis or acute chest symptoms or the liver could be the chief organ involved. Spontaneous resolution of the enlargement was possible; but transfusion with packed erythrocytes might be necessary.

Gutteridge, Newland and Sequeira's (1985) patient was a 26-year-old West-Indian female who was admitted to hospital with fever, abdominal discomfort, jaundice and an enlarging liver which over the next 5 days reached the pelvic brim. The haemoglobin fell to 5.7 g/dl and the reticulocyte count rose to 44%. Exchange transfusion was carried out. Liver biopsy revealed that the hepatic sinusoids contained sickled cells; non-caseating granulomas were conspicuous, too. Cultures were negative for acid-fast bacilli and no specific infecting organism of any sort could be identified. The granulomas were thought possibly to represent a macrophage response to the abnormal surface of sickled cells.

Cirrhosis. According to Serjeant (1974a, p. 93), cirrhosis is uncommon in Hb-SS patients and where it has occurred there has frequently been a history of multiple blood transfusions; he concluded that the available evidence did not establish it as a primary complication.

Viral hepatitis. Hb-SS patients suffer from viral hepatitis but probably not more frequently than do Hb-AA individuals living in the same environment. Barrett-Connor (1968b) referred to six patients with sickle-cell disease and 10 with sickle-cell trait who had been in hospital within a 7-year period with a diagnosis of hepatitis. The clinical, laboratory and liver-biopsy findings were similar to those of Hb-AA patients with hepatitis except for the severe degree of hyperbilirubinaemia in the Hb-SS patients; this was interpreted as a reflection of a heavy bilirubin load on an acutely damaged liver. Barrett-Connor suggested, too, that chronic liver disease may in some Hb-SS patients be the consequence of past unrecognized viral hepatitis rather than being necessarily brought about by intrahepatic sickling.

INVOLVEMENT OF THE EYES

The eye is the site of important pathological changes in sickle-cell disease. Obstruction and obliteration of retinal vessels is all too frequent, presumably as the result of intravascular sickling, sludging of blood and eventual vaso-occlusion. The consequence of the vaso-occlusion is the development of avascular areas in the periphery of the retina, while at the margins of these areas new vessels proliferate and form, too, abnormal arteriovenous anastomoses, a process referred to as proliferative sickle retinopathy (Fig. 11.14). Retinal tears and separation may result. The new vessels tend to bleed and to lead to vitreous haemorrhage and transient impairment of vision,

and the retinal tears and detachment may result in permanent blindness. The retinal lesions are not confined to Hb-SS patients: in fact, they affect (for reasons which are obscure) with even greater frequency Hb-SC and Hb-S/β^+-thalassaemia patients (see Serjeant, 1985a).

That the retina of the eye may be affected in sickle-cell disease has been known for many years. Harden (1937) was one of the first authors to call attention to this possibility. Amongst subsequent important contributions to the literature are papers by Edington and Sarkies (1952), Henry and Chapman (1954), Lieb, Geeraets and Guerry (1959), Welch and Goldberg (1966), Condon and Serjeant (1972), Armaly (1974), Condon and Serjeant (1980) and Hayes, Condon and Serjeant (1981).

Edington and Sarkies (1952) described two male patients, aged 16 and 22 years, respectively, in whom they had detected retinal micro-aneurisms. Neither was significantly anaemic but there was reason to believe that both were homozygous for Hb S. One patient had two small aneurisms well out to the periphery of the left fundus: the other patient had a morula-shaped aneurism as well as a smaller one on the right side and, on the left side, there had been haemorrhage into the vitreous.

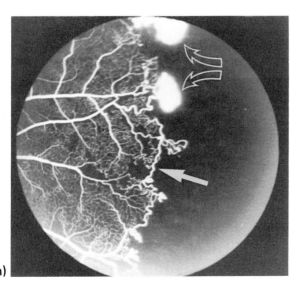
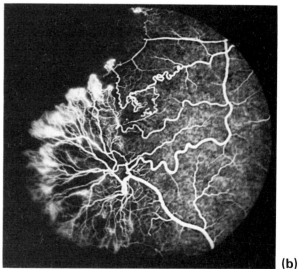

(a)   (b)

Fig. 11.14 Retinal changes in two patients with sickle-cell disease, as revealed by fluorescein angiography.
(a) The angiogram shows the lesions of proliferative sickle retinopathy in a 31-year-old Hb-SS patient. The dark area to the right of the field represents avascular retina. The curved arrows show leaking dye; the straight arrow shows an abnormal arteriovenous communication.
(b) The angiogram shows large proliferative lesions in the retina of a 26-year-old patient with Hb-SC disease.
[Reproduced by permission from Serjeant (1985a).]

Lieb, Geeraets and Guerry (1959) studied the retinae of 65 patients: 46 of 51 Hb-SS patients and all nine Hb-SC patients showed fundal changes, compared with three out of nine Hb-AS individuals. Welch and Goldberg (1966) likened the distinctive arteriovenous anastomoses sometimes to be seen in the periphery of the retina to 'sea-fans' (see p. 149). Condon and Serjeant (1972) reported on the retinae of 76 Hb-SS patients, and concluded that a whitened periphery and evidence of peripheral vascular disease were almost always present.

Condon and Serjeant (1980) reported on 313 Hb-SS patients whom they had followed for 1–8 years. Signs of proliferative sickle retinopathy (PSR) were present in 68 of them (12%) at first examination and developed in a further 46 (8%) during the period of study. In some patients the lesions regressed as the result of auto-infarction. This happened more often in Hb-SS patients than in Hb-SC patients (in whom PSR was more frequent) (Fig. 11.14).

Hayes, Condon and Serjeant (1981) reviewed 261 Hb-SS patients: 29 had proliferative sickle retinopathy (PSR) and this was present in 14% of patients who were over 40 years of age. Amongst the men, those with a relatively high haemoglobin (> 9 g/dl) and a low Hb-F level (< 5%) appeared to have an increased chance of developing retinal lesions. This relationship did not seem, however, to apply to the women in whom PSR was seen in patients whose haemoglobin was lower and Hb-F level higher than in the men.

Talbot and co-workers (1982, 1983) have examined the eyes of many of the Hb-SS children they have been following as part of their cohort study. Sheathing and peripheral closure of retinal arterioles were common findings and their incidence showed an upward trend with age. (The changes were less frequent in Hb-SC patients.) PSR was, however, not found in in any of the 5–7½-year-olds studied. Talbot et al. (1983) found that retinal vessel closure was correlated with a low total haemoglobin, a low Hb-F percentage, and high reticulocyte and ISC counts.

The vessels of the retina are not the only eye vessels to be affected in sickle-cell disease. Venous sacculations and capillary micro-aneurisms can be seen in the conjunctival vessels if they are looked at with the aid of an ophthalmic microscope and sludging of the blood can be seen, too (Knisely et al., 1947; Fink et al., 1961; Paton, 1961). According to Serjeant, Serjeant and Condon (1972) and Nagpal et al. (1977) the grade of abnormality is significantly correlated with the number of irreversibly sickled cells present.

Knisely and co-workers (1947) had referred to sludged blood in the conjunctival vessels of six patients with sickle-cell anaemia who had been referred to them by Dr L. W. Diggs. They were amongst a large number of human patients suffering from a wide variety of conditions in which the phenomenon had been seen: the erythrocytes were [in their words] 'agglutinated into masses (not rouleaux); this changed the blood from its normal relatively fluid state, to a circulating sludge'.

RENAL ABNORMALITIES

Hyposthenuria

A characteristic finding in Hb-SS disease, and in the Hb-AS trait, is impairment of the ability to concentrate urine (hyposthenuria). The abnormality has been extensively studied. Relatively early reports include those of Etteldorf, Tuttle and Clayton (1952), Kunz et al. (1953, 1954), McCrory, Goren and Gornfeld (1953), Heinemann and Cheung (1957), Levitt et al. (1960) and Schlitt and Keitel (1960a,b). The phenomenon, however, had been recognized well before the 1950s, for as far back as 1924 Sydenstricker had remarked 'the urine of both types of case ['latent' and 'active' cases of sickle-cell anaemia] has a low specific gravity'.

Keitel, Thompson and Itano (1956), in an extensive study, found that in young patients with Hb-SS disease the defect in concentration could be alleviated by multiple transfusions. They concluded that the abnormality was in some way associated with the presence of Hb S (the formation of which would be depressed by transfusion) and that it was not due to anaemia itself, for 69% of Hb-AS subjects had the same defect, although less marked. Statius van Eps and co-workers (1967), found, however, that the beneficial effect of repeated transfusions on renal concentration power appeared to be confined to children; there was little response in a 15-year-old and none at all in a woman aged 40, suggesting the development with time of an irreversible structural defect. Earlier studies by Etteldorf et al. (1955) had in fact shown that renal function becomes progressively impaired as Hb-SS disease patients become older. The hyposthenuria is associated with enuresis and nocturia (Noll, Newman and Gross, 1967), and is normally compensated for by an abnormally high fluid intake (Saxena, Scott and Ferguson, 1966).

Hatch and Diggs (1965) found that patients with Hb-SS disease (or with Hb-SC disease) tended to be in negative fluid balance and that while this could normally be compensated for, the negative balance might become a serious feature in crises. Fluid restriction was in general poorly tolerated.

Hatch, Culberton and Diggs (1967) concluded, as the result of studying 13 patients with Hb-SS disease, that the defect in urinary concentration results from a limitation in maintaining a high concentration of solute in the medullary interstitium of the kidney. Ho Ping Kong and Alleyne (1968, 1971) studied 14 adult Jamaicans with Hb-SS disease and observed a mild defect in urinary acidification, H ion excretion being subnormal in response to ammonium chloride loading. Goosens and co-workers (1972) similarly found that the urine pH was higher than anticipated after acid loading, the titrable acidity being lower in Hb-SS and Hb-SC patients than in the Hb-AS trait and in normal subjects. They concluded that the acidification defect in sickle-cell nephropathy was equivalent to an incomplete form of renal tubular acidosis.

In an interesting microradioangiographic study, Statius van Eps and co-workers (1970) demonstrated that in Hb-SS disease there might be an almost complete absence of the vasa recta of the renal medulla and in Hb-SC disease and Hb-AS trait a reduced number of vasa recta and loss of normal architecture. They suggested that the basic lesion in sickle-cell disease nephropathy is a progressive obliteration of the vasa recta and that this inevitably results in loss of the kidney's concentrating function.

Warrier, Sarnaik and Brewer (1978) concluded as the result of studying 25 Hb-SS children aged between 31–62 months that those with high ISC counts tended to develop hyposthenuria earlier and to a greater degree than those with relatively low counts.

Haematuria

As already referred to, painless haematuria occurs in association with the presence of Hb S in the absence of any additional organic cause. The relative frequency of bleeding from the kidney in Hb-SS disease and in the trait is uncertain. It seems to have been more frequently observed and reported in the trait, *e.g.* by Allen (1964), but the population at risk is, of course, far larger. As in the Hb-AS trait, most of the patients have been young adults. The bleeding is usually recurrent and on cystoscopy will be found typically to be coming from one kidney. In some patients the loss of blood has been severe enough to necessitate blood transfusion or suggest the presence of a renal neoplasm (Abel and Brown, 1948).

Occasionally the loss of blood has been so serious as to raise the question as to whether nephrectomy should be undertaken (Mostofi, Vorder Bruegge and Diggs, 1957; Lucas and Bullock, 1960). Because of the risk of bleeding from the remaining kidney, nephrectomy

clearly should not be carried out except as a last resort. In this connection two other possible lines of treatment should be mentioned. Chaplin (1980) referred to a patient who had failed to respond to multiple single-unit transfusions who, nevertheless, responded to a 6-unit partial exchange transfusion. John and co-workers (1980) described how two patients for whom nephrectomy had been considered (one had Hb-SC disease, the other Hb AS) apparently responded to triglycyl vasopressin given intravenously.

Haematuria in a patient with Hb S may of course be due to causes unconnected with the abnormal haemoglobin. Susmano and Lewy (1969), for instance, described the occurrence of acute post-streptococcal glomerulonephritis in two young children: one had Hb-SS disease, the other Hb-AS trait.

Nephrotic syndrome

A few patients with Hb-SS disease have developed the nephrotic syndrome (Berman and Tublin, 1959; Sweeney, Dobbins and Etteldorf, 1962). The causal relationship, if any, between the two conditions is obscure. However, Strauss and co-workers (1975) and Pardoe and co-workers (1975) have suggested that renal tubular epithelial antigen, released perhaps as the result of renal ischaemia, may lead to the development of specific auto-antibodies with secondary deposition of immune complexes within renal glomeruli and proximal tubular cells: Pardoe *et al.* had studied seven patients who appeared to have developed an immune complex nephritis; four presented with the nephrotic syndrome. Four of these patients died of renal failure, and IgG (and IgM in two patients) and complement component C3 (and C1q, C4 and C5 in two patients) were demonstrated on the glomerular basement membrane.

Markenson and co-workers (1978) described an interesting family in which three out of five siblings developed the nephrotic syndrome: three siblings had Hb SS and two of them had the nephrotic syndrome; the third sibling with the nephrotic syndrome had the thalassaemia trait. In this family at least the occurrence of the nephrotic syndrome and the presence of Hb SS did not seem to be causally related.

Acute renal failure

This seems to be a rare event in patients with Hb-SS disease. Salisbury (1960) described how a female aged 32 years with Hb-SS disease recovered from acute renal failure and acidosis which developed as a sequel to a hypotensive episode following cholecystectomy. Devereux and Knowles (1985) described a similar occurrence in a 25-year-old Nigerian male admitted into hospital in a severe and complicated painful crisis. He, too, eventually made a good recovery. The renal failure was attributed to rhabdomyolysis secondary to muscle ischaemia.

Chronic renal failure

There is some evidence of a gradual deterioration in renal function in the older patients with Hb-SS disease and of relatively low haemoglobin levels in patients who are over 40. The two phenomena are interrelated. According to the data of Morgan and Serjeant (1981), the haemoglobin level and renal creatinine clearance are positively correlated. In a further study of 31 patients, Morgan, Gruber and Serjeant (1982) showed that the link between renal disease and low haemoglobin levels is failure by the patient to produce an adequate amount of erythropoietin.

Acute infarction of the kidney

Granfortuna, Zamkoff & Urrutia (1986) described the occurrence in a 44-year-old Hb-SS female of acute infarction of the left kidney apparently due to occlusion of the renal artery.

GOUT

Adult patients with Hb-SS disease occasionally present with gouty arthritis. Gold and co-workers (1968) followed up their observation of gout and hyperuricaemia in a 53-year-old female by a study of 13 other patients with Hb-SS disease and six with Hb-SC disease. Six of the former and two of the latter had serum uric-acid levels exceeding 6 mg/dl. Increased formation secondary to active erythropoiesis was suggested as the cause. Ball and Sorenson's (1970) metabolic study of a 37-year-old male with gouty arthritis indicated an overproduction of uric acid as well as a diminished excretion which was attributed by them to reduction in the number of nephrons.

Walker and Alexander (1971) concluded that gout was an uncommon complication of Hb-SS disease. However, four out of eight patients studied had serum uric-acid levels >8 mg/dl and in these four patients there was evidence of impaired uric-acid clearance by the kidney. They concluded that raised serum levels may be expected when defective renal function is superimposed on increased production. Diamond and co-workers (1976), while agreeing that gout seldom occurs, were, on the other hand, able to demonstrate in seven young adults who had normal serum uric-acid levels that the excretion of urate by the renal tubules was raised. They concluded that this allowed them to maintain normal serum levels despite an overproduction of uric acid.

Ballou and co-workers (1977), who described the occurrence of clinical gout in two adult female patients, aged 17 and 46 years, respectively, with Hb-SC and Hb-CC disease, listed nine adults with Hb-SS disease, aged between 15 and 53 years, who had been described in the literature as having suffered from gout.

Diamond, Meisel and Holden (1979), in a comprehensive study of uric-acid metabolism in 95 patients with sickle-cell disease aged between 17 months and 45 years, concluded that although urate overproduction commenced in childhood normal serum levels are often maintained into adult life, explaining why clinical gout is uncommon. When the serum levels rise [as in 26 out of 67 adults (39%)], this, it was concluded, is secondary to altered tubular function, perhaps secondary to the sickle-cell disease.

CARDIAC INVOLVEMENT

Cardiac enlargement and an increased cardiac output are almost invariably found in Hb-SS patients. The changes compensate for the chronic anaemia and the often impaired oxygenation in the lungs. Cor pulmonale occasionally develops. Left ventricular failure is unusual; hypertension occurs occasionally as the result of renal damage secondary to sickling; myocardial infarction is rare. It seems likely that compared to the past, cardiac problems will become more important as more and more patients survive into late adult life.

Klinefelter (1942) in an early report had stressed that cardiac enlargement was common and that this affected chiefly the right side of the heart; it was often more severe than in other chronic anaemias of comparable severity; cor pulmonale sometimes developed. Winsor and Burch (1944b) reported on the ECG and cardiac state in 25 patients with active sickle-cell anaemia. The heart was enlarged in 95% and evidence of pulmonary thrombosis was found in six of nine patients on whom a necropsy had been carried out. ECGs showed nothing thought to be characteristic although abnormalities were present in 20%.

Cardiac output was studied by Leight and co-workers (1954) and was found to be generally elevated, although the increase did not seem to be proportional to the degree of anaemia present. ECG findings were described by Lindo and Doctor (1955). As a group, the patients have low arterial oxygen tensions and increased alveolar – arterial oxygen gradients (Becklake et al., 1955; Fowler, Smith and Greenfield, 1957; Sproule, Halden and Miller, 1958; Oduntan, 1969). Repeated occlusion of pulmonary vessels appears to be the likely cause of this.

Shubin and co-workers (1960) studied seven Hb-SS children in detail, including the use of cardiac catheterization. Cardiac output was increased, and there was X-ray evidence of cardiomegaly and of diffuse pulmonary vascularity. Blood and plasma volume were increased in five out of six patients (see p. 78). Ng and co-workers (1967) reported essentially similar findings in 36 Hb-SS children; there was ECG evidence of left ventricular hypertrophy in 22. The haemoglobin level of those with cardiovascular abnormalities was lower than in those without abnormalities.

Pearson and co-workers (1965) made some interesting observations on a 4-year-old boy with Hb-SS disease and the tetralogy of Fallot. Despite the arterial desaturation, his symptoms were similar to those of children with uncomplicated Hb-SS disease. Perhaps the rapid circulation time was helpful. Post-operatively, tricuspid incompetence and congestive cardiac failure were associated with a worsening of his thrombotic symptoms.

Gerry, Baird and Fortuin (1976) evaluated left ventricular function in 23 adult Hb-SS patients by means of echocardiography: the ejection-phase indices were greater than normal. The results in patients over 30 years of age were compared with those in patients less than 30, but no significant differences in left ventricular function were detected. Gerry, Baird and Fortuin concluded that the chronic volume overload was well tolerated. Valuable reviews include those of Lindsay, Meshel and Patterson (1974) and Falk and Hood (1982).

Myocardial infarction. As already referred to, Hb-SS patients seldom suffer from myocardial infarcts. The relative youth of most of the patients no doubt plays a part in their rarity. A few well-authenticated cases, however, have been described. Martin and co-workers (1983) reported that a 25-year-old female presented clinical and ECG evidence of infarction. She died, and at necropsy, although the coronary vessels were free from thrombi, there were areas of coagulation necrosis

and fibrosis in the myocardium. Sludging of blood was thought to have led to ischaemia. Barrett and co-workers (1984) reviewed the incidence of infarction in 108 Hb-SS patients aged 16–60 years. Three were considered to have had infarcts, and this was confirmed in two of them at necropsy. There was, however, no evidence of significant coronary atheroma.

Mitral valve prolapse. Pseudoxanthoma elasticum, a disorder of elastic tissue, has been reported in a few patients in association with sickle-cell disease.

Suerig and Siefert (1964) reported the concurrence of the two disorders in a 24-year-old female and referred to other possible cases. Recently, mitral valve prolapse has been demonstrated to occur frequently in Hb-SS patients and the possibility has been raised that this is a manifestation of a generalized connective tissue disorder. Lippman and co-workers (1985b) compared by means of echocardiography the incidence of mitral valve prolapse in 57 patients with sickle-cell disease (46 Hb SS) with that in 35 patients with a comparable degree of chronic anaemia (resulting from end-stage renal disease): 25% of the sickle-cell disease patients had mitral valve prolapse compared with 3% of the anaemic controls. The possibility was raised that a generalized connective tissue abnormality might be linked genetically with haemoglobin synthesis or be 'an epiphenomenon of the sickling process'. Lippman and co-workers (1985a) biopsied the skin of 32 of these patients and analysed the contained collagen in five ways. Evidence was obtained of an elastic tissue abnormality similar to, but not so severe as, that of pseudoxanthoma elasticum. The possibility that the elastic tissue defect might be genetically linked to the Hb-S defect was, however, considered to be unlikely: it was pointed out that the β-globin gene complex is on chromosome 11 while the type-1 collagen and elastin genes are on chromosomes 17 and 7, respectively.

PULMONARY COMPLICATIONS

Compared with individuals of normal haemoglobin genotype, Hb-SS disease patients, particularly young children, relatively frequently suffer from pulmonary symptoms, and in patients whose symptoms develop acutely it may be difficult to distinguish between pulmonary infection and pulmonary infarction.

It is instructive to refer back to Henderson's (1950) valuable clinical study of 54 cases of sickle-cell anaemia:

the youngest patient was 5 years of age, the oldest 50; their mean age 21.2 years. Fourteen of them had presented with 'pneumonia'; in 13 this was associated with crises of abdominal pain, severe joint pain and jaundice. Fever was prolonged and lasted from 4 to 30 days. Routine examination of sputum failed to reveal any specific 'etiologic agent' and no cold agglutinins developed; the response to antibiotic therapy was inconclusive. 'All cases were confirmed by X-ray' and 'none had the appearance of an infarct'. The 'pneumonia' was noted to clear slowly, and it seems very probable with hindsight that infarction as the result of vascular occlusion played a large role in the pneumonia these patients were thought to have suffered from.

Petch and Serjeant (1970) described a comparison between 28 Hb-SS disease patients and 28 non-Hb-SS disease patients admitted to hospital with a diagnosis of pneumonia. The most striking differences were that the pulmonary lesions tended to recur in the Hb-SS patients and that their fever was prolonged. Thus only five of the Hb-SS patients became afebrile within 48 hours compared with 25 of the non-Hb-SS patients. The Hb-SS patients often, too, gave a past history of similar episodes.

In an important paper, Barrett-Connor (1973) stressed the difficulty of differentiating clinically between infection and infarction resulting from vascular occlusion. Eighty patients were reviewed: there were 175 admissions for acute pulmonary symptoms; in three-quarters no final diagnosis was arrived at but most of the patients were thought to have had pneumonia. As pneumococcal infections might be fulminant, it was recommended that all pulmonary episodes should be treated with antibiotics. Bromberg (1974), too, in a review, emphasized the difficulty in differentiating between infection and infarction.

Acute chest syndrome. Charache, Scott and Charache (1979) defined under the title 'Acute chest syndrome' the occurrence of fever, chest pain, increased leucocytosis and a pulmonary infiltrate demonstrable by X-ray. Fifty-two such episodes were studied in 28 Hb-SS patients aged between 15 and 34 years. Possible bacterial pathogens were identified in less than half the cases, and *Staph. aureus* was the only bacterium in sputum the presence of which accompanied an illness longer than that associated with a normal bacterial flora. There was no evidence of pneumococcaemia in any patient and *Str. pneumoniae* was not present in the sputum in numbers considered to be meaningful. Charache, Scott and Charache concluded that 'pneumonia' in adults suffering from Hb-SS disease is often infarction and they pointed out that their data were similar

to those described many years earlier by Henderson (1950). They made the additional point that in view of the lack of evidence that *Str. pneumoniae* is an important pathogen in the acute chest syndrome in adults the immunization of adults with polyvalent pneumococcal vaccine is unlikely to be helpful in its prevention.

Clearly, pulmonary infections are common, particularly in children, but so, too, are infarcts, particularly in older patients. In some patients infection is probably superimposed on infarction secondary to venous occlusion or embolism, which is the primary event. Infarcts, too, appear to be the pathological basis of the cor pulmonale which may sometimes develop (Yater and Hansmann, 1936; Klinefelter, 1942; Moser and Shea, 1957; Bromberg, 1974; Collins and Orringer, 1982).

The pathological consequences of sickle-cell disease on lung function and arterial blood oxygen saturation, and the harmful effect of pulmonary infection or infarction, or both, have been assessed by detailed tests. The arterial oxygen tension has been shown often to be subnormal and vital capacity to be reduced; the alveolar – arterial oxygen tension difference has been found to be widened in most patients and the pulmonary diffusing capacity commonly reduced (Fowler, Smith and Greenfield, 1957; Bromberg and Jensen, 1967; Femi-Pearse, Gazioglu and Yu, 1970; Miller and Serjeant, 1971; Miller *et al.*, 1973).

Miller and co-workers (1973) reported on studies of cardio-pulmonary responses and gas exchange during progressive exercise in 22 Hb-SS disease adults with haemoglobin levels varying from 4 to 10 g/dl. Their exertional dyspnoea was attributed to hyperpnoea and a maximum breathing capacity reduced by small lung volumes.

Further papers dealing with the occurrence of pulmonary thrombo-embolism in Hb-SS disease and with the difficulty in distinguishing between pulmonary infarction and pulmonary infection in patients presenting with acute chest syndromes include those of Walker, Ballas and Burka (1979), Davies *et al.* (1984), Athanasou *et al.* (1985) and Poncz, Kane and Gill (1985).

CENTRAL NERVOUS SYSTEM INVOLVEMENT

The nervous system is commonly involved in sickle-cell disease. This is probably the result of cerebral infarction brought about by vascular obstruction due to sickling. According to Serjeant (1974a, p. 199), between one-quarter and one-third of hospitalized patients have been or are affected. The literature is extensive, most of the reports dealing with acute incidents. Reviews of the early literature include those of Hughes, Diggs and Gillespie (1940), Margolies (1951), Greer and Schotland (1962) and Portnoy and Herion (1972).

Arena (1935) reported the occurrence of hemiplegia in a 6-year-old boy. Hughes, Diggs and Gillespie (1940) described six patients who had developed neurological symptoms and gave details of two necropsies. In addition, they summarized 25 previous reports of sickle-cell anaemia patients with nervous system manifestations.

According to Margolies (1951), the symptoms and signs are extremely variable: of 28 different symptoms listed, drowsiness, stupor, coma or hemiplegia were the most frequent and delirium the least frequent. Greer and Schotland (1962), reported that 30 out of 86 Hb-SS patients (34.8%) developed neurological complications; they were most frequent in the 6 months to 5 years age-group, and convulsions, meningeal signs and cerebrovascular syndromes were most frequent. Portnoy and Herion (1972) stressed the prevalence of hemiplegia, reporting that this had occurred in 15 out of 89 patients (11%) observed over a 5-year period — 10 times the incidence in Hb-AS subjects. Massive intracranial haemorrhage is a rare event, but it has been recorded (Adeloye, Ogbeide and Odeku, 1970; Falter, Sutton and Robinson, 1973).

Konotey-Ahulu (1972c) described an unusual complication, mental-nerve neuropathy, in five patients (two Hb SS, three Hb SC). A burning sensation in the lower lip was followed by numbness which was slow to clear up.

Rather rarely the symptoms and signs point to the occlusion of large blood vessels. Stockman and co-workers (1972) described how seven patients, 2–17 years of age, were affected in this way. Boros, Thomas and Weiner's (1976) report dealt with 18 Hb-SS patients admitted into hospital in coma.

Powers and co-workers (1978) reviewed the frequency of strokes as part of a large study of 537 sickle-cell disease patients: 33 Hb-SS patients (and two Hb-SC patients) had strokes; 25 of them were less than 20 years of age at the time of their first stroke (9.1% of all patients within this age-range). Children were thought to be at greater risk of cerebral infarction and adults of cerebral haemorrhage; 12 patients died, five of infarction, six of haemorrhage and one (an Hb-SC patient) of fat embolism. Follow-up of patients who had had a stroke indicated a recurrence rate of 67%, 80% of the recurrences occurring within 36 months. No predictive features, such as prior illness, haemoglobin level, Hb-F level or previous neurological symptoms identified patients at risk of strokes.

Arnow and co-workers (1978) described an unusual possible mechanism of cerebral infarction, namely, hypocapnoea leading to carotid vessel constriction following hyperventilation. Their patient was a 19-year-old male who had ingested 9 g of aspirin for a 'cold' over a 36-hour period. He was noticed to be breathing more rapidly than normal before lapsing into deep coma. At necropsy an infarct was found in the cerebellum. Protass (1973) had earlier suggested that the occurrence of a marked left hemiparesis in an 11-year-old girl with Hb-SS disease developing immediately after a period of hyperventilation at the end of an EEG recording might have similarly been the result of multiple areas of cerebral ischaemia or infarction brought about by intravascular sickling.

PRONENESS TO BACTERIAL INFECTIONS

Pneumonia, meningitis and septicaemia

The relatively frequent occurrence of serious bacterial infections in patients with sickle-cell disease has already been referred to. Pulmonary infections, septicaemias, meningitis, osteitis and osteomyelitis all occur at greater frequencies than in the general (Hb AA) population and have been, and still are, a cause of premature death. An important cause of their relatively high incidence is undoubtedly vascular occlusion by sickled cells providing sites where organisms can settle down and proliferate. As already mentioned, the differentiation between infarction and infection as the basis of acute chest syndromes is often difficult. The same is true in the assessment of acute abdominal symptoms and in the differentiation of osteomyelitis from bone infarction.

It is beyond the scope of this book to delve deeply into problems of differential diagnosis. The following selected accounts from the literature, however, give an indication of the incidence and importance of bacterial infections in the life-history of Hb-SS patients and of the species of organisms commonly responsible.

Robinson and Watson (1966) stressed the frequency and importance of meningitis, particularly that due to Str. pneumoniae. Of 252 patients with Hb-SS disease who had been followed for the preceding 10 years, 16 (6.3%) had had meningitis, 11 pneumococcal in type. Six of the patients were small children, 2 years or less in age. In contrast, not one of 31 Hb-SC disease patients and 22 Hb-S/thalassaemia patients had contracted meningitis.

Petch and Serjeant (1970) contrasted the progress and response to treatment of 28 Hb-SS patients admitted to hospital with a diagnosis of pneumonia with that of 28 similar but Hb-AA patients. The most striking differences were in the duration of pyrexia and in the history of previous attacks: 23 of the non-Hb-SS patients were afebrile within 48 hours compared with only five of the Hb-SS patients, while nine out of 28 of the latter gave a history of having suffered from similar episodes.

Kabins and Lerner (1970) described how four young children between 5 and 23 months of age had died of pneumococcal septicaemia within a few hours of the onset of symptoms. Two had been diagnosed previously as having Hb-SS disease; one was known to give a positive test for sickling, and one had Hb-S/thalassaemia. In two of the children there was evidence of intravascular coagulation; in one, at least, the adrenal cortical haemorrhages seen at necropsy were characteristic of the Waterhouse-Friderichsen syndrome. Kabins and Lerner likened the fulminant nature of the infection to that well recognized to occur in young children who had undergone splenectomy (Vol. 1, p. 117).

Barrett-Connor (1971) analysed 250 infections in 166 patients and reviewed the literature. Nearly two-thirds of these patients (seen in Miami) had been admitted to hospital for an infection in an 11-year period, and infections had led to the initial diagnosis of sickle-cell disease in about one-quarter of them. A few patients were particularly prone and 14 of them accounted for nearly one-half of the proved bacterial infections; they could not, however, be distinguished by other clinical or laboratory findings from those who were not so prone. Children less than 4 years of age were at greatest risk and those who had not contracted a severe infection by this age had a much reduced risk subsequently. The commonest infection was presumptive pneumonia, not easily distinguishable from infarction. Osteomyelitis occurred at all ages; this was usually due to Salmonella species but could be due to Str. pneumoniae or Staph. pyogenes. It was common for several sites to be affected. Meningitis, when it occurred, had almost always affected children less than 3 years of age; 70% of the infections were due to Str. pneumoniae. At least 10% of patients had had urinary tract infections; E. coli was the commonest organism and about half the patients had E. coli bacteraemia. Some infections were due to Enterobacter-Klebsiella species and these organisms had also caused arthritis. The frequency of painful crises and of infections was not related in individual patients, but when both occurred together the mortality was high. It was concluded that bacterial infection was the commonest cause of death in Hb-SS disease, particularly in children; and it was suggested that impaired alveolar macrophage phagocytosis, splenic blockade and a reduced production of heat-labile opsonins for Str. pneumoniae had played a part in increasing the patients' susceptibility to infections. Details of 15 deaths were given; nine were associated with severe infections.

Seeler, Metzger and Mufson (1972) reported on 12 episodes of Str. pneumoniae bacteraemia or meningitis in 10 children with Hb-SS disease; seven were less than 2 years of age and two died. Hb-SS disease patients accounted for 7.3% of all children admitted to hospital with pneumococcal infections.

Shulman and co-workers (1972) described the occurrence in five Hb-SS children of Mycoplasma pneumonia and stressed its unusual severity. More than one lung lobe was involved and the total leucocyte counts were unusually high — $23.75–54.65 \times 10^9/l$, the majority of the cells being neutrophils.

Robinson and Halpern (1974) stressed the importance of Str. pneumoniae and E. coli as the causative agents of serious infections in Hb-SS children. Of 457 black children admitted to hospital with serious infections, eight had Hb-SS disease. Two of the Hb-SS children died compared with a 1.5% mortality in Hb-AA and Hb-AS children.

Powars (1975) reviewed the clinical histories of the first 10 years of life of children suffering from Hb-SS disease, based on an experience of 422 patients seen in the Los Angeles area over a 20-year period. Seven children less than 5 years old, who had died of the 'sudden death syndrome', were found in reality to have been homozygous for Hb S and to have had pneumococcal septicaemia [see Kabins and Lerner (1970), referred to above]. Ward and Smith (1976) commented on the relatively high incidence of H. influenzae bacteraemia in Hb-SS children. In their series of 37 patients this was the commonest blood isolate in children less than 3 years old.

Overturf, Powars and Baraff (1977) gave further details of the incidence of bacterial meningitis and septicaemia in children with sickle-cell disease in the Los Angeles area: 15.2% of 323 Hb-SS patients developed meningitis or septicaemia during the period of study, the case fatality being 35% for septicaemia and 10% for meningitis. Str. pneumoniae infection almost exclusively affected Hb-SS children less than 5 years of age. The later experience of the same group of paediatricians has indicated a substantial fall in mortality (in a similar child population not receiving prophylactic penicillin or immunization against Str. pneumoniae). According to Powars et al. (1981), this illustrates the benefit of close medical supervision of a Hb-SS child with fever and the prompt parenteral administration of an antibiotic.

Rogers, Vaidya and Serjeant's (1978) data showed that amongst 135 children with Hb-SS disease, diagnosed at birth and followed for 1–5 years, severe bacterial infections were confined to those whose spleen became palpable at or before they were 1 year of age, particularly in those in whom it was palpable at 6 months. There were 14 serious infections and six deaths, and it was suggested that the increased susceptibility resulted from the existence of functional asplenia (although palpable splenomegaly) before the first encounter with the infection.

McDonald and Eichner (1978) described the occurrence in a 16-year-old male with sickle-cell anaemia of fulminating pneumococcal septicaemia that was associated with disseminated intravascular coagulation and bleeding from the gums and venepuncture sites. Diplococci which had been phagocytosed by neutrophils, as well as some lying free, were seen in blood films.

Details of the clinical presentation of 16 Hb-SS, two Hb-SC and one Hb-SO (Arab) patients who had pneumococcal meningitis were given by Griesemer, Winkelstein and Luddy (1978). Five patients had had recurrent episodes of infection. Although 80% of the episodes had affected children less than 3 years of age, there were four patients aged between 9 and 21 years. The point was made that the clinical characteristics of the meningitis in the patients with a haemoglobinopathy were similar to those in the patients with meningitis and Hb AA who served as controls.

McIntosh and her co-workers (1980) reported on the outcome of a programme of early evaluation and treatment of 22 children with sickle-cell disease (15 Hb SS) who had been identified at birth and whose parents had been urged to bring them to hospital without delay if they developed a fever: 182 such episodes were investigated, the children being then between 6 months and 5 years of age. A definite bacterial cause of their fever was established in 69 of the episodes, septicaemia and/or meningitis being diagnosed in six instances; in 34 episodes the fever had been associated with vaso-occlusive syndromes, and in 79 episodes the cause of the fever was not ascertained. McIntosh et al. emphasized the value and importance of the early intravenous administration of antibiotics active against Str. pneumoniae and H. influenzae to all sickle-cell disease children who develop a high fever.

Lobel and Bove (1982) described the clinical presentation and pathological consequences of septicaemia affecting 22 (10.5%) out of 210 children with sickle-cell disease observed over a 9-year period: 19 of those affected had Hb SS. Children less than $2\frac{1}{2}$ years of age were at the greatest risk and Str. pneumoniae was by far the commonest causal organism. Nine of the children became severely ill within 12 hours, but in 13 the severe phase of their illness was preceded by a prodromal period lasting 1–7 days. Six children died: adrenal haemorrhage was present in all; in three the massive haemorrhage and necrosis was typical of the Waterhouse-Friderichsen syndrome.

Vaccination against pneumococcal infection.
The unusual sensitivity of Hb-SS patients to serious and life-threatening infections with Str. pneumoniae has prompted the use of polyvalent pneumococcal vaccines as a means of preventing infection. Clinical trials, too, have been organized in an attempt to assess the frequency of infection in immunized children and the extent of their immune response to the vaccine. The results have been only moderately encouraging, if not disappointing. The responses to the vaccines have been variable, not only with respect to individual patients but also with respect to the immune response to individual capsular antigens; the responses in children less than 2 years of age have been generally less good than those of older children. Some failures have, too, been reported, i.e. the occurrence of pneumococcal septicaemia and/or meningitis in vaccinated children (Ahonkhai et al., 1979; Overturf, Field and Edmonds, 1979). Reports on the immune responses and of the clinical outcome in quite large numbers of patients include those of Addiego et al. (1976), Amman et al. (1977), Buchanan and Schiffman (1980), Kaplan et al. (1982) and Chudwin et al. (1983).

Amman and co-workers (1977) immunized 77 patients with Hb-SS disease, 19 asplenic patients and 82 age-matched controls by means of a single 50-μg subcutaneous dose of a vaccine of eight polysaccharide types of Str. pneumoniae. When the serum of 52 patients was tested 3–4 weeks later the proportion responding and the magnitude of the response did not differ between the immunized patients and the immunized controls. However, during the next 2 years none of the 77 immunized patients contracted a serious pneumococcal infection compared with eight infections in 106 age-matched unimmunized patients.

John and co-workers (1984) compared the results of immunizing 242 Hb-SS children, aged between 6 months and 3 years, by means of a 14-valent pneumococcal vaccine with injecting them monthly with benzathine penicillin. Within a 5-year period there were 11 serious pneumococcal infections in the vaccinated group — 10 with serotypes present in the vaccine (type 23 in five cases), compared with no pneumococcal infections in the penicillin-treated group, although there were four such infections in the group within 1 year of ceasing to give the penicillin.

Typhoid and paratyphoid

Gendrel and co-workers (1982) reported that in West Africa (Gabon), where Salmonella infections are frequent, the incidence of the Hb-SS genotype in children with typhoid or paratyphoid was 2.2 times as frequent, and that of the Hb-AS genotype 1.7 times as frequent, as in children admitted to hospital for other reasons.

Osteitis and osteomyelitis

One of the consequences of infarction of the bone and bone marrow is that the infarcted areas provide suitable sites for the settling down and proliferation of organisms absorbed from the gut. Various species of Salmonella have most commonly been isolated (Diggs, Pulliam and King, 1937; Vandepitte *et al.*, 1953; Hook *et al.*, 1957; Hughes and Carroll, 1957; Roberts and Hilberg, 1958; de Torregrosa *et al.*, 1960; Hendrickse and Collard, 1960; Adeyokunnu and Hendrickse, 1980; Givner, Luddy and Schwartz, 1981) (Fig. 11.15).

It is quite common for multiple sites to be affected simultaneously. This was the case in nine of the 13 Nigerian infants and children aged between 8 days and 9 years described by Hendrickse and Collard (1960). (One of the children was a non-sickler and the Hb-S status of five of them was unknown.) The bones affected comprised the phalanges, metacarpals, radius, ulna, humerus, metatarsals, femur, tibia and scapula.

According to Givner, Luddy and Schwartz (1981), who reviewed the results of bacterial cultures of bone, blood or both in 84 patients with a major sickle haemoglobinopathy in whom a diagnosis of osteomyelitis had been proved, the infecting organism was a species of Salmonella in 74% of patients in whom the

cultures were positive. The point was made that in striking contrast to these results staphylococci were by far the commonest organism responsible for osteomyelitis in patients who did not suffer from an underlying major haemoglobinopathy.

Mechanisms of increased susceptibility to infections

The cause or causes of the Hb-SS patient's increased susceptibility to infections are of major interest and have been the subject of much investigation. It seems likely that atrophy of the spleen ('auto-splenectomy') is a major factor, with possibly, too, as an additional factor, the overloading of the R.E. phagocytic system with products of the breakdown of haemoglobin.

Listed below are some of the studies which have provided evidence of a failure of splenic function and of impaired immune responses. The abnormalities that have been reported include impaired uptake of colloid particles by the spleen, reduced serum opsonizing activity, decreased serum tuftsin concentration, impaired neutrophil phagocytic activity, inhibition of neutrophil migration, impaired complement activation via the alternative pathway, impaired cell-mediated immune responses and impaired natural killer-cell activity. Whether the impaired immune responses can be explained wholly on splenic atrophy and the chronic haemolytic process is uncertain. Possibly, past blood

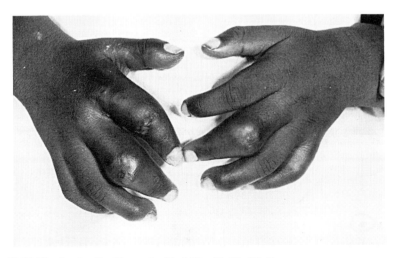

Fig. 11.15 The hands of a 15-month-old child with Hb-SS disease.
Shows dactylitis and signs of *Salm. typhi* osteomyelitis. (Courtesy of Dr Konotey-Ahulu.)

transfusion and infection with lymphotrophic viruses play a part in certain patients. Deficiency of serum immunoglobulins seems unlikely to be a factor. Commonly, IgG and IgA levels are higher than normal, presumably a response to past infections.

Winkelstein and Drachman (1968) reported that the serum opsonizing activity versus *Str. pneumoniae* was impaired in Hb-SS disease: 14 such children were studied when afebrile and free from symptoms and, using normal peripheral-blood polymorphonuclears and the patients' sera, there appeared to be a gross deficiency in a heat-labile serum factor promoting phagocytosis. The impaired activity was attributed to splenic atrophy.

Schwartz and Pearson (1972) injected five Hb-SS children intravenously with 1.0 ml of sheep erythrocytes and followed the response of the heterophile antibody titre. In all five children, three of whom had palpable spleens but with no demonstrable uptake of [^{99m}Tc] sulphur colloid, the antibody response was substantially less than that expected and was similar to the response of asplenic individuals. In contrast, two children with Hb-S/β-thalassaemia and a child with the Hb-AS trait responded normally.

Further evidence of impaired uptake of colloid particles by the spleen was reported by Falter *et al.* (1973) who assessed splenic function and the incidence of infections in 21 Hb-SS children, in 10 healthy (Hb-AA) children and in seven splenectomized (Hb-AA) children. The appearance of the spleen shadow after the injection of [^{99m}Tc] sulphur colloid and the rise in plasma factor-VIII activity after an infusion of adrenalin were assessed. The spleen was not visualized in 15 out of the 21 Hb-SS patients and the shadow was abnormally weak in five patients; and the mean rise in factor-VIII concentration was significantly less than in the normal children and about the same as in the splenectomized children. The incidence of pneumonia and meningitis was significantly increased in those children in whom both tests of splenic function were impaired compared to that in the normal children. Only one patient out of nine who had detectable splenic function had contracted a severe infection.

Dimitrov and co-workers (1972) provided evidence that impairment of neutrophil phagocytic activity may also contribute to proneness to infection. They studied eight Hb-SS patients who gave a history of multiple infections and five additional patients who gave no such history and compared the results of various tests of neutrophil function in the two groups with those in Hb-AS subjects and normal controls. The biochemical responses to the stimulus of phagocytosis appeared to be significantly depressed in the group of patients giving a history of infections compared to the other groups and also to the responses of splenectomized individuals.

Johnston, Newman and Struth (1973) studied the ability of sera from Hb-SS patients to promote the phagocytosis of *Str. pneumoniae* and found that when antibody was present in small amounts and the organisms were not fully sensitized the sera did not fully activate and fix C3 to the bacteria by the alternative pathway.

Wilson, Hughes and Lachmann (1976) reported that the mean complement alternative pathway activity of 29 West-Indian Hb-SS patients was significantly lower than that of healthy controls. In those patients in whom the total alternative pathway activity was subnormal, the activity of factor D (C3 proactivator convertase) was normal but that of factor B (C3 proactivator) was reduced. Wilson, Hughes and Lachmann concluded that deficiency of factor B may contribute to the proneness of Hb-SS patients to severe infections.

Koethe, Casper and Rodey (1976) similarly concluded that there was a partial deficiency of C3PA convertase and suggested that this might be secondary to in-vivo consumption of complement factors as the result of activation by fragments of sickled cells.

Wilson and co-workers (1976) described the interesting association of sickle-cell disease and systemic lupus erythematosus (SLE) in two adult females; they raised the question as to whether the abnormalites and deficiencies in immune function in sickle-cell disease could have played a part in the development of the SLE.

Hand and King (1978) reported on the (heat-labile) opsonizing power of the serum of Hb-SS patients versus Salmonella species. The sera of 12 out of 28 patients were deficient. The serum Ig and antibody levels were normal but some of the sera were deficient in complement function, *e.g.*, the alternative pathway function might be deficient, the C3 level subnormal, or the C4 level slightly reduced. It was concluded that such deficiencies, brought about perhaps by functional asplenia, impaired macrophage function and/or impaired synthesis of complement components, might predispose to Salmonella infection.

Hernández and co-workers (1980) provided some evidence that cell immunity was impaired in sickle-cell anaemia and suggested that this might be a factor in the patients' susceptibility to infections. In an investigation of 20 patients, aged 17–44 years, none of whom had had a recent crisis, they found that phythaemagglutinin (PHA) transformation was decreased in half of them and that some exhibited cutaneous anergy, three out of 15 patients failing to respond to four different antigens.

Bjornson, Lobel and Lampkin (1980) studied 18 sickle-cell disease patients (14 had Hb SS), aged 1 year to 22 years, when free from symptoms and again when admitted to hospital for a painful crisis. Total haemolytic complement activity and the concentration of C3, properdin and IgM were subnormal and were not affected significantly by the onset of a crisis. The activity of other components of the classical and alternative complement pathways was normal or increased and was similarly unaltered by a crisis. No evidence was obtained therefore to suggest that a painful crisis would predispose to microbial infection.

Spirer and co-workers (1980), using a radio-immune assay technique, found the concentration of tuftsin in the serum of 14 Hb-SS patients (and in five with Hb-SC and two with Hb-CC) to be subnormal. [Tuftsin is a phagocytosis-stimulating peptide and its concentration in serum has been looked upon, too, as an indicator of splenic function.] The deficiency was most marked in the Hb-SS patients.

Akenzua and Amiengheme (1981) compared the rates of in-vitro migration of neutrophils obtained from 38 Hb-SS Nigerian children when in steady state and in painful crisis and found that the neutrophils migrated normally in both clinical states. However, it appeared that serum obtained from children when in painful crisis contained an inhibitor active against the migration of the children's own neutrophils as well as against the neutrophils of healthy adults.

Natta and Outschoorn (1984) reported on the serum immunoglobulin profiles of eight adult Hb-SS patients and compared them with those of 11 normal Hb-AA controls. The patients were not in crisis when studied and had not been transfused for many years and had not received any vaccines. The IgG and lgA and C3 concentrations were significantly higher in the patients but the IgM levels were no different from those of the controls. There appeared, however, to be a deficiency of IgG2, and the IgG2:IgG1 ratio was subnormal in all eight patients in which it was measured.

Tapazoglou and co-workers (1985) studied the natural killer-cell activity of peripheral-blood mononuclear cells in 21 Hb-SS patients and found that this was abnormal in those patients who were zinc deficient; they also demonstrated that the killer-cell activity of two normal volunteers declined when they adhered to a zinc-deficient diet. The question was raised as to the clinical significance of zinc deficiency in relation to the susceptibility of Hb-SS patients to viral infections.

Boghossian and co-workers (1985) submitted 30 Hb-SS, nine Hb-SC and five Hb-S/β-thalassaemia patients, and 31 age-matched controls, to a comprehensive study of their defences against infection. A perfusion system was used to study in whole blood the kinetics of the adhesion of leucocytes and their ability to phagocytose, kill and solubilize *Staph. aureus* and *Str. pneumoniae*. The release of lactoferrin from neutrophils was measured; the accumulation of leucocytes at foci of inflammation was visualized through a skin window and the subsequent movement of the cells through a filter was assessed. The concentrations of serum immunoglobulins and of C3 and C4 and total haemolytic complement were estimated. A variety of abnormalities were demonstrated: the rate of migration of neutrophils into filters was slightly reduced and the proportion of monocytes that emigrated from the skin windows, and their rate of migration, were markedly reduced; the adhesion of neutrophils and their ability to kill *Staph. aureus* was

impaired, particularly in the Hb-SS and Hb-S/β-thalassaemia patients; the concentration of IgG and IgA in serum was increased while that of IgM and complement components was normal. The results obtained with the patients and the controls overlapped in all the tests, and Boghossian *et al.* concluded that the defects in phagocytic function which they had observed did not provide a satisfactory explanation for the enhanced susceptibility of the patients to severe infection; their final comment implied that they considered that local infarction caused by intravascular sickling and impaired splenic function were likely to be of more significance.

Ballaster, Abdallah and Prasad (1985) attempted to immunize 16 Hb-SS patients with a polyvalent influenza virus vaccine. The serum IgM responses were subnormal or absent in eight of the patients; their IgG responses, on the other hand, were normal. The results of a ^{99m}Tc spleen scan were available for 11 of the patients. Splenic tissue was not demonstrable in all of the six whose IgM response was subnormal: in contrast, a spleen shadow was present (although in some cases smaller than normal) in four of the five patients whose IgM response was normal.

PREGNANCY

Although at one time considered to be a rare event, pregnancy is now not uncommon in sufferers from Hb-SS disease, but it is still a rather serious occurrence. The patient tends to become more anaemic and there is an increased risk of toxaemia and infection.

The patient's haemoglobin falls to below its usual level and reaches its nadir between 32–34 weeks (as in normal pregnancy). Megaloblastic change is relatively frequent and this can lead to severe anaemia (see p. 105). Painful vaso-occlusive crises are more than usually common, particularly in the third trimester of pregnancy and during the early days of the puerperium. Obstetric complications appear to be unusually frequent and the fetal and maternal death rates are relatively high (see below).

The earlier literature was reviewed by Margolies (1951), who stated that only 50 instances of pregnancy had been reported up to the time of his review. The first comprehensive reports were those of Kobak, Stein and Daro (1941) and Beacham and Beacham (1950). Later papers include those of Adams, Whitacre and Diggs (1953), Eisenstein, Posner and Friedman (1956), Anderson *et al.* (1960), Apthorp, Measday and Lehmann (1963) and Freeman and Ruth (1969).

In West Africa. Hendrickse and Watson-Williams (1966), reporting from Ibadan in Nigeria, painted a gloomy picture. They concluded that fertility was reduced in Hb-SS disease, although not in Hb-SC disease, and that both disorders were a cause of serious morbidity and mortality. Severe anaemia was common, although this could often be alleviated by the administration of folic acid and anti-malarial drugs. The frequency of bone-pain crises was increased, particularly in the third trimester, during labour and in the first few days *post partum*. They reported, too, that occasionally sudden sequestration of blood in the spleen and liver might occur as a terminal event during a bone-pain crisis or in association with severe megaloblastic anaemia and that in such cases exchange transfusion could be life-saving. As compared with Hb-SS disease, Hb-S/β-thalassaemia, Hb-S/high Hb F and Hb-CC disease caused no anxiety. Hendrickse and co-workers (1972) gave further information. Between 1958 and 1969, 39 Hb-SS patients had been followed through 61 pregnancies: there had been seven deaths, associated with severe anaemia, acute sequestration, bacterial infections, bone-pain crises and bone-marrow embolism. Fertility appeared to be low and spontaneous abortion and fetal wastage were high — at least twice that of the general population, and the average birthweight of living infants was low.

Harrison (1982) brought the outlook for mother and infant in Ibadan more up to date: in 1976 the maternal mortality was stated to be 12% in Hb-SS disease (and 6% in Hb-SC disease) and the perinatal death-rate 120 and 34, respectively, per 1000 deliveries.

In the New World. The outlook for Hb-SS mothers and their infants in the United States in the 1960s and earlier was poor. Although there were no deaths amongst the nine Hb-SS West-Indian mothers described by Anderson *et al.* (1960), eight experienced moderate to severe exacerbations of their disease during pregnancy, mostly in the form of painful crises. All their infants survived, although their birthweights were low. (In contrast, five out of seven Hb-SC patients experienced no problems during pregnancy.) Fort and co-workers (1971), nevertheless, came to the conclusion that the outcome of pregnancy did not

justify the risk: in their own experience at Memphis between 1960 and 1969 the maternal mortality had been 10% in Hb-SS patients and 9% in Hb-SC patients — figures they regarded as comparable with other published data; fetal salvage had been as low as 51.5% in Hb-SS patients and 55% in Hb-SC patients (compared with 93% for all deliveries). The experiences described by Horger (1972) and Pritchard *et al.* (1973) were rather similar: fetal loss was high, although the maternal mortality was less.

In the 1970s several centres experimented with exchange transfusion in an attempt to reduce the maternal mortality and fetal loss. Morrison and Wiser (1976a,b) reported significant improvement, *i.e.* fewer spontaneous abortions and fetal and maternal deaths (see, however, below).

Reports published in the 1980s suggested that the outlook for the pregnant Hb-SS mother has continued to improve, although the incidence of complications, *e.g.* pulmonary problems, pre-eclampsia and haematuria, is still considerably higher than in Hb-AA or Hb-AS subjects, and the spontaneous abortion rate and perinatal mortality both remain high (Charache *et al.*, 1980; Milner, Jones and Döbler, 1980).

The value of prophylactic partial exchange transfusion is uncertain, according to Miller *et al.* (1981) and Serjeant (1983). Miller *et al.*, however, recommended that the technique be used in the treatment of pregnant women in crisis or if seriously anaemic.

SURGERY AND ANAESTHESIA

It is well recognized that patients with Hb-SS disease are at special risk from surgical procedures and anaesthesia. Anoxia and hypotension must be avoided at all cost and local or regional anaesthesia employed where practicable rather than a general anaesthetic (Shapiro and Poe, 1955; Browne, 1965; Gilbertson, 1965; Howells *et al.*, 1972; Searle, 1973, etc.). Dehydration, hypothermia and local tissue ischaemia are potentially harmful, and infections, particularly pulmonary ones, must be looked for carefully and if they occur promptly treated. Transfusions should be used with moderation to avoid raising blood viscosity and, if they

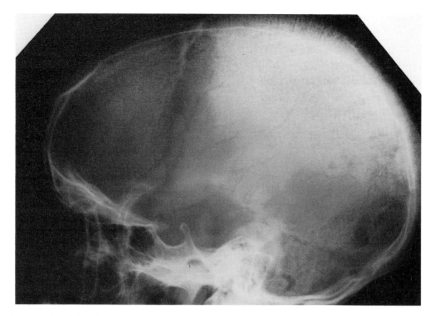

Fig. 11.16 X-ray photograph of the skull of a 24-year-old male with sickle-cell disease.
Shows widening of the diploic space of the skull vault and a 'hair-on-end' appearance. (Reproduced by courtesy of Dr Janet Dacie.)

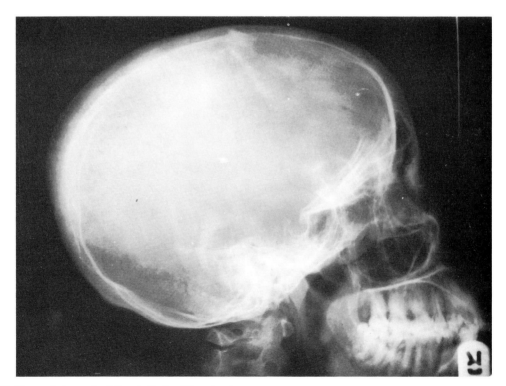

Fig. 11.17 X-ray photograph of the skull of a Ghanaian boy.
Shows widening of the diploic space of the skull vault and occipital bossing. (Reproduced by by courtesy of Dr Konotey-Ahulu.)

are required, blood as fresh as possible should be used to avoid transfusing erythrocytes with a high O_2 affinity, as would be the case if stored blood was used (Serjeant, 1974a, p. 237).

Howells and co-workers (1972) stressed that patients with Hb-SS or Hb-SC disease or Hb-S/thalassaemia are high-risk patients: with the Hb-AS trait, on the other hand, the risk is low, and a few simple precautions are all that are needed.

RADIOGRAPHIC FINDINGS

Skeleton

There is a large literature. Excluding evidence of cardiac enlargement, the most important changes affect the bones (Caffey, 1937; Diggs, Pulliam and King, 1937; Macht and Roman, 1948; Golding, 1956; Middlemiss, 1958; Golding, MacIver and Went, 1959; Ennis, Serjeant and Middlemiss, 1973; Rothschild and Sebes, 1981, etc.). The main abnormalities are irregularity of the bone trabeculae with widening of the medullary cavities and areas of sclerosis. On the other hand, areas of osteoporosis may develop and rarely spontaneous fractures. Aseptic infarcts lead to destruction of the normal bony pattern and sclerosis (Fig. 11.10). Thickening of the diploe of the skull typically occurs and this may lead to a hair-on-end appearance (Figs. 11.16 and 11.17). This is, however, less common than in thalassaemia major (Golding, MacIver and Went, 1959). The vertebrae, viewed laterally, may show a step deformity of their end plates (Fig. 11.18).

Caffey (1937) reported that 10 out of 15 patients with sickle-cell anaemia had a thickened calcarium similar to that seen in erythroblastic anaemia, although there was no obvious vertical striation. Diggs, Pulliam and King (1937) pointed out that two opposing processes take place within the bones and are responsible for the X-ray changes: widening of the medullary spaces due to hyperplasia of the marrow and narrowing of the spaces due to sclerosis.

Middlemiss (1958), reporting from the West Indies, illustrated the consequences of infarcts affecting the hand and the neck of the femur, medullary sclerosis affecting the femur, widened medullary cavities, skull changes, osteoporosis and spontaneous fractures. Later, Ennis, Serjeant and Middlemiss (1973) described the appearances in 61 randomly selected Hb-SS patients. (They pointed out that previous reports may have

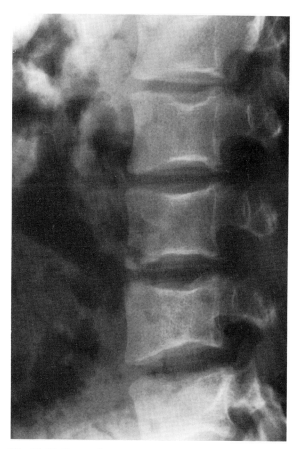

Fig. 11.18 X-ray photograph of thoracic vertebrae of a 19-year-old girl with sickle-cell disease.
Shows a step deformity of vertebral end-plates.
(Reproduced by courtesy of Dr Janet Dacie.)

included patients with Hb-SC disease or Hb-S/thalassaemia or even carriers of the Hb-AS trait.) Osteoporosis was present in 75% of the patients and was most obvious in the skull, tibia and hands, and the bony trabecular pattern was altered in 57%, with wide intratrabecular spaces and thickened trabeculae. Medullary expansion was obvious in 57%, e.g. widening of the diploic space, a flask-shaped deformity of the femur and expansion of the tibia, and occasionally 'squaring', i.e. loss of the lateral concave borders, of the metacarpals. In 36% of the patients there was evidence of past infarction: the femur and tibia were most commonly affected and the lesions were often adjacent to the articular cartilages, i.e. in the head of the femur (Fig. 11.10), with deformity consequent on weight-bearing. In 43% of the patients the vertebrae were abnormal; in two of the patients metacarpals and phalanges were shortened — they gave a history of the hand-foot syndrome. Ennis, Serjeant and Middlemiss concluded that, although few of the X-ray signs of bony disease were pathognomonic of Hb-SS disease, their presence in a black individual made the diagnosis very likely.

Bohrer (1970), reporting from Ibadan, reviewed the localization of 198 acute diaphyseal infarcts in the long bones of 81 patients, 65 of whom had Hb SS, the remainder Hb SC. The infarcts generally affected the whole shaft of the bone in young infants, but were more localized in older infants, children and young adults: 85% were then in the meta-diaphyseal region.

Rothschild and Sebes (1981) stressed the frequency with which erosive disease of the metacarpal heads and carpal bones could be demonstrated in sickle-cell disease and mentioned that in nine out of 100 patients the calcaneus was affected.

Dental bone changes, demonstrable by X-ray, are common, too. Prowler and Smith (1955) found abnormal translucent areas in the mandible and maxillae of all the 11 patients with Hb-SS disease they examined and minimal changes in two out of seven Hb-AS trait subjects. Abnormalities were detected, too, in six out of 10 patients with Hb-SC disease.

Skeletal maturation. X-ray examination has revealed delay. Thus Serjeant and Ashcroft (1973) found that in 81 out of 86 adolescent Hb-SS disease patients seen in Jamaica the maturation of the left radial epiphysis was delayed. The delay was inversely related to the Hb-F percentage, *i.e.* it appeared to be directly related to the proportion of Hb S present.

Spleen

One result of the atrophy and fibrosis of the spleen which is so characteristic of Hb-SS disease is the development sometimes of areas of calcification that can be demonstrated by X-ray (Ehrenpreis and Schwinger, 1952: Hemley, Mellins and Finby, 1963; Seligman, Rosner and Smulewicz, 1973).

Kidneys

As already referred to (p. 35), haematuria is a common accompaniment of sickle-cell disease and of the Hb-AS trait. The bleeding seems to have its origin in renal papillary necrosis, a destructive process that can be demonstrated by X-ray.

Harrow, Sloane and Liebman (1963) demonstrated by intravenous pyelography the existence of cavities in the calyces in five Hb-AS individuals. Akinkugbe (1967), writing from Ibadan, described papillary necrosis in four patients: three had the Hb-AS trait and one Hb-SS disease. Khademi and Marquis (1973) studied eight sickle-cell disease patients by urography as well as by angiography. The main urographic finding was destruction and blunting of the calyces and the most frequent angiographic finding was focal cortical hypertrophy with in three patients areas of cortical thinning and medullary hypertrophy.

BENIGN TYPES OF HOMOZYGOUS SICKLE-CELL DISEASE

In recent years it has been realized that some patients who are undoubtedly homozygous for Hb S suffer from an illness which runs an unexpectedly benign course and that ethnic and other genetic influences can play a part in determining this. In some cases a benign course is associated with high Hb-F levels, in others the concurrent presence of a gene or genes for α-thalassaemia; in still other cases the reason for the mild clinical expression is not obvious.

In Shiite and Kuwaiti Arabs

Gelpi (1970) reported that sickle-cell disease in Shiite Arabs in Saudi Arabia was a relatively benign disorder. Sixty-five unrelated subjects, aged 11–50 years, had been observed over a 10-year period. They had presented with unexplained anaemia, recurrent joint or bone pain and occasionally with abdominal or back pain. None had leg ulcers. Thrombo-embolic and haemolytic or aregenerative crises were rare. The spleen was palpable in 36 and the liver in 20. Three only of the patients had died. Electrophoresis demonstrated a Hb-SS pattern in 54, a Hb-SC pattern in four and a Hb-S >Hb-A pattern in seven. Hb-F concentrations were available in 26: the mean was 10.7% (range 1.4–24.7%). Hb-A_2 levels were >4.5% in nine of 15 subjects tested. Gelpi concluded that sickle-cell disease was frequent in oasis populations; that at least four entities were present — Hb-SS disease, Hb-SC disease and two types of Hb-S/thalassaemia; that the clinical course was generally relatively benign and that many of the patients survived into adult life.

Ali (1970) called attention to a seemingly similar mild variant of Hb-SS disease in Kuwaiti Arabs, which was also associated with unusually high levels of Hb F. Details were given of two families. In the first, four adolescents, aged 10–20 years, were described: their haemoglobin ranged from 8.6 to 13.0 g/dl, with 3–5% reticulocytes; the Hb-F level ranged from 17 to 35%. Electrophoresis demonstrated Hb S and Hb F only, and there was no evidence of thalassaemia in either parent (both of whom were Hb AS). There were two brothers in the second family, aged 25 and 12 years, respectively. Again, electrophoresis demonstrated Hb S and Hb F only. The older brother had a haemoglobin of 12.2 g/dl, with 21% Hb F, and he had never been transfused. The younger brother had recently had an anaemic episode (Hb 7.2 g/dl) and had required transfusion; he had 13% Hb F. Three other mildly affected patients were also mentioned: they had 10–14 g/dl haemoglobin and 20–24% Hb F.

Perrine and co-workers (1972) later reported the results of a larger and more detailed investigation of a group of Shiite Saudi Arabs, who apart from mild skeletal-muscular pain from time to time, were otherwise well and had had few of the other usual complications of sickle-cell disease. This was attributed to their genetic capacity to form large amounts of Hb F. The age of the patients investigated, selected at random from a much larger number, ranged at the time of study between 12 and 56 years. In five of them the spleen was palpable and in six the spleen, at one time palpable, had become impalpable; in seven it had never been felt; in two, calcification within the spleen could be seen on X-ray. Their haemoglobin ranged from 9.0 to 12.3 g/dl and the reticulocyte count was less than 6% in 10 of them. Skeletal changes demonstrable by X-ray were absent, or, if present, 'mild' or 'minimal'. Haemoglobin analysis revealed Hb S, Hb F and Hb A_2 only. The Hb-F level ranged from 4 to 33%, (mean 18.9%) and in two cases was <12%. (The Hb-F level in a 'control' group of 12 Jamaican adults, 12–36 years of age, with Hb-SS disease ranged between 6.2 and 11.5%.)

Perrine et al. (1972) concluded that the patients they had studied were homozygotes for Hb S and that there was no evidence for α-thalassaemia or β-thalassaemia or hereditary persistence of fetal haemoglobin in the families. Both parents of each patient had Hb AS. Although some of the patients were G6PD-deficient, there were no significant differences between these patients and those who were not enzyme-deficient. The clinical histories of the series as a whole were much less severe, and the incidence of complications significantly less frequent, than in the Jamaican adults with relatively mild Hb-SS disease described by Serjeant et al. (1968) (see below). The oxygen affinity of the erythrocytes of

the patients was found to be greater than is usual in Hb-SS disease, due, it was concluded, to the presence of so much Hb F. This, it was thought, might be a factor in keeping the haemoglobin levels and PCVs of the patients relatively high. The benign course of the patients' illness was considered to be due to the presence of the high levels of Hb F reducing the potentiality of the cells to undergo sickling. An interesting difference was demonstrated between the chemical structure of the Hb F of the Saudi-Arabian and Jamaican patients studied. In the former the $^{G}\gamma{:}^{A}\gamma$ ratio (of the two types of γ chains) was found to be similar to that of the Hb F of the normal newborn, whilst the ratio in the Jamaicans corresponded to that usually found in adults forming Hb F.

A further difference in the clinical expression of Hb-SS disease in Saudi Arabs and in Afro-Americans is to be found in the incidence of gallstones. According to Perrine (1973), who reported on 62 Saudi Oasis dwellers, the incidence in this population is only one-quarter to one-sixth that in American blacks.

Further information on the incidence and severity of Hb-SS disease in Saudi Arabs has been provided by Gelpi and King (1976) and Perrine et al. (1978). Gelpi and King screened 391 adult Saudi males for abnormal haemoglobins and found that 48 were AS, two AC and four SS; the four Hb-SS patients were apparently healthy. Perrine and co-workers reported on 270 Saudi Arabs with Hb SS who had been followed up for an average of 10 years. Their illness was generally mild: in 124 of them Hb-SS disease had been diagnosed in the first 3 years of life, 48% because of suspected anaemia, 28% as the result of screening, 19% in the course of the investigation of various illnesses and only 7% as the result of pain that could be attributed to Hb-SS disease. Serious complications occurred much less frequently than would be anticipated in American or Jamaican patients and no leg ulcers developed. The mean haemoglobin levels in children, adult males and adult females were recorded as 9.5 g/dl, 10.6 g/dl and 9.0 g/dl, respectively. The mean Hb-F percentages were high, 25.9, 22.4 and 26.8, respectively. The mortality due to the presence of Hb SS was thought to be only about one-tenth of that expected in Afro-American patients, and the generally benign course of the disease was attributed to the high Hb-F levels.

Two factors explain the high Hb-F levels in the Saudi-Arabian Hb-SS patients: selective survival of F-containing erythrocytes and a high rate of γ-chain synthesis persisting after the neonatal period. Wood and co-workers (1980) compared the γ-chain synthesis as a percentage of the total non-α-chain synthesis in 22 Hb-SS Saudi-Arabian patients and 22 Hb-SS patients of African origin resident in the West Indies: γ-chain synthesis comprised 4.0–19.9% (mean 8.1%) of the total non-α-chain synthesis in the Saudi Arabians compared with <0.3–4.6% (mean 1.7%) in the Africans. In both groups Hb-F percentages were 3–4 times higher in the peripheral blood than the percentages synthesized.

A small group of patients with clinically benign Hb-SS disease (five in all), whose Hb-F levels were not unusually high, were described by Roth *et al.* (1978b) amongst Arabs living near the Sea of Galilee. The physical properties of the Hb S appeared to be identical with those of Afro-American patients, but the group was unusual in having erythrocyte 2,3-DPG levels about twice the normal. Whether the increases were in any way related to the relatively benign course of their illness remains uncertain.

Al-Awamy, Wilson and Pearson (1984) compared splenic function in 24 Hb-SS Saudi patients originating from the Eastern province of the country with that of 22 Afro-American Hb-SS patients: 17 of the Saudi patients had low pocked erythrocyte counts, indicating normal or nearly normal splenic function; in contrast, all the Americans had high pocked cell counts, indicative of markedly impaired splenic function. [Erythrocyte 'pocks' are surface indentations visible by interference phase-contrast microscopy (see also p. 407).] Most of the Saudi patients had a relatively benign illness: they were less anaemic than the Americans and had lower MCVs and higher Hb-F percentages. A minority, however, were severely affected.

In Western Saudi-Arabian and Yemeni Arabs

In contrast to the relatively benign illness of the Saudi and Kuwaiti Arabs in Eastern Saudi Arabia described in the previous sections, Acquaye and co-workers (1985) have described in Saudi and Yemeni Arabs living in Western Saudi Arabia a form of Hb-SS disease which in clinical presentation and haematological findings closely approximates in severity Hb-SS disease as it usually affects Afro-Americans. The Arabian patients were between $1\frac{1}{2}$ and 42 years of age: their mean steady-state haemoglobin was 8.1 g/dl and many of them had suffered from severe anaemia, respiratory and urinary-tract infections and painful infarcts, and some had experienced hepatic crises, the acute chest syndrome, retinal haemorrhage, epistaxis or hemiplegia. The liver was enlarged in 69% and the spleen in 55%. The Hb-F percentage ranged widely, from 1 to 38%: 44 patients had 10% Hb F or less and 27 patients 10% Hb F or more, but the level of Hb F did not seem to have influenced the clinical or haematological expression of their illness except that the low Hb-F group seemed to be more prone to infections.

In Iranians

Haghshenass and co-workers (1977) reported that they had investigated 16 Hb-SS Iranians, aged between 3 and 56 years, whose symptoms were mild. The spleen was palpable in nine of them. Their mean haemoglobin was 10.1 g/dl and mean Hb-F percentage 18 (range 4.9–38). Twenty-nine Hb-AS heterozygotes were also studied; their Hb-F percentage was 1.6 (normal mean 0.6). These interesting findings (similar to those in the Shiites in Saudi Arabia) were thought to indicate the existence in Iranians of a genetically determined ability to produce high levels of Hb F in the presence of Hb-S genes.

In Turks

A further group of Hb-SS patients with a distinctive relatively mild clinical presentation were described by Özsolu and Altinöz (1977) from Ankara. Their report was based on 97 patients aged from infancy to 25 years: their haemoglobin ranged from 3.1 to 11.7 g/dl, mean 7.49 g/dl, and the Hb-F percentage from 1 to 36%, mean 11.5%. There appeared to be no relation between haemoglobin values and Hb-F percentage. The Hb-A$_2$ percentage ranged from 0.7 to 5.5%, mean 2.41%. The patients tolerated their anaemia well and very rarely needed blood transfusion. Their most common complaints were of mild attacks of muscular skeletal pain and of jaundice, and although the group as a whole had experienced most of the well-known complications of Hb-SS disease, including the hand-foot syndrome, painful crises were not common (less than one attack per patient per year) and none of the patients was incapacitated by their illness, and their body habitus was normal. The spleen was palpable in 43%.

In Afro-Americans in the New World

In the West Indies. Hb-SS disease in West Indians has been reported, too, to run not infrequently a relatively benign course. There is, however, no reason to suppose that this is brought about by genetical influences determining unusually high Hb-F levels. Serjeant and co-workers (1968) reported on 60 patients who were over 30 years of age at the time of study. Twenty-eight were males and 32 were females; most were in full-time employment and only two of them were seriously anaemic (haemoglobin <6g/dl persistently). They were of average height and the women had had an average of 2.6 pregnancies. The commonest symptoms were joint and bone pains, ulceration of the leg and jaundice. Six had palpable spleens. The Hb-A$_2$ percentages were low (1.4–2.9%), *i.e.*, there was no evidence that any of them had Hb-S/β-thalassaemia; the Hb-F percentages ranged from <1.0 to 18.2: in 46 the percentage was <10.

In a follow-up paper Serjeant (1975) referred to the above-mentioned 60 patients. Eleven had died, 33 were in reasonable health; in nine their disease interfered with normal activity; five were untraced and the diagnosis in two had been altered to Hb-S/thalassaemia. Serjeant stressed that long survival does not necessarily mean a benign process. However, it did appear that after the age of 30 painful crises and aplastic crises became less frequent and leg ulcers tended to heal. But obstruction to small blood vessels, and the ischaemic changes this leads to, progress, *e.g.* in the eye, and renal function decreases; and the death-rate of Hb-SS disease sufferers aged between 40 and 70 appeared to be about 9 times that of the non-Hb-SS population in Jamaica.

In the United States. American patients, too, have been described whose clinical course has been atypically benign. Jackson, Odom and Bell (1961), in a paper entitled 'Amelioration of sickle cell disease by persistent fetal hemoglobin', described how they had classified 61 Hb-SS patients according to a pathological index based on specific historical and clinical data: 38 patients whose erythrocytes contained 12% or more Hb F had a significantly lower index rating than 23 patients whose cells contained a lesser amount of Hb F. The presence of Hb F was thought to protect the cells from sickling.

Some remarkably long-living patients have also been described. Thus Charache and Richardson (1964), reporting from the Johns Hopkins Hospital, referred to a 55-year-old female black whose Hb-SS disease had not been discovered until she was aged 50. Her haemoglobin comprised 96% Hb S with no increase in Hb A$_2$ or unusual increase in Hb F, and the increase in blood viscosity on deoxygenation was the same as in typical Hb-SS disease. Of 100 other patients studied, only one was in the 50–55-year age-group. Age (within the first four decades) did not seem to affect the haematocrit. Charache and Richardson, in commenting that the pattern of survival in Hb-SS disease was changing for the better, suggested that the then striking differences in the natural history of the disease in Africa and North America reflected the relative freedom (in America) from co-existing parasitic, infective and nutritional disease.

Margolis and co-workers (1973) reported a still older patient — a 71-year-old female black who had been followed for 10 years during which time she had never had a haemolytic or painful crisis. Her Hb-F percentage, however, was relatively high, 12.9, and that of Hb A$_2$ normal, 2.9.

Steinberg and co-workers (1973) reviewed the clinical history and haematological findings in 21 patients, who were 18–56 years of age. They were active and employed and led relatively normal lives; painful crises were infrequent and mild, and some of the patients were free from them. However, their mean haemoglobin level and reticulocyte count and the mean Hb-A$_2$ percentage (2.9) and Hb-F percentage (5.0) did not differ significantly from those of other patients suffering from clinically more severe (and more typical) Hb-SS disease. There was no evidence of admixture with thalassaemia or hereditary persistence of fetal haemoglobin or other haemoglobinopathy. It was suggested that as yet undefined host or environmental factors protect certain individuals from the worst consequences of their disease.

Makler and co-workers (1974) described yet another variant of Hb-SS disease characterized by a mild course and high Hb-F content, with the Hb F being homogeneously distributed in the patients' erythrocytes, as in hereditary persistence of fetal haemoglobin (HPFH) (see p. 436). The patients studied were two black Americans, a male aged 24 and a female aged 29, resident at Colorado Springs at an altitude > 2000 m. The man had been in hospital 4 times for pains in his joints, chest and abdomen. His haemoglobin was 11.2 g/dl and the reticulocyte count 6.4%; electrophoresis revealed 77.7% Hb S, 2.3% Hb A$_2$ and 20% Hb F. His sister had been in hospital only for two normal pregnancies and for sterilization. Her haemoglobin was 10.6 g/dl and reticulocyte count 12.1%; electrophoresis revealed 78.4% Hb S, 2.6% Hb A$_2$ and 19% Hb F. Their parents were both Hb AS and there was no evidence for heterozygosity for thalassaemia or HPFH — their Hb-F levels were 2.5% and 3.5%, respectively. An acid-elution study of the patients' erythrocytes revealed that all stained palely but homogeneously. Makler *et al.* concluded that the high Hb-F levels were determined by a 'new' Hb-F gene which depended for its expression on a defect in the β chain of haemoglobin.

The apparent role of high Hb-F levels in suppressing the worst consequences of being homozygous for Hb S, as exemplified by the studies on the Saudi Arabs, received scant support from the analysis of Powars *et al.* (1980) who compared the clinical histories with the haematological findings in more than 200 Afro-American Hb-SS patients resident in California: 19 were less than 10 years of age and 68% in their second or third decades. Powars and her co-workers failed in fact to demonstrate any relationship between the haematological data, including Hb-F percentage (mean 12 ± 7%), and six out of seven clinical indicators of severity: the only exception was the risk of stroke which appeared to be higher in those with lower levels of Hb F. In a later paper Powars et al (1984) considered the question as to whether there were threshold levels of Hb F that ameliorated the clinical severity of Hb-SS disease. This time their analysis was based on an even larger series of patients, whose follow-up extended up to 11 years. The mean Hb-F percentage of the series was 10 ± 6% with a range of 2–23%. It appeared that a level of 10% or less was associated with an increased risk of serious 'termination' events such as stroke and aseptic necrosis, while a level of 20% or less was associated with an increased frequency of recurrent less serious clinical events such as crises or pulmonary problems. Powers et al. were unable, however, to establish a clear linear trend between Hb-F levels and morbidity; they pointed out that approximately 90% of their patients had Hb-F levels below 20%, the apparent protective threshold.

In Africans in West Africa

Clinically mild cases of Hb-SS disease seem to be rather rare in Africa. According to Fleming (1982), writing about his experience in Nigeria, patients in whom Hb-SS disease is diagnosed for the first time after childhood are likely to give a history of preceding ill health of moderate severity; he mentioned, however, that there are, too, a few patients who present for the first time when they are 'well into adult life' and complain perhaps only of having had occasional rheumatism in the past or admit to having had infrequent pains only after direct and insistent questioning. Konotey-Ahulu (1974), in his comprehensive account of Hb-SS disease in Ghana, although referring to the improving possibility of patients living to adult life, had, however, painted a picture of the clinical course of the disease that was generally far from being benign.

[It is interesting to recall that many years earlier Edington and Lehmann (1955) had described two Africans living in the Gold Coast, who were undoubtedly homozygous for Hb SS, whose history had been very benign indeed: one had 24.2% of Hb F — he had presumably Hb SS plus HPFH; the other (Case 1) had only 5.2% of Hb F and had, therefore, a haemoglobin pattern indicative of typical Hb-SS disease. This man admitted to suffering from 'rheumatism' as a child; while at the 'age of 8 he had had attacks of pain in the larger joints of the limbs accompanied by fever; these attacks occurred about ten times in that year and gradually lessened in frequency and severity until they ceased at the age of 18'.]

Recently, details have been given by Matthew, Rubenstein and Jacobs (1984) of two Cape-Coloured males, aged 41 and 31, respectively, with Hb SS, whose illness had run a mild course. Both had high Hb-F levels, 21% and 15% respectively, and the latter patient had α-thalassaemia, too (−α/−α genotype).

The relationship between the long survival of Hb-SS patients and the concurrent presence of one or two genes for α-thalassaemia has been emphasized by Mears and co-workers (1983), who determined the frequency of α-thalassaemia genotypes in relation to the age of Hb-SS patients living in West Africa, Equatorial Africa or in the United States. This study showed an increase in frequency of the −α gene from 0.18 in patients aged 1–10 years, to 0.27 in those aged 11–20 years, to 0.36 in those over 20 years of age. No such age relationship was demonstrable in Hb-AA individuals who had α-thalassaemia.

In Southern India

A clinically mild form of Hb-SS disease has been described in Southern India by Brittenham et al. (1977). Ninety out of 292 members of a Veddoid ethnic group (31%) were found to have the AS genotype and they were unusual in that the percentage of Hb S was unusually low (19–32%, mean 26%). Seven individuals, aged 1 year to 63 years, were found to be homozygotes (Hb SS): the Hb-F concentration was high in one of them (29%), but only slightly or moderately raised (4–12%) in the remainder. Their illness was clinically mild: only two had had painful crises and the spleen was palpable in three of them. A further and more comprehensive account was given by Brittenham et al. (1979). Fifteen Hb-SS individuals had by then been identified: their Hb-F percentage ranged between 8 and 36% (mean 20%) and the Hb-S percentage ranged between 61 and 90%. In one family one Hb-AS parent probably also had heterocellular HPFH: in the other families HPFH was not demonstrable.

The patients' clinical history was generally mild. As well as interaction with HPFH (in one family), there was evidence of interaction with two genotypes of α-thalassaemia, −α/αα and −α/−α. These interactions were reflected in a trimodal distribution of Hb S in heterozygotes as well as in the degree of microcytosis and hypochromia. The decreased α-chain synthesis resulting from the presence of α-thalassaemia was considered to be a factor in the clinical mildness of the patients' illness.

Kar and co-workers (1986) have, too, given a detailed account of Hb-SS disease as it occurs in Orissa State. [Orissa is situated on the East coast of India, South of Calcutta.] One hundred and thirty-one patients were studied: compared with Jamaican patients, the Indian patients tended to have higher total haemoglobins and erythrocyte counts and higher Hb-F percentages, and lower MCVs, MCHs and reticulocyte counts. The incidence of α-thalassaemia was greater. Palpable spleens were more common, with a later peak age incidence and hypersplenism was relatively frequent. Painful crises and dactylitis were not uncommon but chronic leg ulceration was rare. Kar *et al.* concluded that the manifestations of Hb-SS disease in Orissa were similar to those of Hb-SS patients in the Eastern Province of Saudi Arabia but very different from those of populations of West-African origin.

SICKLE-CELL DISEASE IN THE UNITED KINGDOM

The majority of the patients resident in the United Kingdom who are homozygous for Hb S are blacks of West-Indian or West-African origin, and there is no reason to believe that their clinical presentation and the haematological findings differ in any substantial way from those of Afro-Americans resident in the New World. Amongst the recent and comprehensive clinical studies that have been carried out on patients with Hb-SS disease or other sickle-cell syndromes are those of the following authors: Anionwu *et al.* (1981), a study of 70 patients with sickle-cell disease diagnosed in the London Borough of Brent; Murtaza *et al.* (1981), a review of 171 children with Hb-SS disease admitted to hospital in South London; Davis, Huehns and White (1981), a survey of more than 1300 patients with sickle-cell syndromes seen by haematologists in England and Wales in 1978 and 1979, and Brozović and Anionwu (1984), a review based on 139 Hb-SS and Hb-SC patients seen in the London Borough of Brent from 1964 to 1984 and a comparison of the presentation of

their illness with that of similar patients seen in Jamaica.

CLINICAL DIVERSITY OF SICKLE-CELL DISEASE: A SUMMARY

As has been stressed many times earlier in this Chapter, the degree to which patients who are homozygous for Hb S suffer from their illness varies very widely. At one end of the scale Hb-SS disease is an almost intolerable disorder associated with repeated episodes of severe pain localized to the bones, a marked propensity to serious infections, severe pulmonary and neurological problems and a poor prognosis as to life: at the other end of the scale it is a relatively benign disorder associated with little anaemia and giving rise to few serious symptoms and compatible with a long life. Some of the factors responsible for this diversity in clinical expression are known; amongst them are the concurrent presence of α-thalassaemia and the patient's ability to continue to form Hb F after the neonatal period. But there are other factors, too, that play important roles.

The key to the severity of each individual patient's illness is the readiness with which his or her erythrocytes undergo sickling within local areas of the microvasculature and the extent and duration of the obstruction to the circulation this causes. The many factors, intrinsic and extrinsic to the erythrocyte, which affect the sickling process, are discussed in some detail in Chapter 14 under *Pathogenesis*.

CONCURRENCE OF G6PD DEFICIENCY AND SICKLE-CELL DISEASE

As expected, it is not rare to find evidence for Hb S and G6PD deficiency in the same family. The question arises as to what is the effect of the expression of both abnormalities on the individual. G6PD deficiency could clearly be an unexpected cause of acute haemolysis in a patient (with Hb-SS disease) exposed to oxidant drugs and/or infections, as in the cases described by Smits, Oski and Brody (1969). It has been suggested, however, that the presence of G6PD deficiency may have been, in Africa at least, of selective value for the survival of Hb-SS homozygotes. Naylor and co-workers (1960) in the United States found, however, that the incidence of

G6PD deficiency in HB-SS patients did not differ significantly from that in Hb-AA subjects. Lewis and Hathorn (1965) and Lewis, Kay and Hathorn (1966), on the other hand, reported that in Ghana its incidence in Hb-SS disease patients was about 3 times that in the general population, and they concluded that the enzyme deficiency was beneficial to sufferers from Hb-SS disease [see also Lewis (1967)]. Piomelli and co-workers (1972) came to a similar conclusion based on the study of a small series of cases in the United States. But the way in which G6PD deficiency can possibly help a patient with Hb-SS disease is far from clear. Indeed, Konotey-Ahulu (1972d), in discussing Piomelli and co-workers' observations, stated that in his experience (in Ghana) G6PD deficiency tended to make patients clinically worse so that they needed more frequent hospital admissions. Subsequent studies in the United States in fact failed to confirm that the G6PD A− phenotype occurs more frequently in Hb-SS patients than in Hb-AS or Hb-AA controls (Beutler et al., 1974; Steinberg and Dreiling, 1974).

More recently, Gibbs, Wardle and Serjeant (1980) reported data from the West Indies, based on a study of 120 Hb-S homozygotes, 53 of whom were males and 67 females: 22.6% of the males were G6PD-deficient, a percentage not statistically different from that in the general population and the combined percentage of G6PD-deficient males and females (hemizygotes and heterozygotes) (28.3%) was slightly less than, but not statistically different from, that in the general population. In those aged between 10 and 19 years, however, the percentage of those with abnormal G6PD status (41.7%) was unexpectedly raised. Gibbs, Wardle and Serjeant concluded that, aside from technical explanations, the discrepancies in the literature (which they reviewed) perhaps reflected the different age-groups of the patients studied, but they did not give an explanation for the effect of age which they themselves had observed. Gibbs, Wardle and Serjeant also related the G6PD status of their patients to their haematological and clinical presentation and found no evidence of any effect.

Steinberg and co-workers (1984), reporting on behalf of the Cooperative Study of Sickle Cell Disease, came to the same conclusion, namely, that the presence of the $GdA-$ gene did not enhance the severity of haemolysis or increase the incidence of acute episodes of anaemia or sepsis in Hb-SS patients. They found, moreover, that the prevalence of $GdA-$ did not change significantly when the age of the patients was stratified into decades.

CONCURRENCE OF HEREDITARY SPHEROCYTOSIS AND SICKLE-CELL DISEASE

It is to be expected that rarely a patient carrying a gene or genes for Hb S will suffer from hereditary spherocytosis (HS). In Volume 1 of this book (p. 162) several descriptions of patients with HS who had the Hb-AS trait in addition were mentioned, but no patient who was unequivocally homozygous for Hb S who also had HS was referred to. However, Maurer, Vida and Honig did describe in 1972 a family in which this association had occurred. Five children were born to a Hb-AS mother and a Hb-AS father who also had HS. One child had HS, another the Hb-AS trait and three children (Cases 1–3) had Hb SS plus HS. The child described as Case 1 was transfused at intervals; splenectomy was eventually carried out and her haemoglobin subsequently stabilized at 8–10 g/dl. The child described as Case 2 was reported to have a haemoglobin of 8.4 g/dl and 27% reticulocytes; the spleen was not palpable and she was clinically well. The child described as Case 3 became severely jaundiced soon after birth (bilirubin 16 mg/dl); when 10 months of age he contracted pneumococcal sepsis and meningitis; subsequently he received regular transfusions and the spleen became impalpable. The father and the sibling (without Hb S) underwent splenectomy and were clinically cured (Fig. 11.19).

Babiker and El Seed (1984) have more recently described another family in which HS and the Hb-AS trait have occurred together. The index patient was a 4-year-old Sudanese boy who was anaemic and whose spleen was palpable 5 cm below the costal margin. His haemoglobin was 8.8 g/dl and there were 3% reticulocytes. Many spherocytes could be seen in blood films and osmotic fragility was markedly increased. The sickling test was positive and haemoglobin electrophoresis revealed an AS pattern. The boy's father, and one of his sisters, had the same HS/Hb-AS combination; another sister had typical HS but normal (AA) haemoglobin. The father, aged 35, had had many transfusions when he was young but had not required any for the last 15 years. His spleen was firm to palpation 4 cm below the costal margin but was not visualized by a [99mTc]sulphur colloid scan. Howell-Jolly bodies as well as spherocytes were conspicuous in blood films and it was suggested that the presence of the former and the absence of a [99mTc]sulphur colloid image, despite a normal uptake of the colloid by the liver, indicated splenic hypofunction. It was postulated that the unusually slow circulation of the spherocytes through the spleen pulp, caused by their lack of plasticity, had led to sufficient local hypoxia for sickling to take place and for the spleen to be infarcted, an unusual occurrence in someone with the AS trait (or HS).

CONCURRENCE OF AUTO-IMMUNE HAEMOLYTIC ANAEMIA (AIHA) AND SICKLE-CELL DISEASE

A small number of Hb-SS patients are known to have developed AIHA. Ward, Smith and White's (1979) patient developed acute cold-antibody haemolytic

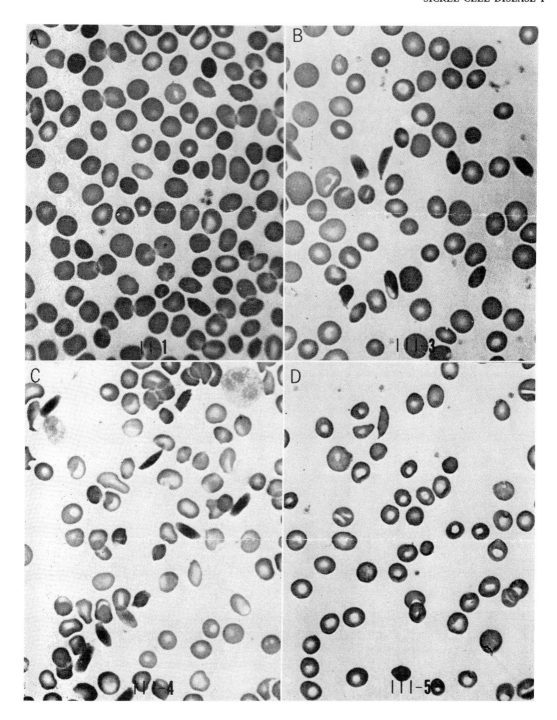

Fig. 11.19 Photomicrographs of blood films of four members of a family carrying genes for both Hb S and hereditary spherocytosis (HS).
Top left: the father who had HS plus Hb-AS trait.
Top right and bottom two photographs: three children who had HS plus Hb-SS disease.
[Reproduced by permission from Maurer, Vida and Honig (1972).]

anaemia in association with pneumonitis. The direct antiglobulin test was positive and many of the erythrocytes presented an unusual appearance. In addition to cells that had sickled or had undergone autoagglutination, many cells showed single or multiple surface protrusions or even fine filaments (as if part of their surface was being shed) when viewed in dried films under the light microscope or by the scanning electron microscope.

Chaplin and Zarkowsky (1981) described one patient, and referred to four others observed within a 10-year period, who had developed warm-antibody AIHA. The patient described in detail was a 19-year-old female who as a child had suffered from juvenile rheumatoid arthritis. An auto-antibody free in her serum and on her erythrocytes was detected in the course of compatibility studies in preparation for a blood transfusion. The direct antiglobulin test was positive with broad-spectrum and anti-γ-globulin sera and an agglutinin as well as several allo-antibodies were demonstrable in her serum. Blood transfusion was followed by acute intravascular haemolysis and haemoglobinuria. She eventually recovered after prednisone therapy had been supplemented with 6-mercaptopurine, during which time the reticulocyte count reached 76%. The four other patients mentioned were three males aged 15–22 years and a female aged 27. Three became severely anaemic and developed very high reticulocyte counts (60–88%). All had positive direct antiglobulin tests and had warm auto-antibodies and several allo-antibodies in their sera. Chaplin and Zarkowsky emphasized the height of the reticulocyte counts [perhaps associated with hypoplasia of the spleen] and noted that when in two patients the reticulocyte counts fell to modest levels (6–16%) the patients then became dangerously anaemic. Corticosteroids were the mainstay of therapy in four of the patients. In patients refractory to steroid (and 6MP) therapy, it was suggested that splenectomy might be justified if radionuclide scanning demonstrated that a 'substantial' amount of splenic tissue was present.

SICKLE-CELL DISEASE COMPLICATED BY A HAEMATOLOGICAL MALIGNANCY

There is no reason to suppose that patients suffering from a sickle-cell disease suffer from malignant disease less frequently than do Hb-AA subjects, if allowance is made for the fact that the great majority of Hb-SS patients are children or relatively young adults.

Stricker and co-workers (1986) have recently reviewed the sparse literature describing the occurrence of haematological malignancies in patients suffering from various types of sickle-cell disease or the sickle-cell trait. They found nine reports of myeloid or lymphoid leukaemia and six reports of lymphoid malignancies; they themselves described four further patients, all adults (two Hb SS, two Hb SC) who developed acute myeloblastic leukaemia, malignant histiocytosis, multiple myeloma and Hodgkin's disease, respectively. Stricker et al. stressed that further epidemiological and cytogenetic data were required before the particular significance (if any) of the concurrence of a haematological malignancy and sickle-cell disease could be assessed.

REFERENCES

ABBASI, A. A., PRASAD, A. S., ORTEGA, J., CONGCO, E. & OBERLEAS, D. (1976). Gonadal function abnormalities in sickle-cell anemia: studies in adult male patients. *Ann. intern. Med.*, **85**, 601–605.

ABEL, M. S. & BROWN, C. R. (1948). Sickle cell disease with severe hematuria simulating renal neoplasm. *J. Amer. med. Ass.*, **136**, 624–625.

ACQUAYE, J. K., OMER, A., GANESHAGURU, K., SEJENY, S. A. & HOFFBRAND, V. (1985). Non-benign sickle cell anaemia in western Saudi Arabia. *Brit. J. Haemat.*, **60**, 99–108.

ADAMS, J. Q., WHITACRE, F. E. & DIGGS, L. W. (1953). Pregnancy and sickle-cell disease. *Obstet. and Gynec.*, **2**, 335–352.

ADDAE, S. (1971). Mechanism for the high incidence of sickle-cell crisis in the tropical cool season. *Lancet*, **ii**, 1256 (Letter).

ADDIEGO, J., SMITH, W. B., MENTZER, W. C., LUBIN, B. & AMMAN, A. J. (1976). Polyvalent pneumococcal polysaccharide immunization in patients with sickle cell anemia. *Pediat. Res.*, **10**, 373 (Abstract).

ADELOYE, A., LUZZATTO, L. & EDINGTON, G. M. (1971). Severe malarial infection in a patient with sickle-cell anaemia. *Brit. med. J.*, **ii**, 445.

ADELOYE, A., OGBEIDE, M. I. & ODEKU, E. G. (1970). Massive intracranial hemorrhage in sickle-cell anemia. *Neurology*, **20**, 1165–1170.

ADEYOKUNNU, A. A. & HENDRICKSE, R. G. (1980). Salmonella osteomyelitis in childhood. A report of 63 cases seen in Nigerian children of whom 57 had sickle cell anaemia. *Arch. Dis. Childh.*, **55**, 175–184.

AGER, J. A. M. & LEHMANN, H. (1958). Observations on some "fast" haemoglobins: K, J, N, and "Barts". *Brit. med. J.*, **i**, 929–931.

AGER, J. A. M., LEHMANN, H. & VELLA, F. (1958). Haemoglobin "Norfolk": a new haemoglobin found in an English family. With observations on the naming of new haemoglobin variants. *Brit. med. J.*, ii, 539–541.

AHONKHAI, V. I., LANDESMAN, S. H., FIKRIG, S. M., SCHMALZER, E. A., BROWN, A. K., CHERUBIN, C. F. & SCHIFFMAN, G. (1979). Failure of pneumococcal vaccine in children with sickle-cell disease. *New Engl. J. Med.*, 301, 26–27.

AKENZUA, G. T. & AMIENGHEME, O. R. (1981). Inhibitor of *in vitro* neutrophil migration in sera of children with homozygous sickle cell gene during pain crisis. *Brit. J. Haemat.*, 47, 345–352.

AKINKUGBE, O. O. (1967). Renal papillary necrosis in sickle-cell haemoglobinopathy. *Brit. med. J.*, iii, 283–284.

AKSOY, M. (1955). Sickle-cell trait in South Turkey. *Lancet*, i, 589–590.

AKSOY, M. (1956). Sickle-cell anemia in South Turkey: a study of fifteen cases in twelve white families. *Blood*, 11, 460–472.

ALAVI, A., BOND, J. P., KUHL, D. E. & CREECH, R. H. (1974).Scan detection of bone marrow infarcts in sickle cell disorders. *J. nucl. Med.*, 15, 1003–1007.

ALAVI, A., SCHUMACHER, R., DORWART, B. & KUHL, D. E. (1976). Bone marrow scan evaluation of arthropathy in sickle cell disorders. *Arch. intern. Med.*, 136, 436–440.

AL-AWAMY, B., WILSON, W. A. & PEARSON, H. A. (1984). Splenic function in sickle cell disease in the Eastern Province of Saudi Arabia. *J. Pediat.*, 104, 714–717.

ALI, S. A. (1970). Milder variant of sickle-cell disease in Arabs in Kuwait associated with unusually high level of foetal haemoglobin. *Brit. J. Haemat.*, 19, 613–619.

ALLEN, T. D. (1964). Sickle cell disease and hematuria: a report of 29 cases. *J. Urol.*, 91, 177–183.

ALLEYNE, S. I., RAUSEO, R. D'H. & SERJEANT, G. R. (1981). Sexual development and fertility of Jamaican female patients with homozygous sickle cell disease. *Arch. intern. Med.*, 141, 1295–1297.

ALLISON, A. C. (1954a). Protection afforded by sickle-cell trait against subtertian malarial infection. *Brit. med. J.*, i, 290–294.

ALLISON, A C. (1954b). Notes on sickle-cell polymorphism. *Ann. hum. Genet.*, 19, 39–51.

ALLISON, A. C. (1954c). The distribution of the sickle-cell trait in East Africa and elsewhere, and its apparent relationship to the incidence of subtertian malaria. *Trans. roy. Soc. trop. Med. Hyg.*, 48, 312–318.

ALLISON, A. C., (1956). The sickle-cell and haemoglobin *C* genes in some African populations. *Ann. hum. Genet.*, 21, 67–89.

ALLISON, A. C. (1957). Malaria in carriers of the sickle-cell trait and in newborn children. *Exp. Parasit.*, 6, 418–447.

ALUOCH, J. R., KILINÇ, Y., AKSOY, M., YÜREGIR, G. T., BAKIOGLU, I., KUTLAR, A., KUTLAR, F. & HUISMAN, T. H. J. (1986). Sickle cell anaemia in Eti-Turks: haematological, clinical and genetic observations. *Brit. J. Haemat.*, 64, 45–55.

AMJAD. H., BANNERMAN, R. M. & JUDISCH, J. M. (1974). Sickling pain and season. *Brit. med. J.*, ii, 54 (Letter).

AMMAN, A. J., ADDIEGO, J., WARA, D. W., LUBIN, B., SMITH, W. B. & MENTZER, W. C. (1977). Polyvalent pneumococcal-polysaccharide immunization of patients with sickle-cell anemia and patients with splenectomy. *New Engl. J. Med.*, 297, 897–900.

ANDERSON, M., WENT, L. N., MacIVER, J. E. & DIXON, H. G. (1960). Sickle-cell disease in Pregnancy. *Lancet*, ii, 516–521.

ANDERSON, W. W. & WARE, R. L. (1932). Sickle cell anemia. *Amer. J. Dis. Child.*, 44, 1055–1070.

ANIONWU, E., WALFORD, D., BROZOVIĆ, M. & KIRKWOOD, B. (1981). Sickle-cell disease in a British urban community. *Brit. med. J.*, 282, 283–286.

ANTONARAKIS, S. E., BOEHM, C. D., SERJEANT, G. R., THEISEN, C. E., DOVER, G. J. & KAZAZIAN, H. H. JNR (1984). Origin of the β^S-globin gene in blacks: the contribution of recurrent mutation or gene conversion or both. *Proc. natn. Acad. Sci. U.S.A.*, 81, 853–856.

APTHORP, G. H., MEASDAY, B. & LEHMANN, H. (1963). Pregnancy in sickle-cell anaemia. *Lancet*, i, 1344–1346.

ARENA, J. M. (1935). Vascular accident and hemiplegia in a patient with sickle cell anemia. *Amer. J. Dis. Child.*, 19, 722–723.

ARMALY, M. (1974). Ocular manifestations in sickle cell disease. *Arch. intern. Med.*, 133, 670–679.

ARNOW, P. M., PANWALKER, A., GARVIN, J. S. & RODRIGUEZ-ERDMANN, F. (1978). Aspirin, hyperventilation, and cerebellar infarction in sickle cell disease. *Arch. intern. Med.*, 138, 148–149.

ASHCROFT, M. T., SERJEANT, G. R. & DESAI, P. (1972). Heights, weights and skeletal age of Jamaican adolescents with sickle cell anaemia. *Arch. Dis. Childh.*, 47, 519–524.

ATHANASOU, N., HATTON, C., McGEE, J. O'D. & WEATHERALL, D. J. (1985). Vascular occlusion and infarction in sickle cell crisis and the sickle chest syndrome. *J. clin. Path.*, 38, 659–664.

ATTAH, E. B. & EKERE, M. C. (1975). Death patterns in sickle cell anemia. *J. Amer. med. Ass.* 233, 889–890.

BABIKER, M. A., EL-HAZMI, M. A. F., AL-JOBORI, A. M., OBEID, H. & BAHAKIM, H. M., (1985). Splenic function in children with sickle cell disease: two different patterns in Saudi Arabia. *Scand. J. Haemat.*, 35, 191–193.

BABIKER, M. A. & EL SEED, F. AL R. A. (1984). A family with sickle cell trait and hereditary spherocytosis. *Scand. J. Haemat.*, **33**, 54–58.

BAKIOGLU, I., HATTORI, Y., KUTLAR, A., MATHEW, C. & HUISMAN, T. H. J. (1985). Five adults with mild sickle cell anemia share a β^S chromosome with the same haplotype. *Amer. J. Hemat.*, **20**, 297–300.

BALL, G. V. & SORENSON, L. B. (1970). The pathogenesis of hyperuricemia and gout in sickle cell anemia. *Arth. Rheum.*, **13**, 846–848.

BALLESTER, O. F., ABDALLAH, J. M. & PRASAD, A. S. (1985). Impaired IgM antibody responses to an influenza virus vaccine in adults with sickle cell anemia. *Amer. J. Hemat.*, **20**, 409–412.

BALLOU, S. P., KAHN, M. A., KUSHNER, I. & HARRIS. J. W. (1977). Secondary gout in hemoglobinopathies: report of two cases and review of the literature. *Amer. J. Hemat.*, **2**, 397–402.

BARRETT, O'N., SAUNDERS, D. E., McFARLAND, D. E. & HUMPHRIES, J. O'N. (1984). Myocardial infarction in sickle cell anemia. *Amer. J. Hemat.*, **16**, 139–147.

BARRETT-CONNOR, E. (1968a). Cholelithiasis in sickle-cell anemia. *Amer. J. Med.*, **45**, 889–898.

BARRETT-CONNOR, E. (1968b). Sickle cell disease and viral hepatitis. *Ann. intern. Med.*, **69**, 517–527.

BARRETT-CONNOR, E. (1971). Bacterial infection and sickle cell anemia. An analysis of 250 infections in 166 patients and a review of the literature. *Medicine (Baltimore)*, **50**, 97–112.

BARRETT-CONNOR, E. (1973). Pneumonia and pulmonary infarction in sickle cell anemia. *J. Amer. med. Ass.*, **224**, 997–1000.

BEACHAM, W. D. & BEACHAM, D. W. (1950). Sickle-cell disease and pregnancy. *Amer. J. Obstet. Gynec.*, **60**, 1217–1228.

BEAVEN, G. H. & GRATZER, W. B. (1959). A critical review of human haemoglobin variants. Part I: methods of separation and characterization; Part II: individual haemoglobins. *J. clin. Path.*, **12**, 1–24, 101–115.

BECKLAKE, M. R., GRIFFITHS, S. B., McGREGOR, M., GOLDMAN, H. I. & SCHREVE, J. P. (1955). Oxygen dissociation curves in sickle cell anemia and in subjects with the sickle cell trait. *J. clin. Invest*, **34**, 751–755.

BEET, E. A. (1946). Sickle cell disease in the Balovale district of Northern Rhodesia. *E. Afr. med. J.*, **23**, 75–86.

BEET, E. A. (1949). The genetics of the sickle-cell trait in a Bantu tribe. *Ann. Eugen.*, **14**, 279–284.

BEET, E. A. (1947). Sickle cell disease in Northern Rhodesia. *E. Afr. med. J.*, **24**, 212–222.

BERMAN, L. B. & TUBLIN, I. (1959). The nephropathies of sickle-cell disease. *Arch. intern. Med.*, **103**, 602–606.

BESSIS, M. & DELPECH, G. (1981). Discovery of the red blood cell with notes on priorities and credits of discoveries, past, present and future. *Blood Cells*, 7, 447–480.

BESSIS, M. & DELPECH, G. (1982). Sickle cell shape

and structure: images and concepts (1840–1980). *Blood Cells*, **8**, 359–435.

BEUTLER, E., DERN, R. J. & FLANAGAN, C. L. (1955). Effect of sickle-cell trait on resistance to malaria. *Brit. med. J.*, **i**, 1189–1191.

BEUTLER, E., JOHNSON, C., POWARS, D. & WEST, C. (1974). Prevalence of glucose-6-phosphate dehydrogenase deficiency in sickle cell disease. *New Engl. J. Med.*, **290**, 826–828.

BJORNSON, A. B., LOBEL, J. S. & LAMPKIN, B. C. (1980). Humoral components of host defense in sickle cell disease during painful crisis and asymptomatic periods. *J. Pediat.*, **96**, 259–262.

BLANK, J. P. & GILL, F. M. (1981). Orbital infarction in sickle cell disease. *Pediatrics*, **67**, 879–881.

BOGHOSSIAN, S. H., WRIGHT, G., WEBSTER, A. D. B. & SEGAL, A. W. (1985). Investigations of host defence in patients with sickle cell disease. *Brit. J. Haemat.*, **59**, 523–531.

BOHRER, S. P. (1970). Acute long bone diaphyseal infarcts in sickle cell disease. *Brit. J. Radiol.*, **43**, 685–697.

BOROS, L., THOMAS, C. & WEINER, W. J. (1976). Large cerebral vessel disease in sickle cell anaemia. *J. Neurol. Neurosurg. Psychiat.*, **39**, 1236–1239.

BRAIN, P. (1952). Sickle-cell anaemia in Africa. *Brit. med. J.*, **ii**, 880 (Letter).

BRECHER, G. (1981). A red cell discovery of the 20th century: hemoglobin. S. *Blood Cells*, **7**, 481–483.

BRITISH COLONIAL MEDICAL RESEARCH COMMITTEE (1957). Terminology of the hereditary haemoglobinopathies with haemoglobin variants. *Brit. med. J.*, **i**, 1235.

BRITISH MEDICAL JOURNAL (1960). Nomenclature of abnormal haemoglobins. *Brit. med. J.*, **ii**, 1155 (Leading article).

BRITTAIN, H. P., DE LA TORRE, A. & WILLEY, E. N. (1966). A case of sickle-cell disease with an abscess arising in an infarct of the liver. *Ann. intern. Med.*, **65**, 560–563.

BRITTENHAM, G., LOZOFF, B., HARRIS, J. W., MAYSON, S. M., MILLER, A. & HUISMAN, T. H. J. (1979). Sickle cell anemia and trait in Southern India: further studies. *Amer. J. Hemat.*, **6**, 107–123.

BRITTENHAM, G., LOZOFF, B., HARRIS, J. W., SHARMA, V. S. & NARASIMHAM, S. (1977). Sickle cell anemia and trait in a population in Southern India. *Amer. J. Hemat.*, **2**, 25–32.

BRODY, J. I., LEVISON, S. P. & CHUNG-JA JUNG (1977). Sickle trait and hematuria associated with von Willebrand syndromes. *Ann. intern. Med.*, **86**, 529–533.

BROMBERG, P. A. (1974). Pulmonary aspects of sickle cell disease. *Arch. intern. Med.*, **133**, 652–657.

BROMBERG, P. A. & JENSEN, W. N. (1967). Arterial oxygen unsaturation in sickle cell disease. *Amer. Rev. resp. Dis.*, **96**, 400–407.

BROWN, C. H. III (1972). Bone marrow necrosis. A

study of seventy cases. *Johns Hopk. med. J.*, **131**, 189–203.

BROWNE, R. A. (1965). Anaesthesia in patients with sickle-cell anaemia. *Brit. J. Anaesth.*, **37**, 181–188.

BROZOVIĆ, M. & ANIONWU, E. (1984). Sickle cell disease in Britain. *J. clin. Path.*, **37**, 1321–1326.

BUCHANAN, G. R. & GLADER, B. E. (1977). Benign course of extreme hyperbilirubinemia and sickle cell anemia: analysis of six cases. *J. Pediat.*, **91**, 21–24.

BUCHANAN, G. R. & GLADER, B. E. (1978). Leukocyte counts in children with sickle cell disease. *Amer. J. Dis. Child.*, **132**, 396–398.

BUCHANAN, G. R. & SCHIFFMAN, G. (1980). Antibody responses to polyvalent pneumococcal vaccine in infants with sickle cell anemia. *J. Pediat.*, **96**, 264–266.

BUNN, H. F. & FORGET, B. G. (1986). *Hemoglobin: Molecular Genetics and Clinical Aspects.* 690 pp. W .B. Saunders, Philadelphia.

BUNN, H. F., FORGET, B. G. & RANNEY, H. M. (1977). *Human Hemoglobins.* 432 pp. W. B. Saunders, Philadelphia, London, Toronto.

CABANNES, R., DUZER, A., PORTIER, A., MASSONAT, J., SENDRA, L. & BUHR, J. L. (1956). Hémoglobines anormales chez l'Algérien musulman. *Sang*, **27**, 580–585.

CAFFEY, J. (1937). The skeletal changes in chronic hemolytic anemias (erythroblastic anemia, sickle cell anemia and chronic hemolytic icterus). *Amer. J. Roentgenol.*, **37**, 293–324.

CAMPBELL, J. H. & CUMMINS, S. D. (1951). Priapism in sickle cell anemia. *J. Urol.*, **66**, 697–703.

CARRINGTON, H. T., FERGUSON, A. D. & SCOTT, R. B. (1958). Studies in sickle-cell anemia. XI. Bone involvement simulating aseptic necrosis. *J. Dis. Child.*, **95**, 157–163.

CASPER, J. T., KOETHE, S., RODEY, G. E. & THATCHER, L. G. (1976). A new method for studying splenic reticuloendothelial dysfunction in sickle cell disease patients and its clinical application: a brief report. *Blood*, **47**, 183–188.

CHAPLIN, H. JNR (1980). Hematuria in hemoglobin S disorders. *Arch. intern. Med.*, **140**, 1573–1574 (Editorial).

CHAPLIN, H. JNR, & ZARKOWSKY, H. S. (1981). Combined sickle cell disease and autoimmune hemolytic anemia. *Arch. intern. Med.*, **141**, 1091–1093.

CHAPMAN, A. Z., REEDER, P. S., FRIEDMAN, I. A. & BAKER, L. A. (1954). Gross hematuria in sickle cell trait and sickle cell C-hemoglobin disease. *J. Lab. clin. Med.*, **44**, 778–779.

CHARACHE, S. & RICHARDSON, S. N. (1964). Prolonged survival of a patient with sickle cell anemia. *Arch. intern. Med.*, **113**, 844–849.

CHARACHE, S., SCOTT, J. C. & CHARACHE, P. (1979). 'Acute chest syndrome' in adults with sickle cell anemia: microbiology, treatment, and prevention. *Arch. intern. Med.*, **139**, 67–69.

CHARACHE, S., SCOTT, J., NIEBYL, J. & BONDS, D. (1980). Management of sickle cell disease in pregnant patients. *Obstet. and Gynec.*, **55**, 407–410.

CHARMOT, G., REYNAUD, R. & BERGOT, J. (1963). Cryoglobulinaemia and cold agglutinins in painful crises of sickle-cell anaemia. *Lancet*, ii. 540.

CHERNOFF, A. I. (1955). The human hemoglobins in health and disease. *New Engl. J. Med.*, **253**, 322–331, 365–374, 416–423.

CHERNOFF, A. I., MINNICH, V. & CHONGCHAREONSUK, S. (1954). Hemoglobin E, a hereditary abnormality of human hemoglobin. *Science*, **120**, 605–606.

CHERNOFF, A. I., SHAPLEIGH, J. B. & MOORE, C. V. (1954). Therapy of chronic ulceration of the legs associated with sickle cell anemia. *J. Amer. med. Ass.*, **155**, 1487–1491.

CHODORKOFF, J. & WHITTEN, C. F. (1963). Intellectual status of children with sickle cell anemia. *J. Pediat.*, **63**, 29–35.

CHOREMIS, C., ZERVOS, N., CONSTANTINIDES, V. & ZANNAS, L. (1951). Sickle-cell anaemia in Greece. *Lancet*, i, 1147–1149.

CHUDWIN, D. S., WARA, D. W., MATTHAY, K. K., CAULFIELD, M. H., SCHIFFMAN, G., MENTZER, W. C. & AMMANN, A. J. (1983). Increased serum opsonic activity and antibody concentration in patients with sickle cell disease after pneumococcal polysacchoride immunization. *J. Pediat.*, **102**, 51–54.

CLINOPATHOLOGIC CONFERENCE (AACH, R. & KISSANE, J., EDS) (1970). A patient with sickle cell anemia surviving forty-eight years. *Amer. J. Med.*, **48**, 226–234.

COHEN, S. M., MILLER, B. W. & ORRIS, H. W. (1947). Fatal sickle cell anemia in a one-month-old infant. *J. Pediat.*, **30**, 468–472.

COLLINS, F. S. & ORRINGER, E. P. (1982). Pulmonary hypertension and cor pulmonale in the sickle hemoglobinopathies. *Amer. J. Med.*, **73**, 814–821.

COMMITTEE FOR CLARIFICATION OF THE NOMENCLATURE OF CELLS AND DISEASES OF THE BLOOD AND BLOOD-FORMING ORGANS (1950). Third report. *Amer. J. clin. Path.*, **20**, 562–579.

CONDON, P. I. & SERJEANT, G. R. (1972). Ocular findings in homozygous sickle cell anemia in Jamaica. *Amer. J. Ophthal.*, **73**, 533–543.

CONDON, P. I. & SERJEANT, G. R. (1980). Behaviour of untreated proliferative sickle retinopathy. *Brit. J. Ophthal.*, **64**, 404–411.

CONLEY, C. L. (1980). Sickle-cell anemia — the first molecular disease. In: *Blood, Pure and Eloquent: a Story of Discovery, of People, and of Ideas* (ed. by M. M. Wintrobe), pp. 318–371. McGraw-Hill Book Co., New York.

CONN, H. O. (1954). Sickle-cell trait and splenic infarction associated with high-altitude flying. *New Engl. J. Med.*, **251**, 417–420.

CONRAD, M. E., PERRINE, G. M., BARTON, J. C. & DURANT, J. R. (1980). Provoked priapism in sickle cell anemia. *Amer. J. Hemat.*, **9**, 121–122.

COOK, J. E. & MEYER, J. (1915). Severe anemia with remarkable elongated and sickle-shaped red blood cells and chronic leg ulcer. *Arch. intern. Med.*, **16**, 644–651.

COOLEY, J. C., PETERSON, W. L. & JERNIGAN, J. P. (1954). Clinical triad of massive splenic infarction, sicklemia trait and high altitude flying. *J. Amer. med. Ass.*, **154**, 111–113.

COOLEY, T. B. & LEE, P. (1926). The sickle cell phenomenon. *Amer. J. Dis. Child.*, **32**, 334–340.

COOPER, M. R. & TOOLE, J. F. (1972). Sickle-cell trait: benign or malignant? *Ann. intern. Med.*, **77**, 997–998 (Editorial notes).

CORRIGAN, J. C. & SCHILLER, I. W. (1934). Sickle cell anemia. A report of eight cases, one with necropsy. *New Engl. J. Med.*, **210**, 410–417.

CRONE, R. I., JEFFERSON, S. C., PILEGGI, V. J. & LOWRY, E. C. (1957). Gross hematuria in sickle-cell trait: a report of eight cases. *Arch. intern. Med.*, **100**, 597–603.

DAESCHNER, C. W. III, MATUSTIK, M. C., CARPENTIERI, U. & HAGGARD, M. E. (1981). Zinc and growth in patients with sickle cell disease. *J. Pediat.*, **98**, 778–780.

DANFORD, E. A., MARR, R. & ELSEY, E. C. (1941). Sickle cell anemia with unusual bone changes. *Amer. J. Roentgenol.*, **45**, 223–226.

DAVIES, S. C., LUCE, P. J., WIN, A. A., RIODAN, J. F. & BROZOVIC, M. (1984). Acute chest syndrome in sickle-cell disease. *Lancet*, i, 36–38.

DAVIS, L. R., HUEHNS, E. R. & WHITE, J. M. (1981). Survey of sickle-cell disease in England and Wales. *Brit. med. J.*, **283**, 1519–1521.

DE SILVA, C. C., BULUGAHAPITIYA, D. T. D., DE SILVA, J., WICKREMASINGHE, R. L. & JONXIS, J. H. P. (1962). Sinhalese family with haemoglobin S. *Brit. med. J.*, i, 1519–1521.

DE TORREGROSA, M. V., DAPENA, R. B., HERNANDEZ, H. & ORTIZ, A. (1960). Association of salmonella-caused osteomyelitis and sickle-cell disease: report of three cases. *J. Amer. med. Ass.*, **174**, 354–356.

DELBROUCK, J. (1958). Contribution a la génétique de la sicklémie. Maintien de la fréquence élévée de sicklémie au Congo belge. *Ann. Soc. belge Méd. trop.*, **38**, 103–134.

DELIYANNIS, G. A. & TAVLARAKIS, N. (1955a). Sickling phenomenon in Northern Greece. *Brit. med. J.*, ii, 299–301.

DELIYANNIS, G. A. & TAVLARAKIS, N. (1955b). Compatibility of sickling with malaria. *Brit. med. J.*, ii, 301–302.

DESFORGES, J. F. & WANG, M. Y. F. W. (1966). Sickle cell anemia. *Med. Clin. N. Amer.*, **50**, 1519–1532.

DEVEREUX, S. & KNOWLES, S. M. (1985). Rhabdomyolysis and acute renal failure in sickle cell anaemia. *Brit. med. J.*, **290**, 1707.

DIAMOND, H. S., MEISEL, A. D. & HOLDEN, D. (1979). The natural history of urate overproduction in sickle cell anemia. *Ann. intern. Med.*, **90**, 752–757.

DIAMOND, H. S., MEISEL, A., SHARON, E., HOLDEN, D. & CACATIAN, A. (1976). Hyperuricosuria and increased tubular secretion of urate in sickle cell anemia. *Amer. J. Med.*, **59**, 796–802.

DIGGS, L. W. (1956). The crisis in sickle cell anemia. Hematologic studies. *Amer. J. clin. Path.*, **26**, 1109–1118.

DIGGS, L. W. (1965). Sickle cell crises (Ward Burdick Award Contribution). *Amer. J. clin. Path.*, **44**, 1–19.

DIGGS, L. W., AHMANN, C. F. & BIBB, J. (1933). Incidence and significance of the sickle cell trait. *Ann. intern. Med.*, **7**, 769–778.

DIGGS, L. W. & CHING, R. E. (1934). Pathology of sickle cell anemia. *Sth. med. J. (Bgham, Ala.)*, **27**, 839–844.

DIGGS, L. W. & FLOWERS, E. (1971). Sickle cell anemia in the home environment. Observations on the natural history of the disease in Tennessee children. *Clin. Pediat.*, 10, 679–700.

DIGGS, L. W., PULLIAM, H. N. & KING, J. C. (1937). The bone changes in sickle cell anemia. *Sth. med. J. (Bgham, Ala.)*, 30, 249–259.

DIMITROV, N. V., DOUVES, F. R., BARTOLOTTA, B., NOCHUMSON, S. & TOTH, M. A. (1972). Metabolic activity of polymorphonuclear leukocytes in sickle cell anaemia. *Acta haemat. (Basel)*, **47**, 283–291.

DREYFUSS, F. & BENYESCH, M. (1951). Sickle-cell trait in Yemenite Jews. *Nature (Lond.)*, **167**, 950.

EDINGTON, G. M. (1953). Sickle-cell anaemia in the Accra district of the Gold Coast. A review of twenty cases. *Brit. med. J.*, ii, 957–961.

EDINGTON, G. M. (1959). Some observations on the abnormal haemoglobin diseases in Ghana. In: *Abnormal Haemoglobins. A Symposium*, pp. 290–299. Blackwell Scientific Pullications, Oxford.

EDINGTON, G. M. & LEHMANN, H. (1954). Haemoglobin G: a new haemoglobin found in a West African. *Lancet*, ii, 173–174.

EDINGTON, G. M. & LEHMANN, H. (1955). Expression of the sickle-cell gene in Africa. (1955). *Brit. med. J.*, i, 1308–1311.

EDINGTON, G. M. & LEHMANN, H. (1956). Sickle-cell trait and malaria in Africa. *Bull. Wld Hlth Org.*, **15**, 837–842.

EDINGTON, G. M. & SARKIES, J. W. R. (1952). Two cases of sickle-cell anaemia associated with retinal microaneurisms. *Trans. roy. Soc. trop. Med. Hyg.*, **46**, 59–62.

EFFIONG, C. E. (1982). Sickle-cell disease in childhood. In: *Sickle-Cell Disease: a Handbook for the General Clinician* (ed. by A. F. Fleming), pp. 57–72. Churchill Livingstone, Edinburgh.

EGDAHL, R. H., MARTIN, W. W & HILKOVITZ, G.

(1963). Splenectomy for hypersplenism in sickle cell anemia. *J. Amer. med. Ass.*, **186**, 745–748.

EHRENPREIS, B. & SCHWINGER, H. N. (1952). Sickle cell anemia. *Amer. J. Roentgenol.*, **68**, 28–36.

EISENSTEIN, M. I., POSNER, A. C. & FRIEDMAN, S. (1956). Sickle-cell anemia in pregnancy. A review of the literature with additional case histories. *Amer. J. Obstet. Gynec.*, **72**, 622–634.

EL-HAZMI, M. A. F. (1982). Haemoglobin disorders: a pattern for thalassaemia and haemoglobinopathies in Arabia. *Acta haemat. (Basel)*, **68**, 43–51.

EMMEL, V. E. (1917). A study of the erythrocytes in a case of severe anemia with elongated and sickle-shaped red blood corpuscles. *Arch. intern. Med.*, **20**, 586–598.

EMOND, A. M., COLLIS, R., DARVILL, D., HIGGS, D. R., MAUDE, G. H. & SERJEANT, G. R. (1985). Acute splenic sequestration in homozygous sickle cell disease: natural history and management. *J. Pediat.*, **107**, 201–206.

EMOND, A. M., HOLMAN, R., HAYES, R. I. & SERJEANT, G. R. (1980). Priapism and impotence in homozygous sickle cell disease. *Arch. intern. Med.*, **140**, 1434–1437.

ENDE, N., PIZZOLATO, P. & ZISKIND, J. (1955). Sicklemia. *Ann. intern. Med.*, **42**, 1065–1075.

ENNIS, J. T., SERJEANT, G. R. & MIDDLEMISS, H. (1973). Homozygous sickle cell disease in Jamaica. *Brit. J. Radiol.*, **46**, 943–950.

ESPINOZA, L. R., SPILBERG, I. & OSTERLAND, C. K. (1974). Joint manifestations of sickle cell disease. *Medicine (Baltimore)*, **53**, 295–305.

ETTELDORF, J. N., SMITH, J. D., TUTTLE, A. H. & DIGGS, L. W. (1955). Renal hemodynamic studies in adults with sickle cell anemia. *Amer. J. Med.*, **18**, 243–248.

ETTELDORF, J. N., TUTTLE, A. H. & CLAYTON, C. W. (1952). Renal studies in pediatrics. I. Renal hemodynamics in children with sickle cell anemia. *Amer. J. Dis. Child.*, **83**, 185–191.

FALK, R. H. & HOOD, W. B. JNR (1982). The heart in sickle cell anemia. *Arch. intern. Med.*, **142**, 1680–1684.

FALTER, M. L., ROBINSON, M. G., KIM, O. S., GO, S. C. & TAUBKIN, S. P. (1973). Splenic function and infection in sickle cell anemia. *Acta haemat. (Basel)*, **50**, 154–161.

FALTER, M. L., SUTTON, A. L. & ROBINSON, M. G. (1973). Massive intracranial hemorrhage in sickle-cell anemia. *Amer. J. Dis. Child.*, **125**, 415–416.

FELDENZER, J., MEARS, J. G., BURNS, A. L., NATTA, C. & BANK, A. (1979). Heterogeneity of DNA fragments associated with the sickle-globin gene. *J. clin. Invest.*, **64**, 751–755.

FEMI-PEARSE, D., GAZIOGLU, K. M. & YU, P. N. (1970). Pulmonary function studies in sickle cell disease. *J. appl. Physiol.*, **28**, 574–577.

FERGUSON, A. D. & SCOTT, R. B. (1959). Studies in sickle-cell anemia. XII. Further studies on hepatic function in sickle-cell anemia. *Amer. J. Dis. Child.*, **97**, 418–425.

FESSAS, PH. (1959). The hereditary anaemias in Greece. In: *Abnormal Haemoglobins: a Symposium* (ed. by J. H. P. Jonxis and J. F. Delafresnaye), pp. 260–270. Blackwell Scientific Publications, Oxford.

FINK, A. J., FUNAHASHI, T., ROBINSON, M. & WATSON, R. J. (1961). Conjunctival blood flow in sickle-cell disease: preliminary report. *Arch. Ophthal. (Chicago)*, **66**, 824–829.

FLEMING, A. F. (1982). Sickle-cell disease during and after puberty. In: *Sickle-Cell Disease: a Handbook for the General Clinician* (ed. by A. F. Fleming), pp. 73–89. Churchill Livingstone, Edinburgh.

FORT, A. T., MORRISON, J. C., BERRERAS, L., DIGGS, L. W. & FISH, S. A. (1971). Counseling the patient with sickle cell disease about reproduction: pregnancy outcome does not justify the risk! *Amer. J. Obstet. Gynec.*, **111**, 324–327.

FOWLER, N. O., SMITH, O. & GREENFIELD, J. C. (1957). Arterial blood oxygenation in sickle cell anemia. *Amer. J. med. Sci.*, **234**, 449–458.

FOY, H., BRASS, W., MOORE, R. A., TIMMS, G. L., KONDI, A. & OLOUCK, T. (1955). Two surveys to investigate the relation of sickle-cell trait and malaria. *Brit. med. J.*, **ii**, 1116–1119.

FOY, H. & KONDI, A. (1951). Sickle-cell anaemia in Africans. *Lancet*, **ii**, 451–452 (Letter).

FOY, H. & KONDI, A. (1952). Sickle-cell trait in Africans. *Brit. med. J.*, **ii**, 41–42.

FOY, H. KONDI, A. & ALEXANDRIDES, C. (1951). Sickle-cell trait and sickle-cell anaemia. *Trans. roy. Soc. trop. Med. Hyg.*, **44**, 729–740.

FOY, H., KONDI, A. & BRASS, W. (1951). Sickle-cell disease of Africans in Kenya. *E. Afr. med. J.*, **28**, 1–5.

FRAZIER, C. W. & RICE, C. E. (1950). Neonatal sickle cell anemia. *J. Amer. med. Ass.*, **143**, 1065–1067.

FREEMAN, M. G. & RUTH, G. U. (1969). SS disease, SC disease and CC disease — obstetric considerations and treatment. *Clin. Obstet. Gynecol.*, **12**, 134–156.

FRIEDMAN, M. J. (1978). Erythrocytic mechanism of sickle cell resistance to malaria. *Proc. natn. Acad. Sci. U.S.A.*, **75**, 1994–1997.

FRIEDMAN, M. J. & TRAGER, W. (1981). The biochemistry of resistance to malaria. *Scient. Amer.*, **244**, 112–120.

GARLICK, J. P. (1960). Sickling and malaria in South-West Nigeria. *Trans. roy. Soc. trop. Med. Hyg.*, **54**, 146–154.

GASTON, M. H., VERTER, J. I., WOODS, G., PEGELOW, C., KELLEHER, J., PRESBURY, G., ZARKOWSKY, H., VICHINSKY, E., IYER, R., LOBEL, J. S., DIAMOND, S., HOLBROOK, C. T., GILL, F. M., RITCHEY, K. & FALLETTA, J. M., FOR THE PROPHYLACTIC PENICILLIN STUDY GROUP. (1986). Prophylaxis with oral penicillin in children with sickle cell anemia. A randomized trial. *New Engl. J. Med.*, **314**, 1593–1599.

GELFAND, M., CHRISTIE, F. & SEYMOUR, A. (1962). Sickle cell anaemia in a heterozygote. *J. trop. Med. Hyg.*, **65**, 143–145.

GELPI, A. P. (1967). Glucose-6-phosphate dehydrogenase deficiency, the sickling trait, and malaria in Saudi Arab children. *J. Pediat.*, **71**, 138–146.

GELPI, A. P. (1970). Sickle cell disease in Saudi Arabs. *Acta haemat. (Basel)*, **43**, 89–99.

GELPI, A. P. (1973). Migrant populations and the origin of the sickle-cell gene. *Ann. intern. Med.*, **79**, 258–264.

GELPI, A. P. & KING, M. C. (1976). Screening for abnormal hemoglobins in the Middle East: new data on hemoglobin S and the presence of hemoglobin C in Saudi Arabia. *Acta haemat. (Basel)*, **56**, 334–337.

GELPI, A. P. & PERRINE, R. P. (1973). Sickle cell disease and trait in white populations. *J. Amer. med. Ass.*, **224**, 605–608.

GENDREL, D., RICHARD-LENOBLE, D., VALETTE, H., KOMBILA, M., MAKANGA-BOUTOTO, H., TOURE, R. & GALLOITT, A. (1982). Salmonella infections and hemoglobin S. *J. Pediat.*, **101**, 68–69.

GERRY, J. L., BAIRD, M. G. & FORTUIN, N. J. (1976). Evaluation of left ventricular function in patients with sickle cell anemia. *Amer. J. Med.*, **60**, 967–972.

GIBBS, W. N., WARDLE, J. & SERJEANT, G. R. (1980). Glucose-6-phosphate dehydrogenase deficiency and homozygous sickle cell disease in Jamaica. *Brit. J. Haemat.*, **45**, 73–80.

GILBERTSON, A. A. (1965). Anaesthesia in West African patients with sickle-cell anaemia, haemoglobin SC disease and sickle-cell trait. *Brit. J. Anaesth.*, **37**, 614–622.

GIVNER, L. B., LUDDY, R. E. & SCHWARTZ, A. D. (1981). Etiology of osteomyelitis in patients with major sickle hemoglobinopathies. *J. Pediat.*, **99**, 411–413.

GOLD, M. S., WILLIAMS, J. C., SPIVACK, M. & GRANN, V. (1968). Sickle cell anemia and hyperuricemia. *J. Amer. med. Ass.*, **206**, 1572–1573.

GOLDING, J. S. R. (1956). The bone changes in sickle cell anaemia. *Ann. roy. Coll. Surg. Engl.*, **19**, 296–314.

GOLDING, J. S. R., MacIVER, J. E. & WENT, L. N. (1959). The bone changes in sickle-cell anemia and its genetic variants. *J. Bone Joint Surg.*, **41-B**, 711–718.

GOLDMAN, S. M., CHAPMAN, A. Z. & CROSS, R. R. JNR (1955). The hematuria of abnormal hemoglobin diseases. *Arch. Surg.*, **71**, 881–884.

GOODWIN, W. E., ALSTON, E. F. & SEMANS, J. H. (1950). Hematuria and sickle cell disease: unexplained gross unilateral renal hematuria in negroes, coincident with the blood sickling trait. *J. Urol.*, **63**, 79–96.

GOOSSENS, J. P., STATIUS, VAN EPS, L. W., SCHOUTEN, H. & GITERSON, A. L. (1972). Incomplete renal tubular acidosis in sickle cell disease. *Clin. chim. Acta*, **41**, 149–156.

GRAHAM, G. S. & McCARTY, S. H. (1927). Notes on sickle cell anemia. *J. Lab. clin. Med.*, **12**, 536–547.

GRAHAM, G. S. & McCARTY, S. H. (1930). Sickle cell (meniscocytic) anemia. *Sth. med. J. (Bgham, Ala.)*, **23**, 598–607.

GRANFORTUNA, J., ZAMKOFF, K. & URRUTIA, E. (1986). Acute renal infarction in sickle cell disease. *Amer. J. Haemat.*, **23**, 59–64.

GREEN, R. L., HUNTSMAN, R. G. & SERJEANT, G. R. (1971). The sickle-cell and altitude. *Brit. med. J.*, **iv**, 593–595.

GREEN, T. W., CONLEY, C. L. & BERTHRONG, M. (1953). The liver in sickle cell anemia. *Bull. Johns Hopk. Hosp.*, **92**, 99–127.

GREER, M. & SCHOTLAND, D. (1962). Abnormal hemoglobin as a cause of neurological disease. *Neurology*, **12**, 114–123.

GRIESEMER, D. A., WINKELSTEIN, J. A. & LUDDY, R. (1978). Pneumococcal meningitis in patients with a major sickle hemoglobinopathy. *J. Pediat*, **92**, 82–84.

GROVER, V. (1947). The clinical manifestations of sickle cell anemia. *Ann. intern. Med.*, **26**, 843–851.

GUERI, M. & SERJEANT, G. R. (1970). Leg ulcers in sickle-cell anaemia. *Trop. geog. Med.*, **22**, 155–160.

GUTTERIDGE, C., NEWLAND, A. C. & SEQUEIRA, J. (1985). Hepatic sequestration in sickle cell anaemia. *Brit. med. J.*, **290**, 1214–1215 (Letter).

HAGGARD, M. E. & SCHNEIDER, R. G. (1961). Sickle cell anemia in the first 2 years of life. *J. Pediat.*, **58**, 785–790.

HAGHSHENASS, M., ISMAIL-BEIGI, F., CLEGG, J. B. & WEATHERALL, D. J. (1977). Mild sickle-cell anaemia in Iran associated with high levels of fetal haemoglobin. *J. med. Genet.*, **14**, 168–171.

HAHN, E. V. (1928). Sickle cell (drepanocytic) anemia. With report of a second case successfully treated by splenectomy and further observations on the mechanism of sickle-cell formation. *Amer. J. med. Sci.*, **175**, 206–217.

HAHN, E. V. & GILLESPIE, E. B. (1927). Sickle cell anemia. Report of a case greatly improved by splenectomy. Experimental study of sickle cell formation. *Arch. intern. Med.*, **39**, 233–254.

HAMMEL, C. F., DeNARDO, S. J., DeNardo, C. L. & LEWIS, J. P. (1973). Bone marrow and bone mineral scintigraphic studies in sickle cell disease. *Brit. J. Haemat.*, **25**, 593–598.

HAND, W. L. & KING, N. L. (1978). Serum opsonization of Salmonella in sickle cell anemia. *Amer. J. Med.*, **64**, 388–395.

HANDLER, C. E. & PERKIN, G. D. (1982). Sickle cell trait and multiple cerebral infarctions. *J. roy. Soc. Med.*, **75**, 550–553.

HARDEN, A. S. JNR (1937). Sickle cell anemia: changes in the vessels and in the bones. *Amer. J. Dis. Child.*, 54, 1045–1051.

HARGROVE, M. D. JNR (1970). Marked increase in serum bilirubin in sickle cell anemia: a report of 6 patients. *Amer. J. dig. Dis.*, 15, 437–442.

HARRISON, K. A. (1982). Sickle-cell disease in pregnancy. In: *Sickle-Cell Disease: a Handbook for the General Clinician* (ed. by A. F. Fleming), pp. 90–99. Churchill Livingstone, Edinburgh.

HARROW, B. R., SLOANE, J. A. & LIEBMAN, N. C. (1963). Roentgenologic demonstration of renal papillary necrosis in sickle-cell trait. *New Engl. J. Med.*, 268, 969–976.

HASEN, H. B. & RAINES, S. L. (1962). Priapism associated with sickle cell disease. *J. Urol.*, 88, 71–76.

HATCH, F. E. JNR., CULBERTON, J. W. & DIGGS, L. W. (1967). Nature of the renal concentrating defect in sickle cell disease. *J. clin. Invest*, 46, 336–345.

HATCH, F. E. & DIGGS, L. W. (1965). Fluid balance in sickle-cell disease. *Arch. intern. Med.*, 116, 10–17.

HATTON, C. S. R., BUNCH, C. & WEATHERALL, D. J. (1985). Hepatic sequestration in sickle cell anaemia. *Brit. med. J.*, 290, 744–745.

HATTORI, Y., KUTLAR, F., KUTLAR, A., MCKIE, V. C. & HUISMAN, T. H. J. (1986). Haplotypes of β^S chromosomes among patients with sickle cell anemia from Georgia. *Hemoglobin*, 10, 623–642.

HAWKER, H., NEILSON, H., HAYES, R. J. & SERJEANT, G. R. (1982). Hematological factors associated with avascular necrosis of the femoral head in homozygous sickle cell disease. *Brit. J. Haemat.*, 50, 29–34.

HAYES, R. J., CONDON, P. I. & SERJEANT, G. R. (1981). Haematological factors associated with proliferative retinopathy in homozygous sickle cell disease. *Brit. J. Ophthal.*, 65, 29–35.

HEGYI, T., DELPHIN, E. S., BANK, A., POLIN, R. A. & BLANC, W. A. (1977). Sickle cell anemia in the newborn. *Pediatrics*, 60, 213–216.

HEINEMANN, H. O. & CHEUNG, M. W. (1957). Renal concentrating mechanism in sickle-cell anemia. *J. Lab. clin. Med.*, 49, 923–927.

HELDRICH, F. J. (1951). Sickle cell anemia: report of a case in a newborn infant. *J. Pediat.*, 39, 90–93.

HEMATOLOGY STUDY SECTION, NATIONAL INSTITUTES OF HEALTH (1953). Statement concerning a system of nomenclature for the varieties of human hemoglobin. *Blood*, 8, 386–387.

HEMLEY, S. D., MELLINS, H. Z. & FINBY, N. (1963). Punctate calcifications of the spleen in sickle cell anemia. *Amer. J. Med.*, 34, 483–485.

HENDERSON, A. B. (1950). Sickle cell anemia. Clinical study of 54 cases. *Amer. J. Med.*, 9, 757–765.

HENDRICKSE, J. P. DE V., HARRISON, K. A., WATSON WILLIAMS, E. J., LUZZATTO, L. & AJABOR, L. N. (1972). Pregnancy in homozygous sickle-cell anaemia. *J. Obstet. Gynaec. Brit. Cmwlth*, 79, 396–409.

HENDRICKSE, J. P. DE V. & WATSON-WILLIAMS, E. J. (1966). The influence of hemoglobinopathies on reproduction. *Amer. J. Obstet. Gynec.*, 94, 739–748.

HENDRICKSE, R. G. & COLLARD, P. (1960). Salmonella osteitis in Nigerian children. *Lancet*, i, 80–82.

HENRY, M. D. & CHAPMAN, A. Z. (1954). Vitreous hemorrhage and retinopathy associated with sickle-cell disease. *Amer. J. Opthal.*, 38, 204–209.

HERNÁNDEZ, P., CRUZ, C., SANTOS, M. N. & BALLESTER, J. M. (1980). Immunologic dysfunction in sickle cell anaemia. *Acta haemat. (Basel)*, 63, 156–161.

HERRICK, J. B. (1910a). Peculiar elongated and sickle-shaped red blood corpuscles in a case of severe anemia. *Trans. Ass. Amer. Phycns*, 25, 553–561.

HERRICK, J. B. (1910b). Peculiar elongated and sickle-shaped red blood corpuscles in a case of severe anemia. *Arch. intern. Med.*, 6, 517–521.

HILKOVITZ, G. & JACOBSON, A. (1961). Hepatic dysfunction and abnormalities of the serum proteins and serum enzymes in sickle-cell anemia. *J. Lab. clin. Med.*, 57, 856–867.

HILKOVITZ, G. & MARTIN, W. W. JNR (1961). Sickle cell anemia. Comment on diagnosis and a report on splenectomy in two sisters. *Arch. intern. Med.*, 108, 109–113.

HO PING KONG, H. & ALLEYNE, G. A. O. (1968). Defect in urinary acidification in adults with sickle-cell anaemia. *Lancet*, ii, 954–955.

HO PING KONG, H. & ALLEYNE, G. A. O. (1971). Studies in acid excretion in adults with sickle-cell anaemia. *Clin. Sci.*, 41, 505–518.

HOOK, E. W., CAMPBELL, C. G., WEENS, H. S. & COOPER, G. R. (1957). Salmonella osteomyelitis in patients with sickle-cell anemia. *New Engl. J. Med.*, 257, 403–407.

HORGER, E. O. (1972). Sickle cell and sickle cell-hemoglobin C disease during pregnancy. *Obstet. and Gynec.*, 39, 873–879.

HOWELLS, T. H., HUNTSMAN, R. G., BOYS, J. E. & MAHMOOD, A. (1972). Anaesthesia and sickle-cell haemoglobin. With a case report. *Brit. J. Anaesth.*, 44, 975–987.

HUCK, J. G. (1923). Sickle cell anemia. *Johns Hopk. Hosp. Bull.*, 34, 335–344.

HUEHNS, E. R. & SHOOTER, E. M. (1965). Human haemoglobins. *J. med. Genet.*, 2, 48–90.

HUGHES, J. G. & CARROLL, D. S. (1957). Salmonella osteomyelitis complicating sickle cell disease. *Pediatrics*, 19, 184–191.

HUGHES, J. G., DIGGS, L. W. & GILLESPIE, C. E. (1940). The involvement of the nervous system in sickle-cell anemia. *J. Pediat.*, 17, 166–184.

HUISMAN, T. H. J. (1958). Abnormal haemoglobins. *Clin. chim. Acta*, 3, 201–225.

HUISMAN, T. H. J. (1963). Normal and abnormal human hemoglobins. *Adv. clin. Chem.*, 6, 231–361.

HUTCHINSON, R. M., MERRICK, M. V. & WHITE, J. M. (1973). Fat embolism in sickle cell disease. *J. clin. Path.*, **26**, 620–622.

INGRAM, V. M. (1956). A specific chemical difference between the globins of normal human and sickle-cell anaemia haemoglobin. *Nature (Lond.)*, **178**, 792–794.

INGRAM, V. M. (1957). Gene mutations in human haemoglobin: the chemical difference between normal and sickle cell haemoglobin. *Nature (Lond.)*, **180**, 326–328.

INGRAM, V. M. (1959). Chemistry of the abnormal human haemoglobins. *Brit. med. Bull.*, **15**, 27–32.

INTERNATIONAL HEMOGLOBIN INFORMATION CENTER (1986). Alphabetical hemoglobin variant list. *Hemoglobin*, **10**, 329–351.

INTERNATIONAL SOCIETY OF HAEMATOLOGY (1965). Recommendations on the nomenclature of abnormal haemoglobins. *Brit. J. Haemat.*, **11**, 121–122.

ISRAEL, R. H. & SALIPANTE, J. S. (1979). Pulmonary infarction in sickle cell trait. *Amer. J. Med.*, **66**, 867–869.

ITANO, H. A. (1951). A third abnormal hemoglobin associated with hereditary hemolytic anemia. *Proc. natn. Acad. Sci. U.S.A.*, **37**, 775–784.

ITANO, H. A. (1955). Clinical states associated with alterations of the hemoglobin molecule. *Arch. intern. Med.*, **96**, 287–295.

ITANO, H. A. (1956). The hemoglobins. *Ann. Rev. Biochem.*, **25**, 331–348.

ITANO, H. A. (1957). The human hemoglobins: their properties and genetic control. *Advanc. protein Chem.*, **12**, 215–268.

ITANO, H. A., BERGREN, W. R. & STURGEON, P. (1954). Identification of a fourth abnormal human hemoglobin. *J. Amer. chem. Soc.*, **76**, 2278.

ITANO, H. A., BERGREN, W. R. & STURGEON, P. (1956). The abnormal human hemoglobins. *Medicine (Baltimore)*, **35**, 121–159.

ITANO, H. A. & NEEL, J. V. (1950). A new inherited abnormality of human hemoglobin. *Proc. natn. Acad. Sci. U.S.A.*, **36**, 613–617.

IVY, R. E. & HOWARD, F. H. (1953). Sickle-cell anemia with unusual bone changes. *J. Pediat.*, **43**, 312–315.

JACKSON, J. F., ODOM, J. L. & BELL, W. N. (1961). Amelioration of sickle cell disease by persistent fetal hemoglobin. *J. Amer. med. Ass.*, **177**, 867–869.

JELLIFFE, D. B., STUART, K. L. & WILLS, V. G. (1954). The sickle cell trait in Jamaica. *Blood*, **9**, 144–152.

JENKINS, M. E., SCOTT, R. B. & BAIRD, R. L. (1960). Studies in sickle cell anemia. XVI. Sudden death during sickle cell anemia crises in young children. *J. Pediat.*, **56**, 30–38.

JIMENEZ, C. T., SCOTT, R. B., HENRY, W. L., SAMPSON, C. C. & FERGUSON, A. D. (1966). Studies in sickle cell anemia. XXVI. The effects of homozygous sickle cell disease on the onset of menarche, pregnancy, fertility, pubescent changes, and body growth in Negro subjects. *Amer. J. Dis. Child.*, **111**, 497–504.

JOHN, A. B., RAMLAL, A., JACKSON, H., MAUDE, G. H., WAIGHT SHARMA, A. & SERJEANT, G. R. (1984). Prevention of pneumococcal infection in children with homozygous sickle cell disease. *Brit. med. J.*, **288**, 1567–1570.

JOHN, E. G., SCHADE, S. G., SPIGOS, D. G., CORT, J. H. & ROSENTHAL, I. M. (1980). Effectiveness of triglycyl vasopressin in persistent hematuria associated with sickle cell hemoglobin. *Arch. intern. Med.*, **140**, 1589–1593.

JOHNSTON, R. B., JNR, NEWMAN, S. L. & STRUTH, S. G. (1973). An abnormality of the alternate pathway of complement activation in sickle-cell disease. *New Engl. J. Med.*, **288**, 803–808.

JONES, S. R., BINDER, R. A. & DONOWHO, E. M. JNR (1970). Sudden death in sickle-cell trait. *New Engl. J. Med.*, **282**, 323–325.

JORDAN, R. A. (1957). Cholelithiasis in sickle cell disease. *Gastroenterology*, **33**, 952–958.

KABINS, S. A. & LERNER, C. (1970). Fulminant pneumococcemia and sickle cell anemia. *J. Amer. med. Ass.*, **211**, 467–471.

KAN, Y. W. & DOZY, A. M. (1978). Polymorphism of DNA sequence adjacent to human β-globin structural gene: relationship to sickle mutation. *Proc. natn. Acad. Sci. U.S.A.*, **75**, 5631–5635.

KAN, Y. W. & DOZY, A. M. (1980). Evolution of the S and C genes in world populations. *Science*, **209**, 388–391.

KAPLAN, J., FROST, H., SARNAIK, S. & SCHIFFMAN, G. (1982). Type-specific antibodies in children with sickle cell anemia given polyvalent pneumococcal vaccine. *J. Pediat.*, **100**, 404–406.

KAR, B. C., SATAPATHY, R. K., KULOZIK, A. E., KULOZIK, M., SIRR, S., SERJEANT, B. E. & SERJEANT, G. R. (1986). Sickle cell disease in Orissa State, India. *Lancet*, **ii**, 1198–1201.

KARAYALCIN, G., IMRAN, M. & ROSNER, F. (1972). Priapism in sickle cell disease: report of five cases. *Amer. J. med. Sci.*, **264**, 289–293.

KARAYALCIN, G., ROSNER, F., KIM, K. Y., CHANDRA, P. & ABALLI, A. J. (1975). Sickle cell anemia — clinical manifestations in 100 patients and review of the literature. *Amer. J. med. Sci.*, **269**, 51–68.

KEELEY, K. & BUCHANAN, G. R. (1982). Acute infarction of long bones in children with sickle cell anemia. *J. Pediat.*, **101**, 170–175.

KEITEL, H. G., THOMPSON, D. & ITANO, H. A. (1956). Hyposthenuria in sickle cell anemia: a reversible renal defect. *J. clin. Invest.*, **35**, 998–1007.

KENDREW, J. C., WATSON, H. C., STRANDBERG, B. E., DICKERSON, R. E., PHILLIPS, D. C. & SHORE, V. C. (1961). The amino-acid sequence of sperm whale myoglobin. A partial determination by X-ray methods, and its correlation with chemical data. *Nature (Lond.)*, **190**, 666–670.

KENNEDY, A. P., WALSH, D. A., NICHOLSON, R., ADAMS, J. G. III & STEINBERG, M. H. (1986). Influence of HbS levels upon the hematological and clinical characteristics of sickle cell trait. *Amer. J. Hemat.*, **22**, 51–54.

KHADEMI, M. & MARQUIS, J. R. (1973). Renal angiography in sickle-cell disease. A preliminary report correlating the angiographic and urographic changes in sickle-cell nephropathy. *Radiology*, **107**, 41–46.

KLINEFELTER, H.F: (1942). The heart in sickle cell anemia. *Amer. J. med. Sci.*, **203**, 34–51.

KLION, F. M., WEINER, M. J. & SCHAFFNER, F. (1964). Cholestasis in sickle cell anemia. *Amer. J. Med.*, **37**, 829–832.

KNISELY, M. H., BLOCK, E. H., ELIOT, T. S. & WARNER, L. (1947). Sludged blood. *Science*, **106**, 431–440.

KNOCHEL, J. P. (1969). Hematuria in sickle cell trait. The effect of intravenous administration of distilled water, urinary alkalinization, and diuresis. *Arch. intern. Med.*, **123**, 160–165.

KOBAK, A. J., STEIN, P. J. & DARO, A. F. (1941). Sickle-cell anemia in pregnancy. A review of the literature and report of six cases. *Amer. J. Obstet. Gynec.*, **41**, 811–823.

KOETHE, S. M., CASPER, J. T. & RODEY, G. E. (1976). Alternative complement pathway activity in sera from patients with sickle cell disease. *Clin. exp. Immunol.*, **23**, 56–60.

KONOTEY- AHULU, F. I. D. (1965a). Sicklaemic human hygrometers. *Lancet*, i, 1003–1004.

KONOTEY-AHULU, F. I. D. (1965b). Torrential epistaxis with symmetrical facial-skin ulceration in sickle-cell anaemia. *Brit. med. J.*, ii, 859–860.

KONOTEY-AHULU, F. I. D. (1968). Hereditary qualitative and quantitative erythrocyte defects in Ghana: an historical and geographical survey. *Ghana med. J.*, **7**, 118–119.

KONOTEY-AHULU, F. I. D. (1971). Computer assisted analysis of data on 1,697 patients attending the sickle cell/haemoglobinopathy clinic of Korle Bu Teaching Hospital, Accra, Ghana. Clinical features: I. Sex, genotype, age, rheumatism and dactylitis frequencies. *Ghana med. J.*, **10**, 241–260.

KONOTEY-AHULU, F. I. D. (1972a). Balanced polymorphism and hereditary qualitative and quantitative erythrocyte defects. *Ghana med. J.*, **11**, 274–285.

KONOTEY-AHULU, F. I. D. (1972b). Sickle-cell trait and altitude. *Brit. med. J.*, i, 177–178 (Letter).

KONOTEY-AHULU, F. I. D. (1972c). Mental-nerve neuropathy: a complication of sickle-cell crisis. *Lancet*, ii, 388 (Letter).

KONOTEY-AHULU, F. I. D. (1972d). Glucose-6-phosphate dehydrogenase deficiency and sickle-cell anemia. *New Engl. J. Med.*, **287**, 887–888 (Letter).

KONOTEY-AHULU, F. I. D. (1972e). The pathogenesis of sickle-cell crisis in Ghana. *Ghana med. J.*, **11**, 304–305.

KONOTEY-AHULU, F. I. D. (1974). The sickle cell diseases. Clinical manifestations including the "sickle crisis". *Arch. intern. Med.*, **133**, 611–619.

KRAMER, M. S., ROOKS, Y., WASHINGTON, L. A. & PEARSON, H. A. (1980). Pre- and postnatal growth and development in sickle cell anemia. *J. Pediat.*, **96**, 857–860.

KUNZ, H. W., MELLIN, G. W., CHEUNG, M. W. & PRATT, E. L. (1953). Impairment of urinary concentration in sickle-cell anemia. *Amer. J. Dis. Child.*, **86**, 512 (Abstract).

KUNZ, H. W., PRATT, E. L., MELLIN, G. W. & CHEUNG, M. W. (1954). Impairment of urinary concentration in sickle cell anemia. *Pediatrics*, **13**, 352–356.

KUTLAR, A., HATTORI, Y., BAKIOGLU, I., KUTLER, F., KAMEL, K. & HUISMAN, T. H. J. (1985). Hematological observations on Arabian SS patients with a homozygosity or heterozygosity for a β^S chromosome with haplotype 31. *Hemoglobin*, **9**, 545–557.

LACHMAN, B. S., LAZERSON, J., STARSHAK, R. J., VAUGHTERS, F. M. & WERLIN, S. L. (1979). The prevalence of cholelithiasis in sickle cell disease as diagnosed by ultrasound and cholecystography. *Pediatrics*, **64**, 601–603.

LAMBOTTE, C. (1962). Hand-foot syndrome in sickle-cell disease. *Amer. J. Dis. Child.*, **104**, 200–201 (Letter).

LAMBOTTE-LEGRAND, J. and C. (1951). L'anémie à hématies falciformes chez l'infant indigène du Bas-Congo. *Ann. Soc. belge Méd. trop.*, **31**, 207–234.

LAMBOTTE-LEGRAND, J. and C. (1952). L'anémie à hématies falciformes en Afrique Noire. *Sang*, **23**, 560–568.

LAMBOTTE-LEGRAND, J. and C. (1955a). Anémie drépanocytaire et homozygotisme (à propos de 300 cas). *Ann. Soc. belge Méd. trop.*, **35**, 47–51.

LAMBOTTE-LEGRAND, J. and C. (1955b). Le pronostic de l'anémie drépanocytaire au Congo Belge (à propos de 300 cas et de 150 décès). *Ann. Soc. belge Méd. trop.*, **35**, 53–57.

LAMBOTTE-LEGRAND, J. and C. (1958). Notes complémentaires sur la drépanocytose. I. Sicklémie et malaria. *Ann. Soc. belge Méd. trop.*, **38**, 45–53.

LEHMANN, H. (1953). The sickle-cell trait: not an essentially negro feature. *Man*, **53**, 9–10.

LEHMANN, H. (1954). Distribution of the sickle cell gene. A new light on the origin of the East Africans. *Eugen. Rev.*, **46**, 101–123.

LEHMANN, H. (1956). Human haemoglobins. *St. Bart's Hosp. J.*, **60**, 237–242.

LEHMANN, H. (1956–57). Variations of haemoglobin synthesis in man. *Acta genet. (Basel)*, **6**, 413–429.

LEHMANN, H. (1959a). Variations in human haemoglobin synthesis and factors governing their inheritance. *Brit. med. Bull.*, **15**, 40–46.

LEHMANN, H. (1959b). Distribution of variations in human haemoglobin synthesis. In: *Abnormal Haemoglobins. A Symposium* (ed. by J. H. P. Jonxis and J. F. Delafresnaye), pp. 202–215. Blackwell Scientific Publications, Oxford.

LEHMANN, H. (1959c). The maintenance of the haemoglobinopathies at high frequency. A consideration of the relation between sickling and malaria and of allied problems. In: *Abnormal Haemoglobins. A Symposium* (ed. by J. H. P. Jonxis and J. F. Delafresnaye), pp. 307–321. Blackwell Scientific Publications, Oxford.

LEHMANN, H. (Chairman) (1966). Haemoglobinopathies and allied disorders. Report of a WHO Scientific Group. *Wld Hlth Org. tech. Rep. Ser.*, No. 338. 40 pp. WHO, Geneva.

LEHMANN, H. (1984). Sickle cell anemia 35 years ago: reminiscence of early African studies. *Amer. J. ped. Hemat./Oncol.*, **6**, 72–76.

LEHMANN, H. & CARRELL, R. W. (1969). Variations in the structure of human haemoglobin: with particular reference to the unstable haemoglobins. *Brit. med. Bull.*, **25**, 14–23.

LEHMANN, H. & CASEY, R. (1982). Human haemoglobin. In: *Comprehensive Biochemistry*, Vol. 19B, Part II, pp. 347–417. Elsevier Scientific Publishing, Amsterdam.

LEHMANN, H. & CUTBUSH, M. (1952). Sickle-cell trait in Southern India. *Brit. med. J.*, **i**, 404–405.

LEHMANN, H. & HUNTSMAN, R. G. (1974). *Man's Haemoglobins, including the Haemoglobinopathies and their Investigation.* 478 pp. North-Holland Publishing Co., Amsterdam, Oxford.

LEHMANN, H. & KYNOCH, P. A. M. (1976). *Human Hemoglobin Variants and their Characteristics.* 241 pp. North-Holland Publishing Co., Amsterdam, New York, Oxford.

LEHMANN, H., MARANJIAN, G. & MOURANT, A. E. (1963). Distribution of sickle-cell haemoglobin in Saudi Arabia. *Nature (Lond.)*, **198**, 492–493.

LEHMANN, H. & RAPER, A. B. (1956). Maintenance of high sickling rate in an African community. *Brit. med. J.*, **ii**, 333–336.

LEIGHT, L., SNIDER, T. H., CLIFFORD, G. O. & HELLEMS, H. K. (1954). Hemodynamic studies in sickle cell anemia. *Circulation*, **10**, 653–662.

LEIKIN, S. L. & McCOO, J. W. JNR (1958). Sickle-cell anemia in infancy. *J. Dis. Child.*, **96**, 51–57.

LEVIN, W. C. (1958). "Asymptomatic" sickle cell trait. *Blood*, **13**, 901–907 (Editorial).

LEVIN, W. C., BAIRD, W. D., PERRY, J. E. & ZUNG, W. W. K. (1957). The experimental production of splenic sequestration of erythrocytes in patients with sickle cell trait. *J. Lab. clin. Med.*, **50**, 926 (Abstract).

LEVITT, M. F., HAUSER, A. D., LEVY, M. S. & POLEMEROS, D. (1960). The renal concentrating defect in sickle cell disease. *Amer. J. Med.*, **29**, 611–622.

LEWIS, R. A. (1967). Sickle-cell anaemia in G.-6-P.D. deficiency. *Lancet*, **i**, 852–853 (Letter).

LEWIS, R. A. & HATHORN, M. (1965). Correlation of S hemoglobin with glucose-6-phosphate dehydrogenase deficiency and its significance. *Blood*, **26**, 176–180.

LEWIS, R. A., KAY, R. W. & HATHORN M. (1966). Sickle cell disease and glucose-6-phosphate dehydrogenase. *Acta haemat. (Basel)*, **36**, 399–411.

LIACHOWITZ, C., ELDERKIN, J., GUICHIRIT, I., BROWN, H. W. & RANNEY, H. M. (1958). Abnormal hemoglobins in negroes of Surinam. *Amer. J. Med.*, **24**, 19–24.

LIE-INJO, L. E. (1957). Sickle cell gene in Indonesia. *Nature (Lond.)*, **179**, 381.

LIEB, W. A., GEERAETS, W. J. & GUERRY, D. III (1959). Sickle-cell retinopathy. Ocular and systemic manifestations of sickle-cell disease. *Acta ophthal.*, Suppl. 58, 44 pp.

LINDO, C. L. & DOCTOR, L. R. (1955). The electrocardiogram in sickle-cell anemia. *Amer. Heart J.*, **50**, 218–224.

LINDSAY J. JNR, MESHEL, J. C. & PATTERSON, R. H. (1974). The cardiovascular manifestations of sickle cell disease. *Arch. intern. Med.*, **133**, 643–651.

LIPPMAN, S. M., ABERGEL, R. P., GINZTON, L. E., UITTO, J., TANAKA, K. R., MIYAMOTO, E. K. & LAKS, M. M. (1985a). Mitral value prolapse in sickle cell disease: manifestation of a generalized connective tissue disorder. *Amer. J. Hemat.*, **19**, 1–12.

LIPPMAN, S. M., GINZTON, L. E., THIGPEN, T., TANAKA, K. R. & LAKS, M M. (1985b). Mitral valve prolapse in sickle cell disease. Presumptive evidence for a linked connective tissue disorder. *Arch. intern. Med.*, **145**, 435–438.

LOBEL, J. S. & BOVE, K. E. (1982). Clinicopathologic characteristics of septicemia in sickle cell disease. *Amer. J. Dis. Child.*, **136**, 543–547.

LUCAS, W. M. & BULLOCK, W. H. (1960). Hematuria in sickie cell disease. *J. Urol.*, **83**, 733–741.

LUND, H. G., CORDONNIER, J. J. & FORBES, K. A. (1954). Gross hematuria in sickle cell disease. *J. Urol.*, **71**, 151–158.

LUZZATTO. L. (1981). Sickle cell anaemia in tropical Africa. *Clinics Haemat.*, **10**, 757–784.

LUZZATTO, L., NWACHUKU-JARRETT, E. S. & REDDY, S. (1970). Increased sickling of parasitised erythrocytes as mechanism of resistance against malaria in the sickle-cell trait. *Lancet*, **i**, 319–321.

McCALL, I. W., DESAI, P., SERJEANT, B. E. & SERJEANT, G. R. (1977). Cholelithiasis in Jamaican patients with homozygous sickle cell disease. *Amer. J. Hemat.*, **3**, 15–21.

McCRORY, W. W., GOREN, N. & GORNFELD, D. (1953). Demonstration of impairment of urinary concentration ability on "Pitressin-resistance" in children with sickle-cell anemia. *Amer. J. Dis. Child.*, **86**, 512–513 (Abstract).

McDONALD, C. R. & EICHNER, E. R. (1978). Concurrent primary pneumococcemia, disseminated intravascular coagulation, and sickle cell anemia. *Sth. med. J.* (*Bgham, Ala.*), **71**, 858–860.

McINTOSH, S., ROOKS, Y., RITCHEY, A. K. & PEARSON, H. A. (1980). Fever in young children with sickle cell disease. *J. Pediat.*, **96**, 199–204.

MACKEY, J. P. & VIVARELLI, F. (1954). Sickle-cell anaemia. *Brit. med. J.*, **i**, 276 (Letter).

McSWEENEY, J. E. J., MERMANN, A. C. & WAGLEY, P. F. (1947). Cold hemagglutinins in sickle cell anemia. *Amer. J. med. Sci.*, **214**, 542–544.

MACHT, S. H. & ROMAN, P. W. (1948). The radiological changes in sickle-cell anemia. *Radiology*, **51**, 697–707.

MAKLER, M. T., BERTHRONG, M., LOCKE, H. R. & DAWSON, D. L. (1974). A new variant of sickle-cell disease with high levels of foetal haemoglobin homogeneously distributed within red cells. *Brit. J. Haemat.*, **26**, 519–526.

MANIATIS, A., BERTLES, J. F. & WETHERS, D. L. (1977). Cold agglutinins and sickle-cell disease. *Lancet*, **i**, 50 (Letter).

MANN, J. R., COTTER, K. P., WALKER R. A., BIRD. G. W. G. & STUART, J. (1975). Anaemic crisis in sickle cell disease. *J. clin. Path.*, **28**, 341–344.

MARGOLIES, M. P. (1951). Sickle cell anemia. A composite study and survey. *Medicine (Baltimore)*, **30**, 357–443.

MARGOLIS, K., COHEN, I. M., RUDMAN, M. S. & DAWSON, R. B. (1973). Long survival in sickle-cell disease. *Lancet*, **i**, 1510–1511 (Letter).

MARKENSON, A. L., CHANDRA, M., LEWY, J. E. & MILLER, D. R. (1978). Sickle cell anemia, the nephrotic syndrome and hypoplastic crisis in a sibship. *Amer. J. Med.*, **64**, 719–723.

MARSDEN, P. D. & SHAH, K. K. (1964). Artificially induced oedema in sickle cell anaemia. *J. trop. Med. Hyg.*, **67**, 31–34.

MARTIN, C. R., COBB, C., TATTER, D., JOHNSON, C. & HAYWOOD, L. J. (1983). Acute myocardial infarction in sickle cell anemia. *Arch. intern. Med.*, **143**, 830–831.

MASON, V. R. (1922). Sickle cell anemia. *J. Amer. med. Ass.*, **79**, 1318–1320.

MATTHEW, C., RUBENSTEIN, R. & JACOBS, P. (1984). Mild clinical course in two South African cases of sickle-cell anaemia. *Acta haemat. (Basel)*, **71**, 247–250.

MAURER, H. S., VIDA, L. N. & HONIG, G. R. (1972). Homozygous sickle cell disease with coexistent hereditary spherocytosis in three siblings. *J. Pediat.*, **80**, 235–242.

MEARS, J. G., BELDJORD, C., BENABADJI, M., BELGHITI, Y. A., BADDOU, M.-A., LABIE, D. & NAGEL, R. L. (1981a). The sickle gene polymorphism in North Africa. *Blood*, **58**, 599–601.

MEARS, J. G., LACHMAN, H. M., CABANNES, R., AMEGNIZAN, K. P. E., LABIE, D. & NAGEL, R. L.

(1981b). Sickle gene: its origin and diffusion from West Africa. *J. clin. Invest.*, **68**, 606–610.

MEARS, J. G., LACHMAN, H. M., LABIE, D. & NAGEL, R. L. (1983). Alpha-thalassemia is related to prolonged survival in sickle cell anemia. *Blood*, **62**, 286–290.

MIDDLEMISS, J. H. (1958). Sickle-cell anemia. *J. Fac. Radiol. (Lond.)*, **9**, 16–24.

MILLER, J. M., HORGER, E. O. III, KEY, T. C. & WALKER, E. M. JNR (1981). Management of sickle hemoglobinopathies in pregnant patients. *Amer. J. Obstet. Gynec.*, **141**, 237–241.

MILLER, G. J. & SERJEANT, G. R. (1971). An assessment of lung volumes and gas transfer in sickle-cell anaemia. *Thorax*, **26**, 309–315.

MILLER, G. J., SERJEANT, G. R., SIVAPRAGASAM, S. & PETCH, M. C. (1973). Cardio-pulmonary responses and gas exchange during exercise in adults with homozygous sickle-cell disease (sickle-cell anaemia). *Clin. Sci.*, **44**, 113–128.

MILNER, P. F. (1974). The sickling disorders. *Clinics Haemat.*, **3**, 289–331.

MILNER, P. F., BROWN, M. & YODER, G. A. (1982). Bone marrow infarction in sickle cell anemia: correlation with hematologic profiles. *Blood*, **60**, 1411–1418.

MILNER, P. F., JONES, B. R. & DÖBLER, J. (1980). Outcome of pregnancy in sickle cell anemia and sickle cell-hemoglobin C disease. *Amer. J. Obstet. Gynec.*, **138**, 239–245.

MINTZ, A. A., CHURCH, G. & ADAMS, E. D. (1955). Cholelithiasis in sickle cell anemia. *J. Pediat.*, **47**, 171–177.

MINTZ, A. A. & PUGH, D. P. (1970). Choledocholithiasis in sickle cell anemia. *Sth. med. J. (Bgham, Ala.)*, **63**, 1498 (Abstract).

MONTGOMERY, R. D. (1960). Tetanus as a complication of sickle-cell disease. *Trans. roy. Soc. trop. Med. Hyg.*, **54**, 385–388.

MOO-PENN, W. R., SCHMIDT, R. M., JUE, D. L., BECHTEL, K. C., WRIGHT, J. M., HORNE, M. K. III, HAYCROFT, G. L., ROTH, E. F. JNR & NAGEL, R. L. (1977). Hemoglobin S Travis: a sickling hemoglobin with two amino acid substitutions [β6 (A3) Glutamic acid→Valine and β142 (H20) Alanine→Valine]. *Europ. J. Biochem.*, **77**, 561–566.

MORGAN, A. G., GRUBER, C. & SERJEANT, G. R. (1982). Erythropoietin and renal function and sickle-cell disease. *Brit. med. J.*, **285**, 1686–1688.

MORGAN, A. G. & SERJEANT, G. R. (1981). Renal function in patients over 40 with homozygous sickle-cell disease. *Brit. med. J.*, **282**, 1181–1183.

MORRISON, J. C. & WISER, W. L. (1976a). The effect of maternal partial exchange transfusion on the infants of patients with sickle cell anemia. *J. Pediat.*, **89**, 286–289.

MORRISON, J. C. & WISER, W. L. (1976b). The use of prophylactic partial exchange transfusion in pregnancies associated with sickle cell hemoglobinopathies. *Obstet. and Gynec.*, **48**, 516–520.

MOSER, K. M. & SHEA, J. G. (1957). The relationship between pulmonary infarction, cor pulmonale and the sickle states. *Amer. J. Med.*, **22**, 561–579.

MOSTOFI, F. K., VORDER BRUEGGE, C. F. & DIGGS, L. W. (1957). Lesions in kidneys removed for unilateral hematuria in sickle-cell disease. *Arch. Path.*, **63**, 336–351.

MOTULSKY, A. G. (1973). Frequency of sickling disorders in U.S. blacks. *New Engl. J. Med.*, **288**, 31–33.

MUIRHEAD, E. E., HALDEN, E. R. & WILSON, B. J. (1956). Recurrent crises in sickle cell anemia responding to cholecystectomy: a syndrome apparently based on cholecysto- and choledocho-stasis. *Amer. J. Med.*, **20**, 953–954 (Abstract).

MURAYAMA, M. & NALBANDIAN, R. M. (1973). *Sickle Cell Hemoglobin: Molecule to Man.* 198 pp. Little, Brown & Co., Boston.

MURPHY, J. R. (1973). Sickle cell hemoglobin (Hb AS) in black football players. *J. Amer. med. Ass.*, **225**, 981–982.

MURTAZA, L. N., STROUD, C. E., DAVIS, L. R. & COOPER, D. J. (1981). Admissions to hospital of children with sickle-cell anaemia: a study in south London. *Brit. med. J.*, **282**, 1048–1051.

NAGEL, R. L., FABRY, M. E., PAGNIER, J., WAJCMAN, H., BAUDIN, V. & LABIE, D. (1984). Two hematologically and genetically distinct forms of sickle cell anemia in Africa: the Senegal and Benin type. *Blood*, **64**, No. 5 (Suppl. 1), 51a (Abstract 116).

NAGEL, R. L., FABRY, M. E., PAGNIER, J., ZOHOUN, I., WAJCMAN, H., BAUDIN, V. & LABIE, D. (1985). Hematologically and genetically distinct forms of sickle cell anemia in Africa. The Senegal type and the Benin type. *New Engl. J. Med.*, **312**, 880–884.

NAGPAL, K. C., ASDOURIAN, G. K., GOLDBAUM, M. H., RAICHAND, M. & GOLDBERG, M. F. (1977). The conjunctival sickling sign, hemoglobin S, and irreversibly sickled erythrocytes. *Arch. Ophthal. (Chicago)*, **95**, 808–811.

NAGPAL, K. C., ASDOURIAN, G. K., PATRIANAKOS, D., GOLDBERG, M. F., RABB, M. F., GOLDBAUM, M. & RAICHAND, M. (1977). Proliferative retinopathy in sickle cell trait. *Arch. intern. Med.*, **137**, 325–328.

NATTA, C. L. & OUTSCHOORN, I. M. (1984). IgG2 deficiency in sickle cell anaemia. *Scand. J. Haemat.*, **33**, 129–134.

NAYLOR, J., ROSENTHAL, I., GROSSMAN, A., SCHULMAN, I. & HSIA, D. Y.-Y. (1960). Activity of glucose-6-phosphate dehydrogenase in erythrocytes of patients with various abnormal hemoglobins. *Pediatrics*, **36**, 285–292.

NEEL, J. V. (1947). The clinical detection of the genetic carriers of inherited disease. *Medicine (Baltimore)*, **26**, 115–153.

NEEL, J. V. (1949). The inheritance of sickle cell anemia. *Science*, **110**, 64–66.

NEEL, J. V. (1951). The inheritance of the sickling phenomenon with particular reference to sickle cell disease. *Blood*, **6**, 389–412.

NEEL, J. V. (1953). Data pertaining to the population dynamics of sickle cell disease. *Amer. J. hum. Genet.*, **5**, 154–167.

NEEL, J. V. (1957). Human hemoglobin types. Their epidemiologic implications. *New Engl. J. Med.*, **256**, 161–171.

NEEL. J. V. (1958). Genetic control of hemoglobin synthesis. *Proc. sixth Congress int. Soc. Hematol. Boston*, p. 665. Grune and Stratton, New York.

NG, M. L., LIEBMAN, J., ANSLOVAR, J. & GROSS, S. (1967). Cardiovascular findings in children with sickle cell anemia. *Dis. Chest*, **52**, 788–799.

NOLL, J. B., NEWMAN, A. J. & GROSS, S. (1967). Enuresis and nocturia in sickle cell disease. *J. Pediat.*, **70**, 965–967.

OBER, W. B., BRUNO, M. S., WEINBERG, S. B., JONES, F. M. JNR & WEINER, L. (1960). Fatal intravascular sickling in a patient with sickle-cell trait. *New Engl. J. Med.*, **263**, 947–949.

O'BRIEN, R. T., MCINTOSH, S., ASPNES, G. T. & PEARSON, H. A. (1976). Prospective study of sickle cell anemia in infancy. *J. Pediat..* **89**, 205–210.

O'BRIEN, R. T., PEARSON, H. A., GODLEY, J. A. & SPENCER, R. P. (1972). Splenic infarct and sickle-(cell) trait. *New Engl. J. Med.*, **287**, 720 (Letter).

ODUNTAN, S. A. (1969). Blood gas studies in some abnormal haemoglobin syndromes. *Brit. J. Haemat.*, **17**, 535–541.

ONWUBALILI, J. K. (1983). Sickle-cell anaemia: an explanation for the ancient myth of reincarnation in Nigeria. *Lancet*, ii, 503–505.

OSEGBE, D. N., AKINYANJU, O. & AMAKU, E. O. (1981). Fertility in males with sickle cell disease. *Lancet*, ii, 275–276.

OVERTURF, G. D., FIELD, R. & EDMONDS, R. (1979). Death from type 6 pneumococcal septicemia in a vaccinated child with sickle cell disease. *New Engl. J. Med.*, **300**, 143.

OVERTURF, G. D., POWARS, D. & BARAFF, L. F. (1977). Bacterial meningitis and septicemia in sickle-cell disease. *Amer. J. Dis. Child.*, **131**, 784–787.

OWEN, D. M., ALDRIDGE, J. E. & THOMPSON, R. B. (1965). An unusual hepatic sequela of sickle cell anemia: a report of five cases. *Amer. J. med. Sci.*, **249**, 175–185.

OZSOLU, S. & ALTINÖZ, N. (1977). Sickle-cell anaemia in Turkey. Evaluation of 97 cases (with parents' findings). *Scand. J. Haemat.*, **19**, 85–92.

PAGNIER, J., BAUDIN, V., LABIE, D., WAJCMAN, H., JAEGER, G & GIROT, R. (1986). Sickle cell anemia in Bantu speaking Africa. *Hemoglobin*, **10**, 73–76.

PAGNIER, J., MEARS, J. G., DUNDA-BELKHODJA, O., SCHAFFER-REGO, K. E., BELDJORD, C., NAGEL, R. L. & LABIE, D. (1984). Evidence for the multicentric origin of the sickle cell hemoglobin gene in Africa. *Proc. natn. Acad. Sci., U.S.A.*, **81**, 1771–1773.

PAGNIER, J., MEARS, J. G., NAGEL, R. L. & LABIE, D. (1983). The multicentric origin of the hemoglobin S gene in Africa. *Blood*, **62**, No. 5 (Suppl. 1), 59a (Abstract 138).

PARDO, V., STRAUSS, J., KRAMER, H., OZAWA, T. & McINTOSH, R. M. (1975). Nephropathy associated with sickle cell anemia: an autologous immune complex nephritis. II. Clinicopathologic study of seven patients. *Amer. J. Med.*, **59**, 650–659.

PATERSON, J. C. S. & SPRAGUE, C. C. (1959). Observations on the genesis of crises in sickle cell anemia. *Ann. intern. Med.*, **50**, 1502–1507.

PATON, D. (1961). The conjunctival sign of sickle-cell disease. *Arch. Ophthal. (Chicago)*, **66**, 90–94.

PAULING, L. (1953–54). Abnormality of hemoglobin molecules in hereditary hemolytic anemias. *Harvey Lectures*, **49**, 216–241.

PAULING, L., ITANO, H. A., SINGER, S. J. & WELLS, I. C. (1949). Sickle cell anemia, a molecular disease. *Science*, **110**, 543–548.

PAULING, L., ITANO, H. A., WELLS, I. C., SCHROEDER, W. A., KAY, L. M., SINGER, S. J. & COREY, R. B. (1950). Sickle cell anemia hemoglobin. *Science*, **111**, 459 (Abstract).

PEARSON, H. A., CORNELIUS, E. A., SCHWARTZ, A. D., ZELSON, J. H., WOLFSON, S. L. & SPENCER, R. P. (1970). Transfusion-reversible functional asplenia in young children with sickle-cell anemia. *New Engl. J. Med.*, **283**, 334–337.

PEARSON, H. A., SCHIEBLER, G. L., KROVETZ, L. J., BARTLEY, T. D. & DAVID, J. K. (1965). Sickle-cell anemia associated with tetralogy of Fallot. *New Engl. J. Med.*, **273**, 1079–1083.

PEARSON, H. A., SPENCER, R. P. & CORNELIUS, E. A. (1969). Functional asplenia in sickle-cell anemia. *New Engl. J. Med.*, **281**, 923–926.

PERRINE, R. P. (1973). Cholelithiasis in sickle cell anemia in a Caucasian population. *Amer. J. Med.*, **54**, 327–332.

PERRINE, R. P., BROWN, M. J., CLEGG, J. B., WEATHERALL, D. J. & MAY, A. (1972). Benign sickle-cell anaemia. *Lancet*, **ii**, 1163–1167.

PERRINE, R. P., PEMBREY, M. E., JOHN, P., PERRINE, S. & SHOUP, F. (1978). Natural history of sickle cell anemia in Saudi Arabs. A study of 270 subjects. *Ann. intern. Med.*, **88**, 1–6.

PETCH, M. C. & SERJEANT, G. R. (1970). Clinical features of pulmonary lesions in sickle-cell anaemia. *Brit. med. J.*, **iii**, 31.

PIOMELLI, S., REINDORF, C. A., ARZANIAN, M. T. & CORASH, L. M. (1972). Clinical and biochemical interactions of glucose-6-phosphate dehydrogenase deficiency and sickle-cell anemia. *New Engl. J. Med.*, **287**, 213–217.

PLACHTA, A. & SPEER, F. D. (1952). Sickle cell disease, benign and malignant (review, analysis and evaluation of the literature). *Bull. N.Y. med. Coll.*, **15**, 1–16.

PLATT, O. & NATHAN, D. G. (1981). Sickle cell disease. In: *Hematology of Infancy and Childhood* (ed. by D. G. Nathan and F. A. Oski), 2nd edn, pp. 687–725. W. B. Saunders, Philadelphia.

PLATT, O. S., ROSENSTOCK, W. & ESPELAND, M. A. (1984). Influence of sickle hemoglobinopathies on growth and development. *New Engl. J. Med.*, **311**, 7–12.

PONCZ, M., KANE, E. & GILL, F. M. (1985). Acute chest syndrome in sickle cell disease: etiology and clinical correlates. *J. Pediat.*, **107**, 861–866.

PORTER, F. S. & THURMAN, W. G. (1963). Studies of sickle cell disease. Diagnosis in infancy. *Amer. J. Dis. Child.*, **106**, 35–42.

PORTIER, A., CABANNES, R. & DUZER, A. (1959). The frequency of distribution of abnormal haemoglobin conditions in Algeria. In: *Abnormal Haemoglobins. A Symposium* (ed. by J. H. P. Jonxis and J. F. Delafresnaye) pp. 279–289. Blackwell Scientific Publications, Oxford.

PORTNOY, B. A. & HERION, J. C. (1972). Neurological manifestation in sickle-cell disease, with a review of the literature and emphasis on the prevalence of hemiplegia. *Ann. intern. Med.*, **76**, 643–652.

POWARS, D. R. (1975). Natural history of sickle cell disease — the first ten years. *Seminars Hemat.*, **12**, 267–285.

POWARS, D., OVERTURF, G., WEISS, J., LEE, S. & CHAN, L. (1981). Pneumococcal septicemia in children with sickle cell anemia. Changing trend of survival. *J. Amer. med. Ass.*, **245**, 1839–1842.

POWARS, D. R., SCHROEDER, W. A., WEISS, J. N., CHAN, L. S. & AZEN, S. P. (1980). Lack of influence of fetal hemoglobin levels or erythrocyte indices on the severity of sickle cell anemia. *J. clin. Invest*, **65**, 732–740.

POWARS, D. R., WEISS, J. N., CHAN, L. S. & SCHROEDER, W. A. (1984). Is there a threshold level of fetal hemoglobin that ameliorates morbidity in sickle cell anemia? *Blood*, **63**, 921–926.

POWARS, D., WILSON, B., IMBUS, C., PEGELOW, C. & ALLEN, J. (1978). The natural history of stroke in sickle cell disease. *Amer. J. Med.*, **65**, 461–471.

PRITCHARD, J. A., SCOTT, D. E., WHALLEY, P. J., CUNNINGHAM, F. G. & MASON, R. A. (1973). The effects of maternal sickle cell hemoglobinopathies in sickle cell trait on reproductive performance. *Amer. J. Obstet. Gynec.*, **117**, 662–670.

PROTASS, L. M. (1973). Possible precipitation of cerebral thrombosis in sickle-cell anemia by hyperventilation. *Ann. intern. Med.*, **79**, 451 (Letter).

PROWLER, J. R. & SMITH, E. W. (1955). Dental bone changes occurring in sickle-cell diseases and abnormal haemoglobin traits. *Radiology*, **65**, 762–769.

RAPER, A. B. (1949). The incidence of sicklaemia. *East Afr. med. J.*, **26**, 281–282(Letter).

RAPER, A. B. (1950). Sickle-cell disease in Africa and America — a comparison. *J. trop. Med. Hyg.*, **53**, 49–53.

RAPER, A. B. (1955). Malaria and the sickling trait. *Brit. med. J.*, **i**, 1186–1189.

RAPER, A. B. (1956). Sickling in relation to morbidity from malaria and other diseases. *Brit. med. J.*, **i**, 965–966.

RATCLIFF, R. G. & WOLF, M. D. (1962). Avascular necrosis of the femoral head associated with sickle cell trait (AS hemoglobin). *Ann. intern. Med.*, **57**, 299–304.

REDWOOD, A. M., WILLIAMS, E. M., DESAI, P. & SERJEANT, G. R. (1976). Climate and painful crisis of sickle-cell disease in Jamaica. *Brit. med. J.*, **i**, 66–68.

REEVES, J. D., LUBIN, B. H. & EMBURY, S. H. (1984). Renal complications of sickle cell trait are related to the percent of Hb S. *Blood*, **64**, No. 5 (Suppl. 1), 52a (Abstract 118).

RHINESMITH, H. S., SCHROEDER, W. A. & PAULING, L. (1957). A quantitative study of the hydrolysis of human dinitrophenyl (DNP) globin. The number and kind of polypeptide chains in normal adult hemoglobin. *J. Amer. chem. Soc.*, **79**, 4682–4686.

RINGELHANN, B. & KONOTEY-AHULU, F. I. D. (1971). The removal of heat-damaged and ^{51}Cr-labelled red cells in haemoglobinopathies. *Brit. J. Haemat.*, **21**, 99–112.

ROBERTS, A. R. & HILBURG, L. E. (1958). Sickle cell disease with salmonella osteomyelitis. *J. Pediat.*, **52**, 170–175.

ROBINSON, M. G. & HALPERN, C. (1974). Infections, *Escherichia coli* and sickle cell anemia. *J. Amer. med. Ass.*, **230**, 1145–1148.

ROBINSON, M. G. & WATSON, R. J. (1966). Pneumococcal meningitis in sickle-cell anemia. *New Engl. J. Med.*, **274**, 1006–1008.

ROGERS, D. W., CLARKE, J. M., CUPIDORE, L., RAMLAL, A. M., SPARKE, B. R. & SERJEANT, G. R. (1978). Early deaths in Jamaican children with sickle cell disease. *Brit. med. J.*, **i**, 1515–1516.

ROGERS, D. W., VAIDYA, S. & SERJEANT, G. R. (1978). Early splenomegaly in homozygous sickle-cell disease: an indicator of susceptibility to infection. *Lancet*, **ii**, 963–965.

ROSSI, E. C., WESTRING, D. W., SANTOS, A. S. & GUTIERREZ, J. (1964). Hypersplenism in sickle cell anemia. *Arch. intern. Med.*, **114**, 408–412.

ROTH, E. F. JNR, FRIEDMAN, M., UEDA, Y., TELLEZ, I., TRAGER, W. & NAGEL, R. L. (1978a). Sickling rates of human AS red cells infected in vitro with *Plasmodium falciparum* malaria. *Science*, **202**, 650–652.

ROTH, E. F. JNR, RACHMILEWITZ, E. H., SCHIFTER, A. & NAGEL, R. L. (1978b). Benign sickle cell anemia in Israeli-Arabs with high red cell 2,3 diphosphoglycerate. *Acta haemat. (Basel)*, **59**, 237–245.

ROTHSCHILD, B. M. & SEBES, J. I. (1981). Calcaneal abnormalities and erosive bone disease associated with sickle cell anemia. *Amer. J. Med.*, **71**, 427–430.

ROTTER, R., LUTTGENS, W. F., PETERSON, W. L., STOCK, A. E. & MOTULSKY, A. G. (1956). Splenic infarction in sicklemia during airplane flight: pathogenesis, hemoglobin analysis and clinical features of six cases. *Ann. intern. Med.*, **44**, 257–270.

ROWE, C. W. & HAGGARD, M. E. (1957). Bone infarcts in sickle-cell anemia. *Radiology*, **68**, 661–668.

RUSSELL, W. M. (1962). Sickle-cell anaemia at age of 7 weeks. *Brit. med. J.*, **ii**, 1517–1518.

SALISBURY, P. F. (1960). Recovery from acute renal failure and acidosis in sickle-cell disease. *J. Amer. med. Ass.*, **174**, 356–358.

SAMUELS, L. D. & STEWART, C. (1970). Estimation of spleen size in sickle cell anemia. *J. nucl. Med.*, **11**, 12–14.

SARNAIK, S., SLOVIS, T. L., CORBETT, D. P., EMAMI, A. & WHITTEN, C. F. (1980). Incidence of cholelithiasis in sickle cell anemia using the ultrasonic gray-scale technique. *J. Pediat.*, **96**, 1005–1008.

SAXENA, U. H., SCOTT, R. B. & FERGUSON, A. D. (1966). Studies in sickle cell anemia. XXV. Observations on fluid intake and output. *J. Pediat.*, **69**, 220–224.

SCHLITT, L. & KEITEL, H. G. (1960a). Pathogenesis of hyposthenuria in persons with sickle cell anemia or the sickle cell trait. *Pediatrics*, **26**, 249–254.

SCHLITT, L. E. & KEITEL, H. G. (1960b). Renal manifestations of sickle cell disease: review. *Amer. J. med. Sci.*, **239**, 773–778.

SCHNEIDER, R. G. (1956). Incidence of electrophoretically distinct abnormalities of hemoglobin in 1550 Negro hospital patients. *Amer. J. clin. Path.*, **26**, 1270–1276.

SCHNEIDER, R. G. & HAGGARD, M. E. (1957). A new haemoglobin variant exhibiting anomalous electrophoretic behaviour. *Nature (Lond.)*, **180**, 1486–1487.

SCHROEDER, W. A. & MATSUDA, G. (1958). N-terminal residues of human fetal hemoglobin. *J. Amer. chem. Soc.*, **80**, 1521.

SCHUMACHER, H. R., ANDREWS, R. & McLAUGHLIN, G. (1973). Arthropathy in sickle-cell disease. *Ann. intern. Med.*, **78**, 203–211.

SCHWARTZ, A. D., (1972). The splenic platelet reservoir in sickle cell anemia. *Blood*, **40**, 678–683.

SCHWARTZ, A. D. & PEARSON, H. A. (1972). Impaired antibody response to intravenous immunization in sickle cell anemia. *Pediat. Res.*, **6**, 145–149.

SCOTT, R. B., BANKS, L. O., JENKINS, M. E. & CRAWFORD, R. P. (1951). Studies in sickle-cell anemia. II. Clinical manifestations of sickle-cell anemia in children. *J. Pediat.*, **34**, 460–471.

SCOTT, R. B., FERGUSON, A. D., JENKINS, M. E. & CLARK, H. M. (1955). Studies in sickle-cell anemia. VIII. Further observations on the clinical manifestations of sickle-cell anemia in children. *Amer. J. Dis. Child.*, **90**, 682–691.

SEARLE, J. F. (1973). Anaesthesia in sickle cell states: a review. *Anaesthesia*, **28**, 48–58.

SEARS, D. A. (1978). The morbidity of sickle cell trait. A review of the literature. *Amer. J. Med.*, **64**, 1021–1036.

SEELER, R. A. (1973). Non-seasonality of sickle-cell crisis. *Lancet*, **ii**, 743 (Letter).

SEELER, R. A., METZGER, W. & MUFSON, M. A. (1972). *Diplococcus pneumoniae* infections in children with sickle cell anemia. *Amer. J. Dis. Child.*, **123**, 8–10.

SEELER, R. A. & SHWIAKI, M. Z. (1972). Acute splenic sequestration crises (ASSC) in young children with sickle cell anemia. Clinical observations in 20 episodes in 14 children. *Clin. Pediat. (Philadelphia)*, **11**, 701–704.

SELIGMAN, B. R., ROSNER, F. & SMULEWICZ, J. J. (1973). Splenic calcification in sickle cell anemia. *Amer. J. med. Sci.*, **265**, 495–499.

SERJEANT, G. R. (1970). Irreversibly sickled cells and splenomegaly in sickle-cell anaemia. *Brit. J. Haemat.*, **19**, 635–641.

SERJEANT, G. R. (1974a). *The Clinical Features of Sickle Cell Disease*. 357 pp. North-Holland Publishing Company, Amsterdam, Oxford.

SERJEANT, G. R. (1974b). Leg ulceration in sickle cell anemia. *Arch. intern. Med.*, **133**, 690–694.

SERJEANT, G. R. (1975). Five-year follow-up of Jamaican adults with sickle cell anaemia. *Brit. med. J.*, **ii**, 20–21.

SERJEANT, G. R. (1981). Observation on the epidemology of sickle cell disease. *Trans. roy. Soc. trop. Med. Hyg.*, **75**, 228–233.

SERJEANT, G. R. (1983). Sickle haemoglobin and pregnancy. *Brit. med. J.*, **287**, 628–630.

SERJEANT, G. R. (1985a). Sickle cell disease. In: *Recent Advances in Haematology*, 4 (ed. by A. V. Hoffbrand), pp. 89–108. Churchill Livingstone, Edinburgh.

SERJEANT, G. R. (1985b). *Sickle Cell Disease*. 478 pp. Oxford University Press.

SERJEANT, G. R. & ASHCROFT, M. T. (1971). Shortening of the digits in sickle cell anaemia. A sequela of the hand-foot syndrome. *Trop. geog. Med.*, **23**, 341–346.

SERJEANT, G. R. & ASHCROFT, M. T. (1973). Delayed skeletal maturation in sickle cell anemia in Jamaica. *Johns Hopk. med. J.*, **132**, 95–102.

SERJEANT, G. R., GALLOWAY, R. E. & GUERI, M. C. (1970). Oral zinc sulphate in sickle-cell ulcers. *Lancet*, **ii**, 891–892.

SERJEANT, G. & GUERI, M. (1970). Sickle cell trait and leg ulceration. *Brit. med. J.*, **i**, 820 (Letter).

SERJEANT, G. R., MAY, H., PATRICK, A. & SLIFER, E. D. (1973). Duodenal ulceration in sickle cell anaemia. *Trans. roy. Soc. trop. Med. Hyg.*, **67**, 59–63.

SERJEANT, G. R., RICHARDS, R., BARBAR, P. R. H & MILNER, P. F. (1968). Relatively benign sickle-cell anaemia in 60 patients aged over 30 in the West Indies. *Brit. med. J.*, **iii**, 86–91.

SERJEANT, G. & SERJEANT, B. (1972). Sickle-cell anaemia before Herrick. *Lancet*, **i**, 746–747 (Letter).

SERJEANT, G. R., SERJEANT, B. E. & CONDON, P. I. (1972). The conjunctival sign in sickle cell anemia: a relationship with irreversibly sickled cells. *J. Amer. med. Ass.*, **219**, 1428–1431.

SHAPIRO, M. P. & HAYES, J. A. (1984). Fat embolism in sickle cell disease. Report of a case with brief review of the literature. *Arch. intern. Med.*, **144**, 181–182.

SHAPIRO, N. D. & POE, M. F. (1955). Sickle-cell disease: an anesthesiological problem. *Anesthesiology*, **16**, 771–780.

SHELLEY, W. M. & CURTIS, E. M. (1958). Bone marrow and fat embolism in sickle cell anemia and sickle cell-hemoglobin C disease. *Bull. Johns Hopk. Hosp.*, **103**, 8–25.

SHERMAN, I. J. (1940). The sickling phenomenon, with special reference to differentiation of sickle-cell anemia from the sickle-cell trait. *Bull. Johns Hopk. Hosp.*, **67**, 309–324.

SHUBIN, H., KAUFMAN, R., SHAPIRO, M. & LEVINSON, D. C. (1960). Cardiovascular findings in children with sickle cell anemia. *Amer. J. Cardiol.*, **6**, 875–885.

SHUKLA, R. N. & SOLANKI, B. R. (1958). Sickle-cell trait in Central India. *Lancet*, **i**, 297–298.

SHUKLA, R. N., SOLANKI, B. R. & PARANDE, A. S. (1958). Sickle cell disease in India. *Blood*, **13**, 552–558.

SHULMAN, S. T., BARTLETT, J., CLYDE, W. A. JNR & AYOUB, E. M. (1972). The unusual severity of mycoplasmal pneumonia in children with sickle-cell disease. *New Engl. J. Med.*, **287**, 164–167.

SHURAFA, M., PRASAD, A. S., RUCKNAGEL, D. L. & KAN, Y. W. (1982). Long survival in sickle cell anemia. *Amer. J. Hemat.*, **12**, 357–365.

SINGER, K. (1955). Hereditary hemolytic disorders associated with abnormal hemoglobins. *Amer. J. Med.*, **18**, 633–652.

SMITH, C. H. (1957). The abnormal hemoglobins: clinical and hematologic aspects. *J. Pediat.*, **50**, 91–113.

SMITH, E. W. & CONLEY, C. L. (1955). Sicklemia and infarction of the spleen during aerial flight. Electrophoresis of the hemoglobin in 15 cases. *Bull. Johns Hopk. Hosp.*, **96**, 35–41.

SMITS, H. L., OSKI, F. A. & BRODY, J. I. (1969). The hemolytic crisis of sickle cell disease: the role of glucose-6-phosphate dehydrogenase deficiency. *J. Pediat.*, **74**, 544–551.

SOUSA, C. M., CATOE, B. L. & SCOTT, R. B. (1962). Studies in sickle cell anemia. XIX. Priapism as a complication in children. *J. Pediat.*, **60**, 52–54.

SPECTOR, D., ZACHARY, J. B., STERIOFF, S. & MILLAN, J. (1978). Painful crises following renal transplantation in sickle cell anemia. *Amer. J. Med.*, **64**, 835–839.

SPIRER, Z., WEISMAN, Y., ZAKUTH, V., FRIDKIN, M. & BOGAIR, N. (1980). Decreased serum tuftsin concentrations in sickle cell disease. *Arch. Dis. Childh.*, **55**, 566–567.

SPROULE, B. J., HALDEN, E. R. & MILLER, W. F. (1958). A study of cardiopulmonary alterations in patients with sickle cell disease and its variants. *J. clin. Invest.*, **37**, 486–495.

STAMATOYANNOPOULOS, G. & NUTE, P. E. (1974). Genetic control of haemoglobins. *Clinics Haemat.*, **3**, 251–287.

STATIUS VAN EPS, L. W., PINEDO-VEELS, C., DE VRIES, G. H. & DE KONING, J. (1970). Nature of concentrating defect in sickle-cell nephropathy. *Lancet*, i, 450–452.

STATIUS VAN EPS, L. W., SCHOUTEN, H., LA PORTE-WIJSMAN, L. W., & STRUYKER BOUDIER, A. M. (1967). The influence of red blood cell transfusions on the hyposthenuria and renal hemodynamics of sickle cell anemia. *Clin. chim. Acta*, **17**, 449–461.

STEINBERG, M. H. & DREILING, B. J. (1974). Glucose-6-phosphate dehydrogenase deficiency in sickle-cell anemia: a study in adults. *Ann. intern. Med.*, **80**, 217–220.

STEINBERG, M. H., DREILING, B. J., MORRISON, F. S. & NECHELES, T. F. (1973). Mild sickle cell disease. Clinical and laboratory studies. *J. Amer. med. Ass.*, **224**, 317–321.

STEINBERG, M. H., WEST, S., GALLACHER, D. & THE COOPERATIVE STUDY OF SICKLE CELL DISEASE (1984). Effects of G-6-PD deficiency upon sickle cell anemia. *Blood*, **64**, No. 5 (Suppl. 1), 53a (Abstract 124).

STEPHENS, C. G. & SCOTT, R. B. (1980). Cholelithiasis in sickle cell anemia: surgical or medical management. *Arch. intern. Med.*, **140**, 648–651.

STEVENS, M. C. G., HAYES, R. J. & SERJEANT, G. R. (1981). Body shape in young children with homozygous sickle cell disease. *Pediatrics*, **71**, 610–614.

STOCKMAN, J. A., NIGRO, M. A., MISHKIN, M. M. & OSKI, F. A. (1972). Occlusion of large cerebral vessels in sickle-cell anemia. *New Engl. J. Med.*, **287**, 846–849.

STRAUSS, J., PARDO, V., KOSS, M. N., GRISWOLD, W. & McINTOSH, R. M. (1975). Nephropathy associated with sickle cell anemia: an autologous immune complex nephritis. I. Studies on nature of glomerular-bound antibody and antigen identification in a patient with sickle cell disease

and immune deposit glomerulonephritis. *Amer. J. Med.*, **58**, 382–387.

STRAUSS, M. B. (1964). Of medicine, men and molecules: wedlock or divorce? *Medicine (Baltimore)*, **43**, 619–624.

STRICKER, R. B., LINKER, C. A., CROWLEY, T. J. & EMBURY, S. H. (1986). Hematologic malignancy in sickle cell disease: report of four cases and review of the literature. *Amer. J. Hemat.*, **21**, 223–230.

SUERIG, K. C. & SIEFERT, F. E. (1964). Pseudoxanthoma elasticum and sickle cell anemia. *Arch. intern. Med.*, **113**, 135–141.

SUSMANO, S. & LEWY, J. E. (1969). Sickle cell disease and acute glomerulonephritis. *Amer. J. Dis. Child.*, **118**, 615–618.

SWEENEY, M. J., DOBBINS, W. T. & ETTELDORF, J. N. (1962). Renal disease with elements of the nephrotic syndrome associated with sickle cell anemia. A report of 2 cases. *J. Pediat.*, **60**, 42–51.

SYDENSTRICKER, V. P. (1924). Further observations on sickle cell anemia. *J. Amer. med. Ass.*, **83**, 12–17.

SYDENSTRICKER, V. P., MULHERIN, W. A. & HOUSEAL, R. W. (1923). Sickle cell anemia: report of two cases in children, with necropsy in one case. *Amer. J. Dis. Child.*, **26**, 132–154.

TALBOT, J. F., BIRD, A. C., RABB, L. M., MAUDE, G. H. & SERJEANT, G. R. (1983). Sickle cell retinopathy in Jamaican children: a search for prognostic factors. *Brit. J. Ophthal.*, **67**, 782–785.

TALBOT, J. F., BIRD, A. C., SERJEANT, G. R. & HAYES, R. J. (1982). Sickle cell retinopathy in young children in Jamaica. *Brit. J. Ophthal.*, **66**, 149–154.

TALIAFERRO, W. H. & HUCK, J. G. (1923). The inheritance of sickle-cell anemia in man. *Genetics*, **8**, 594–598.

TANAKA, K. R., CLIFFORD, G. O. & AXELROD, A. R. (1956). Sickle cell anemia (homozygous S) with aseptic necrosis of femoral head. *Blood*, **11**, 998–1008.

TAPAZOGLOU, E., PRASAD, A. S., HILL, G., BREWER, G. J. & KAPLAN, J. (1985). Decreased natural killer cell activity in patients with zinc deficiency with sickle cell disease. *J. Lab. clin. Med.*, **105**, 19–22.

THOMAS, A. N., PATTISON, C. & SERJEANT, G. R. (1982). Causes of death in sickle-cell disease in Jamaica. *Brit. med. J.*, **285**, 633–635.

TOPLEY, J. M., ROGERS, D. W., STEVENS, M. C. G. & SERJEANT, G. R. (1981). Acute splenic sequestration and hypersplenism in the first five years in homozygous sickle cell disease. *Arch. Dis. Childh.*, **56**, 765–769.

TROWELL, H. C., RAPER, A. B. & WELLBOURN, H. F. (1957). The natural history of homozygous sickle-cell anaemia in Central Africa. *Quart. J. Med.*, **26**, 401–422.

TUCK, S. M., STUDD, J. W. W. & WHITE, J. M. (1983). Pregnancy in women with sickle cell trait. *Brit. J. Obstet. Gynaec.*, **90**, 108–111.

VANDEPITTE, J. (1954). Aspects quantitatifs et génétiques de la sicklanémie à Léopoldville. *Ann. Soc. belge Méd. trop.*, **34**, 501–516.

VANDEPITTE, J. (1959). The incidence of haemoglobinoses in the Belgian Congo. In: *Abnormal Haemoglobins. A Symposium* (ed. by J. H. P. Jonxis and J. F. Delafresnaye), pp. 271–278. Blackwell Scientific Publications, Oxford.

VANDEPITTE, J., COLAERT, J., LAMBOTTE-LEGRAND, J. and C. & PERIN, F. (1953). Les ostéites à Salmonella chez les sicklanémiques. À propos de 5 observations. *Ann. Soc. belge Méd. trop.*, **33**, 511–522.

VANDEPITTE, J. & DELAISSE, J. (1957). Sicklémie et paludisme. Aperçu du problème et contribution personnelle. *Ann. Soc. belge Méd. trop.*, **37**, 703–735.

VANDEPITTE, J. M., ZUELZER, W. W., NEEL, J. V. & COLAERT, J. (1955). Evidence concerning the inadequacy of mutation as an explanation of the frequency of the sickle cell gene in the Belgian Congo. *Blood*, **10**, 341–350.

VERAS, S., DÉMÉTRIADÈS, T. & MANIOS, S. (1953). L'anémie falciforme en Macédoine. *Sang*, **24**, 613.

WADE, L. J. & STEVENSON, L. B. (1941). Necrosis of the bone marrow with fat embolism in sickle cell anemia. *Amer. J. Path.*, **17**, 47–54.

WAINSCOAT, J. S., BELL, J. I., THEIN, S. L., HIGGS, D. R., SERJEANT, G. R., PETO, T. E. A. & WEATHERALL, D. J. (1983). Multiple origin of the sickle mutation: evidence from β^S globin gene cluster polymorphism. *Mol. Biol. Med.*, **1**, 191–197.

WALKER, B. R. & ALEXANDER, F. (1971). Uric acid excretion in sickle cell anemia. *J. Amer. med. Ass.*, **215**, 255–258.

WALKER, B. W., BALLAS, S. K. & BURKA, E. R. (1979). The diagnosis of pulmonary thromboembolism in sickle cell disease. *Amer. J. Hemat.*, **7**, 219–232.

WALTERS, J. H. & LEHMANN, H. (1956). Distribution of the S and C haemoglobin variants in two Nigerian communities. *Trans. roy. Soc. trop. Med. Hyg.*, **50**, 204–208.

WARD, J. & SMITH, A. L. (1976). *Hemophilus influenzae* bacteremia in children with sickle cell disease. *J. Pediat.*, **88**, 261–262.

WARD, P. C. J., SMITH, C. M. & WHITE, J. G. (1979). Erythrocyte ecdysis: an unusual morphologic finding in a case of sickle cell anemia with intercurrent cold-agglutinin syndrome. *Amer. J. clin. Path.*, **72**, 479–485.

WARRIER, R., SARNAIK, S. & BREWER, G. J. (1978). Irreversibly sickled cells and hyposthenuria in sickle cell anemia. *Blood*, **52**, No. 5 (Suppl. 1), 52a (Abstract).

WARTH, J. A. & RUCKNAGEL, D. L. (1983). The increasing complexity of sickle cell anemia. In: *Progress in Hematology*, Vol. XIII (ed. by E. B.

Brown), pp. 25–47. Grune and Stratton, New York.

WATSON, H. C. & KENDREW, J. C. (1961). Amino-acid sequence of sperm whale myoglobin. Comparison between the amino-acid sequences of sperm whale myoglobin and of human haemoglobin. *Nature (Lond.)*, **190**, 670–672.

WATSON, R. J. (1956). Hemoglobins and disease. *Advanc. intern. Med.*, **8**, 305–355.

WATSON, R. J., BURKO, H., MEGAS, H. & ROBINSON, M. (1963). The hand-foot syndrome in sickle-cell disease in young children. *Pediatrics*, **31**, 975–982.

WATSON, R. J., LICHTMAN, H. C. & SHAPIRO, H. D. (1956). Splenomegaly in sickle cell anemia. *Amer. J. Med.*, **20**, 196–206.

WEATHERALL, D. J. & CLEGG, J. B. (1981). *The Thalassaemia Syndromes*, 3rd edn. 875 pp. Blackwell Scientific Publications, Oxford.

WEENS, H. S. (1945). Cholelithiasis in sickle cell anemia. *Ann. intern. Med.*, **22**, 182–191.

WELCH, R. B. & GOLDBERG, M. F. (1966). Sickle-cell hemoglobin and its relation to fundus abnormality. *Arch. Ophthal.*, **75**, 353–362.

WENT, L. N. & MacIVER, J. E. (1958). Sickle-cell anaemia in adults and its differentiation from sickle-cell thalassaemia. *Lancet*, **ii**, 824–826.

WHALLEY, P. J., PRITCHARD, J. A. & RICHARDS, J. R. JNR (1963). Sickle cell trait and pregnancy. *J. Amer. med. Ass.*, **186**, 1132–1135.

WHITE, J. C. (1952–53). Human haemoglobins. In: *Lectures on Scientific Basis of Medicine*, Vol. II, pp. 287–322. Athlone Press, London.

WHITE, J. C. & BEAVEN, G. H. (1954). A review of the varieties of human haemoglobin in health and disease. *J. clin. Path.*, **7**, 175–200.

WHITE, J. M. (1983). The approximate gene frequency of sickle haemoglobin in the Arabian peninsula. *Brit. J. Haemat.*, **55**, 563–564 (Letter).

WHITE, J. M. & DACIE, J. V. (1971). The unstable hemoglobins: molecular and clinical features. In: *Progress in Hematology*, Vol. VII (ed. by E. B. Brown and C. V. Moore), pp. 69–109. Grune and Stratton, New York.

WHITTEN, C. F. (1961). Growth status in sickle-cell anemia. *Amer. J. Dis. Child.*, **102**, 355–364.

WILSON, W. A., HUGHES, G. R. V. & LACHMANN, P. J. (1976). Deficiency of factor B of the complement system in sickle cell anaemia. *Brit. med. J.*, **i**, 367–369.

WILSON, W. A., NICHOLSON, G. D., HUGHES, G. R. V., AMIN, S., ALLEYNE, G. & SERJEANT, G. R. (1976). Systemic lupus erythematosus and sickle-cell anaemia. *Brit. med. J.*, **i**, 813.

WINKELSTEIN, J. A. & DRACHMAN, R. H. (1968). Deficiency of pneumococcal serum opsonizing activity in sickle-cell disease. *New Engl. J. Med.*, **279**, 459–466.

WINSLOW, R. M. & ANDERSON, W. F. (1983). The hemoglobinopathies. In: *The Metabolic Basis of*

Inherited Disease, 5th edn (ed. by J. B. Stanbury, J. B. Wyngaarden, D. S. Fredrickson, J. L. Goldstein and M. S. Brown), pp. 1666–1710. McGraw-Hill Book Company, New York.

WINSOR, T. & BURCH, G. E. (1944a). The habitus of patients with sickle cell anemia. *Hum. Biol.*, **16**, 99–114.

WINSOR, T. & BURCH, G. E. (1944b). The electrocardiogram and cardiac state in active sickle-cell anemia. *Amer. Heart J.*, **29**, 685–696.

WINTROBE, M. M. (1956). *Clinical Hematology*, 4th edn, p. 680. Kimpton, London.

WOOD, J. B., CLEGG, J. B. & WEATHERALL, D. J. (1977). Developmental biology of human hemoglobins. In: *Progress in Hematology*, Vol. X (ed. by E. B. Brown), pp. 43–90. Grune and Stratton, New York.

WOOD, W. G., PEMBREY, M. E., SERJEANT, G. R., PERRINE, R. P. & WEATHERALL, D. J. (1980). Hb-F synthesis in sickle cell anaemia: a comparison of Saudi Arab cases with those of African origin. *Brit. J. Haemat.*, **45**, 431–445.

WORRELL, V. T. & BUTERA, V. (1976). Sickle-cell dactylitis. *J. Bone Joint Surg.*, **58**, 1161–1163.

YATER, W. M. & HANSMANN, G. H. (1936). Sickle-cell anemia: a new cause for cor pulmonale. Report of two cases with numerous disseminated occlusions of the small pulmonary arteries. *Amer. J. med. Sci.*, **191**, 474–484.

ZUELZER, W. W., NEEL, J. V. & ROBINSON A. R. (1956). Abnormal hemoglobins. *Progr. Hemat.*, **1**, 91–137. Grune and Stratton, New York.

Sickle-cell disease II: haematological findings and laboratory diagnosis of homozygous sickle-cell disease and sickle-cell trait; screening programmes for haemoglobinopathies

BLOOD PICTURE IN HOMOZYGOUS SICKLE-CELL DISEASE

Erythrocyte count

Patients in a steady state are as a rule moderately to severely anaemic. The erythrocyte count is usually between 2.0 and $3.5 \times 10^{12}/l$. Age, however, influences the count. If followed from birth (Fig. 12.1), the count, which is then virtually normal, falls quite steeply to a minimum at 2–3 months (as does the count of a Hb-AA infant); it then rises a little to a peak at about 6 months and then falls slowly and steadily to reach a minimum at about 5–6 years (Serjeant et al., 1981a). Serjeant and his co-workers' valuable data (quoted above) were based on a cohort study of 125 Hb-SS newborns each matched with two Hb-AA controls born on the same day. There was no obvious difference between males and females.

After the age of 6 years the erythrocyte count

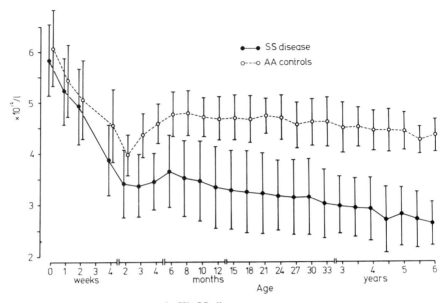

Fig. 12.1 Effect of age on the erythrocyte count in Hb-SS disease.
Data derived from 125 Hb-SS newborns matched with two controls born on the same day. [Reproduced by permission from Serjeant *et al.* (1981a).]

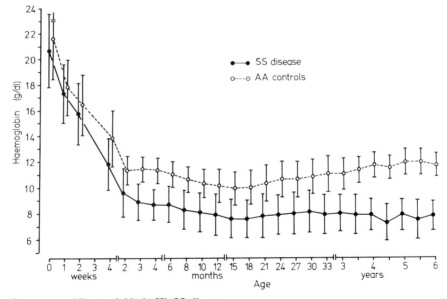

Fig. 12.2 Effect of age on total haemoglobin in Hb-SS disease.
Data derived from 125 Hb-SS newborns matched with two controls born on the same day. [Reproduced by permission from Serjeant *et al.* (1981a).]

hardly alters in females, but in males it increases in adolescence, reaches a plateau and then tends to decrease after the age of 40 (Serjeant, 1985, p. 85). The rise in adolescence seems likely to be hormonal in origin.

Haemoglobin

There is considerable variation from patient to patient but the haemoglobin is usually in the region of 8 g/dl. There are, however, age-related changes (Fig. 12.2). According to the data provided by Hayes *et al*. (1985), based on a large number of West-Indian Hb-SS patients, the haemoglobin of males rises steeply in adolescence and reaches a maximum between 25 and 39 years, 1–3 g/dl higher than in the 10–14 age-group, only to fall slightly after the age of 40. In females the haemoglobin hardly alters between the ages of 5 and 40. Hayes *et al*. made the interesting suggestion that the fall in haemoglobin in males over 40

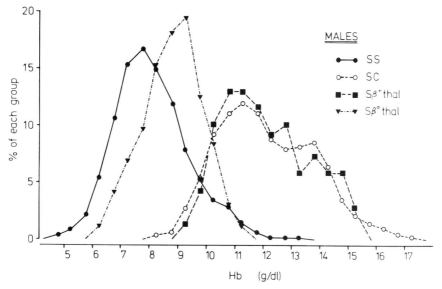

Fig. 12.3 Distribution of haemoglobin levels in male patients, aged between 5 and 40 years, in steady state suffering from a sickle-cell syndrome.
Jamaican data. [Reproduced by permission from Serjeant (1985).]

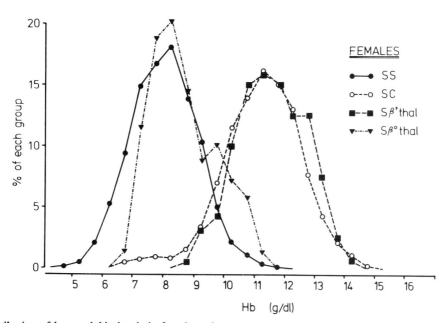

Fig. 12.4 Distribution of haemoglobin levels in female patients, aged between 5 and 40 years, in steady state suffering from a sickle-cell syndrome.
Jamaican data. [Reproduced by permission from Serjeant (1985).]

years of age might be associated with the development of unappreciated renal failure.

Serjeant (1981) had provided some interesting comparisons between the haemoglobin levels of large numbers of iron-sufficient patients, 5 years of age or older, suffering from one or other of the four main types of Hb-S disease endemic in Jamaica, namely, Hb-SS disease, Hb-SC disease, Hb-S/β^+-thalassaemia and Hb-S/β^0-thalassaemia. His data well illustrate the relative severity of anaemia in the four categories of patients, and also how wide the inter-patient differences are (Figs. 12.3 and 12.4).

Plasma volume and total blood volume

In Hb-SS disease the plasma volume is substantially increased so that, despite a low erythrocyte volume, the total blood volume is normal or even above normal (Jenkins, Scott and Ferguson, 1956; Sproule, Halden and Miller, 1958; Erlandson, Shulman and Smith, 1960; Shubin et al., 1960; Barreras, Diggs and Lipscomb, 1966; Steinberg, Dreiling and Lovell, 1977) (Fig. 12.5).

Erlandson, Shulman and Smith (1960) studied eight Hb-SS patients: their total blood volume ranged between 80.6 and 92.6 ml/kg (normal mean 70 $\pm$ 10 ml/kg) and their plasma volume between 61.7 and 73.2 ml/kg (normal mean 45 $\pm$ 10 ml/kg). Erlandson, Shulman and Smith concluded that in Hb-SS disease the increase in plasma volume tended to be greater than in patients with other chronic haemolytic anaemias. In two patients in painful crisis the plasma volume was found to be substantially reduced (and the erythrocyte volume slightly reduced) compared to when the patients were well.

Steinberg, Dreiling and Lovell (1977) reported on 14 adult Hb-SS patients aged between 18 and 62 (mean 27.4) years. Their plasma volume ranged between 46.1 and 77.4 ml/kg (mean 55.0 $\pm$ 7.6 ml/kg).

The cause of the unusual increase in plasma volume in Hb-SS disease is obscure, particularly as the spleen in most patients, except that of small children, is usually so small.

Absolute values

Mean corpuscular volume (MCV). The MCV is generally within or close to the normal range (Diggs and Bibb, 1939); however, in the most anaemic patients it tends to be a little above

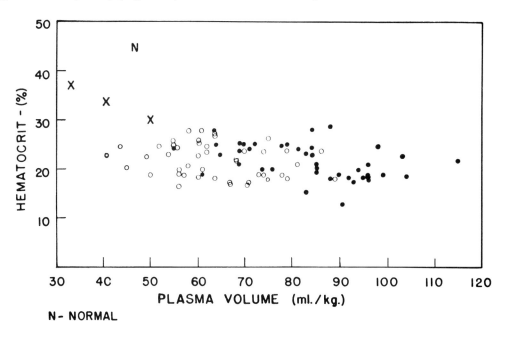

Fig. 12.5 Plasma volume in hereditary haemolytic anaemias.
Results of 40 estimations in 12 patients with sickle-cell anaemia, 46 estimations in 20 patients with thalassaemia and three patients with hereditary spherocytosis. [Reproduced by permission from Erlandson, Schulman and Smith (1960).]

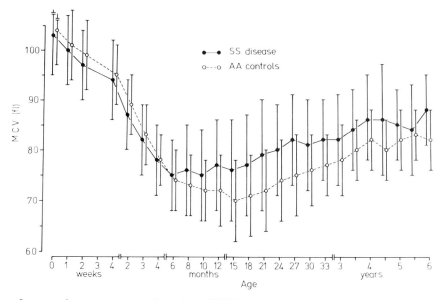

Fig. 12.6 Effect of age on the mean corpuscular volume (MCV).
Jamaican data derived from 125 Hb-SS newborns matched with two controls born on the same day. [Reproduced by permission from Serjeant *et al.* (1981a).]

normal. There is an age-related effect (Fig. 12.6). After the age of 5 years the MCV increases slightly up to the age of 25–29, particularly in females (Serjeant, 1985b, p. 86).

Mean corpuscular haemoglobin (MCH) and haemoglobin concentration (MCHC). These are, too, usually within the normal range (Diggs and Bibb, 1939; Itano, Bergren and Sturgeon, 1956). There are small changes with age that parallel those of the MCV. Significant reductions in MCH result from the presence of one or two genes for α-thalassaemia, *i.e.*, in Hb-SS patients with the $-\alpha/\alpha\alpha$ or $-\alpha/-\alpha$ genotype (see p. 447).

Mean corpuscular diameter (MCD) and thickness (MCT). As long ago as 1937 Erickson and co-workers described the erythrocytes of eight patients with 'sicklemia with anemia' as having a reduced thickness, increased diameter and increased diameter:thickness ratio. Diggs and Bibb (1939) carried out Price Jones curves on 10 patients whose films contained less than 5% of elongated cells. The MCD varied between 7.8 and 9.5 μm, with a mean of 8.7 μm, compared with a mean of 7.6 μm in a control series of five medical students. Further data were provided by Westerman, Pierce and Jensen (1964) based on a study of MCD, MCT, MCV and surface area of the erythrocytes

of 10 Hb-SS disease patients. The MCD was significantly greater, the MCT significantly less and the mean surface area significantly greater than in normal cells of comparable age. The MCV was about the same. Westerman, Pierce and Jensen also reported that Hb-SS erythrocytes contained more lipids (phospholipids and cholesterol) than did control normal cells.

Reticulocyte count

The count is typically raised in steady-state patients and usually ranges between 5 and 20%. Counts above 30% are unusual. In Diggs and Bibb's (1939) 42 patients, the average count was 15%; however, they had 'often observed' counts above 25%, and one patient had had a count as high as 87%. According to Hayes *et al.* (1985), there is a tendency for the count to decline with age.

Relationship between the MCV and other haematological features and the clinical expression of Hb-SS disease

Serjeant, Foster and Serjeant (1981) contrasted a range of haematological features in 55 Hb-SS

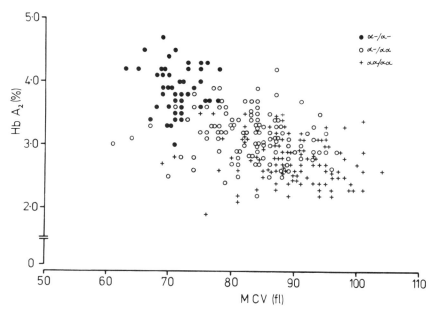

Fig. 12.7 Relationship between mean corpuscular volume (MCV) and haemoglobin-A$_2$ percentage, according to α-globin genotype.
Jamaican data. [Reproduced by permission from Higgs *et al.* (1982).]

patients whose MCV was low (<80 fl) with those of 55 patients, matched for age, sex and Hb-F levels, whose MCV was high (>95 fl). The microcytic patients had a higher mean haemoglobin, PCV, erythrocyte count and Hb-A$_2$ percentage and lower mean reticulocyte count and ISC percentage than the other group. However, the clinical features were similar in each group, except that splenomegaly persisted longer in the microcytic group. It was suggested that the higher blood viscosity resulting from the higher haemoglobin levels balanced in the microcytic patients the rheological advantages of decreased intravascular sickling. The microcytosis was thought to be due to iron deficiency in some patients and in others to the presence of two genes for α-thalassaemia (−α/−α). In Figure 12.7 is illustrated the relationship between MCV and Hb A$_2$ (Serjeant, 1981). The tendency for low MCVs to be associated with a high Hb A$_2$ is the result apparently of the concurrent presence of homozygosity for the −α thalassaemia gene.

Erythrocyte morphology

This varies considerably from patient to patient. In dried stained blood films the characteristic feature is the presence of cells that are conspicuously elongated and have sharp or rounded ends and which are often but not always slightly bent. These are of course the cells noted by Herrick (1910) as being sickle-shaped (Fig. 11.1, p. 2) from which sickle-cell disease takes its name: they are in fact 'irreversibly sickled cells (ISC)', *i.e.* cells which have not reverted to discs on exposure to atmospheric air. Other cells are more like oats in shape; still other cells are intermediate in form between oat-shaped cells and elliptical cells. The proportion of cells present that are sickled or oat-shaped varies considerably from patient to patient but is more or less constant in each individual (Figs. 12.8–12.12). Serjeant, Serjeant and Milner (1969), Serjeant and Serjeant (1972) and Serjeant (1974, p. 68) have published data on ISC counts based on their West-Indies experience. The percentage varied from 0 to 40% with a mean of 12.4%, and was found to be highly significantly inversely correlated with the level of Hb F. The count is diminished, as is the MCV and MCH, if the patient carries a gene or genes for α-thalassaemia. In general the higher the proportion of sickled cells present the more likely is the patient to be seriously affected clinically.

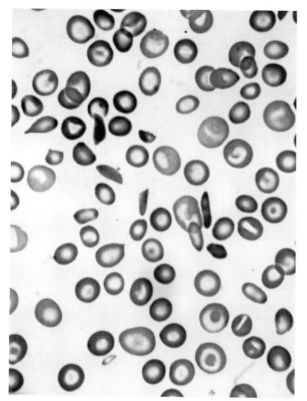

Fig. 12.8 Peripheral-blood film of a Hb-SS patient.
Shows sickled cells, macrocytes, target cells and cell fragments. × 700.

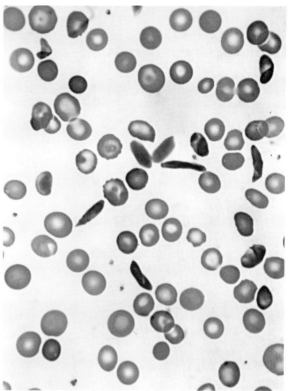

Fig. 12.9 Peripheral-blood film of a Hb-SS patient.
Shows sickled cells and also some contracted spherocyte-like cells. × 700.

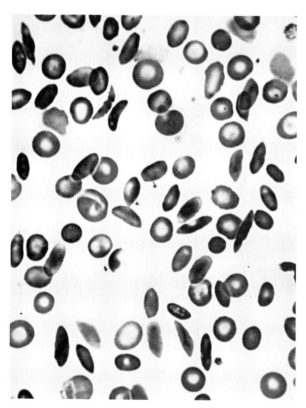

Fig. 12.10 Peripheral-blood film of a Hb-SS patient.
Shows many sickled and oat-shaped cells. Small Pappenheimer bodies can be seen in some of the cells. × 700.

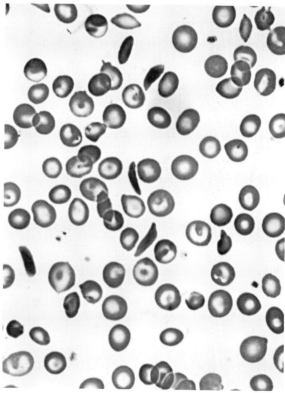

Fig. 12.11 Peripheral-blood film of a Hb-SS patient.
Shows sickled cells and moderate numbers of target cells. × 700.

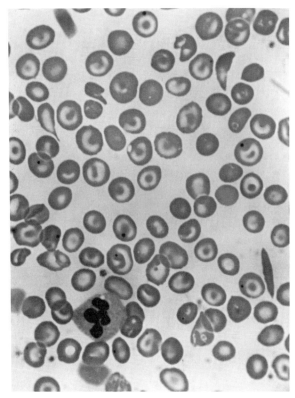

Fig. 12.12 Peripheral-blood film of a Hb-SS patient.
Shows a small number of sickled cells. Target cells and
Howell-Jolly bodies are unusually conspicuous. × 700.

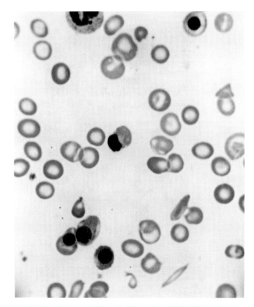

Fig. 12.13 Peripheral-blood film of a Hb-SS patient.
Shows an unusual number of normoblasts. The patient
had suffered from severe bone-marrow infarction. × 700.

Aside from the presence of sickled cells, blood
films from Hb-SS patients show many other interesting features. Anisocytosis is moderate to
marked and there is considerable variation in
staining (anisochromasia); occasional irregularly-
contracted cells are present and a few cells may
resemble spherocytes; macrocytes are often
conspicuous as well as polychomasia — a reflection of the reticulocyte count — and a few or even
many of the cells are target cells; normoblasts can
usually be seen. The progressive atrophy of the
spleen, which is so characteristic of Hb-SS
disease, affects the blood picture: in relation to the
erythrocytes, the consequences include hypochromia due to flattening of the cells, an increased
number of target cells and normoblasts, the presence of occasional siderocytes and Howell-Jolly
bodies and possibly an increased number of
sickled cells. Large but transient increases in the
number of circulating normoblasts may be seen

following the resolution of an aplastic crisis
(Fig. 12.19), and also accompanying massive
infarction of the bone marrow (Fig. 12.13).

Although the presence of sickled cells in peripheral blood films is a characteristic of Hb-SS
disease, sickled cells may be found too, in films
made from the blood of some patients with Hb-
S/thalassaemia. They are absent, or at least rarely
seen, in Hb-SC disease; they have, however, been
reported in Hb-SO disease (Milner et al., 1970).

'Blister cells'. As already referred to (Vol. 1, p. 72),
Barreras, Diggs and Bell (1968) described an interesting
variant of the sickle-cell anaemia blood picture which
they had noticed in six adult patients who were seriously
ill with pulmonary emboli. Their blood films were characterized by the presence of 'blister cells' — erythrocytes with blebs, blisters or bubbles on their surface
(described as resembling 'a round or conical basket with
a handle giving the appearance of a cell with a large
vacuole at one pole but with intact cell membrane').
Other irregularly-contracted cells, of thorn, helmet or
triangular shape, were present, too, as well as spherical,
crenated, burr and fragmented cells. The blood picture
was regarded as a form of microangiopathic haemolytic
anaemia resulting from (partial) occlusion of pulmonary
vessels. Barreras, Diggs and Bell reported, too, that
they had observed small numbers of blister cells in the
films of 14 patients with pulmonary embolism who did
not have sickle-cell anaemia.

Later, Karayalcin, Imran and Rosner (1972) described two patients, one Hb-SS, the other Hb-SC, both with pulmonary infarction, in whom they had similarly found 'blister' cells in their blood films. In the Hb-SS patient, who died 3 days after admission to hospital, 21–23 per 1000 erythrocytes were blister cells; in the Hb-SC patient the blister cells, at first 15 per 1000 erythrocytes, disappeared progressively over a 3-week period during which time the patient was making a clinical recovery from the pulmonary infarction.

'Pitted' cells. According to Caspar and co-workers (1976) and Pearson and co-workers (1979) the number of erythrocytes containing pits (pocks) demonstrable by Normarsky optics (differential interference contrast microscopy) is greatly increased in Hb-SS disease, as it is generally after splenectomy (see Vol. 1, p. 89).

Pearson *et al.* (1979), who reported on 28 Hb-SS disease children, found that the percentage of cells containing pocks increased steadily with age, so that when they were aged 6–8 years most had more than 12%, *i.e.* a percentage in the asplenic range.
Sills and Oski (1979) reported similar findings. In 21 Hb-SS children the pit-cell count ranged between 3.6 and 67.1% (mean 30.8 ± 17.2%): in children less than 3 years old the mean count was 14.0%; in the 11–18-year-old group the mean was 42.4%. Sills and Oski concluded that calculating the percentage of erythrocytes in which single or multiple pits could be seen provided a simple means of assessing splenic function.

Erythrophagocytosis. A small number of monocytes that have phagocytosed erythrocytes can be found in the peripheral blood of some Hb-SS patients (Diggs, 1932).

Solanki (1985) carried out 500-cell differential leucocyte counts in duplicate on 27 Hb-SS patients who were in a steady state. Erythrophagocytosis (EP) was detected in 10 of them (37%). The proportion of leucocytes acting as erythrophages varied from 1 to 6 per 100 (1 to 10 per 100 monocytes). No evidence of EP was found in a control series of normal blood films or in the films of nine splenectomized patients. Solanki suggested that the EP is the result of monocytes recognizing that amongst the population of erythrocytes there are cells the surface of which has undergone changes (indicative of senescence) that have made them ripe for removal from the circulation (see Vol. 1, p. 24). It was thought that atrophy of the spleen was likely to increase the number of such cells present in the peripheral blood.

Intra-erythrocytic inclusions in Hb-SS and

Hb-AS blood. In addition to the Howell-Jolly bodies and siderotic granules found in some of the erythrocytes in Hb-SS blood (p. 82), which appear to be associated with the gradual loss of splenic function, other types of inclusion can be seen, for instance, if unstained films are viewed by dark-field microscopy.

Schneider and co-workers (1972) reported that more than 25% of the erythrocytes of all 74 Hb-SS patients studied contained visible small inclusions compared with only three out of 63 Hb-AA subjects. Smaller percentages of inclusion-containing cells were found in blood films from other Hb-AA, Hb-AS, Hb-AC, Hb-S/thalassaemia Hb-C/thalassaemia and Hb-CC subjects. The haemoglobin content of the residues left after haemolysis (*i.e.* the cell membranes) paralleled the amount of material which could be seen under dark-field illumination, and it was concluded that, although some of the visible particles represented reticulum, siderotic granules, basophilic stippling, Howell-Jolly bodies or vacuoles (associated with functional asplenia), most of the material was precipitated haemoglobin (demonstrable by its reaction with benzidine) resulting from accelerated degradation of the abnormal haemoglobin.
The results of a later and more comprehensive study were reported by Kim *et al.* (1980). They examined the erythrocytes of 101 individuals aged between 10 months and 68 years, who carried a gene or genes for Hb S, Hb C, α- or β-thalassaemia or Hb O in various combinations: 40 of the patients had Hb SS, 21 with less than 10% Hb F and 19 with more than 10% Hb F, and 21 had Hb AS. Inclusions were looked for by dark-field microscopy and also in films after acid elution and staining, as used to demonstrate Hb F (soluble haemoglobin elutes leaving inclusions visible); in addition, the amount of membrane-associated denatured haemoglobin (MADH) was measured. The highest percentage of cells with inclusions (>25% of cells) and the highest amounts of MADH were found in the 21 Hb-SS patients who had a low percentage of Hb F, and in the solitary Hb-SO Arab patient (Fig. 12.14). Lower percentages of cells with inclusions were found in Hb-SS/α-thalassaemia, Hb-S/β⁰-thalassaemia and in Hb-SC patients and in Hb-SS patients with high Hb F. In clinically mild disorders, *e.g.*, in Hb-S/β⁺-thalassaemia, Hb-CC disease and Hb-AC and Hb-AS traits, the results were similar to those in the Hb-AA controls. The acid-elution method appeared to be the better of the two methods used for visualizing inclusions, and the results paralleled those of the MADH estimations. Of 56 patients with Hb SS or Hb SC, those with other evidence of functional asplenia had higher percentages of cells with inclusions and larger amounts of MADH than did those with functioning spleens. The presence of inclusions seemed to be independent of the presence of ISCs.

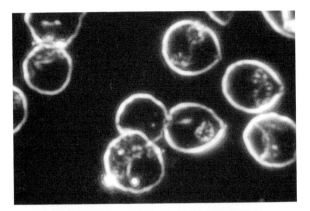

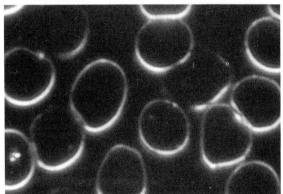

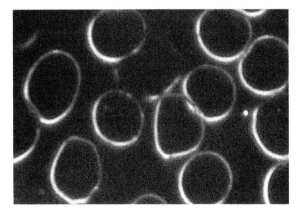

Fig. 12.14 Inclusions within erythrocytes demonstrated by dark-field microscopy.

Top: the patient was a 3-year-old child with Hb-SS disease. Howell-Jolly bodies were present in the peripheral blood and no splenic uptake of [^{99m}Tc]sulphur colloid was demonstrable. There was 0.15% of membrane-associated denatured haemoglobin.

Middle: the patient was 11 years old and had Hb-SC disease. There was 0.09% of membrane-associated denatured haemoglobin.

Bottom: the patient was a 24-year-old woman with the Hb-AS trait. There was 0.03% of membrane-associated denatured haemoglobin.

[Reproduced by permission from Kim *et al*. (1980).]

Effect of age on the blood picture in Hb-SS disease

The cohort study data of Serjeant and co-workers (1981a) has already been referred to. Davis (1976) had earlier described the changes in blood picture in a West-Indian population in London. His data were based on the analysis of 174 blood samples collected from 75 infants and children and young adolescents up to the age of 16. His figure illustrates the gradual fall in haemoglobin and Hb-F percentage and the rise in ISC count from <1% in the first year to 2.4–9.2% subsequently. The reticulocyte count was in the 7.5–12.3% range after the first year. Howell-Jolly bodies, virtually absent in the first year, were present in 0.17–0.43% of the erythrocytes in subsequent years. The percentage of target cells fluctuated between 0.2 and 4.9% and showed no definite trend with age.

Changes in erythrocyte morphology during pain crises in Hb-SS patients

Warth and Rucknagel (1983, 1984) studied, using a technique of arabinogalactan density-gradient centrifugation, the erythrocytes of nine Hb-SS patients in 10 episodes of pain crisis and compared their observations with observations made when the same patients were free from pain, 5–331 days after the crisis. The erythrocytes in five density-separated layers were classified using Nomarsky (interference) optics into nine categories, ranging from normal discocytes to echinocytic ISCs. Crises were found to be associated with the appearance of an increased percentage of echinocytic ISCs and of echinocytes that were not ISCs, especially in the denser gradient layers. These were replaced by normal discocytes in pain-free periods, suggesting that the echinocytic cells had been eliminated. Warth and Rucknagel concluded that pain crises occur in association with echinocytic change and that this may be induced by oxidant injury and quoted previous observations, *e.g.*, low GSH levels, as evidence of this (see p. 207). In an abstract, Warth, Near and Weinstein (1983) reported finding in sickle-cell anaemia blood 'sequestrocytes', erythrocytes similar to the 'blister cells' produced by severe oxidative damage on normal erythrocytes and as seen in G6PD deficiency.

Automated image processing analysis has also been used to determine whether painful crises in Hb-SS patients are associated with significant changes in erythrocyte morphology. Westerman and Bacus (1983) used a system that separated erythrocytes into 14 possible classes based on six measurements — size, haemoglobin content, central pallor, shape (circularity), shape (elongation) and shape (spicularity). Class 7 (elongated cells) and class 8 (irregular-shaped cells) were equated with ISCs — they comprised 3.5–43.5% of the cells and corresponded well with estimates based on visual inspection of films. Fifteen patients were studied when free from symptoms and seven again when in painful crisis: 1000 cells were assessed on each occasion and a differential count carried out. An interesting (but not unexpected) finding was that the percentage of each cell type was typical for each individual patient and was generally stable. During crises the macrocyte:normocyte ratio increased in six out of seven patients (which was thought to reflect a marrow response to increased haemolysis), but the mean percentage of ISCs did not change consistently compared with the mean percentage during asymptomatic periods, although the individual counts varied more than normally during crises. Westerman and Bacus concluded that their observations indicated that the relationship between vaso-occlusive episodes and the ISC count was not as close as had been thought (see also p. 213).

Rodgers, Schechter and Noguchi (1985), who used the phthalate method of Danon and Marikovsky (1964) to separate Hb-SS blood into subpopulations according to density, reported that in several patients the onset of a painful crisis was heralded 12–24 hours previously by the disappearance of the most dense fraction of cells.

High-density erythrocytes

An interesting method of studying the erythrocytes in sickle-cell disease is to centrifuge blood at a high speed in a Percoll-Stractan gradient (Corash et al., 1974; Vettore, De Matteis and Zampini, 1980). In this way not only have Hb-SS erythrocytes been shown to be more heterogeneous than normal with respect to density but a very dense fraction that is not present in normal blood has also been found to separate out (Fabry and Nagel, 1982a,b).

Fabry and Nagel (1982a) emphasized that the proportion of very dense cells varies from patient to patient and that this variability is functionally significant as the size of the high-density population is a reflection of the MCHC and the number of irreversibly sickled cells present. Fabry and Nagel (1982b) described how they had used the technique to study the effect of deoxygenation on erythrocyte density, a controversial topic. Hb-AA cells were found to become less dense, i.e. to swell, when deoxygenated: Hb-SS cells either became more dense, i.e. shrank, or maintained a constant density and volume when deoxygenated, depending upon the pH and amount of K^+ present and on whether the cells reversibly sickled or were irreversibly sickled. ISCs became denser when deoxygenated under all experimental conditions: reversibly sickled cells became denser when deoxygenated at a pH less than 7.25, a potentially serious change as this would result in an increase in MCHC and enhance the polymerization of Hb S; above pH 7.4 (or if the K^+ concentration was high) reversibly sickled cells maintained a constant density. Fabry and Nagel concluded that as sicklers vary with respect to the distribution of cells amongst density classes this heterogeneity would contribute to diversity in clinical severity.

Fabry and her co-workers (1983, 1984a) subsequently studied the effect of the occurrence of a painful crisis on the density distribution of erythrocytes of 11 Hb-SS patients. In 12 out of 14 crises they observed a reduction in the percentage of dense cells [mostly (60–80%) ISCs, but including deformed cells and dense discocytes, and referred to as fraction IV]: in the two most extreme cases the percentage fell from 36% to 9% and from 43% to 13%, respectively. In six patients studied for up to 14 months during which time they were free from crises, the fraction-IV percentage was steady ±5% in five patients and steady ±7% in the remaining patient. Fabry et al. suggested that during crises dense cells are removed by the R.E. cell system or by selective sequestration in areas of vaso-occlusion or by both mechanisms. Fabry and co-workers (1984b) reported on the influence of α-gene deletion (i.e. the concurrent presence of α-thalassaemia) on the percentage of dense cells (F4) present in 100 Hb-SS patients: αα/αα patients had a higher F4 percentage (mean 24 ± 15%) than −α/αα patients (mean 12 ± 8%): in addition, the percentages of F4 and Hb F were found to be inversely correlated. As the result of a further study of 36 adult Hb-SS patients, Billett and co-workers (1985) reported that the percentage of F4 cells (although a measure of the least rheologically competent cells present) did not predict the incidence of painful crises; they concluded, therefore, that micro-circulatory and other factors were more important in clinical vaso-occlusion.

Weems and Lessin (1984), who employed the phthalate ester micro-capillary tube centrifugation method of Danon and Marikovsky (1964) in a study of 27 Hb-SS patients, came to the same conclusion, namely that although all the patients could be seen to have increased dense fractions these could not be definitely correlated with their clinical state.

Lawrence, Fabry and Nagel (1985) measured the 'red-cell distribution width' (RDW) by means of a Coulter counter in 12 Hb-SS patients during 17 painful crises; they also estimated the proportion of very dense cells present (fraction 4 as separated on a Percoll-Stractan gradient). The two measurements were found to decrease in parallel, and Lawrence, Fabry and Nagel pointed out that the easily obtained RDW could be used as an objective laboratory means of monitoring the course of a painful crisis.

Effect of acute splenic sequestration and hypersplenism on the blood picture

As already mentioned (p. 28), acute splenic

sequestration of erythrocytes associated with rapid enlargement of the spleen is a not uncommon complication in young children with Hb-SS disease. This results in a rapid and sometimes serious fall in the haemoglobin concentration in the peripheral blood. Topley and co-workers (1981) recorded a mean fall of 3.2 g/dl (range 0.8–7.3 g) in 71 episodes affecting West-Indian children. This was associated with a mean increase in reticulocyte count of 10% and a rise in normo-blast count, too. The platelet count averaged $232 \times 10^9/l$ in 13 episodes, a count about half that expected. In chronic hypersplenism platelet counts well below $100 \times 10^9/l$ have been recorded (see p. 28).

Erythrocyte osmotic fragility

This is usually moderately diminished in sickle-cell disease (Diggs, 1932; Diggs and Bibb, 1939), but there may be a small tail of unusually fragile cells. On incubation at 37°C for 24 hours, the majority of the erythrocytes become still more resistant but at the same time the proportion of unusually fragile cells increases. The results are essentially the same whether or not the actual tests are carried out on oxygenated or deoxygenated blood (Harris *et al.*, 1956).

In an interesting report on the OF of sickle-cell anaemia blood after incubation for 24 hours at 37°C, Schroeder, Powars and Chan (1981) stated that if heparin was used as anticoagulant there were three different responses to the incubation. In 17 patients the concentration of saline producing 50% lysis ($NaCl_{50}$) decreased; in 12 patients there was little change, while in 13 patients the $NaCl_{50}$ increased — in the last group the Hb-F percentage was relatively high and the clinical course of the patients' illness appeared to be less severe than that of the patients in the other two groups.

Erythrocyte mechanical fragility

This is significantly raised above the normal when Hb-SS disease blood, equilibrated with room air, is tested. When deoxygenated, the increase in fragility is greater still (Diggs and Bibb, 1939; Ham and Castle, 1940; Shen, Castle and Fleming, 1944; Harris *et al.*, 1956).

Expression of I and i antigens on erythrocytes

As in thalassaemia (p. 411), the Ii antigens are expressed unusually strongly both in Hb-SS disease and in the Hb-AS trait. Maniatis, Frieman and Bertles (1977) used an anti-i serum and two anti-I sera of slightly different specificities and compared the agglu-tinability of the erythrocytes from 36 normal adults, 18 Hb-SS disease patients and 27 Hb-AS trait subjects, using a sensitive, quantitative autoanalyser system. They found that the agglutinability by anti-i of Hb-SS cells was intermediate between that of cord-blood cells and normal adult cells and that of Hb-AS cells was slightly greater than that of the normal cells, with some overlap. The findings using the anti-I sera were similar using an anti-I^F serum, but the differences were not statistically significantly different using an anti-I^D serum. There appeared to be no correlation between the Hb-F content and i reactivity.

In a subsequent study, Maniatis, Papayannopoulou and Bertles (1979) used a technique of single-cell immunofluorescence to determine the expression of Ii antigens and Hb F in 15 Hb-SS patients, in 40 carriers of the Hb-AS trait and in normal adult and newborn controls. In the Hb-SS patients 4.7–51.5% (mean 25.9%) of the erythrocytes reacted with the anti-i serum compared with 1–18% (mean 2.3%) in the Hb-AS carriers and 1–15.5% (mean 2.2%) in the Hb-AA adult controls. Using the anti-I serum the results were: Hb-SS patients, 63–90% (mean 78.1%); Hb-AS carriers 22–95% (mean 59.1%) and in the Hb-AA controls 18–80% (mean 47.3%). The differences between the results with the Hb-SS and Hb-AA cells using both the anti-i and anti-I sera were highly significant. The percentage of Hb-F-reacting cells in 11 Hb-SS patients ranged from 6 to 45%. Most cells reacted with a single antiserum but some reacted doubly, *e.g.* to anti-F and anti-i sera. However, there seemed to be no correlation between the percentages of i- and F-reacting cells. This study on individual cells confirmed that the i and I antigens are both expressed unusually strongly on the surface of Hb-SS erythrocytes.

In a more recent study, Basu and co-workers (1984) have explored the possible mechanism of the increased expression of the I and i antigens on the surface of Hb-SS erythrocytes. Using an immuno-electron-microscopic technique, they were able to demonstrate that both antigens are present at an unusually high density, implying an altered exposure of the transmembrane protein 3 on which the antigens are carried. According to Basu *et al.*, such exposure could be relevant to the accelerated removal of Hb-SS cells from the circulation, for band 3 is thought to be a major participant in the non-immune binding of IgG on erythrocytes (Victoria, Mahan and Masouredis, 1982) and also to be immunologi-cally related to the so-called senescent antigen (Kay *et al.*, 1983).

HAEMOGLOBIN IN HOMOZYGOUS SICKLE-CELL DISEASE

Haemoglobin S

The majority (75–95%) of the haemoglobin in Hb-SS disease is Hb S, with a varying but usually small percentage of Hb F and a normal or slightly raised percentage of Hb A_2; Hb A is absent (Pauling *et al.*, 1949; Wells and Itano, 1951) (Table 13.2, p. 134). This Hb-S plus Hb-F and Hb-A_2 pattern, although very suggestive of (homozygous) Hb-SS disease is not absolutely diagnostic of it, as Hb A may be absent in some cases of Hb-S/thalassaemia, *i.e.* in Hb-S/β^0-thalassaemia. Hb-SD disease and Hb-S/HPFH (hereditary persistence of fetal haemoglobin) also need to be excluded.

Haemoglobin F

Bianco (1948) seems to have been the first to have demonstrated an unusually increased resistance to denaturation by alkali of the haemoglobin in the Hb-AS trait ('falcemia') as well as in one patient with microdrepanocytic disease. Subsequently, in America, following the discovery of Hb S, detailed measurements of fetal-type haemoglobin were carried out in cases of sickle-cell disease by Singer and his collaborators and others (Singer, Chernoff and Singer, 1951; Itano, 1952; Singer and Chernoff, 1952; Singer and Fisher, 1952, 1953; Chernoff, 1953). As in thalassaemia, the conclusion was reached that the fetal-type haemoglobin present was in fact identical with normal Hb F (Chernoff, 1953; Itano, 1953c).

Singer and Fisher (1952) investigated 87 patients who had presented with unquestionable clinical and haematological evidence of sickle-cell disease. The erythrocytes of three of them contained no Hb F by the method used; in the others the proportion ranged from 2 to 24%. Singer and Fisher concluded as the result of transfusion experiments that the erythrocyte population of patients with sickle-cell disease was probably composed of three fractions: cells containing Hb S but little or no Hb F; cells containing Hb S and Hb F, and cells containing Hb F with little or no

Hb S. The corpuscles containing most Hb S had the shortest survival *in vivo* when transfused to normal recipients and the greatest sensitivity to mechanical trauma *in vitro*, and the cells containing most Hb F the longest survival *in vivo* and the greatest resistance to trauma *in vitro*.

Reed, Bradley and Ranney (1965) studied the effect of the amelioration of anaemia on the synthesis of Hb F in sickle-cell disease. Two Hb-SS patients (group-A and group-A_2B) were transfused with compatible group-O normal blood so as to maintain near normal haemoglobin levels over a 4-month period. The mean Hb-F percentage in the haemoglobin within the recipients' erythrocytes was measured from time to time after separating the cells by differential agglutination: it rose initially and then declined to pre-transfusion levels, but it did not disappear. These experiments confirmed the supposition that cells containing Hb F circulate for relatively long periods and also that controlling anaemia did not stop Hb F from being formed.

Later work (see below) has largely confirmed the correctness of the measurements of Hb F carried out in the early 1950s. There are, however, some interesting ethnically based differences. The age of the patient has, too, an important effect, the percentage being very high soon after birth and then declining (Fig. 12.15); it stabilizes after about 6 years. The level finally achieved differs quite widely from patient to patient, and there is some evidence that genetic factors influence this (see p. 89). There is also evidence that the higher the Hb-F level the less severely affected the patient is likely to be (see p. 48).

Heterogeneous distribution of Hb F. Shepard, Weatherall and Conley (1962), using the method of Betke and Kleihauer (1958), established that Hb F was heterogeneously distributed in the erythrocytes in Hb-SS disease, in contrast to its homogeneous distribution in hereditary persistence of fetal haemoglobin (HPFH). Eight patients were examined in whom the proportion of Hb F varied from 1.5 to 21% of the total haemoglobin present. In the cases in which the Hb-F concentration exceeded 7%, some cells stained darkly, some palely and most stained within a broad range of intermediate densities.

Variation in Hb-F percentage: patient-to-patient differences. Bickers (1966) recorded Hb-F levels of 3.1–13.6% in 62 patients with Hb-SS, aged 5–42 years.

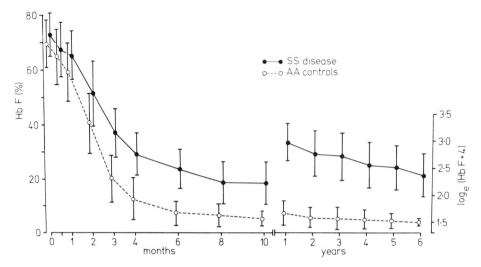

Fig. 12.15 Fall in Hb-F percentage according to age in a series of 266 Hb-SS newborns matched with 243 Hb-AA controls born on the same day.
Jamaican data. [Reproduced by permission from Mason *et al.* (1982).]

The proportion of males over the age of 15 years who had high levels was smaller than that of females of comparable age, and the suggestion was made that males tended to cease forming excessive amounts of Hb F after puberty.

Huisman and co-workers (1972) reported on Hb-F (and Hb-A₂) percentages in 58 patients considered to have Hb-SS disease. The majority of the patients were American blacks. In all but nine of them the Hb-F percentage exceeded 2%; the range was 0.5–33%, the highest value being in an Arab boy aged 10. (Three other Arab patients had high values of 9.5, 18 and 30%, respectively.) Up to the age of 20 years, the percentages tended to decrease with age, and six females between the ages of 20 and 47 had higher values than eight males in the same age-group. Wrightstone and Huisman (1974) recorded similar Hb-F percentages: 0.6–19.8% (mean 6.6%) in 120 Hb-SS black Americans, 5 years of age and older, and 17.5–28.0% in four Hb-SS Arabs.

Serjeant's (1974) estimates were based on 414 Jamaican patients, 221 females and 193 males. The mean for the whole group was 5.58 ± 3.6% and the levels were higher in the females (mean 6.05 ± 3.9%) than in the males (mean 4.93 ± 1.95%). There appeared, however, to be no significant differences between the two sexes until after puberty, after which the levels in the females were generally higher, as had been observed by Bickers (1966) (see above).

Post-natal decline in Hb-F percentage. Davis (1976) studied 75 Hb-SS infants and children in London: they were aged between 4 days and 16 years and 174 blood samples were collected from

them within a 3-year period. Davis found that the high Hb-F percentages present in the first few months of life fell to a mean value of 13.8% by the end of the first year and fell more gradually subsequently: the mean at 10 years was 6.38% and that between 12 and 16 years 5.13%.

Mason and co-workers (1982) provided detailed data on the extent and rapidity of the post-natal decline in the Hb-F percentage in Hb-S homozygotes. Their study was based on 266 Hb-SS and 243 Hb-AA infants who were unselected and who were observed on a regular follow-up basis, not just when admitted to hospital. The largest part of the fall in post-natal Hb-F percentage was found to occur during the first year. No sex difference was obvious in the Hb-SS children, although in the Hb-AA children the levels were slightly higher in females.

Hb-F percentage and clinical severity. Serjeant (1975) reported that the Hb-F level in patients with Hb-SS disease was inversely correlated with the percentage of irreversibly sickled cells (ISCs) present. Both measurements, however, varied widely in individual patients — from 1 to 20% Hb F and from 0 to 40% ISCs. Dover and coworkers (1978) pointed out that the above inverse correlation applied only to the 30% or so of patients with Hb F in excess of 7%. They stressed that the whole-blood Hb-F level reflected the result of three independent processes: the proportion of cells forming Hb F, the amount produced by the Hb-F-producing cells and the possible preferential survival of Hb-F-containing cells. They made the point, too, that scarcely two patients are alike and that it was this heterogeneity which explains the paradox that Hb F protects against irreversible sickling (and cell destruction), yet at low levels the whole-blood Hb-F percentage is not well correlated with the number of ISCs present.

Pembrey and co-workers (1978) gave details of Hb-F percentages in 237 Hb-SS Arabs living in the oases of Eastern Saudi Arabia. The mean Hb-F percentage and percentage of F cells were far higher, 25.56 and 33–98, respectively, than in the black African Hb-SS population in the New World. The percentage of Hb F in AS and AA subjects was, in contrast, similar to that of American blacks. The distribution of Hb F was heterocellular and the high Hb-F levels did not seem to be associated with the presence of α-thalassaemia, HPFH or G6PD deficiency, although it seemed probable that the high levels were genetically determined. The degree of haemolysis, as indicated by the reticulocyte count, and the Hb-F percentage appeared to be inversely correlated.

Further evidence supporting the concept that a high Hb-F level helps to protect a Hb-SS individual from the worst consequences of his illness was provided by Stevens et al. (1981). One hundred and forty-six children were followed at intervals from birth up to 2 years of age and when each child was 6 months old its Hb-F percentage was estimated; this ranged from 5 to 45. The mean Hb-F level was found to be relatively low in children with early palpable splenomegaly, in those who suffered from dactylitis, in those who developed acute splenic sequestration and in those who died before reaching 2 years of age.

Effect of Hb-F concentration on erythrocyte indices. Milner and co-workers (1986) reported on the effect of Hb F (and α-thalassaemia) on erythrocyte indices in a series of 102 American black patients with Hb-SS disease. Irrespective of α-globin genotype, patients with high Hb-F levels (>10 g/l) had higher mean haematocrit, total haemoglobin, MCV and MCH than the patients with low Hb-F levels (<10 g/l). In patients without α-thalassaemia the Hb-F concentration was positively correlated with the MCV and MCH;

those with high levels of Hb F had macrocytosis (mean MCV 99.7 ± 6.2 fl).

Genetic control of Hb-F percentage. Recent studies have provided firm evidence that genetic influences are responsible for the unusually high levels of Hb F that persist after infancy in individual Hb-SS patients and in certain ethnic groups.

Dover, Boyer and Pembrey (1981) reported that the percentage of Hb-F-containing reticulocytes is closely correlated in Hb-SS sibling pairs and also that the F-cell levels in parents and the F-reticulocyte levels in their children are similarly correlated; they concluded that the same genes regulate F-cell-production in non-anaemic persons as in their anaemic children.

Mason and co-workers (1982) observed that the rate of decline in the Hb-F percentage during the first 6 years of the life of Hb-SS children was related to the Hb-F percentages in their parents: their data indicated that a high parental Hb-F level always determined a high level in their children.

Milner and co-workers (1984) concluded that a high Hb-F percentage in a Hb-SS child is determined by a factor linked to the β^S gene of one parent. Twenty Hb-SS patients, members of seven large families, had relatively high Hb-F percentages: in five of the families one Hb-AS parent had a much higher Hb-F percentage and F-cell count than the other; in one family both parents had high values, and in the remaining family both parents had borderline values. Seven of 14 Hb-AS siblings, but only one of eight normal Hb-AA siblings, had Hb-F percentages and F-cell counts above the normal range.

The data of Boyer et al. (1984), however, pointed to the existence of genes affecting between-patient differences in Hb-F percentages that are separate from the β-globin gene cluster. They had contrasted the percentage of Hb-F-bearing reticulocytes in 59 Hb-SS sib pairs, 40 resident in Jamaica and 19 in the United States. The percentage of F reticulocytes varied from 2 to 50. While in many instances the percentages were comparable in the pairs, in 12 Jamaican and three American sibships there were major differences. Miller and co-workers (1984, 1986) approached the problem from a different angle. They prepared cultures from the peripheral blood of Saudi-Arabian Hb-SS patients and their parents, and measured Hb-F production in BFUE. Mean Hb-F production per erythroblast was significantly higher in the Saudi patients than in a control series of erythroblasts derived from cultures prepared from American patients. Furthermore, the data indicated that the high Saudi Hb-F production was inherited from at least one parent despite low levels of Hb-F in the parent's peripheral blood. Analysis of DNA polymorphism within the β-globin gene cluster on chromosome 11 provided further evidence of a genetic influence, for a distinctive haplotype was found on at least one chromosome of all the Hb-SS and Hb-AS patients tested who had high Hb-F percentages.

Wainscoat and co-workers' (1985) Jamaican data have also provided an interesting insight into the molecular-genetic basis of high Hb-F levels. Ten Hb-SS patients, members of the same family, had unusually high Hb-F percentages, namely, 9.3 to 23.6. Each patient was found to possess a chromosome characterized by a β-gene cluster haplotype which is very rare in Jamaicans. The particular interest of this finding is that this haplotype is the one that is common in Hb-SS patients in Eastern Saudi Arabia where a high Hb-F level is the rule rather than the exception (see above). Wainscoat *et al.* suggested that the haplotype could be taken as a genetic marker for high Hb-F production.

Heterogeneity of the γ chain of Hb F

Huisman and co-workers (1972) reported on the chemical heterogeneity of Hb F in a variety of haemoglobin disorders. In 70% of the Hb-SS patients they had studied the $^G\gamma:^A\gamma$ ratio was between 2:3 and 1:1, a range similar to that for the traces of Hb F found in the blood of normal Hb-AA adults. Twelve Hb-SS patients had a higher ratio, approximately 3:1, similar to that of the Hb F of the normal newborn; eight patients had intermediate values. The results of a subsequent study of Hb-SS patients, and Hb-S heterozygotes, were detailed by Gardiner *et al.* in 1982. Both genotypes could be separated into two groups, a low $^G\gamma$ group (40% of $^G\gamma$ chains) and a high $^G\gamma$ group (60% of $^G\gamma$ chains). It seemed as if the normal switch from the newborn $^G\gamma:^A\gamma$ ratio of 7:3 to the adult value of 4:6 had failed to take place in approximately 22% of homozygotes or heterozygotes for Hb S resident in Georgia.

Glycosylated haemoglobin

As already referred to (Vol. 1, p. 23), haemoglobin reacts normally with glucose to form a series of minor (Hb A_1) components, the levels of which are apparently decreased in association with increased haemolysis. Elseweidy and Abraham (1984) studied 29 patients with Hb-SS disease as well as patients suffering from Hb-SC disease or Hb-S/β-thalassaemia. The mean glycosylated haemoglobin (GHb) percentage was significantly less

than normal in the Hb-SS patients but normal in the other two groups. Within each group, however, the Hb-F and the GHb percentages were directly correlated, and a similar relationship between Hb-F and GHb percentages was found when the measurements were made on erythrocyte populations separated according to densities. Elseweidy and Abraham suggested that Hb F influences the extent of glycosylation through its effect on erythrocyte survival, *i.e.* by the cells with high Hb-F levels having a relatively long life-span. The subsequent data of Alayash *et al.* (1986) are consistent with this conclusion: they had studied 30 Hb-SS patients from the Eastern Province of Saudi Arabia whose disease was generally mild. The mean Hb-F percentage in these patients was 12.0 ± 4.8 and the mean GHb percentage 4.36 ± 0.83, a figure that was approximately 90% of that of a control Hb-AA Saudi population whose mean Hb-F percentage was 0.8 and mean GHb percentage 4.85 ± 0.51.

Haemoglobin A_2

Hb-A_2 levels are within the normal range or slightly elevated in Hb-SS disease. They are affected significantly by concurrent iron deficiency, which lowers the percentage slightly, or by the presence of α-thalassaemia which raises the level (Fig. 13.7, p. 141).

Serjeant, Mason and Serjeant (1978) reported on a large study which included 160 Hb-SS infants. The Hb-A_2 percentage climbed steadily from the low levels present at birth in an identical fashion in Hb-SS and normal infants; the percentage reached slightly more than 2% on average at 1 year of age and remained at that level thereafter. Hayes and co-workers (1985) found that the Hb-A_2 levels remained unchanged in patients aged between 5 and 66 years. The mean was 2.95% in males and the level throughout was slightly (approximately 0.1%) higher in males than in females. Huisman and co-workers (1972) and Wrightstone and Huisman (1974) had earlier reported (in a much smaller series of black Americans) slightly raised levels in both Hb-SS and Hb-AS subjects, the majority of their figures being above their upper limit of normal (3.0%).

OXYGEN AFFINITY OF THE ERYTHROCYTES

Patients with sickle-cell disease have blood with decreased O_2 affinity, *i.e.* the O_2-dissociation curve is displaced to the right (Becklake *et al.*, 1955; Fraimow *et al.*, 1958; Rodman *et al.*, 1959; Bromberg, Jensen and McDonough, 1967; Cawein *et al.*, 1969; Charache *et al.*, 1970; Sinet and Pocidalo, 1981) (see Vol. 1, Fig. 2.5). The O_2 affinity of purified Hb S is, however, the same as that of Hb A (Allen and Wyman, 1954).

Bromberg, Jensen and McDonough (1967) studied 22 patients with Hb-SS disease: in all but three of them the $p_{50}O_2$ at pH 7.4 and 37°C (25–42 mm Hg) was greater than the normal mean (25.2 mm Hg) + 2 SD. The $p_{50}O_2$ and total haemoglobin present and the $p_{50}O_2$ and Hb-F percentage were both inversely correlated.

According to Charache and co-workers (1970), although Hb-SS erythrocytes contain more 2,3-DPG than normal, this increase is by itself insufficient to explain the decreased O_2 affinity. They suggested that other organic phosphates as well as inorganic ions, and also perhaps the state of aggregation of the haemoglobin molecule, play a part in this. From the patient's point of view, decreased O_2 affinity is helpful as it facilitates transmission of oxygen from the blood to the tissues but it is harmful, too, in that it promotes sickling.

Seakins and co-workers (1973) also found in 15 patients no correlation between $p_{50}O_2$ and 2,3-DPG concentration. A strong correlation was, however, demonstrated between $p_{50}O_2$ and MCHC, *i.e.* the largest right-shifts in the O_2-dissociation curve were associated with the highest MCHCs, as found in irreversibly sickled cells. As is well recognized (see Vol. 1, p. 19), 2,3-DPG levels *do* influence the O_2-dissociation curve of haemoglobin. Experimentally, too, it can be shown that at any given O_2 tension more Hb-S-containing cells sickle if the 2,3-DPG concentration is increased, and *vice versa*. According to Jensen *et al.* (1973), however, the enhancement of sickling by 2,3-DPG is in part independent of its influence on the O_2 affinity of haemoglobin.

Milner (1974) reviewed the whole problem of oxygen transport in Hb-SS disease and discussed the possibility of controlling sickling by shifting the dissociation curve to the left (see p. 254).

According to May and Huehns (1975), polymerization of reduced Hb S and a high haemoglobin concentration are mainly responsible for the low oxygen affinity of Hb-SS cells. Rossi-Bernardi and co-workers (1975) similarly concluded that the marked right-shift in the O_2-dissociation curve was not due to an effect of pH, pCO_2 or 2,3-DPG content or to an intrinsically altered O_2 affinity of Hb S; the most likely explanation was considered to be the presence within the cell of aggregates of deoxygenated Hb-S molecules.

Ueda, Nagel and Bookchin (1979) reported that the Bohr effect — a shift in O_2 equilibrium with change in pH — is increased in sickle-cell anaemia. This would result in an unusually large decrease in oxygen affinity as the erythrocytes traverse capillaries servicing actively metabolizing tissue, increasing the risk of the cells sickling.

FERROKINETICS AND ERYTHROKINETICS

Ranney and Kono (1959) administered ^{59}Fe to three patients with the Hb-S trait and found that the rate of incorporation of the radio-iron into the Hb-S and Hb-A components of their haemoglobin was approximately the same.

There is no evidence, too, that erythropoiesis itself is ineffective in uncomplicated Hb-SS disease. According to Finch (1972), the mean erythrocyte production rate in a series of 20 Hb-SS patients was 4–5 times the normal and the plasma iron turnover 2–9 times the normal. The mean plasma iron level was 118 $\mu g/dl$. The above findings were found to be almost exactly the same as those in a series of 15 patients with hereditary spherocytosis.

LEUCOCYTES

The leucocyte count is usually raised above the normal in Hb-SS disease (Diggs, 1932; Boggs, Hyde and Srodes, 1973); it may reach $20–30 \times 10^9/l$ or even higher when haemolysis is active or in association with painful crises. The leucocytosis is then chiefly due to an increase in polymorphonuclears, associated with a slight or moderate shift to the left; a few myelocytes may be present (Diggs, 1932).

The occurrence of splenic atrophy probably plays a part in raising the total count.

Boggs, Hyde and Srodes (1973) used DF[32]P to study granulocyte kinetics in eight Hb-SS patients, none of whom were in crisis or had suffered recently from a crisis. The size of the circulating granulocyte pool was high normal or abnormally high in all the patients. The total pool was, however, not increased to the same extent, suggesting a shift from marginated to circulating granulocytes. The half-disappearance time of the granulocytes was unusually short, indicating an increased granulocyte turnover rate.

Buchanan and Glader (1978) reported a detailed study of leucocyte counts in children with various types of sickle-cell disease, with particular reference to differences in the neutrophil response to vaso-occlusive crises and bacterial infections. Their patients included 55 children with Hb-SS disease in a steady state, 35 in vaso-occlusive crises and 16 with acute bacterial infections. The total counts were 7.4–20.6 (mean 12.3) $\times 10^9/l$ in the steady-state children, 9.4–36.0 (mean 16.4) $\times 10^9/l$ in the vaso-occlusive children, and 5.5–44.8 (mean 22.0) $\times 10^9/l$ in the bacterial-infection children. An important difference between the vaso-occlusive and infection groups was that only in the latter were the numbers of non-segmented neutrophils markedly raised. Their presence in large numbers (0.27–12.0, mean $4.58 \times 10^9/l$) was held to be a valuable pointer to acute infection.

Occasionally many normoblasts are present in the peripheral blood — perhaps particularly in association with bone-marrow infarction or in pulmonary infarction, and in such cases they may comprise a substantial proportion of the total 'leucocyte' count.

Leucocyte (neutrophil) alkaline phosphatase (LAP or NAP)

Wajima and Krauss (1968) reported that LAP activity might be subnormal in sickle-cell disease. Thirteen Hb-SS patients with normal total leucocyte counts had LAP scores slightly but not significantly less than those of normal Hb-AA controls. Remarkably, the scores were found not to increase in association with leucocytoses of 10–20 $\times 10^9/l$, irrespective of whether the patients were in steady state or in a painful crisis. This contrasted with the substantial increase in score observed in a series of tuberculous patients who had developed leucocytoses.

Wajima and Kraus's interesting finding was confirmed by Rosner and Karayalcin (1974), who found that the mean score in 50 Hb-SS patients was 41 ± 34 Kaplan units, compared with 68 ± 54 units in 50 Hb-AS individuals and 71 ± 52 units in 50 Hb-SS controls. None of their patients was, however, in crisis at the time the tests were carried out. The question of response to vaso-occlusive crisis and infection was, however, considered by Wajima and Kraus (1975), who studied 41 sickle-cell anaemia patients. The LAP scores were found to be normal or subnormal irrespective of whether the patients were in steady state or in crisis; the scores, however, rose in the presence of infection.

Rosenbloom, Odell and Tanaka (1980), who were dealing primarily with pituitary-adrenal axis function in sickle-cell anaemia, studied eight patients in and out of crisis: their LAP scores were on the low side and did not increase in the crises. No explanation for the low LAP scores and their failure to respond to stressful situations, except infection, seems to be forthcoming.

Nitroblue tetrazolium (NBT) test. Walters and Reddy (1974) assessed the value of the NBT test as a possible means of differentiating between thrombotic crises and infections. The percentage of reacting polymorphonuclears was approximately the same in 24 Hb-SS patients not in crisis as in 22 patients in crisis. However, the percentages increased substantially in patients with pneumonia or septicaemia. Wajima's (1975) results were, however, different. Based on a study of 44 patients, he concluded that the NBT test did *not* differentiate between patients with or without infection. The patients generally had low base-line NBT positivity and their polymorphonuclears responded poorly to in-vitro stimulation. It was suggested that the failure to respond was linked to impaired neutrophil function and a defective complement system (see p. 43).

PLATELETS

The platelet count is commonly significantly raised in Hb-SS disease patients in a steady state, probably partly in consequence of splenic atrophy. Mean counts between $320 \times 10^9/l$ and $473 \times 10^9/l$ have been recorded (Diggs, 1932; Green, Kwaan and Duiz, 1970; Haut, Cowan and Harris, 1973; Freedman and Karpatkin, 1975; Leslie et al., 1975; Kenny, George and Stuart, 1980). Thrombocytopenia has, however, been reported in association with massive splenomegaly (see p. 28). Platelet survival has been shown to be normal or greater than normal in steady-state patients but less than normal in patients in crisis.

Haut, Cowan and Harris (1973) measured by a ^{51}Cr technique the survival of autologous platelets in the circulation of seven sickle-cell disease patients (five Hb SS) and found that the survival was normal or even above normal (mean life-span 10.1 ± 0.6 days) during an uncomplicated phase of their illness; during a crisis in three patients, the survival was found, however, to be reduced to approximately one-third (mean life-span 3.2 ± 0.3 days).

Haut, Cowan and Harris (1973) calculated that in patients with sickle-cell disease who were not in crisis the production of platelets was normal or raised to about 1.5 times the normal and that in those in crisis it was raised to 2–3 times the normal. Platelets derived from patients not in crisis or during crisis were found to be normally aggregable by ADP or thrombin. In contrast, platelets obtained during a post-crisis thrombocytosis were hyperaggregable, perhaps because of the presence of many young platelets.

Freedman and Karpatkin (1975) found that the

megathrombocyte count (as estimated in a Coulter Counter) in eight adult Hb-SS asymptomatic patients was 2–3 times the normal. They suggested that this was due to lack of splenic sequestration. During three crises in two of the patients the count, however, fell significantly.

van der Sar (1970) reported that the platelet count might rise to very high levels and even exceed $1000 \times 10^9/l$ following recovery from an aplastic crisis. Rises to $850 \times 10^9/l$ and to more than $1000 \times 10^9/l$ were observed in patients with an infarctive bone crisis and a pulmonary infarct, respectively.

Platelet aggregation. The question of significant changes in platelet aggregation in sickle-cell disease is controversial, perhaps because of differences in the techniques employed by different observers, genuine variability between patients and the varying activity of their disease at the time the measurements were carried out.

Gruppo and co-workers (1977) carried out tests of platelet function serially in 13 patients with sickle-cell disease and found evidence of impaired aggregation in the presence of epinephrine, ADP and collagen in four of them tested during a painful crisis and in almost half of them tested when they were free of symptoms.

Kenny, George and Stuart (1980) reported on the tests of platelet function they had carried out in 16 patients, aged between 15 and 42 years, who were in a steady state — 12 were Hb SS, three Hb-S/β-thalassaemia and one Hb SC. A lower than normal aggregation threshold with ADP was demonstrated as well as a significant increase in microaggregate formation. The results in 12 splenectomized Hb-AA patients, however, were similar, and Kenny, George and Stuart concluded that the platelet hyperactivity *in vitro* that they had demonstrated, and the increased microaggregate formation *in vivo*, were the consequences of the presence in the circulation of a young metabolically active platelet population which in the Hb-SS patients was one of the consequences of autosplenectomy; it reflected in their view the absence of splenic pooling of young active platelets rather than chronic intravascular activation of platelets in the microcirculation. They conceded, however, that the increased number of active platelets in the circulation could lead to aggregation in areas of stasis during vaso-occlusive crises.

Mehta and Mehta (1980) studied a younger Hb-SS population, aged between 6 and 17 years. They found that the aggregation responses to epinephrine and ADP were subnormal irrespective of whether the patients were in a steady state or were suffering or recovering from a vaso-occlusive crisis. The percentage of circulating platelet aggregates was normal in the steady-state patients but was markedly increased in five out of six of the patients in crisis. Recovery from their crises was associated with a decline in the percentage of platelet aggregates. Mehta and Mehta concluded that in-vivo activation may result in the circulation of 'tired' platelets (as the result of endogenous activation) that had become refractory to stimulation by epinephrine or ADP.

Mehta (1980) reported on plasma β-thromboglobulin (β-TG) levels in a series of Hb-SS children, aged between 6 and 18 years: 19 were in steady state, five had pneumonia and five had acute bone pain attributed to vaso-occlusion. The β-TG (a protein released from the α-granules of platelets as a result, it is thought, of platelet activation) was measured by radio-immune assay. The mean level in the steady-state patients was significantly higher than that in a control series of 12 age-matched normal children, but there was considerable overlap and most of the results were within the normal range; three of the children with pneumonia and four of the children in crisis gave results well above normal. Platelet aggregation *in vitro* with epinephrine and ADP was found (as before) to be subnormal in all three groups of patients and not to be influenced by their clinical state. The above data indicate that plasma β-TG levels are increased in a minority of Hb-SS patients in a steady state; they were substantially higher than normal in the majority of the small series of patients with infections or in vaso-occlusive crisis. Mehta came to the conclusion that platelets were being activated in Hb-SS patients even in steady state and that this explained the decreased in-vitro aggregability that she had demonstrated.

Buchanan and Holtkamp (1983), who measured by radio-immune assay the plasma concentrations of β-thromboglobulin (β-TG) and platelet factor 4 (PT_4) in 43 Hb-SS patients, aged between 1 year and 17 years, in a steady state and in 24 patients in severe vaso-occlusive crisis, concluded, however, as the result of their own observations that platelet activation *in vivo* in Hb-SS children is minimal or at least not greatly enhanced. They found that the β-TG levels tended to be higher than normal in the steady-state patients but did not rise significantly during crises; the PT_4 levels were within the normal range in most of the patients in a steady state (although higher than normal in a minority) and normal, too, in most of those who were in crisis. The ratios of plasma β-TG to PF_4, thought to reflect in-vivo activation of platelets better than the absolute concentration of each protein, were not significantly different in either group of patients from the ratios in the controls. Platelet 5-hydroxytryptamine (5-HT) was also estimated and found to be the same in the two groups of patients as in the controls.

Further evidence in favour of in-vivo platelet activation was reported by Westwick et al. (1983). Compared with normal controls matched for age, sex and race, the number of platelets circulating as aggregates and the plasma β-thromboglobulin and platelet factor-4 levels were significantly raised in seven Hb-SS patients in steady state studied at least twice during a 6-week period. *In vitro*, the patients' platelets aggregated more in response to low doses of ADP and needed more prostacyclin to inhibit ADP-induced aggregation than did control platelets.

Harbury (1984) suggested that during crises platelets become activated by ADP and ATP leaking from damaged erythrocytes and concluded that activated platelets contribute to the solidity of the partial vascular obstruction brought about by sickling.

COAGULATION AND FIBRINOLYSIS

Interesting abnormalities have been reported, and there is evidence indicating mild continued activation of the coagulation and fibrinolytic systems in sickle-cell disease patients in a quiescent steady state and increased activation in patients suffering from vaso-occlusive crises or infections (Henstell, Kligerman and Irwin, 1965; Abildgaard, Simone and Schulman, 1967; Mahmood, Macintosh and Shaper, 1967; Green, Kwaan and Duiz, 1970; Mattii, Weinger and Sise, 1973; Gordon *et al.*, 1974; Rickles and O'Leary, 1974; Leslie *et al.*, 1975; Stathakis *et al.*, 1975; Alkjaersig *et al.*, 1976; Ittyerah *et al.*, 1976; Leichtman and Brewer, 1978; Richardson *et al.*, 1979; Sarji *et al.*, 1979) (see also p. 220 under *Pathogenesis*).

Henstell, Kligerman and Irwin (1965) studied 39 patients, 24 with Hb SS and 15 with Hb AS or Hb SC. There appeared to be a defect in the serum component in the thromboplastin generation test in all the Hb-SS patients and in four of the 15 heterozygotes. This could not be accounted for by deficiencies of factors IX, X, XI or XII, and excess anti-thrombin activity was postulated.

Abildgaard, Simone and Schulman (1967) studied 30 children with Hb-SS disease and found that their mean factor-VIII level was 2.34 times the normal (range 0.69–8.0). The results in six patients in painful crisis did not differ from those of the majority who were in a quiescent phase of their disease. Transfusions were found to be followed by a lowering of the factor-VIII levels, and it was suggested that this was brought about by reducing the rate of haemolysis. No explanation for the raised factor-VIII activity was forthcoming and its relationship, if any, with the thrombotic and vaso-occlusive phenomena of sickle-cell disease was thought to be speculative.

Mahmood, Macintosh and Shaper (1967) studied 13 Hb-SS disease children in crisis and found that their dilute blood-clot lysis times were prolonged compared

with normal controls and with patients with Hb-SS disease who had mild symptoms and did not require admission to hospital; in seven of the 13 children the lysis time exceeded 24 hours. The question was posed (but not answered) as to whether the lengthened lysis times were connected with the genesis of the crises or were a consequence of the crises.

Green, Kwaan and Duiz (1970) also reported reductions in plasma fibrinolytic activity, and it was suggested that this might have resulted from intravascular sickling leading to endothelial damage and decreased production of plasminogen activator.

Mattii, Weinger and Sise (1973) reported on 16 patients: four were Hb SS, four Hb SC and one Hb-S/thalassaemia. Fibrin split products (FDP) were detected in increased amounts in two out of 22 samples from patients not in crisis and in two out of nine samples from patients in crisis. Fibrinogen turnover was, nevertheless, found to be shortened in all five patients studied in crisis and in all seven studied out of crisis. The findings were thought to be suggestive of chronic disseminated intravascular coagulation (DIC), but the generally low values for FDP were notable and unexplained.

Gordon and co-workers (1974) found that the response of fibrinolytic activity to exercise and local heating was normal in 38 children with sickle-cell disease, all studied in asymptomatic periods; 23 had Hb SS. The fibrinogen concentration was observed to rise in crises; the platelet count, however, tended to fall and this was attributed to local vascular trapping of platelets and the sequestration by the spleen of damaged platelets. They considered that there was no evidence of DIC.

Rickles and O'Leary (1974) compared platelet counts, factor-VIII activity and plasma fibrinolytic activity in sickle-cell disease patients in steady asymptomatic state, in crisis and when suffering from an infection. The platelet count was raised in all three states as was factor-VIII activity (to the greatest extent in patients in crisis); the euglobulin lysis time was delayed in crises and markedly delayed in infected patients, but was normal in asymptomatic patients. Rickles and O'Leary concluded that what they had observed, and the changes that had been recorded in the literature, were secondary phenomena consequent on occlusion of small blood vessels and the resultant damage to their endothelial cell lining.

Leslie and co-workers (1975) studied 117 Jamaican patients with Hb-SS disease in steady state and 40 normal controls. They had higher than normal factor-VIII levels and platelet counts, shorter thrombin times, lower factor-V and plasminogen levels and raised levels of fibrin degradation products (FDP). The fibrinogen levels were normal. The data (excluding the high factor-VIII levels) were thought to indicate continuous activation of the coagulation and fibrinolytic systems, even in the absence of painful crises.

Alkjaersig and co-workers (1976) reported on three

patients who had been studied weekly for 1½–2 years. In crisis there was evidence of intravascular fibrin formation and fluctuation in platelet numbers. At the onset of a crisis, or just before, there was an increase in high mol. wt. fibrinogen complexes which reached a peak 2–3 times the original level at approximately 1 week from the start of the crisis. The subsidence of a crisis was associated with a fall in high mol. wt. fibrinogen complexes and an increase in fibrinogen first derivative (an early breakdown product). The platelet count fell at the onset of a crisis, only to rise again to 2–3 times its original level about 2 weeks later. During asymptomatic periods the findings were approximately normal.

Ittyerah and co-workers (1976) assayed the factor-XIII concentration in the plasma in four Hb-SS patients over a 1½–2-year period during which time they experi-

enced several painful crises. During steady state the factor-XIII level tended to be subnormal; it fell further at the onset of a crisis, only to rise substantially following resolution of the crisis (Fig. 12.16). The changes were interpreted as supporting the concept that in the early stages of a crisis fibrin deposition and/or thrombosis occur and enhance the role of sickled erythrocytes in leading to vascular occlusion and organ infarction.

Leichtman and Brewer (1978) provided further evidence of intravascular coagulation during painful crises in Hb-SS patients. They measured fibrinopeptide A (FPA) levels — an indicator of in-vivo thrombin activity — in 21 plasma samples obtained from eight sickle-cell anaemia patients during painful crises and found the levels to be more than 4 SD above the normal mean value. In contrast, the FPA levels in seven out of 10 samples derived from 10 patients during pain-free periods were normal. They suggested that it was platelet activation, as the result of the exposure of subendothelial structures following endothelial damage induced by sickled erythrocytes, that acted as the trigger for low-grade and localized intravascular coagulation.

Sarji and co-workers (1979), who studied Hb-SS patients who were not in crisis, found that both the antigen and procoagulant activities of factor VIII were significantly above normal. They also found that the aggregation of platelets by ADP, epinephrine or collagen was decreased and that aggregation by ristocetin was absent or preceded by a lag phase.

Richardson and co-workers (1979) concluded that the platelet activation, hypercoagulability and hyperviscosity that occurred during painful crises in sickle-cell disease were secondary changes arising from vascular stasis, the precipitating infection, if present, and an acute-phase protein reaction. Although secondary, the changes might, in their view, contribute to vascular occlusion in vessels already partially occluded by sickled cells. They studied in great detail seven patients with Hb SS and one with Hb-S/thalassaemia. When in steady state the patients were found to have increased factor-VIII and plasma heparin-neutralizing activity, raised anti-thrombin III and increased blood viscosity, but reduced factor-V activity. Nine episodes of painful crises were followed closely: on the first day plasma fibrinogen and whole-blood viscosity were significantly raised, and this was followed over the next 2 days by a fall in platelet count. Evidence of coagulation activation during the first 3 days of the crisis was provided by a further rise in plasma fibrinogen, elevated cryofibrinogen and a fall in anti-thrombin III activity. The rise in fibrinogen became maximal on the 4th–5th day of the crises and blood viscosity reached its peak on the 6th–8th day. A rebound rise in platelet count occurred on the 9th–14th day. Richardson et al. made the important point that a very similar sequence of changes occurred in a series of 20 white Hb-AA patients whom they had studied during localized bacterial or viral infections.

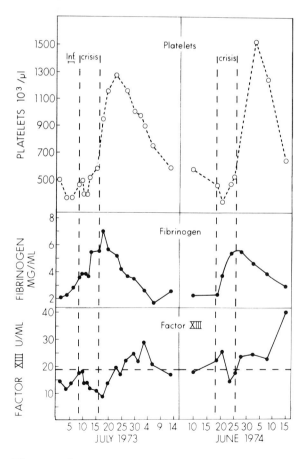

Fig. 12.16 Changes in platelet count, fibrinogen concentration and factor-XIII activity accompanying two vaso-occlusive crises in a patient suffering from sickle-cell disease.

[Reproduced by permission from Ittyerah et al. (1976).]

MISCELLANEOUS BIOCHEMICAL CHANGES

Plasma bilirubin

Most Hb-SS disease patients are jaundiced. According to Serjeant (1974, p 87) the mean total bilirubin level was 3.1 mg/dl in 410 patients in a steady state; 28.3% of the patients, however, had less than 2 mg/dl and were not clinically jaundiced. Age and sex did not appear to influence the level. Most of the bilirubin is unconjugated. Henderson (1950) had stressed, however, the frequency with which direct-reacting pigment can be demonstrated: the direct test was positive in 20 out of 51 samples, the highest values being found in patients with the largest and most tender livers. As already referred to on page 30, pigment gall-stones are commonly formed; occasionally they cause obstruction to the flow of bile, and deep jaundice may result from this.

Plasma proteins

According to Fenichel, Watson and Eirich (1950), abnormalities in the plasma protein pattern are frequently found. Thirteen out of 15 patients with sickle-cell disease had decreased concentrations of albumin, 12 had elevated γ-globulin concentrations and three raised concentrations of β globulin. The plasma fibrinogen level was high in eight out of 10 of these patients. It was suggested that the changes might be non-specific reactions secondary to tissue breakdown and that this occurred particularly in the liver as the result of vascular obstruction due to sickling.

Similar studies were carried out by Allamanis (1955). In infants less than 2 years of age the plasma proteins were usually normal. In older children the concentrations of albumin and α_1, α_2 and β globulins were found to be decreased and that of γ globulin was increased.

Robinson and Sathiapalan (1965) reported that they had failed to find in 26 children with Hb-SS disease living in New York any excess of cryoprecipitable plasma proteins, irrespective of whether the children were in crisis.

Evans and Reindorf (1968) measured serum immunoglobulin levels in 24 children and 15 adults with sickle-cell disease living in New York. IgG, IgM and IgA levels were normal in children less than 4 years of age, but they were all elevated in older children. IgA levels were marginally raised in adults. The raised concentrations were thought to be determined by liver disease or infections.

Gavrilis, Rothenberg and Guy (1974) reported on serum IgG levels in 21 adult patients with sickle-cell disease (13 Hb SS, six Hb SC and two Hb-S/thalassaemia). The IgG levels were moderately raised and the IgA levels markedly so. The IgM levels were variable, and in cases in which the spleen was small, or after splenectomy (1 case), the levels were subnormal.

Plasma haem pigments

As is discussed on page 225, there is every reason to believe that erythrocyte destruction takes place in sickle-cell disease in many organs of the body — wherever in fact erythrocyte sickling leads to vascular occlusion. This being so, the typical consequences of intravascular haemolysis — haemoglobin bound to haptoglobin and free in the plasma, methaemalbuminaemia and haemosiderinuria — should be found. The relevant studies that have been carried out have shown this to be true.

Crosby and Dameshek (1951) in their classic paper on haemoglobinaemia and associated haemosiderinuria included two children with sickle-cell anaemia amongst the 23 patients with haemolytic anaemia they studied: the children's plasma haemoglobin was recorded as 16 and 21 mg/dl, respectively, their urinary haemosiderin as 1 plus.

Lathem and Jensen (1959) studied eight patients with Hb-SS disease and seven with the Hb-AS trait. They concluded that the ability of their plasma to bind added haemoglobin was normal in the trait but was much reduced or absent in Hb-SS disease (and in one patient with Hb-CC disease). On the other hand, normal plasma bound Hb S and Hb C normally. Lathem and Jensen (1962) reported on further studies on nine patients with Hb-SS disease. The mean haem pigment concentration was 17 mg/dl, 15 mg of which was methaemalbumin. Most of the patients had little or no haemoglobin free in the plasma or bound to haptoglobin, and after experimental infusion of haemoglobin in solution little was bound to protein; in eight patients the glomerular clearance and tubular absorption of haemoglobin appeared to be normal.

Upshaw and co-workers (1963) and Iuchi, Diggs and Upshaw (1964) reported rather similar findings; namely, that the plasma haem pigment concentration (as measured with benzidine) was considerably raised (about 6–10 times the normal mean), although varying widely from patient to patient. Haptoglobin was saturated with haemoglobin, and the sera contained methaemalbumin and also some free haemoglobin. The occurrence of painful crises did not in general affect the levels.

Stutman and Shinowara (1965) carried out longitudinal studies of plasma haem pigments in three patients. The concentrations of total haem pigments, and of haematin measured separately, were abnormally high but fluctuated considerably; the average values in samples taken during painful crises did not differ from those taken in clinically asymptomatic periods. Exposure to cold was, however, followed by significant increases.

Neely and co-workers (1969) measured plasma haemoglobin and lactic dehydrogenase (LDH) levels in sickle-cell disease patients in a steady state and in crisis. When they were in a steady state, the plasma haemoglobin concentration and LDH activity were about twice the normal, but on the first day of a febrile painful crisis one or both were 4–5 times the normal. Isozymes I and II of LDH then predominated (as is found normally when there is intravascular haemolysis). However, there were wide fluctuations from patient to patient, so much so that the measurements appeared to be of limited value in distinguishing painful crises from other complicating illnesses.

Wochner and co-workers (1974), using ^{125}I-haemopexin, studied its metabolism in two patients with Hb-SS disease as well as in several patients with porphyria and in normal controls. The plasma concentration of haemopexin and the absolute amount circulating were low in the Hb-SS disease patients and its fractional catabolic rate was accelerated, indicating increased haem binding.

Myoglobinaemia

Roth and co-workers (1980) compared the plasma myoglobin concentration in 17 steady-state Hb-SS patients with that of 30 patients in crisis. The mean value was substantially and significantly higher in those in crisis compared to that of the patients in a steady state. Roth *et al.* suggested that measuring plasma myoglobin might help in the diagnosis of a crisis. They did not claim, however, that the test was infallible.

Erythrocyte sedimentation rate (ESR)

It is well known that the ESR of Hb-SS patients is abnormally low (Bunting, 1939; Diggs and Bibb, 1939; Winsor and Burch, 1944). The reason for this is that sickled cells do not form rouleaux. Jan, Usami and Smith (1981) have more recently studied the effect of variation of pO_2 and haematocrit and demonstrated that retardation of the ESR, as the result of inhibition of aggregation, only takes place when the pO_2 is reduced below 40 mm Hg; they pointed out that to interpret an ESR result it was necessary to know both the pO_2 and haematocrit of the sample.

Plasma lipids

Westerman, Pierce and Jensen (1964), in a study of 10 Hb-SS patients, found that the levels of total lipids, phospholipids and cholesterol were all significantly less than normal, as has been observed in other anaemic patients. Sasaki and co-workers (1983) have more recently reported on the plasma and erythrocyte lipids of 57 Hb-SS patients, aged between 1 year and 18 years, who were free from major complications when investigated. Total cholesterol and phospholipid concentrations were significantly lower than normal, but otherwise the plasma lipid profile was normal. Plasma glycerol was, however, 8 times normal. The low plasma cholesterol values were similar to those of 12 control patients with miscellaneous (mostly haemolytic) anaemias, and while it was conceded that the cause of the hypolipidaemia in Hb-SS disease was unknown, the increased rate of erythrocyte production, necessitating an increased utilization of lipids for erythrocyte membrane synthesis, could be a factor.

Acid-base balance

According to Henderson (1950), Greenberg and Kass (1958) and Barreras and Diggs (1964) and other observers (*e.g.* Olver, 1969), patients in painful crises usually suffer from a metabolic acidosis, associated with a clear reduction of plasma bicarbonate, and this suggests that acidosis is often an important factor in the genesis of the crisis. It has been shown, too, that the deliberate production of acidosis, as for instance by the administration of ammonium chloride, leads to an increase in the percentage of sickled cells in the blood and to the development of painful crises (Barreras and Diggs, 1964). It has long been known, too, that lowering the pH *in vitro* enhances sickling (Hahn and Gillespie, 1927). However, it has to be added that the role of acidosis *in vivo* in precipitating painful crises remains uncertain, for careful studies carried out on 10 adult Jamaicans by Ho and Alleyne (1969) provided no clear evidence of any differences between their blood pH, total CO_2 and pCO_2 when they were in crisis and when they had recovered.

IRON DEFICIENCY

Hb-SS patients do not seem to become overloaded with iron unless they have received many transfusions: on the contrary, iron deficiency is not uncommon. There is some evidence that a moderate degree of iron deficiency may be of clinical benefit to the patient by lowering the MCHC, as pointed out by Greenberg, Kass and Castle in 1957 (see also p. 99).

Iron deficiency seems to be prevalent irrespective of the patients' domicile, as the following recent reports show.

Anderson (1972) reported that of 15 pregnant Jamaican women with sickle-cell syndromes (7 Hb SS) eight had no stainable iron in their bone-marrow aspirates.

Peterson and co-workers (1975) studied 39 patients with Hb-SS disease, aged between 12 and 52 years. In 28 of them stainable iron could be seen in bone-marrow aspirates; their mean serum iron concentration was 100.9 μg/dl and mean total iron-binding capacity (TIBC) 309.9 μg/dl (normal). In 11 of them iron could not be seen in bone-marrow aspirates; their mean serum iron concentration was 75.7 μg/dl and TIBC 309.7 μg/dl. Despite these normal or rather low values for serum iron and TIBC, serum-ferritin levels were markedly raised in both groups, means 749 μg/l and 533 μg/l, respectively, indicating substantial reserves of iron, much perhaps not readily available for erythropoiesis.

According to O'Brien (1978), the serum-ferritin concentration was normal in 11 out of 15 Hb-SS patients who were less than 20 years of age. Davies and co-workers (1984) had studied 31 adult Hb-SS patients (in all of whom globin-chain synthesis was balanced). Twelve of the patients had never been transfused (Group I); 14 had received up to 4 units of blood (Group II), while five had been 'hypertransfused' and had received a mean total of 17.3 litres within a 6-month to 2-year period (Group III). The Group-III patients had high serum-ferritin concentrations, and higher MCVs and MCHs, than the patients in the other two groups. The serum ferritin was less than normal in eight patients in Groups I and II and higher than normal in seven patients in Groups II and III; in the remaining 16 patients the serum ferritin was normal.

Rao and Sur (1980) found that all 25 Indian Hb-SS patients, aged between 2 and 16 years (80% of whom had not been transfused) had subnormal serum iron levels and low transferrin saturation; three children had no iron demonstrable in marrow aspirates and the remaining patients were judged to have reduced iron stores in their marrow.

Oluboyede (1980) reported on 40 Nigerian women, 22 with Hb SS and 18 with Hb SC: 63% of those who were pregnant and 50% of those who were not pregnant had depleted iron stores, as judged from bone-marrow aspirates and serum-ferritin measurements.

Vichinsky and co-workers (1981) had studied 50 Hb-SS patients aged from 1 year to 27 years, and 20 Hb-SC patients aged from 1 year to 30 years, in San Francisco: 16% of those who had not been transfused were found to be iron-deficient; their mean age was 2.4 years.

In the United Kingdom, Davies, Henthorn and Brozović (1983) found that 10 out of 37 patients with sickle-cell syndromes were iron-deficient. They pointed out, as had Vichinsky et al., the importance of differentiating between iron deficiency and α- or β-thalassaemia as causes of microcytosis. Later, Davies and co-workers (1984), in an investigation confined to adults, found evidence of iron deficiency in eight out of 26 Hb-SS patients who had never been transfused or had received not more than 4 units of blood. Seven patients had higher than normal serum-ferritin levels; four belonged to a group that had been hypertransfused.

Rao and co-workers (1984) investigated 60 Hb-SS adults of both sexes attending a hospital in Chicago. In 17 of them (28%), 11 men and six women, in whom there appeared to be no evidence of blood loss from the gastro-intestinal tract, iron could not be demonstrated in the bone marrow.

The cause of the iron deficiency in Hb-SS patients has not always been obvious: in some patients chronic blood loss has clearly played an important part; in others this, or a poor intake of iron, does not seem to have been responsible. Loss of iron in the urine, continuously over a long period of time, seems a possible explanation, and there is some evidence that this indeed happens. Thus Washington and Boggs (1975) found that 27 out of 31 Hb-SS patients excreted abnormally high amounts of iron; the mean daily excretion was 510 μg compared with a normal mean of 88 μg. However, there appeared to be no correlation between the amount of iron excreted and the patients' age, history of past transfusions and serum iron levels, implying that the daily excretion did not reflect the presence or absence of iron overload. The amount excreted by individual patients varied considerably from day to day and did not appear to be related to the occurrence of painful crises: on the other hand, it was markedly increased in two patients in haemolytic crisis and it was concluded that the amount excreted reflected the intensity of intravascular haemolysis.

Iron deficiency and the well-being of the patient

As already referred to, Greenberg, Kass and Castle (1957) made the point that an important factor in determining the severity of a patient's symptoms was the intracellular concentration of Hb S: they concluded that an MCSHC (mean corpuscular sickle haemoglobin concentration) of 15–18 g/dl was likely to be associated with mild haemolytic anaemia, while an MCSHC greater than 20 g/dl would lead to significant anaemia, bony lesions and painful crises.

More recently, Lincoln, Aroesty and Morrison (1973) argued that the relationship between MCHC, iron deficiency and the clinical features of sickle-cell disease deserved further study. Writing from California, they suggested that as malnourishment with consequent iron deficiency became less common in the black population, the incidence of severe sickle-cell anaemia would increase; they also suggested that the complications that affect Hb-SS women in pregnancy might in part be the consequence of routine iron supplementation.

Some recent observations have provided support for these interesting hypotheses.

Haddy and Castro (1982) referred to four patients, three Hb SS and one Hb SC, who were overtly iron-deficient as the result of blood loss. Two of them who had experienced no painful crises when iron-deficient began having crises again after treatment with iron, and

one of them, a 6-year-old girl, experienced two painful crises for the first time within 4 months of the start of intramuscular iron therapy, during which time the MCHC had risen from 25.6 g/dl to 33.6 g/dl.

Castro and Haddy (1983) subsequently described how ^{51}Cr erythrocyte auto-survival studies were carried out on one of these patients, a 45-year-old female with uterine bleeding, before and after several months of effective iron therapy (and hysterectomy). The ^{51}Cr T_{50} decreased from 15.9 days before treatment to 5.2 days after treatment (Fig. 12.17). Other changes included a more than doubling of serum LDH, a 5-fold increase in serum bilirubin and a rise in ISC count from 0.3 to 7.7%. In contrast, the Hb-F percentage decreased from 6.5 to 1.7 after correction of the iron deficiency.

Rao and co-workers (1983) described the effect of giving iron orally to a 46-year-old male Hb-SS patient who was iron-deficient for no obvious reason. Before treatment with iron, the MCHC was 27.6 g/dl and very few sickled cells were present in blood films; after 6 weeks of therapy the MCHC had risen to 33.6 g/dl and the sickle-cell count had risen from 0.02 to 2.2%. *In vitro*, the patient's erythrocytes, when iron-deficient, required a substantially lower oxygen tension to sickle than the erythrocytes of six Hb-SS patients who were not iron-deficient.

ZINC DEFICIENCY

There is evidence that Hb-SS disease patients tend to have subnormal plasma, erythrocyte and neutrophil zinc levels and that this apparent zinc deficiency impairs the healing of skin ulcers, dark adaptation and the patients' growth. The cause of the deficiency is not entirely clear, but an abnormal loss of zinc in the urine, together with impaired nutrition, appear to be important factors.

As already referred to (p. 27), Serjeant, Galloway and Gueri (1970) reported that oral zinc sulphate appeared to accelerate the healing of leg ulcers in Hb-SS patients; they found, too, that the mean serum zinc concentration of 34 such patients was significantly lower than that of healthy Hb-AA relatives. Karayalcin and co-workers (1974) measured the plasma zinc concentration in 50 Hb-SS patients, as well as in 50 Hb-AS carriers and in 50 Hb-AA individuals and similarly found that the mean level in the Hb-SS patients was significantly subnormal, with the Hb-AS carriers giving intermediate values. In a report from Nigeria, however, Kapu, Fleming and Ezem (1976) found no differences between the plasma zinc levels in Hb-SS, Hb-AS and Hb-AA 'non-élite' Nigerians; the values in 'élite' Nigerians and in Europeans were, however, higher. The

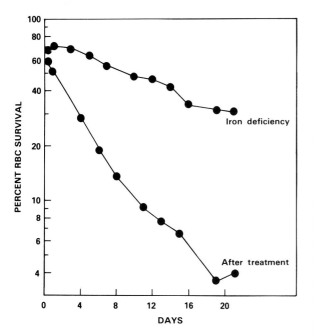

Fig. 12.17 Survival of the ^{51}Cr-labelled erythrocytes of a Hb-SS patient measured when iron-deficient (as the result of metrorrhagia) and after she had been treated with iron.
[Reproduced by permission from Castro and Haddy (1983).]

lowest value in the whole series was in a plasma sample from a Hb-SS patient with leg ulceration — which is apparently rarely seen in West-African patients.

Zinc deficiency in Afro-Americans seems, however, to be a reality and to be of clinical significance. Thus delayed dark adaptation (Warth et al., 1981), impaired delayed hypersensitivity (Ballester and Prasad, 1983) and impairment of growth, both with respect to height and weight (Prasad and Cossack, 1984), have been reported.

Daeschner and co-workers (1985) studied blood lymphocyte function in sickle-cell disease children with or without zinc deficiency, as well as a series of normal controls. The percentage of B and T cells in the peripheral blood of the patients was found not to differ from that of the normal controls and to be independent of zinc deficiency. However, the absolute numbers in both groups of patients were raised, probably as a response to repeated infections. The increase was found to be less marked in the zinc-deficient patients. In addition, the T cells of zinc-deficient patients were found to be significantly less responsive to PHA mitogen than the control normal cells or the cells of the patients who were not zinc-deficient.

APLASTIC (HYPOPLASTIC) CRISES

As in other haemolytic anaemias (see Vol. 1, pp. 96 and 164), a sudden failure of erythropoiesis can lead to rapidly increasing anaemia in patients with Hb-SS disease, so much so that blood transfusion may be required urgently. In the great majority of cases the failure of erythropoiesis seems to be brought about by the action of a parvovirus acting on erythroid progenitor cells. The result may be the virtual disappearance of developing erythroblasts from the bone marrow leading perhaps to an absence of reticulocytes from the peripheral blood. Fortunately, the inhibition of erythropoiesis is typically only temporary, and if the patient can be supported by transfusion, if necessary, during the period of reticulocytopenia (which may last for up to 7–10 days) the marrow will recover completely and the patient will be none the worse. Second attacks seldom, if ever occur. Aplastic crises of the type referred to above seemed at one time to be rare events; in recent years, however, they appear to have become more common. Most, but not all, of those affected have been children and it is quite common for more than one member of a family to be affected almost simultaneously or successively.

As mentioned above, the reticulocyte count may fall to zero. Erythroblasts may be almost absent from the marrow at the start of the crisis; the marrow, however, becomes intensely erythroblastic in the early recovery phase; 'giant' erythroblasts may be present in small numbers (Vol. 1, Fig. 3.46). Typically, the reticulocytopenia is unaccompanied by neutropenia or thrombocytopenia. Recovery is accompanied by a sharp reticulocyte peak in the peripheral blood which may be preceded by an outpouring of normoblasts (Fig. 12.19) and a polymorphonuclear leucocytosis. Atypical lymphocytes may be present at an early stage [see p. 102 (Saarinen et al., 1986)].

Case reports. In 1950, Singer, Motulsky and Wile described two siblings, a 9-year-old boy and an 11-year-old girl suffering from sickle-cell disease, both of whom had respiratory infections, in whom there was an abrupt increase in the severity of their anaemia. This was found to be associated with reticulocytopenia and temporary cessation of erythropoiesis in the bone marrow (Fig. 12.18). In 1951, Chernoff and Josephson reported four more instances of similar aplastic crises in sickle-cell disease; in three patients the

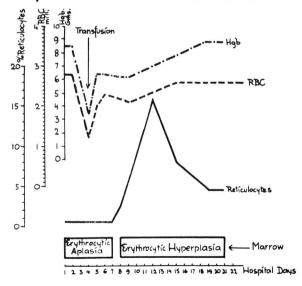

Fig. 12.18 Course of events in an aplastic crisis in a 9-year-old boy with sickle-cell anaemia.
[Reproduced by permission from Singer, Motulsky and Wile (1950).]

initiating cause seemed to be an upper respiratory tract infection and in one patient infection with *Salm. cholera-suis*.

Subsequent descriptions of aplastic or hypo-plastic crises include those reported by Diggs (1956), Leikin (1957), Miesch, Baxter and Levin (1957), Hilkovitz (1960), MacIver and Parker-Williams (1961), Charney and Miller (1964), van der Sar (1967), Hammond, Shore and Movassaghi (1968), Mann *et al.* (1975), Markenson *et al.* (1978), Helmer *et al.* (1979), Serjeant *et al.* (1981), Anderson *et al.* (1982), Rao *et al.* (1983), Evans *et al.* (1984) and Saarinen *et al.* (1986).

Familial incidence

More than one member of a family were affected at about the same time or successively in the reports of Leikin (1957), Hilkovitz (1960), MacIver and Parker-Williams (1961), Mann *et al.* (1975) and Markenson *et al.* (1978). Serjeant (1985, p. 75) made the interesting comment that if one sibling in a family suffers from an aplastic crisis there is a 50% chance of another (Hb-SS) sibling developing a similar crisis within 3 weeks, if aged under 16 and living in the same house. Evans and co-workers' (1984) report of a Hb-SS child who developed an aplastic crisis after being in contact in hospital with a HS child who became reticulocytopenic and needed two transfusions illustrates the infectivity of parvovirus. Both children were shown to have formed human parvo-virus specific IgM antibody, indicating recent infection in each case.

These familial occurrences led to the realization that the cause of the crises was almost certainly an infectious agent. It was not, however, until 1981 that any such agent could be identified. Then Pattison and co-workers presented convincing evidence that six Hb-SS children admitted to hospital in hypoplastic crisis were infected by a parvovirus (see below).

As already mentioned, aplastic crises appear to occur more commonly in Hb-SS disease than was at one time thought. Thus, although Diggs (1956), who reviewed the histories of 166 patients admitted to hospital in Memphis 747 times in clinical crises, had found that only one of these admissions was for a true aplastic crisis, MacIver and Parker-Williams (1961) considered

that the syndrome was not uncommon in Jamaica. They had seen 12 such cases, 10 within 7 months. Mann and co-workers (1975), too, who reported on 13 children with Hb-SS disease admitted to hospital 16 times for episodes of acute anaemia, found that 10 out of the 16 episodes appeared to be attributable to reticulocyto-penia. By 1981, Serjeant and co-workers were able to report that they had records of 112 children in Jamaica who had had aplastic crises since 1952 and that most of the crises had occurred in five periods, namely 1956, 1960, 1965–67, 1971–73 and 1980. Anderson and co-workers (1982), too, reported that of the nine aplastic crises that they had seen between April 1979 and May 1981 seven had occurred in 1980.

Although most of the case reports mentioned above have been concerned with aplastic crises in children, adults are not exempt. The patient described by Miesch, Baxter and Levin (1957) was a male aged 25 and van der Sar's (1967) four patients, studied in Curaçao, were females aged between 17 and 29. The patient of Helmer *et al.* (1979), in whom they were able to demonstrate the the extent of the erythroid aplasia by scintigraphy using ^{111}indium chloride, was a female aged 20, while the seven patients described by Rao *et al.* (1983) were young men and women aged between 17 and 23.

Role of parvovirus infection

The demonstration that an infective agent similar to parvovirus B19 might be responsible for the aplastic crises affecting six Hb-SS children in London (Pattison *et al.*, 1981) provided the stimulus for the reinvestigation of serum samples that had been stored from 28 patients who had suffered from aplastic crises in Jamaica in 1979 and 1980. Evidence for infection with a parvo-virus-like agent was found in 24 of the patients; viral antigen was detected in two of them and evidence of sero-conversion (a serum negative for antibody becoming positive) in nine. All the remaining samples — sera withdrawn when the patient was convalescent — were positive for anti-body, and there was evidence to suggest that the virus was similar to parvovirus B19 (Serjeant *et al.*, 1981).

The general effect of parvovirus infection seems to be similar to that of other common viral infections, and pyrexia, chills, sore throat, cough, vomiting, diarrhoea, myalgia and abdominal pain have all been described in a variety of combinations. There is evidence that infection with parvovirus-like agents is in fact extremely common and that many individuals are infected without any clinical signs or symptoms being discernible. Thus Serjeant and co-workers (1981b) reported, using the technique of counter-current immunoelectrophoresis, that antibody against parvovirus B19 was present in 17% of 48 Hb-AA sera used as controls, and Anderson *et al.* (1982), using the same technique, were able to demonstrate antibody in the sera of 30% of healthy blood donors, despite the fact that they found that in some individuals antibody becomes no longer detectable 12–24 months after infection.

More recent studies which clearly implicate parvovirus infection and bone-marrow erythroid aplasia include those of Mortimer *et al.* (1983), Evans *et al.* (1984), Kelleher *et al.* (1984), Young *et al.* (1984) Gowda *et al.* (1985) and Saarinen *et al.* (1986).

Mortimer *et al.* and Young *et al.* were able to demonstrate that the virus inhibited erythropoietic colony formation *in vitro*, with the late erythroid progenitor cells being particularly sensitive. They were able to show that fresh serum from a patient with HS in aplastic crisis was potent in inhibiting erythroid colony formation even at a 10^{-4} dilution and that the inhibiting action could be neutralized by serum containing antibody to the virus. They reported, too, that acute-phase sera from eight patients suffering from other viral infections, tested in the same system, failed to affect erythroid colony formation significantly. They emphasized that the SPL (serum parvovirus-like) virus is the first virus to be identified as being definitely cytotoxic to human haemopoietic cells.

It is interesting to record that in in-vitro work carried out before the role of parvovirus had been discovered, Lutton and co-workers (1980) had found that serum taken from one Hb-SS patient when in an aplastic crisis inhibited erythroid colony formation while a similar sample taken 2 months later failed to do this. Lutton *et al.* also reported that bone marrow taken from five Hb-SS patients 2–6 days after the onset of a crisis was well able to respond, by forming colonies in a plasma-clot system, when stimulated by erythropoietin. They concluded that the defect in erythropoiesis in Hb-SS patients in hypoproliferative crises might in some cases be due to a circulating inhibitor.

Recently, Saarinen and co-workers (1986) described how an 'epidemic' of acute erythroblastopenic crises affected, between May and August 1984, 26 patients suffering from a hereditary haemolytic anaemia who lived in N.E. Ohio. They were between 2 and 23 years old: 20 had Hb-SS disease, four Hb-SC disease, one Hb-S/ β-thalassaemia and one HS. Twenty-two of the patients needed blood transfusion. Reticulocytosis developed 2–14 days after presentation; in one patient (who was not transfused) the reticulocyte peak was preceded by a normoblast peak (Fig. 12.19). There appeared to be no arrest of platelet production — counts

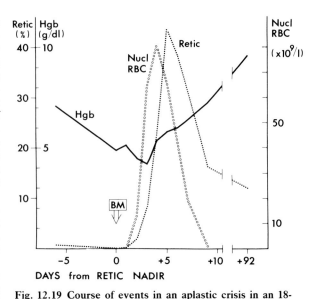

Fig. 12.19 Course of events in an aplastic crisis in an 18-year-old Hb-SS patient who had refused to be transfused.
The reticulocyte peak in the peripheral blood on recovery was preceded by a normoblast peak. [Reproduced by permission from Saarinen *et al.* (1986).]

less than $150 \times 10^9/l$ were recorded in only two of the patients. Thrombocytosis was, however, a regular feature after recovery, with counts between 509 and $1133 \times 10^9/l$ in 13 patients. A short-lived neutropenia ($<1 \times 10^9/l$ neutrophils) was noted in four of 23 patients: many, however, developed a leucocytosis on recovery; in nine the total counts exceeded $25 \times 10^9/l$, the maximum being $47.3 \times 10^9/l$. In several patients atypical lymphocytes were to be seen in the peripheral blood: in five out of 23 there were more than 10%; up to 5% plasma cells were present in four out of 23 patients. In nine of 23 patients there were more than 5% of eosinophils. Viral studies provided evidence of infection with human parvovirus B19. In five patients in acute phase $10^8–10^{12}$ viral particles per ml serum were demonstrable by electron microscopy; highly viraemic sera inhibited erythroid colony formation; B19-specific IgM was detected in 24 out of 26 sera and B19-specific IgG in 21 out of 32 sera.

Causes of aplastic crises other than parvovirus

Although infection with parvovirus appears to be by far the most common cause of aplastic or hypoplastic crises in Hb-SS patients, other infections may be responsible.

Miesch, Baxter and Levin's (1957) patient was a 25-year-old Hb-SS male who was submitted to laparotomy for possible appendicitis. The appendix was removed but was considered to be normal and mesenteric adenitis was diagnosed. In retrospect it appeared likely that the patient had suffered from an abdominal crisis and that the appendectomy had precipitated (in some way) an acute erythroblastopenic crisis.

The patient reported by Megas, Papadaki and Constantinides (1961), a boy aged 4 years, died of *Salm. typhimurium* septicaemia. He had 5.3 g/dl haemoglobin and a total leucocyte count of $3 \times 10^9/l$, of which only 12% were mature polymorphonuclears. Reticulocytes appeared to be absent from the peripheral blood, and his marrow, although cellular, contained only a few normoblasts — the erythroid:myeloid ratio was 1:15.

Charney and Miller (1964), in summarizing the clinical and haematological findings in nine Hb-SS children who had developed severe reticulocytopenia (0.0–2.6% reticulocytes), recorded that one child had streptococcal septicaemia and three pneumococcal pneumonia or pneumococcal upper respiratory tract infections.

Mann and co-workers (1975) found evidence of Mycoplasma infection in two patients and cold agglutinins active at room temperature in 11 other patients, all of whom had episodes of acute anaemia; one further patient had staphylococcal osteomyelitis, pneumonia and septicaemia.

Serjeant (1985, p. 77) commented that it was a common experience for the reticulocyte count and haemoglobin level to fall during many infections in Hb-SS patients and mentioned in particular pneumonia, urinary tract infections and septicaemia.

An unusual case of bone-marrow hypoplasia was reported by Kim *et al.* (1975): their patient was a boy aged 10 who was receiving anticonvulsant drugs for a stroke and who developed severe pancytopenia (1.5% reticulocytes, $1.8 \times 10^9/l$ leucocytes and $20 \times 10^9/l$ platelets) which lasted for about 3 weeks. Pardoll and co-workers (1982) reported another remarkable case in which an aplastic crisis appeared to be the consequence of extensive bone-marrow necrosis — the patient suffered from Hb-S/β^0-thalassaemia.

Erythropoietin and aplastic crises

Hammond, Shore and Movassaghi (1968) described

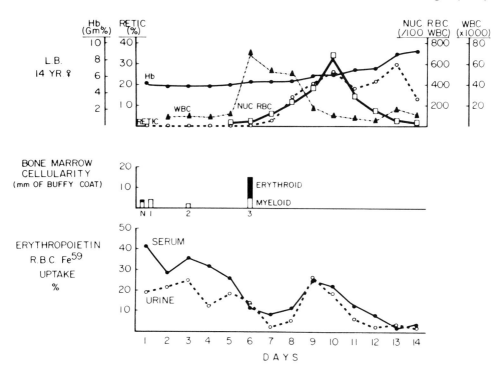

Fig. 12.20 **Relationship between serum and urine erythropoietin levels during the course of an aplastic crisis affecting a 14-year-old Hb-SS female.**
[Reproduced by permission from Hammond, Shore and Movassaghi (1968).]

as part of a comprehensive report on the production, utilization and excretion of erythro-poietin (EP) in various anaemias serial obser-vations, using a polycythaemic mouse assay, on the serum and urinary EP levels in a 14-year-old female with sickle-cell anaemia who experienced and recovered from an acute aplastic crisis (Fig. 12.20). A reciprocal relationship between the EP level and bone-marrow erythroid activity was established. This was also well shown when the serum EP levels in 31 patients with Hb-SS disease were plotted against the patients' haemoglobin level: increased EP activity was found in the serum of patients with a haemoglobin less than 9.5 g/dl, which became progressively more marked in the more anaemic patients (Fig. 12.21).

Haddy and co-workers (1979) reported on assays for erythropoietin, using a mouse test, that they had carried out on 37 patients with Hb-SS: 11 were free from symp-toms, 11 had an infection (eight had pneumonia) and 12 were in a vaso-occlusive crisis. In these three groups the mean haemoglobin, haematocrit, reticulocyte count and plasma erythropoietin level were similar:in contrast, the plasma erythropoietin level was extremely high in two out of three patients tested in an aplastic crisis.

McGonigle and co-workers (1985) measured by means of a radio-immune assay the serum erythropoietin (EP) levels in 30 patients, aged between 2 and 18 years, suffering from haemolytic anaemia: 24 had Hb-SS disease, five Hb-SC disease and one HS. They found a clear inverse exponential relationship between the EP concentration and the haematocrit and a positive corre-lation between the EP concentration and reticulocyte count. (Five children with Fanconi's hypoproliferative anaemia were also studied: their EP levels were all higher than those of the haemolytic anaemia patients.)

Sherwood and co-workers (1986) concluded that sickle-cell disease patients have relatively low serum EP levels compared with those of patients with a compar-able degree of anaemia not associated with a haemoglo-binopathy. They themselves had studied 28 patients with Hb-SS disease and two with Hb-S/β$^+$-thalassaemia, aged between 1 year and 17 years. Of the 13 anaemic patients who served as controls, eight had a haematological malignancy. An exponential relationship between serum EP and the degree of anaemia was estab-lished for both groups of patients. However, in the haemoglobinopathy patients the EP levels rose sharply only when the patient's haemoglobin level was less than 9 g/dl, whereas in the control anaemic patients the rise took place at about the 12 g/dl level. The response to anaemia was noted to be more blunted in the older sickle-cell disease patients than in the younger patients, and it was suggested that renal damage might be responsible for the haemoglobinopathy patients' rela-tively poor EP response to anaemia.

MEGALOBLASTIC HAEMOPOIESIS

Folate deficiency. While deficiency of vitamin B$_{12}$ is unusual and megaloblastic anaemia due to

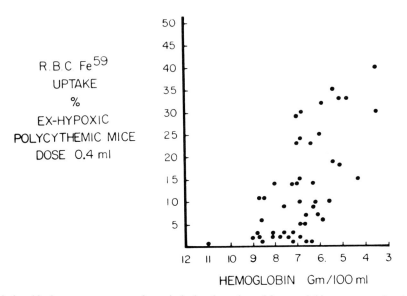

Fig. 12.21 **Relationship between serum erythropoietin levels and total haemoglobin concentration in 31 patients with Hb-SS disease.**
[Reproduced by permission from Hammond, Shore and Movassaghi (1968).]

this cause in Hb-SS patients must be rare, folate deficiency of sufficient severity to affect haemopoiesis is quite common. Small children living in poor social and economic conditions are particularly prone to this, but adults may be affected, too. The basic cause seems to be the hyperplastic marrow's increased demand for folate (as in other haemolytic anaemias in which there is active erythropoiesis), coupled with poor nutrition and in some instances, too, the increased demand for the vitamin associated with infection or pregnancy.

Affected patients present with degrees of anaemia that are unusual in uncomplicated Hb-SS disease. The bone marrow will show all degrees of megaloblastic change and peripheral blood films unusual degrees of anisocytosis, poikilocytosis and macrocytosis and possibly, too, circulating megaloblasts.

The first reports of megaloblastic anaemia complicating sickle-cell disease date from the 1950s and early 1960s (Zuelzer and Rutsky, 1953, their Case 2; Miesch, Baxter and Levin, 1957; Jonsson, Roath and Kirkpatrick, 1959; Oliner and Heller, 1959; Pierce and Rath, 1962), and it was not long before it was shown that in reality it was quite common to find in Hb-SS patients clinical or laboratory evidence of folate deficiency.

MacIver and Went (1960) found that five out of 50 Jamaican infants with megaloblastic anaemia had Hb-SS disease: they responded dramatically to treatment with folic acid. Watson-Williams (1962) reported that 43 out of 405 patients newly diagnosed in Ibadan as having sickle-cell disease showed signs of megaloblastic anaemia. The patients' height and weight, as well as their blood picture, improved following treatment with folic acid.

In the United States, Pearson and Cobb (1964) found that folate deficiency, as indicated by a low *L. casei* serum assay and by FIGLU excretion, was frequent in Hb-SS disease: almost one-third of 25 patients (2–29 years of age) had low serum levels and the majority an increased FIGLU excretion. The patients, however, were considered to show no clear haematological evidence of megaloblastic change. Shojania and Gross (1964), in a similar study, reported that of 24 children with chronic haemolytic anaemia (19 had Hb-SS disease) more than half were folate-deficient, as shown by serum folate levels.

Lindenbaum and Klipstein (1963) described how they investigated a 27-year-old female with Hb-SS disease and a well-marked megaloblastic anaemia and found that her requirement for folate was apparently much greater than in normal people. It appeared that her stores of folate were markedly depleted: she failed to respond to the doses of folic acid that folic-acid-deficient patients usually respond to; folic acid was cleared from the plasma abnormally rapidly, and it was only after she was given 1000 μg of folic acid daily by mouth that her megaloblastic haemopoiesis was replaced by normoblastic and her serum folate concentration increased substantially. Lindenbaum and Klipstein included in their paper a valuable review of the reported cases of megaloblastic anaemia complicating various types of haemolytic anaemia: in their tabulation were 21 cases of Hb-SS disease and two cases of Hb-SC disease. Alperin (1967), too, in a detailed study of a 16-year-old Hb-SS male who had had three episodes of megaloblastic anaemia, found that as much as 500 μg a day of orally administered folic acid were required to prevent relapse.

Lopez, Shimizu and Cooperman (1973) reported another interesting study. Their patient was a 10-year-old Hb-SS male living in New York who had suffered from four episodes of folate deficiency in $2\frac{1}{2}$ years. It appeared that neither impaired intestinal absorption nor excessive loss of the vitamin in the urine was responsible and he was on a diet which would have been adequate in folate content for a normal child. The interesting observation was made that in each of the four episodes failure to gain weight preceded the haematological changes of folate deficiency.

Liu's (1974, 1975) data suggested that folate deficiency, as judged by serum and erythrocyte folate levels, was not uncommon in the 1970s in the American black population, at least in Georgia and Kentucky: thus while 51% of Hb-SS patients had a serum folate level less than 5 ng/ml, similar values were found in 26% of Hb-AS subjects and in 27.5% of Hb-AA subjects (Liu, 1975). According to Liu (1974), folate deficiency does not contribute significantly to the retarded growth of Hb-SS patients.

Vitamin-B$_{12}$ deficiency. As already mentioned, megaloblastic anaemia caused by deficiency of vitamin B$_{12}$ in patients with Hb-SS disease must be a rarity. (The author does not know of a well-authenticated case.) Estimations of serum B$_{12}$ levels in black Africans have shown slightly subnormal levels, but no results have been reported that are near the levels found in overt B$_{12}$ deficiency (Osifo *et al.*, 1983; Osifo, Lukanmbi and Adeyokunnu, 1984). Higher than normal levels of two of the serum transcobalamins (TC I and TC II) were found in association with higher than normal total leucocyte and neutrophil counts.

Dyserythropoiesis of uncertain cause

Osamo and Eyetsimitan (1976) reported from Benin, Nigeria, that they had observed three patients with sickle-cell anaemia in whom dyserythropoiesis in the bone marrow, including erythroblast multinuclearity, suggested Di Guglielmo's disease. They gave details of one boy aged 6 years. The three patients improved on conservative management and it seemed as if the dys-erythropoiesis was secondary, but to what could not be established.

BLOOD PICTURE IN SICKLE-CELL TRAIT

The Hb-AS trait, although leading to a positive sickling test, has generally been considered to be not normally associated with anaemia or any abnormality detectable by a routine blood exam-ination. Blood films and absolute values, too, have usually been considered to be normal. Recent evidence (see below) suggests, however, that this view may not be strictly correct.

As far back as 1933, Diggs, Ahmann and Bibb had stated that the majority of persons with the sickle-cell trait are not anaemic; and the majority of subsequent workers who have compared the haematological findings in Hb-AS carriers with those of normal Hb-AA American blacks living in the same socio-economic circum-stances have similarly concluded that the prevalence of anaemia is the same in the two groups (e.g., Brown et al., 1972; Polednak and Janerich, 1975).

An exception to the above generalization is the report of Yip and Nelson (1981) based on a study in Minnea-polis of 47 Hb-AS children (mean age 59.6 months) and 94 Hb-AA age-matched black controls. The mean haemoglobin concentration of the Hb-AS children was 0.5 g/dl lower than that of the controls, a difference that was statistically significant ($P < 0.01$). Both the trait children and the controls tended to be anaemic when compared to a reference scale for healthy non-iron-deficient white children: the prevalence of anaemia (a value < 2 SD below the reference mean) was calculated to be 19% for the trait children compared with 6% for the control group. In contrast, in the course of an inter-esting study on the prevalence and causes of anaemia in a different ethnic community in another part of the world — Arabs in a South Lebanon village — Hershko and co-workers (1982) found that iron-deficiency anaemia was less frequent (an incidence of 1.3%) in individuals with the Hb-AS trait than in the normal population in which the incidence was 10.3%. Increased iron absorption by the Hb-AS individuals was suggested as one possible cause.

Some recent studies have revealed differences in absolute values between individuals with the Hb-AS trait and normal Hb-AA controls. Sheehan and Frenkel (1983) and Maggio, Gagliono and Siciliano (1984), who studied adult males (in whom iron deficiency was considered to be unlikely), reported finding that the MCV of Hb-AS individuals tended to be significantly less than that of Hb-AA controls. Castro and Scott (1985) similarly found a small but statistically significant reduction in MCV in the Hb-AS trait. They had studied 150 Hb-AS black individuals (of both sexes and of a range of ages, mostly young adults and pre-school children) and as controls 2136 Hb-AA blacks of similar sex and age distribution: they found, in addition to the reduction in MCV, a small but significant reduction in MCH and a small increase in erythrocyte count. There were, however, no significant differences in haemo-globin, haematocrit and MCHC; on these criteria, therefore, the incidence of anaemia in the two groups was the same.

Osmotic fragility. In line with the reductions in MCV and MCH referred to above, Diggs and Bibb (1939) had reported that osmotic resistance is increased in the Hb-AS trait.

Erythrocyte life-span. The erythrocytes of healthy carriers of the Hb-AS trait have a normal life-span *in vivo*. This has been shown to be so by the Ashby method and by ^{51}Cr and DF^{32}P (Singer at al., 1948; Callender et al., 1949; Barbedo and McCurdy, 1974; Sears, 1978). However, according to Basu, Woodruff and Pettit (1963), even slight pyrexia (99–101°F) may cause transient increased haemolysis, associated with some accumulation of ^{51}Cr in the spleen.

Hb-AS blood stores well under routine blood-bank conditions for up to 17 days at least and survives normally in normal recipients (Levin and Truax, 1960). It is interesting to recall that Syden-stricker (1924) had come to a similar conclusion many years previously: he had transfused a normal recipient with blood from an individual with latent sickle-cell anaemia (*i.e.*, with Hb AS) and had detected the transfused cells in the recipient by testing for in-vitro sickling 23 days later.

Haemoglobin

Ratio of Hb S to Hb A. About 22–45% of the haemoglobin in Hb-AS subjects is Hb S (Wells and Itano, 1951; Zuelzer, Neel and Robinson, 1956). Significant intrafamily differences in the proportion of Hb S and Hb A exist (Neel, Wells and Itano, 1951). Neel (1952) explained this by suggesting that other genes (not necessarily those for abnormal haemoglobins) might influence significantly the amount of Hb S formed as the result of the presence of the gene for Hb S.

Tondo and Sulzano (1962) investigated 1014 Brazilian blacks and found that 5.9% of them carried the Hb-AS trait. The percentage of Hb S varied from 24.9 to 50.7, mean 41.1 ± 5.9 and there was some indication of a trimodal frequency, with peaks at 32–34%, 42–44% and 48–50%.

Wrightstone, Huisman and van der Sar (1968), who reported on the percentage of Hb S in 63 Hb-AS individuals, similarly reported a wide range of values, namely 25–47%. The data, in their view, did not exclude the possibility that in the state of Georgia, at least, only one modality was present with respect to Hb-S percentages; they conceded, however, that more than one modality related to familial factors might exist in other areas of the world.

The relatively low proportion of Hb S compared with Hb A in the erythrocytes of Hb-AS heterozygotes can in theory be explained in more than one way: one possibility is that the synthesis of β^S chains occurs more slowly than that of the normal β^A chains; another is that the β^S chains after synthesis are unstable; another is that the assembly of the completed chains into the Hb-S tetramer is less rapid than in the case of Hb A; still another possibility is that cells containing relatively high proportions of Hb S are selectively removed from the circulating blood after leaving the bone marrow. The early work in relation to this problem was reviewed by White (1971) and Sarup and White (1974).

Heywood, Karon and Weissman (1964), in studies on reticulocytes from bone marrow and peripheral blood, concluded that the ratio of haemoglobins in Hb-AS heterozygotes (and also in Hb-AD, Hb-AC and Hb-SC heterozygotes) was an accurate reflection of the rates at which the haemoglobins were being synthesized.

Boyer, Hathaway and Garrick (1964) concluded that β^S (and β^0) mRNA is less stable than β^A mRNA and that this instability is a major factor determining the final Hb-A/Hb-S ratio in the peripheral blood.

More recent studies have shown conclusively that in some families at least an important modifying factor is the presence of a gene or genes for α-thalassaemia. In 1974 DeSimone and co-workers reported that they had compared the $\alpha : \beta$-chain synthesis ratios in reticulocytes obtained from eight Hb-AS individuals. Three had a high proportion of Hb S (40–42%); five had a low proportion (26–32%). In the former the rate of α-chain synthesis approximated closely to that of the β chain; in the latter it was 66–80% of that of the β chain.

Abraham and Huisman (1977) studied the affinity *in vitro* of α chains for β chains in artificial mixtures of α chains and several different types of variant β chains. In the case of Hb S they found that α chains preferred to assemble with β^A chains rather than with β^S chains: they made the point that such preference of assembly is a major post-translational control mechanism regulating the level of a β-chain variant in heterozygotes with Hb A.

The proportion of Hb S to Hb A in individual Hb-AS subjects remains, it is thought, constant after the first 1 year or so of life. However, concurrent severe iron deficiency or megaloblastic anaemia can influence this. Thus the Hb-S percentage rose from 30 to 42% as the result of iron therapy in an iron-deficient patient described by Levere, Lichtman and Levine (1964) and from 10.6 to 38.5%, with a correspondingly marked reduction in the solubility of the reduced haemolysate, in a patient being treated for megaloblastic anaemia by Heller *et al.* (1963). Whether the synthesis of Hb S is abnormally slowed in such cases or whether there is a disproportionate destruction of cells containing the highest percentages of Hb S remains uncertain.

A recent technical advance has enabled the proportion of Hb S to Hb A in individual erythrocytes in heterozygotes to be determined. Anyaibe and co-workers (1983) reported that, using the technique of single-cell electrophoresis, they had been able to show that the relative proportions of Hb S and Hb A in heterozygotes varied widely from cell to cell. They found, too, that approximately 7% of cells in AS heterozygotes contained apparently Hb A alone — a finding consistent with the known failure of a small proportion of a heterozygote's cells to sickle at zero O_2 tension (Allison, 1956). Anyaibe, Castro and Headings (1985), who had applied the technique to the blood of 30 Hb-AS individuals, reported considerable differences between the heterozygotes in the way in which Hb S was distributed in their erythrocyte population.

Hb F. This is present in normal amounts in infants who have the Hb-S trait. In older children and adults Hb F is usually absent or, at the most, present only in traces (Chernoff, 1953; White and Beaven, 1959). Abnormally high concentrations of Hb F are suggestive of Hb-S/β-thalassaemia (see p. 134).

Hb A_2. The percentage of Hb A_2 appears to be slightly increased in Hb-AS subjects. Wrightstone, Huisman and van der Sar (1968) found that the mean Hb-A$_2$ percentage in 63 Hb-AS heterozygotes was 3.5, with a range of 2.3–4.2. This contrasted with their data on 50 Hb-AA individuals whose mean percentage was 2.8, with a range of 1.9–3.6. Almost identical figures have been more recently reported by Francina et al. (1982): the mean Hb-A$_2$ percentage in their 99 Hb-AS subjects was 3.52 ± 0.57 compared with 2.52 ± 0.55 in 100 Hb-AA subjects, a statistically significant difference ($P < 0.001$). They suggested that

the difference could be explained either by the β^S chains having less affinity for α chains than β^A chains, thus increasing the availability of α chains for combination with δ chains, or by the β^S chains undergoing more proteolysis than β^A chains.

Reeves, Berard and Reeves (1983) similarly reported slightly raised Hb-A$_2$ percentages in black Hb-AS subjects: mean 3.4 ± 0.3 compared with a mean of 3.1 ± 0.3 in black Hb-AA controls.

LABORATORY DIAGNOSIS OF SICKLE-CELL DISEASE AND TRAIT; DEMONSTRATION OF THE PRESENCE OF HAEMOGLOBIN S

The laboratory diagnosis of a sickle-cell disease or sickle-cell trait depends upon the demonstration of Hb S. This is generally straightforward and easy. Leaving aside the recognition of ISCs in films of peripheral blood, the presence of Hb S can be deduced by demonstrating that many of the patient's erythrocytes sickle in vitro when deoxygenated. Its presence can be confirmed by submitting a haemolysate to electrophoresis, or other techniques such as iso-electric focusing and column chromatography, and observing an abnormal band of haemoglobin running in the expected position of Hb S. A strong band in the expected position of Hb S on routine haemoglobin electrophoresis, and the apparent absence of Hb A, however, does not necessarily mean that the patient is homozygous for Hb S. Noronha and Honig (1979), for instance, in an interesting discussion on the diagnosis of Hb-SS disease in two white American children, listed 13 other sickle syndromes in which the haemoglobin pattern on routine electrophoresis is difficult or impossible to distinguish from that of Hb-SS disease without further study. [Some of the syndromes are of course very uncommon.]

Descriptions of the techniques that are appropriate for the clear separation of Hb S from other abnormal haemoglobins and Hb A are beyond the scope of this book, as are the methods of chain and peptide separation and amino-acid analysis necessary for the precise chemical diagnosis of Hb S.

Sickling tests in all their forms are relatively time-consuming and require the use of a microscope; and they are thus somewhat inappropriate when many samples of blood need to be tested as in large-scale studies into the frequency of Hb S in populations. For this reason the possibility of using the diminished solubility of Hb S when deoxygenated more directly in tests for its presence has been explored, and a number of tests based on this characteristic have been elaborated (see below). As in all laboratory tests, careful standardization, controls and quality assessment are necessary. Reviews and monographs that give good accounts of the laboratory diagnosis of Hb S include those of Efremov and Huisman (1974), Lehmann and Huntsman (1974). Huisman (1979) and Serjeant (1985).

Early observations on the sickling test

Sickling was originally brought about by keeping a fluid preparation of blood in a sealed container. Under these circumstances deoxygenation takes place gradually and the erythrocytes were observed to undergo progressive distortion within minutes or hours, the process being noted to occur considerably faster in Hb-SS disease than in the Hb-AS trait (Figs. 12.22–12.24). The next advance was the observation that sickling could be accelerated by adding a reducing agent to the cell suspension, e.g., sodium metabisulphite and vitamin C (Daland and Castle, 1948), sodium

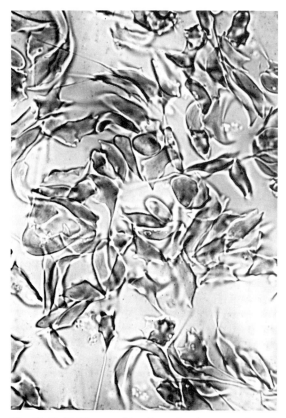

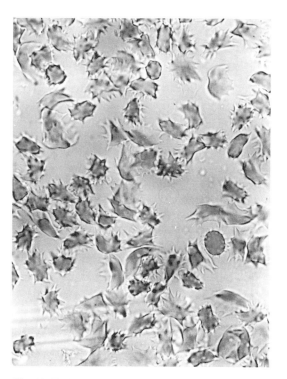

Fig. 12.23 Holly-leaf sickling resulting from the deoxygenation of Hb-AS trait blood.

Fig. 12.22 Sickling resulting from the deoxygenation of Hb-SS disease blood.

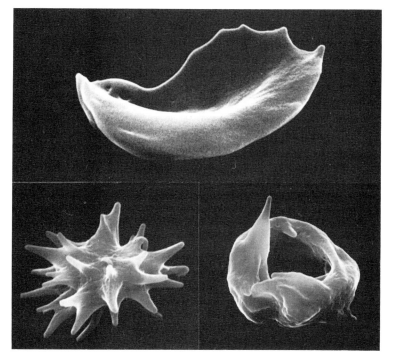

Fig. 12.24 Sickled cells as viewed by a scanning electron microscope.

Top: a deoxygenated discocyte.

Bottom left: a deoxygenated echinocyte.

Bottom right: a deoxygenated stomatocyte.

(Reproduced by courtesy of Professor Marcel Bessis.)

dithionite at pH 6.8 (Itano and Pauling, 1949) or sodium hydrosulphite (Williams and Mackey, 1949). Early, too, in the history of the sickling test it was found that sickling was retarded if the temperature was lowered below 37°C (Syden-stricker et al., 1923; Sherman, 1940) and that it fails to occur at 4°C (Bessis et al., 1954). Robinson (1945) demonstrated that the addition of cultures of various bacteria to blood hastened sickling, and Singer and Robin (1948) reported that the addition of a culture of B. subtilis at 37°C could bring it about within 15 minutes.

The chemical reducing agents, although they have proved to be potent and valuable, have the disadvantage that they are relatively unstable in solution. Unawareness of this has led to error. Other possible sources of error pointed out by Schneider, Alperin and Lehmann (1967), which apply, too, to sickling in sealed whole-blood preparations without added reducing agent, include artifacts produced by drying of the cell suspension, increased plasma viscosity, the presence of transfused normal erythrocytes, contamination with bacteria, exposure to heat and the presence of marked poikilocytosis.

Isaacs (1950) produced a type of 'sickling' by suspending normal erythrocytes in highly viscous gelatin solutions, and 'false' sickle cells were observed by Shapiro (1958) to develop in sealed preparations kept for 8–24 hours. These curious spiculated forms, which developed first at the edges of the cell suspensions, were described as being more noticeable in the blood of women than of men; they were observed to develop, too, in the blood of various domestic animals.

Tests based on the diminished solubility of deoxygenated haemoglobin S

As also referred to on page 109, Itano (1953a,b) had published basic data on the differences in solubility of naturally-occurring mixtures of human haemoglobins after reduction. Goldberg (1958) extended this work and demonstrated that a solubility test, modified slightly from that of Itano (1953b) could give highly reproducible results. Huntsman and co-workers (1970) reported similarly. Subsequently, several solubility tests for the diagnosis of sickle-cell disease have been commercially marketed. Solubility is generally

judged by its effect on the observer's ability to read black print through a standard depth of solution, and some of the tests, at least, have proved highly successful and accurate.

Canning and Huntsman (1970) and Ballard and co-workers (1970) recorded complete concordance in results when large series of Hb-AS blood samples were tested by a commercially available solubility test and a microscopically read sickling test. Loh (1971) concluded in a similar study that the solubility test was in fact more sensitive than a microscopically read metabisulphite test in detecting the Hb-AS trait. Powell and Beach (1971) tested 88 specimens and found complete concurrence between the results using a modification of the Sickledex test employing Microtiter plates containing 96 wells, the standard Sickledex test and electrophoresis.

Nalbandian and co-workers (1971) explored the possibility of assessing haemoglobin solubility by an automated technique. In a system capable of making 120 determinations in 1 hour they found that Hb AS could be accurately demonstrated but they were unable to distinguish Hb AS from Hb SS. A similar study was carried out by Canning et al. (1972). They found that although Hb AA could be distinguished from Hb AS, Hb AS could not be separated from Hb SC, nor Hb AS from Hb SS with a high content of Hb F. It was found to be advisable, too, to adjust the haemoglobin level in the sample to at least 10 g/dl. Konotey-Ahulu (1972) stressed the difficulty of distinguishing between Hb AS and Hb SC in visually read tests, and made the point that this was important in Ghana where the incidence of Hb-SC disease was about the same as that of Hb-SS disease (about 1% of all births).

Schmidt and Wilson (1973) reviewed the performance of several commercially available solubility tests. Some performed very well, others less well by giving too many false negatives. False positives were possible also, e.g., in dysproteinaemias or as the result of hyperlipidaemia. False negatives mostly occurred with markedly anaemic blood samples (Hb <7 g/dl), with the blood of patients who had recently received a large transfusion or with the blood of infants less than 6 months of age (see p. 111), or as the result of the reagents being inactive.

The Murayama test

Nalbandian and co-workers (1970), who stated that 17 abnormal haemoglobins were known that gave a similar pattern to that of Hb S on electrophoresis at pH 8.0–8.9, described what they referred to as a single specific test for Hb S — the Murayama test. The basis of this test is that haemolysates containing Hb S gel at 37°C when deoxygenated; and that when such a gel is placed in ice-water it liquefies. Liquefication signifies a positive test and, according to Nalbandian et al., this is characteristic of haemolysates containing Hb S (or Hb C Harlem).

Visualization of Hb S within individual erythrocytes

This has been attempted by differential elution and by the use of specific antisera. Yakulis and Heller (1964) described how they had been able to pretreat films with 2.48 M-phosphate buffer and sodium dithionate so that the haemoglobin in cells containing Hb A, Hb F, Hb C or Hb D was completely eluted with the result that the cells were virtually colourless when subsequently stained; in contrast, the haemoglobin in Hb-SS cells was not eluted and stained well and that in Hb-AS cells stained in an intermediate fashion.

Headings and co-workers (1975) used fluorescent-labelled antisera raised against Hb A, Hb S and Hb F and were able to identify the corresponding haemoglobins in cells suspended in agar. Papayannopoulou and co-workers (1976) used similarly labelled antibodies against Hb S and Hb F. They were able to apply the method to fixed films of peripheral blood and bone marrow. Hb-AS and Hb-SS cells reacted strongly and to a similar degree of brightness; cord-blood Hb-AS cells also reacted but to varying degrees. In bone marrow, normoblasts containing Hb S fluoresced more brightly than did mature erythrocytes. When the anti-Hb-F antibody was applied to normoblasts only 5–10% reacted compared with about 25% of adult erythrocytes in the peripheral blood, indicating the preferential survival of cells containing Hb F.

SCREENING PROGRAMMES FOR HAEMOGLOBINOPATHIES

In children and adults. The emphasis has been on the development of simple, economically cheap but reliable techniques that will provide presumptive evidence at least of the presence of the Hb-AS trait and Hb-SS and Hb-SC disease.

Barnes, Komarmy and Novack (1972) used haemolysates prepared from unwashed erythrocytes collected into heparinized microhaematocrit tubes, which were then submitted to 10-minute cellulose acetate electrophoresis; each test was calculated to cost not more than 10 U.S. cents.

Greenberg, Harvey and Morgan (1972) used a solubility test estimated to cost 3–4 U.S. cents. Of 482 samples of finger-prick blood, 33 were found to give positive results, i.e., opacity rather than translucency; all the samples were found later to sickle in isotonic sodium metabisulphite solution.

Garrick, Dembure and Guthrie (1973) submitted haemolysates, prepared by elution of spots of blood collected on filter paper, to cellulose acetate and citrate-agar electrophoresis. Eluates from the filter-paper spots were used, too, for solubility testing. The material cost of each screen was calculated to be 3 U.S. cents. One advantage of allowing the blood to be tested to dry on filter paper is that spots can be more easily dispatched to the laboratory by post than can liquid blood; they can, if necessary, according to Garrick, Dembure and Guthrie be kept in the 'freezer' for up to 3 months in the case of specimens from children more than 4 months of age and from adults, and for 6 weeks in the case of specimens from newborn infants.

Outside the Western hemisphere, it is desirable to employ screening techniques that are sensitive to the presence of Hb D and Hb E, as well as Hb S and Hb C. Stuart and his co-workers (1973), for instance, in Birmingham (U.K.), screened 6835 school children who were mainly of West-Indian or Asian origin by using starch-gel electrophoresis at pH 8.6 as the primary test and agar-gel electrophoresis at pH 6.2 to discriminate between Hb S and Hb D and between Hb C and Hb E. The haemolysates they tested were derived from blood collected into heparinized capillary tubes: 574 haemoglobinopathies were detected.

A consideration of the ethics and desirability of screening a population for the presence of Hb S, or other abnormal inherited trait, is beyond the scope of this book. Suffice it to say that the writer feels that it is highly desirable that anyone carrying a potentially dangerous genetically transmittable trait should be aware of this fact and should be informed of the likelihood of transmitting the trait to the next generation. A particularly thoughtful and sympathetic account of the problem in relation to Hb S and the black population in the United States was written by Rucknagel (1974).

In the newborn. It is less easy to diagnose the Hb-AS trait or Hb-SS disease in newborn infants than in older children and adults. This is due to the small percentage of Hb S present at birth. According to Schneider and Haggard (1955), the Hb-S percentage in a series of newborn 'sicklemic' infants varied from not demonstrable by free electrophoresis to 21, and increased to adult levels by $4\frac{1}{2}$–7 months. The result of this is that, although sickling will take place at birth when a cord-blood sample is deoxygenated, it takes place far less readily than in later life (Scott; Crawford and Jenkins, 1948; Watson, Stahman and Bilello, 1948; Schneider and Haggard, 1955; Shields *et al.*, 1958).

Watson, Stahman and Bilello found in a series of newborn infants that from 0.5 to 29.5% of their erythrocytes sickled, compared with 84–100% of the cells in the blood of their mothers. One infant's blood was studied at frequent intervals: the proportion of cells that sickled increased from 6% at birth to 90% at 4 months.

The reluctance of cord blood to sickle readily, even if the infant is homozygous for Hb S, means that the diagnosis of Hb-S trait or Hb-SS disease is best made by other means. Three techniques have been widely used as screening tests: electrophoresis on cellulose acetate paper or in citrate agar gel and separation by thin-layer iso-electric focusing. Each technique has had its advocates. Yawson, Huntsman and Metters (1970) compared the value of electrophoresis on paper, cellulose acetate and in starch gel with that in agar gel in studying 50 infants born of mothers known to carry the Hb-S or Hb-C trait. The results with agar gel were found to be superior to those using the other media. Additional experience led Huntsman, Metters and Yawson (1972) to the same conclusion. [The potential value of agar-gel electrophoresis in the demonstration of Hb C and Hb S in neonatal blood was implicit in the early reports of Robinson *et al.* (1957) and Marder and Conley (1959), respectively.]

Schroeder, Jakway and Powars (1973) and Powars, Schroeder and White (1975) used a microcolumn chromatographic method to screen cord blood. Powars, Schroeder and White found that it was possible within 2 hours to distinguish between Hb AS and Hb SS and between Hb AC, Hb SC and Hb CC. Hb SS and Hb CC could be distinguished, too, but the test failed to distinguish between Hb-C/thalassaemia and Hb-S/thalassaemia and Hb-S/HPHF (hereditary persistence of fetal haemoglobin).

Pearson and co-workers (1974) carried out rapid agar-gel electrophoresis at pH 6.2. Hb A, Hb F, Hb S and

Hb C were clearly separated: 61 newborn blacks and Puerto Ricans gave a FAS pattern (6.8% of those tested), six (0.2%) a FS (Hb-SS) pattern and 16 a FAC pattern.

Serjeant and her co-workers (1974) and Serjeant and Serjeant (1979) reported that they had found cellulose acetate electrophoresis both cheap and satisfactory and considered the method 'eminently suitable' for cord-blood screening. They used the buffer system described by Serjeant *et al.* (1974). They had detected 225 cases of Hb-SS disease in the course of 67 000 consecutive cord-blood samples in Jamaica. Henthorn, Anionwu and Brozovic (1984) described how they had tested 3165 cord-blood specimens in London, using the same cellulose acetate technique, and found that the results were satisfactory. The incidence of an abnormal haemoglobin at birth was 6.9% and the cost of each test was computed to be 30p.

Friedman and co-workers (1978) described how they had exploited the known increased susceptibility of Hb S to denaturation by mechanical stress (see p. 223) in a shaking test. Blood was obtained from 187 2–7-day-old black neonates by heel puncture and haemolysates were submitted to both agar-gel electrophoresis and the shaking test. The results were concordant and there was no overlap in the shaking test between the percentage of haemoglobin that precipitated in the samples containing Hb S and those containing Hb F and Hb A only. Friedman *et al.* stressed the reliability, simplicity and cheapness of the test but added that it needed careful standardization.

Galacteros and co-workers (1980) described how they had used a thin-layer iso-electric focusing technique (TLIF) (Basset *et al.*, 1978) in the screening of cord-blood samples for abnormal haemoglobins. In their hands it proved to be more successful than electrophoresis on cellulose acetate or in citrate agar gel: thus 100 abnormal haemoglobins were detected by TLIF compared with 70 by cellulose acetate and 80 by cellulose acetate and citrate agar combined. The TLIF technique was approximately twice as successful as the other two techniques in detecting Hb Bart's and this almost entirely explained its overall superiority in detecting abnormal haemoglobins.

REFERENCES

ABILDGAARD, C. F., SIMONE, J. V. & SHULMAN, I. (1967). Factor VIII (antihaemophilic factor) activity in sickle-cell anaemia. *Brit. J. Haemat.*, **13**, 19–27.

ABRAHAM, E. C. & HUISMAN, T. H. J. (1977). Differences in affinity of variant β chains for α chains: a possible explanation for the variation in the percentage of β chain varaints in heterozygotes. *Hemoglobin*, **1**, 861–873.

ALAYASH, A. I., DAFALLAH, A., AL-HUSAYNI, H., AL-ALI, A. K., AL-QUORAIN, A., OMER, A. H. S., WILSON, M. T., BONAVENTURA, J. & CASHON, R.

(1986). Glycosylated hemoglobin levels in a benign form of sickle cell anemia in Saudi Arabia. *Acta haemat. (Basel)*, **75**, 160–164.

ALKJAERSIG, N., FLETCHER, A., JOIST, H. & CHAPLIN, H. JNR (1976). Hemostatic alterations accompanying sickle cell pain crises. *J. Lab. clin. Med.*, **88**, 440–449.

ALLAMANIS, J. (1955). Paper electrophoresis of serum proteins in Cooley's anemia and sickle cell anaemia. *Acta paediat. (Uppsala)*, **44**, 122–127.

ALLEN, D. W. & WYMAN, J. JNR (1954). Équilibre de

l'hémoglobine de drepanocytose avec l'oxygène. *Rev. Hémat.*, **9**, 155–157.

ALLISON, A. C. (1956). Observations on the sickling phenomenon and on the distribution of different haemoglobin types in erythrocyte populations. *Clin. Sci.*, **15**, 497–510.

ALPERIN, J. B. (1967). Folic acid deficiency complicating sickle cell anemia. A study on the response to titrated doses of folic acid. *Arch. intern. Med.*, **120**, 298–306.

ANDERSON, M. F. (1972). The iron status of pregnant women with hemoglobinopathies. *Amer. J. Obstet. Gynec.*, **113**, 895–900.

ANDERSON, M. J., DAVIS, L. R.', HODGSON, J., JONES, S. E., MURTAZA, L., PATTISON, J. R., STROUD, C. E. & WHITE, J. M. (1982). Occurrence of infection with a parvovirus-like agent in children with sickle cell anaemia during a two-year period. *J. clin. Path.*, **35**, 744–749.

ANYAIBE, S., CASTRO, O. & HEADINGS, V. (1985). Distributions of hemoglobins A and S among erythrocytes of heterozygotes. *Hemoglobin*, **9**, 137–155.

ANYAIBE, S., WILSON, P., SCOTT, R. & HEADINGS, V. (1983). Relative proportions of human hemoglobins A, S, C in individual erythrocytes of heterozygotes. *Hemoglobin*, **7**, 227–244.

BALLARD, M. S., RADEL, E., SAKHADEO, S. & SCHORR, J. B. (1970). A new diagnostic test for hemoglobin S. *J. Pediat.*, **76**, 117–119.

BALLESTER, O. F. & PRASAD, A. S. (1983). Anergy, zinc deficiency, and decreased nucleoside phosphorylase activity in patients with sickle cell anemia. *Ann. intern. Med.*, **98**, 180–182.

BARBEDO, M. M. R. & McCURDY, P. R.(1974). Red cell life span in sickle cell trait. *Acta haemat. (Basel)*, **51**, 339–343.

BARNES, M. G., KOMARMY, L. & NOVACK, A. H. (1972). A comprehensive screening program for hemoglobinopathies. *J. Amer. med. Ass.*, **219**, 701–705.

BARRERAS, L. & DIGGS, L. W. (1964). Bicarbonates, pH and percentage of sickled cells in venous blood of patients in sickle cell crisis. *Amer. J. med. Sci.*, **247**, 710–718.

BARRERAS, L., DIGGS, L. W. & BELL, A. (1968). Erythrocyte morphology in patients with sickle cell anemia and pulmonary emboli. *J. Amer. med. Ass.*, **203**, 569–573.

BARRERAS, L., DIGGS, L. W. & LIPSCOMB, A. (1966). Plasma volume in sickle cell disease. *Sth. med. J. (Bgham, Ala.)*, **59**, 456–458.

BASSET, P., BEUZARD, Y., GAREL, M. C. & ROSA, J. (1978). Isoelectric focusing of human hemoglobin: its application to screening, to the characterization of 70 variants, and to the study of modified fractions of normal hemoglobins. *Blood*, **51**, 971–982.

BASU, A. K., WOODRUFF, A. W. & PETTITT, L. E. (1963). Effect of pyrexia on sicklaemic states.

Lancet, **ii**, 1088–1090.

BASU, M. K., LEE, M. M., MANIATIS, A. & BERTLES, J. F. (1984). Characteristics of I and i antigen receptors on the membrane of erythrocytes in sickle cell anemia. *J. Lab. clin. Med.*, **103**, 712–719.

BECKLAKE, M. R., GRIFFITHS, S. B., McGREGOR, M., GOLDMAN, H. I. & SCHREVE, J. P. (1955). Oxygen dissociation curves in sickle cell anemia and in subjects with the sickle cell trait. *J. clin. Invest.*, **34**, 751–755.

BESSIS, M., BRICKA, M., BRETON-GORIUS, J. & TABUIS, J. (1954). New observations on sickle cells, with special reference to their agglutinability. *Blood.* **9**, 39–45.

BETKE, K. & KLEIHAUER, E. (1958). Fetaler und bleibender Blutfarbstoff in Erythrocyten und Erythroblasten von menschlichen Feten und Neugerborenen. *Blut*, **4**, 241–249.

BIANCO, I. (1948). La resistenza emoglobinica nei portatori di microcitemia e di falcemia. *Policlinico, Sez. prat.*, **55**, 103–105.

BICKERS, J. B. (1966). Alkali-resistant hemoglobin in sickle cell disease. *Ann. intern. Med.*, **64**, 1028–1033.

BILLETT, H. H., KIM, K., FABRY, M. E. & NAGEL, R. L. (1985). Dense cell distribution does not predict incidence of sickle cell painful crisis in SS patients. *Blood*, **66**, No. 5 (Suppl. 1), 56a (Abstract 109).

BOGGS, D. R., HYDE, F. & SRODES, C. (1973). An unusual pattern of neutrophil kinetics in sickle cell anemia. *Blood*, **41**, 59–65.

BOYER, S. H., DOVER, G. J., SERJEANT, G. R., SMITH, K. D., ANTONARAKIS, S. E., EMBURY, S. H., MARGOLOT, L., NOYES, A. N., BOYER, M. L. & BIAS, W. B. (1984). Production of F cells in sickle cell anemia: regulation by a genetic locus or loci separate from the β-globin gene cluster. *Blood*, **64**, 1053–1058.

BOYER, S. H., HATHAWAY, P. & GARRICK, M. D. (1964). Modulation of protein synthesis in man: an in vitro study of hemoglobin synthesis by heterozygotes. *Cold Spr. Harb. Symp. quant. Biol.*, **29**, 333–346.

BROMBERG, P. A., JENSEN, W. N. & McDONOUGH, M. (1967). Blood oxygen dissociation curves in sickle cell disease. *J. Lab. clin. Med.*, **70**, 480–488.

BROWN, K., LUBIN, B., SMITH, R. & OSKI, F. (1972). Prevalence of anemia among preadolescent and young adolescent urban black Americans. *J. Pediat.*, **81**, 714–718.

BUCHANAN, G. R. & GLADER, B. E. (1978). Leukocyte counts in children with sickle cell disease. *Amer. J. Dis. Child.*, **132**, 396–398.

BUCHANAN, G. R. & HOLTKAMP, C. A. (1983). Evidence against enhanced platelet activity in sickle cell anaemia. *Brit. J. Haemat.*, **54**, 595–603.

BUNTING, H. (1939). Sedimentation rates of sickled and non-sickled cells from patients with sickle cell anemia. *Amer. J. med. Sci.*, **198**, 191–193.

CALLENDER, S. T. E., NICKEL, J. F., MOORE, C. V. & POWELL, E. O. (1949). Sickle-cell disease: studied by measuring the survival of transfused red cells. *J. Lab. clin. Med.*, **34**, 90–104.

CANNING, D. M., CRANE, R. S., HUNTSMAN, R. G. & YAWSON, G. I. (1972). An automatic screening technique for the detection of sickle-cell haemoglobin. *J. clin. Path.*, **25**, 330–334.

CANNING D. M. & HUNTSMAN, R. G. (1970). An assessment of Sickledex as an alternative to the sickling test. *J. clin. Path.*, **23**, 736–737.

CASPER, J. T., KOETHE, S., RODEY, G. E. & THATCHER, L. G. (1976). A new method for studying splenic reticuloendothelial dysfunction in sickle cell disease patients and its clinical application: a brief report. *Blood*, **47**, 183–188.

CASTRO, O. & HADDY, T. B. (1983). Improved survival of iron-deficient sickle erythrocytes. *New Engl. J. Med.*, **308**, 527 (Letter).

CASTRO, O. & SCOTT, R. B. (1985). Red blood cell counts and indices in sickle cell trait in a black American population. *Hemoglobin*, **9**, 65–67.

CAWEIN, M. J., O'NEILL, R. P., DANZER, L. W., LAPPAT, E. J. & ROACH, T. (1969). A study of the sickling phenomenon and oxygen dissociation curve in patients with hemoglobins SS, SD, SF and SC. *Blood*, **34**, 682–690.

CHARACHE, S., GRISOLIA, S., FIEDLER, A. J. & HELLEGERS, A. E. (1970). Effect of 2,3-diphosphoglycerate on oxygen affinity of blood in sickle cell anemia. *J. clin. Invest.*, **49**, 806–812.

CHARNEY, E. & MILLER, G. (1964). Reticulocytopenia in sickle cell disease. Aplastic episodes in the course of sickle cell disease in children. (1964). *Amer. J. Dis. Child.*, **107**, 450–455.

CHERNOFF, A. I. (1953). Immunologic studies of hemoglobins. II. Quantitative precipitin test using anti fetal hemoglobin sera. *Blood*, **8**, 413–421.

CHERNOFF, A. I. & JOSEPHSON, A. M. (1951). Acute erythroblastopenia in sickle-cell anemia and infectious mononucleosis. *Amer. J. Dis. Child.*, **82**, 310–322.

CORASH, L. M., PIOMELLI, S., CHEN, H. C., SEAMAN, C. & GROSS, E. (1974). Separation of erythrocytes according to age on a simplified density gradient. *J. Lab. clin. Med.*, **84**, 147–151.

CROSBY, W. H. & DAMESHEK, W. (1951). The significance of hemoglobinemia and associated hemosiderinuria, with particular reference to various types of hemolytic anemia. *J. Lab. clin. Med.*, **38**, 829–841.

DAESCHNER, C. W. III, CARPENTIERI, U., GOLDMAN, A. S. & HAGGARD, M. E. (1985). Zinc deficiency and blood lymphocyte function with sickle cell disease. *Scand. J. Haemat.*, **35**, 186–190.

DALAND, G. A. & CASTLE, W. B. (1948). A single and rapid method for demonstrating sickling of the red blood cells: the use of reducing agents. *J. Lab. clin. Med.*, **33**, 1082–1088.

DANON, D. & MARIKOVSKY, Y. (1964). Determination of density distribution of red cell population. *J. Lab. clin. Med.*, **64**, 668–674.

DAVIES, S., HENTHORN, J. & BROZOVIĆ, M. (1983). Iron deficiency in sickle cell anaemia. J. clin. Path., **36**, 1012–1015.

DAVIES, S., HENTHORN, J. S., WIN, A. A. & BROZOVIC, M. (1984). Effect of blood transfusion on iron status in sickle cell anaemia. *Clin. lab. Haemat.*, **6**, 17–22.

DAVIS, L. R. (1976). Changing blood picture in sickle-cell anaemia from shortly after birth to adolescence. *J. clin. Path.*, **29**, 898–901.

DeSIMONE, J., KLEVE, L., LONGLEY, M. A. & SHAEFFER, S. (1974). Unbalanced globin chain synthesis in reticulocytes of sickle cell trait individuals with low concentrations of hemoglobin S. *Biochem. biophys. Res. Commun.*, **59**, 564–569.

DIGGS, L. W. (1932). The blood picture in sickle cell anemia. *Sth. med. J. (Bgham, Ala.)*, **25**, 615–620.

DIGGS, L. W. (1956). The crisis in sickle cell anemia. Hematologic studies. *Amer. J. clin. Path.*, **26**, 1109–1118.

DIGGS, L. W., AHMANN, C. F. & BIBB, J. (1933). Incidence and significance of the sickle cell trait. *Ann. intern. Med.*, **7**, 769–778.

DIGGS, L. W. & BIBB, J. (1939). The erythrocyte in sickle cell anemia. Morphology, size, hemoglobin content, fragility and sedimentation rate. *J. Amer. med. Ass.*, **112**, 695–701.

DOVER, G. J., BOYER, S. H., CHARACHE, S. & HEINTZELMAN, K. (1978). Individual variation in the production and survival of F cells in sickle-cell disease. *New Engl. J. Med.*, **299**, 1428–1435.

DOVER, G. J., BOYER, S. H. & PEMBREY, M. E. (1981). F-cell production in sickle cell anemia: regulation by genes linked to β-hemoglobin locus. *Science*, **211**, 1441–1444.

EFREMOV, G. D. & HUISMAN, T. H. J. (1974). The laboratory diagnosis of hemoglobinopathies. *Clinics Haemat.*, **3**, 527–570.

ELSEWEIDY, M. M. & ABRAHAM, E. C. (1984). The relationship between fetal hemoglobin level and glycosylation in sickle cell disease. *Amer. J. Hemat.*, **16**, 375–381.

ERLANDSON, M. E., SHULMAN, I. & SMITH, C. H. (1960). Studies on congenital hemolytic syndromes. III. Rates of destruction and production of erythrocytes in sickle cell anemia. *Pediatrics*, **25**, 629–644.

EVANS, H. E. & REINDORF, C. (1968). Serum immunoglobulin levels in sickle cell disease and thalassemia major. *Amer. J. Dis. Child.*, **116**, 586–590.

EVANS, J. P. M., ROSSITER, M. A., KUMARAN, T. O. & MARSH, G. W. (1984). Human parvovirus aplasia: case due to cross infection in a ward. *Brit. med. J.*, **288**, 681.

FABRY, M. E., BENJAMIN, L., LAWRENCE, C. & NAGEL, R. L. (1983). An objective sign of painful crisis in sickle cell anemia: concomitant reduction of high density red cells. *Blood*, **62**, No. 5 (Suppl. 1), 56a (Abstract 126).

FABRY, M. E., BENJAMIN, L., LAWRENCE, C. & NAGEL, R. L. (1984a). An objective sign in painful crisis in sickle cell anemia: the concomitant reduction of high density red cells. *Blood*, **64**, 559–563.

FABRY, M. E., MEARS, J. G., PATEL, P., SCHAEFER-REGO, K., CARMICHAEL, L. D., MARTINEZ, G. & NAGEL, R. L. (1984b). Dense cells in sickle cell anemia: the effects of gene interaction. *Blood*, **64**, 1042–1046.

FABRY, M. E. & NAGEL, R. L. (1982a). Heterogeneity of red cells in the sickler: a characteristic with practical, clinical and pathophysiological implications. *Blood Cells*, **8**, 9–15.

FABRY, M. E. & NAGEL, A. L. (1982b). The effect of deoxygenation on red cell density: significance for the pathophysiology of sickle cell anemia. *Blood*, **60**, 1370–1377.

FENICHEL, R. L., WATSON, J. & EIRICH, F. (1950). Electrophoretic studies of the plasma and serum proteins in sickle cell anemia. *J. clin. Invest.*, **29**, 1620–1624.

FINCH, C. A. (1972). Pathophysiologic aspects of sickle cell anemia. *Amer. J. Med.*, **53**, 1–6.

FRAIMOW, W., RODMAN, T., CLOSE, H. P., CATHCART, R. & PURCELL, M. K. (1958). The oxyhemoglobin dissociation curve in sickle cell anemia. *Amer. J. med. Sci.*, **236**, 225–232.

FRANCINA, A., DORLÉAC, E., BAUDONNET, C., JACCOUD, P. & DELAUNAY, J. (1982). Microchromatofocusing of hemoglobins. Increased hemoglobin A_2 percentage in sickle cell trait. *Clin. chim. Acta*, **121**, 261–264.

FREEDMAN, M. L. & KARPATKIN, S. (1975). Elevated platelet count and megathrombocyte number in sickle cell anemia. *Blood*, **46**, 579–582.

FRIEDMAN, S., BACK, B., DELIVORIA-PAPADOPOULOS, M., ATWATER, J., ASAKURA, T. & SCHWARTZ, E. (1978). A simple test for detection of sickle hemoglobin in the neonatal period. *Amer. J. clin. Path.*, **70**, 85–88.

GALACTEROS, F., KLEMAN, K., CABURI-MARTIN, J., BEUZARD, Y., ROSA, J. & LUBIN, B. (1980). Cord blood screening for hemoglobin abnormalities by thin layer isoelectric focusing. *Blood*, **56**, 1068–1071.

GARDINER, M. B., REESE, A. L., HEADLEE, M. E. & HUISMAN, T. H. J. (1982). The heterogeneity of the γ-chain of fetal haemoglobin in HbS heterozygotes. *Blood*, **60**, 513–518.

GARRICK, M. D., DEMBURE, P. & GUTHRIE, R. (1973). Sickle-cell anemia and other hemoglobinopathies. Procedures and strategy for screening employing spots of blood on filter paper as specimen. *New Engl. J. Med.*, **288**, 1265–1268.

GAVRILLIS, P., ROTHENBERG, S. P. & GUY, R. (1974). Correlation of low serum IgM levels with absence of functional splenic tissue in sickle cell disease syndromes. *Amer. J. Med.*, **57**, 542–545.

GOLDBERG, C. A. J. (1958). The ferrohemoglobin solubility test. Its accuracy and precision together with values found in the presence of some abnormal hemoglobins. *Clin. Chem.*, **4**, 146–149.

GORDON, P. A., BREEZE, G. R., MANN, J. R. & STUART, J. (1974). Coagulation fibrinolysis in sickle-cell disease. *J. clin. Path.*, **27**, 485–489.

GOWDA, N., RAO, S., COHEN, B., MILLER, S. & BROWN, A. (1985). Human parvovirus (HPV) infection in sickle cell patients with and without hypoplastic crisis. *Blood*, **66**, No. 5 (Suppl. 1), 59a (Abstract 122).

GREEN, D., KWAAN, H. C. & DUIZ, G. (1970). Impaired fibrinolysis in sickle cell disease. Relation to crisis and infection. *Thrombos. Diathes. haemorrh. (Stuttg.)*, **24**, 10–16.

GREENBERG, M. S., HARVEY, H. A. & MORGAN, C. (1972). A simple and inexpensive screening test for sickle hemoglobin. *New Engl. J. Med.*, **286**, 1143–1144.

GREENBERG, M. S. & KASS, E. H. (1958). Studies on the destruction of red blood cells. XIII. Observations on the role of pH in the pathogenesis and treatment of painful crisis in sickle-cell disease. *Arch. intern. Med.*, **101**, 355–363.

GREENBERG, M. S., KASS, E. H. & CASTLE, W. B. (1957). Studies on the destruction of blood cells. XII. Factors influencing the role of S hemoglobin in the pathologic physiology of sickle cell anemia and related disorders. *J. clin. Invest.*, **36**, 833–843.

GRUPPO, R. A., GLUECK, H. I., GRANGER, S. M. & MILLER, M. A. (1977). Platelet function in sickle cell anemia. *Thromb. Res.*, **10**, 325–335.

HADDY, T. B. & CASTRO, O. (1982). Overt iron deficiency in sickle cell disease. *Arch. intern. Med.*, **142**, 1621–1624.

HADDY, T. B., LUSHER, J. M., HENDRICKS, S. & TROSKO, B. K. (1979). Erythropoiesis in sickle cell anaemia during acute infection and crisis. *Scand. J. Haemat.*, **22**, 289–295.

HAHN, E. V. & GILLESPIE, E. B. (1927). Sickle cell anemia. Report of a case greatly improved by splenectomy. Experimental study of sickle cell formation. *Arch. intern. Med.*, **39**, 233–254.

HAM, T. H. & CASTLE, W. B. (1940). Relation of increased hypotonic fragility and of erythrostasis to the mechanism of hemolysis in certain anemias. *Trans. Ass. Amer. Phycns*, **55**, 127–131.

HAMMOND, D., SHORE, N. & MOVASSAGHI, N. (1968). Production, utilization and excretion of erythroprietin: I. Chronic anaemias. II. Aplastic crisis. III. Erythropoietic effects of normal plasma. *Ann. N. Y. Acad. Sci.*, **149**, 516–527.

HARBURY, C. B. (1984). Platelet activity during sickle crisis. *Blood*, **64**, No. 5 (Suppl. 1), 48a (Abstract 104).

HARRIS, J. W., BREWSTER, H. H., HAM, T. H. & CASTLE, W. B. (1956). Studies on the destruction of red blood cells. X. The biophysics and biology of sickle-cell disease. *Arch. intern. Med.*, **97**, 145–168.

HAUT, M. J., COWAN, D. H. & HARRIS, J. W. (1973). Platelet function and survival in sickle cell disease. *J. Lab. clin. Med.*, **82**, 44–53.

HAYES, R. J., BECKFORD, M., GRANDISON, Y., MASON, K., SERJEANT, B. E. & SERJEANT, G. R. (1985). The haematology of steady state homozygous sickle cell disease: frequency distributions, variation with age and sex, longitudinal observations. *Brit. J. Haemat.*, **59**, 369–382.

HEADINGS, V., BHATTACHARYA, S., SHUKLA, S., ANAIBE, S., EATON, L., CALVERT, A. & SCOTT, R. (1975). Identification of specific hemoglobins within individual erythrocytes. *Blood*, **45**, 263–271.

HELLER, P., YAKULIS, V. J., EPSTEIN, R. B. & FRIEDLAND, S. (1963). Variation in the amount of hemoglobin S in a patient with sickle cell trait and megaloblastic anemia. *Blood*, **21**, 479–483.

HELMER, R. E. III, SAYLE, B. A., ALPERIN, J. B. & GARDNER, F. H. (1979). ^{111}In chloride bone marrow scintigraphy and ferrokinetic studies in a case of sickle cell anemia with transient erythroid aplasia. *Acta haemat. (Basel)*, **61**, 330–333.

HENDERSON, A. B. (1950). Sickle cell anemia. Clinical study of 54 cases. *Amer. J. Med.*, **9**, 757–765.

HENSTELL, H. H., KLIGERMAN, M. & IRWIN, L. E. (1965). Sickle cell disease. A serum defect in the thromboplastin generation test. *Blood*, **25**, 907–920.

HENTHORN, J., ANIONWU, E. & BROZOVIC, M. (1984). Screening cord blood for sickle haemoglobinopathies in Brent. *Brit. med. J.* **289**, 479–480.

HERRICK, J. B. (1910). Peculiar elongated and sickle-shaped red blood corpuscles in a case of severe anemia. *Trans. Ass. Amer. Phycns*, **25**, 553–561.

HERSHKO, C., MOREB, J., GAZIEL, Y., KONIJN, A. M. & RACHMILEWITZ, E. A. (1982). Reduced frequency of iron deficiency anaemia in sickle cell trait. *Scand. J. Haemat.*, **29**, 304–310.

HEYWOOD, J. D., KARON, M. & WEISSMAN, S. (1964). Studies of the in vitro synthesis of heterogenic hemoglobins. *J. clin. Invest.*, **43**, 2368–2376.

HIGGS, D. R., ALDRIDGE, B. E., LAMB, J., CLEGG, J. B., WEATHERALL, D. J., HAYES, R. J., GRANDISON, Y., LOWRIE, Y., MASON, K. P., SERJEANT, B. E. & SERJEANT, G. R. (1982). The interaction of alpha-thalassemia and homozygous sickle-cell disease. *New Engl. J. Med.*, **306**, 1441–1446.

HILKOVITZ, G. (1960). Sickle-cell disease. The "aplastic crisis" and erythroid maturation defect occurring simultaneously in three members of a family. *Arch. intern. Med.*, **105**, 76–82.

HO PING KONG, H. & ALLEYNE, G. A. O. (1969). Acid-base status of adults with sickle-cell anaemia. *Brit. med. J.*, **iii**, 271–273.

HUISMAN, T. H. J. (1979). Sickle cell anemia as a syndrome: a review of diagnostic features. *Amer. J. Hemat.*, **6**, 173–184.

HUISMAN, T. H. J., SCHROEDER, W. A., BOUVER, N. G., MILLER, A., SHELTON, J. R., SHELTON, J. B. & APELL, G. (1972). Chemical heterogeneity of fetal hemoglobin in subjects with sickle cell anemia, homozygous Hb-C disease, SC-disease, and various combinations of hemoglobin variants. *Clin. chim. Acta*, **38**, 5–16.

HUNTSMAN, R. G., BARCLAY, G. P. T., CANNING, D. M. & YAWSON, G. I. (1970). A rapid whole blood solubility test to differentiate the sickle-cell trait from sickle-cell anaemia. *J. clin. Path.*, **23**, 781–783.

HUNTSMAN, R. G., METTERS, J. S. & YAWSON, G. I. (1972). The diagnosis of sickle cell disease in the newborn infant. *J. Pediat.*, **80**, 279–281.

ISAACS, R. (1950). Sickling: a property of all red blood cells. *Science*, **112**, 716–718.

ITANO, H. A. (1952). Abnormal hemoglobins in hemolytic anaemia. *Fed. Proc.*, **11**, 235–236 (Abstract).

ITANO, H. A. (1953a). Solubilities of naturally occurring mixtures of human hemoglobin. *Arch. Biochem.*, **47**, 148–159.

ITANO, H. A. (1953b). Human hemoglobin. *Science*, **117**, 89–94.

ITANO, H. A. (1953c). The identification of fetal hemoglobin in four modifications of sickle cell disease. *Fed. Proc.*, **12**, 224 (Abstract).

ITANO, H. A., BERGREN, W. R. & STURGEON, P. (1956). The abnormal human hemoglobins. *Medicine (Baltimore)*, **35**, 121–159.

ITANO, H. A. & PAULING, L. (1949). A rapid diagnostic test for sickle cell anemia. *Blood*, **4**, 66–68.

ITTYERAH, R., ALKJAERSIG, N., FLETCHER, A. & CHAPLIN, H. (1976). Coagulation factor XIII concentration in sickle-cell disease. *J. Lab. clin. Med.*, **88**, 546–554.

IUCHI, I., DIGGS, L. W. & UPSHAW, J. D. JNR (1964). Benzidine-positive pigments in serum of patients with sickle cell anemia during painful crises. *Ann. intern. Med.*, **60**, 1022–1027.

JAN, K.-M., USAMI, S. & SMITH, J. A. (1981). Influence of oxygen tension and hematocrit reading on ESRs of sickle cells. Role of RBC aggregation. *Arch. intern. Med.*, **141**, 1815–1818.

JENKINS, M. E., SCOTT, R. B. & FERGUSON, A. D. (1956). Studies in sickle cell anemia. VII. Blood volume relationships and the use of a plasma extender in sickle cell disease in childhood: a preliminary report. *Pediatrics*, **18**, 239–247.

JENSEN, M., BUNN, H. F., HALIKAS, G., KAN, Y. W. & NATHAN, D. G. (1953). Effects of cyanate and 2,3-diphosphoglycerate on sickling. Relationship to oxygenation. *J. clin. Invest*, **52**, 2542–2547.

JONSSON, U., ROATH, O. S. & KIRKPATRICK, C. I. F. (1959). Nutritional megaloblastic anemia associated with sickle cell states. *Blood*, **14**, 535–547.

KAPU, M. M., FLEMING, A. F. & EZEM, B. U. (1976). Plasma-zinc in sickle-cell anaemia. *Lancet*, **i**, 920 (Letter).

KARAYALCIN, G., IMRAN, M. & ROSNER, F. (1972). "Blister cells". Association with pregnancy, sickle cell disease, and pulmonary infarction. *J. Amer. med. Ass.*, **219**, 1727–1729.

KARAYALCIN, G., ROSNER, F., KIM, K. Y. & CHANDRA, P. (1974). Plasma-zinc in sickle cell-anaemia. *Lancet*, **i**, 217 (Letter).

KAY, M. M. B., GOODMAN, S. R., SORENSEN, K., WHITFIELD, C. F., WONG, P., ZAKI, L. & RUDLOFF, V. (1983). Senescent cell antigen is immunologically related to band 3. *Proc. natn. Acad. Sci. U.S.A.*, **80**, 1631–1635.

KELLEHER, J. F., LUBAN, N. L. C., COHEN, B. J. & MORTIMER, P. P. (1984). Human serum parvovirus as the cause of aplastic crisis in sickle cell disease. *Amer. J. Dis. Child.*, **138**, 401–403.

KENNY, M. W., GEORGE, A. J. & STUART, J. (1980). Platelet hyperactivity in sickle-cell disease: a consequence of hyposplenism. *J. clin. Path.*, **33**, 622–625.

KIM, H. C., FRIEDMAN, S., ASAKURA, T. & SCHWARTZ, E. (1980). Inclusions in red blood cells containing Hb S or Hb C. *Brit. J. Haemat.*, **44**, 547–554.

KIM, K. Y., KARAYALCIN, G., ROSNER, F. & ABALLI, A. (1975). Pancytopenia in a patient with sickle cell anemia. *Amer. J. Dis. Child.*, **129**, 1195–1196.

KONOTEY-AHULU, F. I. D. (1972). Detecting sickle haemoglobin. *Brit. med. J.*, **iv**, 239 (Letter).

LATHEM, W. & JENSEN, W. N. (1959). Plasma hemoglobin-binding capacity in sickle cell disease. *Blood*, **14**, 1047–1056.

LATHEM, W. & JENSEN, W. N. (1962). The renal excretion of hemoglobin in sickle cell anemia, with observations on spontaneously occurring hemoglobinemia and methemalbuminemia. *J. Lab. clin. Med.*, **59**, 137–146.

LAWRENCE, C., FABRY, M. E. & NAGEL, R. L. (1985). Red cell distribution width parallels dense red cell disappearance during painful crises in sickle cell anemia. *J. Lab. clin. Med.*, **105**, 706–710.

LEHMANN, H. & HUNTSMAN, R. G. (1974). *Man's Haemoglobins, including the Haemoglobinopathies and their Investigation*, completely revised edn. 479 pp. North-Holland Publishing Co., Amsterdam, Oxford.

LEICHTMAN, D. A. & BREWER, G. J. (1978). Elevated plasma levels of fibrinopeptide A during sickle cell anemia pain crisis — evidence for intravascular coagulation. *Amer. J. Hemat.*, **5**, 183–190.

LEIKIN, S. L. (1957). The aplastic crisis of sickle-cell disease. Occurrence in several members of families within a short period of time. *J. Dis. Child.*, **93**, 128–139.

LESLIE, J., LANGLER, D., SERJEANT, G. R., SERJEANT, B. E., DESAI, P. & GORDON, Y. B.

(1975). Coagulation changes during the steady state in homozygous sickle-cell disease in Jamaica. *Brit. J. Haemat.*, **30**, 159–166.

LEVERE, R. D., LICHTMAN, H. C. & LEVINE, J. (1964). Effect of iron-deficiency anaemia on the metabolism of the heterogenic haemoglobins in sickle-cell trait. *Nature (Lond.)*, **202**, 499–501.

LEVIN, W. C. & TRUAX, W. E. (1960). Influence of storage on erythrocyte survival in blood obtained from donors with sickle cell trait. *J. Lab. clin. Med.*, **55**, 94–97.

LINCOLN, T. L., AROESTY, J. & MORRISON, P. (1973). Iron deficiency and sickle-cell disease: a hypothesis. *Lancet*, **ii**, 260–261.

LINDENBAUM, J. & KLIPSTEIN, F. A. (1963). Folic acid deficiency in sickle-cell anemia. *New Engl. J. Med.*, **269**, 875–882.

LIU, Y. K. (1974). Folate deficiency in children with sickle cell anemia. Lack of relationship between folate deficiency and growth retardation in sickle cell anemia. *Amer. J. Dis. Child.*, **127**, 389–393.

LIU, Y. K. (1975). Folic acid deficiency in sickle cell anaemia. *Scand. J. Haemat.*, **14**, 71–79.

LOH, W.-P. (1971). Evaluation of a rapid test tube turbidity test for the detection of sickle cell hemoglobin. *Amer. J. clin. Path.*, **55**, 55–57.

LOPEZ, R., SHIMIZU, N. & COOPERMAN, J. M. (1973). Recurrent folic acid deficiency in sickle cell disease. *Amer. J. Dis. Child.*, **125**, 544–548.

LUTTON, J. D., SCHMALZER, E. A., RAO, A. N., RAO, S. P. & LEVERE, R. D. (1980). Erythroid colony studies on sickle cell anemia in hypoproliferative crisis. *Amer. J. Hemat.*, **8**, 15–21.

McGONIGLE, R. J. S., OHENE-FREMPONG, K., LEWY, J. E. & FISHER, J. W. (1985). Erythropoietin response to anaemia in children with sickle cell disease and Fanconi's hypoproliferative anaemia. *Acta haemat. (Basel)*, **74**, 6–9.

MACIVER, J. E. & PARKER-WILLIAMS, E. J. (1961). The aplastic crisis in sickle-cell anaemia. *Lancet*, **i**, 1086–1089.

MACIVER, J. E. & WENT, L. N. (1960). Sickle-cell anaemia complicated by megaloblastic anaemia of infancy. *Brit. med. J.*, **i**, 775–779.

MAGGIO, A., GAGLIANO, F. & SICILIANO, S. (1984). Hemoglobin phenotype and mean erythrocyte volume in Sicilian people. *Acta haemat. (Basel)*, **71**, 214.

MAHMOOD, A., MACINTOSH, D. M. & SHAPER, A. G. (1967). Fibrinolytic activity in the clinical crisis of sickle-cell anaemia. *Brit. med. J.*, **iii**, 653–654.

MANIATIS, A., FRIEMAN, B. & BERTLES, J. F. (1977). Increased expression in erythrocytic Ii antigens in sickle cell disease and sickle cell trait. *Vox Sang.*, **33**, 29–36.

MANIATIS, A., PAPAYANNOPOULOU, T. & BERTLES, J. F. (1979). Fetal characteristics of erythrocytes in sickle cell anaemia: an immunofluorescence study of individual cells. *Blood*, **54**, 159–168.

MANN, J. R., COTTER, K. P., WALKER, R. A., BIRD, G. W. G. & STUART, J. (1975). Anaemic crisis in sickle cell disease. *J. clin. Path.*, **28**, 341–344.

MARDER, D. J. & CONLEY, C. L. (1959). Electrophoresis of hemoglobin on agar gels. Frequency of hemoglobin D in a negro population. *Bull. Johns Hopk. Hosp.*, **105**, 77–88.

MARKENSON, A. L., CHANDRA, M., LEWY, J. E. & MILLER, D. R. (1978). Sickle cell anemia, the nephrotic syndrome and hypoplastic crisis in a sibship. *Amer. J. Med.*, **64**, 719–723.

MASON, K. P., GRANDISON, Y., HAYES, R. J., SERJEANT, B. E., SERJEANT, G. R., VAIDYA, S. & WOOD, W. G. (1982). Post-natal decline of fetal hemoglobin in homozygous sickle cell disease: relationship to parental Hb F levels. *Brit. J. Haemat.*, **52**, 455–463.

MATII, M. B., WEINGER, R. & SISE, H. S. (1973). Coagulation, fibrinogen survival and fibrin split products in sickle cell disease. *Blood*, **42**, 1004 (Abstract 82).

MAY, A. & HUEHNS, E. R. (1975). The concentration dependence of the oxygen affinity of haemoglobin S. *Brit. J. Haemat.*, **30**, 327–335.

MEGAS, H., PAPADAKI, E. & CONSTANTINIDES, B. (1961). Salmonella septicemia and aplastic crisis in a patient with sickle-cell anemia. *Acta paediat. (Uppsala)*, **50**, 517–521.

MEHTA, P. (1980). Significance of plasma β-thromboglobulin values in patients with sickle cell disease. *J. Pediat.*, **97**, 941–943.

MEHTA, P. & MEHTA, J. (1980). Abnormalities of platelet aggregation in sickle cell disease. *J. Pediat.*, **96**, 209–213.

MIESCH, D. C., BAXTER, M. R. & LEVIN, W. C. (1957). Acute erythroblastopenia: pathogenesis, manifestations, and management. *Arch. intern. Med.*, **99**, 461–473.

MILLER, B. A., SALAMAH, M., AHMED, M., ANTOGNETTI, G., WEATHERALL, D. J. & NATHAN, D. G. (1984). High fetal hemoglobin production in sickle cell anemia (SCA) patients (PTS) from the oases of Saudi Arabia is genetically determined. *Blood*, **64**, No. 5 (Suppl. 1), 51a (Abstract 113).

MILLER, B. A., SALAMAH, M., AHMED, M., WAINSCOAT, J., ANTOGNETTI, G., ORKIN, S., WEATHERALL, D. & NATHAN, D. G. (1986). High fetal hemoglobin production in sickle cell anemia in the Eastern Province of Saudi Arabia is genetically determined. *Blood*, **67**, 1404–1410.

MILNER, P. F. (1974). Oxygen transport in sickle cell anemia. *Arch. intern. Med.*, **133**, 565–572.

MILNER, P. F., GARBUTT, G. J., NOLAN-DAVIS, L. V., JONAH, F., WILSON, L. B. & WILSON, J. T. (1986). The effect of Hb F and α-thalassemia on the red cell indices in sickle cell anemia. *Amer. J. Hemat.*, **21**, 383–395.

MILNER, P. F., LEIBFARTH, J. D., FORD, J., BARTON, B. P., GRENETT, H. E. & GARVER, F. A. (1984).

Increased Hb F in sickle cell anemia is determined by a factor linked to the β^S gene from one parent. *Blood*, **63**, 64–72.

MILNER, P. F., MILLER, C., GREY, R., SEAKING, M., DeJONG, W. W. & WENT. L. N. (1970). Hemoglobin O Arab in four negro families and its interaction with hemoglobin S and hemoglobin C. *New Engl. J. Med.*, **283**, 1417–1425.

MORTIMER, P. P., HUMPHRIES, R. K., MOORE, J. G., PURCELL, R. H. & YOUNG, N. S. (1983). A human parvovirus-like virus inhibits haematopoietic colony formation in vitro. *Nature (Lond.)*, **302**, 426–429.

NALBANDIAN, R. M., HENRY, R. L., NICHOLS, B. M., CAMP, F. R. JNR & WOLF, P. L. (1970). Molecular basis for a simple, specific test for S hemoglobin: the Murayama test. *Clin. Chem.*, **16**, 945–950.

NALBANDIAN, R. M., NICHOLS, B. M., CAMP, F. R. JNR, LUSHER, J. M., CONTE, N. F., HENRY, R. L. & WOLF, P. L. (1971). Automated dithionite test for rapid, inexpensive detection of hemoglobin S and non-S sickling hemoglobinopathies. *Clin. Chem.*, **17**, 1033–1037.

NEEL, J. V. (1952). Perspectives in the genetics of sickle cell disease. *Blood*, **7**, 467–471.

NEEL, J. V., WELLS, I. C. & ITANO, H. A. (1951). Familial differences in the proportion of abnormal hemoglobin present in the sickle cell trait. *J. clin. Invest.*, **30**, 1120–1124.

NEELY, C. L., WAJIMA, T., KRAUS, A. P., DIGGS, L. W. & BARRERAS, L. (1969). Lactic acid dehydrogenase activity and plasma hemoglobin elevations in sickle cell disease. *Amer. J. clin. Path.*, **52**, 167–169.

NORONHA, P. A. & HONIG, G. R. (1979). Sickle cell anemia in two white American children: essential laboratory criteria for diagnosis. *Pediatrics*, **63**, 242–246.

O'BRIEN, R. T. (1978). Iron burden in sickle cell anemia. *J. Pediat.*, **92**, 579–582.

OLINER, H. L. & HELLER, P. (1959). Megaloblastic erythropoiesis and acquired hemolysis in sickle-cell anemia. *New Engl. J. Med.*, **261**, 19–22.

OLUBOYEDE, O. A. (1980). Iron studies in pregnant and non-pregnant women with haemoglobin SS or SC disease. *Brit. J. Obstet. Gynaec.*, **87**, 989–996.

OLVER, R. E. (1969). Severe acidosis during a painful sickle cell crisis. *Proc. roy. Soc. Med.*, **62**, 1097.

OSAMO, N. O. & EYETSIMITAN, W. (1976). Secondary dyserythropoietic activity resembling Di Guglielmo's disease in sickle-cell anaemia. *Brit. med. J.*, **i**, 1126.

OSIFO, 'B. O. A., ADEYOKUNNU, A., PARMENTIER, Y., GERARD, P. & NICHOLAS, J. P. (1983). Abnormalities of serum transcobalamins in sickle cell disease (Hb SS) in black Africa. *Scand. J. Haemat.*, **30**, 135–140.

OSIFO, 'B. O. A., LUKANMBI, F. A. & ADEYOKUNNU, A. (1984). Serum cobalamin concentration in sickle cell disease (Hb SS). *Acta haemat. (Basel)*, **71**, 299–303.

PAPAYANNOPOULOU, T. H., McGUIRE, T. C., LIM, G., GARZEL, E., NUTE, P. E. & STAMATOYANNOPOULOS, G. (1976). Identification of haemoglobin S in red cells and normoblasts, using fluorescent anti-Hb S antibodies. *Brit. J. Haemat.*, **34**, 25–31.

PARDOLL, D. M., RODEHEFFER, R. J., SMITH, R. R. L. & CHARACHE, S. (1982). Aplastic crisis due to extensive bone marrow necrosis in sickle cell disease. *Arch. intern. Med.*, **142**, 2223–2225.

PATTISON, J. R., JONES, S. E., HODGSON, J., DAVIS, L. R., WHITE, J. M., STROUD, C. E. & MURTAZA, L. (1981). Parvovirus infections and hypoplastic crisis in sickle-cell anaemia. *Lancet*, **i**, 664–665 (Letter).

PAULING, L., ITANO, H. A., SINGER, S. J. & WELLS, I. C. (1949). Sickle cell anemia, a molecular disease. *Science*, **110**, 543–548.

PEARSON, H. A. & COBB, W. T. (1964). Folic acid studies in sickle-cell anemia. *J. Lab. clin. Med.*, **64**, 913–921.

PEARSON, H. A., McINTOSH, S., RITCHEY, A. K., LOBEL, J. S., ROOKS, Y. & JOHNSTON, D. (1979). Developmental aspects of splenic function in sickle cell diseases. *Blood*, **53**, 358–365.

PEARSON, H. A., O'BRIEN, R. T., McINTOSH, S., ASPNES, G. T. & YAUNG, M.-M. (1974). Routine screening of umbilical cord blood for sickle cell diseases. *J. Amer. med. Ass.*, **227**, 420–421.

PEMBREY, M. E., WOOD, W. G., WEATHERALL, D. J. & PERRINE, R. P. (1978). Fetal haemoglobin production and the sickle gene in the oases of Eastern Saudi Arabia. *Brit. J. Haemat.*, **40**, 415–429.

PETERSON, C. M., GRAZIANO, J. H., DE CIUTIIS, A., GRADY, R. W., CERAMI, A., WORWOOD, M. & JACOBS, A. (1975). Iron metabolism, sickle cell disease, and response to cyanate. *Blood*, **46**, 583–590.

PIERCE, L. E. & RATH, C. E. (1962). Evidence for folic acid deficiency and genesis of anemic sickle cell crisis. *Blood*, **20**, 19–32.

POLEDNAK, A. P. & JANERICH, D. T. (1975). Hematocrit among blacks with sickle cell trait. *Hum. Biol.*, **47**, 493–504.

POWARS, D., SCHROEDER, W. A. & WHITE, L. (1975). Rapid diagnosis of sickle cell disease at birth by microcolumn chromatography. *Pediatrics*, **55**, 630–635.

POWELL, J. B. & BEACH, D. G. (1971). A modification of the "Sickledex" test for hemoglobin S. *Clin. Chem.*, **17**, 1055–1056.

PRASAD, A. S. & COSSACK, Z. T. (1984). Zinc supplementation and growth in sickle cell disease. *Ann. intern. Med.*, **100**, 367–371.

RANNEY, H. M. & KONO, P. (1959). Studies of the incorporation of Fe^{59} into normal and abnormal hemoglobins. *J. clin. Invest.*, **38**, 508–515.

RAO, K. R. P., PATEL, A. R., ANDERSON, M. J.,

HODGSON, J., JONES, S. E. & PATTISON, J. R. (1983). Infection with parvovirus-like virus and aplastic crisis in chronic hemolytic anemia. *Ann. intern. Med.*, **98**, 930–932.

RAO, K. R. P., PATEL, A. R., HONIG, G. R., VIDA, L. N. & McGINNIS, P. R. (1983). Iron deficiency and sickle cell anemia. *Arch. intern. Med.*, **143**, 1030–1032.

RAO, K. R. P., PATEL, A. R., McGINNIS, P. & Patel, M. K. (1984). Iron stores in adults with sickle cell anemia. *J. Lab. clin. Med.*, **103**, 792–797.

RAO, N. J. & SUR, A. M. (1980). Iron deficiency in sickle cell disease. *Acta paediat. scand.*, **69** 337–340.

REED, L. J., BRADLEY, T. B. JNR & RANNEY, H. M. (1965). The effect of amelioration of anemia on the synthesis of fetal hemoglobin in sickle cell anemia. *Blood*, **25**, 37–48.

REEVES, J. D., BERARD, D. B. & REEVES, A. E. (1983). Hemoglobin concentration, MCV, and HB A$_2$ in sickle cell trait. *Blood*, **62**, No. 5 (Suppl. 1), 60a (Abstract 142).

RICHARDSON, S. G. N., MATTHEWS, K. B., STUART, J., GEDDES, A. M. & WILCOX, R. M. (1979). Serial changes in coagulation and viscosity during sickle-cell crisis. *Brit. J. Haemat.*, **41**, 95–103.

RICKLES, F. R. & O'LEARY, D. S. (1974). Role of coagulation system in pathophysiology of sickle cell disease. *Arch. intern. Med.*, **133**, 635–641.

ROBINSON, A. B., ROBSON, M., HARRISON, A. P. & ZUELZER, W. W. (1957). A new technique for differentiation of hemoglobin. *J. Lab. clin. Med.*, **50**, 745–752.

ROBINSON, G. (1945). A rapid method for detecting the sickle cell trait. *Trans. roy. Soc. trop. Med. Hyg.*, **39**, 264.

ROBINSON, M. G. & SATHIAPALAN, R. (1965). Cryoprecipitable proteins in sickle-cell anaemia. *Lancet*, **ii**, 957–958 (Letter).

RODGERS, G. P., SCHECHTER, A. N. & NOGUCHI, C. T. (1985). Cell heterogeneity in sickle cell disease: quantitation of the erythrocyte density profile. *J. Lab. clin. Med.*, **106**, 30–37.

RODMAN, T., CLOSE, H. P., CATHCART, R. & PURCELL, M. K. (1959). The oxyhemoglobin dissociation curve in the common hemoglobinopathies. *Amer. J. Med.*, **27**, 558–566.

ROSENBLOOM, B. E., ODELL, W. D. & TANAKA, K. R. (1980). Pituitary-adrenal axis function in sickle cell anemia and its relationship to leukocyte alkaline phosphatase. *Amer. J. Hemat.*, **9**, 373–379.

ROSNER, F. & KARAYALCIN, G. (1974). Decreased leukocyte alkaline phosphatase activity in sickle-cell anemia. *Ann. intern. Med.*, **80**, 668–669 (Letter).

ROSSI-BERNARDI, L., LUZZANA, M., SAMAJA, M., ROSSI, F., PERRELLA, M. & BERGER, R. L. (1975). The functional properties of sickle cell blood. *FEBS Lett.*, **59**, 15–19.

ROTH, E. F. JNR, BARDFIELD, P. A., GOLDSMITH, S. J., RADEL, E. & WILLIAMS, J. C. (1980).

Myoglobinemia in sickle cell crisis. *Clin. Res.*, **28**, 322A (Abstract).

RUCKNAGEL, D. L. (1974). The genetics of sickle cell anemia and related syndromes. *Arch. intern. Med.*, **133**, 595–606.

SAARINEN, U. M., CHORBA, T. L., TATTERSALL, P., YOUNG, N. S., ANDERSON, L. J., PALMER, E. & COCCIA, P. F. (1986). Human parvovirus B19-induced epidemic acute red cell aplasia in patients with hereditary hemolytic anemia. *Blood*, **67**, 1411–1417.

SARJI, K. E., EURENIUS, K., FULLWOOD, C. O., SCHRAIBMAN, H. B. & COLWELL, J. A. (1979). Abnormalities of platelet aggregation in sickle cell anemia. Presence of a plasma factor inhibiting aggregation by ristocetin. *Thromb. Res.*, **14**, 283–297.

SARUP, B. M. & WHITE, J. M. (1974). The synthesis of globin peptide chains in sickle-cell disease. *Brit. J. Haemat.*, **27**, 153–161.

SASAKI, J., WATERMAN, M. R., BUCHANAN, G. R. & COTTAM, G. L. (1983). Plasma and erythrocyte lipids in sickle cell anaemia. *Clin. lab. Haemat.*, **5**, 35–44.

SCHMIDT, R. M. & WILSON, S. M. (1973). Standardisation in detection of abnormal hemoglobins. Solubility tests for hemoglobin S. *J. Amer. med. Ass.*, **225**, 1225–1230.

SCHNEIDER, R. G., ALPERIN, J. B. & LEHMANN, H. (1967). Sickling tests. Pitfalls in performance and interpretation. *J. Amer. med. Ass.*, **202**, 419–421.

SCHNEIDER, R. G. & HAGGARD, M. E. (1955). Sickling, a quantitative delayed genetic factor. *Proc. Soc. exp. Biol. Med.*, **89**, 196–199.

SCHNEIDER, R. G., TAKEDA, I., GUSTAVSON, L. P. & ALPERIN, J. B. (1972). Intraerythrocytic precipitations of haemoglobins S and C. *Nature new Biol.*, **235**, 88–90.

SCHROEDER, W. A., JAKWAY, J. & POWARS, D. (1973). Detection of hemoglobins S and C at birth: a rapid screening procedure by column chromatography. *J. Lab. clin. Med.*, **82**, 303–308.

SCHROEDER, W. A., POWARS, D. & CHAN, L. (1981). Anomalous osmotic fragility in sickle cell anemia. *Blood*, **58**, No. 5 (Suppl. 1), 63a (Abstract 164).

SCOTT, R. B., CRAWFORD, R. P. & JENKINS, M. (1948). Incidence of sicklemia in the newborn negro infant. *Amer. J. Dis. Child.*, **75**, 842–849.

SEAKINS, M., GIBBS, W. N., MILNER, P. F. & BERTLES, J. F. (1973). Erythrocyte Hb-S concentration. An important factor in the low oxygen affinity of blood in sickle cell anemia. *J. clin. Invest.*, **52**, 422–432.

SEARS, D. A. (1978). The morbidity of sickle cell trait. A review of the literature. *Amer. J. Med.*, **64**, 1021–1036.

SERJEANT, B. E., FORBES, M., WILLIAMS, L. L. & SERJEANT, G. R. (1974). Screening cord bloods for detection of sickle cell disease in Jamaica. *Clin.*

Chem., **20**, 666–669.

SERJEANT, B. E., MASON, K. P. & SERJEANT, G. R. (1978). The development of haemoglobin A₂ in normal negro infants and in sickle cell disease. *Brit. J. Haemat.*, **39**, 259–265.

SERJEANT, G. R. (1974). *The Clinical Features of Sickle Cell Disease.* 357 pp. North-Holland Publishing Co., Amsterdam, Oxford.

SERJEANT, G. R. (1975). Fetal haemoglobin in homozygous sickle cell disease. *Clinics Haemat.*, **4**, 109–122.

SERJEANT, G. R. (1981). Observations on the epidemiology of sickle cell disease. *Trans. roy. Soc. trop. Med. Hyg.*, **75**, 228–233.

SERJEANT, G. R. (1985). *Sickle Cell Disease.* 478 pp. Oxford University Press.

SERJEANT, G. R., FOSTER, K. & SERJEANT, B. E. (1981). Red cell size and the clinical and haematological features of homozygous sickle cell disease. *Brit. J. Haemat.*, **48**, 445–449.

SERJEANT, G. R., GALLOWAY, R. E. & GUERI, M. C. (1970). Oral zinc sulphate in sickle-cell ulcers. *Lancet*, **ii**, 891–893.

SERJEANT, G. R., GRANDISON, Y., LOWRIE, Y., MASON, K., PHILLIPS, J., SERJEANT, B. E. & VAIDYA, S. (1981a). The development of haematological changes in homozygous sickle cell disease: a cohort study from birth to 6 years. *Brit. J. Haemat.*, **48**, 533–543.

SERGEANT, G. R. & SERJEANT, B. E. (1972). A comparison of erythrocyte characteristics in sickle cell syndromes in Jamaica. *Brit. J. Haemat.*, **23**, 205–213.

SERJEANT, G. & SERJEANT, B. (1979). Neonatal screening for sickle hemoglobin. *Amer. J. clin. Path.*, **72**, 251 (Letter).

SERJEANT, G. R., SERJEANT, B. E. & MILNER, P. F. (1969). The irreversibly sickled cell: a determinant of haemolysis in sickle cell anaemia. *Brit. J. Haemat.*, **17**, 527–533.

SERJEANT, G. R., TOPLEY, J. M., MASON, K., SERJEANT, B. E., PATTISON, J. R., JONES, S. E. & MOHAMED, R. (1981b). Outbreak of aplastic crisis in sickle cell anaemia associated with parvovirus-like agent. *Lancet*, **ii**, 595–597.

SHAPIRO, M. (1958). 'False' sickle cells. *Lancet*, **ii**, 958–959.

SHEEHAN, R. G. & FRENKEL, E. P. (1983). Influence of hemoglobin phenotype on the mean erythrocyte volume. *Acta haemat.* (Basel), **69**, 260–265.

SHEN, S. C., CASTLE, W. B. & FLEMING, E. M. (1944). Experimental and clinical observations on increased mechanical fragility of erythrocytes. *Science*, **100**, 387–389.

SHEPARD, M. K., WEATHERALL, D. J. & CONLEY, C. L. (1962). Semi-quantitative estimation of the distribution of fetal hemoglobin in red cell populations. *Bull. Johns Hopk. Hosp.*, **100**, 293–310.

SHERMAN, I. J. (1940). The sickling phenomenon, with special reference to differentiation of sickle-cell anemia from the sickle-cell trait. *Bull. Johns Hopk. Hosp.*, **67**, 309–324.

SHERWOOD, J. B., GOLDWASSER, E., CHILCOTE, R., CARMICHAEL, L. D. & NAGEL, R. L. (1986). Sickle cell anemia patients have low erythropoietin levels for their degree of anemia. *Blood*, **67**, 46–49.

SHIELDS, G. S., LICHTMAN, H. C., MESSITE, J. & WATSON, R. J. (1958). Studies in sickle cell disease. I. Quantitative aspects of sickling in the newborn period. *Pediatrics*, **22**, 309–318.

SHOJANIA, A. M. & GROSS, S. (1964). Hemolytic anemias and folic acid deficiency in children. *Amer. J. Dis. Child.*, **108**, 53–61.

SHUBIN, H., KAUFMAN, R., SHAPIRO, M. & LEVINSON, D. C. (1960). Cardiovascular findings in children with sickle cell anemia. *Amer. J. Cardiol.*, **6**, 875–885.

SILLS, R. H. & OSKI, F. A. (1979). RBC surface pits in the sickle hemoglobinopathies. *Amer. J. Dis. Child.*, **133**, 526–527.

SINET, M. & POCIDALO, J. J. (1981). Blood-oxygen affinity and sickling in sickle cell disease: effect of prior deoxygenation. *J. Lab. clin. Med.*, **98**, 492–499.

SINGER, K. & CHERNOFF, A. I. (1952). Studies on abnormal hemoglobins. III. The interrelationship of type S (sickle cell) hemoglobin and type F (alkali resistant) hemoglobin in sickle cell anemia. *Blood*, **7**, 47–52.

SINGER, K., CHERNOFF, A. I. & SINGER, L. (1951). Studies on abnormal hemoglobins. I. Their demonstration in sickle cell anemia and other hematologic disorders by means of alkali denaturation. II. Their identification by means of the method of fractional denaturation. *Blood*, **6**, 413–428, 429–435.

SINGER, K. & FISHER, B. (1952). Studies on abnormal hemoglobins. V. The distribution of type S (sickle cell) hemoglobin and type F (alkali resistant) hemoglobin within the red cell population in sickle cell anemia. *Blood*, **7**, 1216–1226.

SINGER, K. & FISHER, B. (1953). Studies in abnormal hemoglobins. VII. The composition of the non-S hemoglobin fraction in sickle-cell anemia blood. A comparative quantitative study by the methods of electrophoresis and alkali denaturation. *J. Lab. clin. Med.*, **42**, 195–204.

SINGER, K., MOTULSKY, A. G. & WILE, S. A. (1950). Aplastic crisis in sickle cell anemia. A study of its mechanism and its relationship to other types of hemolytic crisis. *J. Lab. clin. Med.*, **35**, 721–736.

SINGER, K. & ROBIN, S. (1948). Rapid test for the demonstration of sickle cells and its clinical significance. *J. Amer. med. Ass.*, **136**, 1021–1025.

SINGER, K., ROBIN, S., KING, J. C., & JEFFERSON, R. N. (1948). The life span of the sickle cell and the pathogenesis of sickle cell anemia. *J. Lab. clin. Med.*, **33**, 975–984.

SOLANKI, D. L. (1985). Erythrophagocytosis in vivo in sickle cell anemia. *Amer. J. Hemat.*, **20**, 353–357.

SPROULE, B. J., HALDEN, E. R. & MILLER, W. F. (1958). A study of cardiopulmonary alterations in patients with sickle cell disease and its variants. *J. clin. Invest.*, **37**. 487–495.

STATHAKIS, N. E., PAPAYANNIS, A. G., PAPAYOTAS, P. S. & GARDIKAS, C. (1975). Hypercoagulability and hypofibrinolysis in sickle-cell disease. *Blut*, **31**, 355–360.

STEINBERG, M. H., DREILING, B. J. & LOVELL, W. J. (1977). Sickle cell anemia: erythrokinetics, blood volumes, and a study of possible determinants of severity. *Amer. J. Hemat.*, **2**, 17–23.

STEVENS, M. C. G., HAYES, R. J., VAIDYA, S. & SERJEANT, G. R. (1981). Fetal hemoglobin and clinical severity of homozygous sickle cell disease in early childhood. *J. Pediat.*, **98**, 37–41.

STUART, J., SCHWARTZ, F. C. M., LITTLE, A. J. & RAINE, D. N. (1973). Screening for abnormal haemoglobins: a pilot study. *Brit. med. J.*, **iv**, 284–287.

STUTMAN, L. J. & SHINOWARA, G. Y. (1965). Plasma tetrapyrrole pigments in sickle cell anemia. Long term studies and the effects of low temperatures. *Amer. J. clin. Path.*, **43**, 94–103.

SYDENSTRICKER, V. P. (1924). Further observations on sickle cell anemia. *J. Amer. med. Ass.*, **83**, 12–17.

SYDENSTRICKER, V. P., MULHERIN, W. A. & HOUSEAL, R. W. (1923). Sickle cell anemia: report of two cases in children, with necropsy in one case. *Amer. J. Dis. Child.*, **26**, 132–154.

TONDO, C. V. & SULZANO, F. M. (1962). Abnormal hemoglobins in a Brazilian negro population. *Amer. J. hum. Genet.*, **14**, 401–409.

TOPLEY, J. M., ROGERS, D. W., STEVENS, M. C. G. & SERJEANT, G. R. (1981). Acute splenic sequestration and hypersplenism in the first five years in homozygous sickle cell disease. *Arch. Dis. Childh.*, **56**, 765–769.

UEDA, Y., NAGEL, R. L. & BOOKCHIN, R. M. (1979). An increased Bohr effect in sickle cell anemia. *Blood*, **53**, 472–480.

UPSHAW, J. D., IUCHI, I., DIGGS, L. W. & LYLE, D. (1963). Serum benzidine-positive pigments in sickle cell anemia. *J. Lab. clin. Med.*, **62**, 950–960.

VAN DER SAR, A. (1967). Aplastic sickle cell crisis. A report on four cases. *Trop. geogr. Med.*, **19**, 273–285.

VAN DER SAR, A. (1970). The sudden rise in platelets and reticulocytes in sickle cell crises. *Trop. geogr. Med.*, **21**, 30–40.

VETTORE, L., DE MATTEIS, M. C. & ZAMPINI, P. (1980). A new density gradient system for the separation of human red blood cells. *Amer. J. Hemat.*, **8**, 291–297.

VICHINSKY, E., KLEMAN, K., EMBURY, S. & LUBIN, B. (1981). The diagnosis of iron deficiency in sickle cell disease. *Blood*, **58**, 963–968.

VICTORIA, E. J., MAHAN, L. C. & MASOUREDIS, S. P. (1982). The IgG binding function of the normal red cell plasma membrane: identification of integral polypeptides that bind IgG. *Brit. J. Haemat.*, **50**, 101–110.

WAINSCOAT, J. S., THEIN, S. L., HIGGS, D. R., BELL, J. I., WEATHERALL, D. J., AL-AWAMY, B. H. & SERJEANT, G. R. (1985). A genetic masker for elevated levels of haemoglobin F in homozygous sickle cell disease. *Brit. J. Haemat.*, **60**, 261–268.

WAJIMA, T. (1975). Nitroblue tetrazolium test in patients with sickle-cell anemia. *Amer. J. clin. Path.*, **64**, 608–612.

WAJIMA, T. & KRAUS, A. P. (1968). Low leukocyte alkaline phosphatase activity in sickle cell anemia. *J. Lab. clin. Med.*, **72**, 980–984.

WAJIMA, T. & KRAUS, A. P. (1975). Leukocyte alkaline phosphatase in sickle-cell anemia. *New Engl. J. Med.*, **293**, 918–919.

WALTERS, T. R. & REDDY, B. N. (1974). Sickle cell anaemia and the NBT test. *J. clin. Path.*, **27**, 783–785.

WARTH, J. A., NEAR, K. & WEINSTEIN, R. S. (1983). Sequestrocytes: oxidant injury-induced erythrocytes in sickle cell anemia. *Blood*, **62**, No. 5 (Suppl. 1), 62a (Abstract 150).

WARTH, J. A., PRASAD, A. S., ZWAS, F. & FRANK, R. N. (1981). Abnormal dark adaptation in sickle cell anemia. *J. Lab. clin. Med.*, **98**, 189–194.

WARTH, J. A. & RUCKNAGEL, D. L. (1983). Echinocytic change in sickle cell pain crisis. *Blood*, **62**, No. 5 (Suppl. 1), 62a (Abstract 151).

WARTH, J. A. & RUCKNAGEL, D. L. (1984). Density ultracentrifugation of sickle cells during and after pain crisis: increased dense echinocytes in crisis. *Blood*, **64**, 507–515.

WASHINGTON, R. & BOGGS, D. R. (1975). Urinary iron in patients with sickle cell anemia. *J. Lab. clin. Med.*, **86**, 17–23.

WATSON, J., STAHMAN, A. W. & BILELLO, F. P. (1948). Significance of paucity of sickle cells in newborn negro infants. *Amer. J. med. Sci.*, **215**, 419–423.

WATSON-WILLIAMS, E. J. (1962). Folic acid deficiency in sickle-cell anaemia. *East Afr. med. J.*, **39**, 213–221.

WEEMS, H. B. & LESSIN, L. S. (1984). Erythrocyte density distribution in sickle cell anemia. *Acta haemat. (Basel)*, **71**, 361–370.

WELLS, I. C. & ITANO, H. A. (1951). The ratio of sickle-cell hemoglobin to normal hemoglobin in sicklemics. *J. biol. Chem.*, **188**, 65–74.

WESTERMAN, M. I. & BACUS, J. W. (1983). Red blood cell morphology in sickle-cell anemia as determined by image processing analysis: the relationship to painful crisis. *Amer. J. clin. Path.*, **79**, 667–672.

WESTERMAN, M. P., PIERCE, L. E. & JENSEN, W. N. (1964). Erythrocyte and plasma lipids in sickle cell anemia. *Blood*, **23**, 200–205.

WESTWICK, J., WATSON-WILLIAMS, E. J., KRISHNAMURTHI, S., MARKS, G., ELLIS, V., SCULLY, M. F., WHITE, J. M. & KAKKAR, V. V. (1983). Platelet activation during steady state sickle cell disease. *J. Med*, **14**, 17–36.

WHITE, J. C. & BEAVEN, G. H. (1959). Foetal haemoglobin. *Brit. med. Bull.*, **15**, 33–39.

WHITE, J. M. (1971). The synthesis of abnormal haemoglobins. *Ser. Haemat.*, **4**, 116–132.

WILLIAMS, A. W. & MACKEY, J. P. (1949). Rapid determination of the sickle cell trait by the use of a reducing agent. *J. clin. Path.*, **2**, 141–142.

WINSOR, T. & BURCH, G. E. (1944). Rate of sedimentation of erythrocytes in sickle cell anemia. *Arch. intern. Med.*, **73**, 41–52.

WOCHNER, R. D., SPILBERG, I., IIO, A., LIEM, H. H. & MULLER-EBERHARD, U. (1974). Hemopexin metabolism in sickle-cell disease, porphyrias and control subjects — effects of heme injection. *New Engl. J. Med.*, **290**, 822–826.

WRIGHTSTONE, R. N. & HUISMAN, T. H. J. (1974). On the levels of hemoglobins F and A$_2$ in sickle-cell anemia and some related disorders. *Amer. J. clin. Path.*, **61**, 375–381.

WRIGHTSTONE, R. N., HUISMAN, T. H. J. & VAN DER SAR, A. (1968). Qualitative and quantitative studies of sickle cell hemoglobin in homozygotes and heterozygotes. *Clin. chim. Acta*, **22**, 593–602.

YAKULIS, V. J. & HELLER, P. (1964). An elution test for the visualization of hemoglobin S in blood smears. *Blood*, **24**, 198–201.

YAWSON, G. I., HUNTSMAN, R. G. & METTERS, J. S. (1970). An assessment of techniques for the diagnosis of sickle-cell disease and haemoglobin C disease in cord blood samples. *J. clin. Path.*, **23**, 533–537.

YIP, R. & NELSON, P. E. (1981). Hemoglobin concentration of children with sickle cell trait. *J. Pediat.*, **99**, 257–258.

YOUNG, N. S., MORTIMER, P. P., MOORE, J. G. & HUMPHRIES R. K. (1984). Characterization of a virus that causes transient aplastic crisis. *J. clin. Invest.*, **73**, 224–230.

ZUELZER, W. W., NEEL, J. V. & ROBINSON, A. R. (1956). Abnormal hemoglobins. In: *Progress in Hematology*, Vol. 1 (ed. by L. M. Tocantins), pp. 91–137. Grune and Stratton, New York.

ZUELZER, W. W. & RUTSKY, J. (1953). Megaloblastic anemia of infancy. *Advanc. Pediat.*, **6**, 283–306.

13

Sickle-cell disease III: compound heterozygosity for haemoglobin S and β-thalassaemia or other abnormal β-chain variant haemoglobin or hereditary persistence of fetal haemoglobin; effect of α-thalassaemia or α-chain variant haemoglobins on homozygous sickle-cell anaemia

At a time when Hb S was the only abnormal haemoglobin that had been discovered, cases of 'sickle-cell anaemia' were known in which only one of the parents of the propositus appeared to be a carrier of the sickle-cell trait. Neel (1952) suggested that the most likely explanation was that the 'normal' parents had contributed another gene (or genes) which in combination with a single gene for sickle-cell haemoglobin produced overt sickle-cell anaemia. This suggestion is now known to be correct, and many patients in whom Hb S has been combined with β-thalassaemia or Hb C have been studied as well as a smaller number in whom Hb S has been combined with Hb D, Hb E, Hb O or hereditary persistence of fetal haemoglobin (HPHF). Combinations of Hb S with other abnormal haemoglobins have been reported, too, but they are mostly rare and generally do not produce characteristic clinical or haematological effects.

The combinations of Hb S with β-thalassaemia, Hb C, Hb D, Hb E or Hb O are important for they lead to clinically significant haemolytic syndromes.

SICKLE-CELL THALASSAEMIA (Hb-S/THALASSAEMIA)

History and distribution

This form of sickle-cell disease was described from Sicily by Silvestroni and Bianco (1944–45, 1946, 1952) as 'la malattia micro-drepanocitica' and by Gatto and Russo (1955) as 'thalassodrepanocitosi'. Silvestroni and Bianco (1952) stated that micro-drepanocytic disease could be distinguished from homozygous sickle-cell anaemia by haematological characteristics as well as by genetical studies. Subsequently, Americans of Italian, Sicilian or Greek origin were found to be suffering from the same syndrome (Powell, Rodarte and Neel, 1950; Lawrence, Neel and Itano, 1952; Wasserman, Phelps and Hertzog, 1952; Neel, Itano and Lawrence, 1953; Sturgeon, Itano and Valentine, 1953: Smith and Conley, 1954). Hb-S/thalassaemia was also found to occur in black Americans of African origin (Green and Conley, 1951 (three possible cases); Banks, Scott and Simmons, 1952; Smith and Conley, 1954; Singer, Singer and Goldberg, 1955; Shields et al., 1956).

It was soon found that Hb-S/thalassaemia was widely distributed outside Italy and the United States. Thus it was reported to occur in Kuwait (Walters and Young, 1954), in the United Kingdom (Humble et al., 1954), in Tunisia (Roche et al., 1956), in Greece (Alexandridis, Stamoulis and Tsigalidou, 1956; Choremis and Zannos, 1957), in Southern Turkey (Aksoy and Lehmann, 1957a; Aksoy, 1959), in India (Nail et al., 1957; Shukla and Solanki, 1957; Chatterjea et al., 1958; Chatterjea, 1959), in Jamaica (MacIver, Went and Cruickshank, 1958; Went and MacIver, 1958a), and in Australia in families of Mediterranean extraction (Budtz-Olsen et al., 1961; Cowling, Ungar and Baird, 1965).

According to Serjeant (1974, p. 250), the incidence of Hb-S/thalassaemia in Ghana is about 1 in 800 births and about 1 in 5000 births in the black population in the West Indies and in the United States. In the Jamaican cohort study, the incidence of Hb-S/β$^+$-thalassaemia was about 1 in 3000 and that of Hb-S/β^0-thalassaemia about 1 in 7000 (Serjeant, 1981, 1985, p. 306). The disease is probably most common in Southern Italy and in Greece (where the incidence of β-thalassaemia is especially high).

The early reports referred to above indicated that although Hb-S/thalassaemia is usually a serious disease many patients reach adult life. Typically, the patients are anaemic and slightly to moderately jaundiced and have an enlarged liver and spleen, and they suffer from recurrent bouts of fever and osteo-articular and abdominal pains, and perhaps from chronic ulceration of the leg. As in Hb-SS disease most, if not all, of the patients' symptoms can be attributed to intravascular sickling. Less common complications such as splenic infarction resulting from a flight in an unpressurized aircraft (Rotter *et al.*, 1956) and Salmonella osteomyelitis (Silver, Simon and Clement, 1957) were also referred to in early reports, and it seems likely that the Greek woman aged 49 reported as having sickle-cell anaemia and as having suffered from bone-marrow embolism (Wade and Stevenson, 1941) had in reality Hb-S/thalassaemia.

It is interesting to recall that reports exist in the relatively early literature on sickle-cell disease purporting to describe the occurrence of homozygous sickle-cell anaemia in white families. Significantly, the affected individuals usually had Greek, Italian or Sicilian ancestors (Cooley and Lee, 1929; Rosenfield and Pincus, 1932; Haden and Evans, 1937; Weiner, 1937; Greenwald and Burrett, 1940; Ogden, 1943) and most, if not all, of these patients seem likely in retrospect to have been suffering from Hb-S/thalassaemia. [Reich and Rosenberg (1953) were able to show that this was true in the case of Haden and Evans's patient.]

Early reports of the occurrence of clinically mild forms of Hb-S/thalassaemia

Humble and co-workers (1954) reported some interesting consequences of the marriage of a black with the Hb-AS trait and a Caucasian from Naples who had thalassaemia minor. One of the children, considered to be a double (compound) heterozygote, was anaemic with signs of excessive haemolysis; however, two other brothers, also apparently compound heterozygotes, were only slightly anaemic and showed no signs of overt haemolysis.

Singer, Singer and Goldberg (1955) reported the occurrence of Hb-S/thalassaemia in four female blacks in the United States. They also concluded that the disease might occur in quite mild forms for one of their patients was not anaemic. W. A. Reynolds (1962) similarly reported that two black siblings had a benign form

of the disease, and it is interesting to note that both had quite high levels of Hb A (28–30%) (see later).

In 1955, Silvestroni and Bianco gave further details of the disease, as seen in Sicily. They, too, stressed that the disorder was sometimes a mild one and might not be clinically obvious until late childhood. Ascenzi and Silvestroni (1957), however, described in detail the clinical and morbid anatomical and histological findings of a fatal case. Their patient was a 10-year-old boy from Calabria in the south of Italy; his spleen weighed 1050 g.

Aksoy and Lehmann (1957a) reported that Hb-S/thalassaemia was not infrequent among Eti-Turks living in South Turkey. In this racial group, too, the severity of the disease seems to vary greatly, for in addition to five anaemic patients two individuals were discovered who were not anaemic and were free from symptoms. Aksoy and Lehmann concluded that the clinical effect of being heterozygous for Hb S and thalassaemia probably depended upon the degree to which the presence of the thalassaemia gene suppressed the formation of Hb A.

HETEROGENEITY OF Hb-S/THALASSAEMIA

The accounts of Hb-S/thalassaemia quoted in the preceding paragraphs were all written before the heterogeneity of thalassaemia was appreciated. Now it is known that Hb S may be associated with a whole range of β-thalassaemia variants, and also that the presence of a gene or genes for α-thalassaemia modifies (ameliorates) the expression of homozygous sickle-cell anaemia (see p. 137). It is the heterogeneity of the genes of β-thalassaemia, with their quantitatively different effects on β-globin synthesis, that explains to a large extent why the severity of the clinical expression in compound heterozygotes for Hb S and β-thalassaemia varies so widely (see also p. 130). It is interesting to note, nevertheless, that a similar clinical and haematological expression (phenotype) may result from diverse molecular lesions within the same family (Anagnou *et al.*, 1985).

Serjeant (1985, p. 305) recognized six genetically distinct types of Hb-S/β-thalassaemia: namely, types in which the gene for Hb S is associated with that for β^0-thalassaemia, $\beta^\pm$-thalassaemia, β^+-thalassaemia, $\delta\beta^0$-thalassaemia, $\delta\beta^+$-thalassaemia, and Hb Lepore, respectively. Most well known and well studied are the Hb-S/

β^0-thalassaemia and Hb-S/β^+-thalassaemia combinations (also referred to as the non-Hb-A and Hb-A types, according to whether Hb A is absent or present). In general, and as might be anticipated, the clinical course in Hb-S/β^0-thalassaemia is more severe than in Hb-S/β^+-thalassaemia (Weatherall, 1964a; Serjeant et al., 1973).

Some accounts have associated a benign clinical course in patients not forming Hb A with the presence of a high percentage of Hb F (Stamatoyannopoulos, Sofroniadou and Akrivakis, 1967;

Shaeffer, Moake and Kleve, 1976). In both these reports the patients were adults, males aged 45 and 70 years, respectively; Hb A was absent and 24–27% Hb F was present. Shaeffer, Moake and Kleve (1976) showed that the Hb F was distributed heterogeneously within the erythrocytes, and concluded that this rendered unlikely the presence of a gene for hereditary persistence of fetal haemoglobin. The mollifying influence of high levels of Hb F in Hb-SS disease was referred to on page 48.

Hb-S/β-THALASSAEMIA: FURTHER DETAILS OF THE CLINICAL AND HAEMATOLOGICAL FEATURES

Descriptions of the clinical and haematological features of large numbers of cases are now available. Those of Silvestroni and Bianco (1955), Monti, Feldhake and Schwartz (1964), Weatherall (1964a), Pearson (1969), Serjeant et al. (1973), Weatherall and Clegg (1981) and Serjeant (1985) are particularly valuable.

Silvestroni and Bianco's (1955) account was based on 35 cases studied in Sicily. The expression of the disease, even in this presumably genetically relatively homogeneous population, varied widely. Thus, while half of the patients had been known to be anaemic since early childhood, others had had no symptoms up to the age of 10 years. Osteo-articular crises and leg ulceration were infrequent and anaemia was seldom severe, the haemoglobin being recorded as ranging between 50 and 72%. Mortality, however, seemed to be high and only two of their patients were adults. Some of the children showed signs of physical retardation, and Silvestroni and Bianco made the point that pregnancies seemed to be rarely successful and that miscarriages were frequent.

Weatherall's (1964a) report was based on studies on 16 black Americans. Three had an Hb-S, Hb-F, Hb-A$_2$ pattern on haemoglobin electrophoresis (no Hb A), with 6.4–7.7% Hb F; clinically, they all had a severe illness indistinguishable from that of typical Hb-SS disease. The remaining patients had a milder syndrome. Haemoglobin

electrophoresis gave a Hb-S, Hb-A, Hb-F, Hb-A$_2$ pattern, with 20–30% Hb A and 1.0–6.6% Hb F (except for one patient who had 26%). Weatherall concluded that his data indicated that there were at least two varieties of Hb-S/thalassaemia, the clinical expression of which was related, at least in part, to the presence of absence of Hb A.

The data presented by Monti, Feldhake and Schwartz (1964) were less clear-cut with respect to the effect of the presence of Hb A. Eleven patients had been studied, four not forming Hb A and seven forming about 25% Hb A. Nine were blacks, two were Italians. Two of the four patients not forming Hb A had a mild illness and the three patients who had died all belonged to the group forming Hb A. Pain had been a major symptom in all but one of the patients, and the spleen was palpable in eight of 10 patients (one had been splenectomized). One of the patients forming Hb A had experienced a remarkable anaemic crisis in which the haemoglobin fell to 6 g/dl and the reticulocyte count to less than 1%, while the spleen enlarged to 19 cm below the left costal margin. A bone-marrow aspirate showed intense 'left-shifted' erythropoiesis. On recovery, the haemoglobin rose to 14.5 g/dl and the spleen shrank to 2 cm below the costal margin.

Pearson's (1969) data, based on a study of 14 black children, again indicated a wide range of severity and heterogeneity. Hb A was present in eight patients; in six it could not be demonstrated. The PCVs of the patients forming Hb A were generally higher than in those not forming detectable Hb A; otherwise, the clinical and haematological features of the two series appeared indistinguishable. Sickled cells were seen in the peripheral blood in 10 of the 14 patients, and half of them had experienced painful vaso-occlusive incidents; one had had typical dactylitis. The spleen was palpable in 11 of them. Two children had died in a splenic sequestration crisis (one had 19% Hb A, in the other none was demonstrable). One patient had had three crises of massive splenomegaly associated with severe anaemia, prior to splenectomy. The children's growth, as measured by their height and weight, was subnormal and was similar to that of children with Hb-SS disease. The oxygen-dissociation curve of haemoglobin was shifted to the right, as in Hb-SS disease. In one family the Hb-F level was exceptionally high: it was 18% in a girl whose disease had led to symptoms and 37% in her mother, who also had Hb-S/β-thalassaemia; she, however, was symptom-free.

Hb-S/β-thalassaemia in Jamaica

Serjeant and co-workers (1973) described and contrasted the clinical and haematological features in 56 patients: 17 had no demonstrable Hb A, six had low Hb-A levels (mean 12.9% in males and 12.0% in females) and 33 had high Hb-A levels (mean 24.4% in males and 25.5% in females). Those with low Hb-A levels or no demonstrable Hb A had lower total haemoglobin levels, more rapid haemolysis and a more severe clinical presentation and course: e.g., they required more frequent hospital admissions, had greater enlargement of the liver, spleen and heart and a higher incidence of joint pains, avascular necrosis of bone and leg ulceration. The likely heterogeneity of the series is illustrated by the fact that 13 out of the 56 patients (24%) had Chinese or Indian ancestors.

Taking the series of 56 Jamaican patients as a whole the following clinical facts emerged: their ages ranged from 3 years to 60, 22 being over 30; in 21 of the patients Hb-S/thalassaemia was diagnosed in the course of family studies or as the result of routine investigation for an unrelated event, e.g., pregnancy. Joint pains were the commonest symptom; the hand-foot syndrome, osteomyelitis, leg ulceration, splenic infarction, jaundice or pneumonia were the presenting symptoms or signs of 11 of the patients (20%). The liver was palpable in 33 patients (59%) and the spleen was palpable in 29 (52%); in most cases it did not extend below 5 cm from the costal margin. Two patients, however, had had massive splenomegaly probably associated with a sequestration crisis.

Fifteen patients (27%) gave a history of leg ulcers, which had usually developed when they were between the ages of 10 and 15 years; in seven the ulceration had

persisted for months or years. Five patients gave a history suggestive of the hand-foot syndrome in childhood. Eight gave a history of pneumonia; in two this was probably associated with pulmonary embolism. Two patients had neurological lesions: one had had a subarachnoid haemorrhage associated with hemiparesis and the other a transient sixth nerve palsy which gave rise to diplopia. Other complications recorded by Serjeant (1985) include avascular necrosis of the head of the femur or humerus, aplastic crisis (see p. 135), haematuria and priapism.

Pregnancy

Reports of pregnancy in Hb-S/β-thalassaemia patients have often indicated a high incidence of complications during pregnancy and immediately after delivery, particularly increased anaemia and jaundice, pulmonary infarction and painful vaso-occlusive crises (Brown and Ober, 1958; Henderson et al., 1962; Dunn and Haynes, 1967; Laros and Kalstone, 1971; Hendrickse et al., 1972; Serjeant, 1974, p. 258; Jewett, 1976). The fetal loss rate has also been relatively high. Hendrickse and co-workers (1972), for instance, compared and contrasted the incidence of complications of pregnancy in a relatively large series of Nigerian women suffering from various types of haemoglobinopathy. They concluded that Hb-S/β-thalassaemia patients have a high incidence of increased anaemia, bone-pain crises and an increased risk of post-partum haemorrhage; only one of 13 pregnancies was considered to be free of complications.

Not all reports have, however, been so gloomy. From Africa for instance, Bentsi-Enchill and Konotey-Ahulu (1969) and Konotey-Ahulu and Ringelhann (1969) described how a 40-year-old Ghanaian woman had had 11 successful pregnancies plus one premature delivery, and the experience in Jamaica has been encouraging also. Twenty-one patients in Serjeant and co-workers' (1973) series had been pregnant. There had been 73 pregnancies in all and these were generally well tolerated; and there had been but eight abortions and only one still-birth (average 3.1 live-births per patient). Three patients experienced painful crises before or soon after delivery. According to Serjeant (1985, p. 310) patients who have Hb-S/β$^+$-thalassaemia have larger families than those with Hb-S/β^0-thalassaemia. Serjeant's most recent figures were 75 live-births per 31 β^+ patients compared with 18 live-births per 14 β^0 patients.

Hb-S/β-thalassaemia in West Africa

According to Esan (1970), 0.8% of (Western) Nigerians are carriers of the β-thalassaemia trait. Hb-S/β-thalassaemia has, however, until recently seldom been reported. As referred to in the previous section, Bentsi-Enchill and Konotey-Ahulu (1969) described a Ghanaian woman with Hb-S/thalassaemia who had had 11 successful pregnancies and Esan (1970) mentioned that three Hb-S/thalassaemia patients had been discovered during his survey of thalassaemia syndromes in Nigeria. Subsequently, Bienzle and co-workers (1983) described 20 cases from Liberia, and it seems clear from their description that the clinical expression of the disorder is generally mild. Their patients' haemoglobin ranged from 7.7 to 13.1 g/dl and their reticulocyte count from 2 to 6%. No ISCs were seen in peripheral-blood films and there were few target cells. In every case the disorder was of the β^+ variety, with the percentage of Hb A varying from 11.6 to 37.3; Hb A_2 ranged from 4.0 to 6.4% and Hb F from 0.5 to 18.3%. Bienzle et al. concluded that Hb-S/β-thalassaemia may have been overlooked in West Africa in the past, either because of the lack of symptoms sufficiently severe to bring patients to hospital or, in the case of patients with severe symptoms, because they had been misdiagnosed as suffering from Hb-SS disease. According to Serjeant (1974, 1985), the gene frequencies of Hb-S and β-thalassaemia in Ghana are such that the incidence of Hb-S/β^+- and β^0-thalassaemia should be about 1 in 800 births (compared with approximately 1 in 5000 births in the black population in North America).

Dactylitis

As already referred to, the hand-foot syndrome was described by Serjeant et al. (1973) as a presenting symptom in their series of Jamaican Hb-S/β-thalassaemia patients. Dactylitis, although a common complication in children, appears rarely to affect adults. Rao and co-workers (1980), however, described how a 26-year-old black male from Chicago developed diffuse swelling of the hands accompanied by pyrexia. The swelling subsided slowly and was complete within 3 months. An X-ray taken 2 months after the onset showed multiple small translucent areas in the metacarpals. This patient had not suffered from the hand-foot syndrome as a child but had experienced 4–5 painful crises each year since childhood.

Eye changes

Rudd, Evans and Peeney (1953) described the occurrence in a 22-year-old male West African of haemorrhages in the fundus associated with probable retinal detachment. Latent sickling was demonstrated and although the original diagnosis had been thalassaemia minor, Hb-S/thalassaemia appeared to be more likely.

Goldberg, Charache and Acacio (1971) reported on 14 patients. The most important lesion, seen in nine patients, was a proliferative retinopathy similar to that seen particularly in Hb-SC disease. The retinal changes appeared to be more closely correlated with the percentage of Hb S present than with the general clinical condition of the patients. In the Jamaican patients, reported on by Condon and Serjeant (1972b), proliferative retinopathy was less frequently seen: it was present in only seven of 50 patients. Two syndromes were identified according to the presence or absence of Hb A: with Hb A the overall findings closely resembled those seen in Hb-SC disease; without Hb A the findings were similar to those of Hb-SS disease. Serjeant (1985, p. 261) reported, too, that proliferative retinopathy appeared to be more frequent in the Hb-S/β^+-thalassaemia patients than in the otherwise more seriously affected Hb-S/β^0-thalassaemia patients.

THE SPLEEN IN Hb-S/β-THALASSAEMIA

As the early reports indicated, the spleen is usually easily palpable in adults affected with Hb-S/β-thalassaemia as well as in children. However, according to Serjeant (1985, p. 311), the incidence of splenomegaly tends to decline in β^0 patients as they grow older (as it does in Hb-SS disease); in β^+ patients, however, this does not happen.

Acute sequestration

This does occur; it is a serious event and has led to the patient's death (Pearson, 1969; Serjeant et al., 1973). According to Serjeant (1985), in almost all such cases, the patient has had Hb-S/β^0-thalassaemia. The syndrome almost always affects small children. Solanki and Kletter (1984), however, referred to four adult patients aged between 23 and 44: two had Hb-S/β^+-thalassaemia and two Hb-SC disease.

Infarction of the spleen

Spontaneous. Serjeant and his co-workers (1973) reported that four out of 56 Jamaican patients (one was a child aged 4, three were adults) had experienced spontaneous infarction of the spleen and that one additional patient had been affected while travelling in a pressurized aircraft (see below).

During aeroplane flights. In 1950, Sullivan described as suffering from 'sicklemia' an 18-year-old coloured male who had experienced pain in the left upper quadrant of the abdomen and nausea while in an aeroplane flight over the Rocky Mountains. His blood sickled and the spleen was markedly enlarged, and, although not anaemic, his blood film was described as showing anisocytosis, marked poikilocytosis, hypochromia and slight target-cell formation, and an osmotic fragility test revealed increased resistance. In retrospect, it seems highly likely that this patient was suffering from Hb-S/β-thalassaemia.

Rotter and co-workers (1956) described splenic infarction following aeroplane flights in six black soldiers. Their Case 6 was a 19-year-old male who developed pyrexia and a severe cramping left-sided abdominal pain following a transcontinental flight. He had 12.6 g/dl haemoglobin, and haemoglobin electrophoresis revealed 76% Hb S, 26% Hb A and 3.4% Hb F.

Berthrong and co-workers (1957) reported a similar, but fatal, incident affecting a 42-year-old patient of Greek ancestry whose paper electrophoretic pattern of Hb S and Hb F was considered to be characteristic of the combination of sickle-cell trait and thalassaemia minor.

Ziperman and Graham (1962) described two further cases, one a 19-year-old black with Hb-SC disease and one a 25-year-old black with Hb-S/thalassaemia; they also reviewed the symptoms and signs in 25 previously reported cases and discussed the role of splenectomy in treatment. They concluded that laparotomy should only be undertaken if the diagnosis was in doubt, as all the patients whose history they had reviewed had recovered, regardless of the way they had been treated.

Green, Huntsman and Serjeant (1971) reviewed in an important paper the circumstances under which patients with a haemoglobinopathy had developed crises associated with high-altitude flying. Included among the seven patients whose history they described was a 34-year-old Jamaican woman who developed the signs and symptoms of splenic infarction whilst flying in a pressurized aircraft from Bermuda to London; she had Hb-S/thalassaemia.

Intrathoracic extramedullary erythropoiesis

As already described (Vol. 1, p. 94) extramedullary tumour-like masses of bone marrow occasionally develop in patients who suffer from hereditary anaemias that are accompanied by hyperplasia of the bone marrow. The masses, which are in reality outgrowths of medullary bone marrow, most commonly protrude into the posterior mediastinum. They have been most often seen in adult patients suffering from thalassaemia intermedia (see p. 427) or hereditary spherocytosis. Verani, Olson and Moake (1980), however, described their development in a 72-year-old black woman with Hb-S/β^0-thalassaemia. At necropsy, numerous masses ranging in size up to $8 \times 5 \times 4$ cm were found bilaterally in the thoracic and lumbar paravertebral regions. It is interesting to note that many erythroblasts were present in the peripheral blood (660 per 100 leucocytes). Verani, Olson and Moake cited in a table references to 55 previously described cases. The list included one patient with sickle-cell anaemia (Seidler and Becker, 1964) and one patient with Hb-E/thalassaemia (Da Costa, Loh and Hanam, 1974).

Radiological appearances

These were well described and illustrated in the Jamaican series by Serjeant, Ennis and Middlemiss (1973b). In general, the appearances were similar to, if not indistinguishable from, those seen in Hb-SS and Hb-SC disease. Fourteen of the patients were of the non-Hb-A type and 33 of the Hb-A type; the findings in the former group more closely resembled those in Hb-SS disease while those in the latter more closely resembled those in Hb-SC disease. Expansion of the marrow space and retarded bone age were more common in the non-Hb-A type and cortical thickening was more common in the Hb-A type. Remarkably, however, the radiological findings did not seem to correlate with clinical severity as assessed in retrospect.

Occurrence in identical twins

Joishy, Griner and Rowley (1976) studied identical twins, aged 25, of Italian-American origin who had Hb-S/β-thalassaemia. The results were interesting: although the clinical and haematological expression of their illness was similar in many respects, there were some differences, suggesting non-genetic influences. Similar features included the severity of their anaemia, the erythrocyte indices, blood volume, haemoglobin composition and globin-chain synthesis rates. However, one only of the twins had had an aplastic crisis as a child; one had cardiac decompensation and had had an earlier onset of vaso-occlusive crises. Their ^{51}Cr T$_{50}$ differed slightly but significantly: in one it was 18.5 days, in the other 21 days; and the less severely affected twin had functional asplenia, as demonstrated by a ^{99m}Tc scan and by the presence of Howell-Jolly bodies in her blood film. The more severely affected twin was overweight. Joishy, Griner and Rowley concluded that functional asplenia, and leanness, too, might be beneficial.

COMPARISON OF CLINICAL FEATURES OF Hb-S/β^0-THALASSAEMIA AND Hb-S/β$^+$-THALASSAEMIA

That the clinical course of patients with Hb-S/β$^+$-thalassaemia is often, although not invariably, less severe than in those with Hb-S/β^0-thalassaemia has already been mentioned. Serjeant (1985, p. 313) summarized his West-Indian experience as follows: Hb-S/β^0-thalassaemia is clinically and haematologically similar to Hb-SS disease, though often milder: in contrast, Hb-S/β$^+$-thalassaemia is a very mild condition which is often unrecognized clinically. Amongst the differences in clinical severity between the two catergories of patients that were emphasized by Serjeant were the following: painful crises occur in both types of case, but the crises are mild and infrequent in β$^+$ patients compared with β^0 patients in whom their severity and frequency approximate to that in Hb-SS disease patients; dactylitis is probably more frequent in β^0 patients; leg ulceration is twice as common in β^0 patients; the liver is enlarged more frequently in β^0 patients and splen-

ectomy is more frequently undertaken; hypersplenism and acute splenic sequestration both occur more frequently in β^0 patients; signs of a hyperdynamic circulation and cardiomegaly are found more commonly in β^0 patients; retardation in growth (both height and weight) and in skeletal maturation, and in sexual development, is more marked in β^0 patients. In contrast, proliferative retinopathy occurs more frequently in β$^+$ patients.

SIMILARITIES AND DIFFERENCES BETWEEN Hb-S/β^0-THALASSAEMIA AND Hb-SS DISEASE

Steinberg and Dreiling (1976) compared the clinical and haematological findings of five patients with Hb-S/β^0-thalassaemia with those of five homozygous Hb-SS patients and concluded that, although there were significant differences in blood pictures when each series was considered as a group, it was not always possible to categorize individual patients on the basis of clinical, haematological and electrophoretic data.

Serjeant and co-workers (1979) carried out a similar study on a much larger series of patients — *i.e.*, on 41 patients with Hb-S/β^0-thalassaemia and 123 age-matched Hb-SS patients. The clinical features of the two series differed in only two respects: splenomegaly was more persistent and fetal loss was less frequent in the Hb-S/β^0-thalassaemia patients than in the Hb-SS patients. There were, on the other hand, major differences in the blood picture (see p. 131).

As already referred to (p. 21), Platt, Rosenstock and Espeland (1984) compared the height and weight and sexual maturation of 2115 patients with various sickle haemoglobinopathies — the data were derived from the United States Cooperative Study Group. They found that the Hb-SS and Hb-S/β^0-thalassaemia patients were consistently smaller and less sexually mature than the Hb-SC and Hb-S/β$^+$-thalassaemia patients. For all patients low weight was more pronounced than low height, the differences being more apparent in patients over 7 years of age.

Belhani and co-workers' (1984) report was based on a study carried out on a different ethnic group, namely, 42 patients with Hb-S/β-thalassaemia (31 β^0 and 11 β^+) and 42 with Hb-SS disease, all Algerians. Persistent splenomegaly was more common and painful crises were less frequent in the Hb-S/β-thalassaemia patients than in the Hb-SS disease patients. Belhani *et al.* concluded that Hb-S/β-thalassaemia is more severe in Algerians than in the black population in the Western hemisphere and is of similar severity to that of Italian patients.

BLOOD PICTURE IN Hb-S/β-THALASSAEMIA

Hb-S/β-thalassaemia results in a hypochromic microcytic anaemia of variable severity (Table 13.1). In stained blood films many microcytes, a mild to moderate degree of anisopoikilocytosis, some elliptocytosis and moderate numbers of target cells are characteristic features (Fig. 13.1). Sickled cells are seldom seen in freshly made films but all the erythrocytes will in time sickle *in vitro*. In the more anaemic patients polychromasia and perhaps punctate basophilia may be conspicuous. Osmotic resistance is markedly decreased.

Silvestroni and Bianco (1952) had stressed that microdrepanocytic disease could be distinguished from homozygous sickle-cell anaemia by haematological characteristics as well as by genetical studies, while Went and MacIver (1958a), in comparing the blood picture in Hb-S/thalassaemia and Hb-SS disease, stressed that 'fixed' sickled cells (ISCs) were seldom to be seen in Hb-S/thalassaemia and that, compared with Hb-SS disease, target cells and hypochromia were much more evident in cases of Hb-S/thalassaemia. Aksoy and Erdem (1967) reported that there were two types of Hb-

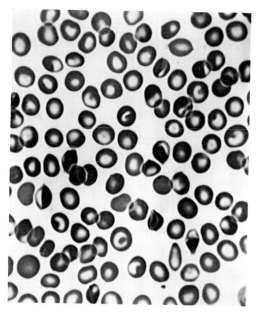

Fig. 13.1 Peripheral-blood film of a Hb-S/β-thalassaemia patient.
Shows moderate anisocytosis, slight hypochromia, some poikilocytes and a few target cells. No well-formed sickled cells are present. × 700.

S/thalassaemia, as judged by MCV, a normocytic type and a microcytic type.

Serjeant and Serjeant (1972) reported detailed steady-state haematological data on 57 Jamaican patients, 16 males and 41 females, suffering from Hb-S/β-thalassaemia. The presence or absence of Hb A appeared to determine a biphasic distribution of values. Thus, those forming Hb A had, compared with those not forming Hb A, higher mean haemoglobin levels (10.7 ± 1.2 g/dl compared with 8.1 ± 1.1 g/dl), higher MCHC (31.5 ± 1.3% compared with 28.8 ± 1.7%), fewer ISCs (0% compared with 1.8 ± 1.9%) and a lower reticulocyte

Table 13.1 Haematological findings in the more important sickle-cell syndromes: a summary.

Disease	Haemoglobin (g/dl)	Erythrocyte count (× 10^{12}/l)	MCV (fl)	MCH (pg)	Reticulocyte count (%)	Sickled cells (ISCs)
Hb-SS	7–9	2.0–3.5	90–100	29–34	5–20	Present
Hb-S/β^0-thal	7–9	3.5–4.5	65–75	18–24	5–10	Rare
Hb-S/β^+-thal	10–12	4.3–5.2	68–78	20–27	3–6	Absent
Hb-SC	10–12	3.5–5.0	75–85	25–30	3–8	Rare
Hb-SD Punjab	7–10	2.0–3.5	90–115	29–34	5–20	Present
Hb-SO Arab	7–9	2.0–3.0	85–105	29–34	5–15	Present

The figures quoted are believed to represent the findings in the majority of the patients in each category. As described in the text, the findings are affected to a major degree by the age of the patient, as well as by the patient's racial origin and by the α-globin genotype.

count (3.2 ± 1.9% compared with 8.6 ± 3.7%). The mean MCV in the patients not forming Hb A was 69.8 ± 7.5 fl and in those forming Hb A it was 72.0 ± 6.6 fl, while the MCH in the patients not forming Hb A was 20.1 ± 2.4 pg and 22.6 ± 2.4 pg in those forming Hb A. Taking the two groups together, the mean erythrocyte counts were markedly and significantlly higher, and

the MCV and MCH and reticulocyte count, significantly lower, than in Hb-SS disease, whilst the values for a comparable series of Hb-SC disease patients fell between the two (except in respect of erythrocyte counts which were similar in the Hb-S/thalassaemia and Hb-SC cases). However, the values of individual patients in each series overlapped (Figs. 13.2 and 13.3).

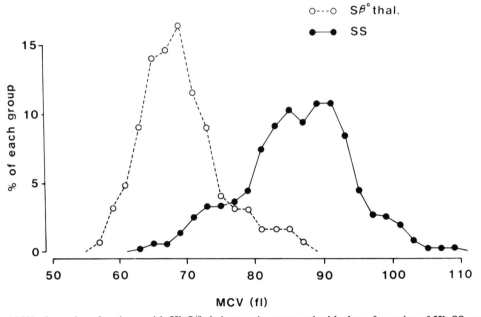

Fig. 13.2 The MCV of a series of patients with Hb-S/β-thalassaemia compared with that of a series of Hb-SS patients. Jamaican data. [Reproduced by permission from Serjeant (1985).]

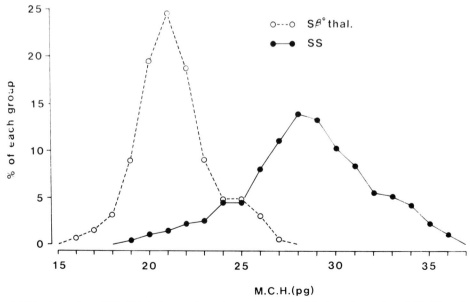

Fig. 13.3 The MCH of a series of Hb-S/β-thalassaemia patients compared with that of a series of Hb-SS patients. Jamaican data. [Reproduced by permission from Serjeant (1985).]

Further studies by Serjeant and his colleagues in Jamaica have confirmed the previously observed differences between the patients forming Hb A (Hb-S/β^+-thalassaemia) and those not forming Hb A (Hb-S/β^0-thalassaemia): the former group have higher values for total haemoglobin, erythrocyte count, MCHC, MCH and MCV and lower percentages of Hb F, Hb A_2 and reticulocytes. These differences are apparent early in life. The Jamaican cohort study included 32 children with Hb-S/β^+-thalassaemia and 14 with Hb-S/β^0-thalassaemia (along with larger numbers of Hb-SS and Hb-SC children). Details of their progress from birth to 5 years of age were given by Stevens et al. (1985). The Hb-F percentage fell similarly in the β^+ and β^0 cases, reaching about 20% at 10 months and falling more slowly thereafter. The Hb-A_2 percentage was closely similar in both groups; it climbed slowly from birth and reached about 4–5% at the 5th year. Total haemoglobin fell steeply after birth: it reached its nadir at about 3–6 months, and remained more or less at that level subsequently; that of the β^+ children was often similar to that of normal (Hb-AA) children (Fig. 13.4). The erythrocyte counts fell in a rather similar fashion, but recovered a little after minimum levels at about 3 months and remained thereafter mostly unchanged at about 4.0–4.5 $\times$ 10^{12}/1. The MCV fell from about 100 fl at birth to a minimum of about 65 fl at 6 months, then rose slightly and stabilized at levels significantly lower than in Hb-SS or Hb-AA children. The MCH followed a similar pattern.

Reticulocytes

Serjeant and Serjeant (1972) reported a mean reticulocyte count of 8.6 $\pm$ 3.7% in 19 Hb-S/thalassaemia patients not forming Hb A and a mean count of 3.2 $\pm$ 1.9% in 31 patients forming Hb A. Steinberg and Dreiling's (1976) figures were similar: in five Hb-S/β^0-thalassaemia patients the mean was 6.6 $\pm$ 3.4% and in seven Hb-S/β^+-thalassaemia patients 2.6 $\pm$ 0.55%.

Stevens and co-workers (1985) traced in their cohort study the changes in reticulocyte count from the children's birth until they were 5 years of age. In the β^+ children the count never exceeded 3%; in the β^0 children, on the other hand, the count reached 5–10% after 3 months. Even so, the mean counts of the β^0 children were less than those of Hb-SS children of comparable age.

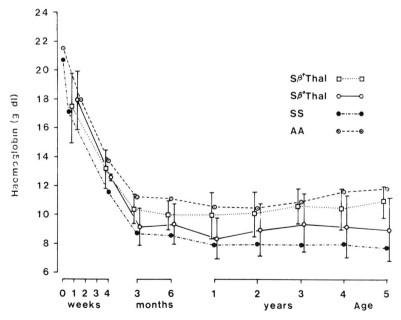

Fig. 13.4 Change in total haemoglobin up to the age of 5 years in a series of patients with Hb-S/β^+-thalassaemia or Hb-S/β^0-thalassaemia compared with Hb-SS patients and normal (Hb-AA) controls.
Jamaican data. [Reproduced by permission from Stevens et al. (1985).]

HAEMOGLOBIN IN Hb-S/β-THALASSAEMIA

Ascenzi and Silvestroni (1953) showed that Italian carriers of the sickle-cell trait and Italian patients with microdrepanocytic disease had within their erythrocytes an abnormal haemoglobin which appeared to be identical with the sickle-cell haemoglobin present in the black Afro-American patients studied in the United States: the sickled cells were birefringent under the polarizing microscope and the haemoglobin when reduced formed tactoids. It is now generally accepted that the chemical, physical and molecular properties of Hb S are the same irrespective of the racial origin of the patient forming the abnormal haemoglobin.

It was originally thought in compound heterozygotes for Hb-S and thalassaemia traits that Hb S, Hb F and Hb A were present together and that the presence of Hb A could be used as an important diagnostic point in differentiating between patients who were compound heterozygotes from those who were Hb-SS homozygotes. It was soon recognized, however, that Hb A might be absent or at any rate present in such small amounts that it was difficult to demonstrate. This was recognized by Zuelzer (1957) and by Singer *et al.* (1957) who pointed out that in such cases the differentiation from homozygous Hb-SS disease could perhaps only be satisfactorily settled by family studies. Earlier, Zuelzer, Neel and Robinson (1956) had reported that the usual finding was for 60–80% of the haemoglobin

present to be Hb S, up to 17% Hb F and the remainder Hb A; they mentioned, however, that three patients had only 22–36% Hb S and were essentially symptom-free. They concluded that it was likely that thalassaemia minor comprised 'two, three or even more different genetic entities'.

Singer and co-workers (1957), too, argued that the wide variation in the amount of Hb S that might be present supported the contention that there was more than one gene for thalassaemia and that the genes differed in their capacity to suppress the formation of Hb A or, alternatively, that modifying genes were responsible.

Went and MacIver (1958a) related the different haemoglobin patterns demonstrable by electrophoresis to the racial origin of the patients: in three Afro-Chinese patients Hb A was absent and there was 10% of Hb F, while in eight Afro-Caucasian or African patients there was 15–27% of Hb A and only small amounts of Hb F. MacIver, Went and Cruikshank (1958) reported similar findings: an absence of Hb A in two patients of mixed Chinese and Asian origin and the presence of Hb A in three families of mixed African and Caucasian origin. Later studies emphasizing the variability of the electrophoretic pattern of Hb-S/β-thalassaemia include those of Koneman, Miale and Mason (1963) and Angelopoulos (1965) who reported five different patterns in seven patients within three Greek families.

Serjeant and co-workers (1973) reported on the haemoglobin patterns of 56 Hb-S/β-thalassaemia patients and considered that the group could be divided into three categories with respect to Hb A, *i.e.*, no Hb A (17 patients), low Hb A (10–14%) (6 patients) and high Hb A (18–30%) (33 patients). The percentage of Hb S in the whole series ranged from 49.5 to over 90; it exceeded 70 in the majority of cases (Table 13.2).

Table 13.2 Haemoglobin percentages in the more important sickle-cell syndromes: a summary.

Haemoglobin genotype	Hb A	Hb S	Hb A_2	Hb F	Hb C	Hb D	Hb O	Hb E
AS	52–75	22–45	2.0–3.5	<1				
SS		75–95	2.0–2.5	2–20				
S/β⁰-thal		70–90	4–6	6–8				
S/β⁺-thal	10–30	50–80	4–6	4–6				
S/HPFH		65–85	1–3.5	14–35				
SC		45–55	<3.5	0.5–5	48–57			
SD Punjab		c 50	1.8–3.5	<5		c 50		
SO Arab		c 50	<3.5	5–28			c 50	
SE		c 60	<3.5	c 1				c 40

The figures quoted are believed to represent the findings in the majority of patients in each category. In the relatively rare syndromes (SD, SO and SE) only very approximate figures can be given. As described in the text, the findings are affected to a major degree by the age of the patient, as well as by the patient's racial origin and by the α-globin genotype.

Hb-F and Hb-A₂ percentages

Wrightstone and Huisman (1974) gave figures for Hb F and Hb A$_2$ in two series of black Americans: in seven Hb-S/β^0-thalassaemia patients Hb F ranged from 7 to 16%, mean 10%, and Hb A$_2$ from 3 to 6.9%, mean 5.8%; and in 20 Hb-S/β$^+$-thalassaemia patients Hb F ranged from 0 to 20%, mean 7%, and Hb A$_2$ from 3 to 8.0%, mean 5.0%.

Serjeant's (1985, p. 307) recent data were based on a large series of West Indians: in 59 Hb-S/β^0 thalassaemia patients the mean Hb-F percentage was 7.0 ± 0.42 and mean Hb-A$_2$ percentage 5.02 ± 0.56, while in 76 Hb-S/β$^+$-thalassaemia patients the mean Hb-F percentage was 5.1 ± 0.42 and the mean Hb-A$_2$ percentage 4.66 ± 0.57.

Belhani and co-workers (1984) measured Hb-F and Hb-A$_2$ percentages in a series of Algerian patients with Hb-S/β-thalassaemia and contrasted the findings with those of patients with Hb-SS disease. The mean Hb-F percentage was 14.33 ± 8.95 in 25 β^0 patients and 6.6 ± 3.78 in seven β$^+$ patients; in 22 Hb-SS patients the mean was 8.5 ± 8.3. The mean Hb-A$_2$ percentage was 4.45 ± 1.03 in 28 β^0 patients and 5.16 ± 0.83 in 10 β$^+$ patients; in 16 Hb-SS patients the mean was 3.3 ± 0.59.

LIFE-SPAN OF ERYTHROCYTES IN Hb-S/β-THALASSAEMIA

The available evidence confirms the supposition that the life-span of the erythrocytes delivered to the peripheral blood is considerably but variably shortened. ^{51}Cr T$_{50}$ times of 10.0–18.8 days in eight patients (Malamos et al., 1963), 7–24 days in six patients (Monti, Feldhake and Schwartz, 1964) and 18.5 and 21 days in identical twins (Joishy, Griner and Rowley, 1976) have been recorded. The longer times were recorded in β$^+$ patients.

Malamos and co-workers (1963) reported that in-vivo counting indicated that erythrocyte destruction takes place to a variable extent in both the spleen and liver, and that the uptake pattern of ^{51}Cr is intermediate between that in Hb-SS disease and that in thalassaemia major in which the spleen is particularly active (Malamos et al., 1961).

APLASTIC CRISES

Aplastic crises have but rarely been recorded in Hb-S/β-thalassaemia.

Monti, Feldhake and Schwartz (1964) referred to two and possibly three such occurrences. One patient was a male aged 33 whose haemoglobin fell to 6 g/dl and the reticulocyte count to less than 1%; his spleen was enlarged to 19 cm below the left costal margin. Erythropoiesis was extremely active and markedly left-shifted. The reticulocyte count rose on the 3rd day and eventually his haemoglobin reached 14.5 g/dl. The spleen had by then shrunk to 2 cm below the left costal margin. The course of his illness suggests acute splenic sequestration associated with a transient inhibition of erythropoiesis; the cause was not established.

Pardoll and co-workers (1982) referred to another remarkable patient, a 20-year-old female, who developed severe anaemia (Hb 4.7 g/dl), reticulocytopenia (0.1% reticulocytes) and thrombocytopenia (43×10^9/l platelets) associated with extensive bone-marrow necrosis.

Serjeant (1985, p. 310) referred to two patients (both with Hb-S/β^0-thalassaemia) who had developed aplastic crises, out of a total of 130 with Hb-S/thalassaemia, but gave no details.

HAEMOGLOBIN CHAIN SYNTHESIS IN Hb-S/β-THALASSAEMIA

The studies that have been carried out have demonstrated a variable degree of failure of β^A-chain production and a relative excess of production of α chains. As in β-thalassaemia heterozygotes, chain synthesis may be balanced in bone-marrow cells although defective in peripheral-blood reticulocytes. As well as being of scientific interest, the measurement of chain synthesis is of practical diagnostic value.

Bank and co-workers (1973) found that β^A-chain production was absent or markedly decreased in symptomatic and anaemic Hb-S/β-thalassaemia patients of black American or Mediterranean origin. In contrast, in relatively asymptomatic mildly anaemic black patients, while an excess of α-chain production could be demonstrated in studies on peripheral-blood reticulocytes, the α- and β-chain synthetic rates were more nearly balanced in bone-marrow cells.

Gill and Schwartz (1973) studied five Hb-S/β-thalassaemia patients as well as four simple heterozygotes for β-thalassaemia. In both groups total β-chain synthesis was decreased in peripheral-blood reticulocytes relative to α-chain synthesis but in bone-marrow cells synthesis was balanced, even in the patients with Hb-S/β-thalassaemia who were moderately severely anaemic. It was concluded that the major mechanism achieving balanced chain synthesis in the bone marrow is its capacity to increase the synthesis of β^S chains.

Steinberg and Dreiling (1976) estimated α:non-α globin-chain synthesis rates in peripheral-blood reticulocytes in Hb-S/β-thalassaemia and in homozygous Hb-SS disease. The ratios were 1.24, 1.42 and 2.87 in three β^0 patients, 1.74 (mean) $\pm$ 0.31 in seven β^+ patients and 1.01 in a Hb-SS patient.

Kim and co-workers (1977) studied three Hb-S/β^0-thalassaemia patients: the $\beta^S + \gamma$:α-chain ratio was 0.48–0.67 (normal Hb-AA controls, 1.01 $\pm$ 0.06) and the radioactive free α-chain pool was markedly raised. They also studied four patients who were carriers of the α-thalassaemia trait as well as being homozygotes for Hb S: the mean $\beta^S + \gamma$: α-chain ratio of the group was 1.26 $\pm$ 0.18. They concluded that measurement of the chain synthesis ratio provides a useful means of differentiating between Hb-S/β-thalassaemia and Hb-S/α-thalassaemia when family studies are not practicable.

Hb-S/$\delta\beta$-THALASSAEMIA

Hb-S/$\delta\beta^0$-thalassaemia

This uncommon condition is characterized by a mild clinical course. Hb A is absent and the Hb-A_2 percentage low. The syndrome was originally reported as affecting Sicilians, Italians and Greeks (Russo, La Grutta and Mollica, 1963; Silvestroni and Bianco, 1964; Stamatoyannopoulos, Sofroniadou and Akrivakis, 1967). Subsequently, it was found in a few black families in the United States (Zelkowitz et al., 1972; Altay, Schroeder and Huisman, 1977; Kinney et al., 1978). In these families, too, the clinical course of the affected compound heterozygotes was a mild one. The basis of the molecular lesion leading to failure to synthesize Hb A *and* Hb A_2 is a deletion affecting the $\gamma\delta\beta$ gene region of chromosome 11 (see p. 511).

Zelkowitz and co-workers (1972) described the occurrence of $\delta\beta$-thalassaemia in three black families. The propositus of their Family C was a compound heterozygote for $\delta\beta$-thalassaemia and Hb S; he was 28 years old and had been admitted to hospital for the investigation of abdominal pain which was shown to be caused by a duodenal ulcer. He was not anaemic; but when aged 21 he had undergone splenectomy for spontaneous rupture of the spleen. Study of his haemoglobin revealed 62% Hb S, 28% Hb F and 2.1% Hb A_2. His father was a compound heterozygote for $\delta\beta$-thalassaemia and Hb C and his mother had the Hb-S trait. Two of his children had the $\delta\beta$-thalassaemia trait; their Hb-F levels were similarly high (23–24%) and this was also

true of his father who had 26% Hb F. In each case the Hb F was distributed unevenly amongst the erythrocytes.

Hb-S/$\delta\beta^+$-thalassaemia

The 38-year-old male described by Russo and Mollica (1962) was mildly anaemic and the liver and spleen were slightly enlarged; clinically, however, he was well. He had 25–32% Hb A, a normal Hb-A_2 percentage, 20–22% Hb F and 47–55% Hb S. Weatherall and Clegg (1981, p. 352) discussed the nature of this interesting family in which Hb S was interacting with two types of thalassaemia — normal A_2 ($\delta\beta$) thalassaemia and high A_2 thalassaemia.

Hb-SS/δ-thalassaemia

Thompson and co-workers (1966) described an unusual patient whom they considered was homozygous for Hb S as well as being a heterozygote for δ-thalassaemia. He was a 38-year-old black American who had a moderately severe haemolytic anaemia, for which he had undergone splenectomy; he had never experienced any painful crises. The ^{51}Cr T_{50} was 12 days. Almost all the haemoglobin was Hb S. No Hb A was demonstrable and there was only 1.4% Hb A_2.

Hb-S/Hb LEPORE

This is an uncommon variant which leads to a haemolytic anaemia associated with hypochromia, microcytosis and anisopoikilocytosis. ISCs may be seen in blood films. The disorder is of very variable severity. Hb Lepore, the result of $\delta\beta$ globin-chain fusion (see p. 442), is usually present at a concentration of approximately 10%. The disorder has been found in Greek, Italian and Jamaican families.

The combination was first reported under the title 'hemoglobin Pylos-hemoglobin S combination' by Stamatoyannopoulos and Fessas (1963) and by Silvestroni and Bianco (1963) as 'la malattia da Hb S-Hb Lepore'. The Greek patients were a girl and a boy, aged 13 and 12 years, respectively, who were members of two different families. Both had a moderate to mild haemolytic anaemia: haemoglobin 8.6 g/dl with 33% reticulocytes and haemoglobin 13.3 g/dl with 7% reticulocytes, respectively. The girl had had no painful episodes and the boy had had only rare attacks; both had palpable spleens. The two sisters, members of a southern Italian family, who were described by Silvestroni, Bianco and

Baglioni (1965) as carrying both Hb S and Hb Lepore (Boston), were more severely affected: one had had bone and joint pains since childhood and had needed transfusions during pregnancies. Their liver and spleen were enlarged.

The Jamaican woman described by Ahern et al. (1972) was 76 years old when investigated; she had lived an active life and had had five successful pregnancies and no abortions, and had not had any symptoms suggestive of a sickling syndrome until she developed a crural ulcer when she was aged 70. She had 10.6 g/dl haemoglobin and 3.5% reticulocytes; the MCV was 78 fl and MCH 27.6 pg. There was 70% Hb S, 11% Hb Lepore, 2.6% Hb A_2 and 10% Hb F. In her blood film there were 1–2% 'fixed sickle cells' (ISCs). The ^{51}Cr erythrocyte survival (? ^{51}Cr T_{50}) was 15 days.

Recently, Stevens and co-workers (1982) described the occurrence of Hb-S/Hb Lepore in a Jamaican family described as being of predominately African origin. Two children were affected: the propositus was a boy aged 8 who was small for his age; he was jaundiced and had a moderately enlarged liver, and his spleen, at first not palpable, later enlarged to 5 cm below the costal margin. He subsequently had three episodes of pneumonia and several attacks of bone pain. The blood picture was compatible with a diagnosis of Hb-SS disease; in particular, 1–2% of ISCs were present. His younger sister was found to have the same disorder: her clinical history was similar and this was also true of her blood picture. On electrophoresis, both children were shown to possess, as well as Hb S, an abnormal haemoglobin component which was identified as being Hb Lepore Boston. Their mother was found to be a carrier of Hb Lepore; their father had the Hb-S trait. Stevens and his co-workers made the important point that the Hb-S/Hb-Lepore combination should be thought of when a patient, whose history and blood picture suggest Hb-SS disease, is found to have one parent whose erythrocytes fail to sickle.

Hb-S/β-THALASSAEMIA PLUS 'Hb G'

Schwartz and co-workers (1957) described the occurrence of Hb S, Hb G and thalassaemia in a family of Italian origin. The propositus, a 28-year-old male, had a severe form of sickle-cell disease; he was known to have had episodes of fever and painful joints and splenomegaly since the age of 4 years. His haemoglobin was 6–8 g/dl and marked anisopoikilocytosis and hypochromia and target cells, sickled cells, spherocytes and normoblasts could be seen in stained blood films. The reticulocyte count was 12%, MCV 84 fl, and MCH 26 pg. His father had the Hb-AS trait and his mother thalassaemia trait and Hb G.

Electrophoresis of the haemoglobin of the propositus revealed Hb S and Hb G (as a minor component) and there was 3.2% Hb F. A brother, thought to be a compound heterozygote for Hb S and Hb G (but not to have thalassaemia), had been well all his life. Schwartz et al. concluded that the presence of Hb G had had no effect on the expression of either Hb S or thalassaemia. The exact nature of 'Hb G' in this family is uncertain.

ASSOCIATION OF Hb-S/β-THALASSAEMIA WITH HEREDITARY ELLIPTOCYTOSIS

van Ros, Seynhaeve and Fiasse (1976) described a Zaïrian family carrying the genes for Hb S, β$^+$-thalassaemia and HE. The propositus, a male child of 7 years who had Hb-S/β$^+$-thalassaemia plus HE, had had a relatively mild clinical course except for bilateral ischaemic necrosis of ribs. He had 9.8 g/dl haemoglobin when he was examined. Haemoglobin analysis revealed 57% Hb S, 34% Hb A, 5.8% Hb A_2 and 4.2% Hb F. A few sickled cells could be seen in blood films. Other siblings had HE alone (90% of elliptical cells) or Hb-S/β$^+$-thalassaemia.

EFFECT OF α-THALASSAEMIA ON SICKLE-CELL DISEASE

It is now realized that the presence of α-thalassaemia affects the haematological findings in sickle-cell disease and has, too, an ameliorating effect on its severity. The degree to which the clinical expression of the disease is affected is, however, somewhat variable.

EARLY REPORTS

Aksoy (1963) described four Turkish patients as suffering from typical severe Hb-S/thalassaemia and, in addition, two patients who were relatively symptom-free and in whom the results of haemoglobin electrophoresis were atypical: they had 51–54% Hb A, 42–47% Hb S and 2.5–4.1% Hb A_2; Hb F was absent. The patients were slightly anaemic: haemoglobin 11.2–13.3 g/dl; the MCV was 81–82 fl, and it was suggested that they were heterozygotes for Hb S and α-thalassaemia. One of them married a man with the Hb-S trait, and one of their children, a boy aged $4\frac{1}{2}$ years, was severely affected; he was considered to be homozygous for Hb S and also to have α-thalassaemia. The MCV was 75.8 fl and the MCH 23.4 pg; the serum iron was 140 μg/dl.

Since this early report, the realization that the α-globin genes are duplicated and the development of techniques by which globin-chain synthesis rates can be measured, and the application of molecular-genetic analysis to clinical problems, have rendered the diagnosis α- thalassaemia, in its various forms, increasingly precise (see p. 513).

Weatherall and co-workers (1969) described a large Saudi-Arabian family in which the propositus was a female child who was considered to be homozygous for Hb-S and also to possess two genes for α-thalassaemia. (Both parents were heterozygotes for Hb-S and α-thalassaemia.) When she was aged 30 months there were, however, no abnormal physical signs; in particular, neither the spleen nor the liver was palpable. The haemoglobin was 8.9 g/dl, MCV 70 fl and MCH 20 pg. Haemoglobin electrophoresis revealed 40.7% Hb S, 43.7% Hb F and 1.6% Hb A_2 and there was 14% Hb Bart's, indicating a marked failure in α-chain synthesis. Chromatographic analysis revealed an absence of β^A chains. The peripheral-blood film was characterized by marked anisocytosis and poikilocytosis and there were many target cells. Other members of the family showed the haematological stigmata of heterozygous α-thalassaemia or Hb-H disease; three had Hb-SS disease, with high Hb-F levels and a relatively mild clinical course.

van Enk and co-workers (1972) described two Hb-SS Ghanaian women who had had six and seven, respectively, successful pregnancies and had had, too, mild symptoms when not pregnant; α-thalassaemia was diagnosed by demonstrating impaired synthesis of α chains. It was suggested that the presence of α-thalassaemia helped to reduce the severity of Hb-SS disease by lowering the concentration of haemoglobin in the erythrocytes and in this way reducing the tendency of the cells to sickle *in vivo*.

RECENT REPORTS

Recent data on the effect of α-thalassaemia on the haematological findings in Hb-SS patients and on the clinical severity of their disease have indicated that although many patients seem to have derived clinical benefit from the presence of one or two genes for α-thalassaemia, this is not always the case.

Honig and co-workers (1978) described five American blacks, aged 5 months to 16 years, with Hb-SS disease, in whom the presumptive presence of a gene for α-thalassaemia did not appear to have a beneficial effect on the clinical expression of their illness. (In each of the four affected families both parents of the propositus had the Hb-AS trait and one parent microcytosis in the absence of iron deficiency.) Leaving aside the 5-month-old infant, the four other children had 84–94% Hb S, 2.3–13.5% Hb F, a MCV of 59–79 fl and 6.2–18.4% reticulocytes. Microcytes, many target cells and some irregularly contracted and oat-shaped forms were conspicuous in blood films. Sickled cells appeared to be absent. A similarly severely affected patient was described by Natta (1978). He was a 15-year-old black whose growth was retarded and who needed transfusions: electrophoresis demonstrated 95.6% Hb S and 3.2% Hb A_2 and there were 16% reticulocytes. The MCV was 86 fl and MCH 28 pg. The α:β^S globin-chain synthesis ratio was 0.5.

It is now realized that α-chain deficiency due to the α-thalassaemia-2 determinant (see p. 458) is quite common in the black population of the United States (and in Africa and the West Indies, too) and that it is the presence of this determinant when homozygous that has a significant influence on the expression of Hb-SS disease.

Felice and co-workers (1979) studied the in-vitro synthesis of the haemoglobin chains in 34 Hb-SS patients and calculated the α:non-α chain-synthesis ratios. Four patients had α:non-α ratios (at 30 minutes) of 0.75 ± 0.1: they were considered to be homozygous for α-thalassaemia; their mean MCV was 65.5 fl. The remaining 30 Hb-SS patients had ratios of 0.90 or above; their MCV increased from 77 to 94 fl parallel with the increase in the ratios to unity (normal). Those with the lowest ratios, mean 0.90, whose mean MCV was 77 fl, were thought to be heterozygous for α-thalassaemia-2. Felice *et al.* concluded that homozygosity for α-thalassaemia ($-\alpha/-\alpha/\beta^S\beta^S$ genotype) leads to clinically mild Hb-SS disease and microcytosis similar to that seen in Hb-S/β^0-thalassaemia. Heterozygosity for α-thalassaemia-2, on the other hand, appeared to have little influence clinically but was associated with slight microcytosis (see also p. 143).

Fich and Rachmilewitz (1981) described from Israel a 23-year-old Hb-SS Arab who complained of severe priapism; his clinical history had previously been a benign one. His haemoglobin was 6.8 g/dl and he had 16.8% reticulocytes and a platelet count of 934×10^9/l. A technetium scan revealed no functioning spleen tissue. Globin-chain synthesis studies demonstrated a relative failure of α-globin synthesis.

The data of Higgs *et al.* (1982) were based on studies carried out on a large number of Jamaican patients: 45

were of the $\alpha-/\alpha-$ genotype, 115 were $\alpha-/\alpha\alpha$ and 105 $\alpha\alpha/\alpha\alpha$ (normal). (Their genotype was determined by restriction-endonuclease DNA analysis.) Higgs and his co-workers were able to demonstrate that the $\alpha-/\alpha-$ patients had a higher erythrocyte count, a higher haemoglobin level and a higher Hb-A$_2$ percentage, but a lower Hb-F percentage, a lower MCH, MCHC and MCV, a lower reticulocyte count and ISC count and a lower serum bilirubin than the $\alpha\alpha/\alpha\alpha$ cases (Figs. 13.5 and 13.6). The results in the $\alpha-/\alpha\alpha$ patients were intermediate. Clinically, the $\alpha-/\alpha-$ patients had had fewer episodes of acute chest syndrome and chronic leg ulceration than the $\alpha\alpha/\alpha\alpha$ patients but more had large spleens than members of the other two groups. Higgs *et al.* concluded that the presence of α-thalassaemia inhibits sickling *in vivo* in Hb-SS disease and may be an important genetic determinant of haematological severity.

Further evidence on the effect of the α-globin genotype on the Hb-SS patient's spleen was provided by Mears *et al.* (1982). Fifteen children were studied: 10 had experienced at least one splenic sequestration crisis and five had splenomegaly persisting beyond the age of 5 years. Six of these patients had the $-\alpha/\alpha\alpha$ genotype and three the $-\alpha/-\alpha$ genotype, a $-\alpha$ chromosome

frequency of 0.40. In 45 age-matched controls, all Hb-SS but without splenic complications, the $-\alpha$ chromosome frequency was significantly less (0.15).

Embury and his co-workers (1982) studied 47 black American Hb-SS patients aged between 4 and 41 years: 25 had four α genes, 18 three α genes and four of them two α genes. The deletion of the genes from four to three to two was associated with a clear progressive decrease in MCH(S)C and in MCH(S), and in MCV, and a rise in MCH(F) and absolute reticulocyte count, and a rise in total haemoglobin and haematocrit. Embury *et al.* concluded that the decreased intra-erythrocytic concentration of Hb S [MCH(S)C] and the increased concentration of Hb F [MCH(F)] were diminishing the degree of haemolysis associated with homozygous sickle-cell disease.

Higgs and co-workers (1984) described four Hb-SS patients in whom the $\alpha\alpha\alpha/\alpha\alpha$ genotype had been identified. The triplicated gene did not, however, seem to affect the clinical or haematological severity of their disease. The genotype did, however, appear to influence the percentage of Hb S (or Hb C) in Hb-AS (and Hb-AC) heterozygotes: in nine Hb-AS subjects the percentage of Hb S was at the upper end of the range of percentages found in randomly selected Hb-AS subjects.

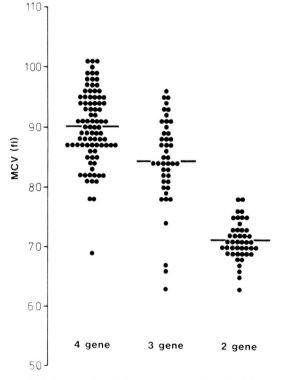

Fig. 13.5 Effect of α-globin genotype on the MCV in a series of Hb-SS patients.

Jamaican data. [Reproduced by permission from Higgs *et al.* (1982).]

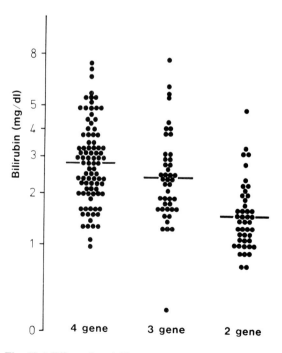

Fig. 13.6 Effect of α-globin genotype on plasma bilirubin in a series of Hb-SS patients.

Jamaican data. [Reproduced by permission from Serjeant (1985).]

Steinberg and co-workers (1983, 1984) summarized the very large experience of the Cooperative Study of Sickle Cell Disease Group. While confirming that the presence of α-thalassaemia (or β^0-thalassaemia) was associated with a low MCV, it was found that neither microcytosis nor the presence of β^0-thalassaemia or α-thalassaemia (proved by globin biosynthesis studies or by α-globin gene mapping) provided clear protection from vaso-occlusive phenomena such as painful episodes, acute chest syndrome and leg ulceration, while the prevalence of aseptic necrosis actually appeared to be increased in patients with Hb-SS/α-thalassaemia and in patients over 20 years of age who had an MCV less than 79 fl. It was concluded that the clinical severity of Hb-SS depends on a complicated relationship between MCV, MCHC, total haemoglobin, Hb-F percentage and perhaps the interaction between the erythrocytes and their environment, and that the crucial determinant is erythrocyte mass; the point was made that while a lowered MCV and MCHC might be of benefit by themselves and lead to a reduction in haemolysis, any consequent rise in haemoglobin might cause a sufficient increase in blood viscosity to impair blood flow in critical regions. In relation to attempts at therapy, it was emphasized that efforts to reduce haemolysis and raise the haematocrit may well promote vaso-occlusive complications unless there is a concurrent reduction in the intracellular concentration of Hb S.

Steinberg and Hebbel (1983), in a review, discussed the importance of α-thalassaemia and other genetic and cellular factors in relation to the clinical diversity and severity of Hb-SS disease.

El-Hazmi (1985) reported on a different ethnic group, namely, 68 Hb-SS Saudi Arabians: 27 had four α genes, 21 three α genes and 20 two α genes. In the $-\alpha/-\alpha$ patients the mean MCV, MCH and Hb-F percentages were significantly lower, and the mean PCV and Hb-A$_2$ levels were significantly higher, than in the Hb-SS patients; the mean erythrocyte counts and haemoglobin levels were higher but not significantly so. The results in the $-\alpha/\alpha\alpha$ patients were intermediate. Serum alkaline phosphatase, SGOT and SGPT activities were highest in the $-\alpha/-\alpha$ patients. Retrospective analysis indicated that the α-thalassaemia patients had had fewer complications and had received fewer transfusions than the Hb-SS patients who were free from α-thalassaemia.

More recently, Stevens and his co-workers (1986), as part of the Jamaican cohort study of Hb-SS children, compared the blood picture from birth of nine $-\alpha/-\alpha$ children and 90 $-\alpha/\alpha\alpha$ children with that of 167 $\alpha\alpha/\alpha\alpha$ controls. The 2α-gene group had lower MCVs from birth, higher erythrocyte counts from 1 month, lower reticulocyte counts from 3 months and higher Hb-A$_2$ percentages from 1 year, compared with the 4α-gene group. The 3α-gene children had intermediate indices which were closer to the 4-gene than the 2-gene group. No differences in total haemoglobin or Hb-F percentage were apparent by 8 years. The most characteristic findings in the 2-gene group were the low MCV and raised Hb-A$_2$ percentage. The low MCV at birth was considered to have some predictive value for α-thalassaemia.

Lie-Injo and her co-workers (1986) reported on the α-gene status of 12 Hb-SS and 30 Hb-AS Malaysian Indians (from Orissa). All 12 Hb-SS patients were either homozygous or heterozygous for α-thalassaemia-2 (α-thal-2) ($-\alpha$ haplotype). Two types of α-thal-2 deletion were shown to be responsible: in nine patients this was of the rightward type; in one it was of the leftward type, and two patients were doubly heterozygous for both genotypes.

Effect of α-thalassaemia on Hb-A$_2$ percentage

Serjeant (1985, p. 91) has reported on the Hb-A$_2$ percentages in Hb-SS Jamaican patients of different α-globin genotype and compared the findings with those in Hb-S/β^0-thalassaemia. The values in the Hb-SS patients with a $-\alpha/-\alpha$ genotype were generally higher than those in patients with the $-\alpha/\alpha\alpha$ or $\alpha\alpha/\alpha\alpha$ genotype; they overlapped the high values found in Hb-S/β^0-thalassaemia (Fig. 13.7).

Effect of α-thalassaemia on the eye lesions in Hb-SS disease

In the West Indies, too, Condon and co-workers (1983) compared the incidence of vaso-occlusion affecting the macular vessels of the retina in 25 pairs of Hb-SS $\alpha\alpha/\alpha\alpha$ and Hb-SS $-\alpha/-\alpha$ patients. They found that, although capillary abnormalities in the perimacular region were significantly less severe in the α-thalassaemia patients, the retina appeared to have been damaged to a similar degree in the two genotypes when assessed by two other criteria.

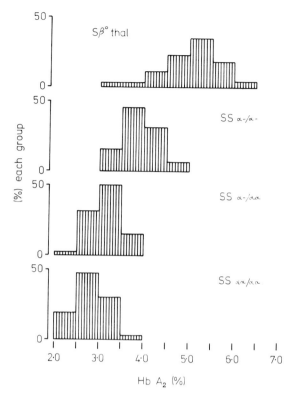

Fig. 13.7 Effect of α-globin genotype on Hb-A$_2$ percentage in a series of Hb-SS patients compared to the Hb-A$_2$ percentages in a series of Hb-S/β-thalassaemia patients.
Jamaican data. [Reproduced by permission from Serjeant (1985).]

Effect of α-thalassaemia on rheology and on Hb-SS erythrocyte density

The effect of α-thalassaemia on rheology in Hb-SS disease was studied by B. Serjeant and her co-workers (1983). Twenty-four Hb-SS $-\alpha/-\alpha$ patients were matched with 24 Hb-SS $\alpha\alpha/\alpha\alpha$ controls. Compared with the controls, the erythrocytes of the $-\alpha/-\alpha$ patients were more deformable, as assessed by passage through 5 μm pores, and the viscosity of whole blood was less at a standard haematocrit level. However, at the patients' own haematocrit levels (higher in the $-\alpha/-\alpha$ patients than in the $\alpha\alpha/\alpha\alpha$ controls) the whole-blood viscosity of the $-\alpha/-\alpha$ patients exceeded that of the controls. Serjeant et al. concluded that any increase in the whole-blood viscosity in $-\alpha/-\alpha$ patients tends to negate the rheological benefit of the increase in erythrocyte deformity and thus would limit the clinical benefit that the patients might otherwise enjoy.

Rodgers and co-workers (1983) compared erythrocyte density and Hb-F content in 16 $\alpha\alpha/\alpha\alpha$ Hb-SS patients and 17 $-\alpha/-\alpha$ Hb-SS patients. The MCHC was less in the $-\alpha/-\alpha$ patients and the percentage of dense cells

far less (0–4.6 compared with 0–31, mean 10 $\pm$ 8). The median density was 1.104 $\pm$ 0.04 in the $\alpha\alpha/\alpha\alpha$ patients compared with 1.097 $\pm$ 0.02 in the $-\alpha/-\alpha$ patients. The percentage of reticulocytes in which Hb F could be demonstrated (F reticulocytes) was the same in the two series and the mean Hb F per cell was less in the $-\alpha/-\alpha$ cases (5.6 $\pm$ 1.8 pg compared with 8.4 $\pm$ 2.2 pg), a reduction proportional to the reduction in total MCH. Rodgers et al. stressed that in attempting to evaluate the mechanisms that contribute to disease severity the cellular distribution of Hb F, and the median cell density and the percentage of very dense cells present, should be taken into account.

Embury and co-workers (1984) studied 45 patients with Hb-SS disease, 29 having four α genes, 13 three α genes and two only two α genes. They found that the percentage of ISCs and of very dense erythrocytes, and the diminished deformability of Hb-SS erythrocytes, varied directly with the α-globin gene number. They attributed the reduced severity of haemolysis in patients with α-thalassaemia to a reduction in the intracellular concentration of Hb S and its retarded polymerization.

Noguchi and co-workers (1985) studied 52 Hb-SS patients, 32 of whom had α-thalassaemia as well (19 $\alpha-/\alpha-$ genotype and 13 $\alpha-/\alpha\alpha$ genotype). The abnormally broad distribution of erythrocyte density, and the high proportion of very dense cells, found in the Hb-SS $\alpha\alpha/\alpha\alpha$ patients were found to be significantly reduced in the Hb-SS $\alpha-/\alpha-$ patients (Fig. 13.8). It was concluded that the reduction in haemolysis that accompanies the presence of α-thalassaemia is brought about by a diminution in the increase in cell density associated with polymerization of Hb S.

Effect of α-thalassaemia on the permeability of the Hb-SS erythrocyte membrane to monovalent cations

Embury, Backer and Glader (1983, 1985) studied the changes in intracellular Na$^+$ and K$^+$ concentration as the result of incubating Hb-SS erythrocytes in vitro under anaerobic conditions. Using blood depleted of ISCs, Hb-SS $-\alpha/-\alpha$ erythrocytes were found to lose less K$^+$ and to gain less Na$^+$ than Hb-SS $\alpha\alpha/\alpha\alpha$ cells, with $-\alpha/\alpha\alpha$ cells giving intermediate values. [The changes in all three α genotypes were far greater than in Hb-AA controls (Fig. 13.9).] The cation changes were found, too, to be inversely related to the ratio of the surface area of the cell membrane to the cell volume. Embury, Backer and Glader concluded that their data indicated that the excess of cell membrane relative to cell volume plays a part in the protective effect of α-thalassaemia and that α-thalassaemia protects the Hb-SS erythrocyte by diminishing erythrocyte K$^+$ and water loss and the increased cellular haemoglobin concentration and reduced deformability consequent on this; they referred to the work of Izumo et al. (1985) who had demonstrated that deoxygenation in vitro, in the absence of added ouabain, results in Hb-SS erythrocyte dehy-

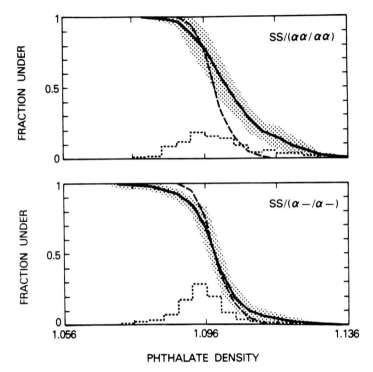

Fig. 13.8 The mean erythroccyte density profile in Hb-SS patients of $-\alpha/-\alpha$ or $\alpha\alpha/\alpha\alpha$ genotype, respectively, expressed as a cumulative frequency.
[Reproduced by permission from Noguchi *et al.* (1985).]

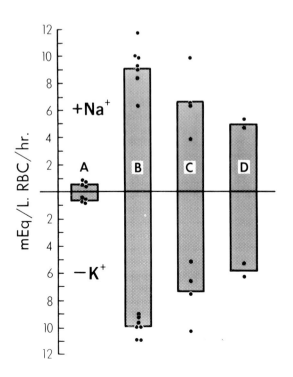

dration and that this could be prevented by blocking Na^+-K^+-ATPase with ouabain. The dehydration was considered by Embury, Backer and Glader (1985) to result from the differential pumping of three Na^+ ions out of the cell for every two K^+ ions pumped in. Embury, Oliver and Kropp (1985), who estimated erythrocyte surface area from the maximum volume attained prior to hypotonic haemolysis, calculated that the surface area:volume ratio increased from 1.29 to 1.41 to 1.45 in the Hb-SS erythrocytes with reduction in α genes from four to three to two. Increased surface area was thought to lead to increased deformability, and it was suggested that membrane redundancy could be a factor in protecting the membrane from deleterious cation losses consequent on stretching caused by Hb-S polymerization.

Fig. 13.9 Changes in net sodium and potassium content of erythrocytes during deoxygenation.
A: data from normal control subjects. B: data from seven Hb-SS patients with four α-globin genes. C: data from four Hb-SS patients with three α-globin genes. D: data from two Hb-SS patients with two α-globin genes.
[Reproduced by permission from Embury, Backer and Glader (1985).]

Effect of α-thalassaemia on erythrocyte life-span in Hb-SS disease

de Ceulaer and co-workers (1983) reported ^{51}Cr auto-survival data derived from 11 Hb-SS patients of $-\alpha/-\alpha$ genotype and from 11 age- and sex-matched Hb-SS ($\alpha\alpha/\alpha\alpha$) controls. The mean ^{51}Cr T_{50} of the $-\alpha/-\alpha$ patients was 13.8 days and that of the $\alpha\alpha/\alpha\alpha$ controls 9.4 days. The mean haemoglobin of the former group was 8.9 g/dl and mean MCV 72 fl, compared with 7.8 g/dl and 92 fl of the latter (control) group.

EFFECT OF α-THALASSAEMIA HAPLOTYPE ON Hb-SS DISEASE AND Hb-AS HETEROZYGOTES

The recent discovery of the diversity in the molecular-genetic basis of α-thalassaemia haplotypes (p. 513) has prompted investigations into whether such differences affect the clinical expression of Hb-S/α-thalassaemia in any significant way. Some evidence on this question is summarized below.

Felice and co-workers (1984b) analysed DNA samples from 345 black children suffering from Hb-SS or Hb-SC disease or Hb-S/β$^+$-thalassaemia and found that 34% were of the $-\alpha/\alpha\alpha$ genotype and 4% were of the $-\alpha/-\alpha$ genotype. In every case the $-\alpha$ haplotype was caused by a 3.7 kb α-gene deletion. The incidence of the deletion appeared to be the same in the three types of sickle-cell disease. Eight patients (2.3%) had a large 10.4 kb deletion involving the zeta-2 gene and the entire inter-zeta DNA region; their MCV was normal (mean 89 fl) and the mean Hb-S percentage in Hb-AS relatives was as high as 41.5%, findings that indicated that the deletion did not affect the expression of the α-globin genes. One patient had a triplicated α gene.

Embury and co-workers (1985) reported that they had identified a black Hb-SS individual who was a $-\alpha/\alpha\alpha$ heterozygote caused by an unusual (leftward) deletion affecting the α-gene complex. This was the only leftward deletion found amongst 255 Hb-SS α-thalassaemia-2 patients. The unusual patient could not be distinguished clinically or haematologically from those whose α-thalassaemia was brought about by the common α-gene haplotype.

EFFECT OF α-THALASSAEMIA ON Hb-SS CHILDREN OF DIFFERENT AGES

Stevens and co-workers (1984) compared the blood picture from birth onwards up to the age of 6 years of a group of 237 Hb-SS West-Indian children of whom 79 were of the $-\alpha/\alpha\alpha$ genotype and nine of the $-\alpha/-\alpha$ genotype. The $-\alpha/-\alpha$ group had, compared with the four gene $\alpha\alpha/\alpha\alpha$ group, a lower MCV from birth onwards, a higher erythrocyte count from 1 month, a lower reticulocyte count from 3 months, a higher Hb-A percentage from 1 year, and a lower but rather variable MCHC. The results in the three gene ($-\alpha/\alpha\alpha$) group were intermediate. There were, however, no differences between the three groups in total haemoglobin or Hb-F percentage up to the age of 6 years.

Felice and co-workers (1985) determined the α-gene numbers in 400 Hb-SS and Hb-SC patients attending sickle-cell clinics in Augusta. The haemoglobin levels of children belonging to the three genotypes, $\alpha\alpha/\alpha\alpha$, $-\alpha/\alpha\alpha$ and $-\alpha/-\alpha$, were about the same up to the age of 5–7 years; later, the haemoglobin levels in the $-\alpha/-\alpha$ children were generally higher than in the $-\alpha/\alpha\alpha$ children, which in turn were higher than in the $\alpha\alpha/\alpha\alpha$ children. The Hb-F percentages in the three genotypes were similar after the age of 7 years in the Hb-SS patients and after 3 years in the Hb-SC patients.

INTERACTION BETWEEN Hb G PHILADELPHIA AND α-THALASSAEMIA WITH Hb-SS DISEASE

Knox-Macaulay and co-workers (1984) reported the occurrence in four Nigerian families of Hb S, Hb G Philadelphia (an α-chain variant) and also of a gene for α-thalassaemia. Four Hb-SS homozygotes were also heterozygotes for Hb G. They presented with the clinical and haematological findings characteristic of Hb-SS disease; the haemoglobin electrophoresis findings were, however, at first sight suggestive of Hb-SC disease.

EFFECT OF α-THALASSAEMIA ON Hb-S HETEROZYGOTES

Steinberg, Adams and Dreiling (1975) showed that the presence of α-thalassaemia affected the percentage of Hb S present in Hb-S heterozygotes. They had studied 14 Hb-AS heterozygotes in whom the Hb-S concentration in the peripheral blood was less than 35% and showed that the mean α:β-chain synthesis ratio was 0.76. In contrast, in Hb-AS heterozygotes with Hb-S percentages greater than 35%, the mean α:β-chain synthesis ratio was approximately 1.0 — they were presumably free from α-thalassaemia.

Huisman (1977) provided further evidence on the effect of α-thalassaemia genes on Hb-S percentages in Hb-S heterozygotes. In 33 individuals presumed to have the normal $\alpha\alpha/\alpha\alpha$ genotype the mean Hb-S percentage was 41.2; in 25 with a $-\alpha/\alpha\alpha$ genotype the mean percentage was 35.4 and in 10 with a $-\alpha/-\alpha$ genotype the mean percentage was 28.1.

Recent data have provided further confirmation of the relationship between α-gene deletion and the haematological indices and globin-chain synthesis ratios in the Hb-AS trait complicated by the concurrent presence of α-thalassaemia.

Wong, Ali and Boyadjian (1981) reported a trimodal distribution of Hb-S percentages as the result of interaction with α-thalassaemia in a series of blacks resident in Canada. The mean percentages were 40.4 in those with the $\alpha\alpha/\alpha\alpha$ genotype, 35.1 in those with the $-\alpha/\alpha\alpha$ genotype and 28.6 in those with the $-\alpha/-\alpha$ genotype. The MCV and MCH of the three groups were directly related to the percentage of Hb S present.

Felice and co-workers (1981) found that the percentage of Hb S and the MCV were directly correlated with the α:non-α globin-chain synthesis ratios in a series of 60 Hb-AS heterozygotes and five Hb-AS heterozygotes with an associated α-chain heterozygosity (ASAG). They stressed, however, that the biosynthetic ratios in individuals with four, three or two active α-globin genes, respectively, overlapped to the extent that this rendered making a diagnosis in individual cases unreliable.

Huisman (1983) summarized his data in an extensive review: in 88 Hb-AS heterozygotes of $\alpha\alpha/\alpha\alpha$ genotype the mean MCV was 85 ± 5.6 fl and the mean Hb-S percentage 41.5 ± 1.9; in 115 Hb-AS heterozygotes of $-\alpha/\alpha\alpha$ genotype the mean MCV 78 ± 5.6 fl and mean Hb-S percentage 35.1 ± 2.1, and in 44 Hb-AS heterozygotes of $-\alpha/-\alpha$ genotype the mean MCV was 71 ± 9.9 fl and the mean Hb-S percentage was 27.3 ± 2.2.

Association of Hb-AS trait and Hb-H disease

This combination has rarely been reported. Brief details of three such occurrences are, however, given below. A characteristic feature is that only about 20% of the haemoglobin is Hb S.

Matthay and co-workers (1979) described a 5-year-old male whose black father had the Hb-AS trait and was thought in addition to be a silent carrier of α-thalassaemia ($-\alpha/\alpha\alpha$). The child's mother was Chinese and had the α-thalassaemia trait ($--/\alpha\alpha$). The child had a microcytic hypochromic anaemia despite ample iron stores. His haemoglobin was 9.4 g/dl, erythrocyte count 5.5–5.8 $\times$ 10^{12}/l, MCV 51 fl and MCH 17 pg. The reticulocyte count was not raised (0.6–0.8%), and Hb-H inclusions were seen in only a very few erythrocytes when the cells were exposed to brilliant cresyl blue. Haemoglobin electrophoresis revealed 66–72% Hb A, 1.9–3.2% Hb A_2, 17–21% Hb S and a trace of Hb Bart's (3% at 31 months). There was 4.0–4.7% Hb F. The α:β+γ globin synthesis ratio was 0.58 when carried out on peripheral blood. Molecular-genetic analysis indicated that the patient possessed only one gene for α globin. The presence of the gene for Hb S was thought to modify the expression of Hb-H disease: the virtual absence of Hb H was attributed to the small number of β^A chains being formed (since one β-globin gene was directing the formation of β^S chains). The low percentage of Hb S was considered to be due to the affinity of α chains for β^A chains being greater than for β^S chains.

A similar occurrence, but in a patient of wholly black parentage, was described by Felice and co-workers (1984a). Their patient was a 5-year-old girl who, having the Hb-AS trait, was found in addition to have a severe hypochromic microcytic thalassaemia-like anaemia: haemoglobin 5.8–9.6 g/dl, erythrocytes 5.21 $\times$ 10^{12}/l, MCV 55 fl and MCH 16.1 pg. Haemoglobin electrophoresis revealed: Hb S 19.9%, Hb A_2 2.5% and Hb H 1.1%: the remainder of the haemoglobin was Hb A and no Hb Bart's was detected. A few erythrocytes developed inclusions after exposure to brilliant cresyl blue. The α: β^A + β^S ratio was 0.23. The patient's mother was shown to be a heterozygote for α-thalassaemia-2; her father could not be studied. The patient was considered to have the $\alpha°\alpha°/\alpha°\alpha$ ($--/-\alpha$) genotype, and molecular-genetic analysis indicated that the $\alpha°\alpha°$ haplotype was associated with deletion of all the α and ζ (zeta) genes.

A further patient was described by Martinez and co-workers (1986). He was a male aged 15 years of black and Chinese origin who was moderately anaemic and had a palpable spleen. His haemoglobin was 10.1 g/dl, erythrocyte count 4.59 × 10^{12}/l, MCV 76 fl, MCH 22 pg and MCHC 29 g/l. His α-globin genotype was −α/−− and the α:β globin synthesis ratio 0.46. The Hb-S percentage was 18.5, Hb F 2.4, Hb A_2 2.4 and Hb Bart's 3.0. No Hb H could be detected by gel electrophoresis or by column chromatography.

ASSOCIATION OF THE GENE FOR Hb S WITH THE GENE(S) FOR HEREDITARY PERSISTENCE OF FETAL HAEMOGLOBIN (HPFH)

As described in Chapter 18 (p. 435), several forms of HPFH exist and lead to relatively high levels of Hb F in the peripheral blood persisting into adult life. HPFH is by itself a benign condition and carriers of the trait generally lead normal lives and are not anaemic. Compound heterozygosity for Hb S and HPFH occurs rather rarely but is well known: according to Serjeant (1985, p. 326), the condition occurs in Jamaica once in approximately every 11 000 births and in the United States once in 25 000 births; its main interest and importance lies in the fact that haemoglobin electrophoresis gives a pattern that can be confused with that of Hb-SS disease or Hb-S/β⁰-thalassaemia (see below).

Physical examination of Hb-S/HPFH individuals reveals as a rule no abnormality, and growth and maturation are generally normal, and pregnancy ordinarily presents no problems.

Blood picture. Patients with Hb-S/HPFH are typically not anaemic, and the MCV and reticulocyte count are usually within the normal range. Anisocytosis is as a rule slight but a few target cells may be present. Sickled cells are absent. Serjeant (1985, p. 327) tabulated data from the cases reported between 1955 and 1963. Application of the Betke-Kleihauer acid elution technique to blood films shows that all the erythrocytes contain Hb F and that it is relatively evenly distributed amongst the cells (pancellular HPFH).

Haemoglobin electrophoresis. This reveals a Hb S, Hb F and Hb A_2 pattern; Hb A is absent (Table 13.2). In the pancellular type of HPFH the Hb-F percentage is between 15 and 35 and that of Hb A_2 normal or slightly subnormal. Wrightstone and Huisman (1974) recorded Hb-A_2 percentages of 1.2–3.6 in 24 patients (mean 2.5%).

Early case reports

Edington and Lehmann (1955a,b) called attention to the fact that the haemoglobin of certain apparently clinically normal individuals might give on electrophoresis a Hb-S, Hb-F pattern (with Hb A not demonstrable) which appeared to be identical with that given by the haemoglobin of homozygous Hb-SS patients. Two West-African families were being studied. The propositus in the first family, a healthy adult male, with this Hb-S, Hb-F pattern had 5.9% Hb F; he had a normal daughter who formed Hb A but not Hb S and had 5% Hb F. The propositus in the second family, also a healthy adult male, formed 26% Hb F; he also had a normal daughter who formed Hb A but not Hb S; she had 24% Hb F. Compound heterozygosity for Hb S and thalassaemia was discussed as a possible explanation for the findings but no conclusion was reached: the absence of target cells in blood films and of microcytosis (the MCV being 81 fl and 89 fl, respectively, in the two propositi) were thought to be against this diagnosis.

A similar condition to that observed by Edington and Lehmann in West Africa was subsequently reported (at first under a variety of tentative names) in black families resident in Jamaica (Went and MacIver, 1958b; MacIver, Went and Irvine, 1961) and in the United States (Griggs and Harris, 1956; Bradley and Conley, 1960; Herman and Conley 1960; Bradley, Brawner and Conley, 1961; Conley et al., 1963; Natta et al., 1974; Altay, Schroeder and Huisman, 1977), as well as in East Africa (Jacob and Raper, 1958). Neel and co-workers (1956) and Thompson and Lehmann (1962) reported further cases from West Africa. None of these patients seems to have been significantly anaemic, except one of two sisters (both with 30% Hb F and 70% Hb S) who was in terminal renal failure (Case 10 of Griggs and Harris, 1956). Conley and co-workers (1963), however, reported that of the 20 Hb-S/HPFH individuals studied at the Johns Hopkins Hospital three gave histories of symptoms possibly attributable to their haemoglobin abnormality — two had had mild joint pains and one aseptic necrosis of the head of a femur.

Went and MacIver (1958b) and Herman and Conley (1960) attributed the benign nature of the combination of Hb S and HPFH to the high intracellular concentration of Hb F making the cells resistant to sickling. Bradley and Conley (1960), Bradley, Brawner and Conley (1961) and Conley and co-workers (1963) pointed out that in Hb-S/HPFH the distribution of Hb F within the erythrocytes is uniform, with the result that all the cells would be protected from sickling at physiological O_2 tensions by the presence of Hb F, in contrast to Hb-SS disease in which the Hb F is heterogeneously distributed within the erythrocyte population so that many cells would contain insufficient Hb F to protect them from sickling even if the overall percentage of Hb F in the blood was relatively high.

Diagnosis of Hb-S/HPFH

This depends upon a consideration of the (generally benign) clinical history of the patient, his/her haematological findings and haemoglobin analysis, and the results of family studies, with one parent positive for HPFH, the other a carrier of Hb S and any children heterozygotes for Hb S or HPFH.

Although in most cases the clinical history of Hb-S/HPFH individuals is a benign one, some of the characteristic vaso-occlusive complications of sickle-cell disease have been recorded. Serjeant, (1985, p. 326) lists, and gives references to, reports of, for instance, mild haemolytic anaemia, splenomegaly, avascular necrosis of the hip, hemiparesis and occlusion of retinal arterioles (Talbot, Bird and Serjeant, 1983). He makes the point, however, that in some patients the distinction between Hb-S/HPFH and Hb-S/δβ-thalassaemia is difficult.

Association of Hb S with heterocellular types of hereditary persistence of fetal haemoglobin

Subsequent to the discovery of the African (pancellular) type of HPFH, other (heterocellular) variants have been described in which the percentage of Hb F formed is less and in which not all the erythrocytes contain demonstrable amounts of Hb F (see p. 437). Families in which clinically mild forms of Hb-S disease have occurred and in which it was suggested that there had been interaction with a heterocellular HPFH gene were described by Stamatoyannopoulos et al. (1975), by Wood, Weatherall and Clegg (1976) and Serjeant, Serjeant and Mason (1977).

HAEMOGLOBIN-S/HAEMOGLOBIN-C DISEASE (Hb-SC DISEASE)

The clinical syndrome associated with compound heterozygosity for Hb S and Hb C was first described in two black American families by Kaplan, Zuelzer and Neel (1951) who used the provisional title 'hemoglobin III' for Hb C. The condition was subsequently found to be not rare in the United States (although less common than homozygosity for Hb S), and it now has a large literature.

Early reports and reviews include those of Neel, Kaplan and Zuelzer (1953), Conley and Smith (1954), Smith and Conley (1954), Hook and Cooper (1958), Smith and Krevans (1959), Tuttle and Koch (1960) and River et al. (1961). Hb-SC disease was soon reported, too, from West Africa (Edington and Lehmann, 1954; Hendrickse, 1958) and from Jamaica (MacIver and Went, 1958) where it has been extensively studied (Serjeant, Ashcroft and Serjeant, 1973; Stevens et al., 1985).

According to Serjeant (1985, p. 296), the expected frequency of Hb-SC disease in the black population of North America is about 1 in 1000 births while in Jamaica the incidence is about 1 in 500 births.

Hb-SC disease has, too, been reported, although rarely, in Europeans, e.g., by Blatrix et al. (1970) in a Sicilian and by Dunstan et al. (1972) in a South-African boy of Dutch and English parentage. Reports of its occurrence in black immigrants to the United Kingdom date from the late 1950s (Bannerman and White, 1957; Diamond, 1959; Black et al., 1972).

CLINICAL FEATURES

Hb-SC disease resembles Hb-SS disease in many respects, but it is generally milder and follows a

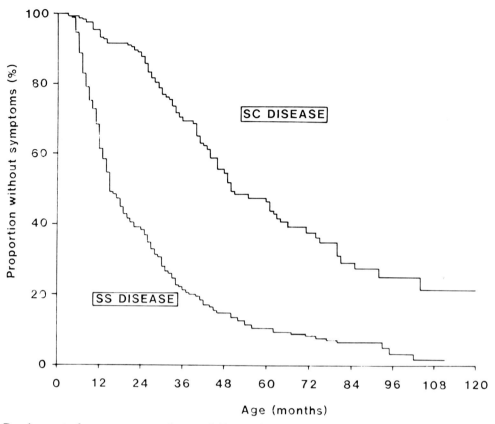

Fig. 13.10 Development of symptoms up to the age of 10 years in a series of Hb-SC patients compared with a series of Hb-SS patients.
Jamaican data. [Reproduced by permission from Serjeant (1985).]

more benign course. Although often diagnosed in childhood, this is not always so, and in some patients symptoms leading to the diagnosis do not arise until well into adult life (Fig. 13.10). Fewer painful vaso-occlusive crises occur than in Hb-SS disease and unexplained haematuria is less frequent. Anaemia is less severe. Growth and fertility are not affected, and pregnancy is on the whole well tolerated. The spleen is usually palpable, irrespective of the age of the patient. The generally benign presentation does not, however, apply to the retina, where serious lesions appear to occur more frequently than in Hb-SS disease (see p. 33).

In Smith and Conley's (1954) important review, details were given of the haematological and clinical findings in 16 patients with atypical sickle-cell disease who on re-evaluation at the Johns Hopkins Hospital were found to have Hb-SC disease; details were also given of 11 cases recorded in the literature. The age at which these patients first suffered from symptoms attributable to Hb-SC disease varied from 2 to 70 years; two of Smith and Conley's patients, aged 13 and 65 years, respectively, had never complained of any symptoms. Smith and Conley concluded that virtually all atypical cases of sickle-cell disease were likely to prove to be genetic variants of the disease.

The clinical histories of a large series of patients were described from Chicago by River *et al.* (1961) (75 patients, 14 months to 65 years of age) and from Jamaica by Serjeant, Ashcroft and Serjeant (1973) (90 patients, 7–87 years of age). The findings in both series were almost identical. Bone, joint or abdominal pains were the commonest presenting symptoms, and 83% of the Jamaican patients had experienced such pains at one time or another. Haematuria, epistaxis and infections were not uncommon in the Chicago series. Almost one-third of the Jamaican patients gave a history of pneumonia; 20% had had leg ulcers, most occurring in patients between the ages of 10 and 15 years. Jaundice was not common, the serum bilirubin being less than 2.0 mg/dl in all but four patients.

In children, Tuttle and Koch (1960) had stressed how variable was the clinical expression. The predominant symptoms were musculo-skeletal pain and painful abdominal crises; two-thirds of their 18 patients had enlargement of the liver and spleen and one-third enlargement of the heart and cardiac murmurs.

In a more recent report Ballas et al. (1982) compared 27 Hb-SC patients studied at Philadelphia with a larger number of Hb-SS patients; they reported that the degree of increased haemolysis and the complications of chronic haemolytic anaemia — cholelithiasis, leg ulcers, and enlargement of the liver and heart — were less severe than in the Hb-SS patients, and that asplenia and its sequelae — an increase in the platelet count and a reduction in serum IgM levels — occurred less frequently. Cerebrovascular accidents occurred with equal frequency, while thrombo-embolic incidents, retinopathy and renal papillary necrosis were more frequent in the Hb-SC patients.

Unusual presentations

Arterial thrombi following atypical pneumonia. Burchmore and co-workers (1962) described the occurrence in a 27-year-old Jamaican female of arterial thrombosis affecting major arteries in the left forearm and leg. A high-titre cold agglutinin was present (titre 2000 at 12°C), and it was suggested that this combined with intravascular sickling had led to the thrombosis.
Pulmonary angiography leading to diagnosis. Bashour and Lindsay (1975) described two adult patients who were investigated by pulmonary angiography to ascertain the cause of pleuritic pain. Abnormalities of vascular perfusion were demonstrated and, in searching for an explanation for this, they were found to be suffering from Hb-SC disease.
TAB vaccination leading to diagnosis. Lecocq and Harper (1963) described how inoculation with TAB vaccine, which was followed in 3 hours or so by a painful crisis, led to the diagnosis of hitherto unsuspected Hb-SC disease in a 30-year-old black female.
Acting as blood donor leading to diagnosis. Murphy, Malhotra and Sweet (1980) described a most unusual and tragic event in which the use of blood from a 21-year-old asymptomatic Caucasian in the form of an exchange transfusion led to (or at least contributed to) the death of an infant of 34 weeks' gestation with hyperbilirubinaemia. The necropsy findings in the infant indicated that death was due to massive intravascular sickling and the donor was subsequently found to have Hb-SC disease.

Renal complications

These are similar to those experienced by Hb-SS patients but they occur possibly less frequently.

Three of the 16 Hb-SC patients described by

Smith and Conley (1954) had gross haematuria, two of them having had many recurrences. Chapman and co-workers (1954) similarly reported that three Hb-SC patients had had 'idiopathic hematuria'. Tuttle and Koch (1960), however, in their report on 18 children with Hb-SC disease stated that none of them gave a history of gross haematuria and none had microscopic haematuria at the time they were under observation; the results of renal function studies carried out on one patient were reported to be similar to those in Hb-SS children.

River and co-workers (1961) in their clinical study of 75 Hb-SC patients aged between 14 months and 65 years described haematuria as being not uncommon. Fourteen patients had experienced haematuria; their average age was 30 and none was less than 20 years of age. All the attacks subsided without surgical intervention. In two patients the bleeding originated from one kidney on one occasion and from the other kidney on another occasion. The urine specific gravity was recorded in 52 patients: it varied from 1.003–1.024, with a mean of 1.011. The hyposthenuria was thought to be similar to that in the Hb-AS trait and less serious than in Hb-SS disease.

Ballas and co-workers (1982) reported that they had demonstrated by intravenous pyelography calyceal blunting, indicative of renal papillary necrosis, in 73% of 15 patients; microscopic haematuria was demonstrated in 7% of their Hb-SC patients compared with 14% of their Hb-SS patients. Urine specific gravity (1.010 ± 0.003) was low and similar in both groups of patients. Serjeant, Ashcroft and Serjeant (1973) stated that only two of their 90 Jamaican patients had experienced haematuria.

Neurological complications

Neurological symptoms and signs, including hemiplegia, convulsions, stupor and coma, have been recorded not infrequently in Hb-SC disease. Their incidence is, however, less than in Hb-SS disease. Important early reviews include those of River et al. (1961) (on neuropsychiatric disease), Greer and Schotland (1962) and Portnoy and Herion (1972).

Fabian and Peters (1984) have more recently reviewed the literature and referred to the incidence of neurological problems in 68 personally studied Hb-SC patients and in 68 age-matched controls. Two of their Hb-SC patients had developed hemiplegia, and the incidence, too, of retinopathy, stupor, coma and seizures was significantly increased. Five patients had become stuporose and comatose; in two of them, aged 35 and 65, respectively, their neurological condition led to the diagnosis, for the first time, of underlying Hb-SC disease.

Eye complications

As already mentioned, eye complications are relatively frequent and important in Hb-SC disease. Early reports stem from the mid-1950s (Smith and Conley, 1954; Hannon, 1956; Goodman, von Sallmann and Holland, 1957). Retinitis proliferans (proliferative sickle retinopathy) and vitreous haemorrhages are the most characteristic lesions (see Fig. 11.4).

Retinal lesions. Hannon (1956) found these lesions on presentation in seven out of 20 Hb-SC disease patients attending the Johns Hopkins Hospital and, not finding similar lesions in larger series of Hb-SS and Hb-AS individuals, concluded that the peculiar retinopathy occurred almost exclusively in Hb-SC disease. Goodman, von Sallmann and Holland (1957) reviewed past work and gave a detailed description of the eye findings in four Hb-SC disease patients: the lesions described included retinitis proliferans, aneurismal vascular dilatations, arborizing vascular networks, focal vascular constriction and dilatation, sheathing and obstruction of arterioles and venules, preretinal haemorrhages, and vitreous and retinal haemorrhages. They also noted 'sausage-like dilatation of fine vessels, with red cells massed in the dilated segments' in the conjunctiva of one patient. They concluded that the retinopathy was the consequence of acute or chronic vascular obstruction; they stressed how relatively frequently the eyes and kidneys are involved together in systemic diseases and instanced as examples hypertension, diabetes and sickle-cell syndromes.

Later and more complete descriptions of the retinal lesions in Hb-SC disease were provided by Welch and Goldberg (1966), Goldberg (1971a,b), Condon and Serjeant (1972a) and Asdourian et al. (1975). Serjeant (1985) devoted a whole chapter to the eye changes in the sickle-cell diseases; he pointed out that the ability to examine the retinal vessels [by, in particular, fluorescent angiography] provides a unique means of observing directly the vaso-occlusive process in sickle-cell disease.

Welch and Goldberg (1966) studied 22 Hb-SC patients at the Johns Hopkins Hospital: 77% of them had some form of retinitis proliferans including arteriovenous 'fans' projecting into the vitreous. They named the fans 'sea fans' from their resemblance to the sea fan *Gorgonia flabellum*, an Alcyonarian polyp. Vitreous haemorrhages were also commonly present. Welch and Goldberg did not observe 'sea fans' in any other type of retinopathy. Goldberg (1971a,b), in a study of 24 Hb-SC patients, listed five stages in the development of 'proliferative sickle retinopathy', ranging from peripheral arteriolar occlusions, present in 91% of the patients, to retinal detachment, present in 8%. Goldberg (1971b) stressed that the lesions were progressive and that they were most frequently seen in 20–30-year-old adults.

Condon and Serjeant (1972a) reported on 70 consecutive West-Indian Hb-SC disease patients and compared the ocular findings with those of 76 Hb-SS patients. Proliferative sickle retinopathy was noted in 63% of the Hb-SC patients compared with 26% of the Hb-SS patients. The higher incidence of the lesions in the Hb-SC patients was considered to be due to their relatively high haemoglobin levels acting as an adverse factor by increasing blood viscosity — lesions were present in 73% of the Hb-SC patients with haemoglobins greater than 12.5 g/dl and only in 15% of those with haemoglobins < 12.5 g/dl. Retinitis proliferans was seen in 38 eyes and typical 'sea fans' in 11 eyes. However, Condon and Serjeant concluded that the presence of 'sea fans' was not pathognomonic of Hb-SC disease.

In a further detailed report on their West-Indian patients, Hayes, Condon and Serjeant (1981) compared the haematological indices in Hb-SC patients who had developed proliferative sickle retinopathy (PSR) with those who had not. [PSR had occurred in 90 out of 243 patients (37%): the lesions were most frequent in the 20–30 year age-group; 68% of the patients aged 45 years or over were affected.] Hayes, Condon and Serjeant's main findings were that the occurrence of PSR was positively related to a high MCV in men and to a low Hb-F percentage in both sexes. The significant relationship to total haemoglobin in men was secondary to the strong age-related upward trend in haemoglobin level.

B. E. Serjeant and her co-workers (1984) reported on still further studies which included measurement of plasma, serum and whole-blood viscosity and erythrocyte deformity (filterability) in 31 age- and sex-matched pairs of Hb-SC patients with and without, respectively, signs of proliferative sickle retinopathy (PSR). The patients with PSR were found to have a significantly higher mean MCH and a lower mean Hb-F percentage, but the viscosity measurements and other haematological indices did not differ. (The mean haemoglobin levels and MCV were higher in the patients with PSR but the differences were not significant.) It was concluded that although there was no evidence of rheological differences at the time the PSR developed, transient differences between the patients with and without PSR could not be excluded. It was suggested that the apparent conflict between greater vascular occlusion in Hb-SS disease and a higher incidence of PSR in Hb-SC disease could be explained by different tendencies to auto-infarction in the two genotypes. The possibility that in rare instances fluorescein angiography might precipitate a painful crisis was raised by Acheson and Serjeant (1985) on the basis of two such occurrences.

Conjunctival lesions. As already mentioned, Goodman, von Sallmann and Holland (1957) had observed local dilatation of blood vessels in the conjunctivae of one of their patients. Paton (1961, 1962) found, using a slit lamp, evidence of multiple short, often comma-shaped, capillary segments, with afferent and efferent limbs often not visible, in 12 out of 15 Hb-SC patients (and in 54 out of 56 Hb-SS patients). Their presence was interpreted as indicating vascular stasis.

Pregnancy

Early observations had suggested that pregnancy was a definite hazard, and Smith and Conley (1954) reported that all five of their pregnant patients had become severely anaemic during the last trimester or *post partum*; two had died of post-partum haemorrhage and one for no obvious cause [see also Smith and Krevans (1959)].

Curtis (1959) reviewed the obstetrical history of 16 Hb-SS patients. During the first two trimesters the incidence of complications was not abnormal; in the last trimester, however, the incidence of complications was high. Pulmonary infarction, preceded by increase in anaemia and bone pain, was experienced by six women and pulmonary infarction was strongly suspected in two others. Three patients died. Curtis stressed how the triad of anaemia, bone pain and pulmonary infarction might in Hb-SC disease be experienced by patients for the first time in pregnancy — in contrast to Hb-SS disease in which a similar sequence was often experienced from early childhood, with no apparent increase in incidence

during pregnancy. Curtis also stressed that once a Hb-SC patient had developed bone marrow and pulmonary infarction in one pregnancy, a further pregnancy would be likely to expose the patient to a similar episode.

Fullerton and Watson-Williams (1962) reporting from Nigeria referred to three patients, one of whom died, who became suddenly severely anaemic shortly after delivery. Necropsy in the fatal case demonstrated striking packing of vessels in the spleen and liver with sickled cells. Seven other patients died having developed severe megaloblastic anaemia (see p. 159). Rywlin, Block and Werner (1963) also reported a fatal case — a patient in crisis with fat and bone-marrow embolization of the lungs; and Chmel and Bertles (1975) described a patient who suffered *post partum* from severe fat embolism but who recovered after an exchange transfusion. This latter patient had been given pitocin, and the question was raised as to whether this was a dangerous drug to use because of its property of causing a fall in the blood flow through the bone marrow.

Further experience has indicated that the mortality and morbidity associated with pregnancy is in reality relatively low (at least in the United States and Jamaica). Pregnancy was well tolerated and there were no maternal deaths amongst the Chicago and Jamaican patients reported, respectively, by River *et al.* (1961) and Serjeant, Ashcroft and Serjeant (1973). Of the Chicago women, all those over 21 had become pregnant, with an average of 3.5 pregnancies and 2.8 live-births per patient. In the Jamaican series, 21 patients over 20 years of age had had 72 pregnancies and 65 live-births; 10 patients had had, however, complications which could be attributed to their Hb-SC disease.

In a more recent report from Philadelphia, Ballas and co-workers (1982) have, however, described a less satisfactory picture: nine out of 16 female patients became pregnant on 34 occasions; five of the pregnancies terminated in spontaneous abortions, two ended in still-births and 10 were associated with perinatal complications.

The possible role of oral contraceptives in increasing the risk of vaso-occlusive complications was raised by the report of Haynes and Dunn (1967) who described two patients who had developed pulmonary embolism.

Infections

Infections are less frequent in Hb-SC patients than in Hb-SS disease (Ballas *et al.*, 1982). They occur, however, more frequently than in Hb-AA individuals.

Septicaemia. Hb-SC children seem rarely to develop overwhelming septicaemia — in contrast to Hb-SS children. Chilcote and Dampier (1984), however, described the clinical history of a 9-year-old girl who died within 12 hours of the onset of symptoms. Blood culture had grown *Str. pneumoniae*, type 18. The spleen was not palpable and a pitted (pocked) erythrocyte count indicated splenic dysfunction: 17% of the cells were pitted compared with 1% or less in normal controls and a mean count of 20% in splenectomized children.

Respiratory infections. Topley and co-workers (1982) reported on a large-scale survey carried out on 139 Hb-SC Jamaican children who had been followed from birth until the age of 6 years. Compared with 247 Hb-AA controls, infection incidence and survival curve analysis revealed a highly significant increase in infections in the Hb-SC children. Respiratory and gastrointestinal infections were the most common, but only the respiratory infections were more frequent in the Hb-SC children. Septicaemia was confined to the Hb-SC children: three had pneumococcal bacteraemia, one *H. influenzae* bacteraemia. The blood pictures in the children with or without a history of severe infection were indistinguishable, but infections appeared to be more common in the children whose spleen had enlarged early in life.

Mycoplasma infection. Chusid, Lachman and Lazerson (1978) described the occurrence of unusually severe Mycoplasma pneumonia in a 7-year-old black boy with Hb-SC disease.

Osteomyelitis. Lohmuller and Marshall (1958) reported infection of the humerus by a paracolon bacillus. Osteomyelitis due to infection with Salmonella is not uncommon. Widen and Cardon (1961) reviewed the reports published between 1925 and 1959 of such infections (involving several Salmonella species) in sickle-cell disease (mostly Hb-SS disease) and themselves reported the occurrence of *Salm. typhimurium* infection in a 15-year-old black American with proved Hb-SC disease. Onuaguluchi and Akande (1966) stressed the importance of Salmonella infections in precipitating severe crises in Hb-SC patients in Nigeria.

Unusual infections. Rodgers, Barrera and Martin (1980) reported that they had isolated from the blood of a 33-year-old black Hb-SC patient an aerobic gram-positive spore-forming organism, *Bacillus cereus*. The gall bladder was thought to be the site of the primary infection. The bacteraemia was associated with an acute haemolytic episode.

Pulmonary infarction

This is a not uncommon complication, and as in Hb-SS disease the distinction between primary infection and primary infarction and infection secondary to infarction may be difficult. According to Serjeant (1985, p. 302), pulmonary embolism secondary to bone-marrow necrosis brought about by bone infarction may be more common in Hb-SC disease than in Hb-SS disease. The occurrence of infarction during pregnancy, and its serious import, was referred to by Curtis (1959) (see p. 150). Chronic pulmonary hypertension secondary to pulmonary arteriolar obstruction has been recorded (Hales, 1983).

THE SPLEEN IN Hb-SC DISEASE

Compared with Hb-SS disease, the spleen is far more commonly palpable, even in adults. It was reported to be enlarged in two-thirds of the Chicago patients described by River *et al.* (1961) and in 51% of the Jamaican patients described by Serjeant, Ashcroft and Serjeant (1973); the latter group noted that the proportionately largest spleens were most commonly found in young patients.

Infarction

Five of the Jamaican patients referred to by Serjeant, Ashcroft and Serjeant (1973) had experienced splenic infarction. Yeung and Lessin (1976) gave details of 13 Hb-SC patients who had been reported to suffer from splenic infarction; in 12 of them this had developed in association with air travel (see below). This was not so, however, in the case of the 18-year-old male Hb-SC patient they had personally studied, whose infarct developed without apparent cause and was subsequently documented both by arteriography and scintillation scanning. Chu and Niederman (1977) described, too, the occurrence at a low altitude of a splenic infarct in a 14-year-old Hb-SC male.

Ballas and co-workers' (1982) data indicated that splenic infarction is by no means rare in Hb-SC patients. They described the state of the spleen in 25 Hb-SC patients aged between 15 and 60 years: 13 had splenomegaly and three a normally sized spleen; nine, however, had asplenia as defined by [^{99m}Tc] sulphur colloid scintigraphy.

Sears and Udden (1985) described in detail the clinical and haematological findings in four episodes of acute splenic infarction affecting three adult Hb-SC patients; they, too, concluded that, despite the paucity of descriptions of acute episodes, splenic infarction is probably not a rare event in Hb-SC adult patients and that it can occur in a subclinical fashion and give rise to symptoms of varying degrees of severity. Small shrunken spleens have been found at necropsy (Lau, 1959; Ober *et al.*, 1959). The spleen of Lau's patient, a black American, measured 3.5 × 4 × 6 cm and weighed only 10 g.

Infarction in aeroplane flights or at high altitudes

Splenic infarction has quite frequently been recorded in Hb-SC patients during flights in unpressurized or partially pressurized aircraft (Doenges, Smith and Wise, 1954; Motulsky, 1954; Smith and Conley, 1955; Coleman and Furth, 1956; Rotter *et al.*, 1956). Green, Huntsman and Serjeant (1971) described how this had happened to four Hb-SC patients; they made the point that Hb-SC patients should avoid air travel as far as possible, even in pressurized aircraft. Patients with Hb-SS disease were thought to be able to travel by air with less risk, possibly because of the likelihood of 'autosplenectomy' having already taken place.

Githens and co-workers (1977) described splenic infarction in four 11–18-year-olds during or immediately following mountain climbing to 9000–12 000 feet and in one 10-year-old boy who had flown in a commercial aircraft from Los Angeles to Denver. All had Hb-SC disease.

Transient asplenism

Joshpe, Rothenberg and Baum (1973) described the unusual history of a 22-year-old female who, following the premature birth of a still-born infant, developed an *E. coli* urinary tract infection accompanied by a painful crisis: the haemoglobin was 9.3 g/dl, with 35% reticulocytes and 11.5 × 10^9/l leucocytes. Numerous sickled cells and normoblasts and Howell-Jolly bodies could be seen in blood films. Although the spleen was then palpable 6 cm below the costal margin, a [^{99m}Tc] sulphur colloid scan revealed only an indistinct small area of radioactivity adjacent to the liver. After clinical recovery, the scan was repeated and a large spleen demonstrated, by which time the Howell-Jolly bodies had disappeared from blood films and only occasional sickled cells could be seen. It was suggested that the splenic microcirculation had been temporarily obstructed by sickled cells.

'Pocked' erythrocyte counts

Evidence that splenic function is commonly partially impaired in Hb-SC disease was provided by Pearson *et al.* (1979) who had measured the percentage of 'pocked' erythrocytes in the peripheral blood of normal children, asplenic children and Hb-SS children, and in five Hb-SC children. The Hb-SC children had counts (3.5 ± 1.9%) above the normal range (0–0.8%), although substantially less than the counts of the Hb-SS children (see p. 83).

Hypersplenism and acute splenic sequestration

Gross enlargement of the spleen seems to be a rare event in Hb-SC disease. Topley, Obeid and Mann (1977), described, however, how the spleen of a West-Indian girl gradually increased in size over a 6-year-period until it reached 13 cm below the left costal margin. Finally, she developed an acute splenic sequestration crisis during which the haemoglobin fell as low as 1.4 g/dl. She died of a cardiac arrest and at necropsy the spleen, which was congested with blood, weighed 2210 g.

An episode of acute splenic sequestration was described by Geola, Kukreja and Schade (1978). Their patient, a 24-year-old male, developed pneumonia and multiple pulmonary thrombo-embolic events; these were associated with rapid enlargement of the spleen to 10 cm below the left costal margin. A [^{99m}Tc]sulphur colloid scan failed to show a significant uptake of colloid. On recovery, sickled cells and erythrocytes containing crystals and microspherocytes appeared in the peripheral blood; these were thought to have been released from the spleen as it diminished in size. Repeat scans then showed a homogeneous uptake of colloid.

Andrews and Buchanan (1984) reported the occurrence of transient episodes of relatively mild acute splenic sequestration in three Hb-SC patients. None of them had been exposed to a high altitude. One patient had developed infectious mononucleosis; the second had had severe epistaxis, resulting in hypovolaemic shock for which he had been transfused; the third had had left upper quadrant pain associated with an enlarging spleen and a falling haemoglobin that had developed without apparent cause.

THE LIVER IN Hb-SC DISEASE

The liver was found to be palpable in 38% of Serjeant, Ashcroft and Serjeant's (1973) Jamaican patients, with enlargement increasing apparently with age. In five other series of patients quoted by Serjeant (1985, p. 303) the percentage of patients recorded as having hepatomegaly varied from 16 [Ballas et al., 1982 (who reported on 25 adults aged from 16 to 60 years)] to 61 [Tuttle and Koch, 1960 (who reported on 18 patients aged from $1\frac{1}{2}$ to 18 years)].

Gallstones. Their incidence is probably less than in Hb-SS disease. River and co-workers (1961) stated that six of their 75 patients were known to have formed gallstones and that three had undergone cholecystectomy. Only one of the six patients was less than 35 years of age. Ballas and co-workers (1982) reported that gallstones were present in 41% of 17 Hb-SC patients as compared with 77% of 43 Hb-SS patients.

BONE NECROSIS

Aseptic necrosis of the femoral head has been repeatedly described (Smith and Conley, 1954; Vandepitte and Colaert, 1955; Lohmuller and Marshall, 1958; Smith and Krevans, 1959; River et al., 1961). Serjeant, Ashcroft and Serjeant (1973) reported radiological evidence of this in 14 out of their 90 patients. Other bones, e.g. the head of humerus, may also be affected. Seeler (1983) recorded a rare occurrence, infarction of the superior orbital rim: this was associated with retrobulbar oedema and severe unilateral exophthalmos, which fortunately resolved spontaneously after about 6 weeks.

BONE-MARROW NECROSIS

As in Hb-SS disease, necrosis of the bone marrow may lead not only to local pain but also to serious disseminated fat and bone-marrow cell embolism. Shelley and Curtis (1958) described this happening to a Hb-SC patient and reviewed the relevant literature, and Ober and co-workers (1959) published detailed necropsy and histological findings in one such case. Charache and Page (1967), too, reviewed the literature and described three patients with sickle-cell disease in whom they had aspirated necrotic (infarcted) bone marrow: one

had Hb-SC disease; she was a woman aged 27 who died in coma.

X-RAY FINDINGS IN Hb-SC DISEASE

Cockshott (1958) and Barton and Cockshott (1962) reported on the findings in a large series of patients in Nigeria. Slight to moderate changes in bone texture were noted in about one-third of the cases; they were interpreted as consistent with the consequences of hyperplasia of the bone marrow, infarction or infection.

Golding, MacIver and Went (1959) investigated 19 Hb-SC patients in Jamaica (and 51 Hb-SS patients). Evidence for avascular necrosis of the head of the femur was commonly found in both disorders but changes secondary to hyperplasia of the bone marrow appeared to be confined to Hb-SS disease.

River and co-workers (1961) reported that X-ray photographs of the skull in 33 patients had failed to demonstrate a hair-on-end appearance; abnormalities were confined to slight thickening of the calvarium and slight stippled osteoporosis, one or both changes being present in eight patients. X-rays of the long bones revealed evidence of cortical sclerosis, coarsened trabeculation, periosteal reactions and bone infarction in a 'surprising' number of patients. The changes were often as severe as in Hb-SS disease. Widening of the medullary canal was absent; evidence of bone infarction was the most striking finding.

Becker (1962) reported on the X-ray changes in the bones of 14 patients with Hb-SC disease studied in Philadelphia. The changes seen were similar to, but less pronounced than, those seen in Hb-SS disease; the frequency of aseptic necrosis of bone was, however, emphasized. X-rays revealed no noteworthy abnormalities in 40% of the patients despite the fact that they had symptoms attributable to their haemoglobinopathy. Reynolds (1962) compared the X-ray findings in 25 Hb-SC patients studied in Dallas with those of 56 Hb-SS patients: no X-ray abnormalities were demonstrable in almost half of the Hb-SC patients. He concluded that X-ray studies did not help in differentiating between the two syndromes.

Serjeant, Ennis and Middlemiss (1973a) reported on 130 adult Jamaican Hb-SC patients. Increased translucency of bone, abnormal trabecular patterns, expansion of the medulla, wide vascular channels and evidence of infarction, both medullary and cortical, were the changes particularly noted; their frequency appeared to increase with age. Avascular necrosis was thought to be the most characteristic lesion. A relatively high haemoglobin level (compared to that in Hb-SS disease) was considered to be a contributory cause (acting by increasing the viscosity of the blood). However, there seemed to be lack of correlation between the clinical severity of the disease and the radiological changes. Serjeant (1974, p. 246) provided a comparison of the radiological findings in 50 Hb-SC patients with those of 50 Hb-SS patients. Evidence of expansion of the bone marrow was more frequent in the Hb-SS patients, but the incidence of medullary or articular infarction was about the same in both groups.

BLOOD PICTURE IN Hb-SC DISEASE

Erythrocytes and haemoglobin; absolute values

The blood picture in Hb-SC disease differs qualitatively and quantitatively from that in Hb-SS disease. Anaemia is less severe than in Hb-SS disease or Hb-S/β-thalassaemia and the reticulocyte count is lower (Table 13.1). Characteristically, sickled cells are rarely met with in films of freshly drawn peripheral blood of Hb-SC patients; as a rule none can be found. Smith and Conley (1954) reported that they had seen them in only a 'few' of their 16 patients. Bunn, Forget and Ranney (1977, p. 277) mentioned (and illustrated) the presence of 'occasional' plump sickled cells. Anisocytosis and poikilocytosis are less conspicuous than in Hb-SS disease but target cells are to be seen in large numbers, 45–80% of the cells being affected according to Kaplan, Zuelzer and Neel (1951) and Smith and Conley (1954) (Fig. 13.11). Few siderocytes are present, in contrast to Hb-SS disease (Kaplan, Zuelzer and Neel, 1951).

The values for MCV and MCH are intermediate between those of Hb-SS and Hb-S/β-thalassaemia patients; the MCHC is strikingly higher than in either of the two other conditions. Osmotic resistance is increased. Mechanical fragility is normal in oxygenated blood but increased after saturation with carbon dioxide (Kaplan, Zuelzer and Neel, 1951).

In vitro, Hb-SC erythrocytes sickle readily. According to Kaplan, Zuelzer and Neel (1951, 1953) the cells sickle as in Hb-SS disease, *i.e.*,

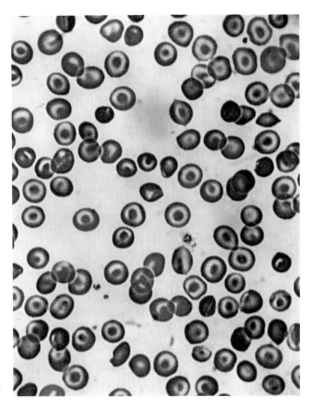

Fig. 13.11 Peripheral-blood film of a patient with Hb-SC disease.
There is slight anisocytosis and poikilocytosis. The great majority of the erythrocytes are target cells. No well-formed sickled cells are present. × 700.

rapidly in the presence of sodium metabisulphite, with virtually all the cells becoming filamentous forms. River *et al.* (1961) remarked, however, that the sickled cells present a picture intermediate between that of Hb-SS disease and Hb-AS trait, with filamentous and 'holly wreath' forms being present in varying proportions.

According to Tuttle and Koch (1960) and Diggs and Bell (1965), the haemoglobin may crystallize intracellularly resulting in characteristic morphological changes. Blood films from 60 Hb-SC disease patients were studied by Diggs and Bell (1965): in 42 of them (70%) varying numbers of erythrocytes contained crystals, the mean being 3.2%, range 0–24%. These cells, which had a distorted contour, contained usually a single dark-staining crystal with parallel sides and bluntly pyramidal or rounded ends. (Diggs and Bell remarked that the cells are more distorted than are the crystal-containing cells seen in Hb-CC disease and stated that they had not observed any crystals in the films of 82 Hb-SS patients.) Diggs and Bell also recorded interesting additional data obtained from their 60 patients, *e.g.*, for sickled cells a mean of 0.6%, range 0–4%; for target cells a mean of 19.9%, range 18–62%, and for other poikilocytes (spherical, oval, folded, single-pointed and bizarre-shaped cells) a mean of 4.5%, range 2.0–18.4%.

Conley (1964), who reported that the haemoglobin within Hb-CC erythrocytes would undergo crystallization when the cells were suspended in hypertonic 3 g/dl NaCl, noted that similar crystals would form in Hb-SC cells when subjected to the same osmotic dehydration, *i.e.*, Hb C will co-crystallize with Hb S, just as Hb C co-polymerizes with Hb S. [Conley (1986, personal communication) suggests that the two phenomena occurring simultaneously are at least in part responsible for the unique clinical features of Hb-SC disease.]

Ringelhann and Khorsandi (1972) also emphasized the ease with which the haemoglobin in Hb-SC erythrocytes crystallizes. They, too, suspended blood in 3 g/dl NaCl and found that 30–40% of Hb-SC cells (and 40–60% of Hb-CC cells) develop intracellular crystals after 3 hours at 37°C.

Schneider and co-workers (1972), who examined air-dried blood films from a large number of patients with various haemoglobinopathies by means of phase or dark-field microscopy, stated that in Hb-SC patients one or more small particles were to be seen in almost every erythrocyte examined, as seen also in Hb-SS homozygotes (see p. 83). Most of the particles appeared to be, or to contain, haemoglobin, *i.e.*, they reacted with benzidine, and their presence was thought to reflect the insolubility (and tendency to precipitate) of Hb C (and Hb S) (see p. 293).

Serjeant and Serjeant (1972) published extensive data on the blood picture in Hb-SC disease based on 97 patients studied in Jamaica. The mean haemoglobin for the series was 11.7 ± 1.7 g/dl, being slightly higher in males (mean 12.4 ± 1.9 g/dl) than in females (mean 11.0 ± 1.1 g/dl); the mean MCHC was 34.8 ± 1.2%, being identical in both sexes, and the mean reticulocyte count was 3.1 ± 1.5%, being slightly higher in females than in males. ISCs were not seen in films of either sex. Data for erythrocyte count, MCV and MCH were available from 57 patients: the mean erythrocyte count in the males was 4.60 ± 0.76 × 10^12/1 and in the females 4.07 ± 0.53 × 10^12/1; the mean MCV (both sexes) was 79.3 ± 6.6 fl and the mean MCH (both sexes) was 27.4 ± 2.4 pg.

Figures for total haemoglobin reported by Konotey-Ahulu (1974) from Ghana were closely similar. The mean haemoglobin of 377 Hb-SC patients in a steady state was 11.20 ± 2.21 g/dl, with a range from 5.25 g/dl

(one patient) to 16.5 g/dl (two patients).

The blood picture data of Bannerman and co-workers (1979), based on 31 adult West-Indian Hb-SC patients, were similar to the data of Serjeant and Serjeant (1972); the study was, however, extended to include measurement of erythrocyte survival as well as erythrocyte, plasma and total blood volumes and oxygen dissociation (see later).

Glader, Propper and Buchanan (1979), who studied 81 sickle-cell syndrome patients in Boston, emphasized that microcytosis was common to Hb-SS, Hb-S/β-thalassaemia and Hb-SC patients. The mean MCV (75.4 ± 6.0 fl) in the 19 Hb-SC patients fell between the mean values for the other two genotypes. All three means were substantially less than that of 22 patients with other types of haemolytic anaemias associated with comparably raised reticulocyte counts. The microcytosis, and the low MCH values, were attributed to the abnormal haemoglobin being synthesized at a reduced rate.

Ballas and co-workers' (1982) data were derived from a comparative study of 27 Hb-SC patients aged between 16 and 60 years and 66 Hb-SS patients aged between 12 and 58 years. Erythrocyte counts, PCV and total haemoglobin were significantly higher in the Hb-SC patients and MCV (mean 78.2 ± 5.1 fl), MCH (mean 27.1 ± 2.5 pg) and reticulocyte count (mean 3.9 ± 2.1%) were significantly lower. In their description of the peripheral-blood film, Ballas *et al.* referred to the numerous target cells and to the presence of microspherocytes and 'so-called fat sickle cells or boat-shaped cells'. No irreversibly sickled cells (ISCs) were seen in their series of 27 patients.

Fabry and co-workers (1982) studied 20 Hb-SC patients and stressed the abnormally high MCHC found in Hb-SC disease. Using Percoll-Stractan density gradients they found that the average MCHC of Hb-SC erythrocytes was 36.4 ± 0.76 g/dl. The cells in the gradient were distributed symmetrically around the average density, but in a little less than half the patients a small proportion (< 5%) of very dense cells was present; these cells were denser than the ISCs of Hb-SS patients. Fabry *et al.* also established that Hb-SC reticulocytes were denser than Hb-AA reticulocytes and that Hb-AC erythrocytes were also abnormally dense (mean HCHC 34.0 g/dl). They demonstrated, too, that reducing the MCHC of Hb-SC erythrocytes by lowering the osmolarity of the medium in which the cells were suspended diminished their oxygen affinity, reduced the viscosity of deoxygenated suspensions, and the rate of sickling, and diminished the deoxygenated-induced K^+ efflux.

Stevens, Maude and Serjeant (1984) compared the development of the blood picture from birth in 166 children with Hb-SC disease with that of 243 Hb-AA children and 266 Hb-SS children. Values for total haemoglobin, erythrocyte and reticulocyte counts and Hb-F percentage followed the same age-related changes, with the findings in the Hb-SC children being intermediate between those of the Hb-AA and Hb-SS children (Fig. 13.12). Two noteworthy features were the high MCHC (calculated from the spun micro-haematocrit) and the low MCV, the latter emerging as early as 2 months (Fig. 13.13). The microcytosis could not be explained on concurrent α-thalassaemia or iron deficiency and was considered to be a feature of Hb-SC disease that could be relevant to its pathogenesis.

The haematological findings in Hb-SC patients, which have been summarized above, correspond closely to the data reported earlier, e.g., by Smith and Conley (1954) and Hook and Cooper (1958) based on smaller series of patients. The high MCHC of Hb-SC disease had been commented on by Schneider et al. (1972).

Normoblastaemia

Nucleated erythrocytes and Howell-Jolly bodies are more frequent in the peripheral blood of Hb-SS patients than in Hb-SC patients. According to Hook and Cooper (1958), however, up to 20–40% of the nucleated cells in the peripheral blood may be normoblasts in Hb-SC patients suffering from painful crises. Ballas and co-workers (1982) reported that Hb-SC patients who have asplenia have more nucleated erythrocytes in their peripheral blood than have those with splenomegaly.

Haemoglobin

The electrophoretic pattern is rather constant. About one-half of the haemoglobin is Hb C (Table 13.2); the remainder is Hb S except for small amounts of Hb F and Hb A_2 (which does not separate from Hb C on routine electrophoresis at an alkaline pH).

Zuelzer, Neel and Robinson (1956) in their

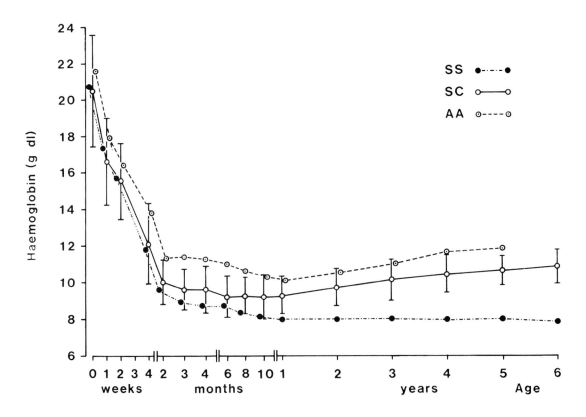

Fig. 13.12 Changes in total haemoglobin up to the age of 6 years in Hb-SC patients compared with the changes in Hb-SS patients and in normal (Hb-AA) controls.
Jamaican data. [Reproduced by permission from Stevens et al. (1985).]

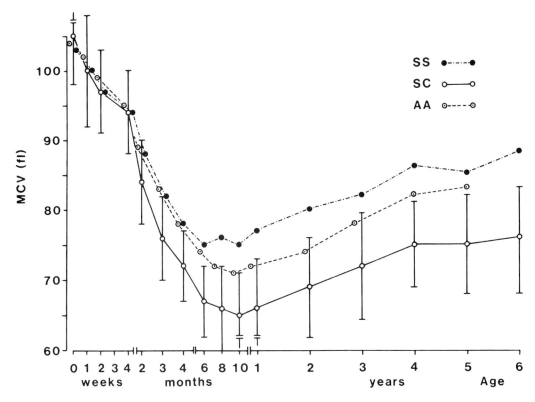

Fig. 13.13 Changes in MCV up to the age of 6 years in Hb-SC patients compared with the changes in Hb-SS patients and in normal (Hb-AA) controls.
Jamaican data. [Reproduced by permission from Stevens *et al*. (1985).]

review stated that the data then available indicated that 50–67% of the haemoglobin in Hb-SC disease was Hb C. Tuttle and Koch (1960) recorded 49–65% Hb C in 18 patients, 9 months to 18 years of age, with 31–51% Hb S. Huisman and co-workers (1972) reported 45–53% Hb S and Bannerman and co-workers (1979) 51.6–65.8% Hb S in 31 adult patients. Ballas and co-workers (1982), who studied 24 patients, reported means for Hb S of 48.4 ± 3.73% and for Hb C of 51.6 ± 3.73%. Serjeant (1985, p. 296) described the electrophoretic pattern in Hb-SC disease as being one in which characteristically Hb S and Hb C are present in approximately equal amounts on alkali and acid agar electrophoresis.

Hb F. Went and MacIver (1958a) recorded 0.7–8.0% Hb F in their series of 45 patients, Tuttle and Koch (1960) 0.9–4.0% Hb F, mean 2.4%, in 18 patients, Serjeant, Ashcroft and Serjeant (1973) a mean of 1.1% Hb F, range

0.3–5.2%, in 89 patients aged 7–87 years, and Wrightstone and Huisman (1974) a mean of 2.5%, range 1.0–7.0%, in 24 patients. Huisman and co-workers (1972) investigated the ratio of $^G\gamma$ to $^A\gamma$ chains in 15 Hb-SC patients. The ratio varied widely, as in Hb-SS patients (see p. 90).

Erythrocyte life-span

This is usually moderately shortened, but may be almost normal.

McCurdy, Mahmood and Sherman (1975) reported detailed laboratory data in nine Hb-SC patients, including erythrocyte life-span studies using ^{51}Cr and DF^{32}P. The ^{51}Cr T$_{50}$ ranged from 10.7 to 20.2 days, mean 15.7 ± 2.7 days, and the erythrocyte life-span, calculated from the DF^{32}P data, ranged from 23.1 to 35.6 days, mean 28.9 days.

Bannerman and co-workers (1979) studied 15 male and 16 female Hb-SC adults in steady state, using ^{51}Cr;

their ages ranged from 17 to 59 years. The ^{51}Cr T_{50s} were similar in the two sexes: 12.6–26.2 days in the males and 12.4–24.6 days in the females. Erythrocyte survival and the mean pitted erythrocyte count both seemed to be independent of whether or not the patient's spleen was palpably enlarged, findings suggesting that the spleen does not [usually] play an important role in the increased haemolysis.

Oxygen dissociation

As in Hb-SS disease, the oxygen-dissociation curve of haemoglobin is shifted in Hb-SC disease to the right of the normal curve, *i.e.*, oxygen is liberated from the haemoglobin unusually readily as the O_2 tension falls.

The shift of the curve appears to be related to the amount of Hb S present. Thus a straight line relationship between the percentage of Hb S and the $p_{50}O_2$ was demonstrated by Cawein *et al.* (1969) in a small series of Hb-SS and Hb-SC patients (and also in Hb-SD and Hb-S/thalassaemia patients). Bannerman and co-workers (1979) in their comprehensive study of 31 adults with Hb-SC disease recorded a relatively narrow $p_{50}O_2$ range: 36.7–43.6 mm Hg, mean 40.5 mm Hg, the curve being consistently shifted to the right.

Haemoglobin synthesis and iron kinetics

Movitt, Mangum and Porter (1963) studied five adult patients. The rate of haemoglobin synthesis was increased in each patient, being 2.2–6.8 g/l blood per day (normal 1.0–1.6 g/l blood per day). The serum iron ranged from 65 to 165 μg/dl and the plasma iron clearance ($T_{\frac{1}{2}}$) was accelerated.

Leucocyte count

The total leucocyte count is within or slightly above the normal range in steady-state patients, but high counts often accompany crises.

Smith and Conley (1954), in their review of patients with sickle-cell variants, stated that the total leucocyte count was usually less than 10×10^9/l; they reported, however, a count of 22×10^9/l in a Hb-SC patient in a severe haemolytic crisis and a count of 59×10^9/l in a patient, who probably had Hb-SC disease, during a haemolytic crisis associated with pregnancy.
Hook and Cooper (1958) studied 16 Hb-SC patients. When asymptomatic, their mean leucocyte count was 9.24×10^9/l. However, much higher counts, even as high as 42.0 and 43.0×10^9/l, were observed in patients in painful crises.

More recently, Ballas and co-workers (1982) recorded that the mean total leucocyte count of 27 Hb-SC patients in a steady state was $8.7 \pm 2.9 \times 10^9$/l, compared with a mean of $13.0 \pm 4.5 \times 10^9$/l in 66 Hb-SS patients. Ballas *et al.* also reported that leucocyte alkaline phosphatase scores were abnormally low in their Hb-SC patients and comparable to the low scores already reported in Hb-SS disease (see p. 92).

Platelet count

This is usually normal but may be raised in patients with shrunken spleens and, conversely, it is subnormal in hypersplenism.

Ballas and co-workers (1982) reported a mean platelet count of $274 \pm 109 \times 10^9$/l in 27 steady-state patients compared with a mean count of $525 \pm 265 \times 10^9$/l in 66 Hb-SS patients. Ballas *et al.* also recorded a mean count of $316 \pm 99 \times 10^9$/l in nine asplenic Hb-SC patients compared with $221 \pm 51 \times 10^9$/l in 13 Hb-SC patients who had splenomegaly.

Miscellaneous biochemical data

Serum bilirubin. The level is normal or moderately raised, and is usually substantially lower than in Hb-SS disease.

Hook and Cooper (1958) recorded a mean of 0.7 mg/dl in 16 Hb-SC patients compared with a mean of 2.2 mg/dl in 36 Hb-SS patients. Tuttle and Koch (1960) recorded a mean of 1.2 mg/dl (range 0.7–2.1 mg/dl) in 13 children. Ballas and co-workers (1982) reported a mean of 1.5 ± 0.84 mg/dl in 25 adult Hb-SC patients, compared with a mean of 3.59 ± 2.22 mg/dl in 64 Hb-SS patients.

Urine urobilinogen. Hook and Cooper (1958) recorded values greater than 5 mg/24 hours in five out of 14 patients, compared with raised values in 14 out of 19 Hb-SS patients.

Serum lactic dehydrogenase. Ballas and co-workers (1982) reported a higher than normal mean of 247 ± 85 units/ml in 27 Hb-SC patients compared with a very high mean of 436 ± 149 units/ml in 53 Hb-SS patients.
Liver function tests. The mean serum albumin concentration and serum alkaline phosphatase and SGOT activities were within the normal range in the Hb-SC patients described by Ballas *et al.* (1982).

Serum uric acid and serum creatinine. Ballas *et al.* (1982) recorded normal mean values.

Serum immunoglobulins. Mean total γ globulin and IgG, IgA and IgM concentrations were all slightly above normal in the patients studied by Ballas *et al.* (1982).

Serum iron and transferrin. The mean values for serum iron concentration, total iron-binding capacity and transferrin saturation were within the normal range in the patients studied by Ballas *et al.* (1982). Serum-ferritin levels were substantially less than in the Hb-SS patients.

APLASTIC CRISES IN Hb-SC DISEASE

These seem to have been seldom reported, although no doubt parvovirus-induced marrow aplasia does occur from time to time. In fact, of the 12 West-Indian children with sickle-cell anaemia reported by MacIver and Parker-Williams (1961) to have had an aplastic crisis, one had Hb-SC disease. On the other hand, none of the 90 Hb-SC patients later reviewed by Serjeant, Ashcroft and Serjeant (1973) developed this complication; all but six were, however, over the age of 12 years.

MEGALOBLASTIC ERYTHROPOIESIS IN Hb-SC DISEASE

Shaldon (1961) recorded the occurrence of megaloblastic erythropoiesis in a 1-year-old Ibo infant with Hb-SC disease who had been receiving pyrimethamine as a prophylactic against malaria.

According to Fullerton and Watson-Williams (1962), megaloblastic erythropoiesis was demonstrable in 30% of 190 pregnant Nigerian women who had Hb-SC disease. This high incidence was attributed to pregnancy increasing the requirement for folates in addition to the increased haemolysis. Severe anaemia developed very rapidly in some of the patients and was the cause of seven deaths.

In the United States and the West Indies, megaloblastic anaemia seems rarely to complicate Hb-SC disease. Thus this was recorded only in one of Serjeant, Ashcroft and Serjeant's (1973) 90 patients — in this patient megaloblastic change which developed *post partum* led to Hb-SC disease being recognized.

α-THALASSAEMIA IN ASSOCIATION WITH Hb-SC DISEASE

As described on page 458, heterozygosity for α-thalassaemia ($-\alpha/\alpha\alpha$ genotype) is a common finding in American blacks and homozygosity ($-\alpha/-\alpha$) is not rare. It is inevitable, therefore, that a significant proportion of Hb-SC patients will be heterozygotes for α-thalassaemia as well and a few will be homozygotes. The presence of α-thalassaemia will affect the haematological findings, as it does in Hb-SS disease. Recent studies suggest, however, that clinical severity is not significantly altered (see later).

Tuttle and Koch (1960) raised the question of the transmission of a variant of thalassaemia ('hereditary microcytosis') to a small girl with Hb-SC disease from her Hb-AS father who had an unexplained low MCV (as had her two siblings). No certain diagnosis, however, was established.

Honig and co-workers (1976) described under the title 'hemoglobin SC-α thalassemia' a patient in whom the concurrence of Hb-SC disease and α-thalassaemia seems to have been highly likely. Their patient was a male member of a black American family in which the father was considered to have the Hb-AS trait plus α-thalassaemia and the mother the Hb-AC trait plus α-thalassaemia. The propositus, when 7 years of age, had 7.9 g/dl haemoglobin, $4.91 \times 10^{12}/l$ erythrocytes, MCV 53 fl, MCH 16.2 pg and 7.2% reticulocytes. Blood films were characterized by marked anisocytosis and poikilocytosis, very flat cells, many target cells, 'safety-pin' cells and a few contracted cells resembling spherocytes; no sickled cells were seen. The α: β + γ chain-synthesis ratio was estimated to be 0.68. Sickling occurred *in vitro*, but to a lesser extent than in typical Hb-SC disease, for at nearly complete O_2 desaturation less than 35% of the erythrocytes had sickled. Although without symptoms, the propositus was considered to be more anaemic, and to have more active haemolysis, than in typical uncomplicated Hb-SC disease. Osmotic fragility was decreased, too, more than is usual in Hb-SC disease. Another sibling had Hb-H disease.

A further possibly similar instance of the interaction between α-thalassaemia and Hb-SC disease was reported by Honig *et al.* (1979). The patient was a child whose erythrocyte indices pointed to the presence of thalassaemia, but neither parent (one Hb AS, the other Hb AC) showed any haematological evidence of thalassaemia. However, globin-chain synthesis was unbalanced in both of them, and it was concluded that they were probably 'silent' carriers of α-thalassaemia.

Three further probable examples of Hb-SC/α-thalassaemia were briefly mentioned by Ballas *et al.*

(1982). Three out of 18 Hb-SC patients in whom globin-chain synthesis was measured gave values within the α-thalassaemia trait range. They had almost exactly equal amounts of Hb S and Hb C in their erythrocytes, indicating that the β^S and β^C chains had an equal affinity for the limited number of α chains available. [This is in contrast to Hb-AS/α-thalassaemia individuals who form substantially less Hb S than Hb A.]

Recent studies have confirmed the supposition that Hb-SC/α-thalassaemia occurs quite frequently and have shown that the presence of α-thalassaemia has in fact little or no effect on the clinical severity of Hb-SC disease. Steinberg and co-workers (1983) investigated the α-globin genotype of 53 Hb-SC adults by means of restriction endo-nuclease gene mapping: ten of the patients were shown to have the $-\alpha/\alpha\alpha$ genotype and four the $-\alpha/-\alpha$ genotype. The patients with α-thalas-saemia had a lower MCV and MCH than those of $\alpha\alpha/\alpha\alpha$ genotype, but total haemoglobin and the reticulocyte percentages were similar irrespective of the presence of α-thalassaemia. No relationship, too, could be identified between the α-globin genotype and the incidence of pain crises, bone lesions, proliferative sickle retinopathy or clinical severity score. Steinberg *et al.* concluded that any benefit or deleterious effect resulting from the presence of α-thalassaemia would be very difficult to substantiate because of the general mildness of the disease.

Hb-SC DISEASE PLUS HEREDITARY SPHEROCYTOSIS (HS)

The presence in the same family of the genes for Hb S and Hb C and for a hereditary haemolytic anaemia other than a haemoglobinopathy would clearly be a rare but not impossible event. Hb-SC disease and HS have in fact been described in the same individual. Thus Thompson and Robertson (1964) described a family in which two siblings were thought to have Hb-SC disease plus HS. Their father had the Hb-AC trait and their mother (probably) the Hb-AS trait plus HS — her brother had undergone splenectomy for HS. The propos-itus, a female aged 23, had 10.6 g/dl haemoglobin with 1.9% reticulocytes. A blood film showed hypochromia, target cells and small round sphero-cytes; osmotic fragility was increased. The spleen was palpable 3 cm below the costal margin. Clini-cally, her illness ran a relatively mild course. The oldest child of the propositus appeared to have Hb-SS disease plus HS (see p. 54).

HAEMOGLOBIN-S/HAEMOGLOBIN-D DISEASE (Hb-SD DISEASE)

A small number of families have been reported in which compound heterozygosity for a Hb D and Hb S has occurred. In some cases, *e.g.*, when the Hb D is Hb D Punjab, the combination leads to a haemolytic anaemia of moderate to quite severe intensity, with sickled cells in the circulation, which clinically closely resembles Hb-SS disease. Almost all the characteristic symptoms of Hb-SS disease have been complained of by individual patients at one time or another. However, symp-toms of vaso-occlusive origin have in general not been serious, sexual development has usually been normal and pregnancy has been well tolerated. According to Serjeant (1974, p. 277) the spleen has been palpable in about one-third of the reported cases. With other (non-reactive) types of Hb D (see p. 298), the Hb-SD individual has been free of symptoms and not anaemic.

Early reports. The first patients to be described with clinically important Hb-SD disease belonged to a family investigated by Itano (1951), and subsequently reported in more detail by Sturgeon, Itano and Bergren (1955). [The two patients studied had previously been described, when small children, by Cooke and Mack (1934) as suffering from sickle-cell anaemia occurring in a white American family, and it is extremely inter-esting to note in retrospect that sickling *in vitro* was recorded by Cooke and Mack to have taken place unusually slowly.] Other early reports include those of Dacie (1954), Stewart and MacIver (1956) and Smith and Conley (1959).

Sturgeon, Itano and Bergren's (1955) patients, a brother and sister, were aged 21 and 23, respectively, when studied; they were of Irish, English and American-Indian ancestry. Their mother had the Hb-AD trait and their father the Hb-AS trait. Both children had mild haemolytic anaemia: the brother suffered from repeated attacks of limb and abdominal pain but his sister, who was only slightly less anaemic, had few complaints. Both had a similar blood picture: there were moderate numbers of sickled cells in the circulation, a moderate degree of anisocytosis and a small number of target cells. The MCV was 113–118 fl; the reticulocyte count was 7.2–8.1%. The brother's spleen had been removed in infancy; his sister's was not palpable. Their haemoglobin was later studied in detail by Babin, Jones and Schroeder (1964) and named Hb D Los Angeles $(\alpha_2\beta_2^{121 \; Glu \; NH_2})$; it was subsequently found to be identical with Hb D Punjab (see p. 298).

Dacie's (1954) patient was a white girl, 9 years of age, who had been in hospital twice previously for pyrexia of unexplained origin. She was moderately anaemic: haemoglobin, 8.4 g/dl and erythrocytes 2.0 × 10^{12}/l. There were 9% reticulocytes. The MCV was 100 fl and the MCHC 32%. Osmotic fragility was decreased. Blood films showed marked anisocytosis and anisochromasia and oat- and sickled-shaped cells were present (Fig. 13.14). The child's father was born in Jamaica, as he believed of Irish, French, English and Scottish ancestors: he had, nevertheless, the Hb-AS trait. The mother was English, but she had remote ancestors who were Austrian and Spanish; she had the Hb-AD trait.

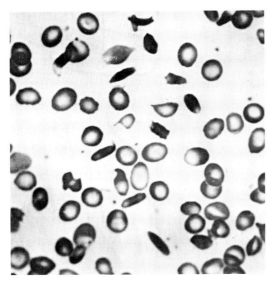

Fig. 13.14 Peripheral-blood film of a patient with Hb-SD disease.
There is a moderate degree of anisocytosis and poikilocytosis, as well as moderate numbers of oat-shaped and sickled cells. × 700.

Stewart and MacIver's (1956) patient was a woman aged 32 who complained of ulceration of the ankles. Her mother, who was English, had the Hb-AD trait and her father was a black West African; he was dead but presumably had contributed the gene for Hb S. The propositus was anaemic: she had 8.7 g/dl haemoglobin and her erythrocytes underwent filamentous sickling *in vitro*. She died of pyelonephritis; at necropsy the spleen was found to be extremely small in size ($1\frac{3}{4} \times \frac{1}{4} \times \frac{3}{4}''$).

Smith and Conley's (1959) patient was a white young man aged 20. His ancestors had come from England. His main complaint was of recurrent episodes of pain in the back and limbs which he had had since childhood. He also had had attacks of 'pneumonia' and transient ulcers of the legs. He had a haemolytic anaemia, but this had not been serious enough to stop him being an athlete. Four family members on his mother's side had oval erythrocytes. Smith and Conley pointed out that patients with Hb-SD disease may have long clinical remissions and may even not be anaemic. They attributed the bone pains and pulmonary manifestations to occlusion of vessels by sickled cells and possibly to emboli of fat and bone-marrow cells and remarked that in their patient the symptoms were as severe as in Hb-SS disease, although the concentration of intracellular Hb S was much less.

A further account of this patient when he was aged 29 has been provided by Charache and Page (1967). He was admitted to hospital acutely ill and tender to palpation over the sternum and lumbar spine. Necrotic bone marrow was aspirated from the sternum.

Further case reports. Additional cases of symptomatic Hb-SD disease have been described in a variety of racial groups, *e.g.*, by Arends, Layrisse and Rincon (1959) in a Portuguese child, by McCurdy and Gieschen (1960) in a black American, by Figueroa and Arends (1963) in a Venezuelan child, by Cawein *et al.* (1966) in four unrelated black American adults, by Ringelhann *et al.* (1967) in two small girls born to a Ghanaian mother and an English father, by Ozsoylu (1969) in a family of Spanish and Mexican origin and by Uriarte, Atencio and Colombo (1973) in a Cuban child whose father was a mestizo and his mother Spanish.

The four patients described by Cawein *et al.* (1966) had signs of chronic haemolytic anaemia but none of them had experienced painful vaso-occlusive crises. Their haemoglobins ranged from 5.7 to 9.9 g/dl, MCV 99 to 133 fl, reticulocyte counts 14 to 40%, and serum bilirubin 2.1 to 5.3 mg/dl. Sickled cells were present in the blood films of each patient and normoblasts, too, were present in variable numbers — 1–168 per 100 leucocytes. Electrophoresis revealed 25–77% Hb S, the remainder of the haemoglobin being Hb D, and there appeared to be no correlation between the percentage of Hb S and clinical severity. *In vitro*, the rate of sickling was distinctly slower than in Hb-SS disease.

Ozsoylu (1969) described a family in which four siblings had Hb-SD disease; their father had Hb AD and their mother Hb AS. The propositus, who had a severe haemolytic anaemia, developed a transient aplastic crisis in which the haemoglobin fell to 3.1 g/dl and the reticulocyte count to less than 0.1%. All four siblings had high Hb-F levels (13–20%).

Uriate, Atencio and Colombo's (1973) patient was an infant; at 3 months of age the haemoglobin was 4.5 g/dl and the spleen was palpable 11 cm, and the liver 6 cm, below the costal margin. Splenectomy was eventually carried out and was followed by a series of infections. Subsequently, however, the haemoglobin stabilized at about 5–7 g/dl, with 6–18% reticulocytes, and transfusions were required only during infective episodes.

The clinical history of a similarly severely affected child has more recently been reported by Kelleher et al. (1984). Their patient was a small black boy, who during the first 2 years of his life had suffered from acute splenic sequestration, pneumococcal sepsis, aplastic crisis and functional asplenia. The point was made that Hb-SD children should receive the same close and comprehensive medical care as Hb-SS patients.

Not all patients with the Hb-S/Hb-D combination suffer from overt increased haemolysis. One reason for this is that there are several types of 'Hb D' which vary in the way they interact with Hb S (see below).

Watson-Williams and co-workers (1965) described from Ibadan a Yoruba male who was not anaemic and yet whose haemoglobin on electrophoresis migrated as a single band simulating Hb SS. His haemoglobin was 14.8 g/dl, reticulocyte count less than 1% and the ^{51}Cr T$_{50}$ 28 days. The erythrocytes sickled in vitro, but peripheral-blood films were normal and no sickled cells were seen. The Hb D was eventually identified as a 'new' haemoglobin and named Hb D Ibadan (β 87$^{\text{Thr} \rightarrow \text{Lys}}$). Hb F was not demonstrated and the proportion of Hb S present was much less than 50%, namely 20%. The solubility of the haemoglobin mixture was greater than that found in symptomatic Hb-SD disease and was in the upper range of that found in the Hb-AS trait. Watson-Williams et al. stressed that Hb D Ibadan should be looked upon as unusual rather than abnormal.

Restrepo and Londoño (1965) described a rather similar case, a 40-year-old female, a member of a black Colombian family, who had had 11 pregnancies and except for mild osteo-articular pains had always been in good health. The liver was palpable 6 cm below the costal margin but the spleen could not be felt. Her haemoglobin was 12.4 g/dl, MCV 83 fl, reticulocytes 1.4%, bilirubin 0.6 mg/dl, serum iron 100 μg/dl and the ^{51}Cr T$_{50}$ 27 days. Some poikilocytes and target cells

were seen in films but no sickled cells. On electrophoresis her haemoglobin was found to consist of 47.5% Hb S, 47.5% Hb D and 5% Hb F. The exact nature of this Hb D was not, however, established.

According to Bunn, Forget and Ranney (1977, p. 279), at least nine haemoglobins with the electrophoretic properties of Hb D had up to that time been found in combination with Hb S, but only two of them — Hb D Punjab and Hb Lepore — lead in compound heterozygotes to overt symptomatic haemolytic anaemia. Bunn, Forget and Ranney stated, too, that another 12 haemoglobin variants had a similar electrophoretic mobility to Hb D but had not yet been reported with Hb S in the same individual.

Life-span of erythrocytes

The ^{51}Cr T$_{50}$ in the 18-year-old black described by McCurdy and Gieschen (1960) was 16 days, equivalent to a mean life-span of 23 days.

Haemoglobin

The haemoglobin in Hb-SD disease migrates at pH 8.6 as a single band simulating homozygous Hb-SS disease. Hb A is absent. Hb D (i.e. Hb D Punjab), however, clearly separates from Hb S on electrophoresis in citrate agar at pH 6.2: it then migrates like Hb A. The percentage of the haemoglobin which is Hb S was reported by Cawein et al. (1966) to range in their four patients from 25 to 77, almost all the remainder being Hb D. Schneider and co-workers (1968) reported that Hb S and Hb D were present in about equal amounts in their patient. The amount of Hb F present has generally been small — Ozsoylu's (1969) patients had exceptionally high percentages (13–20%).

Blood picture

The blood picture is very similar to that of Hb-SS disease (Table 13.1). Serjeant (1985, p. 320), who tabulated data from 18 cases, including five unpublished Jamaican cases, gave a haemoglobin range of 5.7–10.7 g/dl [excluding the patient of Restrepo and Londoño (1965)]; there were

3.0–40% reticulocytes; the MCV ranged from 81 to 133 fl (in 10 cases > 100 fl) and the MCHC from 28 to 36 g/dl. Moderate anisocytosis and poikilocytosis, with target cells and some sickled and oat-shaped cells, are to be seen in stained films (Fig. 13.14).

Sickling *in vitro.* Erythrocytes from patients with Hb-SD disease sickle more slowly than do Hb-SS cells, so that at first sight sickling may appear not to be taking place in a sealed preparation of blood to which no reducing agent has been added. If a reducing agent is added, however, unequivocal sickling occurs. Cawein and co-workers (1966) reported that 60% of the Hb-SD cells of one patient sickled when exposed for 40 minutes at 37°C to a mixture of 1% O_2, 5% CO_2 and 94% N_2 compared with almost 100% of Hb-SS cells.

HAEMOGLOBIN-S/HAEMOGLOBIN-E DISEASE (Hb-SE DISEASE)

Because of the marked differences in the geographical distribution of Hb S and Hb E (Figs. 11.3 and 16.8), their presence in one individual is not likely to occur often. This combination has, however, occurred and it results in chronic haemolytic anaemia of generally mild intensity. The small number of patients reported have, however, had few symptoms.

Aksoy and Lehmann (1957b) described an Eti-Turk family in which two members, a 70-year-old woman and one of her sons, had a mild hypochromic microcytic anaemia. Their only physical complaints were occasional joint and bone pains. The affected son's spleen was slightly enlarged. Some target cells were present but otherwise their blood films were not remarkable. Both subjects had slightly raised reticulocyte counts (3.5–4%) and raised serum bilirubin levels (1.2–1.6 mg/dl). Their erythrocytes sickled *in vitro* and their haemoglobin was found to consist of approximately 40% Hb E and 60% Hb S.

Aksoy (1960) described a further Turkish family with the same Hb S plus Hb-E combination. The propositus was a 63-year-old woman; she complained of vague abdominal discomfort and was pale. The spleen was palpable about 3 cm below the left costal margin. An X-ray of the skull showed fine osteoporosis. She had 8.4 g/dl haemoglobin and there were 3% reticulocytes; the MCV was 97 fl and numerous target cells and a few sickled cells, as well as anisocytosis and polychromasia, could be seen in blood films. Electrophoresis revealed an Hb S plus Hb-E pattern with more Hb S than Hb E.

Altay, Niazi and Huisman (1976–77) described the occurrence of the Hb-SE combination in a black family resident in Georgia. The propositus was a female aged 20: she had no symptoms attributable to a haemoglobinopathy and had 12.7 g/dl haemoglobin, $4.66 \times 10^{12}/l$ erythrocytes, an MCV of 71 fl, 34.6% Hb A_2 + E, 1.3% Hb F and 64.2% Hb S. In-vitro globin-chain synthesis gave a $\beta^E:\beta^S$ ratio of 1:1.75. The gene frequency of Hb E in black populations was quoted as 0.0001 and the Hb-SE combination frequency was calculated to be approximately 1 in 100 000.

More recently, Hardy and Ragbeer (1985) described briefly two small Saudi children, aged 1 year and 6 years, respectively, who had inherited Hb E from their father and Hb S from their mother. They showed, however, little or no evidence of increased haemolysis; they were barely anaemic (haemoglobins 11.9 and 11.8 g/dl), their spleen was not palpable, and they had reticulocyte counts within the normal range. There was, on the other hand, definite microcytosis (MCV 61 and 66 fl), osmotic resistance was increased, and target cells were conspicuous in blood films.

HAEMOGLOBIN-S/HAEMOGLOBIN-O DISEASE (Hb-SO DISEASE)

A small number of patients have been described who have been compound heterozygotes for Hb-S and Hb-O Arab ($\beta^{121 \ Glu \ \rightarrow \ Lys}$). They have had a moderately severe haemolytic anaemia and have suffered from many of the physical complaints characteristic of Hb-SS disease, *e.g.*, recurrent osteo-articular and abdominal pains, the hand-foot syndrome, leg ulceration, pneumonia, pneumococcal septicaemia, haematuria and splenic sequestration (Ramot *et al.*, 1960; Ibrahim and Mustafa,

1967; Milner *et al.*, 1970; Javid, 1973; Kendall and Barr, 1973; McCurdy, Mahmood and Sherman, 1975; Charache *et al.*, 1977; Kazazian *et al.*, 1978; Gilman and Abel, 1980).

Blood films show anisocytosis and poikilocytosis and target cells and sickled cells, a picture indistinguishable from that of Hb-SS disease. *In vitro*, the erythrocytes sickle readily.

A presumptive diagnosis of Hb-SO disease can be made by electrophoresis: at pH 8.6 Hb O Arab migrates like Hb C, a characteristic that has led to the misdiagnosis of Hb-SO disease as Hb-SC disease. At pH 6.2, however, Hb O can be clearly separated from Hb C as it then migrates like Hb S.

The patients studied by Ramot *et al.* (1960) were an Arab boy aged 8 years and his younger sister. The boy had a palpable spleen and had had vaso-occlusive symptoms. Their father had Hb AO and their mother Hb AS. The haemoglobin of both children gave what appeared to be a Hb S plus Hb O plus Hb A pattern on electrophoresis. [The apparent presence of Hb A was not explained.] The boy had 7.0 g/dl haemoglobin, with 32% reticulocytes; the MCV was 100 fl. The girl had 8.6 g/dl haemoglobin, and 8% reticulocytes; her MCV was 110 fl. The boy had 10% Hb F and the girl 28%. Considerable anisopoikilocytosis and occasional sickled cells could be seen in blood films.

Ibrahim and Mustafa's (1967) patients were a Sudanese man aged 27 and his sister aged 15; their father had Hb AS and their mother Hb AO. Both patients had had osteo-articular symptoms — an infarcted head of the humerus and swollen hands, respectively. They were moderately severely anaemic, with some megaloblastic changes in the marrow. Electrophoresis of the haemoglobin of the propositus gave a Hb S plus Hb O pattern with 5.5% Hb F; Hb A was absent. Ibrahim and Mustafa stated that the incidence of Hb S in the Northern Sudanese was 2% and that of Hb O 0.1%; they considered that their patients had a relatively mild form of sickle-cell disease and equated it with Hb-SC disease.

Milner and co-workers (1970) reported Hb-SO disease in four members of four unrelated Jamaican families. Their clinical course appeared to be comparable to that seen in Hb-SD disease and to be rather more severe than in Hb-SC disease from which they had at one time been thought to be suffering. Their haemoglobins ranged from 7.0 to 8.7 g/dl, MCV 76 to 86 fl and reticulocytes from 2.9 to 13.0%; the serum bilirubin was 1.0–2.0 mg/dl. The O_2 affinity of the Hb-SO erythrocytes was reduced and comparable to that of Hb-SS cells; it was outside the range for Hb-SC cells. Milner *et al.*, demonstrated, too, that the natural mixture of 57% Hb S plus 43% Hb O gelled at 19.7 g/dl concen-

tration, which is 4.4 g/dl less than the gelling of 100% Hb S under the same circumstances; furthermore, the minimum gelling concentrations of all Hb-SO mixtures tested, containing 33% Hb S upwards, were less than that of Hb S alone.

Javid (1973) described Hb-SO disease in a black American female, aged 18, who also, at the time of investigation, had viral hepatitis. Her haemoglobin was 7.9 g/dl, MCV 100 fl, with 13.6% reticulocytes. The serum bilirubin was 13.2 mg/dl (9 mg direct). Slight anisocytosis, many target cells and a few sickled cells could be seen in blood films. Javid quoted data [including those of Milner *et al.* (1970)] on the minimum concentration of Hb S, in mixtures with another haemoglobin, necessary for in-vitro gelling. Of the six different 50:50 mixtures quoted, that of Hb S plus Hb O required the lowest concentration of Hb S (21 g/dl) for gelling. This was considered by Javid to be compatible with the generally rather severe clinical picture of Hb-SO disease.

Gilman and Abel (1980) described a 32-month-old white girl with Hb-SO disease who had experienced three life-threatening episodes of splenic sequestration during which her haemoglobin had fallen to 3.9, 2.8 and 4.2 g/dl, respectively. A [^{99m}Tc]sulphur colloid scan revealed impaired uptake of the radionuclide by an enlarged (12.5 cm) spleen. Splenectomy was followed by stabilization of the haemoglobin at 7.5–8.5 g/dl. The spleen weighed 125 g.

COMPOUND HETEROZYCOSITY FOR Hb S AND Hb C HARLEM

Moo-Pen and co-workers (1975) have described a 35-year-old black female who gave a history typical of Hb-SS disease: she had had numerous vaso-occlusive crises in adolescence and early adult life but they had become less frequent as she became older. Her haemoglobin was 9.0 g/dl and sickled cells could be seen in blood films. Electrophoresis demonstrated that she had 49.9% Hb S and 43.6% Hb C Harlem. [Hb C Harlem is characterized by two substitutions in the β-globin chain: $β_2^{6 \text{ Glu} \rightarrow \text{Val}}$, as in Hb S, plus $B_2^{73 \text{ Asp} \rightarrow \text{Asn}}$.] Two children were heterozygotes for Hb A and Hb C Harlem and one had the Hb-AS trait. They appeared to be clinically normal.

COMPOUND HETEROZYGOSITY FOR Hb S AND NON-REACTING β-CHAIN VARIANTS

Quite a large number of families have now been

described in which some members have been compound heterozygotes for Hb S and a β-chain variant which does not react significantly with Hb S, as do, for instance, Hb C, Hb D and Hb O. Such variants behave as harmless substitutes for Hb A: the affected individuals are not significantly anaemic; their clinical story and haematological findings (except for their haemoglobin electrophoretic patterns) are those of the Hb-AS trait.

The recorded combinations include the following (in chronological order): Hb S plus Hb K (O'Gorman et al., 1963; Ringelhann et al., 1971); Hb S plus Hb J Baltimore (Weatherall, 1964b); Hb S plus Hb Korle-Bu (Konotey-Ahulu et al., 1968); Hb S plus Hb Richmond (Efremov et al., 1969); Hb S plus Hb Osu-Christianborg (Konotey-Ahulu et al., 1971; McCurdy et al., 1974); Hb S plus Hb Ocho Rios (Beresford, Clegg and Weatherall, 1972); Hb S plus Hb J Bangkok (Gunay et al., 1974); Hb S plus Hb G Galveston (McCurdy et al., 1974); Hb S plus Hb Pyrgos (Tatsis, Sofroniadou and Stergiopoulos, 1976) and Hb S plus Hb Cambden (Honig et al., 1980). None of the patients described in the above reports had symptoms which could with certainty be attributed to their abnormal haemoglobin. Unexplained microcytosis and hypochromia were, however, present in the Hb-S/Hb-J Baltimore and Hb-S/Hb-Pyrgos patients; the Hb-S/Hb-Cambden patient was also microcytic, but in this case it seemed likely that he had α-thalassaemia also.

Hb-SJ disease. The patient described by Went and MacIver (1959) as a compound heterozygote for Hb S and Hb J was a Jamaican male with a fair complexion aged 42. He had had a partial gastrectomy for a duodenal ulcer and was considered to have a mild compensated haemolytic anaemia: his haemoglobin was 11.7 g/dl, with 4% reticulocytes, and the MCV was 90 fl.

COMPOUND HETEROZYGOSITY FOR Hb S AND AN UNSTABLE HAEMOGLOBIN

Steinberg and co-workers (1974) described two adult black females who were Hb-S heterozygotes whose second haemoglobin was Hb Hope ($\beta^{136\ Gly} \rightarrow {}^{Asp}$), a slightly unstable variant: they were slightly anaemic and the ^{51}Cr T_{50} was reported to be 16 days and 18 days, respectively. There was, however, no other evidence of haemolytic anaemia. The second patient described by Honig et al. (1980), a pregnant black Hb-S heterozygote aged 16, also had a slightly unstable second

haemoglobin, namely, Hb Tacoma ($\beta^{30\ Arg} \rightarrow {}^{Ser}$). Her haemoglobin was 11.9 g/dl and there were 2.2% reticulocytes.

More recently, Rhoda and co-workers (1986) have described the occurrence of compound heterozygosity for Hb S and Hb Siriraj, a slightly unstable β-chain variant ($\alpha_2\beta_2^{7\ Glu} \rightarrow {}^{Lys}$). The propositus was a 51-year-old black living in Martinique; he had considered himself healthy and had been free from vaso-occlusive crises. His spleen was, however, slightly enlarged and he had 'Grade II sickle-cell retinitis'. Of nine children, four had the Hb-S trait (41–47% Hb S), five the Hb-Siriraj trait (32–35% Hb Siriraj). Although he had 15.8 g/dl haemoglobin, there was evidence of slightly increased haemolysis. Serum haptoglobins were absent and he had 2.8% reticulocytes. The effect of reduction in O_2 tension in producing sickling indicated that Hb Siriraj interacts with Hb S in a manner similar to that of Hb A.

EFFECT OF α-CHAIN VARIANTS ON THE EXPRESSION OF Hb S

A small number of reports are now available of patients homozygous for Hb S who were at the same time heterozygous for an α-chain variant. Three such combinations are referred to below. With Hb Memphis ($\alpha^{23\ Glu} \rightarrow {}^{Gln}$) the expression of the Hb-SS disease appears to be reduced; in contrast, the presence of Hb Stanleyville II ($\alpha^{78\ Asn} \rightarrow {}^{Lys}$) and Hb G Philadelphia ($\alpha^{68\ Asn} \rightarrow {}^{Lys}$) appears to have had little or no effect.

Hb-SS/Hb-Memphis disease

Kraus and co-workers (1967) described two black patients with Hb-SS/Hb-Memphis disease, a man aged 73 and his niece aged 33. Clinically, the male propositus had had joint pains as an adolescent and leg ulcers, but neither patient had had painful crises nor other symptoms attributable to their Hb-SS disease. They were, however, anaemic; their haemoglobin was 7.3 g/dl and 9.5 g/dl, respectively; their reticulocyte count was 2.4% and 4.5%, and the ^{51}Cr T_{50} of the propositus was 6.9 days. According to Kraus et al., the findings in these patients illustrated how the vaso-occlusive complications of sickle-cell disease and the increased haemolysis are brought about by different mechanisms. They attributed the paucity of their patients' symptoms to the higher than usual concentration of Hb S required for haemoglobin to gel on deoxygenation. The viscosity of their whole blood on deoxygenation was, too, closer to that of normal (Hb-AA) blood than to Hb-SS blood.

Cooper and co-workers (1973) described a third case of Hb-SS/Hb-Memphis disease. Their patient was a black American, aged 53, who had had mild musculo-skeletal pains but no painful crises. He had had hyposthenuria and his spleen was not palpable (or demonstrable by isotopic techniques); sludging was not seen in the conjunctival vessels. He had, however, a moderately severe haemolytic anaemia: haemoglobin 9.5 g/dl, with 5–24% reticulocytes, and the ^{51}Cr T_{50} was 11 days. Many sickled cells could be seen in blood films and Howell-Jolly bodies and normoblasts were present, too. X-rays of his skeleton revealed osteoporotic and osteolytic changes but no evidence of infarction. The viscosity of his blood was similar to that in the Hb-AS trait and significantly less than in typical Hb-SS disease. Cooper et al. commented on the fact that, despite the absence of clinical episodes of infarction, the spleen had, nevertheless, atrophied, and they concluded that it must be especially sensitive to the thrombotic effect of sickled cells. They remarked, too, that the findings in their patient emphasized that infarction and haemolysis were independent processes in sickle-cell disease.

Hb-SS/Hb-Stanleyville II disease

The patient described by Hall-Craggs et al. (1964), a male Nilotic child from Uganda appeared clinically and haematologically to have typical Hb-SS disease, with dactylitis and severe anaemia.

Hb-SS/Hb-G Philadelphia disease

The history and haematological findings of Pugh, Monical and Minnich's (1964) patient, a black American aged 29, also appeared to be indistinguishable from those of typical Hb-SS disease. More recently, a further patient, a black American boy, was described by Charache et al. (1977) with the same combination. Clinically, he, too, had been thought to have Hb-SS disease. Electrophoresis of his haemoglobin, however, revealed two bands which were at first thought to indicate Hb-SC disease. But the presence of irreversibly sickled cells in peripheral-blood films and the failure of crystals to develop intracellularly when the erythrocytes were suspended in 3 g/dl NaCl were against this diagnosis. Eventually, the band which was present in addition to that of Hb S was identified as a Hb-G/Hb-S hybrid $\alpha_2^G \beta_2^S$. The patient's father, who was a heterozygote for both Hb S and Hb G, was clinically normal, i.e., the Hb G did not interact with the Hb S. On electrophoresis, four haemoglobin components could be demonstrated: Hb A ($\alpha_2^A \beta_2^A$), Hb G ($\alpha_2^G \beta_2^A$), Hb S ($\alpha_2^A \beta_2^S$) and a Hb-G/Hb-S hybrid ($\alpha_2^G \beta_2^S$). Target cells could be seen in his blood film.

Another family in which Hb S and Hb G Philadelphia co-existed was described by Lie-Injo, Wang and Burnett (1968). The propositus, a male black aged 45, was a heterozygote for Hb S and Hb G. His haemoglobin was 12.3 g/dl (after iron therapy) and the reticulocyte count was 2.1%. The MCV was 62.2 fl and MCH 22.8 pg. A few target cells, but no sickled cells, could be seen in peripheral-blood films. Sickling took place slowly in vitro. The patient's two children were also heterozygotes for Hb S and Hb G; they, too, had a microcytic hypochromic anaemia but without any evidence of increased haemolysis.

A further patient, who was also a heterozygote for Hb S and Hb G, was described by Wrightstone, Hubbard and Huisman (1974). In this instance the haemoglobin was Hb G Georgia. The patient, a black American boy aged 7 years, had a hypochromic anaemia. This, however, seemed to be the consequence of epistaxis and again there was no evidence of increased haemolysis. According to McCurdy et al. (1975), the presence of Hb G Philadelphia leads to impaired synthesis of α chains similar to that of α-thalassaemia. This would lead to a low MCH and microcytosis.

REFERENCES

ACHESON, R. & SERJEANT, G. (1985). Painful crises in sickle cell disease after fluorescein angiography. Lancet, i, 1222 (Letter).

AHERN, E. J., AHERN, V. N., AARONS, G. H., JONES, R. T. & BRIMHALL, B. (1972). Hemoglobin Lepore$_{Washington}$ in two Jamaican families: interaction with beta chain variants. Blood, 40, 246–256.

AKSOY, M. (1959). Abnormal haemoglobins in Turkey. In: Abnormal Haemoglobins, A Symposium (ed. by J. H. P. Jonxis and J. F. Delafresnaye), pp. 216–235. Blackwell Scientific Publications, Oxford.

AKSOY, M. (1960). The hemoglobin E syndromes. II. Sickle-cell–hemoglobin E disease. Blood, 15, 610–613.

AKSOY, M. (1963). The first observation of homozygous hemoglobin S-alpha thalassemia disease and two types of sickle cell thalassemia disease: (a) sickle cell-alpha thalassemia disease, (b) sickle cell-beta thalassemia disease. Blood. 22, 757–769.

AKSOY, M. & ERDEM, S. (1967). The thalassaemia

syndromes. VI. Two subtypes of sickle cell-beta thalassaemia disease: (a) normocytic type of sickle cell-beta thalassaemia disease; (b) microcytic type of sickle cell-beta thalassaemia disease. *Acta haemat. (Basel)*, **37**, 181–188.

AKSOY, M. & LEHMANN, H. (1957a). Sickle-cell–thalassaemia disease in South Turkey. *Brit. med. J.*, i, 734–738.

AKSOY, M. & LEHMANN, H. (1957b). The first observation of sickle-cell haemoglobin E disease. *Nature (Lond.)*, **179**, 1248–1249.

ALEXANDRIDIS, K., STAMOULIS, V. & TSIGALIDOU, V. (1956). Der Erbgang der Mittelmeer-Hämopathien. *Kongr. europ. Ges. Hämat., Freiburg, 1955*, pp. 676–686. Springer-Verlag, Berlin.

ALTAY, C., NIAZI, G. A. & HUISMAN, T. H. J. (1976–77). The combination of Hb S and Hb E in a black female. *Hemoglobin*, **1**, 100–102.

ALTAY, C., SCHROEDER, W. A. & HUISMAN, T. H. J. (1977). The $^{G}\gamma$-$\delta\beta$-thalassemia and $^{G}\gamma$-β^0-HPFH conditions in combination with β thalassemia and Hb S. *Amer. J. Hemat.*, **3**, 1–14.

ANAGNOU, N. P., PAPAYANNOPOULOU, T., STAMATOYANNOPOULOS, G. & NIENHUIS, A. W. (1985). Structurally diverse molecular deletions in the β-globin gene cluster exhibit an identical phenotype on interaction with the β^S-gene. *Blood*, **65**, 1245–1251.

ANDREWS, J. & BUCHANAN, G. R. (1984). Mild splenic sequestration crises in sickle-hemoglobin C disease. *Clin. Pediat.*, **23**, 354–355.

ANGELOPOULOS, B. (1965). Genetic and electrophoretic studies in three Greek families inheriting the traits for both sickling and thalassemia. *Blut.* **11**, 18–25.

ARENDS, T., LAYRISSE, M. & RINCON, A. R. (1959). Sickle cell–haemoglobin D disease in a Portuguese child. *Acta haemat. (Basel)*, **22**, 118–126.

ASCENZI, A. & SILVERSTRONI, E. (1953). On the optical properties of the hemoglobin in microdrepanocytic disease. *Blood*, **8**, 1061–1066.

ASCENZI, A. & SILVESTRONI, E. (1957). Étude anatomo-clinique d'un cas de maladie microdrépanocytique. *Acta haemat. (Basel)*, **18**, 205–218.

ASDOURIAN, G., NAGPAL, K. C., GOLDBAUM, M., PATRIANAKOS, D., GOLDBERG, M. F. & RABB, M. (1975). Evolution of the retinal black sunburst lesion in sickling haemoglobinopathies. *Brit. J. Ophthal.*, **59**, 710–716.

BABIN, D. R., JONES, R. T. & SCHROEDER, W. A. (1964). Hemoglobin D$_{Los\ Angeles}$: $\alpha_2\beta_2^{121\ glu\ NH_2}$ *Biochim. biophys. Acta*, **86**, 136–143.

BALLAS, S. K., LEWIS, C. N., NOONE, A. M., KRASNOW, S. H., KAMARULZAMAN, E. & BURKA, E. R. (1982). Clinical, hematological and biochemical features of Hb SC disease. *Amer. J. Hemat.*, **13**, 37–51.

BANK, A., DOW, L. W., FARACE, M. G., O'DONNELL, J. V., FORD, S. & NATTA, C. (1973). Changes in globin synthesis with erythroid cell maturation in sickle thalassemia. *Blood.* **41**, 353–357.

BANKS, L. O., SCOTT, R. B. & SIMMONS, J. (1952). Studies in sickle cell anemia. Inheritance factor, including effect of interaction of genes for sicklemia and thalassemia. *Amer. J. Dis. Child.*, **84**, 601–608.

BANNERMAN, R. H. O. & WHITE, J. C. (1957). Sickle-cell disease and pregnancy. *J. Obstet. Gynaec. Brit. Emp.*, **64**, 682–690.

BANNERMAN, R. M., SERJEANT, B., SEAKINS, M., ENGLAND, J. M. & SERJEANT, G. R. (1979). Determinants of haemoglobin level in sickle cell–haemoglobin C disease. *Brit. J. Haemat.*, **43**, 49–56.

BARTON, C. J. & COCKSHOTT, W. P. (1962). Bone changes in hemoglobin SC disease. *Amer. J. Roentgenol.*, **88**, 523–532.

BASHOUR, T. L. & LINDSAY, J. JNR (1975). Hemoglobin S-C disease presenting as acute pneumonitis with pulmonary angiographic findings in two patients. *Amer. J. Med.*, **58**, 559–560.

BECKER, J. A. (1962). Hemoglobin S-C disease. *Amer. J. Roentgenol.*, **88**, 503–511.

BELHANI, M., MORLE, L., GODET, J., BACHIR, D., HENNI, T., ZERHOUNI, F., BENSENOUCI, A. & COLONNA, P. (1984). Sickle cell β-thalassaemia compared with sickle cell anaemia in Algeria. *Scand. J. Haemat.*, **32**, 346–350.

BENTSI-ENCHILL, K. K. & KONOTEY-AHULU, F. I. D. (1969). Thirteen children from twelve pregnancies in sickle-cell thalassaemia. *Brit. med. J.*, iii, 762.

BERESFORD, C. H., CLEGG, J. B. & WEATHERALL, D. J. (1972). Haemoglobin Ocho Rios (β52(D3) aspartic acid → alanine): a new β-chain variant of haemoglobin A found in combination with haemoglobin S. *J. med. Genet.*, **9**, 151–153.

BERTHRONG, M., DONALD, J. H., PEREZ-MESA, C. & GANEM, G. (1957). Necropsy findings in a white man with thalassemia minor-sickle cell trait with fatal crisis precipitated by airplane flight. *Amer. J. Path.*, **33**, 590–591.

BIENZLE, U., KAPPES, R., REIMER, A., FELDHEIM, M., TISCHENDORF, F. W. & KOHNE, E. (1983). Sickle cell-β^+-thalassaemia. A haematological and clinical study in Liberia. *Blut*, **47**, 279–285.

BLACK, A. J., CONDON, P. I., GOMPELS, B. M., GREEN, R. L., HUNTSMAN, R. G. & JENKINS, G. C. (1972). Sickle-cell haemoglobin C disease in London. *J. clin. Path.*, **25**, 49–55.

BLATRIX, C., DE TRAVERSE, P. M., COQUELET, M. L., ISRAEL, J., PELLETIER, P. & FERRARA, G. (1970). La double hétérozygotie hémoglobinose C-thalassémie dans la race blanche. *Presse méd.*, **78**, 1791–1792.

BRADLEY, T. B. JNR, BRAWNER, J. N. III & CONLEY, C. L. (1961). Further observations on an inherited anomaly characterized by persistence of fetal hemoglobin. *Bull. Johns Hopk. Hosp.*, **108**, 242–257.

BRADLEY, T. B. JNR & CONLEY, C. L. (1960). Studies of inherited disorder manifested by persistence of fetal hemoglobin. *Trans. Ass. Amer. Phycns*, **73**, 72–79.

BROWN, D. E. & OBER, W. B. (1958). Sickle-cell thalassemia (microdrepanocytic disease) in pregnancy. *Obstet. and Gynec.*, **75**, 773–784.

BUDTZ-OLSEN, O. E., BELL, K., HILLCOAT, B. L. & NEWOOMBE, R. L. G. (1961). Sickle-cell thalassaemia disease in a family with intermarriage of siblings. *Med. J. Aust.*, **ii**, 902–904.

BUNN, H. F., FORGET, B. G. & RANNEY, H. M. (1977). *Human Hemoglobins*. W. B. Saunders, Philadelphia, London, Toronto.

BURCHMORE, J. W., BUCKLE, R. M., LEHMANN, H. & JENKINS, W. J. (1962). Agglutinating-sickling arterial thrombosis. An unusual case of sickle-cell haemoglobin-C disease. *Lancet*, **ii**, 1008–1010.

CAWEIN, M. J., LAPPAT, E. J., BRANGLE, R. W. & FARLEY, C. H. (1966). Hemoglobin S-D disease. *Ann. intern. Med.*, **64**, 62–70.

CAWEIN, M. J., O'NEILL, R. P., DANZER, L. A., LAPPAT, E. J. & ROACH, T. (1969). A study of the sickling phenomenon and oxygen dissociation curve in patients with hemoglobins SS, SD, SF and SC. *Blood*, **34**, 682–690.

CHAPMAN, A. Z., REEDER, P. S., FRIEDMAN, I. A. & BAKER. L. A. (1954). Gross hematuria in sickle cell trait and sickle cell C-hemoglobin disease. *J. Lab. clin. Med.*, **44**, 778–779.

CHARACHE, S. & PAGE, D. L. (1967). Infarction of bone marrow in the sickle cell disorders. *Ann. intern. Med.*, **67**, 1195–1200.

CHARACHE, S., ZINKHAM, W. H., DICKERMAN, J. D., BRIMHALL, B. & DOVER, G. J. (1977). Hemoglobin SC, SS/G$_{Philadelphia}$ and SO$_{Arab}$ diseases. Diagnostic importance of an integrative analysis of clinical, hematologic and electrophoretic findings. *Amer. J. Med.*, **62**, 439–446.

CHATTERJEA, J. B. (1959). Haemoglobinopathy in India. In: *Abnormal Haemoglobins. A Symposium* (ed. by J. H. P. Jonxis and J. F. Delafresnaye), pp. 322–339. Blackwell Scientific Publications, Oxford.

CHATTERJEA, J. B., SWARUP, S., GHOSH, S. K. & RAY, R. N. (1958). Hb.S-thalassaemia disease in India. *J. Indian med. Ass.*, **30**, 4–8.

CHILCOTE, R. R. & DAMPIER, C. (1984). Overwhelming pneumoccal septicemia in a patient with HbSC disease and splenic dysfunction. *J. Pediat.*, **104**, 734–736.

CHMEL, H. & BERTLES, J. F. (1975). Hemoglobin S/C disease in a pregnant woman with crisis and fat embolization syndrome. *Amer. J. Med.*, **58**, 563–566.

CHOREMIS, C. & ZANNOS, L. (1957). Microdrepanocytic disease in Greece. *Blood*, **12**, 454–460.

CHU, J.-Y. & NIEDERMAN, L. G. (1977). Splenic sequestration syndrome in sickle/hemoglobin C disease at low altitude. *J. Pediat.*, **91**, 350–351 (Letter).

CHUSID, M. J., LACHMAN, B. S. & LAZERSON, J. (1978). Severe Mycoplasma pneumonia and vesicular eruption in SC hemoglobinopathy. *J. Pediat.*, **93**, 449–451.

COCKSHOTT, W. P. (1958). Haemoglobin SC disease. *J. Fac. Radiol. (Lond.)*, **9**, 211–216.

COLEMAN, W. A. & FURTH, F. W. (1956). Splenic infarction in a patient with sickle-cell-hemoglobin-C disease. Report of a case occurring following air travel. *Arch. intern. Med.*, **98**, 247–249.

CONDON, P. I., MARSH, R. J., MAUDE, G. H., HIGGS, D. R., WEATHERALL, D. J. & SERJEANT, G. R. (1983). Alpha thalassaemia and the macular vasculature in homozygous sickle cell disease. *Brit. J. Ophthal.*, **67**, 779–781.

CONDON, P. I. & SERJEANT, G. R. (1972a). Ocular findings in hemoglobin SC disease in Jamaica. *Amer. J. Ophthal.*, **74**, 921–931.

CONDON, P. I. & SERJEANT, R. G. (1972b). Ocular findings in sickle cell thalassemia in Jamaica. *Amer. J. Opthal.*, **74**, 1105–1109.

CONLEY, C. L. (1964). Pathophysiological effects of some abnormal hemoglobins. *Medicine (Baltimore)*, **43**, 785–787.

CONLEY, C. L. & SMITH, E. W. (1954). Clinical features of genetic variants of sickle cell disease. *Trans. Ass. Amer. Phycns*, **67**, 261–267.

CONLEY, C. L., WEATHERALL, D. J., RICHARDSON, S. N., SHEPARD, M. K. & CHARACHE, S. (1963). Hereditary persistence of fetal hemoglobin: a study of 79 affected persons in 15 negro families in Baltimore. *Blood*, **21**, 261–281.

COOKE, J. V. & MACK, J. K. (1934). Sickle-cell anemia in a white American family. *J. Pediat.*, **5**, 601–607.

COOLEY, T. B. & LEE, P. (1929). Sickle cell anemia in a Greek family. *Amer. J. Dis. Child.*, **38**, 103–106.

COOPER, M. R., KRAUS, A. P., FELTS, J. H., RAMSEUR, W. L., MYERS, R. & KRAUS, L. M. (1973). A third case of hemoglobin Memphis/sickle cell disease. Whole blood viscosity used as a screening test. *Amer. J. Med.*, **55**, 535–541.

COWLING, D. C., UNGAR, B. & BAIRD, C. W. (1965). Sickle cell thalassaemia: a report of four cases in three Mediterranean families living in Australia. *Med. J. Aust.*, **ii**, 75–79.

CURTIS, E. M. (1959). Pregnancy in sickle cell anemia, sickle cell-hemoglobin C disease, and variants thereof. *Amer. J. Obstet. Gynec.*, **77**, 1312–1323.

DA COSTA, J. L., LOH, Y. S. & HANAM, E. (1974). Extramedullary hemopoiesis with multiple tumor-simulating mediastinal masses in hemoglobin-E thalassemia disease. *Chest*, **65**, 210–212.

DACIE, J. V. (1954). *The Haemolytic Anaemias:*

Congenital and Acquired, p. 146. Churchill, London.

DE CEULAER, K., HIGGS, D. R., WEATHERALL, D. J., HAYES, R. J., SERJEANT, B. E. & SERJEANT, G. R. (1983). α-thalassaemia reduces the hemolytic rate in homozygous sickle-cell disease. *New Engl. J. Med.*, **309**, 189–190 (Letter).

DIAMOND, M. P. (1959). Five cases of sickle-cell haemoglobin-C disease. *Lancet*, ii, 322–324.

DIGGS, L. W. & BELL, A. (1965). Intraerythrocytic hemoglobin crystals in sickle cell-hemoglobin C disease. *Blood*, **25**, 218–223.

DOENGES, J. P., SMITH, E. W. & WISE, S. P. III (1954). Splenic infarction following air travel and associated with the sickling phenomenon. *J. Amer. med. Ass.*, **156**, 955–957.

DUNN, J. M. & HAYNES, R. L. (1967). Sickle cell thalassemia in pregnancy. *Amer. J. Obstet. Gynec.*, **97**, 574–575.

DUNSTON, T., ROWLAND, R., HUNTSMAN, R. G. & YAWSON, G. (1972). Sickle-cell haemoglobin C disease and sickle-cell beta thalassaemia in White South Africans. *S. Afr. med. J.*, **46**, 1423–1426.

EDINGTON, G. M. & LEHMANN, H. (1954). A case of sickle cell-haemoglobin C disease and a survey of haemoglobin C incidence in West Africa. *Trans. roy. Soc. trop. Med. Hyg.*, **48**, 332–336.

EDINGTON, G. M. & LEHMANN, H. (1955a). Expression of the sickle-cell gene in Africa. *Brit. med. J.*, i, 1308–1311.

EDINGTON, G. M. & LEHMANN, H. (1955b). Expression of the sickle-cell gene in Africa. *Brit. med. J.*, ii, 1328 (Letter).

EFREMOV, G. D., HUISMAN, T. H. J., SMITH, L. L., WILSON, J. B., KITCHENS, J. L., WRIGHTSTONE, R. N. & ADAMS, H. R. (1969). Hemoglobin Richmond, a human hemoglobin which forms asymmetric hybrids with other hemoglobins. *J. biol. Chem.*, **244**, 6105–6116.

EL-HAZMI, M. A. F. (1985). Clinical manifestations and laboratory findings of sickle cell anaemia in association with α-thalassaemia in Saudi Arabia. *Acta haemat. (Basel)*, **74**, 155–160.

EMBURY, S. H., BACKER, K. & GLADER, B. E. (1983). Red blood cells (RBC) monovalent cation permeability as a function of α-globin gene number in homozygous sickle cell anemia (Hb-SS). *Blood*, **62**, No. 5 (Suppl.1), 55a (Abstract 124).

EMBURY, S. H., BACKER, K. & GLADER, B. E. (1985). Monovalent cation changes in sickle erythrocytes: a direct reflection of α-globin gene number. *J. Lab. clin. Med.*, **106**, 75–79.

EMBURY, S. H., CLARK, M. R., MONROY, G. & MOHANDAS, N. (1984). Concurrent sickle cell anemia and α-thalassaemia. Effect on pathological properties of sickle erythrocytes. *J. clin. Invest.*, **73**, 116–123.

EMBURY, S. H., DOZY, A. M., MILLER, J., DAVIS, J. R. JNR, KLEMAN, K. M., PREISLER, H., VICHINSKY, E., LANDE, W. N., LUBIN, B. H.,

KAN, Y. W. & MENTZER, W. C. (1982). Concurrent sickle-cell anemia and α-thalassaemia: effect on severity of anemia. *New Engl. J. Med.*, **306**, 270–274.

EMBURY, S. H., GHOLSON, M. A., GILLETTE, P., RIEDER, R. F. & THE NATIONAL COOPERATIVE STUDY OF SICKLE CELL DISEASE. (1985). The leftward deletion α-thal-2 haplotype in a black subject with hemoglobin SS. *Blood*, **65**, 769–771.

EMBURY, S. H., OLIVER, M. & KROPP, J. (1985). The beneficial effect of α thalassemia on sickle cell anemia (SCA) is related to increased membrane redundancy. *Blood*, **66**, No. 5 (Suppl. 1), 58a (Abstract 119).

ESAN, G. J. F. (1970). The thalassaemia syndromes in Nigeria. *Brit. J. Haemat.*, **19**, 47–56.

FABIAN, R. H. & PETERS, B. H. (1984). Neurological complications of hemoglobin SC disease. *Arch. Neurol.*, **41**, 289–292.

FABRY, M. E., DHANANJAYA, K. K., RAVENTOS-SUAREZ, C., CHANG, H. & NAGEL, R. L. (1982). SC erythrocytes have an abnormally high intracellular hemoglobin concentration. Pathophysiological consequences. *J. clin. Invest.*, **70**, 1315–1319.

FELICE, A. E., ALTAY, C. A., MILNER, P. F. & HUISMAN, T. H. J. (1981). The occurrence and identification of α-thalassemia-2 among hemoglobin S heterozygotes. *Amer. J. clin. Path.*, **76**, 70–73.

FELICE, A. E., CLEEK, M. P., MCKIE, K., MCKIE, V. & HUISMAN, T. H. J. (1984a). The rare α-thalassemia-1 of blacks is a ζα-thalassemia-1 associated with deletion of all α- and ζ-globin genes. *Blood*, **63**, 1253–1257.

FELICE, A. E., MCKIE, V. C., MCKIE, K. & HUISMAN, T. H. J. (1984b). Deletions and duplications of α or ζ genes in children with sickle cell anemia. *Blood*, **64**, No. 5 (Suppl. 1), 47a (Abstract 100).

FELICE, A. E., MARINO, E. M., MCKIE, K. M. & MCKIE, V.C. (1985). Developmental hematology of SS and SC disease in association with α-thalassaemia-2. *Blood*, **66**, No. 5 (Suppl. 1), 59a (Abstract 121).

FELICE, A. E., WEBBER, B., MILLER, A., MAYSON, S. M., HARRIS, H. F., HENSON, J. B., GRAVELY, M. E. & HUISMAN, T. H. J. (1979). The association of sickle cell anemia with heterozygous and homozygous α-thalassemia-2. In vitro HB chain synthesis. *Amer. J. Hemat.*, **6**, 91–106.

FICH, A. & RACHMILEWITZ, E. A. (1981). Priapism in a non-black with sickle cell anemia associated with α-thalassemia. *Amer. J. Hemat.*, **10**, 313–315.

FIGUEROA, E. & ARENDS, T. (1963). Enfermedad por drepanocitosis y hemoglobina D complicada con anemia megaloblatica en un niño Venezolano. *Arch. venez. Pueric.*, **26**, 494–503.

FULLERTON, W. T. & WATSON-WILLIAMS, E. J. (1962). Haemoglobin SC disease and megaloblastic anaemia of pregnancy. *J. Obstet. Gynaec. Brit. Cmwlth*, **69**, 729–735.

GATTO, I. & RUSSO, G. (1955). Ricerche ematologiche nella thalassodrepanocitosi. *Pediatria (Napoli)*, **63**, 560–586.

GEOLA, F., KUKREJA, S. C. & SCHADE, S. E. (1978). Splenic sequestration with sickle cell-C disease. *Arch. intern. Med.*; **138**, 307–308.

GILL, F. M. & SCHWARTZ, E. (1973). Synthesis of globin chains in sickle β-thalassemia. *J. clin. Invest*, **52**, 709–714.

GILMAN, P. A. & ABEL, A. S. (1980). Acute splenic sequestration in hemoglobin sickle O-Arab disease. *Johns Hopk. Hosp. med. J.*, **146**, 285–288.

GITHENS, J. H., GROSS, G. P., EIFE, R. F. & WALLNER, S. F. (1977). Splenic sequestration syndrome at mountain altitudes in sickle/hemoglobin C disease. *J. Pediat.*, **90**, 203–206.

GLADER, B. E., PROPPER, R. D. & BUCHANAN, G. R. (1979). Microcytosis associated with sickle cell anemia. *Amer. J. clin. Path.*, **72**, 63–64.

GOLDBERG, M. F. (1971a). Classification and pathogenesis of proliferative sickle retinopathy. *Amer. J. Ophthal.*, **71**, 649–665.

GOLDBERG, M. F. (1971b). Natural history of untreated proliferative sickle retinopathy. *Arch. Ophthal.*, **85**, 428–437.

GOLDBERG, M. F., CHARACHE, S. & ACACIO, I. (1971). Ophthalmologic manifestations of sickle cell thalassemia. *Arch. intern. Med.*, **128**, 33–39.

GOLDING, J. S. R., MacIVER, J. E. & WENT, L. N. (1959). The bone changes in sickle cell anaemia and its genetic variants. *J. Bone Jt Surg.*, **41B**, 711–718.

GOODMAN, G., VON SALLMAN, L. & HOLLAND, M. G. (1957). Ocular manifestations of sickle-cell disease. *Arch. Ophthal. (Chicago)*, **58**, 655–682.

GREEN, R. L., HUNTSMAN, R. G. & SERJEANT, G. R. (1971). The sickle-cell and altitude. *Brit. med. J.*, **4**, 593–595.

GREEN, T. W. & CONLEY C. L. (1951). Occurrence of symptoms of sickle cell disease in the absence of persistent anemia. *Ann. intern. Med.*, **34**, 849–855.

GREENWALD, L. & BURRETT, J. B. (1940). Sickle-cell anemia in a White family. *Amer. J. med. Sci.*, **199**, 768–774.

GREER, M. & SCHOTLAND, D. (1962). Abnormal hemoglobin as a cause of neurological disease. *Neurology*, **12**, 114–123.

GRIGGS, R. C. & HARRIS, J. W. (1956). The biophysics of the variants of sickle-cell disease. *Arch. intern. Med.*, **97**, 315–326.

GUNAY, U., PAULI, C., SHAMSUDDIN, M., MASON, R. G., HEINZE, W. J. & HONIG, G. R. (1974). Sickle hemoglobin in combination with Hb J^{Bangkok} ($\alpha_2^A\beta_2^{56\ gly \to asp}$). *Blood*, **44**, 683–690.

HADEN, R. L. & EVANS, F. D. (1937). Sickle cell anaemia in the white race. Improvement in two cases following splenectomy. *Arch. intern. Med.*, **60**, 133–142.

HALES, C. A. (1983). Case records of the Massachusetts General Hospital. *New Engl. J. Med.*, **309**, 1627–1636.

HALL-CRAGGS, M., MARSDEN, P. D., RAPER, A. B., LEHMANN, H. & BEALE, D. (1964). Homozygous sickle-cell anaemia arising from two different haemoglobins S. Interaction of haemoglobins S and Stanleyville-II. *Brit. med. J.*, ii, 87–89.

HANNON, J. F. (1956). Vitreous hemorrhages associated with sickle-cell hemoglobin C disease. *Amer. J. Ophthal.*, **42**, 707–712.

HARDY, M. J. & RAGBEER, M. S. (1985). Homozygous HbE and HbSE in a Saudi family. *Hemoglobin*, **9**, 47–52.

HAYES, R. J., CONDON, P. I. & SERJEANT, G. R. (1981). Haematological factors associated with proliferative retinopathy in sickle cell–haemoglobin C disease. *Brit. J. Ophthal.*, **65**, 712–717.

HAYNES, R. L. & DUNN, J. M. (1967). Oral contraceptives, thrombosis, and sickle cell hemoglobinopathies. *J. Amer. med. Ass.*, **200**, 994–996.

HENDERSON, A. B., POTTS, E. B., BURGESS, D. & WHITE, F. (1962). Sickle-cell thalassemia disease and pregnancy: a case study. *Amer. J. med. Sci.*, **244**, 605–611.

HENDRICKSE, J. P. DE V., HARRISON, K. A., WATSON-WILLIAMS, E. J., LUZZATTO, L. & AJABOR, L. N. (1972). Pregnancy in abnormal haemoglobins CC, S-thalassaemia, SF, CF, double heterozygotes. *J. Obstet. Gynaec. Brit. Cmwlth*, **79**, 410–415.

HENDRICKSE, R. G. (1958). Sickle cell haemoglobin C disease and homozygous haemoglobin C disease in Nigerian children. *W. Afr. med. J.*, **7**, 80–90.

HERMAN, E. C. JNR & CONLEY, C. L. (1960). Hereditary persistence of fetal hemoglobin. A family study. *Amer. J. Med.*, **29**, 9–17.

HIGGS, D. R., ALDRIDGE, B. E., LAMB, J., CLEGG, J. B., WEATHERALL, D. J., HAYES, R., GRANDISON, Y., LOWRIE, Y., MASON, K. P., SERJEANT, B. E. & SERJEANT, G. R. (1982). The interaction of alpha-thalassemia and homozygous sickle-cell disease. *New Engl. J. Med.*, **306**, 1441–1446.

HIGGS, D. R., CLEGG, J. B., WEATHERALL, D. J., SERJEANT, B. E. & SERJEANT, G. R. (1984). Interaction of the ααα globin gene haplotype and sickle haemoglobin. *Brit. J. Haemat.*, **57**, 671–678.

HONIG, G. R., GUNAY, U., MASON, R. G., VIDA, L. N. & FERENC, C. (1976). Sickle cell syndromes. I. Hemoglobin SC-α thalassemia. *Pediat. Res.*, **10**, 613–620.

HONIG, G. R., KOSHY, M., MASON, R. G. & VIDA, L. N. (1978). Sickle cell syndromes. II. The sickle cell anemia -α-thalassemia syndrome. *J. Pediat.*, **92**, 556–561.

HONIG, G. R., MASON, R. G., SHAMSUDDIN, M.,

VIDA, L. N., RAO, K. R.P. & PATEL, A. R. (1980). Two new sickle cell syndromes: Hb S, Hb Camden, and α-thalassemia; and Hb S in combination with Hb Tacoma. *Blood*, 55, 655–660.

HONIG, G. R., MASON, R. G., TREMAINE, L. M. & VIDA, L. N. (1979). Sickle cell syndromes. III. Silent-carrier α-thalassemia in combination with hemoglobin S and hemoglobin C. *Pediat. Res.*, 13, 1109–1111.

HOOK, E. W. & COOPER, G. R. (1958). The clinical manifestations of sickle cell-hemoglobin C disease and sickle cell anemia. *Sth. med. J. (Bgham, Ala.)*, 51, 610–626.

HUESTIS, D. W., GERSTBREIN, H. L., COOPER, W. M. & CHAPMAN, W. L. (1959). Sickle cell — hemoglobin C disease. *Lab. Invest.*, 8, 736–760.

HUISMAN, T. H. J. (1977). Trimodality in the percentages of the β chain variants in heterozygotes: the effect of the number of active Hb_α structural loci. *Hemoglobin*, 1, 349–382.

HUISMAN, T. H. J. (1983). Percentages of abnormal hemoglobins in adults with a heterozygosity for an α-chain and/or a β-chain variant. *Amer. J. Hemat.*, 14, 393–404.

HUISMAN, T. H. J., SCHROEDER, W. A., BOUVER, N. G., MILLER, A., SHELTON, J. R., SHELTON, J. B. & APELL, G. (1972). Chemical heterogeneity of fetal hemoglobin in subjects with sickle cell anemia, homozygous Hb-C disease, SC-disease, and various combinations of hemoglobin variants. *Clin. chim. Acta*, 38, 5–16.

HUMBLE, J. G., ANDERSON, I., WHITE, J. C. & FREEMAN, T. (1954). A family illustrating the double inheritance of the sickle cell trait and of Mediterranean anaemia. *J. clin. Path.*, 7, 201–208.

IBRAHIM, S. A. & MUSTAFA, D. (1967). Sickle-cell haemoglobin Ò disease in a Sudanese family. *Brit. med. J.*, ii, 715–717.

ITANO, H. A. (1951). A third abnormal hemoglobin associated with hereditary hemolytic anemia. *Proc. natn. Acad. Sci. U.S.A.*, 37, 775–784.

IZUMO, H., WILLIAMS, M., ROSA, R., HOFFMAN, N., FLIER, J. & EPSTEIN, F. H. (1985). Na-K-ATPase and ion fluxes in sickle cell anemia: implications for therapy. *Clin. Res.*, 33, 343A (Abstract).

JACOB, G. F. & RAPER, A. B. (1958). Hereditary persistence of foetal haemoglobin production, and its interaction with the sickle-cell trait. *Brit. J. Haemat.*, 4, 138–149.

JAVID, J. (1973). Hemoglobin SO_{Arabia} disease in a Black American. *Amer. J. med. Sci.*, 265, 266–274.

JEWETT, J. E. (1976). Sickle-cell trait, thalassemia, G-6-PD deficiency and puerperal pulmonary embolism. *New Engl. J. Med.*, 295, 1076–1077.

JOISHY, S. K., GRINER, P. F. & ROWLEY, P. T. (1976). Sickle β-thalassemia: identical twins differing in severity implicate non genetic factors influencing course. *Amer. J. Hemat.*, 1, 23–33.

JOSHPE, G., ROTHENBERG, S. P. & BAUM, S. (1973). Transient functional asplenism in sickle cell-C disease. *Amer. J. Med.*, 55, 720–722.

KAPLAN, E., ZUELZER, W. W. & NEEL, J. V. (1951). A new inherited abnormality of hemoglobin and its interaction with sickle cell hemoglobin. *Blood*, 6, 1240–1259.

KAPLAN, E., ZUELZER, W. W. & NEEL, J. V., (1953). Further studies on hemoglobin C. II. The hematologic effects of hemoglobin C alone and in combination with sickle cell hemoglobin. *Blood*, 8, 735–746.

KAZAZIAN, H. H. JNR, DOVER, G. L., LIGHTBODY, K. L. & PARK, I. J. (1978). Prenatal diagnosis in a fetus at risk for hemoglobin S-O_{Arab} disease. *J. Pediat.*, 93, 502–504.

KELLEHER, J. F. JNR, PARK, J. O. K., KIM, H. C. & SCHROEDER, W. A. (1984). Life-threatening complications in a child with hemoglobin SD–Los Angeles disease. *Hemoglobin*, 8, 203–213.

KENDALL, A. G. & BARR, R. D. (1973). Haemoglobinopathies in Kenya. *Trans. roy. Soc. trop. Med. Hyg.*, 67, 770–781.

KIM, H. C., WEIERBACH, R. G., FRIEDMAN, S. & SCHWARTZ, E. (1977). Detection of sickle α- or $β^0$-thalassemia by studies of globin biosynthesis. *Blood*, 49, 785–792.

KINNEY, T. R., FRIEDMAN, SH., CIFUENTES, E., KIM, H. C. & SCHWARTZ, E. (1978). Variations in globin synthesis in deta-beta-thalassaemia. *Brit. J. Haemat.*, 38, 15–32.

KNOX-MACAULAY, H. H. M., FLEMING, A. F., LAMB, J., & MBA, E. C. (1984). Haemoglobin G Philadelphia and its interaction with haemoglobin S and alpha-thalassaemia in Nigerians. *Clin. lab. Haemat.*, 6, 113–121.

KONEMAN, E. W., MIALE, J. B. & MASON, A. (1963). Current biochemical and genetic concepts in the diagnosis of sickle cell-thalassemia. A study of 8 families. *Amer. J. clin. Path.*, 40, 1–20.

KONOTEY-AHULU, F. I. D. (1974). The sickle cell diseases. Clinical manifestations including the "sickle crisis". *Arch. intern. Med.*, 133, 611–619.

KONOTEY-AHULU, F. I. D., GALLO, E., LEHMANN, H. & RINGELHANN, B. (1968). Haemoglobin Korle-Bu (β73 aspartic acid → asparagine): showing one of the two amino acid substitutions of haemoglobin C Harlem. *J. Med. Genet.*, 5, 107–111.

KONETEY-AHULU, F. I. D., KINDERLERER, J. L., LEHMANN, H. & RINGELHANN, B. (1971). Haemoglobin Osu-Christianborg: a new β chain variant of haemoglobin A (β52(D3) aspartic acid → asparagine) in combination with haemoglobin S. *J. med. Genet.*, 8, 302–305.

KONOTEY-AHULU, F. I. D. & RINGELHANN, B. (1969). Sickle-cell anaemia, sickle-cell thalassaemia, sickle-cell haemoglobin C disease, and asymptomatic haemoglobin C thalassaemia in one Ghanaian family. *Brit. med. J.*, i, 607–612.

KRAUS, A. P., MIYAJI, T., IUCHI, I. & KRAUS, L. M.

(1967). Hemoglobin Memphis/S. A new variant of sickle-cell anemia. *Trans. Ass. Amer. Phycns*, **80**, 297–304.

LAROS, R. K. JNR, & KALSTONE, C. E. (1971). Sickle cell β-thalassemia and pregnancy. *Obstet. and Gynec.*, **37**, 67–71.

LAU, F. Y. K. (1959). Pulmonary infarction and atrophy of the spleen associated with sickle-cell hemoglobin C disease. *New Engl. J. Med.*, **260**, 907–911.

LAWRENCE, J. S., NEEL, J. V. & ITANO, H. A. (1952). Hemolytic anemia presumably due to coexistence of the genes for thalassemia and sickling. *Trans. Ass. Amer. Phycns*, **65**, 203–213.

LECOCQ, F. R. & HARPER, J. Y. JNR (1963). Sickle-cell hemoglobulin C crisis precipitation by fever therapy. *Arch. intern. Med.*, **111**, 149–152.

LIE-INJO, L. E., HASSAN, K., JOISHY, S. K. & LIM, M. L. (1986). Sickle cell anemia associated with α-thalassemia in Malaysian Indians. *Amer. J. Hemat.*, **22**, 265–274.

LIE-INJO, L. E., WANG, A. C. & BURNETT, R. C. (1968). Another family showing the interaction of the genes for Hb G and Hb S. *Acta haemat. (Basel)*, **40**, 286–298.

LOHMULLER, H. W. & MARSHALL, J. F.(1958). Hemoglobin C-S disease complicated by paracolon osteomyelitis. *Arch. intern. Med.*, **101**, 761–764.

McCURDY, P. R. & GIESCHEN, M. M. (1960). Clinical and physiologic studies in a Negro with sickle-cell haemoglobin D disease. *New Engl. J. Med.*, **262**, 961–964.

McCURDY, P. R., LORKIN, P. A., CASEY, R., LEHMANN, H., UDDIN, D. E. & DICKSON, L. G. (1974). Hemoglobin S-G(S-D) syndrome. *Amer. J. Med.*, **57**, 665–670.

McCURDY, P. R., MAHMOOD, L. & SHERMAN, A. S. (1975). Red cell life span in sickle cell-hemoglobin C disease with a note about sickle cell-hemoglobin O$_{ARAB}$. *Blood*, **45**, 273–279.

McCURDY, P. R., SHERMAN, A. S., KAMUZORA, H. & LEHMANN, H. (1975). Globin synthesis in subjects doubly heterozygous for hemoglobin G-Philadelphia and hemoglobin S or C. *J. Lab. clin. Med.*, **85**, 891–897.

MacIVER, J. E. & PARKER-WILLIAMS, E. J. (1961). The aplastic crisis in sickle-cell anaemia. *Lancet*, **i**, 1086–1089.

MacIVER, J. E. & WENT, L. N. (1958). Further observations on abnormal haemoglobins in Jamaica. *W. Indian med. J.*, **7**, 109–122.

MacIVER, J. E., WENT, L. N. & CRUICKSHANK, E. K. (1958). Sickle cell-thalassemia disease in Jamaica. *Blood*, **13**, 359–366.

MacIVER, J. E., WENT, L. N. & IRVINE, R. A. (1961). Hereditary persistence of foetal haemoglobin: a family study suggesting allelism of the F gene to the S and C haemoglobin genes. *Brit. J. Haemat.*, **7**, 373–381.

MALAMOS, B., BELCHER, E. H., GYFTAKI, E. & BINOPOULOS, D. (1961). Simultaneous radioactive tracer studies of erythropoiesis and red-cell destruction in thalassaemia. *Brit. J. Haemat.*, **7**, 411–429.

MALAMOS, B., BELCHER, E. H., GYFTAKI, E. & BINOPOULOS, D. (1963). Simultaneous radioactive tracer studies of erythropoiesis and red-cell destruction in sickle-cell disease and sickle-cell haemoglobin/thalassaemia. *Brit. J. Haemat.*, **9**, 487–498.

MARTINEZ, G., FERREIRA, R., HERNANDEZ, A., DI RIENZO, A. & COLOMBO, B. (1986). Association of Hb H disease with sickle-trait. *Hemoglobin*, **10**, 421–425.

MATTHAY, K. K., MENTZER, W. C., DOZY, A. M., KAN, Y. W. & BAINTON, D. F. (1979). Modification of hemoglobin H disease by sickle trait. *J. clin. Invest.*, **64**, 1024–1032.

MEARS, J. G., SCHOENBRUN, M., SCHAEFER, K. E., BESLAK, M. & RADEL, E. (1982). Frequent association of alpha thalassemia with splenic sequestration crisis and splenomegaly in sickle cell (SS) subjects. *Blood*, **60**, No. 5 (Suppl. 1), 47a (Abstract 115).

MILNER, P. F., MILLER, C., GREY, R., SEAKINS, M., DEJONG, W. W. & WENT, L. N. (1970). Hemoglobin O Arab in four negro families and its interaction with hemoglobin S and hemoglobin C. *New Engl. J. Med.*, **283**, 1417–1425.

MONTI, A., FELDHAKE, C. & SCHWARTZ, S. O. (1964). The S-thalassemia syndrome. *Ann N.Y. Acad. Sci.*, **119**, 474–484.

MOO-PEN, W., BECHTEL, K., JUE, D., CHAN, M. S., HOPKINS, G., SCHNEIDER, N. J., WRIGHT, J. & SCHMIDT, R. M. (1975). The presence of hemoglobin S and C Harlem in an individual in the United States. *Blood*, **46**, 363–367.

MOTULSKY, A. G. (1954). Sicklemia. *J. Amer. med. Ass.*, **155**, 388 (Letter).

MOVITT, E. R., MANGUM, J. F. & PORTER, W. R. (1963). Sickle cell-hemoglobin C disease. Quantitative determination of iron kinetics and hemoglobin synthesis. *Blood*, **21**, 535–545.

MURPHY, R. J. C., MALHOTRA, C. & SWEET, A. Y. (1980). Death following an exchange transfusion with hemoglobin SC blood. *J. Pediat.*, **96**, 110–112.

NAIL, S. K., KOTHARI, B. V., JHAVERI, C. L., SUKUMARAN, P. K. & SANGHVI, L. D. (1957). Fatal hemolytic anemia presumably due to the combination of sickle cell and thalassemia gene. *Indian J. med. Sci.*, **11**, 244–249

NATTA, C. (1978). Failure of the α-thalassemia gene to decrease the severity of sickle cell anemia. *Blood*, **51**, 1163–1168.

NATTA, C. L., NIAZI, G. A., FORDS, S. & BANK, A. (1974). Balanced globin chain synthesis in hereditary persistence of fetal hemoglobin. *J. clin.*

Invest., **54**, 433–438.

NEEL, J. V. (1952). Perspectives in the genetics of sickle cell disease. *Blood*, **7**, 467–471.

NEEL, J. V., HIERNAUZ, J., LINHARD, J., ROBINSON, A., ZUELZER, W. W. & LIVINGSTONE, F. B. (1956). Data on the occurrence of haemoglobin C and other abnormal haemoglobins in some African populations. *Amer. J. hum. Genet.*, **8**, 138–150.

NEEL, J. V., ITANO, H. A. & LAWRENCE, J. S. (1953). Two cases of sickle cell disease presumably due to the combination of the genes for thalassemia and sickle cell hemoglobin. *Blood*, **8**, 434–443.

NEEL, J. V., KAPLAN, E. & ZUELZER, W. W. (1953). Further studies on hemoglobin C. I. A description of three additional families segregating for hemoglobin C and sickle cell hemoglobin. *Blood*, **8**, 724–734.

NOGUCHI. C. T., DOVER, G. J., RODGERS, G. P., SERJEANT, G. R., ANTONARAKIS, S. E., ANAGNOU, N. P., HIGGS, D. R., WEATHERALL, D. J. & SCHECHTER, A. N. (1985). Alpha thalassemia changes erythrocyte heterogeneity in sickle cell disease. *J. clin. Invest.*, **75**, 1632–1637.

OBER, W. B., BRUNO, M. S., SIMON, R. M. & WEINER, L. (1959). Hemoglobin S-C disease with fat embolism. Report of patient dying in crisis; autopsy findings. *Amer. J. Med.*, **27**, 647–658.

OGDEN, M. A. (1943). Sickle cell anemia in the White race, with report of cases in two families. *Arch. intern. Med.*, **71**, 164–182.

O'GORMAN, P., ALLSOPP, K. M., LEHMANN, H. & SUKUMARAN, P. K. (1963). Sickle-cell haemoglobin K disease. *Brit. med. J.*, **ii**, 1381–1382.

ONUAGULUCHI, G., & AKANDE, E. O. (1966). Severe crises with jaundice in young non-pregnant adults with sickle-cell haemoglobin-C disease. *Lancet*, **i**, 737–739.

OZSOYLU, S. (1969). Haemoglobin S-D disease in a Turkish family. *Scand. J. Haemat.*, **6**, 10–14.

PARDOLL, D. M., RODEHEFFER, R. J., SMITH, R. R. L. & CHARACHE, S. (1982). Aplastic crisis due to extensive bone marrow necrosis in sickle cell disease. *Arch. intern. Med.*, **142**, 2223–2225.

PATON, D. (1961). The conjunctival sign of sickle-cell disease. *Arch. Ophthal.*, **66**, 90–94.

PATON, D. (1962). The conjunctival sign of sickle-cell disease. *Arch. Ophthal.*, **68**, 627–632.

PEARSON, H. A. (1969). Hemoglobin S-thalassaemia syndrome in Negro children. *Ann. N.Y. Acad. Sci.*, **165**, 83–92.

PEARSON, H. A., MCINTOSH, S., RITCHEY, A. K., LOBEL. J. S., ROOKS, Y. & JOHNSTON, D. (1979). Developmental aspects of splenic function in sickle cell diseases. *Blood*, **53**, 358–365.

PLATT, O. S., ROSENSTOCK, W. & ESPELAND, M. A. (1984). Influence of sickle hemoglobinopathies on growth and development. *New Engl. J. Med.*, **311**, 7–12.

PORTNOY, B. A. & HERION, J. C. (1972).

Neurological manifestations in sickle-cell disease, with a review of the literature and emphasis on the prevelance of hemiplegia. *Ann. intern. Med.*, **76**, 643–652.

POWELL, W. N., RODARTE, J. G. & NEEL, J. V. (1950). The occurrence in a family of Sicilian ancestry of the traits for both sickling and thalassemia. *Blood*, **5**, 887–897.

PUGH, R. P., MONICAL, T. V. & MINNICH, V. (1964). Sickle cell anemia with two adult hemoglobins — Hb S and HbG$_{Philadelphia}$/S. *Blood*, **23**, 206–215.

RAMOT, B., FISHER, S., REMEZ, D., SCHNEERSON, R., KAHANE, D., AGER, J. A. M. & LEHMANN, H. (1960). Haemoglobin O in an Arab family. Sickle-cell haemoglobin O trait. *Brit. med. J.*, **ii** 1262–1264.

RAO, K. R. P., PATEL, A. R., SHAH, P. C. & VOHRA, R. M. (1980). Sickle cell dactylitis. *Arch. intern. Med.*, **140**, 439 (Letter).

REICH, R. S. & ROSENBERG, N. J. (1953). Aseptic necrosis of bone in Caucasians with chronic hemolytic anemia due to combined sickling and thalassaemia traits. *J. Bone Joint Surg.*, **35A**, 894–904.

RESTREPO, A. M. & LONDOÑO, O. G. (1965). Sickle cell hemoglobin D disease in a Negro Colombian patient. *Ann. intern. Med.*, **62**, 1301–1306.

REYNOLDS, J. (1962). Roentgenographic and clinical appraisal of sickle cell-hemoglobin C disease. *Amer. J. Roentgenol.*, **88**, 512–522.

REYNOLDS, W. A. (1962). Benign sickle cell-thalassemia disease and cryptic thalassemia in a Negro family. *Ann. intern. Med.*, **57**, 121–128.

RHODA, M. D., AROUS, N., GAREL, M. C., MAZARIN, M., MONPLAISIR, N., BRACONNIER, F., ROSA, J., COHEN-SOLAL, M. & GALACTEROS, F. (1986). Interaction of hemoglobin Siriraj with hemoglobin S: a mild sickle cell syndrome. *Hemoglobin*, **10**, 21–31.

RINGELHANN, B. & KHORSANDI, M. (1972). Hemoglobin crystallization test to differentiate cells with Hb SC and CC genotype from SS cells without electrophoresis. *Amer. J. clin. Path.*, **57**, 467–470.

RINGELHANN, B., KONOTEY-AHULU, F. I. D., TALAPATRA, N. C., NKRUMAH, F. K., WILTSHIRE, B. G. & LEHMANN, H. (1971). Haemoglobin K Woolwich ($\alpha_2\beta_2$ 132 lysine → glutamine) in Ghana. *Acta haemat. (Basel)*, **45**, 250–258.

RINGELHANN, B., LEWIS, R. A., LORKIN, P. A., KYNOCH, P. A. M. & LEHMANN, H. (1967). Sickle cell haemoglobin D Punjab disease: S from Ghana and D from England. *Acta haemat. (Basel)*, **38**, 324–331.

RIVER, G. L., ROBBINS, A. B., SCHWARTZ, S. O. & FELDHAKE, C. (1961). S-C hemoglobin: a clinical study. *Blood*, **18**, 385–416.

ROCHE, J., DERRIEN, Y., DIACONO, G., DURIEUX, J., LAURENT, G., REYNAUD, J., ROUX, M. & BRANGIER, J. (1956). Coexistence des tares sicklémique et thalassémique dans une famille tunisienne. Conséquences hématologiques. *Rev. Hémat.*, **11**, 26–48.

RODGERS, G. M., BARRERA, E. JNR & MARTIN, R. R. (1980). *Bacillus cereus* bacteremia and hemolytic anemia in a patient with hemoglobin SC disease. *Arch. intern. Med.*, **140**, 1103–1104.

RODGERS, G. P., DOVER, G. J., NOGUCHI, C. T., SERJEANT, G. R., ANTONARAKIS, S. E., ANAGNOU, N. P., HIGGS, D. R. & SCHECTER, A. N. (1983). α thalassemia changes cell density and hemoglobin F in sickle cell disease. *Blood*, **62**, No. 5 (Suppl. 1), 60a (Abstract 144).

ROSENFIELD, S. & PINCUS, J. B. (1932). The occurrence of sicklemia in the White race. *Amer. J. med. Sci.*, **184**, 674–682.

ROTTER, R., LUTTGENS, W. F., PETERSON, W. L., STOCK, A. E. & MOTULSKY, A. G. (1956). Splenic infarction in sicklemia during airplane flight: pathogenesis, hemoglobin analysis and clinical features of six cases. *Ann. intern. Med.*, **44**, 257–270.

RUDD, C., EVANS, P. J. & PEENEY, A. L. P. (1953). Ocular complications in thalassaemia minor. *Brit. J. Ophthal.*, **37**, 353–358.

RUSSO, G., LA GRUTTA, A. & MOLLICA, A. (1963). Sulla eterogeneita della thalassemia. Contributo casistico ed interpretazione biochimica e genetica. *Riv. pediat. sicil.*, **18**, 239–241.

RUSSO, G. & MOLLICA, F. (1962). Sickle cell haemoglobin and two types of thalassaemia in the same family. *Acta haemat. (Basel)*, **28**, 329–340.

RYWLIN, A. M., BLOCK, A. L. & WERNER, C. S. (1963). Hemoglobin C and S disease in pregnancy. Report of a case with bone marrow and fat embolism. *Amer. J. Obstet. Gynec.*, **86**, 1055–1059.

SCHNEIDER, R. G., TAKEDA, I., GUSTAVSON, L. P. & ALPERIN, J. B. (1972). Intraerythrocytic precipitations of haemoglobins S and C. *Nature new Biol.*, **235**, 88–90.

SCHNEIDER, R. G., UEDA, S., ALPERIN, J. B., LEVIN, W. C., JONES, R. T. & BRIMHALL, B. (1968). Hemoglobin D Los Angeles in two Caucasian families: hemoglobin SD disease and hemoglobin D thalassemia. *Blood*, **32**, 250–259.

SCHWARTZ, H. C., SPAET, T. H., ZUELZER, W. W., NEEL, J. V., ROBINSON, A. R. & KAUFMAN, S. F. (1957). Combinations of hemoglobin G, hemoglobin S and thalassemia occurring in one family. *Blood*, **12**, 238–250.

SEARS, D. A. & UDDEN, M. M. (1985). Splenic infarction, splenic sequestration, and functional hyposplenism in hemoglobin S-C disease. *Amer. J. Hemat.*, **18**, 261–268.

SEELER, R. A. (1983). Exophthalmos in hemoglobin SC disease. *J. Pediat.*, **102**, 90–91.

SEIDLER, R. C. & BECKER, J. A. (1964). Intrathoracic extramedullary hematopoiesis. *Radiology*, **83**, 1057–1059.

SERJEANT, B. E., MASON, K. P., CONDON, P. I., HAYES, R. J., KENNY, M. W., STUART, J. & SERJEANT, G. R. (1984). Blood rheology and proliferative retinopathy in sickle cell–haemoglobin C disease. *Brit. J. Ophthal.*, **68**, 325–328.

SERJEANT, B. E., MASON, K. P., KENNY, M. W., STUART, J., HIGGS, D. R., WEATHERALL, D. J., HAYES, R. J. & SERJEANT, G. R. (1983). Effect of alpha thalassaemia on the rheology of homozygous sickle cell disease. *Brit. J. Haemat.*, **55**, 479–486.

SERJEANT, G. R. (1974). *The Clinical Features of Sickle Cell Disease*. 357 pp. North-Holland Publishing Company, Amsterdam, Oxford.

SERJEANT, G. R. (1981) Observations on the epidemiology of sickle cell disease. *Proc. roy Soc. trop. Med. Hyg.*, **75**, 228–233.

SERJEANT, G. R. (1985). *Sickle Cell Disease*. 478 pp. Oxford University Press.

SERJEANT, G. R., ASHCROFT, M. T. & SERJEANT, B. E. (1973). The clinical features of haemoglobin SC disease in Jamaica. *Brit. J. Haemat.*, **24**, 491–501.

SERJEANT, G. R., ASHCROFT, M. T., SERJEANT, B. E. & MILNER, P. F. (1973). The clinical features of sickle-cell/β thalassaemia in Jamaica. *Brit. J. Haemat.*, **24**, 19–30.

SERJEANT, G. R., ENNIS, J. T. & MIDDLEMISS, J. H. (1973a). Haemoglobin SC disease in Jamaica. *Brit. J. Radiol.*, **46**, 935–950.

SERJEANT, G. R., ENNIS, J. T. & MIDDLEMISS, H. (1973b). Sickle cell β thalassaemia in Jamaica. *Brit. J. Radiol.*, **46**, 951–959.

SERJEANT, G. R. & SERJEANT, B. E. (1972). A comparison of erythrocyte characteristics in sickle cell syndromes in Jamaica. *Brit. J. Haemat.*, **23**, 205–213.

SERJEANT, G. R., SERJEANT, B. E. & MASON, K. (1977). Heterocellular hereditary persistence of fetal haemoglobin and homozygous sickle-cell disease. *Lancet*, **i**, 795–796 (Letter).

SERJEANT, G. R., SOMMEREUX, A.-M., STEVENSON, M., MASON, K. & SERJEANT, B. E. (1979). Comparison of sickle cell-β^0 thalassaemia with homozygous sickle cell disease. *Brit. J. Haemat.*, **41**, 83–93.

SHAEFFER, J. R., MOAKE, J. L. & KLEVE, L. (1976). Sickle cell-β^0 thalassaemia variant with high hemoglobin F and mild clinical course. *Amer. J. Med.*, **61**, 437–438.

SHALDON, S. (1961). Megaloblastic erythropoiesis associated with sickle cell anaemia. *Brit. med J.*, **i**, 640–641.

SHELLEY, W. M. & CURTIS, E. M. (1958). Bone marrow and fat embolism in sickle cell anemia and sickle cell-hemoglobin C disease. *Bull. Johns Hopk. Hosp.*, **103**, 8–25.

SHIELDS, G. S., WETHERS, D., GAVIS, G. & WATSON, R. J. (1956). Hemoglobin-S-thalassemia disease. Report of a case in a negro child. *Amer. J. Dis.*

Child., **91**, 485–489.

SHUKLA, R. N. & SOLANKI, B. R. (1957). Inherited chronic hemolytic anemia. Interaction of hemoglobin 'S' with thalassemia. *Indian J. med. Sci.*, **11**, 722–727.

SILVER, H. K., SIMON, J. L. & CLEMENT, D. H. (1957). Salmonella osteomyelitis and abnormal hemoglobin disease. *Pediatrics*, **20**, 439–447.

SILVESTRONI, E. & BIANCO, I. (1944–45). Micro-drepanocito-anemia in un sogetto di razza bianca. *Boll. Accad. med. Roma*, **70**, 347–351.

SILVESTRONI, E. & BIANCO, I. (1946). Una nuova entita nosologica: "la malattia micro-drepanocitica". *Haematologica*, **29**, 455–488.

SILVESTRONI, E. & BIANCO, I. (1952). Genetic aspects of sickle cell anemia and microdrepanocytic disease. *Blood*, **7**, 429–435.

SILVESTRONI, E. & BIANCO, I. (1955). New data on microdrepanocytic disease. *Blood*, **10**, 623–632.

SILVESTRONI, E. & BIANCO, I. (1963). Una nuova varietà di anemia drepanocitica: la malattia da Hb S-Hb Lepore. *Progr. Med. (Napoli)*, **19**, 545–548.

SILVESTRONI, E. & BIANCO, I. (1964). Un caso di malattia microdrepanocitica da Hb S e varietà di microcitemia con quota normale di Hb A_2 e quota elevata di Hb F. *Progr. med. (Napoli)*, **20**, 509–513.

SILVESTRONI, E., BIANCO, I. & BAGLIONI, C. (1965). Interaction of hemoglobin Lepore with sickle cell trait and microcythemia (thalassemia) in a southern Italian family. *Blood*, **25**, 457–469.

SINGER, K., JOSEPHSON, A. M., SINGER, L., HELLER, P. & ZIMMERMAN, H. J. (1957). Studies on abnormal hemoglobins. XIII. Hemoglobin S-thalassemia disease and hemoglobin C-thalassemia disease in siblings. *Blood*, **12**, 593–602.

SINGER, K., SINGER, L. & GOLDBERG, S. R. (1955). Studies on abnormal hemoglobins. XI. Sickle cell-thalassemia disease in the negro. The significance of the S+A+F and S+A patterns obtained by hemoglobin analysis. *Blood*, **10**, 405–415.

SMITH, E. W. & CONLEY, C. L. (1954). Clinical features of the genetic variants of sickle cell disease. *Bull. Johns Hopk. Hosp.*, **94**, 289–318.

SMITH, E. W. & CONLEY, C. L. (1955). Sicklemia and infarction of the spleen during aerial flight. Electrophoresis of the hemoglobin in 15 cases. *Bull. Johns Hopk. Hosp.*, **96**, 35–41.

SMITH, E. W. & CONLEY, C. L. (1959). Sickle cell-hemoglobin D disease. *Ann. intern. Med.*, **50**, 94–105.

SMITH, E. W. & KREVANS, J. R. (1959). Clinical manifestations of hemoglobin C disorders. *Bull. Johns Hopk. Hosp.*, **104**, 17–43.

SOLANKI, D. L. & KLETTER, G. G. (1984). Acute splenic sequestration crises (ASSC) in adults with sickle cell disease. *Blood*, **64**, No. 5 (Suppl. 1), 53a (Abstract 122).

STAMATOYANNOPOULOS, G. & FESSAS, PH. (1963). Observations on hemoglobin "Pylos": the hemoglobin Pylos-hemoglobin S combination. *J. Lab. clin. Med.*, **62**, 193–200.

STAMATOYANNOPOULOS, G., SOFRONIADOU, G. C. & AKRIVAKIS, A. (1967). Absence of hemoglobin A in a double heterozygote for F-thalassemia and hemoglobin S. *Blood*, **30**, 772–776.

STAMATOYANNOPOULOS, G., WOOD, W. G., PAPAYANNOPOULOU, TH. & NUTE P. E. (1975). A new form of hereditary persistence of fetal hemoglobin in blacks and its association with sickle cell trait. *Blood*. **46**, 683–692.

STEINBERG, M. H., ADAMS, J. G. III & DREILING, B. J. (1975). Alpha thalassaemia in adults with sickle-cell trait. *Brit. J. Haemat.*, **30**, 31–37.

STEINBERG, M. H., ADAMS, J. G., THIGPEN, J. T., MORRISON, F. S. & DREILING, B. J. (1974). Hemoglobin Hope ($\alpha_2\beta_2^{136\text{-gly-asp}}$)-S disease; clinical and biochemical studies. *J. Lab. clin. Med.*, **84**, 632–642.

STEINBERG, M. H., COLEMAN, M. B., ADAMS, J. G., RIEDER, E., PLATICA, O., CEDENO, M., MILNER, P., WEST, S., ROSENSTOCK, W. & THE COOPERATIVE STUDY OF SICKLE CELL DISEASE (1983). Effects of α-thalassemia and microcytosis upon the hematological and vaso-occlusive severity of sickle cell anemia. *Blood* **62**, No. 5 (Suppl. 1), 61a (Abstract 148).

STEINBERG, M. H. & DREILING, B. J. (1976). Clinical, hematologic and biosynthetic studies in sickle cell-β^0-thalassemia: a comparison with sickle cell anemia. *Amer. J. Haemat.*, **1**, 35–44.

STEINBERG, M. H. & HEBBEL, R. P. (1983). Clinical diversity of sickle cell anemia: genetic and cellular modulation of disease severity. *Amer. J. Hemat.*, **14**, 405–416.

STEINBERG, M. H., ROSENSTOCK, W., COLEMAN, M. B., ADAMS, J. G., PLATICA, O., CEDENO, M., RIEDER, R. F., WILSON, J. T., MILNER, P., WEST, S. & THE COOPERATIVE STUDY OF SICKLE CELL DISEASE (1984). Effects of thalassemia and microcytosis on the hematologic and vasoocclusive severity of sickle cell anemia. *Blood*, **63**, 1353–1360.

STEVENS, M. C, G., LEHMANN, H., MASON, K. P., SERJEANT, B. E. & SERJEANT, G. R. (1982). Sickle cell-Hb Lepore$_{Boston}$ syndrome. Uncommon differential diagnosis of homozygous sickle cell disease. *Amer. J. Dis. Child.*, **136**, 19–22.

STEVENS, M. C. G., MAUDE, G. H., BECKFORD, M., GRANDISON, Y., MASON, K., SERJEANT, B. E., TAYLOR, B., TOPLEY, J. M. & SERJEANT, G. R. (1985). Haematological change in sickle cell–haemoglobin C disease and in sickle cell–beta thalassaemia: a cohort study from birth. *Brit. J. Haemat.*, **60**, 279–292.

STEVENS, M. C. G., MAUDE, G. H., BECKFORD, M., GRANDISON, Y., MASON, K., TAYLOR, B., SERJEANT, B. E., HIGGS, D. R., TEAL, H., WEATHERALL, D. J. & SERJEANT, G. R. (1986). α-thalassemia and the hematology of homozygous sickle cell disease in childhood. *Blood.* **67**, 411–414.

STEVENS, M. C. G., MAUDE, G. H., HIGGS, D. R., WEATHERALL, D. J. & SERJEANT, G. R. (1984). Alpha thalassemia and the hematology of homozygous sickle cell disease in childhood. *Blood*, **64**, No. 5 (Suppl. 1), 54a (Abstract 125).

STEVENS, M. C. G., MAUDE, G. H. & SERJEANT, G. R. (1984). The hematology of Hb SC disease in childhood. *Blood*, **64**, No. 5 (Suppl. 1), 54a (Abstract 126).

STEWART, J. W. & MacIVER, J. E. (1956). Sickle-cell/haemoglobin-D disease in a Mulatto girl. *Lancet*, **i**, 23–25.

STURGEON, P., ITANO, H. A. & BERGREN, W. R. (1955). Clinical manifestations of inherited abnormal hemoglobins. I. The interaction of hemoglobin-S with hemoglobin-D. *Blood*, **10**, 389–404.

STURGEON, P., ITANO, H. A. & VALENTINE, W. N. (1953). Chronic hemolytic anemia associated with thalassemia and sickling traits. *Blood*, **7**, 350–357.

SULLIVAN, B. H., JNR (1950). Danger of airplane flight to persons with sicklemia. *Ann. intern. Med.*, **32**, 338–342.

TALBOT, J. F., BIRD, A. C. & SERJEANT. G. R. (1983). Retinal changes in sickle cell/hereditary persistence of fetal hemoglobin syndrome. *Brit. J. Ophthal.*, **67**, 777–778.

TATSIS, B., SOFRONIADOU, K. & STERGIOPOULOS, C. I. (1976). Hemoglobin Pyrgos $\alpha_2\beta_2^{83(EF7)Gly \rightarrow Asp}$. A new hemoglobin variant in double heterozygosity with hemoglobin S. *Blood*, **47**, 827–832.

THOMPSON, G. R. & LEHMANN, H. (1962). Combination of high levels of haemoglobin F with haemoglobin A, S, and C in Ghana. *Brit. med. J.*, **i**, 1521–1523.

THOMPSON, R. B., HEWITT, B. JNR, ORD, E., ODOM, J. & BELL, W. N. (1966). A new thalassemic syndrome: homozygous hemoglobin S disease delta thalassemia. *Acta haemat. (Basel)*, **36**, 412–417.

THOMPSON, R. B. & ROBERTSON, M. G. (1964). Three inherited intra-erythrocytic defects: hereditary spherocytosis, Hb S and Hb C. *Acta haemat. (Basel)*. **32**, 233–238.

TOPLEY, J. M., CUPIDORE, L., VAIDYA, S., HAYES, R. J. & SERJEANT, G. R. (1982). Pneumococcal and other infections in children with sickle cell–hemoglobin C (SC) disease. *J. Pediat.*, **101**, 176–179.

TOPLEY, J. M., OBEID, D. & MANN, J. R. (1977). Acute splenic sequestration crisis preceded by hypersplenism in haemoglobin SC disease. *Brit. med. J.*, **i**, 617–618.

TUTTLE, A. H. & KOCH, B. (1960). Clinical and hematological manifestations of hemoglobin CS disease in children. *J. Pediat.*, **56**, 331–342.

URIARTE, A., ATENCIO, R. P. & COLOMBO, B. (1973). Haemoglobin D Punjab in a Cuban family and its interaction with haemoglobin S. *Acta haemat. (Basel)*, **50**, 315–320.

VANDERPITTE, J. & COLAERT, J. (1955). Un cas de syndrome falciforme dû à l'interaction de deux hémoglobines anormales C et S. *Ann. Soc. belge Méd. trop.*, **35**, 457–464.

VAN ENK, A., LANG, A., WHITE, J. M. & LEHMANN, H. (1972). Benign obstetric history in women with sickle-cell anaemia associated with α-thalassaemia. *Brit. med. J.*, **iv**, 524–526.

VAN ROS, G., SEYNHAEVE, V. & FIASSE, L. (1976). β^+-thalassaemia, haemoglobin S and hereditary elliptocytosis in a Zaïrian family. Ischaemic costal necroses in a child with sickle cell β^+-thalassaemia *Acta haemat. (Basel)*, **56**, 241–252.

VERANI, R., OLSON, J. & MOAKE, J. L. (1980). Intrathoracic extramedullary hematopoiesis. Report of a case in a patient with sickle-cell disease — β-thalassemia. *Amer. J. clin. Path.*, **73**, 133–136.

WADE, L. J. & STEVENSON, L. D. (1941). Necrosis of the bone marrow with fat embolism in sickle cell anemia. *Amer. J. Path.*, **17**, 47–54.

WALTERS, J. H. & YOUNG, N. A. F. (1954). Micro-drepanocytic disease associated with megaloblastic anaemia of pregnancy. *Trans. roy. Soc. trop. Med. Hyg.*, **48**, 253–260.

WASSERMAN, C. F., PHELPS, V. R. & HERTZOG, A. J. (1952). Chronic hemolytic anemia in a white child due to thalassemia and sicklemia, with a genealogic survey. *Pediatrics*, **9**, 286–289.

WATSON-WILLIAMS, E. J., BEALE, D., IRVINE, D. & LEHMANN, H. (1965). A new haemoglobin, D Ibadan (β-87 threonine → lysine), producing no sickle-cell haemoglobin D disease with haemoglobin S. *Nature (Lond.)*, **205**, 1273–1276.

WEATHERALL, D. J. (1964a). Biochemical phenotypes of thalassemia in the American negro population. *Ann. N.Y. Acad. Sci.*, **119**, 450–462.

WEATHERALL, D. J. (1964b). Hemoglobin J$_{(Baltimore)}$ coexisting in a family with hemoglobin S. *Bull. Johns Hopk. Hosp.*, **114**, 1–12.

WEATHERALL, D. J. & CLEGG, J. B. (1981). *The Thalassaemia Syndromes.* 875 pp. Blackwell Scientific Publications, Oxford.

WEATHERALL, D. J., CLEGG, J. B., BLANKSON, J. & McNEIL, J. R. (1969). A new sickling disorder resulting from interaction of the genes for haemoglobin S and α-thalassaemia. *Brit. J. Haemat.*, **17**, 517–526.

WEINER, S. B. (1937). Sickle-cell anemia in Italian child. A case report. *J. Mt Sinai Hosp.*, **4**, 88–91.

WELCH, R. B. & GOLDBERG, M. F. (1966). Sickle-cell hemoglobin and its relation to fundus abnormality. *Arch. Ophthal.*, **75**, 353–362.

WENT, L. N. & MacIVER, J. E. (1958a). Sickle-cell anemia in adults and its differentiation from sickle-cell thalassaemia. *Lancet*, **ii**, 824–826.

WENT, L. N. & MacIVER, J. E. (1958b). An unusual type of hemoglobinopathy resembling sickle cell thalassemia in a Jamaican family. *Blood*, **13**, 559–568.

WENT, L. N. & MacIVER, J. E. (1959). Sickle-cell/haemoglobin-J disease. *Brit. med. J.*, ii, 138–139.

WIDEN, A. L. & CARDON, L. (1961). Salmonella typhimurium osteomyelitis with sickle cell-hemoglobin C disease: review and case report. *Ann. intern. Med.*, **54**, 510–521.

WONG, S. C., ALI, M. A. M. & BOYADJIAN, S. E. (1981). Sickle cell traits in Canada. Trimodal distribution of Hb S as a result of interaction with α-thalassaemia gene. *Acta haemat. (Basel)*, **65**, 157–163.

WOOD, W. G., WEATHERALL, D. J. & CLEGG, J. B. (1976). Interaction of heterocellular hereditary persistence of foetal haemoglobin with β thalassaemia and sickle cell anaemia. *Nature (Lond.)*, **264**, 247–249.

WRIGHTSTONE, R. N., HUBBARD, M. & HUISMAN, T. H. J. (1974). Hemoglobin S-Gα Georgia disease: a case report. *Acta haemat. (Basel)*, **51**, 315–320.

WRIGHTSTONE, R. N. & HUISMAN, T. H. J. (1974). On the levels of hemoglobins F and A_2 in sickle-cell anemia and some related disorders. *Amer. J. clin. Path.*, **61**, 375–381.

YEUNG, K.-Y. & LESSIN, L. S. (1976). Splenic infarction in sickle cell-hemoglobin C disease. Demonstration by selective splenic arteriogram and scintillation scan. *Arch. intern. Med.*, **136**, 905–911.

ZELKOWITZ, L., TORRES, C., BHOOPALAM, N., YAKULIS, V. J. & HELLER, P. (1972). Double heterozygous βδ-thalassemia in negroes. *Arch. intern. Med.*, **129**, 975–979.

ZIPERMAN, H. H. & GRAHAM. J. L. (1962). Abdominal crises associated with sicklemia and airplane flights. A report of two cases. *Amer. J. Surg.*, **103**, 269–271.

ZUELZER, W. W. (1957). Hemoglobinopathies. *Fed. Proc.*, **16**, 769–773.

ZUELZER, W. W., NEEL, J. V. & ROBINSON, A. R. (1956). Abnormal hemoglobins. *Progr. Hemat.*, **1**, 91–137. Grune and Stratton, New York.

14

Sickle-cell disease IV: pathology, the sickling phenomenon and pathogenesis

FINDINGS AT NECROPSY

The usual gross findings at necropsy are the signs of anaemia and cardiac failure, hepatomegaly and haemosiderosis and often, too, evidence of infection. The spleen is characteristically small and fibrotic, but may be enlarged in young children, and there may be evidence of infarction of other organs. The bone marrow is hyperplastic and increased in extent. Diggs (1973) published a full review of the anatomical lesions of sickle-cell disease based on necropsies performed in Memphis, other pathological material, and data extracted from an extensive literature. Serjeant (1985), too, dealt with the pathology of sickle-cell disease in considerable detail, and some of his illustrations are reproductions of photographs provided by Dr Diggs. It is only possible in the present text to provide a summary of the main findings and of certain key publications.

Early reports

The first published record of the findings *post mortem* in a case of sickle-cell disease appears to be that of Sydenstricker, Mulherin and Houseal (1923). This is a remarkably good account: the small size of the spleen was mentioned and was regard as the consequence of repeated haemorrhages. The distribution of many 'brown granules' in the liver and kidney was thought to be strongly in favour of a haemolytic origin for the patient's anaemia. In films of bone marrow made *post mortem* filiform erythrocytes of up to 49 μm in length were noted. Graham (1924), too, recounted in detail the post-mortem findings in a 30-year-old male suffering from sickle-cell anaemia who had been admitted to hospital with a tentative diagnosis of acute meningitis. There were no gross lesions in the brain but *Str. haemolyticus* was grown from his blood. The spleen was atrophic.

Hein, McCalla and Thorne (1927) summarized the most prominent post-mortem findings in a 20-year-old male who had died of peritonitis following a perforated duodenal ulcer as 'extreme splenic atrophy and general signs of increased hemolysis'. Another relatively early and detailed account is that of Diggs and Ching (1934). This was based on necropsies carried out on four patients with severe sickle-cell disease and on 30 patients with the sickle-cell trait.

Diggs (1935), in describing siderofibrosis of the spleen, referred to reports on 33 cases; his own observations were based on 19 spleens. He concluded that, if left alone, patients 'will in effect "splenectomize" themselves without the benefit of surgery'. He illustrated a spleen that weighed as little as 2.4 g and described it as a 'small, hard, nodular organ of dull gray'. Bridges (1939) recorded an even smaller spleen: it weighed 1.5 g. The patient was a 4-year-old child.

Kimmelstiel (1948) described in detail the necropsy findings in an 11-year-old female who died following cholecystectomy for the clinical picture of 'acute surgical abdomen'. Post-mortem examination revealed diffuse bilateral cortical necrosis of the kidney and diffuse ischaemic infarctions of the liver and gall bladder and multiple large foci of necrosis in the brain. The spleen was not grossly recognizable: in its place was 'an ill-defined area of thickening at the inferior surface of the diaphragm which measured 2 × 2 × 0.5 cm'.

Edington (1955) reviewed the findings in 40 necropsies carried out at Accra in West Africa; 13 were on pregnant patients who had died suddenly. Not all Edington's patients were homozygous for Hb S; some certainly had Hb-SC disease. His report, however, contains much of interest. He grouped pathological findings into two categories: those associated with haemolysis, *e.g.*, jaundice and siderosis, and those due to thrombi leading to infarction of the lungs, spleen and elsewhere. In five of Edington's patients the spleen was reduced to a small fibrous mass; in others it was congested. In pregnant patients who had died severely anaemic, the pallor of their organs contrasted sharply with the dark red blood of the fetus.

Ascenzi and Silvestroni (1957) described in detail the histological findings in a 10-year-old boy who died of microdrepanocytic disease (Hb-S/thalassaemia).

Cause of death

Infections rank high as an immediate cause of death. Thus they were responsible for nine of the 15 deaths amongst a series of 100 patients studied in Baltimore by Charache and Richardson (1964).

Serjeant and his colleagues (Thomas, Pattison and Serjeant, 1982; Serjeant, 1985) have provided valuable information as to the mortality in the West-Indian Hb-SS population. The age at death and its causes were reviewed in 241 fatal cases. [The age distribution at death was similar in the West-Indian and Memphis cases (Diggs, 1973) and in cases collected from the world literature.] The risk of death was at its highest in children under 5 years of age, particularly in infants during their second 6 months of life. In the Jamaican cohort study, 6% of the children died within the first year and a further 10% during the next 9 years. There was a later peak at death at 20–24 years, partly due to deaths during pregnancy.

Acute splenic sequestration and pneumonia were the principal causes of the early mortality in Jamaica (and pneumococcal septicaemia and meningitis in the United States). The acute chest syndrome was responsible for 20–30% of deaths before the age of 10 and became a major cause of death after this age: lung infections were mainly responsible in young children; embolism became more important as the patients became older. Renal failure was mostly a problem after the age of 20; acute pyelonephritis and the nephrotic syndrome were, however, responsible for the deaths of some children. Cardiovascular problems led to the deaths of seven patients under the age of 20 and of six patients older than 30. Pregnancy was responsible for the deaths of 10 women, aged 15–28 years, and aplastic crises for the deaths of seven children.

Parfrey, Moore and Hutchins (1985) reviewed the causes of death of 74 sickle-cell disease patients at the Johns Hopkins Hospital. Infection was the most frequent precipitating cause (26%). Amongst other causes were uraemia (12%), sequestration crisis (12%) and emboli derived from necrotic bone marrow (9%). No sufficient cause of death was identified in 22%; 27% of the patients had died during a pain crisis, 60% were free from a pain crisis at the time of death. A clear cause of death was apparent in almost all (92%) of the patients who died but were not suffering from a pain crisis but a clear cause was found in only 11 out of 20 patients (55%) who had died during a pain crisis. Parfrey, Moore and Hutchins concluded that their data provided an affirmative answer to the question as to whether a pain crisis by itself led sometimes to the patient's death.

GROSS AND MICROSCOPIC PATHOLOGICAL CHANGES

Bone marrow

As in other haemolytic anaemias and in thalassaemia, sickle-cell anaemia is associated with expansion and hyperplasia of the red bone marrow. In young Hb-SS children red marrow occupies the medullary spaces throughout the bony skeleton, and it is to be found even in the small bones of the hands and feet; in older children the red marrow retreats to the juxta-articular medullary spaces of the long bones and the central skeleton. The widening of the diploic spaces of the skull bones and the expansion of the facial bones in the growing child are brought about by the spacial requirement of the bone marrow within the bones. Diggs (1967), in a review of the bone and joint lesions in sickle-cell disease, illustrated the extension of red marrow into the long bones and also the replacement of the marrow in infarcted areas by necrotic and fibrous tissue. As Serjeant (1985, p. 67) pointed out, the location of bone pain is linked to the presence of active marrow within the affected bones; hence the occurrence of the hand-foot syndrome in small children.

Microscopic findings.

Erythropoietic cells predominate; fat cells tend to disappear. Erythropoiesis is typically normoblastic. However, megaloblastic change occurs from time to time (see p. 104).

Sickled cells are usually more conspicuous in films of aspirated bone marrow than in the peripheral blood. As already mentioned, Sydenstricker, Mulherin and Houseal (1923) noted, too, the presence of long filiform erythrocytes in post-mortem films. Vandepitte and Louis (1953) called attention to similar structures in wet preparations of biopsied bone marrow in sickle-cell disease, but not in the trait.

Bone-marrow necrosis. This has already been referred to as a cause of bone pain and as a source of fat or marrow-cell embolism. The cells in aspirated necrotic marrow have poorly defined outlines, scanty cytoplasm and smudged nuclei, and there is heavy background protein staining. Charache and Page (1967), who aspirated infarcted marrow from three patients (one Hb SS, the others Hb SC and Hb SD, respectively), suggested that this would be a common finding, if looked for, in patients in crisis. Brown (1972), in a review of 66 cases of bone-marrow necrosis observed *post mortem*, found that four patients had Hb-SS disease (most of the remainder had died of gram-negative infections). Three of the Hb-SS disease patients were in crisis and had complained of bone pain, and thrombi containing sickled cells were found in the areas of necrosis; one patient had had Hb-SS disease and typhoid, and three patients had had Hb-SC disease.

Aplastic crises. The findings in sickle-cell disease are similar to those in hereditary spherocytosis (see Vol. 1, pp. 96 and 164).

Megaloblastic change. This has been referred to on page 104.

Spleen

The contracted spleen of sickle-cell disease results from a more or less complete replacement of its normal structure by iron-impregnated fibrous tissue; crystals of calcium salts may be present in addition (Bennett, 1929a,b; Bridges, 1939; Edington, 1955). Diggs (1935) described a siderofibrotic spleen as being composed of 'wide-whitish fibrous tissue strands, flecked with yellow and brown; [he added that] the residual pulp is partitioned off into localized units and varies in color, depending upon the degree of congestion, fibrosis and pigmentation'. In enlarged congested spleens, as in young subjects with Hb-SS disease and in Hb-SC disease, the spleen pulp is stuffed with enormous numbers of very tightly packed sickled cells with the result that the sinusoids are compressed and appear as 'tiny chinks in a sea of blood' (Edington, 1955). Perifollicular haemorrhages are sometimes a conspicuous feature. Erythrophagocytosis may be discernible.

Rich (1928) had pointed out that 'pools of blood partly or completely surrounding the Malpighian bodies' were a characteristic finding in the spleen of patients with sickle-cell disease or the trait, and he interpreted this as being due to a congenital malformation of the splenic sinuses allowing a free escape of blood into the pulp. The concept was not accepted and it is now generally agreed that the pooling of blood in the spleen pulp, particularly around the periphery of the Malpighian bodies, is due to sickling of the erythrocytes and their consequent inability to escape through the stomata into the venous sinuses of the spleen (Tomlinson, 1945). The blood trapped within the spleen undergoes lysis in time and eventually all that is left of the spleen is the type of fibrous remnant referred to above.

Klug, Kaye and Jensen (1982) have more recently reported on the transmission and scanning electron-microscopic appearances of spleens surgically removed from patients with sickle-cell anaemia. In sickle-cell anaemia the basal lamina surrounding the endothelial cells lining the sinuses was thickened, and the cells themselves were characterized by flattening and loss of nuclei. Erythrocytes were frequently to be seen adhering to endothelial cells, particularly at inter-endothelial cell apatures.

Liver

Major pathological changes are not uncommon. As already mentioned, liver enlargement is a common finding (p. 31). The histopathological findings in most patients at necropsy indicate recurrent vascular obstruction leading to liver-cell necrosis and the processes of regeneration and repair. Unequivocal cirrhosis occurs only rarely; a major degree of haemosiderosis is, too, uncommon except in patients who have received many transfusions.

Green, Conley and Berthrong (1953) reported on 21 necropsies: unequivocal cirrhosis was found in four patients, but in many of the others there were active or healed areas of necrosis. The necrosis was attributed to vascular obstruction brought about by impacted masses of sickled cells or by Kupffer cells swollen as the result of phagocytosing erythrocytes.

Edington (1955), in his study of 40 cases in West Africa, reported only one instance of cirrhosis. However, increased fibrosis was noted in two other patients, central atrophy in two patients and focal necrosis in one. The parenchymal cells were relatively unaffected. The most striking feature was erythrophagocytosis by Kupffer cells, some of which were distended with as many as 20–30 sickled erythrocytes. The sinusoids were generally dilated and congested, and in four instances a fibrin network was present in the sinusoids in which sickled erythrocytes were enmeshed. Areas of extramedullary erythropoiesis were noted in eight instances. Edington made the interesting observation that in three necropsies in which the spleen was enlarged and engorged with blood there was no evidence of erythrophagocytosis in the liver.

Bogoch and co-workers (1955) described in detail the clinical, biochemical, histological and histochemical findings in four patients, investigated by needle biopsy, who had presented with the signs and symptoms of liver disease: one patient was diagnosed as having hepatitis, one haemochromatosis (he had received many transfusions) and two portal cirrhosis. Foci of degenerating and necrotic parenchyma cells in the patient with hepatitis were attributed to local ischaemia resulting from obstruction of hepatic sinuses by clumps of sickled cells.

Further details of liver pathology in sickle-cell disease were given by Song (1955, 1957). Song (1957) reviewed 31 necropsies. Some evidence of liver damage was present in all. The lesions were interpreted as being due to impairment of the circulation leading to stagnation of sickled cells and to the formation of thrombi composed of agglutinated and hyalinized sickled cells, and ultimately to anoxic necrosis of liver cells. The liver sinuses were generally dilated, and the parenchyma showed various degrees of necrosis, atrophy, siderosis and fibrosis. The degree of fibrous-tissue proliferation was considered to justify the diagnosis of cirrhosis in nine instances.

Walters (1958) reported on liver-biopsy studies carried out on 16 sickle-cell disease patients in Nigeria. The most striking finding, present in every specimen, was wide dilatation of the sinusoids, with the presence within their lumen of a delicate foam-like reticulum. Walters considered that the reticulum was composed of fibrin; it appeared to be in continuity with the longitudinal fibres of the sinusoidal walls and in time to be incorporated into them. Walters suggested that this process of intrasinusoidal deposition of fibrin could explain how, in advanced cases, the liver cells were separated by a wide zone of coarse fibrous tissue from the endothelial walls of patent, though narrowed, sinuses.

Rosenblate, Eisenstein and Holmes (1970) described the ultrastructural findings in liver tissue aspirated by means of a Menghini needle in 12 successive patients, in all of whom at least two chemical tests of liver function had given abnormal results. The biopsies were carried out 4–19 days after the onset of the crises leading to their admission to hospital. The ultrastructural changes in each patient resembled those produced in experimental animals by hypoxia. The hepatocytes appeared to be in various stages of degeneration, and it was concluded that the aggregation of sickled cells, fibrin and platelets in the sinuses had interfered with their nutrition. The Kupffer cells were hypertrophied and contained ingested sickled cells.

A more recent report by Bauer, Moore and Hutchins (1980) has added to the accumulating knowledge of the way in which the liver is damaged in sickle-cell disease. Their data were derived from necropsies carried out on 70 patients (57 Hb SS, 12 Hb SC and one Hb-S/thalassaemia) at the Johns Hopkins Hospital. They ranged in age from 5 months to 75 years (mean age 21 years). The livers of 64 patients (91%) were enlarged and contained Kupffer cells distended with phagocytosed erythrocytes. The liver sinusoids of 19 patients (27%) were markedly distended with sickled erythrocytes and appeared obstructed. Areas of focal necrosis of liver parenchyma cells were present in 24 patients (34%) and evidence of portal fibrosis and nodular repair in 14 patients (20%). In seven patients (10%) cirrhosis of unknown causation was present and three additional patients had cirrhosis associated with haemochromatosis; 30 other patients had a pathological degree of iron accumulation in parenchymal cells. Bauer, Moore and Hutchins concluded that the spectrum of unexplained liver injury found in sickle-cell disease patients is best explained as a consequence of repeated intravascular

sickling and massive Kuppfer cell enlargement as the result of erythrophagocytosis, leading to local obstruction of the sinusoids with resulting hypoxia, fibrosis and repair.

Kidneys

Bauer (1940) referred to a 10-year-old female with sickle-cell disease in whom massive necrosis of the renal cortex was found at necropsy.

Edington (1955), whose description was based on necropsy material derived from 40 West Africans suffering from sickle-cell disease, reported that the glomerular tufts were congested; this appeared often to lead to thrombosis, as some of the glomeruli were partially or even completely fibrosed.

Further details of the renal changes occurring in the early and late stages of Hb-SS disease were given by Bernstein and Whitten (1960), Pitcock et al. (1970) and Buckalew and Someren (1974). Congestion and glomerular engorgement and focal ischaemic changes lead eventually to sclerosis. Papillary necrosis and vascular engorgement of the submucosa of the renal pelvis are the pathological bases for haematuria. The proximal tubular cells are usually heavily loaded with iron.

Nephrotic syndrome. Berman and Tublin (1959) reported on a renal biopsy carried out on a 9-year-old male with sickle-cell disease suffering from the nephrotic syndrome: the glomeruli varied in appearance from the normal to completely hyalinized and many were distended by masses of sickled cells.

McCoy (1969) and Walker, Alexander and Birdsall (1971) described and discussed the light-microscopic and ultrastructural appearances of the kidneys in sickle-cell nephropathy and the nephrotic syndrome. The lesions were considered to be similar to those seen in proliferative glomerular nephritis and in the nephrotic syndrome induced by saccharated iron oxide.

Lungs

The basic changes leading to infarcts in the lungs appear most often to be occlusion of small blood vessels secondary to impaction of sickled erythrocytes. Diggs (1969) summarized the extent and nature of pulmonary lesions based on an experience of 72 necropsies (62 Hb-SS disease). Emboli, infarcts, effusions and adhesions were the main findings. Gross infarcts were demonstrated in 12 patients. The emboli were usually formed of sickled cells and fragments of clot, but some contained fat and fragments of cellular bone marrow.

Brain

Wertham, Mitchell and Angrist (1942) described the presence in the brain of five sickle-cell anaemia patients of diffusely distributed small necrotic lesions based on vascular obstruction; in one patient there was evidence of extensive fat embolism. Baird and co-workers (1964), too, reported on the brains of five Hb-SS children who had died with neurological symptoms and signs; infarcts and areas of perivascular haemorrhage were diffusely distributed.

Stockman and co-workers (1972) stressed that in sickle-cell anaemia patients with major signs and symptoms of cerebral involvement large vessels may be occluded. In six out of seven such patients investigated by cerebral angiography, large cerebral arteries, including the internal carotid, were found to be partially or completely occluded.

Dactylitis

Weinberg and Currarino (1972) described the necropsy findings in an infant aged 9 months who died with sickle-cell dactylitis. The bone marrow, medullary trabeculae and inner layer of cortical bone in the affected digits were extensively infarcted, the periosteum was elevated and new bone was being formed beneath it; the osteochondral junction was disorganized. The findings were similar to those seen in rabbits when the medullary blood supply was completely interrupted experimentally while that of the periosteum was spared.

Distribution of iron

As already referred to (p. 97), some patients with sickle-cell disease appear to be iron-deficient despite having a life-long chronic haemolytic anaemia which might have been expected to result in increased iron absorption from the gastrointestinal tract. More commonly, the body iron burden appears to be normal as judged by serum-ferritin levels, unless the patients are receiving regular transfusions.

Natta, Creque and Navarro (1985) pointed out that assessment of the iron status of Hb-SS patients by inspection of appropriately stained aspirated bone marrow is an unreliable way of assessing body iron. In a 37-year-old man with a high serum-ferritin concentration, bone marrow obtained at necropsy was found to be devoid of stainable iron, despite grossly increased iron stores in the liver and in a small infarcted spleen and a moderate amount of iron in renal tubular cells.

THE SICKLING PHENOMENON

As already referred to (p. 3), the sickling of erythrocytes *in vitro* appears to have been first noticed by Emmel (1917) when a 'culture preparation' of the blood from a 'case of severe anemia with elongated and sickle-shaped red blood corpuscles' was kept at room temperature. The next significant advance was the recognition by Sydenstricker (1924) that sickling occurred faster in 'active' cases than in 'latent' cases.

Early studies: the relationship between oxygen tension and sickling

In 1927 was published the classic paper of Hahn and Gillespie who were the first to relate sickle-cell formation *in vitro* to a reduction in the partial pressure of oxygen. They concluded that sickling was a reversible phenomenon which depended on whether the haemoglobin was combined with oxygen or dissociated and that the discoid form of the cell was stable when the haemoglobin was combined and that the distorted form was stable when the haemoglobin was dissociated. They added that 'the failure of corpuscles which have lost their hemoglobin to undergo sickle cell formation is consistent with our hypothesis relating the distortion to the hemoglobin'.

Twenty-two years were to pass before this hypothesis was proved to be correct.

Hahn and Gillespie's conclusions received support from in-vivo studies of Scriver and Waugh (1930), who, in a study of the effect of venous stasis on the number of sickled cells in blood withdrawn from below a tourniquet, found that the number definitely increased if the partial pressure of oxygen was reduced below 40–45 mm Hg. They concluded that anoxia after death was the cause of the large masses of sickled cells which might be seen *post mortem*.

The above-mentioned pioneer studies on the relationship between oxygen tension and sickling have been repeatedly confirmed and elaborated. Diggs (1932) and Sherman (1940), like Sydenstricker (1924) by implication, distinguished clearly between the behaviour of erythrocytes from subjects with 'sicklemia' (sickle-cell trait) or sickle-cell anaemia, respectively. Sherman (1940) observed that, in order for sickling to occur, oxygen tension had to be reduced far more in sickle-cell trait than in sickle-cell anaemia.

Murphy and Shapiro (1944) described the effect of oxygen tension, the concentration of reticulocytes and the nature of the suspending medium on the process of sickling and, referring to Sherman's (1940) observation of the birefringence of sickled cells, wrote that it suggests 'that certain molecules of the cell become reorientated when the cell undergoes sickling'. They stressed the extent to which cells varied in their proneness to sickle: they noted that more and more sickled as the O_2 tension was reduced until, if the amount of combined haemoglobin (oxyhaemoglobin) was reduced to a sufficient minimum, all the cells sickled.

Lange, Minnich and Moore (1950, 1951), working with mixtures of oxygen and nitrogen with 10% of added carbon dioxide, found that sickle-cell anaemia (Hb-SS) erythrocytes sickled in 4–6% oxygen while sickle-cell trait (Hb-AS) cells did not sickle until the percentage of oxygen was less than 2%. They also noticed that Hb-AS cells sickled at pH 6.0 or less when exposed to 2% oxygen, while those of Hb-SS disease sickled at a pH as high as 7.25.

Harris and co-workers (1956) reported on the relationship between oxygen (O_2) tension and sickling *in vitro*, and on the effect of O_2 tension on blood viscosity and erythrocyte mechanical fragility. They showed that in sickle-cell disease sickling could take place at physiological O_2 tensions, *e.g.*, at 40 mm Hg, while in the sickle-cell trait an unphysiological tension of 10 mm Hg or less was required. They also found that O_2 tensions at which tactoid formation could be induced in solutions of Hb S were limited to the tensions that caused sickling of intact cells. They concluded that lowering the pH increased sickling by facilitating the deoxygenation of haemoglobin.

Griggs and Harris (1956) compared the findings in Hb-SC disease and Hb-S/thalassaemia with those in Hb-SS disease. They found that, while in Hb-SS disease (with 90–100% of Hb S) an O_2 tension of 60 mm Hg might produce sickling *in vitro*, in Hb-SC disease or Hb-S/thalassaemia (with 50–80% of Hb S) a tension of 40 mm Hg was required, and in Hb-AS trait (with 24–48% Hb S) a tension of less than 10 mm Hg. They concluded that the most sensitive index of sickling was an increase in mechanical fragility (? due to the formation of intracellular small tactoids), then tactoid formation in haemoglobin solutions and finally (as the least sensitive index) overt sickling and viscosity changes which ran parallel to each other.

Allison (1956) also studied the sickling process in detail. He found that at a physiological pH sickling of Hb-SS disease erythrocytes took place at 40 mm Hg O_2 tension, when about 45% of the haemoglobin was deoxygenated. Individual cells varied in their sensitivity to sickling, some not sickling until the tension was reduced to 20 mm Hg or less. Allison also observed that the cells from Hb-SC and Hb-S/thalassaemia patients reacted in a way intermediate between those of patients with Hb-SS disease and carriers of the Hb-AS trait; he concluded that sickling took at least 2 minutes to take place and that this fact had an important bearing on the possibility of harmful consequences *in vivo* (see p. 220). Sickling was found to be inhibited at 4°C.

Greenberg, Kass and Castle (1957) showed that a positive correlation exists between the ease with which sickling and increases in blood viscosity take place when blood is deoxygenated and the concentration of Hb S in the erythroctes; they showed, too, that at 60 mm Hg O_2 tension a small fall in pH, *e.g.*, from 7.5 to 7.0, results in a marked increase in the percentage of sickled cells. Greenberg and Kass (1958) observed that a fall in pH *in vivo*, as could be produced by the administration of ammonium chloride, might precipitate a painful crisis.

Harris (1959), in an important and extensive review (350 references), described in detail almost all that was known of the sickling phenomenon up to the time of writing and examined the role of physical and chemical factors in bringing it about.

Factors other than oxygen tension affecting sickling: cellular hydration, MCHC, CO_2 and pH, and temperature

Perillie and Epstein (1963) showed that when erythrocytes containing Hb S are immersed in hypertonic solutions they undergo sickling even at the O_2 tension of room air and at normal body temperature and pH; they suggested that cellular dehydration was responsible.

Guy, Gavrilis and Rothenberg (1973) reported the opposite phenomenon — that the percentage of cells that sickled when deoxygenated diminished in parallel with decrease in the salt concentration of the suspending medium. Irreversibly sickled cells (ISCs) were found not to be affected.

Rampling (1975) discussed the mechanisms by which CO_2 enhances sickling and fall in temperature inhibits it. CO_2 was considered to act in a complex fashion by affecting pH and 2,3-DPG concentration as well as the oxygen affinity of Hb S; fall in temperature was thought to affect pH and to block hydrophobic bonds necessary for polymer formation.

Bookchin, Balazs and Landau (1976) had studied the effect on sickling of varying the pH and intracellular haemoglobin concentration. Small increases in pH were found to inhibit sickling; small reductions, on the other hand, promoted sickling more than could be accounted for by the Bohr effect. Sickling was found to be correlated with the minimum gelling concentration (see p. 195). Osmotic shrinkage of erythrocytes resulted in a large fall in O_2 affinity and a marked increase in sickling, so much so that the O_2 affinity and sickling of Hb-AS cells resembled that of unaltered Hb-SS cells if the MCHC was raised to 40%. Bookchin, Balazs and Landau pointed out that partial deoxygenation combined with osmotic shrinkage, as found *in vivo* in the renal medulla, would promote sickling at that site.

Zarkowsky and Hochmuth (1977) reported on experiments they had carried out on the effect of pH on sickling. The suspension of cells to be tested were exposed to sodium dithionite and sickling recorded on videotape. The sickling time of Hb-AS and Hb-SC cells

was progressively reduced when the pH was lowered from 7.4 to 6.8 but that of Hb-SS cells was much less affected unless the cells were suspended in a hypotonic medium.

Further studies on the effect of the water content of Hb-S-containing cells and sickling were reported by Clark *et al.* (1980) (see p. 202).

Ueda and Bookchin (1984) reported that varying the CO_2 tension affects several properties of Hb-SS cells quite differently from its effect on Hb-AA cells and that the extent of the differences is dependent on pH: these differences include an increase in the O_2 affinity of Hb-SS blood when the pCO_2 is raised from 40 to 80 mm Hg at normal or raised pH levels.

Effect of 2,3-DPG. Jensen and Nathan (1972) reported that a high concentration of DPG increased, and a low concentration decreased, the sickling of Hb-S- containing cells at any given pO_2. They considered that this was brought about by DPG affecting the oxygen affinity of the haemoglobin as well as by an additional direct mechanism. Nagel and Bookchin's (1974) conclusions were similar: namely, that DPG promoted gelling of deoxyHb S not only by lowering the concentration of haemoglobin required for gelling but also by inducing a structural change in the molecule.

Zarkowsky and Hochmuth (1977) also reported that decrease in DPG was associated with a marked increase in sickling time.

SICKLING: MORPHOLOGICAL CHANGES

Emmel (1917) had observed that hair-like processes might develop when cells sickled as the result of being 'cultured' *in vitro*, and Sydenstricker, Mulherin and Houseal (1923) described how filiform cells up to 40 μm in length might be seen in films of bone-marrow cells made *post mortem*. Diggs, Ahmann and Bibb (1933) illustrated how sickling develops with the passage of time in sealed moist preparations of sickle-cell anaemia and sickle-cell trait blood. Sickling occurred more slowly in the case of the trait, but at 24 hours the appearances were much the same.

Diggs and Bibb (1939) described in detail the changes in morphology that develop when erythrocytes containing Hb S are allowed to remain sealed under a coverslip (see Figs. 12.22 and 12.23). They pointed out that although the distorted cells are referred to as 'sickled cells', the term is inappropriate except for cells that are 'narrow, pointed and curved'. They concluded that the truly sickle-shaped cell is a degenerative form.

Sherman (1940) described how partial deoxygenation (90% N_2, 10% O_2) may lead to the development of 'holly wreath' forms, cells with an irregular sharply pointed central zone.

Details of the sequence of changes, as viewed under the light microscope, when cells undergo reversible sickling in sealed preparations were also well described and illustrated by Ponder (1945, 1948). He reported that the membrane at one side of a cell becomes thicker and an area on the opposite side thinner; thinning continues until a breach occurs; then the newly formed ends separate and stretch the cell substance in the biconcavity so formed, so that eventually this appears as a thin almost invisible fringe lying within the bicon-cavity of a sickle-shaped cell. The first stage, in which the cell thickens on one side and thins at the opposite side, takes, according to Ponder (1948); 1–2 minutes; the remainder of the transformation after the break in continuity takes only 1 second or so. As the points of the sickle separate each extends outward and may form a filament 10 μm or more in length. On reoxygenation, the process is reversed, and the long filaments break off and contract forming rods and globules floating free in the suspending medium. Ponder stressed how the shape changes in individual cells vary and that sometimes the preliminary thickening in the membrane takes place in two or three places simultaneously, resulting in the formation of very bizarre-shaped cells; he considered that the 'holly wreath' forms described by Sherman (1940) were sickled cells that had undergone crenation. Later authors (e.g. Rebuck, Sturrock and Monaghan, 1950; Lessin, Jensen and Klug, 1972; Hellerstein and Bunthrarungroj, 1974) have often referred realistically to very bizarre-shaped cells as 'holly leaf' forms.

Bessis and co-workers (1954) noted that sickling is almost completely inhibited at 4°C: at this temperature the 'shape of the cell remains almost circular, there is no development of spicules, and the hemoglobin in the interior becomes rearranged so as to form two or three large and irregularly shaped masses'.

These early studies have been confirmed and extended by later work. Jensen (1969), who studied sickling under the scanning electron microscope, observed that sickled cells, which had developed long thin spicules when sickled, may lose the spicules on reoxygenation, whilst cells which when sickled had assumed less extreme forms (e.g. holly wreath or oat-shaped cells) revert to normal without fragmentation. Jensen and Lessin (1970) pointed out that during sickling the haemoglobin becomes unevenly distributed so that the cell membrane of opposite sides of the cell can make contact in places and seal, thus facilitating fragmentation without loss of cell contents. Padilla, Bromberg and Jensen (1973), using cine-photomicrography to record the events that occur during deoxygenation and reoxygenation, found that the repetitive sickling of single cells does not always result in the same deformity; and although this sometimes takes place without an apparent loss of membrane, the process may result in the shedding of microspherules and permanent cell deformation.

Ham and his co-workers (1968), in the course of experiments on the effect of heat on erythrocytes, submitted oxygenated discoid Hb-SS cells to a temperature of 49°C. The progressive budding and microspherocyte formation which resulted was similar to that observed with Hb-AA cells. When sodium metabisulphate was added to the heated cells, only about half of them sickled; many of the spherical cells did not sickle, while in some only a few processes developed.

Reticulocytes sickle, but less readily than adult erythocytes (Scriver and Waugh, 1930; Diggs and Bibb, 1939; Watson, 1948; Grasso, Sullivan and Sullivan, 1975a). Normoblasts sickle, too, but even less readily than do reticulocytes (Diggs and Bibb, 1939; Watson, 1948). Pointed and sickled normoblasts are, nevertheless, occasionally to be seen in films of peripheral blood (Diggs and Bibb, 1939). According to Grasso, Sullivan and Sullivan (1975b) sickled normoblasts are not found in preparations of bone marrow fixed immediately after aspiration. However, when purposely deoxygenated, 10–20% of the more mature normoblasts form polymer visible in electron micrographs. The cells even then show at the most minimal alteration in shape.

Clark and co-workers (1980) reported on the effect of the water content of Hb-SS erythrocytes on sickling morphology and showed that cells that were severely dehydrated during sickling retained their sickle shape even after prolonged reoxygenation. However, when the water content of the cells was allowed to increase by reducing the osmolarity of the suspending medium the cells unsickled. On the other hand, cells dehydrated before being deoxygenated failed to form the extended spicules characteristic of cells with a normal water content that have undergone sickling; this, it was suggested, is due to the haemoglobin being so concentrated that it behaves as a semi-solid.

Allan and co-workers (1982) reported further studies on the loss of cell membrane that takes place when Hb-S-containing erythrocytes sickle. As recorded by Padilla, Bromberg and Jensen (1973), this may result in the shedding of microspherules and permanent cell deformation. Allan *et al.* found that when Hb-SS cells are sickled *in vitro* as much as 2–3% of their lipid may be lost as spectrin-free haemoglobin-containing spicules in the form of rods and microspheres. The rods, which contain polymerized Hb S, eventually degrade to chains of microvesicles of approximately. 0.1 μm diameter. The material shed

appears to be derived from the distal parts of the spicules which develop when a cell sickles. Allan *et al.* were able to demonstrate by electron microscopy similar material free in the blood of Hb-SS patients but not in normal blood; its composition was the same as that of the spicules shed *in vitro*. Allan *et al.* concluded that the spicules developing when a cell sickles, which are almost free of spectrin and actin, are formed of polymerized Hb S extending through gaps in the actin-spectrin framework of the cells' cytoskeleton and causing herniation of the lipid bilayer part of the membrane; they suggested that the rod-like spicules are released on reoxygenation because the haemoglobin in the spicules fails to depolymerize under conditions in which the haemoglobin in the body of the cell does, thus allowing the membrane to fuse around the 'necks' of the spicules.

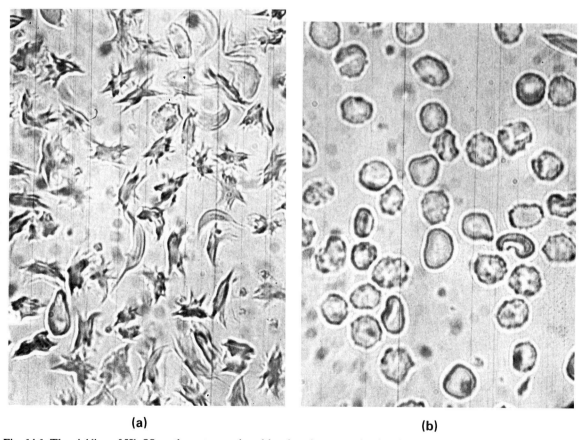

(a)   (b)

Fig. 14.1 The sickling of Hb-SS erythrocytes produced by slow deoxygenation by nitrogen (a) and rapid deoxygenation by 2% sodium dithionite (b).
[Reproduced by permission from Asakura and Mayberry (1984).]

Method of deoxygenation and extent and type of sickling

Bookchin and co-workers (1984) described how altering the nature and osmolarity of the suspending medium affected the sickling of Hb-AS erythrocytes: for instance, in plasma 6–20% of the cells were found to sickle; in iso-osmotic Hepes buffered saline 8–10%, in iso-osmotic sodium phosphate buffered saline 36–46% and in iso-osmotic sodium phosphate 74–85%; in hypo-osmotic sodium phosphate buffered saline 8%, and in hypo-osmotic sodium phosphate 4–5%.

Asakura and Mayberry (1984) described how the method of deoxygenation of Hb-SS erythrocytes affects the speed and type of morphological change. A high yield (90%) of sickled cells was obtained if Hb-SS blood was deoxygenated slowly in nitrogen (N_2) gas; in contrast, exposure to 2% sodium dithionite achieved rapid deoxygenation but a lower yield of sickled cells and a high percentage of irregularly-shaped ('mosaic') cells (Fig. 14.1). Mosaic cells also developed when deoxygenation with nitrogen was carried out rapidly; and only about 20% of the mosaic cells changed to sickled forms when submitted to prolonged incubation at 37°C. If, however, the mosaic cells were cooled, 'desickled' and deoxygenated again slowly with N_2, most converted to sickled cells. (The mosaic form was thought to result from the precipitation of rapidly deoxygenated Hb S.) Sodium dithionite was found to reduce intracellular Hb S faster than did sodium metabisulphite, explaining the higher yield of sickling obtained with metabisulphite than with dithionite. Acidification and shaking, as well as rise in temperature, were all shown to accelerate sickling. Asakura and Mayberry's paper contains an interesting table of the time required for sickling (< 1 second to 15 minutes) as recorded by different observers, from Ponder (1948) to Zarkowsky and Hochmuth (1975).

Ultrasonic absorption properties of sickled cells

Shung and co-workers (1979) described how the sickling of erythrocytes results in an increase in the absorption of ultrasound. In their experiments they were able to show how the absorption was closely related to oxygen tension and how increase in pH decreased the absorption. They concluded that the technique provided a rapid and non-subjective means of assessing sickling.

MECHANISM OF SICKLING

Early studies

The actual mechanism of sickling has been the subject of much research. Sherman in 1940 was the first to observe that cells which underwent sickling become birefringent. Pauling and his co-workers (1949) suggested that under conditions of reduced oxygen tension the molecules of Hb S undergo a partial alignment within the cells and that elongation of the cells in one axis and distortion follows from this. Harris (1950) suggested that linkage of individual molecules leads to the formation of long tactoids (liquid crystalline masses). He found that the decreased solubility of Hb S brought about by deoxygenation results in solutions becoming more viscous. This was, however, dependent on the concentration of Hb S. At concentrations less than 10 g/dl viscosity did not increase; above this concentration, viscosity increased until at 24 g/dl a gel-like state resulted. Microscopy of the viscous solutions revealed spindle-shaped bodies, 1–15 μm in length, which were birefringent; they disappeared when the solutions were oxygenated and reappeared when they were deoxygenated. Harris pointed out the similarity in shape between the spindle-shaped tactoids and sickled erythrocytes (Figs. 14.2 and 14.3).

Perutz and Mitchison (1950) showed that reduced Hb S is far less soluble than reduced Hb A. Whereas the solubility of reduced Hb A was found to be about one-half of that of oxygenated Hb A, the solubility of reduced Hb S was no more than one-hundredth of that of oxygenated Hb S. They suggested that the sickle shape and birefringence of the distorted cells results from crystallization of the haemoglobin within the cell membranes. Further differences between Hb A and Hb S were described by Perutz, Liquori and Eirich (1951). Using a slightly different technique, they found that the solubility of reduced Hb S was about one-tenth of that of reduced Hb A. As a result of other experiments they concluded that

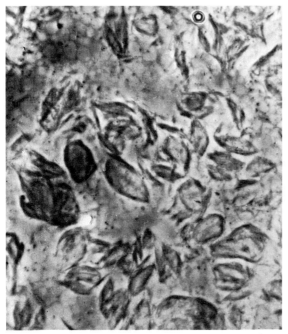

Fig. 14.2 Haemoglobin tactoids formed in a stroma-free solution of deoxygenated Hb S.
A phase photomicrograph. Magnification as in Figure 14.3. [Reproduced by permission from Harris (1950).]

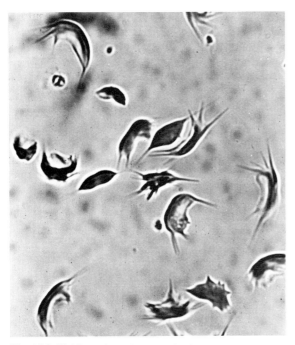

Fig. 14.3 Sickling of erythrocytes in the deoxygenated whole blood of a Hb-SS patient.
A phase photomicrograph. Magnification as in Figure 14.2. [Reproduced by permission from Harris (1950).]

the solubility of reduced Hb S is only one-seventh of that required to keep the haemoglobin in solution in the cell.

The differences in solubility between Hb S and Hb A provide one method for the distinction between the Hb-AS trait and Hb-SS disease, as the observed solubility seems to be a direct reflection of the proportion of Hb S present (see p. 110). Itano (1953a,b) found that the solubility of the haemoglobin varied with the genotype: that in Hb-AS trait was the most soluble, then that in Hb-SC disease, then that in Hb-S/thalassaemia; least soluble was that in Hb-SS disease.

Singer and Singer (1953), in studies in which they measured the minimum concentration of Hb S which would cause solutions of haemoglobin, when deoxygenated, to undergo gelling, observed that the 'gelling point' was modified by the presence of other types of haemoglobin. In Hb-AS trait, for instance, the presence of Hb A appeared to diminish the minimal concentration of Hb S required for gelling; Hb C reduced this still further. Singer and Singer made the point that sickling depends not only on the presence of Hb S but also on its interaction with other haemoglobins.

The hypothesis that the haemoglobin in sickled cells is in the form of tactoids of reduced haemoglobin was generally accepted. Harris and his co-workers (1956) had pointed out that the slight loss of cell water which takes place when a cell sickles, the appearances on electron microscopy and the results of X-ray-scattering studies failed to support the hypothesis of a crystalline structure for the sickled cell. Optical studies led Bessis and co-workers (1958) also to support the concept of gel formation rather than that of actual crystallization.

Molecular orientation of Hb S in sickled cells.

The observation that sickled cells are birefringent (Sherman, 1940) led to the concept of a linear arrangement of Hb-S molecules when deoxygenated. Electron microscopy confirmed this supposition, although there was, at least at first, some divergence of views as to the nature of the structures seen.

Rebuck, Sturrock and Monaghan (1950) in early electron-microscopic studies reported a patchy aggregation of haemoglobin and incipient intracellular crystallization within sickled cells; they considered that the 'holly leaf' form is brought about by aggregation of haemoglobin in the entire corpuscular rim, accompanied by angulation.

Dervichian and co-workers (1952) concluded, as the result of X-ray studies, that the haemoglobin in sickled cells is unlikely to be in a crystalline state. Bessis, Bricka and Breton-Gorius (1953) and Bessis *et. al.* (1954), using the technique of gold-shadowing electron microscopy, observed striations parallel to the long axis of sickled cells. These were interpreted as being produced by 'little rods of hemoglobin viewed through the surface of the cell, but seen in relief' (Bessis *et al.*, 1954).

Rebuck, Sturrock and Monto (1955) again attributed the cell distortion to aggregation of haemoglobin and described how the haemoglobin is eccentrically massed in cells showing peripheral spicules.

Bessis and his co-workers (1958) reported that the appearance of sickled erythrocytes when viewed by phase and interference microscopy differs from those of human and rat erythrocytes in which the haemoglobin was crystalline. Under the polarizing microscope sickled cells were found to be associated with birefringence which could, it was thought, be produced by a mass of little crystals; under the electron microscope, however, the appearances, a 'ramifying feltwork', were considered to be compatible with the hypothesis that the haemoglobin had undergone gelification.

Ponder (1958), too, argued against the possibility that the haemoglobin in sickled cells is crystalline; the available evidence he considered pointed to the haemoglobin being in the form of an orientated gel.

Later work has indicated that the changes that take place in sickling cells in fact fall short of crystal formation, contrary to the interpretation advanced by Stetson (1966) on the basis of an electron-microscopic study. It is now clear that deoxygenation, instead of causing the haemoglobin to form crystals, causes the pathological Hb-S molecules to be stacked linearly in the form of long filaments and that it is the formation of these filaments that distort the erythrocytes so that they assume a bizarre sickled shape. The gradual build-up of knowledge in this field makes a fascinating story of which an outline is given below.

Murayama (1964) discussed the molecular ways in which a binding site on the abnormal Hb-S β chain, acting as a key, could bind to an α chain when the molecule is deoxygenated, thus achieving linear stacking of the truncated tetrahedrons formed by the four globin chains of each molecule. It was suggested that the key comprised

an intramolecular hydrophobic bond between the two terminal valyl residues, the first residue and the abnormal sixth (Glu → Val) residue of Hb S. On oxygenation the linear stacking of the molecules would 'crumble' when the 'keys' on the β chain underwent an architectural alteration. Murayama (1965, 1967) demonstrated that sickled cells would orient themselves perpendicular to magnetic lines of force, a finding consistent with the evidence from measurements of dichroism in polarized light which indicated that deoxygenated Hb-S molecules are stacked along the long axis of the molecules and that the haem plates are perpendicular to the molecules' long axis (Murayama, Olson and Jennings, 1965). Murayama (1966, 1967), in reviews, summarized the above data and interpreted the filaments demonstrable in electron micrographs as hollow cables formed of six Hb-S monofilaments (Fig. 14.4 and 14.5).

Interesting light was shed on the molecular rearrangements leading to sickling by the observations of Krauss *et al.* (1966) on the interaction between Hb S and certain other naturally-occurring haemoglobins, *i.e.* Hb Memphis, Hb C Harlem and Hb Korle-Bu. Hb Memphis is remarkable as it stems from two amino-acid substitutions, one in the α chain (α 23 Glu → Gln) and one in the β chain (β6 Glu → Val), the same mutation as in Hb S. Hb Memphis gels less readily than does Hb S on deoxygenation, the inference being that the α-chain substitution interferes with the molecular interactions brought about by the Hb-S substitution as the result of deoxygenation (Kraus *et al.*, 1966) [see also Benesch *et al.*, 1979 (p. 196)]. (Compound heterozygotes for Hb S and Hb Memphis have a much milder haemolytic anaemia than do Hb-SS homozygotes.)

Hb C Harlem results from two substitutions within the same chain: β6 Glu → Val, as in Hb S, and β73 Asp → Asn (Bookchin, Nagel and Ranney, 1967). This haemoglobin, too, although relatively insoluble when deoxygenated, gels less readily than does Hb S, suggesting that the β73 substitution also impedes in some way the molecular interaction brought about by the β6 substitution. Hb Korle-Bu (Konotey-Ahulu *et al.*, 1968) has the same β73 substitution as does Hb C Harlem but it lacks the substitution at the β6 position. Like Hb F (as opposed to Hb A) it fails to participate in gelling with Hb S, thus providing further evidence of the importance of the β73 position as a site of interaction of Hb-S molecules when deoxygenated (Bookchin, Nagel and Ranney, 1970).

White (1968) demonstrated numerous electron-dense filaments and rods in sickled cells and concluded that the degree to which a cell becomes

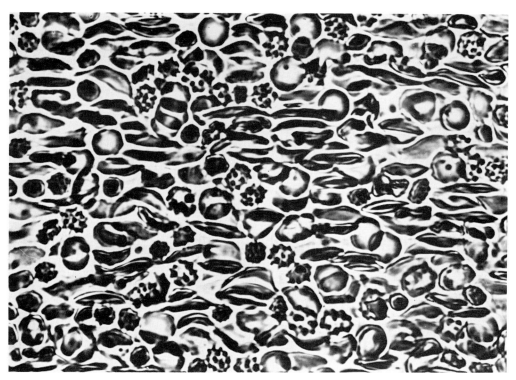

Fig. 14.4 Magnetically oriented sickled erythrocytes.
The magnetic lines of force run from top to bottom. The sickled cells are oriented with their long axes perpendicular to the lines of force. [Reproduced by permission from Murayama (1967).]

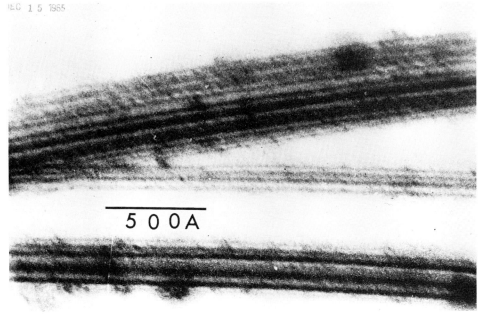

Fig. 14.5 Electron micrograph of Hb-S microtubules.
[Reproduced by permission from Murayama (1967).]

distorted is related to the amount of Hb S converted to rod forms and to the extent to which the rods become arranged parallel to the long axis of the cell. The rods, interpreted as polymers of Hb S, were considered to be similar to, although not morphologically identical with, protein microtubular polymers.

Döbler and Bertles (1968) carried out studies on sickled cells in venous blood that had been fixed for EM study anaerobically without loss or gain of oxygen. Fibrils could be demonstrated in some of the sickled cells identical with those produced in discoidal cells that had undergone sickling *in vitro*. Bertles and Döbler (1969) reviewed previous work and contrasted the appearances in irreversibly sickled cells (ISCs) with those in cells that reversibly sickled. Aberrant appearances in ISCs suggested that their membrane had been damaged. Deoxygenation of non-ISCs led to the appearance of loosely arranged filaments having a tendency to lie parallel within cell protruberances and in the cells' long axis. The question was raised as to whether formation of the filaments leads to a cell being distorted or whether a cell's distortion dictates how the filaments are arranged.

Bessis, Döbler and Mandon (1970) published some excellent photographs of sickled cells as seen by scanning electron microscopy (*e.g.* Fig. 12.24, p. 109). Very long filamentous spicules were demonstrated, as well as sickled cells undergoing echinocytosis. Bessis and Döbler (1970) showed that in ultra-thin sections of sickled cells the (micro-) filaments present might be oriented radially in the centre of the cell although arranged parallel to the long axis of spicules; they were never seen to be bound to cell membrane. The cells were referred to as being distorted to 'holly leaf' or sickle shape by the growing filaments. In sections of echinocytes the filaments were seen to be arranged in three dimensions, penetrating pre-existing spicules and eventually elongating them.

White and Heagan (1970a) reported on the EM appearances of stroma-free gels of deoxygenated Hb S. Rods identical to those seen in intact sickled cells were the basic structural units. The radiating elements seen in EM preparations of crystallizing Hb S were different from the rods seen in gels and intact cells. White and Heagan (1970b) compared the fine structure of gels of oxyHb S and deoxyHb S and oxyHb A, as produced in phosphate buffer with added sodium metabisulphite. The gels of deoxyHb S were formed of solid rods; those of oxyHb S, oxyHb A and deoxyHb A contained masses of hollow polymers identical in arrangement to microtubules.

Lessin, Jensen and Klug (1972), in a well-illustrated review, discussed the then current knowledge of the ultrastructure of sickled cells as revealed by freeze-etching, scanning and thin-section electron microscopy. Magdoff-Fairchild, Swerdlow and Bertles (1972) compared the X-ray diffraction patterns given by deoxygenated and oxygenated Hb-S-containing erythrocytes. As compared with oxygenated cells and haemoglobin solutions, the diffraction patterns obtained with the deoxygenated cells and haemoglobin solutions showed a distribution of intensities characteristic of patterns produced by regularly arranged fibres.

Finch and co-workers (1973) and Bertles (1974) reviewed the likely ultrastructure of the linear arrangement of deoxygenated molecules of Hb S. It was concluded that deoxyHb S aggregates in long straight fibres which may extend through most of the length of the cell; X-ray diffraction and EM studies had shown that each fibre is a long tubular structure made up of six filaments wound around a hollow core. 'Each of these six filaments is composed of Hb-S molecules, like beads on a string; and the filaments are in register so that the fiber is in effect a stack of disks, each disk being of six Hb-S molecules in a planar hexagon. A small successive rotation of each disk generates the six helices' (Bertles, 1974). In relation to the mechanism of the molecular rearrangement consequent on deoxygenation, Bertles wrote: 'Deoxygenation alters the spatial relationships within individual hemoglobin molecules'; also that their movement 'apparently suffices to bring certain surface regions of any one deoxygenated Hb-S molecule into line with receptor regions on a neighboring molecule'.

White in his 1974 review concluded that the sickling phenomenon which takes place in intact cells and the gelling of cell-free solutions of Hb S result from a sol-gel transformation in which solid rods of Hb-S polymers arrange themselves in parallel fashion; he considered that the polymers are unique in that they differ in molecular organization from haemoglobin aggregates, microtubules and crystals.

Grasso, Sullivan and Sullivan (1975a,b) compared the EM appearances of adult Hb-SS-containing erythrocytes with those of reticulocytes and normoblasts withdrawn from bone marrow and processed without further deoxygenation: some of the reticulocytes had a highly ordered pattern similar to that of adult cells (but for the presence, too, of organelles); in others the pattern was less organized and in some cells the haemoglobin in the bulk of the cytoplasm was not polymerized. These differences were considered to reflect the differences in the concentration of haemoglobin in individual cells. The EM appearances of the normoblasts were normal, but 10–20% of them (the mature forms) showed evidence of haemoglobin polymerization on deoxygenation.

More recent EM studies have provided further information as to the way in which deoxyHb-S molecules are arranged in fibres.

Ohtsuki and co-workers (1977) reported that their optical and digital analysis of electron micrographs had revealed an arrangement of Hb-S molecules similar to that described by Finch *et al.* (1973). The fibres appeared to be composed of stacked discs each formed of six haemoglobin molecules: the fibres had an outer diameter of 160–170 Å and an inner diameter of 60 Å and formed a helix composed of 56 discs per helical turn.

Finch (1978) provided a brief review in which he summarized the rather conflicting results then available (on Hb-S fibre size and the number of strands per fibre) and stressed the need in in-vitro work for the material to be examined at as near physiological conditions as possible. It is certainly possible that the structure of fibres of deoxyHb S, as revealed by electron microscopy, will vary according to the way in which deoxygenation is brought about, as do the morphological appearances of sickling when viewed under the light microscope at modest magnifications (see p. 189). The work of Dykes, Crepeau and Edelstein (1978, 1979) did in fact lead them to a conclusion as to the arrangement of the molecules in Hb-S fibres which differed from that of Finch *et al.* (1973) and Ohtsuki *et al.* (1977): 3-dimensional reconstruction suggested to them that Hb-S fibres, 20 nm (200 Å) in diameter, are composed of an inner helical core of four strands surrounded by an outer helix of 10 strands, giving 14 strands per fibre in all (Figs. 14.6 and 14.7). Crepeau and co-workers (1978) later conceded that, while the 14-stranded structure is the predominant form of Hb S in sickled cells, 6-stranded fibres become stabilized under certain conditions.

Garrell, Crepeau and Edelstein (1979) carried out thin-section electron microscopy after a tannic acid embedding procedure which gave improved resolution and observed patterns which were consistent with the previously described 14-strand structure of Hb-S fibres.

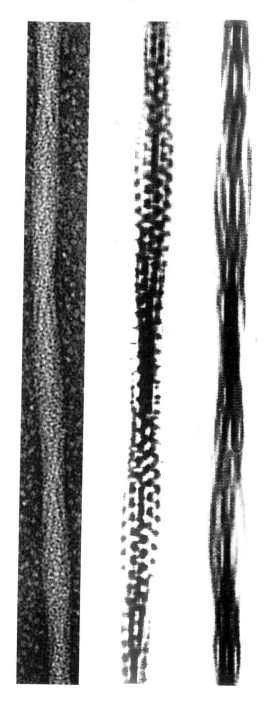

Fig. 14.6 Negatively stained image and reconstruction of a fibre of Hb S.

Left: micrograph of a fibre prepared from a sickled cell by direct lysis. Negative stain.

Centre: two-dimensional reconstruction of a fibre of Hb S using computer reconstruction techniques.

Right: two-dimensional reconstruction as in centre, but with only the maxima of layer lines 1–6 of the Fourier transform used.

[Reproduced by permission from Dykes, Crepeau and Edelstein (1978).]

The relationship between fibres and crystals of deoxygenated Hb S was investigated by Magdoff-Fairchild and Chiu (1979). Using X-ray diffraction techniques,

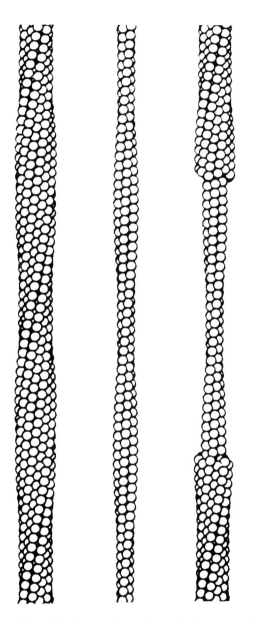

Fig. 14.7 Solid sphere models of the helical elements of a fibre of Hb S.

Left: the outer strands.

Centre: the inner strands, in alignment with the outer strands.

Right: a cutaway version showing both the inner and outer strands in proper juxtaposition.

[Reproduced by permission from Dykes, Crepeau and Edelstein (1978).]

they obtained patterns that were similar in most respects. The conclusion was reached that the specific molecular interactions that cause the aggregation leading to sickling are the same as those that lead to the formation of crystals.

Maugh (1981) ably reviewed the new understanding of sickle-cell disease that has been brought about as the result of the previous decade's fruitful research, much of which has been summarized above.

Kaperonis, Handley and Chien (1986), too, have reported on the relationship between fibre formation and crystallization. Hb-SS blood was studied that had been stored in capillaries from 1 to 132 days. Fibres with a fibre-to-fibre periodicity of 18.6 nm were demonstrated by electron microscopy from Day 1 onward. Between Days 65 and 132, crystals of haemoglobin developed extracellularly with a lattice periodicity of 9.63 nm, and it was suggested that the crystals formed via a stage of fibre dissolution rather than by progressive alignment and direct fusion of existing fibres.

Sickling times of individual erythrocytes

The time taken for erythrocytes containing Hb S to sickle when exposed to reduced oxygen tension has an important clinical bearing (see p. 220). Changes in fact take place rapidly, the rate of change depending upon the degree of deoxygenation, the concentration of Hb S present, the temperature and other factors, too, including the speed of deoxygenation and, *in vitro*, the means by which it is brought about (see p. 188).

Messer and Harris (1970) passed suspensions of Hb-SS, Hb-SC, Hb-S/thalassaemia and Hb-AS erythrocytes through Millepore filters at a constant rate of flow and studied the effect of the sudden addition of sodium dithionite on the filterability of the suspensions. This decreased almost immediately (in 0.12 second) on the deoxygenation of Hb-SS and Hb-S/thalassaemia cells, but more slowly with Hb-SC cells (0.5 second) and much more slowly with Hb-AS cells (5 seconds). It took much longer for morphological abnormalities to be recognizable under the light microscope (4 seconds in the case of Hb-SS cells). On sudden reoxygenation, the decreased filterability of all types of cells was abolished within 0.12 second.

Rampling and Sirs (1973) reported an even faster reaction time, finding the first morphological signs of sickling of Hb-SS cells 0.03 second after exposure to dithionite.

Not all Hb-SS erythrocytes sickle at the same speed. This was illustrated by the data of Zarkowsky and Hochmuch (1975), obtained by recording the process of sickling on film and videotape when the cells were suddenly deoxygenated to zero pO_2 by sodium dithionite. An initial lag phase was followed by a phase of rapid deformation. The T_{50} for the sickling of Hb-SS cells was approximately 2.0 seconds (range 1–8 seconds) and for Hb-AS cells 70 seconds (range 8–185 seconds). Increasing the buffer's osmolarity resulted in shorter times, and decreasing it in longer times. In Hb-SS blood, fractionated by centrifugation, the T_{50} decreased progressively from top (T_{50} 3.34 seconds) to bottom (T_{50} 1.4 seconds) parallel with the increase in MCHC. A rise in pH above 7.4 and fall in temperature lengthened the T_{50}.

Hahn, Messer and Bradley (1976) studied by means of electron microscopy the rapidity with which Hb S underwent polymerization when Hb-SS erythrocytes were exposed to a degree of hypoxia as might be found in the capillary circulation. Some erythrocytes were found 0.5–1.0 second after exposure to an oxygen tension of 4.7 kPa to be indistinguishable from oxygenated cells. Most, however, appeared abnormal; there were areas of increased electron density in some and randomly oriented short fibres could be seen in others; the fibres were not, however, highly ordered and tightly packed until at least 15 seconds had elapsed, at which time most of the cells were still normally shaped when viewed under the light microscope. On reoxygenation, the return of reversibly sickled cells to a normal shape lagged behind the disappearance of fibres demonstrable by electron microscopy. The rate of polymer formation was found to be greatly influenced by the concentration of Hb S present. With relatively light cells (MCHC 31 g/dl), fibres were not observed within 40 seconds of deoxygenation; with relatively dense cells (MCHC 36 g/dl), on the other hand, they were visible in 3 seconds.

AGGREGATION OF Hb-S MOLECULES AND GELLING OF Hb-S SOLUTIONS

One of the consequences of the molecular aggregation which occurs when Hb S is deoxygenated is that haemoglobin in solution undergoes gelification (Singer and Chernoff, 1952; Singer and Singer, 1953). The sol–gel transformation is temperature sensitive — it is inhibited at low temperatures and markedly dependent, too, upon the haemoglobin being present in sufficient concentration.

Singer and Singer (1953) reported on the phenomenon of gelling in considerable detail; they considered that the gelling phenomenon indicated the presence of S haemoglobin and that it did not occur with any other type of human haemoglobin. The lowest Hb-S concentration of a haemolysate was designated as its 'lowest gelling point'. Singer and Singer showed that the lowest gelling points in haemolysates derived from the sickle-cell trait, the 'C variant' (Hb C plus Hb S) and from sickle-cell anaemia (Hb S plus Hb F) differed distinctly; and they used the demonstrable differencs in the lowest gelling points as a basis for a diagnostic gelling test to distinguish between sickle-cell anaemia, sickle-cell trait and atypical, e.g. 'C variant', cases.

Following Singer and Singer's (1953) pioneer studies, the exact circumstances under which gelling of Hb S takes place, and the effect of the presence of other haemoglobins on the process, have been the subjects of much research.

Charache and Conley (1964) studied a variety of combinations of Hb S with another haemoglobin. Hb D Punjab was notable in that Hb-SD erythrocytes behaved similarly to Hb-SS cells in relation to increase in blood viscosity on deoxygenation despite the relatively low concentration of Hb S in the Hb-SD cells. An order of reactivity was established: Hb D Punjab > Hb C > Hb J Baltimore = Hb A > Hb F.

Haemoglobin interaction was further investigated by Bertles, Rabinowitz and Döbler (1969, 1970), who concluded that while Hb A and Hb C can participate in the filamentous fine structure characteristic of sickling, Hb F cannot; i.e., γ chains cannot bind to (interact with) deoxygenated molecules of Hb S. They worked with cell-free haemolysates, made mixtures, deoxygenated them and measured the proportion of each haemoglobin in the resultant gels after submitting the gels to electrophoresis. Electron microscopy of mixtures of Hb D and Hb C and of Hb S and Hb A revealed bundles of parallel filaments similar to those found in gels derived from pure deoxygenated Hb S.

Kinetics and mechanism of gelation

Minton (1973) suggested that aggregation of deoxygenated Hb-S molecules took place in two steps: a linear polymerization of haemoglobin tetramers into filaments followed by a side-to-side aggregation of the filaments. The second step was thought to result in the sol-gel change.

Hofrichter, Ross and Eaton (1974) defined two stages in the process of gelation: a delay period and then a sigmoid progress curve. The delay time was found to be exquisitely sensitive to the concentration of deoxyHb S present and to temperature: e.g., a decrease in concentration of Hb S from 23 g/dl to 22 g/dl increased the delay time by a factor of 4 and a 1°C rise in the 20–30°C range almost halved the delay time. Extrapolation of their in-vitro data to conditions *in vivo* led Hofrichter, Ross and Eaton to conclude that small changes in haemoglobin concentration and physiological changes in O_2 saturation would produce changes in delay time sufficiently great for it to be an extremely important variable in determining the clinical course of sickle-cell disease.

Bookchin and Nagel (1974) tabulated, in a valuable review on the interaction between human haemoglobins, the minimum concentration of Hb S required for gelling to take place in the presence of other haemoglobins: the concentration varied from 41 g/dl in a mixture of 40% Hb S and 60% Hb F to 32 g/dl in a mixture of 40% Hb S and 60% Hb A. (The minimum gelling concentration of Hb S alone was reported as 23–24 g/dl.) Bookchin and Nagel related the clinical severity of the sickling syndromes to the nature of the haemoglobin interacting with Hb S and to the extent to which the combinations facilitated gelling and sickling.

Moffat (1974) investigated the gelation behaviour of mixtures of Hb S and other haemoglobins and concluded that differences in gelation behaviour in haemoglobin mixtures are due to the formation of mixed hybrid tetramers produced by the association of unlike dimers.

Harris and Bensusan (1975) investigated by the continuous monitoring of viscosity the kinetics of the sol–gel transformation of Hb S brought about by deoxygenation; they experimented, too, with various combinations of haemoglobin. Using Hb S an initial lag phase was found to be followed by a gradual and minor increase in viscosity, then a rapid and major increase (to as much as 180 times the initial value), then a moderately rapid decrease, and finally equilibrium at approximately 50% of the maximum viscosity reached. The duration of the lag phase, the rate of increase in viscocity and the maximum change were greatly influenced by haemoglobin concentration and temperature. Adding Hb A or Hb F to Hb S lengthened the lag phase and attenuated the rate of increase in viscosity and its magnitude; adding Hb C to Hb S resulted in a different curve of increase, without the final phase of decrease as seen with Hb S. The results with Hb S in solution paralleled the effects of haemoglobin concentration, temperature, haemoglobin admixture, 2,3-DPG concentration and ionic strength on the sickling of intact cells and on the minimum gelling point of Hb S. The curious final decrease in viscosity, observed with Hb S, was thought possibly to be due to the lateral association of deoxyHb-S fibres, i.e., to a process of consolidation.

Eaton, Hofrichter and Ross (1976), in an interesting review, stressed the paramount importance of the concentration of Hb S, in addition to the degree of deoxygenation and temperature, on the gelling process: experimentally, variation in these three factors would result in gelling delay times of from less than 1 second to many hours or days, while a 20% decrease in Hb-S concentration would increase the delay time by a factor of approximately 250! Eaton, Hofrichter and Ross stressed, too, the possible significance of the delay time of gelation in relation to the clinical severity of sickle-cell disease; they pointed out that the capillary transit time would normally be about 1 second, and the O_2 saturation at the venous end of the capillary normally less than 75%, and they postulated that crises occur when the delay time for sickling (gelling) is shortened and capillary transit times are long enough to increase the probability of sickling taking place in the microcirculation. Hofrichter, Ross and Eaton (1976) measured by a new technique the delay time and extent of gelation in the same sample: their main conclusion was that, while the amount of polymer formed is roughly proportional to the supersaturation of Hb S, the delay time, i.e. the rate of polymer formation, is proportional to a high power of Hb-S solubility.

Magdoff-Fairchild and co-workers (1976) reported on thermodynamic aspects of the polymerization of deoxygenated Hb S, measuring its solubility at varying pH and temperature and at a range of concentrations.

Benesch and co-workers (1977, 1979), knowing that the presence of a naturally-occurring amino-acid substitution in the α chains of Hb-S molecules had been reported to inhibit the polymerization of Hb-S when deoxygenated, prepared in the laboratory a series of hybrid tetramers of haemoglobin containing the Hb-S substitution in the β chains and one of 14 different substitutions in the α chains. The solubility of the hybrid haemoglobins was measured after deoxygenation, and Benesch et al. were able to show that while surface mutations in certain regions of the α chain decreased the insolubility of native deoxyHb S mutations in other regions had no effect. Thus substitution of histidine for aspartic acid at the α-47 position caused some inhibition of polymerization (i.e. increased the solubility) of Hb S, while the substitution of tyrosine for aspartic acid at the α-75 position, and alanine for aspartic acid at the α-6 position, potentiated polymerization. This work thus confirmed that substitutions in the α chains could affect Hb-S fibre formation and gelling; and at the same time it threw some light on the mechanisms of the self-association of molecules of Hb S.

Benesch and co-workers (1980) reported further details of the extent to which the presence of Hb A, Hb A_2 and Hb F affected the gelling of Hb S when deoxygenated. In each case the additional haemoglobin was found to be incorporated into the gel and to increase the solubility of Hb S; Hb F was found to be particularly effective.

The intracellular polymerization of Hb S and its relevance to sickle-cell disease was dealt with by Noguchi and Schechter (1981) in a comprehensive review: they referred to the recent work that has demonstrated the existence of Hb-S polymer in some cells at high oxygen saturation and also to the existence of cells carrying significant amounts of deoxyHb S which do not show morphological evidence of sickling. They emphasized that deoxygenation leads to a continuum of cellular changes and that only with severe and prolonged deoxygenation do large domains of highly ordered polymer form which cause the cell to sickle. Noguchi and Schechter stressed that while cells containing large amounts of ordered polymer are likely to be caught in capillaries and venules, other cells containing polymer, although not obviously deformed, probably have difficulty in traversing the narrow constrictions presented by precapillary arterioles. Noguchi, Torchia and Schechter (1980, 1982) gave details of the relationship between oxygen tension and polymer formation as revealed by the technique of ^{13}C nuclear magnetic resonance. With Hb-SS cells polymer was detected at greater than 90% O_2 saturation; the amount of polymer increased, with decreasing O_2 saturation, to approximately 70% of the total haemoglobin at complete deoxygenation. In contrast, in Hb-AS cells no polymer was detected at greater than 60% O_2 saturation and approximately 40% polymer at complete deoxygenation. The relationship between polymer formation as a function of O_2 saturation was found to be roughly hyperbolic, reflecting the continuous nature of polymer formation, while that for sickle formation was sigmoidal.

Chien and co-workers (1982) reported on the quantitative relationship between deoxygenation and the rheological behaviour of Hb-SS cell suspensions and concentrated solutions of Hb S at different conditions of shear. At low O_2 saturation the viscoelastic property of Hb-SS cell suspensions was increasingly determined by the concentration of the intracellular Hb S; the data, too, indicated that Hb-S aggregates can be dispersed by shear stress. Briehl (1982) found that the relationship between the delay time of gelation of deoxyHb S and shear was a complicated one: on the one hand, intra-erythrocytic shear was found to accelerate gelation; on the other, shear was found to convert a solid gel to a viscous one.

Adachi and Asakura (1982) found that the aggregation of Hb S when deoxygenated was greatly influenced by the concentration of phosphate buffer in which the haemoglobin was dissolved.

Danish and Harris (1983) studied the gelation of Hb-S solutions in dilute phosphate buffer, as measured in a microviscometer. They concluded that microaggregates are formed early in the lag phase, that stirring favours the formation of the microaggregates, and that the aggregation becomes stable if the shearing is stopped.

Nischio and co-workers (1983), using a laser light-scattering technique, were able to demonstrate the aggregation of Hb S in single Hb-SS cells; they showed, too, that the aggregation dispersed on reoxygenation and suggested that the technique might prove of use in the testing of anti-sickling drugs.

Wenger and Balcerzak (1984) reported a further study on the kinetics of Hb-S polymerization. Temperature changes were used to induce polymerization or depolymerization of Hb-S solutions, and the occurrence of gelation was determined by viscosity change or spectrophotometrically. Agitation of the sample was found to accelerate gelling and to reduce the delay time.

Embury and co-workers (1985) used differential polarization imaging microscopy to detect aligned polymer (AP) within individual Hb-S-containing cells. With this technique the presence of polymer is indicated by linear dichroism. No polymer was detected by this means in oxygenated Hb-AA and Hb-SS cells. On the other hand, with deoxygenated Hb-SS cells the signals due to AP were given by several types of cells: those with multiple domains of AP; those with AP, unaligned polymer and unpolymerized haemoglobin, and normal discocytes with AP arranged concentrically around the cells' periphery.

Brittenham, Schechter and Noguchi (1985) presented an interesting analysis of the role of Hb-S polymerization in relation to the haemolytic and clinical severity in 12 different sickling syndromes, calculating the degree of intracellular Hb-S polymerization (the polymer fraction), in relation to O_2 saturation, from knowledge of the MCHC and the proportions of Hb S, Hb F, Hb A_2 and Hb A present. They concluded that the polymer fraction present was indeed the primary determinant of both haemolytic and clinical severity and accounted for approximately 80% of patient-to-patient variability. In general, the lower the polymer fraction the higher the haemoglobin level was found to be in the different syndromes.

Birefringence of Hb-S solutions

Mizukami and co-workers (1986) studied the birefringence of thin layers of Hb-S solutions as an indication of polymer formation. When the solutions were deoxygenated slowly, birefingence appeared at Hb-S concentrations greater than 24 g/dl and its magnitude increased as the concentration of haemoglobin was increased. The magnitude of birefringence, however, decreased as the rate of deoxygenation was increased. Experiments in which erythrocyte ghosts were added to purified Hb-S solutions suggested that the ghosts served as templates on which large Hb-S polymers could form at relatively high rates of deoxygenation.

IRREVERSIBLY SICKLED CELLS (ISCs)

The sickled erythrocytes seen in films made from Hb-SS blood that has been allowed to dry in the air are irreversibly sickled cells (ISCs). They have lost their ability to revert to a normal shape despite exposure to oxygen at atmospheric tension (> 100 mm Hg).

As seen in dried and stained blood films or scanning electron micrographs, ISCs differ in appearance from the sickled cells that form *in vitro* when Hb-SS blood is deoxygenated: they have a smoother contour, lack terminal spikes and may be simply elongated or oat-shaped rather than sickled-shaped (Fig. 14.8). As already referred to and illustrated (p. 80 and Figs. 12.8–12.12), ISCs are present in variable numbers in the peripheral blood of Hb-SS patients and may comprise up to 40% or even 50% of the erythrocyte population; they are rarely absent. Only small numbers are likely to be found in Hb-S/β-thalassaemia or none at all, and they are rarely present in Hb-SC disease or Hb-SE disease. ISCs are, however, regularly present in Hb-SD disease (Fig. 13.14) and in Hb-SO disease.

The presence of sickled cells that failed to revert to a normal disc-like shape when the peripheral blood of sickle-cell anaemia patients was exposed to atmospheric air was commented on by Scriver and Waugh (1930) and Diggs and Bibb (1939) and subsequently by Murphy and Shapiro (1944, 1945) and Shen, Fleming and Castle (1949).

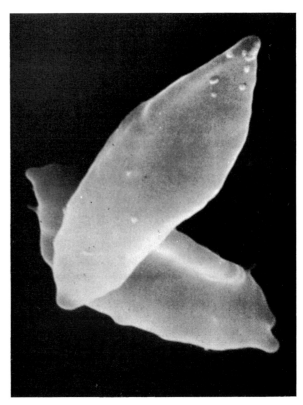

Fig. 14.8 Scanning electron micrograph of two irreversibly sickled cells.
(Reproduced by permission of Dr J. G. White.)

Scriver and Waugh (1930) studied in detail a 7-year-old black girl in Montreal whom they had diagnosed as suffering from sickle-cell anaemia and confirmed the relationship between oxygen tension and sickling that had been previously demonstrated by Hahn and Gillespie (1927). Their patient was found to have approximately 10% of sickled cells in the peripheral blood when films were made in the ordinary way and allowed to dry in air. A similar percentage was noted in sealed cover-slip preparations immediately after preparation; after 24 hours, however, the percentage was noted to have increased to over 80%. Scriver and Waugh then attempted to make permanent preparations of the blood which had been sealed and allowed to stand; they found, however, that on exposure to air (whilst the films were drying) most of the sickled cells reverted to the normal form. Only approximately 10% of the cells in the dried films remained sickled and this suggested to them 'the possibility that they represent the original sickle cells and are of a more persistent character'. Scriver and Waugh thus undoubtedly described irreversibly sickled cells, although they did not name them as such. They made and recorded another interesting observation: namely, that the O_2-dissociation curve of their patient's blood was distinctly shifted to the right. [Much later work on the relationship between O_2-dissociation curves, anaemia and 2,3-DPG concentration is summarized on pages 18–20 (Vol. 1).]

Diggs and Bibb (1939), too, undoubtedly described irreversibly sickled cells but they, too, did not use this title. They pointed out that cells that are elliptic or oat- or crescent-shaped at the time of preparation of a test for sickling do not undergo changes similar to those undergone by round or oval cells: they described them as having 'evidently already passed through the process, have lost their filaments and finlike appendages and have become irreparably changed in shape'. They noted, too, their presence in the pleural and peritoneal cavities of three patients with 'sicklemia' (Hb-AS trait) who had no sickled cells in the peripheral blood. The sickled cells from the cavities 'would not round up on exposure to air' and were described as 'irrevocably sickled'.

Murphy and Shapiro (1944, 1945), similarly appear not to have used the term 'irreversibly sickled cells'. However, in describing what happens to a cell when it sickled, they wrote: 'its flexibility is lost and it appears as fixed and rigid as a crystal of ice as it moves about and abuts against cells and fixed objects' (Murphy and Shapiro, 1944). Later, they wrote that the sickling threshold decreases with age until the cell becomes 'permanently sickled' and that the cell becomes 'all the more unalterably sickled as it approaches senility' (Murphy and Shapiro, 1945).

Shen, Fleming and Castle (1949), on the other hand, did use the term 'irreversibly sickled cells'. They noted that the sickled cells seen in films allowed to dry in air did not show the filaments produced when previously normal cells sickled *in vitro*. They suggested that the cells became irreversibly sickled because of previous periods of intermittent or continuous stagnation in tissue capillaries and they noted that such cells rarely stained as reticulocytes. They found when the

blood of four patients was incubated for up to 24 hours at 37.5°C in the absence of oxygen that many of the cells which were not reticulocytes eventually lost their ability to revert to their previously disc-like shape. Reticulocytes, on the other hand, retained to a considerable extent their ability to do this.

ISCs are more mechanically fragile than are non-sickled cells (Shen, Castle and Fleming, 1944; Lange, Minnich and Moore, 1951) and haemolysis *in vivo* has been shown to be positively correlated with the ISC count (Serjeant, Serjeant and Milner, 1969; McCurdy and Sherman, 1978; etc.) (see p. 222). The content of Hb F in ISCs has been shown to be on the whole less than that in cells capable of reversible sickling.

Bertles, Roth and Anku (1967) and Bertles and Milner (1968) measured the optical density of individual cells stained by the Betke-Kleihauer technique and found that the mean values for Hb F in ISCs were consistently less than half that in non ISCs. In blood fractionated by centrifugation, the percentage Hb F as measured by alkali resistance, fell off markedly in the heaviest fractions containing more than 90% ISCs. Bertles and Milner (1968) concluded that the synthesis of Hb F was least in those cells which were destined to become irreversibly sickled and that ISCs suffered preferential destruction. They also adduced from labelling experiments that the non-ISC to ISC transformation might take place early in a cell's life-span, *i.e.* soon after the cell had been released from the bone marrow.

Jensen, Bromberg and Barefield (1969) exposed ISCs to a hypotonic medium and reported that the cells became ovoid and then spherical before lysing. When the ghosts were resuspended in an isotonic medium they assumed their original distorted shape, and Jensen, Bromberg and Barefield concluded that ISCs result from permanent membrane changes.

Chien, Usami and Bertles (1970), who studied blood fractionated by centrifugation, concluded that the MCV of ISCs was reduced and the MCHC raised. However, the MCH of the top fraction and the bottom fraction which contained 50–70% ISCs was identical.

As already referred to (p. 28), Serjeant (1970) concluded, based on his experience of 325 Jamaican patients aged between 12 and 60 years, that a low ISC count was associated with persistence of splenomegaly. The count, too, was found not to increase with age and to be unaffected by splenectomy. It was negatively correlated with the Hb-F percentage, although varying widely in patients who had low Hb-F levels.

That ISCs can result solely from the presence of Hb S independently of any abnormality in the

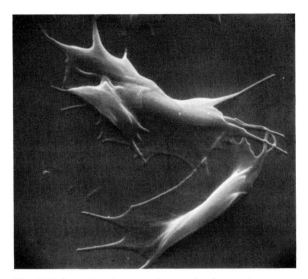

Fig. 14.9 Scanning electron micrograph of normal erythrocyte membrane: Hb-S hybrid cells after deoxygenation with sodium dithionite.

[Reproduced by permission from Clark and Shohet (1976).]

erythrocyte membrane was illustrated by the ingenious experiments of Clark and Shohet (1976). Hybrid erythrocytes formed of normal membranes, but containing Hb S, sickled on deoxygenation and became ISCs after prolonged anoxia (Fig. 14.9); in contrast, hybrid cells formed of the erythrocyte membranes of Hb-SS patients, but containing Hb A, did not sickle under any conditions of deoxygenation.

The interrelationships between the ISC count and other blood indices have been clearly established by the report of Serjeant and his co-workers (1978) from the West Indies. A review of 515 Hb-SS patients revealed that their ISC counts were positively correlated with total MCH and MCHC and Hb-S MCH and MCHC and negatively correlated with total Hb and Hb-F percentage; it seemed, too, that a low MCHC probably determined low ISC counts at any Hb-F level.

The importance of MCHC on the deformability of ISCs was again emphasized by Clark, Mohandas and Shohet (1980). Using an ektacytometer they were able to demonstrate the profound influence of MCHC and intracellular viscosity on the deformability of well-oxygenated ISCs: they reported that virtually undeformable cells became totally deformable when osmolarity

was reduced from 290 to 130 m-osM and concluded that cellular dehydration rather than altered membrane properties is the primary determinant of the decreased deformability of ISCs; they stressed that fully oxygenated ISCs were undeformable. Eaton, Jacob and White (1979), in a valuable and comprehensive review, provided a summary of the general characteristics of the ISC and of its morphology, rheology and life-span, its formation *in vivo* and *in vitro*, the composition of its membrane and the nature of its membrane defect, and the implications that the presence of ISCs has for the therapy of Hb-SS disease.

Palek and Liu (1979) suggested the following sequence of events: polymerization of intracellular and membrane-bound deoxyHb S leads to deformation of the spectrin cytoskeleton, independently of erythrocyte Ca^{2+} and ATP; then follows a marked increase in membrane permeability for monovalent and divalent cations leading to a net Ca^{2+} gain and dehydration; next a Ca^{2+} ATP-dependent rearrangement of spectrin takes place resulting in a rigid ISC.

Clark and her co-workers (1980) concluded that the phenomenon of fixed sickling is dependent on severe ion and water loss, that the membrane of ISCs is more deformable than had previously been thought and that the idea that an elevated Ca^{2+} content of the membrane directly causes increased rigidity is probably wrong, excess calcium acting in their view on the basis of the Gardos effect.

Allan and co-workers (1981) reported on the relationship between ISC formation and the release from the cells of microvesicles. The blood of 17 Hb-SS patients was incubated at 37°C for up to 96 hours. ISCs developed and free microvesicles were liberated equivalent in some cases to a loss of up to 10% of the total cell phospholipid. Ca^{2+} ions were found not to be required for the formation of the microvesicles; Ca^{2+}, however, accelerated the process. Allan *et al.* suggested that ISCs formed *in vivo* are less spiculated than cells sickled *in vitro* because they have lost spicules in the form of microvesicles.

Bessis, Feo and Jones (1982) studied the relationship between pO_2 and the deformability of Hb-AS and Hb-SS erythrocytes, using an automated ektacytometer. Hb-AS cells were found to give a pO_2 versus deformability curve which varied from patient to patient: the cells were found to be normally deformable at a pO_2 of 5 mm Hg upwards at a pH of 7.3, but a lower pH (*e.g.* 7.1) and a rise in osmolarity induced loss of deformability at pO_2 tensions of up to 40 mm Hg. Hb-SS blood also exhibited patient-to-patient differences and marked heterogeneity, too, within an individual patient's erythrocyte population. Five fractions were separated by centrifugation and were shown to give characteristic responses, specific for each patient, to pO_2 change, pH and osmolarity. ISCs and the densest discocytes, with an MCHC of 37 g/dl, were found to be non-deformable. The ektacytometric method was considered to be potentially valuable in the assessment of anti-sickling drugs.

Westerman and Allan (1983) studied the formation of ISCs by inducing cell shrinkage, ion loss, Ca^{2+} accumulation and membrane loss singly or in combination by treating the cells with the ionophore valinomycin, the ionophore A23187 plus Ca^{2+} or hypertonic saline. Their data pointed to loss of water as an important factor in bringing about the irreversible sickling of Hb-SS cells. Endogenously-formed ISCs were found not to release microvesicles when treated with the ionophore A23187 nor to release spicules as the result of repeated deoxygenation-reoxygenation. It was suggested that this is because such cells have already lost in vivo that portion of their membrane which is susceptible to removal by these means.

Nash, Johnson and Meiselman (1984) employed a micropipette technique to measure cell surface area, volume, membrane shear elastic modulus and time constant for viscoelastic shape recovery and used these measurements to calculate membrane surface viscosity. Their data suggested that ISCs are formed by a two-stage process: (1) accelerated loss of volume leading to increased cytoplasmic and effective membrane viscosity, and (2) a sharp rise in membrane rigidity thought to be linked with structural alteration to the membrane. They concluded that the rheological properties of Hb-SS blood depend upon the presence of poorly deformable reversibly sickled cells as well as the presence of ISCs.

Counting sickled cells in blood samples

A sickle-cell count comprises reversibly sickled cells as well as irreversibly sickled cells (ISCs) and unless precautions are taken to withdraw samples of blood without allowing exposure to air, followed by fixation, as for instance in formalin in isotonic saline, counting will give an erroneous result. The sickled cells seen in films of blood allowed to dry in air are ISCs.

Jensen, Rucknagel and Taylor (1960) reported the results of a carefully conducted study into the percentage of sickled cells present in venous and arterial blood of 10 Hb-SS patients and two Hb-SC patients. The blood was collected anaerobically and fixed in formal-saline. The percentage O_2 saturation of the blood samples was also estimated. As expected the arterial blood samples

(obtained by femoral puncture) contained fewer sickled cells than the venous samples (obtained by catheterization from eight sites). Although the percentage of sickled cells differed considerably between the patients, the percentage present in the venous samples obtained from different sites was relatively constant in individual patients despite moderate differences in oxygen content. None of the patients had more than 30% sickled cells, and there was no obvious correlation between the sickled-cell percentage and the clinical severity of their illness.

The question of the relationship between oxygen tension in vivo and the proportion of erythrocytes which undergo sickling was reinvestigated by Serjeant, Petch and Serjeant (1973). They studied 10 patients and estimated the percentage of sickled cells (total, reversibly sickled and irreversibly sickled) in formal-saline-fixed blood obtained from five sites by venous catheterization and compared the percentage with that in brachial artery blood exposed to air or 100% oxygen. The ISC count was steady and constant in all areas, but there was a general tendency for the reversibly sickled cell count in the venous samples to increase with fall in O_2 saturation. Inhalation of 100% oxygen produced a fall in the total percentage count in pulmonary artery (venous) and brachial artery blood in nine out of the 10 patients studied. Serjeant, Petch and Serjeant made the point that a negative correlation between O_2 saturation and percentage sickled cells is apparent when the data of single individuals are studied but may be lost when the data of several patients whose susceptibility to sickling differs are pooled.

Clark and co-workers (1982) had suggested that as it was difficult to carry out ISC counts accurately, cell density should be measured as an alternative. By means of a simple 2-step density gradient analysis of whole blood centrifuged in a microhaematocrit, the proportion of high-density cells was shown to be closely correlated with the percentage of morphologically identified ISCs; measurement of cell deformability by means of an ektacytometer was also shown to be closely correlated with the ISC count.

Rodgers, Noguchi and Schechter (1984) also questioned the accuracy of ISC counts; they pointed out that a very high partial pressure of O_2 is required for full saturation of Hb-SS erythrocytes with oxygen and that exposure of blood to carbon monoxide gives a more accurate measure of the percentage of sickled cells that are in a truly irreversible state. Data from 10 patients were quoted: blood exposed to room air (90.9% O_2 saturation), mean ISC count 14.7%, range 6.4–28.4%; blood exposed to 100% oxygen (97.5% O_2 saturation), mean ISC count 9.9%, range 5.0–13.4%; blood exposed to carbon monoxide (100% CO saturation), mean ISC count 6.6%, range 2.6–13.5%

CATION CONTENT, CATION PERMEABILITY AND CELL WATER OF SICKLED CELLS

It has been repeatedly shown that the sickling phenomenon is associated with changes in cellular cation content: namely, a relatively small increase in intracellular Na^+ accompanied by a relatively large loss of intracellular K^+. The net result is a fall in Na^+ plus K^+, some loss of cell water and a rise in MCHC. Sickled cells have, too, been reported to accumulate increased amounts of calcium, an element which is normally present in erythrocytes at only very low concentration. The cause and mechanism of the cation changes associated with sickling and their relevance to water content, MCHC and the rigidity of sickled cells, in particular ISCs, and their significance in relation to the vaso-occlusive and haemolytic phenomena of sickle-cell disease, have been closely studied.

Early reports. In 1944 Murphy and Shapiro stated that a single preliminary test using radioactive potassium had shown that the erythrocytes of a sickle-cell disease patient were about twice as permeable to K^+ as were control normal cells.

Tosteson, Shea and Darling (1952), Tosteson, Carlsen and Dunham (1955) and Tosteson (1955) reported that Hb-SS cells, when deoxygenated, lose K^+ and gain Na^+ and that the changes could not be accounted for by the increased amounts of intercellular plasma lying between centrifuged sickled cells. They concluded that sickling accelerated the transport of Na^+ and K^+ by a non-diffusion, presumed carrier, process.

Clarkson and Maizels (1955) observed that when sickle-cell anaemia blood was deoxygenated the amount of Na^+ that could be easily exchanged was increased and that the rate constant for the influx of Na^+ other than

that which is easily exchanged was approximately doubled.

Bartlett and co-workers (1955), who studied a 30-year-old patient with sickle-cell anaemia, found no evidence of any abnormality in carbohydrate metabolism: the utilization of glucose and the formation of lactate, and the uptake of inorganic [^{32}P] phosphate, were normal, irrespective of whether the erythrocytes were exposed to O_2 or N_2.

Adams (1957) reviewed the then available information on erythrocyte Na^+ and K^+ in sickle-cell anaemia and himself studied 10 patients with sickle-cell anaemia, 17 with the sickle-cell trait and 17 normal subjects. Significant alteration in Na^+ to K^+ ratios were observed. However, it was concluded that the changes were not the result of cellular electrolyte shifts but were produced by an increase in intercellular plasma in the centrifuged deoxygenated samples. Later work, summarized below, has, however, shown that this conclusion was erroneous and that when Hb-SS cells sickle there is a genuine loss of K^+ and gain of Na^+.

More recent reports. Statius van Eps and co-workers (1971) reported on the erythrocyte Na^+ and K^+ concentration in 27 Hb-SS patients, four Hb-SC patients and 25 normal control subjects. (No details of the sickle-cell disease patients were given except that they were said to be free of symptoms.) The mean Na^+ concentration was found to be elevated by 52% and the mean K^+ concentration to be reduced by 12%.

Masys, Bromberg and Balcerzak (1974) studied the cell volume changes accompanying the deoxygenation of Hb-SS, Hb-SC and Hb-AA erythrocytes: (1) using ^{131}I-albumin as a plasma marker so that movement of water in and out of the erythrocytes could be measured by the alteration in the concentration of the radio-label, and (2) measuring the distribution of cell volumes of glutaraldehyde-fixed oxygenated or deoxygenated erythrocytes by means of a Coulter Model B counter. The Hb-AA cells were found to swell when deoxygenated, but the Hb-SS cells shrank considerably, as did the Hb-SC cells to a lesser extent. On incubation of deoxygenated Hb-SS blood for up to 90 minutes, substantial amounts of K^+ were found to transfer from cell to plasma.

Glader and co-workers (1976) compared the cation, water and ATP content of ISCs formed *in vivo* with those of ISCs developed *in vitro* by depletion of ATP in the presence of Ca^{2+}. *In vitro*, the cells became depleted of K^+ and were markedly dehydrated. The findings in ISCs formed *in vivo* and separated from blood by centrifugation were similar: namely, very low K^+, low Na^+ plus K^+, a low MCV and low ATP.

Glader and Nathan (1978) reported detailed studies on alterations in cation permeability during sickling. Sickled (Hb-SS) cells incubated under 100% nitrogen for 4 hours lost K^+ and gained an equivalent amount of Na^+. No ISCs resulted. However, many ISCs developed when a cell suspension was incubated for 24 hours in a glucose-free Na^+ medium containing Ca^{2+}. The cells at the end of the incubation had a high Na$^+$ and a very low K$^+$ content and were depleted in cations and water. On the other hand, when the cells were incubated in 100% nitrogen in a glucose-free K$^+$ medium containing Ca^{2+}, there were no major changes in cation and water content and no ISCs formed. Glader and Nathan concluded that the formation of ISCs reflected the loss of K$^+$ and water in ATP-depleted cells in the presence of Ca^{2+}; also that it appeared unlikely that it was the accumulation of Ca^{2+} in the cell membrane that was alone responsible for the injury to the membrane — for ISCs did not develop in K$^+$-containing media. They, suggested, however, that the Ca^{2+} accumulation would lead to K$^+$ loss exceeding Na$^+$ gain, with consequent cell dehydration which could not be rectified by the Na$^+$, K$^+$-ATPase cation pump. In a further study, Glader and co-workers (1978) investigated the relationship between cation and other changes and the number of ISCs present in the peripheral blood of Hb-SS patients. The extent of the reduction in total Na$^+$ plus K$^+$ and in MCV was found to be positively correlated with the percentage of ISCs in the samples analysed. The ISCs, too, were found to be grossly depleted of ATP. The Na$^+$ concentration did not appear to be correlated with the ISC percentage.

Clark, Morrison and Shohet (1978) measured active cation transport in Hb-SS disease blood fractionated into reticulocytes, discoidal cells and ISCs. Active transport was decreased in the ISCs although ouabain-sensitive ATPase activity appeared normal.

Roth, Nagel and Bookchin (1981) reported that pH affects sickling and the passage of K$^+$ efflux across the cell membrane in an opposite manner: i.e., it increases K$^+$ efflux in a linear manner but diminishes sickling. They concluded that in testing possible anti-sickling drugs both intracellular and extracellular pH need to be controlled, if K$^+$ efflux is used as a reflection of the extent of intracellular Hb-S polymer formation.

The cause of the abnormal cation leaks in sickled cells remains unexplained. Rossi, Mohandas and Clark (1984) suggested that the K$^+$ leak could result from 'localized membrane stress imposed by growing bundles of Hb S polymer inside the cell'; they had found, that K$^+$ efflux was substantially greater in cells suspended in an isotonic medium than in a hypertonic medium in which deoxygenated Hb-SS cells do not form the long spicules of aggregated Hb S characteristic of cells deoxygenated in an isotonic medium (Clark et al., 1980).

Mohandas, Rossi and Clark (1986) described in detail the experiments they had carried out to test the hypothesis that the membrane distortion associated with sickling is directly related to the cation permeability changes that accompany sickling. Hb-SS erythrocytes were separated on Stractan density gradients into high and low MCHC cell populations. These were deoxygenated when suspended in media of varying osmolarity. When initially low MCHC cells were deoxygenated, the resulting increase in cation fluxes was found to be suppressed when the MCHC was increased by increasing the osmolarity of the suspending medium. This suppression was associated with inhibition of the cellular distortion. In contrast, deoxygenation of initially high MCHC cells had little effect on cation permeability and resulted in little cellular distortion. Reducing the MCHC of these cells by decreasing the osmolarity of the suspending medium resulted, however, in an increase in both cation permeability and in cellular distortion. Mohandas, Rossi and Clark concluded that their experimental data did in fact lend support to the hypothesis that membrane distortion is directly related to increased cation permeability.

Intra-erythrocytic pH

Lam, Lin and Ho (1979) measured the intra-erythrocytic pH in five adult Hb-SS and five Hb-AA subjects by means of ^{31}P nuclear magnetic resonance. The mean pH of the Hb-SS cells was 7.14 compared with 7.29 of the Hb-AA cells. The 2,3-DPG concentration in the fresh Hb-SS blood was 30% above normal but fell much faster than normal on incubation. The difference between the pH of the Hb-SS and Hb-AA cells was, nevertheless, found to remain constant, even after depletion of the DPG. Lam, Lin and Ho concluded that the low pH and higher than normal DPG concentration were intrinsic properties of Hb-SS blood, both of which promoted polymerization of Hb-SS molecules.

Kaperonis, Bertles and Chien (1979) similarly reported that the intracellular pH of Hb-SS cells was slightly but significantly lower than that of Hb-AA cells. They had studied nine Hb-SS patients and seven Hb-AA controls and measured whole-blood pH as well as the intracellular pH of erythrocytes separated into top, middle and bottom fractions by centrifugation. The whole-blood pH was similar in both groups, but the pH of the Hb-SS cells in each fraction was significantly less than that of the Hb-AA cells, the lowest pH of each genotype being in the bottom fraction of densest cells. Kaperonis, Bertles and Chien pointed out that as the densest cells have the lowest 2,3-DPG : haemoglobin ratio, the low pH cannot be due to the intracellular organic phosphate; they proposed instead that it is the result of a redistribution of ions caused by progressive alterations in the cell membranes in vivo.

Role of calcium

Eaton and co-workers (1973) reported that the mean Ca^{2+} content of Hb-SS erythrocytes was about 7.5 times the normal and that ISCs contained about twice as much Ca^{2+} as did cells of normal morphology. Studies with ^{45}Ca showed that the inward leak of Ca^{2+} was about 10 times the normal in oxygenated Hb-SS cells and was about 40 times the normal when the cells were deoxygenated (Fig. 14.10). Eaton et al. concluded that in Hb-SS disease an excess of Ca^{2+} accumulated in the cell membrane during sickling and probably 'fixed' it in a sickled shape and that this process would eventually produce ISCs; they suggested that the accumulation of Ca^{2+} plus progressive metabolic depletion could explain the diminished filterability of oxygenated Hb-SS cells. Experiments with a Ca^{2+} ionophore were thought to support this concept (Eaton et al., 1975).

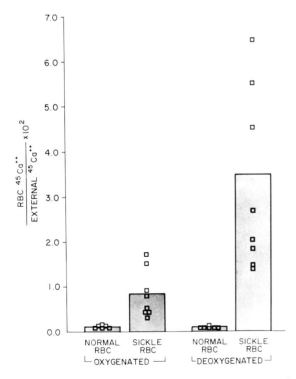

Fig. 14.10 Calcium leak into oxygenated and deoxygenated sickled erythrocytes.
Expressed as percentage of external $^{45}Ca^{2+}$ entering the cells during $1\frac{1}{2}$ hours' incubation at 37° C. The horizontal bars represent the means. [Reproduced by permission from Eaton et al. (1973).]

Palek (1973) reported similarly, but the differences observed between Hb-SS cells and normal cells were much less dramatic. The Ca^{2+} content of Hb-SS erythrocytes (as measured by atomic absorption spectrophotometry) was found to be 2.6 times greater than that of normal cells and 1.7 times that of the cells from patients with other types of haemolytic anaemia and comparable reticulocyte counts. When Hb-SS disease cells sickled, ^{45}Ca was rapidly taken up and there was a further uptake if the cells were depleted of ATP. With normal cells, restoration of ATP was followed by a rapid extrusion of Ca^{2+}, but this did not happen with Hb-SS cells. ^{45}Ca was not rapidly taken up when Hb-SS cells were incubated in the presence of oxygen.

Schrier and co-workers (1975) studied ^{45}Ca efflux and endocytosis in the resealed erythrocyte ghosts of five patients with Hb-SS disease. They concluded that although Ca^{2+} is probably present in Hb-SS ghosts in one pool accessible to the Ca^{2+} pump, its inaccessibility in other juxtamembrane pools probably accounts for the rigidity of Hb-SS erythrocytes and their ghosts.

Several more recent studies (see below) have confirmed that erythrocyte calcium levels are abnormally raised in sickle-cell disease and that ISCs are particularly highly loaded with calcium. Flux studies with ^{45}Ca have shown that calcium uptake is excessive, and there is some evidence that the Ca^{2+} plus Mg^{2+}-ATPase — the calcium pump — and calmodulin, the pump activator, act normally, but that some abnormal property of the cell membrane prevents calmodulin activating the pump in the normal way.

Palek, Thomas and Ozog (1977) measured erythrocyte Ca^{2+} and Ca^{2+} movement in Hb-SS erythrocytes by atomic absorption spectrophotometry: the mean Ca^{2+} content was approximately 2.5 times that of control cells and 2.0 times that of the mean value given by 18 patients suffering from other types of haemolytic anaemia. The dense Hb-SS cell fraction, rich in ISCs, had a higher Ca^{2+} content than the light fraction. The ^{45}Ca studies indicated an abnormally high influx into Hb-SS cells. This was thought to relate to the sickling change because the excessive influx did not occur if sickling was prevented by carbon monoxide and because the heightened influx was observed, too, but to a lesser degree, with Hb-AS cells that had undergone sickling.

Steinberg (1978) reported on similar studies carried out on the blood of 31 patients (26 Hb SS) suffering from sickle-cell disorders of different clinical severity. In Hb-SS disease the Ca^{2+} uptake was found to be increased under both oxygenated and deoxygenated conditions; it was directly correlated with the number of ISCs present and inversely correlated with the intracellular K^+ concentration. No relationship was established, however, between the severity of disease score and Ca^{2+} levels, Ca^{2+} flux and ISC count.

Eaton and co-workers (1978) reported on experiments in which they had exposed normal and Hb-SS erythrocytes to small amounts of calcium in the presence of an ionophore (a monocarboxylic acid which allows the free passage of divalent cations, especially Ca^{2+}, across membranes). Calcium accumulation, achieved in this way, was found to lead to a decrease in cell water, K^+, ATP and osmotic fragility — all characteristics of ISCs. Also, Ca^{2+} loading caused a marked decrease in the O_2 affinity of Hb-SS cells (but not of normal cells), another hallmark of ISCs. The ionophore-induced Ca^{2+} accumulation of deoxygenated Hb-SS cells was found, too, to result in the temporary retention of the sickled shape following reoxygenation, despite an absence of detectable intracellular Hb-S fibres.

Jain and Shohet (1981) demonstrated that Ca^{2+}-loaded erythrocytes were more sensitive than normal cells to lipid peroxidation after exposure to a peroxidant threat; they suggested that loading with calcium could be a factor in the peroxidation of lipid found in sickled cells.

Wiley and McCulloch (1982) reviewed the mechanisms controlling the transport of calcium through the erythrocyte membrane and the effect of drugs thereon, as well as the findings in the clinical syndromes, of which Hb-SS disease is but one, in which the Ca^{2+} flux is known to be abnormal.

Bookchin and Lew (1983), in their review of erythrocyte membrane abnormalities in Hb-SS disease, concluded that the hypothesis that attributes cellular dehydration and rigidity to the cells' increased Ca^{2+} content is 'inconsistent with experience'. They quoted preliminary evidence in support of the view that 'the paradoxical failure of intracellular Ca^{2+} to cause its well-known effects may be due to compartmentalization of the increased calcium inside concealed inside-out vesicles, which are more numerous in SS cells than in normal red cells'.

Ortiz, Lew and Bookchin (1986) investigated the relationship between the amount of calcium in the membrane of Hb-SS erythrocytes and leak of potassium. They obtained, however, no evidence of a Ca^{2+}-sensitive K^+ channel activity in oxygenated Hb-SS cells, but their data did not exclude the possibility of brief activation of K^+ channels during deoxygenation-induced polymerization of Hb S, thereby contributing to the dehydration of the deoxygenated cells.

Ca^{2+}, Mg^{2+}-ATPase (the calcium pump). Gopinath and Vincenzi (1979) reported that the Ca^{2+}, Mg^{2+}-ATPase in Hb-SS erythrocytes responded less than normally to the activator protein (calmodulin) and that both young and old Hb-SS cells responded similarly.

Litosch and Lee (1980) found that resealed Hb-SS erythrocytes preloaded with ^{45}Ca retained approximately 4 times more ^{45}Ca than did normal cells and that diminution in Ca^{2+}, Mg^{2+}-ATPase pump activity — estimated to be 84% of the normal — could not explain this; they concluded that the retention of Ca^{2+} was a reflection of an alteration in the Ca^{2+}-binding properties of the cell membrane.

Dixon and Winslow (1981) prepared Ca^{2+}, Mg^{2+}-ATPase from Hb-AA, Hb-AS and Hb-SS individuals and calmodulin from Hb-SS and Hb-AA ghosts. They found that calmodulin prepared from either source failed to stimulate the ATPase of Hb-SS cells and they concluded that the accumulation of Ca^{2+} in Hb-SS cells was probably not the result of an abnormality of the calmodulin but more likely to be due to an abnormal property of the membrane preventing the calmodulin from interacting at the ATPase sites in the membrane.

Luthra and Sears (1982) reported the Ca^{2+}-ATPase activity in haemolysates of Hb-SS erythrocytes was greater than that in haemolysates prepared from normal Hb-AA cells. (This was true, too, of Mg^{2+} and Na^+, K^+-ATPase activities.) The highest ATPase activity was found in low-density (young) Hb-SS cells, but its activity exceeded the normal in cells of all the density fractions tested. Luthra and Sears concluded that the high Ca^{2+} levels found in Hb-SS cells could not be explained by any failure of the calcium pump.

Effect of sickling on cellular ATP content and role of metabolic depletion in ISC formation

The ATP content of ISCs has been the subject of some controversy. It seems that the processes leading to irreversibility of sickling can take place in the presence of normal amounts of ATP but that the oldest ISCs, at least, may have a markedly reduced concentration.

Prankerd (1955) reported on studies carried out on two patients with sickle-cell disease, one a black female, the other a white male. Sickling in vitro was found to be associated with a slowing of uptake of ^{32}P, a fall in ATP and a diminution in the specific activity of intracellular prosphate esters and a rise in the specific activity of intracellular orthophosphate.

Jensen, Shohet and Nathan (1973) considered the proposition that irreversibility of sickling is a consequence of failure of cellular metabolism. However, they found that only if ATP is almost completely depleted are sickled cells unable to revert to discs. If Ca^{2+} was omitted, ISCs were not generated despite metabolic depletion.

Lessin and Wallas (1973) concluded that ISCs were generated as the result of prolonged hypoxia and that the membrane lesion in ISCs was induced by membrane–haemoglobin interaction, independently of cellular ATP levels. In an experimental system, ATP levels were maintained for the first 16 hours of incubation (under 95% N_2). ISCs, however, developed before this — slowly for the first 12 hours and then more rapidly. Membrane-bound haemoglobin, in the form of microaggregates demonstrable by electron microscopy, increased in amount slowly during the first 16 hours and then rapidly during the final 8 hours of incubation.

Glader and Müller (1975) concluded that dehydration *per se* could induce irreversible membrane injury, *i.e.*, ISC formation, independently of cellular energy status or Ca^{2+} content.

Weed and Bessis (1975) attempted to measure the ATP content of individual ISCs by means of the luciferin-luciferase reaction. The cell's ATP content, as visualized under the phase-contrast microscope, was very low compared with the mean values for the whole erythrocyte population and non-ISCs, respectively. Glader and co-workers (1976), too, reported that a low ATP was a characteristic of ISCs formed *in vivo*. Clark, Unger and Shohet (1978), however, were unable to confirm that the ATP content of ISCs was markedly reduced. They separated Hb-SS blood into seven fractions by centrifugation and found that the ATP level in the cells in the heaviest fractions, containing a high proportion of ISCs, did not differ significantly from that in the cells in the lighter fractions containing few ISCs.

AUTO-OXIDATION OF THE Hb-SS ERYTHROCYTE MEMBRANE

The possibility that auto-oxidation of the erythrocyte membrane is a factor leading to shortening of the life-span of Hb-SS erythrocytes has received increasing attention in recent years. Evidence in favour of this has been based on measurements of erythrocyte and plasma vitamin-E concentrations and of intracellular GSH and of the activity of GSH peroxidase, catalase and superoxide dismutase (enzymes which protect against oxidative damage), as well as on the assessment of the spontaneous generation of oxygen and hydroxyl radicals and of the accumulation of denaturation products of haemoglobin within the cell membrane. The sensitivity of Hb-SS erythrocytes to oxidant stress *in vitro* has, too, been explored. Reports dealing with the results of such studies are summarized below, and there now seems little doubt but that cell membrane oxidant damage, as well as lipid peroxidation, contribute to the increased haemolysis that is a feature of severe forms of sickle-cell disease.

Nair, McCullough and Das (1977) reported that they had measured superoxide dismutase (SOD) activity and membrane peroxidation following peroxide threat in both the ISC and reversible sickle-cell (RSC) fractions of sickle-cell anaemia blood. Both fractions were found to possess abnormally high levels of SOD activity and to be highly susceptible to oxidation injury. The high SOD activity was considered to be a defence mechanism against oxidative stress. Das and Nair (1980), who studied up to 20 adult Hb-SS patients, reported that sickled erythrocytes contained less GSH peroxidase and catalase activity, but more SOD activity and 'peroxidation potential', than did normal control erythrocytes; fluorescent lipid pigment and malonyldialdehyde, suggestive of membrane lipid peroxidation, were also demonstrable. Heinz bodies, too, were to be seen by transmission electron microscopy in some erythrocyte membranes.

Chiu and Lubin (1979) reported on vitamin-E levels in 54 Hb-SS patients, The concentration of the vitamin in both plasma and erythrocytes was significantly lower than in controls; in contrast, GSH peroxidase activity was found to be greater than normal. Chiu, Lubin and Shohet (1979) studied the effect of sickling on the susceptibility of the lipid in Hb-SS erythrocytes to peroxidation by H_2O_2 (as indicated by the formation of malonyldialdehyde) and also the effect of sickling on the reaction of cells to trinitrobenzenesulphonic acid (TNBS), a probe identifying aminophospholipids on the cell surface. They found that when Hb-SS cells were sickled by deoxygenation the susceptibility to peroxidation and the binding on of TNBS were markedly increased. The data were held to imply that a rearrangement of the membrane lipids takes place during sickling, and Chiu, Lubin and Shohet suggested that in ISCs such reorganization becomes permanent.

Zimmerman and Natta (1981) found that the whole-blood GSH peroxidase activity in 21 black Hb-SS patients was significantly increased compared to that in normal blacks; they studied in addition 21 other blacks suffering from various other haemoglobinopathies (of whom 13 had α- thalassaemia trait or Hb-H disease) and found high values in most of these patients, too.

The role of spontaneous oxygen radical generation by sickled erythrocytes and of auto-oxidation as a mechanism of membrane damage, which might be crucial for adhesion to endothelial cells, was considered by Hebbel and his co-workers in a series of communications and papers (Hebbel, Eaton and Steinberg, 1981; 1982; Hebbel *et al.*, 1982; Rank *et al.*, 1983) and summarized in a recent review (Hebbel, 1985).

Wetterstroem and Brewer (1981) had studied the erythrocytes of 29 sickle-cell disease patients and concluded that the cells' capacity to withstand oxidant stress was less than normal. The mean erythrocyte GSH content was subnormal despite the young age of the cells; GSH reductase activity was normal but that of GSH peroxidase was raised. There was, too, a significant negative correlation between the patients' ISC counts and the cells' GSH content.

Hebbel, Eaton and Steinberg (1981, 1982) demonstrated that the spontaneous generation of oxygen and hydroxyl radicals by fresh Hb-SS erythroctes was abnormally high and that H_2O_2 formation and superoxide activity were increased. Haemichrome (HC), a denatured product of ferric haemoglobin, was also demonstrable. This was considered to be the 'footprint' of erythrocyte auto-oxidation and to indicate, and perhaps facilitate and accelerate, the occurrence of membrane damage; the amount of membrane-bound HC was thought to correlate positively with erythrocyte adherence to endothelium and with clinical severity. Details of the work and conclusions summarized above were given by Hebbel et al. (1982).

Further information on haemichrome (HC) in Hb-SS erythrocytes was provided by Campwala and Desforges (1982), who had studied the blood of five Hb-SS patients and eight normal Hb-AA controls. Washed membranes of the highest density Hb-AA cells (separated on a Stractan gradient) contained much more HC than did Hb-AA cells of lesser density. Similar preparations obtained from both high- and low-density Hb-SS cells contained 3–4 times as much HC as that present in the membranes of the whole population of Hb-AA cells (and about the same as that in the membranes of the highest density Hb-AA cells). Campwala and Desforges concluded that, while in Hb-AA blood the presence of HC in the membranes of the heaviest cells was a reflection of loss of enzyme-reducing systems due to ageing, in the Hb-SS cell population it was formed in consequence of the presence of an abnormal haemoglobin rather than of ageing.

Brewer and co-workers (1983) studied the relationship between GSH levels and the formation of Heinz bodies in response to oxidant stress in 39 Hb-SS patients: the mean GSH concentration was low and Heinz-body formation was increased. The low GSH levels were attributed to increased consumption secondary to the production of active oxygen radicals.

Rank and co-workers (1983) reported that the redox status of Hb-SS erythrocyte membrane thiols is abnormal, i.e. they had evidence of intramolecular thiol oxidation; they considered that this would contribute to the impaired survival of the erythrocytes in vivo.

Beretta and co-workers (1983) compared the antioxidant system in the erythrocytes of 20 Hb-AS heterozygotes with that in 68 Hb-AA controls. GSH levels were similar, but superoxide dismutase and GSH peroxidase activities were increased and catalase activity decreased in the Hb-AS subjects.

Lachant, Davidson and Tanaka (1983) investigated the possibility of failure of the pentose phosphate shunt in Hb-SS disease as a potential mechanism of the formation of Heinz bodies and the peroxidation of the erythrocyte membrane. Fourteen patients with sickle-cell disease were studied (12 had Hb-SS), as well as 50 patients with non-enzymopenic increased haemolysis and 43 normal controls. In Hb-SS disease G6PD activity and pentose phosphate (HM) shunt activity after methylene blue stimulation were found to be increased and GSH reductase activity was decreased. The GSH concentration was subnormal and Heinz-body formation after exposure to acetylphenyhydrazine was increased. Enzymes in the pentose phosphate shunt and the EM pathway were individually estimated: no differences were detected between the Hb-SS patients and patients with other types of haemolytic anaemia except that in the former group G6PD activity was increased and GSH reductase activity reduced. The findings in Hb-SS disease were considered to indicate continuous oxidant stress, and the following sequence of events was postulated; oxygen-free radicals are generated due to the instability of Hb S; the detoxification of the free radicals is suboptimal due to the low concentration of GSH as the result of impaired pentose phosphate shunt function; haemoglobin is oxidized to haemichrome; the presence of oxygen-free radicals and haemichrome leads to further denaturation of Hb S and the peroxidation of cell membranes inadequately protected by vitamin E.

Wetterstroem and co-workers (1984) studied the relationship between GSH levels and Heinz-body formation and the presence of ISCs in 39 Hb-SS patients. The GSH concentrations, expressed in relation to either haemoglobin or cell water, were significantly decreased, and a weak but significant correlation was demonstrated between the GSH level and ISC count. In five Stractan gradient separated fractions the percent of abnormal cells present was negatively correlated with the GSH concentration. Wetterstroem et al. also found that Heinz-body formation in response to oxidant stress was increased, with, surprisingly, more Heinz bodies developing in cells which were not ISCs than in ISCs.

Jain and Shohet (1984) discussed the role of the peroxidation of membrane lipids in the genesis of ISCs and reported that 2–3 times as much malonyldialdehyde (MDA) as normal was generated by Hb-SS blood as the result of 24 hours' incubation under aerobic conditions. In untreated ISC-enriched Hb-SS blood, obtained by the use of Stractan density gradients, a novel phospholipid, an MDA adduct, was demonstrated. This was not found in Hb-AA erythrocytes and its presence was considered to indicate that ISCs had undergone lipid peroxidative damage and accumulation of MDA in vivo. Jain and Shohet referred to their earlier work (Jain and Shohet, 1981) which had indicated that loading erythrocytes with calcium (as occurs spontaneously in Hb-SS disease) increases the vulnerability of erythrocyte membranes to lipid peroxidation.

Schacter and co-workers (1985) have provided further evidence as to whether the very variable severity of symptoms in Hb-SS patients is related to the intracellular activity of the antioxidant enzyme superoxide dismutase (SOD). Hb-AA blacks were found to have more SOD activity than Hb-AA white controls (? a racial difference). Nevertheless, it was established that the black Hb-SS patients, with moderate or severe symptoms, had less SOD activity than control blacks or Hb-SS patients with mild symptoms. The correlation of SOD activity and the severity of symptoms was shown not to be a function of age or sex and was unrelated to Hb-F percentage or reticulocyte count. Schacter *et al.* concluded that their observations supported the hypothesis that oxidant damage to erythrocytes contributes to the severity of the Hb-SS patient's disease. The SOD activity findings were not, however, supported by MDA measurement, perhaps, it was suggested, because MDA was likely to be elevated only transiently or locally.

Rank, Carlsson and Hebbel (1985) have provided direct evidence of an abnormal redox status of membrane-protein thiols in Hb-SS disease. They used thiol-disulphide exchange chromatography to determine the partition of SDS-solubilized proteins into gel bound (reduced thiol) and filtrate (oxidized/blocked thiol) fractions and found that in Hb-SS patients significantly increased amounts of the membrane proteins were in the filtrate fraction, indicating abnormal intramolecular oxidation of thiols.

Hebbel (1986) reviewed the relationship between antioxidants and erythrocyte membrane vulnerability. In relation to sickle cells, he suggested that the excess iron in the membrane in the form of haem (see p. 211) may play an important role in the cells' excessive generation of oxidants.

ERYTHROCYTE LIPIDS IN Hb-SS DISEASE

Early studies on erythrocyte and plasma lipids in sickle-cell disease were reviewed by Westerman, Pierce and Jensen (1964). They themselves had studied 10 patients, aged between 16 and 42 years, considered to have sickle-cell anaemia: total lipids appeared to be highly significantly increased when related to volume, number of cells or surface area, compared with values in normal young erythrocytes and there were less significant increases in phospholipids and cholesterol. Westerman, Pierce and Jensen also measured cell diameter, thickness, volume and surface area and concluded that sickle-cell disease erythrocytes had a larger mean diameter and were thinner and had a larger surface area than control normal young erythrocytes, thus confirming the much earlier data of Erickson *et al.* (1937) who had reported that sickle-cell erythrocytes were 'thinner and more discoid' when compared with a randomly aged population. Westerman, Pierce and Jensen pointed out that the lower than normal plasma total lipid, phospholipid and cholesterol concentrations that they had observed in their sickle-cell anaemia patients had been observed in patients suffering from other types of haemolytic anaemia.

In a later paper, Westerman, Diloy-Puray and Streczyn (1979) reinvestigated the relationship between cell age and irreversibility of sickling and membrane lipid concentration; they measured total phospholipid, cholesterol and sialic acid in the top, middle and bottom fractions of the centrifuged blood of 10 Hb-SS patients and compared the results with measurements made on similar fractions of the blood of normal control subjects and reticulocyte-rich Hb-AA patients. The conclusion was reached that the high total lipid content of Hb-SS cell membranes could be explained by the generally younger cell age and that the low values found in ISCs were no lower relatively than in similarly aged populations of normal cells. [In interpreting these data, the increase in erythrocyte surface area, and accompanying increase in phospholipid and cholesterol, resulting from splenic atrophy or splenectomy (see Vol. 1, p. 87) has to be taken into account.]

Rate of lipid synthesis. Lane, Ballas and Burka (1976) used [^{14}C] glycerol to study the de-novo rate of lipid synthesis by Hb-SS and Hb-AA reticulocytes. In the absence of sickling, the rates of synthesis were similar in the two genotypes. However, when sickling was induced by deoxygenation the rate of synthesis by the Hb-SS cells was substantially increased (mean 69%) above the control values. According to Lane, Ballas and Burka, damage to cell membranes leads to increase in lipid synthesis and they concluded that their findings further support the concept that the erythrocyte membrane lesions of sickle-cell disease are secondary to the sickling process.

Distribution of phospholipids in the Hb-SS cell membrane

Lubin and co-workers (1981a,b) reported on the organization of phospholipids in the membranes of Hb-SS erythrocytes. Compared with normal Hb-AA cells, the outer leaflet of the cell membrane of deoxygenated reversibly sickled cells, and of ISCs, was found to be enriched in phosphatidylethanolamine, in addition to containing some phosphatidylserine. These changes were compensated for by reduction in the amount of phosphatidylcholine present. In contrast to the

ISCs, in which the distribution of phospholipids was abnormal irrespective of oxygen tension, reoxygenation of reversibly sickled cells almost completely restored the organization of the lipids to normal. Lubin *et al.* concluded that the process of sickling induces an abnormality in the organization of the membrane lipids, which becomes permanent in the ISCs; they suggested, too, that the presence of phosphatidylserine in the outer leaflet of the membrane may be a factor in bringing about the adhesion of Hb-SS erythrocytes to endothelial cells.

Schwartz and co-workers (1983a) set out to investigate the binding of Hb-AA, Hb-AS and Hb-SS erythrocytes to artificial membranes of known lipid composition. They used liposomes containing acidic phospholipids and found that Hb-SS cells bound significantly more liposomes and that the binding was increased under hypoxic conditions. Schwartz *et al.* suggested that the translocation of phosphatidylserine and phosphatidylethanolamine to the outlet leaflet of the Hb-SS erythrocyte membrane contributes to the increased binding. ISCs were, however, found to be less capable of binding liposomes than discoid erythrocytes, a finding indicating that other factors are involved. Schwartz *et al.* concluded that liposomes can be used as sensitive probes in the investigation of the Hb-SS cell membrane.

Zachowski and co-workers (1985) compared the diffusion rates of the aminophospholipids through the Hb-SS cell membrane, using spin-labelled analogues; they calculated that the transverse diffusion rate of phosphatidylserine was diminished by 41% and that of phosphatidylethanolamine by 14% in Hb-SS cells compared with Hb-AA cells, and they concluded that the deformity of sickled cells is not entirely due to its contained haemoglobin or to alteration to its cytoskeletal proteins but also in part due to perturbation in the selective transport of the aminophospholipids.

Wagner and co-workers (1985) in a review, discussed the role of the membrane proteins, particularly spectrin and protein 4.1, in maintaining the distribution of phospholipids; they discussed, too, the distribution of the phospholipids in sickled cells and how vesiculation leads to loss of phospholipids (see also p. 220); and also the pathological consequences of vesiculation, including the role of vesicles in hypercoagulability and the effect of the vesicles in impairing the phagocytic function of RE cells with consequent increased susceptibility to infections.

ERYTHROCYTE MEMBRANE PROTEINS IN Hb-SS DISEASE

Normally, spectrin and actin form a self-supporting fibrillar, lattice-like protein network at the inner face of the erythrocyte membrane. Triton X-100 extraction can remove all the integral proteins of the membrane and most of the lipids and leave behind a residue (ghost) composed mostly of spectrin and actin (see Vol. 1. pp. 12–14).

Whether the membrane proteins are abnormal in Hb-SS disease has been the subject of considerable research. In an early study of four patients whose erythrocytes were subjected to SDS polyacrylamide gel electrophoresis (PAGE), Durocher, Conrad and Payne (1974) could discern no difference in the major protein groups between the Hb-SS patients and normal controls.

Riggs and Ingram (1975) compared the SDS PAGE patterns of 10 Hb-SS patients with those of 15 Hb-AA controls. PAS staining of the three major glycoproteins was subnormal in the Hb-SS patients and appeared to be associated with a marked reduction in sialic acid content. The changes did not seem to be correlated with the proportion of ISCs present. Ballas and Burka (1980), who studied the erythrocyte membranes of 22 adult Hb-SS patients, found that their SDS PAGE patterns were normal.

Findings in ISCs

Lux and John (1975) and Lux, John and Karnovsky (1976) described how ISCs submitted to triton extraction formed ISC-shaped residues. (All the membrane-associated Hb S was removed by the triton.) However, when reversibly sickled cells were treated in the same way, the residues were not sickle-shaped, and it was suggested that ISCs had acquired a defect in their spectrin–actin lattice, perhaps associated with increased Ca^{2+} and reduced ATP, and that it was this that was maintaining the ISCs' shape.

Palek (1977) and Palek and Liu (1979), in reviews, have discussed how the permanent sickled shape of the ISC is brought about: they concluded that the polymerization of intracellular and membrane-bound deoxy Hb S is followed by a permanent deformation of the actin–spectrin cytoskeleton — independent of change in erythrocyte Ca^{2+} and ATP — and by a marked increase in membrane permeability for monovalent and divalent cations, with a marked influx of Ca^{2+} and a net Ca^{2+} gain, with resultant cellular dehydration. Then a characteristic Ca^{2+}, ATP-dependent rearrangement of spectrin takes place resulting in a sphero-echinocytic ISC with a further increase in membrane rigidity.

Smith and co-workers (1980) reported on a comparison of the deformability and the properties of membrane spectrin between the erythrocytes of the llama, human ISCs, elliptocytes from non-haemolytic hereditary elliptocytosis (HE) and normal erythrocytes. The deformability of the human ISCs was found to be greatly reduced compared to the normal; the extractability of spectrin was reduced but casein kinase activity (a measure of spectrin kinase) was increased.

Abnormal spectrin–ankyrin interaction

The binding of spectrin to ankyrin has been found to be defective in Hb-SS membranes. Platt, Falcone and Lux (1983, 1985) studied a series of patients suffering from various sickle-cell syndromes of whom eight were Hb-SS homozygotes. Inside-out vesicles (IOVs) derived from Hb-SS erythrocytes were found to bind on approximately 50% less ankyrin than did control (Hb-AA) IOVs. This did not seem to be related to the reticulocyte count. On the other hand, the data suggested that the abnormality parallels clinical severity: thus the IOVs of the Hb-SS patient who had fewest symptoms had the highest binding capacity of the series, while IOVs of patients with the Hb-AS trait or Hb-SS disease plus high Hb F or with Hb-S/β^+-thalassaemia bound normally; on the other hand, IOVs from the patient with symptomatic Hb-S/$\beta°$-thalassaemia bound abnormally. It was found, however, that when ankyrin derived from Hb-SS erythrocytes was isolated and studied in solution (as opposed to when in situ in IOVs), it bound normally to spectrin. Platt, Falcone and Lux concluded that the presence of Hb S, or perhaps the metabolic consequence of sickling, damages the protein skeleton, and that this damage alters the cell surface and leads to abnormal cell-to-cell interactions which may be related to clinical severity.

Phosphorylation and protein kinase activity in Hb-SS cell membranes

Beutler, Quinto and Johnson (1976) estimated the rate of phosphorylation in the membranes of erythrocytes derived from patients with various types of haemolytic anaemia. In four patients with Hb-SS disease phos-

phorylation was found to be more impaired after 60 minutes' incubation than in HS. The exact significance of these observations was, however, not determined.

Hosey and Tao (1976) reported that one or more polypeptides designated 4.5–4.8 act as substrates for GTP-using kinases in Hb-SS cell membranes but not in normal cell membranes. They suggested that phosphoryl acceptor sites are uncovered as the consequence of sickling or that the substrate specificity of the kinases is decreased: and they raised the question as to whether abnormal membrane phosphorylation plays a part in altered cation transport.

Delaunay, Galand and Boivin (1982) studied nine Hb-SS patients: their membrane proteins were submitted to SDS PAGE after first labelling erythrocyte ghosts with [γ-^{32}P]ATP. Decreased labelling of the spectrin bands appeared to be related to the presence of Hb-SS disease, rather than to a young cell population. However, Delaunay, Galand and Boivin recalled that similar decreased labelling had been observed in other conditions associated with major changes in erythrocyte shape.

Fairbanks and co-workers (1983) measured autophosphorylation and the casein kinase and cAMP-stimulated histone kinase activity in the erythrocyte membranes of eight Hb-SS patients and of control patients suffering from other anaemias associated with a young cell population. Their findings led them to conclude that the altered phosphorylation patterns they had observed could be best explained by the presence of young cells within the erythrocyte populations.

Polyamines in Hb-SS cell membranes. Natta and Kremzner (1982) studied four Hb-SS patients and reported that the polyamines, spermidine and spermine, were present in higher concentration in erythrocyte stroma and lysate derived from Hb-SS cells than in stroma and lysate from Hb-AA cells. Whether this was a phenomenon associated solely with a young cell population was left undecided.

Binding of Hb S to erythrocyte membranes

More haemoglobin can be demonstrated to be within the cell membranes of Hb-SS cells than of normal erythrocytes. In an early report, Klipstein and Ranney (1960) described how they had found that the erythrocyte membranes of Hb-AS (and Hb-AC) heterozygotes contained the abnormal haemoglobin in a higher proportion, compared to Hb A, than in water-soluble or whole haemolysate haemoglobin. The suggestion was made that this might result from the difference in charge between the abnormal haemoglobin and Hb A.

As already referred to (p. 83), Schneider and co-workers (1972) demonstrated that small intraerythrocytic particles, demonstrable by dark-field microscopy, are more frequently visible in Hb-SS erythrocytes than in cells of Hb-AA (or Hb-AS) genotypes, and they showed, too, by the reaction of the particles with benzidine that most of them contain haemoglobin. They also measured the haemoglobin content of post-haemolysis erythrocyte residues and found that the haemoglobin content of the membranes of Hb-SS cells (expressed in mg per ml cells) was more than 10 times that of Hb-AA cells. The nature of the haemoglobin found in membranes and its relationship in Hb-SS disease to the presence of ISCs has been investigated subsequently. Fischer and co-workers (1975), for instance, considered that most of the haemoglobin in the erythrocyte membranes in Hb-SS blood is in ISCs.

Asakura and co-workers (1977) investigated the nature of the haemoglobin present in membranes and found that most of it, in both Hb-SS cells and Hb-AA cells, is oxyhaemoglobin; however, there is, too, a small amount, which is not removed by washing, which is denatured and is in the form of haemichrome. The haemichrome fraction in Hb-SS cells amounts to only approximately 0.2% of the total haemoglobin but this is about 5 times as much as is present in Hb-AA cells. Asakura *et al.* considered as possible factors in the denaturation of the haemoglobin the mechanical trauma of repeated passages through the microcirculation and the repeated conformational changes taking place when Hb S oscillates between the oxy and deoxy form. According to Shaklai, Sharma and Ranney (1981), Hb S is bound to erythrocyte membranes more avidly than is Hb A, and they suggested, in the presence of very high intracellular concentrations of Hb S, that the increased affinity and binding of Hb S to the membranes may be of importance in pathogenesis.

Sears and Luthra (1983) studied thoroughly washed erythrocyte ghosts derived from 16 Hb-SS patients and 13 Hb-AA controls and found that the content of total protein, total globin and haemoglobin was significantly greater in the Hb-SS ghosts than in the controls. The blood of eight Hb-SS patients was separated into three fractions by centrifugation and this led to the finding that membrane-bound globin and haemoglobin were present in greater amount in the densest fraction.

Free haem in Hb-SS erythrocytes

Liu, Zhai and Palek (1984), referring to the often reported presence of micro Heinz-body inclusions in Hb-SS erythrocytes, looked for the presence of free haem (hemin) in the cytosol of Hb-SS cells and found at least 4 times as much as in the cytosol of normal Hb-AA cells. The amount of haem demonstrable in the Hb-SS cells was increased by shaking to an extent almost double that which occurred with Hb-AA cells.

PATHOGENESIS OF SICKLE-CELL DISEASE

Early ideas on pathogenesis

Ham and Castle (1940) reported that the viscosity of the whole blood of five patients with sickle-cell anaemia was 40–115% greater when it was deoxygenated than when it was fully oxygenated. They suggested that this happened, too, *in vivo*, and that it could set in motion a vicious cycle of further deoxygenation, more intense sickling and a still greater increase in viscosity and that the consequent slowing of the circulation led to local thrombus formation. Erythrostasis in the spleen and other organs was, in their view, an important factor, too, in the genesis of increased haemolysis.

Bauer (1940) had come to much the same conclusion as had Ham and Castle, namely, that the essential pathogenetic mechanism was 'stagnation and conglutination of disfigured red corpuscles' and that this occurred particularly, but not exclusively, in organs in which the rate of blood flow, and in consequence the oxygen tension, was unusually low. The consequences of the stagnation were listed by Bauer as '(1) thrombosis; (2) ischemia, necrosis and fibrosis, and (3) resolution of the red blood cells with subsequent anemia'. He also suggested that as anaemia, in his view, was not the most dangerous consequence of sickling, sickle-cell disease was a more logical term than sickle-cell anaemia.

Shen, Castle and Fleming (1944) demonstrated that sickled cells were unusually easily lysed by mechanical trauma. Murphy and Shapiro (1944) stressed, too, that they were very rigid cells. In their own words: when a cell becomes sickled 'its flexibility is lost and it appears as fixed and rigid as a crystal of ice as it moves about and abuts against cells and fixed objects'. They concluded that it was the sickled cells' increased rigidity that led to blockage of capillaries.

Singer (1951), in a valuable early review on sickle-cell anaemia, emphasized the importance of increased haemolysis in pathogenesis.

These early views, and the reported relationship between oxygen tension and sickling — in particular the pioneer descriptions of Hahn and Gillespie (1927), Scriver and Waugh (1930) and Sherman (1940) (see p. 3) — have been shown by much subsequent work to be substantially correct. The difference in the degree to which the oxygen tension has to be lowered to produce sickling was found to explain why the consequences of having the Hb-AS trait are so very much less than those of homozygosity for Hb S: in the latter state sickling takes place at physiological degrees of deoxygenation while in the trait this is not so.

Harris and co-workers (1956) and Griggs and Harris (1956) brought together in important papers many observations on the consequences of sickling in Hb-SS anaemia and in other forms of sickle-cell disease, and on the relationship between sickling and increases in blood viscosity and mechanical fragility. A vicious cycle was thought to occur in organs where the circulation was slowed: in such circumstances deoxygenation led to sickling; this caused slowing of the circulation; this led to decrease in pH due to accumulation of carbon dioxide and this made the sickling worse by facilitating deoxygenation; the result was arrest of the circulation by plugs of sickled cells; local thrombosis was the consequence. The impacted cells were thought to undergo lysis *in situ* or, if they escaped into the circulation, to circulate as mechanically fragile irreversibly sickled cells. The stagnating erythrocytes were considered also to undergo deleterious metabolic changes which led to a reduction in their life span, that is if they managed to circulate again; and the small tails of unusually fragile cells in osmotic fragility tests were thought to be caused by the presence of metabolically damaged cells.

Allison's (1956) work appeared to explain how homozygosity for Hb S is compatible with life despite the fact that sickling can take place at about the normal O_2 tension of mixed venous blood (approximately 40 mm Hg). Significantly, he found that 2 minutes was the minimum time required for sickling *in vitro* at an equivalent O_2, tension, a length of time much longer than the 15 seconds or so for which erythrocytes would normally be exposed to such a low O_2 tension while they were making their way from the venous end of capillaries to the lungs where they would become rapidly reoxygenated.

Allison (1957) described how deoxygenation of a stroma-free solution of Hb S resulted in an increase in its viscosity and concluded that Hb S formed mixed molecular aggregates with Hb A or Hb C when the haemoglobins in solution were deoxygenated.

Greenberg, Kass and Castle (1957) showed that the clinical phenomena associated with the presence of Hb S could be correlated with the mean corpuscular concentration of Hb S (the MCSHC): individuals with an MCSHC of less than 15 g/dl were not anaemic and did not have painful crises; those with an MCSHC of 15–18 g/dl had a mild haemolytic anaemia, while those with an MCSHC of 20 g/dl or more had severe anaemia, bony lesions and painful crises. *In vitro*, Greenberg, Kass and Castle showed how closely viscosity (and sickling) were correlated with MCSHC: viscosity rose sharply as the MCSHC exceeded 10 g/dl. Lowering the pH to 6.8–7.0 increased viscosity and it was pointed out how in-vivo increases in viscosity were likely to be greatest at sites of erythroconcentration and where the blood pH was low. Greenberg and Kass (1958) dealt with the role of pH and other metabolic changes in the genesis of crises. Metabolic acidosis was considered to induce crises by facilitating sickling either locally or generally; and this was also suggested as a mechanism by which anaesthesia could precipitate a crisis.

Rubenstein (1961) pointed out that the high viscosity of Hb-SS blood relative to that of normal blood of the same PCV was further increased by a fall in temperature; he suggested that, in addition to pO_2, pCO_2 and pH, the temperature of the tissue through which the blood was circulating was a factor in the localization of sickling lesions.

Charache and Conley (1964) contrasted the effect of deoxygenation on viscosity, on haemoglobin solubility and on the rate of sickling in a range of sickling disorders. The results of the three laboratory measurements ran parallel. The severity of the patients' illness appeared to be correlated with the rate of increase in the viscosity of their blood on deoxygenation, this being determined by the content of Hb S and the degree of interaction with any other haemoglobin. The viscosity of deoxygenated blood was found to be directly proportional to the proportion of sickled cells present and to be greater with filamentous sickling than when 'holly leaf' forms were present; it was found, too, to increase in proportion to the square of the PCV, and this was considered by Charache and Conley probably to explain the occasional occurrence of vascular occlusive episodes in patients with heterozygous sickling disorders who were not anaemic.

Dintenfass (1964) set about to compare the internal viscosity of Hb-AA, Hb-AS and Hb-SS cells using a cone-to-cone viscometer and erythrocytes that had been packed after centrifugation at 15 000 **g**. The viscosity of the packed Hb-AA, Hb-AS and Hb-SS cells steadily increased in that order when the haemoglobin was oxygenated; when deoxygenated, however, the viscosity of the Hb-SS cells was shown to be as much as 200–1000 times greater than that of the Hb-AA cells. Dintenfass concluded that 'whenever sickle cells appear, their internal rigidity causes the blood to behave as a highly viscous suspension' and that if sickling takes place at high haematocrit levels, as are known to exist in the microcapillary circulation as the result of plasma skimming, this alone could cause localized stoppage of the circulation.

LATER STUDIES: IMPORTANCE OF BLOOD VISCOSITY

Ham and co-workers (1968) studied the effect of deoxygenation and hypertonicity on the viscosity of erythrocyte suspensions. Over a range of PCVs the increase in viscosity of Hb-AS cells was found to be much greater on deoxygenation than that of normal cells, and it was noted that suspension of the cells in hypertonic saline impaired their deformability and impeded their passage through microfilters. It was suggested in relation to the kidney lesion of Hb-AS trait individuals that the increase in viscosity within the vasa recta resulting from hypertonicity at normal PCVs slowed the circulation to such a degree that the local deoxygenation and lowered pH reached the critical level for sickling to occur.

Chien, Usami and Bertles (1969, 1970) demonstrated, under experimental conditions in which the PCVs, shear rate and suspending medium were varied, that the viscosity of blood containing irreversibly sickled cells (ISCs) always exceeded that of normal cells. The viscosity of oxygenated Hb-SS blood was found to be increased and this was attributed mainly but not entirely to the presence of ISCs. Chien, Usami and Bertles concluded that the flow of Hb-SS blood through the microcirculation *in vivo* was likely to be impaired even under conditions of full oxygenation.

Klug, Lessin and Radice (1974) stressed the importance of the presence of ISCs, even in well-oxygenated blood, in causing an increase in blood viscosity; this they attributed to the combined effects of the increased internal viscosity and the increased membrane rigidity of the cells. They were able to study, and to record by microcinematography, in the anaesthetized living rat, previously exchanged-transfused with Hb-SS cells, how sickled cells became held up in mesenteric vessels, particularly at capillary junctions, when the animal breathed air of low oxygen content.

Harris and Bensusan (1975) studied the kinetics of sol-to-gel transformation of solutions of Hb S by continuously monitoring the viscosity changes induced by deoxygenation. The changes, which appeared to occur in five phases, could be demonstrated to be affected by haemoglobin concentration, temperature and admixture with haemoglobins other than Hb S.

Usami, Chien and Bertles (1975) studied the effect of deoxygenation on the deformability of Hb-SS cells by a microsieving technique using polycarbonate filters having pores of 5 μm in diameter and established a clear relationship between pO$_2$ and resistance to flow. Usami and co-workers (1975) stressed in analysing the rheological disturbances of Hb-SS blood that both the deformability of the cells and the medium in which the cells are suspended have to be taken into account.

Murphy, Wengard and Brereton (1976), in studies on the influence of PCV and hypertonicity, etc. on the increase in viscosity produced by the deoxygenation of Hb-SS blood, found that its viscosity was disproportionately reduced by the addition of Hb-AA cells, *e.g.*, when one volume of Hb-AA cells was added to three volumes of Hb-SS cells the viscosity of the latter was reduced by 50%.

Chien (1977) again pointed out that the viscosity of oxygenated Hb-SS-containing blood was greater than that of Hb-AA blood at the same PCV. Microsieving was found to be a more sensitive way of detecting reduced deformability than viscometry. Chien also stressed that the anaemia found in sickle-cell diseases tended to compensate for the presence of Hb S by facilitating (by reduction in whole-blood viscosity) the blood flow through, and the delivery of oxygen to, the tissues. Self, McIntire and Zanger (1977) emphasized the importance of the 'optimum hematocrit', defined as the PCV at which the flow of haemoglobin through the tissues is maximized.

Klug and Lessin (1977) reported further details of their experiments with rats, and described how Hb-SS-containing discocytes, if unable to pass through critical-sized capillaries, underwent sickling 20–30 seconds after the flow of blood came to a standstill.

LaCelle (1977) perfused arterioles in the mouse cremaster muscle at constant pressure and showed that Hb-SS erythrocytes are able to initiate capillary occlusion at normal intracapillary pO_2.

Rieber, Veliz and Pollack (1977) pointed out that while crises are episodic in Hb-SS disease, the molecular abnormality is constant in individual patients. In seeking an answer to this paradox, they measured the filterability and proneness to sickle of their patients' blood quantitatively during crises and subsequently; they found that recovery from a crisis was associated with increased filterability and decreased susceptibility to sickle — presumably because of loss of some of the most abnormal erythrocytes during the crisis.

Further data on the deformability of sickled cells were reported by Havell, Hillman and Lessin (1978). They used micropipettes and negative pressure, recorded continuously, to determine what they referred to as membrane rigidity and total cell deformability. With ISCs both measurements were markedly increased, and they concluded that an ISC membrane abnormability plays a part in the abnormal rheology of Hb-SS disease blood. Smith and co-workers (1981) in similar studies, using micropipettes and a Nucleopore filter of average pore size 3.0 μm, found that ISCs could be separated into 'hard' and 'soft' cells according to their apparent deformability. The morphology of the two categories of cell did not seem to differ and their haemoglobin composition and concentration were similar, too. However, their deformability differed

markedly: that of the soft cells appeared to be almost normal, while the hard cells were far less deformable. The proportion of hard ISCs varied from 5 to 20% in the peripheral blood of the patients studied, and it was these cells — which were thought to have undergone an irreversible membrane change — which were held to play an important part in the increased viscosity of Hb-SS disease whole blood.

Kenny and co-workers (1981) studied the erythrocyte filterability of eight patients in 10 vaso-occlusive crises, using a positive pressure, washed-cell method (Kenny, Meakin and Stuart, 1981). They obtained evidence of decrease in filterability on the first day of a crisis which persisted until the 6–7th day. The percentage of ISCs did not, however, alter significantly.

Horne (1981) in a review referred to sickle-cell anaemia as an aberration of blood rheology due to loss of normal erythrocyte deformability; he discussed the principles governing the flow of blood through small calibre vessels and how the flow could be compromised by the intra-erythocytic aggregation of Hb-S molecules.

Additional in-vivo observations of the rheological behaviour of human Hb-SS erythrocytes in the microcirculation of the cremaster muscle of rats and mice were reported by Lipowsky, Usami and Chien (1982). In rather similar studies of the mesoappendix microvasculature of rats, Baez, Kaul and Nagel (1982) noted that deoxygenated Hb-SS cells could tenaciously adhere to venular and arteriolar endothelium and that even oxygenated Hb-SS cells might loosely adhere if the flow-rate was slow. As expected, perfusion with Hb-SS cells resulted in a marked increase in peripheral resistance and a significant fall in blood flow. Baez, Kaul and Nagel also observed and recorded cinematographically the changes in shape that Hb-SS and Hb-AA cells undergo during their passage through small vessels. Oxygenated cells of both genotypes were seen to be able to assume an elongated sausage shape during passage through pre-capillary sphincters of 2.8–3.1 μm internal diameter. Oxygenated Hb-SS cells occasionally occluded capillary orifaces; this happened more often with deoxygenated Hb-SS cells and it led to impaction by succeeding cells.

Schmid-Schönbein and Heidtmann (1982) stressed the importance of plasma factors in the altered flow behaviour of Hb-SS blood — in particular, the concentration of fibrinogen and other high molecular weight proteins which together markedly affect plasma viscosity as well as promote erythrocyte rouleaux formation.

The rheology of sickled cells was the subject of interesting symposia published, with Discussions, in *Blood Cells* in 1977 (Vol. 3, pp. 223–312), and in *Blood Cells* in 1982 (Vol. 8, pp. 9–184), at which many of those whose contributions have been summarized above were present.

Gulley and co-workers (1982) demonstrated, using an ektacytometer, how much the deformability of normal erythrocytes is affected by their state of hydration. (To raise the ion and water content, the cells were incubated in a medium containing lithium carbonate; to decrease the ion and water content the cells were exposed to the K ionophore, valinomycin.) A rise or fall in cell hydration, compared to the normal, decreased cell deformability. The deformability of fresh, well-oxygenated Hb SS blood was found to be well below that of Hb-AA blood; it improved markedly, however, when the volume of the cells was increased by hydration. Gulley *et al.* concluded that Hb-SS cells are suboptimally hydrated and that their abnormal rheology is in part at least the result of cell dehydration.

Schmid-Schönbein (1982) reviewed the response of Hb-S-containing erythrocytes to deformation in great detail and described experimental studies using artificial glass capillaries.

Kaul and co-workers (1983) emphasized the heterogeneity of the Hb-SS patient's erythrocyte population and the bearing this had on the clinical severity of his illness. The blood of six Hb-SS patients was separated on a Percoll-Renograffin density gradient into four fractions (I–IV): in order of increasing density the populations comprised mainly reticulocytes, discocytes, dense discocytes and ISCs, respectively. The viscosity of the fractions was assessed by means of a cone-plate viscometer and their haemodynamic characteristics in a Baez rat mesoappendix preparation. Fraction I, rich in reticulocytes, was found to have a higher viscosity than anticipated from the MCHC; the other fractions (when oxygenated) showed a moderate increase in viscosity parallel with the increase in MCHC. When deoxygenated, all four fractions nearly doubled their viscosity. The rat mesentery preparation gave, however, a different picture: when oxygenated, the fractions behaved as predicted from the viscosity measurements; when deoxygenated on the other hand, the resistance to flow increased dramatically, particularly that of Fraction III (dense discocytes) and Fraction IV (mainly ISCs). Kaul *et al.* concluded that the varying distribution of cell densities in the blood of Hb-SS patients would have an important influence on the circulation of blood through small blood vessels.

Evans, Mohandas and Leung (1984) reported on the static (time-independent) and dynamic (time-dependent) deformability of Hb-SS and normal (Hb-AA) erythrocytes which they had separated into subpopulations using Stractan density gradients. Individual erythrocytes were tested for their extensional and bending rigidities by means of micromechanical manipulation. The extensional rigidity of Hb-SS cells was found to increase with increasing haemoglobin concentration while that of normal cells was independent of cell hydration. Hb-SS cells exhibited inelastic behaviour at much lower haemoglobin concentrations than normal cells. The dynamic rigidity of both types of cell

increased to the same extent with increasing haemoglobin concentration. Evans, Mohandas and Leung concluded that increased haemoglobin concentration, perhaps particularly increased subjacent to the cell membrane, plays a major role in determining the rigidity of Hb-SS cells. Irreversible membrane changes, too, result from cell dehydration and these plus increased haemoglobin concentration were together thought to exert a major influence on the cells' circulation within the small blood vessels of the body.

Reports illustrating the effect of changes in blood viscosity on the clinical well-being of Hb-SS patients

Three revealing reports are quoted below.

Anderson and co-workers (1975) recorded how the gradual development of multiple myeloma in a 34-year-old patient led to the increasingly frequent occurrence of vaso-occlusive crises over an 18-month period. This was attributed to the IgG paraprotein increasing the whole-blood viscosity.

Spector and co-workers (1978) reported in a 34-year-old female a similar increase in the occurrence of painful crises. The mechanism was, however, different. The patient had chronic renal failure and was eventually successfully transplanted. Her PCV rose subsequently, and it seemed likely that this was the factor which caused, by increasing whole-blood viscosity, the increased incidence of vaso-occlusive episodes.

Charache, de la Monte and Macdonald (1982) described the fatal effect on a patient of the accidental chronic inhalation of carbon monoxide (CO). This caused a substantial increase in her haemoglobin and PCV and hence in the viscosity of her blood, and this, in association with a reduction in the anti-sickling effect of the CO when she was removed from the CO-contaminated air in her home, appeared to lead to her death from 'cardio-pulmonary arrest'. Charache, de la Monte and Macdonald stressed how, in a very real sense, patients are protected from the dangerous consequences of hyperviscosity by increased haemolysis and the anaemia it leads to.

Changes in Hb-SS erythrocyte deformability in vaso-occlusive crises

As already referred to (p. 214), there is evidence that whole-blood viscosity increases in Hb-SS patients during crises and that the viscosity increases in parallel with rises in the concentration of plasma fibrinogen. Rieber, Veliz and Pollack (1977), who measured in eight Hb-SS patients erythrocyte filterability and the susceptibility of the erythrocytes to sickle *in vitro*, found that recovery from a crisis is associated with an increase in filterability and a decreased tendency of the cells to sickle on deoxygenation.

Kenny and co-workers (1981) reported on serial studies in which erythrocyte deformability, plasma viscosity and whole-blood viscosity were measured daily during the duration of 10 vaso-occlusive crises. Erythrocyte deformability, measured by means of a 5-μm polycarbonate membrane and positive pressure, was found to be reduced on Day 1 of the crisis, but the ISC count and the plasma and whole-blood viscosity did not increase significantly until Day 5, in parallel with the acute-phase rise in plasma fibrinogen. Lucas and co-workers (1985), using a modified gravity filtration method which they considered to be more physiological, measured erythrocyte deformability in eight Hb-SS patients in painful crises. A significant loss of filterability was demonstrated on Day 2, but in this series no increase in ISC count. The loss of filterability was considered likely to be due to the presence in the circulation of rheologically altered cells released from the sites of micro-circulatory stasis. An interesting collateral finding was that the erythrocyte filterability of six patients who were free of symptoms was found to vary considerably over a period of time; this appeared to be independent of the ISC count. Lucas et al. concluded that the fluctuations in observed filterability were likely to be secondary to the occurrence of clinically occult vaso-occlusive events affecting the microcirculation.

ADHERENCE OF SICKLED CELLS TO ENDOTHELIAL CELLS

Recently, it has been reported that sickled erythrocytes have an abnormally great tendency to adhere to vascular endothelium and to macrophages, and it has been suggested that these properties play important roles in the pathogenesis of vaso-occlusive crises and in the cells' abnormally short life-span. The reports of Hebbel et al. (1978) and Hoover et al. (1979) aroused considerable interest: it seemed that adhesion to endothelium might indeed explain how Hb-SS cells were retained long enough in small calibre blood vessels for sickling to take place and for vaso-occlusion

to result. Research has been focused particularly on the circumstances under which adhesion takes place and the reasons why Hb-S-containing cells adhere abnormally.

Hebbel and co-workers (1978), knowing that Hb-SS cell membranes had been reported to be deficient in sialic acid, tested the erythrocytes derived from 10 Hb-SS and 10 Hb-AA blood samples to see whether the two types of cells differed in their ability to adhere to cultured human umbilical-cord endothelial cells. Hb-SS cells were in fact found to adhere abnormally readily; adhesion increased with cell density but was not confined to ISCs. Hebbel et al. reported that EM studies of the localization of cationized ferritin had suggested that the cells abnormal adherence was the consequence of 'an abnormality of HbS RBC membrane topography'. [It should be added that Clark et al. (1981) reported that they had found no difference in the density or distribution of negative charges on the surface of oxygenated Hb-AA or Hb-SS cells.]

Hoover and co-workers (1979) reported similarly, but used a different technique, testing the adhesion of ^{51}Cr-labelled erythrocytes to endothelial cells cultured from calf aorta. Hb-SS erythrocytes were found to adhere better than Hb-AA cells and Hoover et al. suggested that enhanced adhesion might be partially responsible for the blockage of capillaries in sickle-cell anaemia.

Hebbel and co-workers (1980b) described in detail the work of Hebbel et al. (1978) referred to above. Normal and Hb-SS erythrocytes in suspension were allowed to settle on to the cultured human endothelial cells, and it was found that whereas normal erythrocytes could be quite easily washed away from the endothelial cells, sickled cells adhered abnormally and remained stuck to the surface of the endothelial cells despite multiple washes. Adhesion was found not to be enhanced by deoxygenation; it was, however, diminished by enzymatic removal of sialic acid from the erythrocytes. Hebbel et al. concluded that abnormal adherence to vascular endothelium could be a pathogenetic factor in microvascular occlusion.

Hebbel and co-workers (1980a) studied 33 Hb-SS patients with the aim of determining whether the severity of their disease (as judged by the frequency of microvascular occlusions) could be correlated with the abnormal adherence of their sickled cells to cultured vascular endothelium. They found that this was, in fact, so. On the other hand, the clinical indices of severity were not correlated with the haemoglobin level, percentage of ISCs or Hb F, or reticulocyte count.

Hebbel, Moldow and Steinberg (1981) gave further details of their work. They reported that although the adherence of sickled cells to cultured vascular endothelium had been found to vary from patient to patient and to be correlated with the incidence and severity of vaso-occlusive episodes, for individual patients the development of an acute vaso-occlusive crisis was found not to be accompanied by an increase in the inherent propensity of their sickled cells to adhere to the endothelium. It was shown, however, that plasma factors, such as acute-phase proteins and fibrinogen, known to be increased in infections, enhanced adherence; and also that sickled cells adhered more avidly to endothelium if it was damaged, or under hyperosmolar conditions. It was concluded that changes in the plasma environment of sickled cells in the microcirculation could help to precipitate crises by facilitating interaction between sickled cells and endothelium. It was pointed out also that endothelial damage secondary to endotoxaemia and/or the activation of complement might precipitate crises by facilitating the adherence of sickled cells. It was finally suggested that adherence to endothelium might be the initiating factor in vaso-occlusion and that by impeding the blood flow the adhesions could bring about stasis and secondary sickling and thus set in train organ infarction and clinical crisis. Hb-AS trait erythrocytes were found to adhere abnormally to endothelial cells under hyperosmolar conditons, and it was suggested that this might be important in bringing about local vaso-occlusive damage in the kidneys.

Hebbel and co-workers (1982) reviewed the role of erythrocyte/endothelial interactions and the pathogenesis of sickle-cell disease; adherence was considered to be a factor which initiated vaso-occlusion either by primarily occluding small blood vessels or by slowing the blood flow sufficiently for secondary sickling to take place.

Burns, Wilkinson and Nagel (1983, 1985), accepting that Hb-SS erythrocytes adhere to endothelial cells abnormally readily under static conditions, set out to investigate the adhesion of cells in flowing systems. They perfused human umbilical-cord veins with suspensions of ^{51}Cr-labelled erythrocytes at ambient O_2 tensions at a rate of 1 ml per minute and found that with undamaged endothelium only a small and similar percentage of Hb-AA and Hb-SS cells adhered; they obtained the same result using a continuous closed loop system. Scanning electron microscopy confirmed that adhesion was sparse and focal. Using another approach, Burns, Wilkinson and Nagel perfused erythrocytes through fibronectin-coated glass capillaries in which endothelial cells had been cultured. Again, adherence was minimal and the result was the same with Hb-AA and Hb-SS cells. However, when the experiments were repeated using capillaries with multiple bends, so that vortex flow increased the probability of cells coming into contact with endothelium, more Hb-SS cells than Hb-AA cells adhered. Burns, Wilkinson and Nagel (1985) concluded that Hb-SS cells become trapped in the microcirculation because of a complex combination of haemodynamic forces, plasma factors and erythrocyte membrane pecularities, rather than simply because of the cells' propensity to adhere to vascular endothelium.

Smith and La Celle (1981) reported that they had used microprobes to ascertain the minimal force required to shear the erythrocytes of sickle-cell anaemia patients from the surface of cultured endothelial cells. Approximately 3% of reversibly sickled cells adhered, and a wide range of force was found to be required for the freeing of individual cells, the upper limit being about 5000 times that required for simple deformation of the cell membrane. Smith and La Celle concluded that adhesion to vascular endothelium in places of low shear could contribute to vaso-occlusion.

Mohandas and Evans (1983) and Mohandas, Evans and Kukan (1984) used a micropipette technique to measure the adherence to endothelium of individual erythrocytes. The vast majority of Hb-SS cells were found to adhere strongly compared with a minority of normal cells which adhered but weakly. The source of plasma in which the cells were suspended was shown to have an important effect: thus when Hb-SS cells were suspended in normal plasma, less than 20% adhered; while the adherence of normal cells in sickle-cell anaemia plasma was only moderately increased. Mohandas, Evans and Kukan (1984) concluded that both membrane and plasma factors contributed to adhesion and that changes in plasma were likely to play an important role in the development of vaso-occlusive crises.

Mohandas and Evans (1984) and Mohandas et al.

(1985) had experimented with different suspending media. Hb-SS cells suspended in EDTA plasma were found not to adhere to vascular endothelium while cells from the same source adhered when citrate or heparin had been used as anticoagulant. Mohandas and Evans concluded that Ca^{2+}, as well as collagen-binding plasma proteins, played a crucial role in adhesion; they also reported that irregularly-shaped deformable cells were 4–6 times more adherent than discoid cells, while ISCs were least adherent.

Mohandas et al. (1985), using the micropipette technique, distinguished three ways in which erythrocytes adhered to endothelial cells: (1) adherence but no area of strong contact, (2) adherence by one small area of strong contact, and (3) adherence by a large area of strong contact. Much more force was found to be required to detach single cells from endothelium when the force was applied tangentially than when the force was applied in a direction normal to the endothelial surface.

Wautier and co-workers (1983a,b, 1985) investigated the adhesion to cultured human umblical-cord endothelial cells of erythrocytes derived from 30 patients with sickle-cell syndromes (22 had Hb-SS disease). Compared with normal Hb-AA cells, significantly more Hb-S-containing cells adhered, but the cells from diabetic patients adhered abnormally, too. Fibrinogen added to the system increased adherence and a higher percentage of cells adhered when the patients were in crisis than when they were in health, particularly if the crisis accompanied an inflammatory condition. Young erythrocytes, labelled with $[^3H]$leucine, were found to adhere more readily than the population, of mixed ages, labelled with ^{51}Cr. Wautier et al. (1985) concluded, however, that the abnormal adherence of Hb-SS cells could not be explained on the basis of an increased population of young cells.

Barabino and co-workers (1985) similarly studied the effect of age on the adhesion of Hb-SS cells to cultured human umbilical-cord endothelial cells. Young (less dense) cells were found in fact to be more adherent than older cells and it was thought that the adhesion of these young cells to endothelium in vivo could contribute to vaso-occlusion by lengthening the transit of older cells through the microcirculation.

Hebbel, Schwartz and Mohandas (1985) have stressed the complexity of the mechanisms resulting in the adhesion of Hb-SS erythrcytes to vascular endothelium, as well as to monocytes, macrophages and model membranes. In their view, adherence to endothelium may be brought about by aberrant electrostatic forces in conjunction with a major contribution from factors in the plasma environment; abnormal translocation of aminophospholipid in the Hb-SS cell membrane is implicated in the adhesion of Hb-SS cells to monocytes and liposomes; adherence to macrophages may be brought about by abnormal amounts of IgG on the Hb-SS cell surface and/or by the surface being modified by lipid peroxidation. Hebbel, Schwartz and Mohandas concluded that, regardless of mechanisms, the available data suggest that the adherence of Hb-SS cells to endothelium correlates with the severity of vaso-occlusive crises and may contribute to patient-to-patient differences and to the temporal variations in clinical severity.

Wautier and co-workers (1986) demonstrated that adhesion of Hb-SS erythrocytes to endothelial cells is associated with an increased liberation by the cells of prostacyclin (PGI_2), as indicated by the release of 6-keto-prostaglandin F_{1a}. They interpreted this as indicating that an abnormal degree of adhesion damages the cells to which the erythrocytes adhere. The amount of 6-keto-prostaglandin F_{1a} released correlated with the extent of the adhesion.

ABNORMAL MICROVASCULAR ACTIVITY

There is evidence that the reaction of an individual Hb-SS patient's minute blood vessels to internal and external stimuli and to the occurrence of sickling itself probably plays an important role in determining the occurrence and severity of vaso-occlusive crises. Nagel and Fabry (1985), in an interesting review on the 'many pathophysiologies' of sickle-cell anaemia, stressed that the presence of relatively rigid very dense cells and ISCs is not by itself a major determinant of vaso-occlusions. They concluded that crises are most frequently initiated by a disturbance in the microcirculation, which in the presence of cells with a potentiality to sickle leads to vascular obstruction.

The possibility that abnormal vasoconstriction might be a factor had been investigated by Lin et al. (1983) who compared the serum concentration of a small molecular weight vasoactive factor (VAF) in a series of seven Hb-SS patients and 14 Hb-AA controls. (The assay method they used was based on measuring the coronary artery flow-rate in the isolated perfused rabbit heart.) The serum VAF concentration in the Hb-SS patients was found to be significantly greater than in the controls, and the serum of the Hb-SS patients was found, too, to be more active in inducing platelet aggregation. Lin *et al.* concluded that VAF (thought normally to decrease prostacyclin synthesis by vascular tissue) might contribute to the pathogenesis of vaso-occlusive crises by its action in promoting vasoconstriction and platelet aggregation.

Rodgers and co-workers (1983, 1984) provided evidence of abnormal vasomotor activity and periodicity in the flow of the blood in the microcirculation of the skin. They used a laser-Doppler blood-flow monitor capable of the non-invasive instantaneous and continuous measurement of blood flow and found in a series of six Hb-SS patients in a stable state that the blood flow in the forearm underwent local, large (approximately 50%) amplitude oscillations with a periodicity of 7–10 seconds (Fig. 14.11). They found, too, when the blood content of Hb S was reduced in two patients to less than 40% by exchange-transfusion with normal blood, that the local rhythmic variation in resting blood flow markedly diminished or disappeared. Rodgers *et al.* (1984) considered in detail the factors controlling the blood flow through small vessels and suggested that in Hb-SS patients increase in intravascular pressure, caused by the presence of abnormally rigid erythrocytes, may elicit 'in phase "myogenic" oscillation'; they suggested, too, that the oscillations in blood flow which they had observed reflected the phased

rhythmic flow through large groups of neighbouring capillaries and that the phased flow could be compensatory in that sudden surges of flow might help to overcome microvascular obstruction. The threshold for determining the rhythmic flow would depend, in their view, on the haematocrit, the distribution of Hb S in individual cells and the extent to which the Hb S was polymerized.

The role of vascular tone in an artificially-perfused microvascular system with intact innervation was explored by Kaul, Fabry and Nagel (1985). They concluded that sickle-cell-induced vaso-occlusion depends on vascular tone as well as on the cells' density, the pO_2 and the perfusion pressure.

ROLE OF Hb-SS CELLS IN THROMBUS FORMATION

The question arises as to whether Hb-SS cells themselves play any special role in generating thrombi within the small blood vessels which they occlude. The answer is that laboratory observations suggest that they probably do, but that, not unexpectedly, the underlying mechanisms are complicated.

McKeller and Dacie (1958), in the course of searching for a reason why patients with paroxysmal nocturnal haemoglobinuria commonly

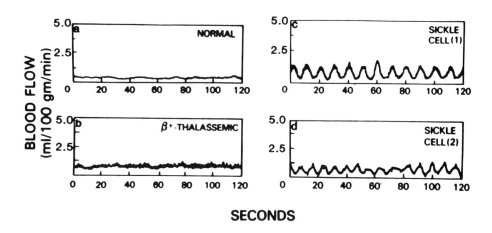

SECONDS

Fig. 14.11 Typical patterns of resting forearm cutaneous blood capillary flow in a normal subject, in two patients with Hb-SS disease and in one patient with β⁺-thalassaemia.
[Reproduced by permission from Rodgers *et al.* (1984).]

suffer from venous thrombosis, found that when their citrated blood was incubated *in vitro* at 37°C material with thromboplastic activity was liberated from the erythrocytes into the plasma. The same happened, too, with the blood of three patients with sickle-cell anaemia. The material was liberated independently of the presence of platelets or the onset of haemolysis.

The phenomenon was more fully investigated by Bradlow (1961) who convincingly demonstrated that a large proportion of the material liberated, which he considered had platelet-like coagulant properties and was probably composed of phospholipid, was derived from reticulocytes. This work suggested that the abnormally large number of circulating reticulocytes is a factor in the predisposition of patients with various types of haemolytic anaemia, including sickle-cell anaemia, to develop venous thrombosis.

Further evidence that sickled cells may themselves play a specific accelerating role in blood coagulation, irrespective of the presence of reticulocytes, was published by Chiu *et al.* (1981) and Lubin *et al.* (1981a,b). Sickled cells added to platelet-poor plasma, to which Russell's viper venom had been added, shortened its recalcification time by approximately 30%, while normal erythrocytes and oxygenated reversibly sickled cells did not do this. This effect was attributed to a rearrangement of membrane phospholipids consequent on sickling (see p. 208). According to Chiu *et al.* and Lubin *et al.*, it is the exposure of excess phosphatidylethanolamine and of phosphatidylserine in the outer leaflet of the membrane that is likely to be responsible for the ability of sickled cells to accelerate the clotting of plasma.

Stuart and Sills (1981) have produced some evidence that impaired production of prostacyclin (PGI$_2$) may be implicated in the formation of thrombi in Hb-SS patients. (Prostacyclin, formed by endothelial cells, is anti-aggregatory and anti-thrombotic.) Stuart and Sills had found that plasma derived from Hb-SS patients was less effective in stimulating the formation of prostacyclin by umbilical artery endothelium than control samples of plasma derived from normal subjects or patients with chronic haemolytic anaemias other than Hb-SS disease or from splenectomized individuals.

Evidence pointing to the existence in patients with Hb-SS disease of chronic intravascular coagulation has already been discussed (see p. 94). Further positive evidence was provided by Gordon *et al.* (1983) who showed that the mean coagulant and antigen titres of Hageman factor (a contact factor) in a series of 22 Hb-SS children were abnormally low and that the titres were further reduced in vaso-occlusive crises. Evidence of platelet activation in vaso-occlusive crises was reported by Billett *et al.* (1984). In eight out of 11 crises they found raised blood levels of β-thromboglobulin and platelet factor 4 either at the time of admission of the patients or subsequently.

According to Burns (1985), Hb-SS cells have a greater than normal affinity to adsorb purified fibrinogen in solution and to bind more readily than Hb-AA cells to fibrin. Burns suggested that binding to fibrin at sites of anoxia-produced endothelial cell damage might lead to plugging of small blood vessels and be a factor in the production of vaso-occlusive crises.

SICKLING *IN VIVO*: WHY DOES IT HAPPEN? A SUMMARY

In this short section an attempt will be made to summarize why sickling of sufficient severity to lead to local vaso-occlusive lesions takes place *in vivo* in Hb-SS disease. The problem is to reconcile the relatively slow process of sickling produced *in vitro* as the result of exposing blood to 40 mm Hg partial pressure of oxygen (approximately the normal pO_2 of mixed venous blood) with the rapidity with which erythrocytes normally traverse the capillary and venous system of the body (in about 15 seconds). The fact that sickling does take place *in vivo* seems to depend essentially on three factors which favour its occurrence. These are (1) the abnormal tendency of Hb-SS cells to adhere to vascular endothelium, (2) the increased viscosity of Hb-SS blood, and (3) the diminished O$_2$ affinity of Hb S. Together they slow the blood's passage through the microcirculation sufficiently to lead to rapid deoxygenation and sickling.

The factors which affect the viscosity of Hb-SS-containing blood and diminish its O$_2$ affinity have already been extensively discussed: in summary, they include the PCV, the concentration of Hb S within the cell, the rigidity of the cell's content and of its membrane, the number of ISCs present, intracellular pH, the Bohr effect and the concentration of 2,3-DPG.

How long it actually takes for Hb-SS blood to traverse capillaries must vary greatly from organ to organ: for instance, the transit time seems likely to be much greater in the spleen than in the heart and probably prolonged, too, in the liver and bone marrow. It seems likely that it is this organ-to-organ difference in capillary transit time which determines which organ will suffer from vaso-occlusive lesions and which will escape.

Clinically, crises occur when the circulation of blood through the minute blood vessels of organs in which the transit time is normally nearly critical for sickling is further slowed by an extraneous event or events which alone or collectively lead to a sufficient impairment of the circulation to initiate a vicious cycle: *e.g.*, developing sickling leads to a further increase in the blood's viscosity, to a further slowing of the circulation, to a greater degree of sickling, to further retardation of blood flow, to a fall in pH, to more extensive sickling and finally to cessation of blood flow leading to local infarction and pain. The events which precipitate crises tend to vary from individual to individual, but infections, fever, acidosis, anoxia and dehydration are well-known initiators of crises, and perhaps, also, exposure to cold (see p. 22).

As mentioned above, these extraneous events act ultimately by impairing the microcirculation locally, either directly, as with anoxia or dehydration, or indirectly, as for instance, by their effect on the plasma proteins, especially perhaps fibrinogen. The basic background to sickling is, of course, the intracellular concentration of Hb S, which is constant (after the first year or so of life) in each individual patient.

ERYTHROCYTE LIFE-SPAN IN SICKLE-CELL DISEASE

Measurements have demonstrated that the life-span of the erythrocytes is considerably dimin-ished in Hb-SS disease and diminished to a minor degree in Hb-SC disease and Hb-S/β-thalassaemia. Normal erythrocytes transfused to patients with any of the sickle haemoglobinopathies characteristically survive normally.

As long ago as 1924, Sydenstricker had concluded that when anaemia was present in 'active' cases of sickle-cell anaemia this was due to excessive blood destruction. As already referred to (p. 3), he recognized latent and active phases of the disease (in a ratio of 9:1 in his series) and stated that active phases had been observed in the children and grandchildren of persons presenting in the latent phase. He transfused the blood of one such latent case into a normal recipient and followed its survival by subjecting the recipient's blood to a sickling test at intervals after the transfusion. Sickled cells were still present 23 days after the transfusion and Sydenstricker concluded that they were surviving normally.

The first direct measurements of the life-span *in vivo* of the erythrocytes in Hb-SS disease were reported by Singer *et al.* (1948) and Callender *et al.* (1949). Using the Ashby technique, marked differences in the survival of the transfused cells were observed: a proportion of the cells disappeared rapidly from the circulation; others were eliminated far more slowly. Singer and Fisher (1952) correlated the difference in survival time with the relative amounts of Hb S and Hb F present and concluded that the cells containing the greatest amount of Hb F survived the longest.

The life-span of Hb-SS-containing erythrocytes was also estimated in pioneer studies by London *et al.* (1949) using [^{15}N]glycine. In an adult male in steady state (haemoglobin 10.8 g/dl) the curve of elimination of labelled erythrocytes from the peripheral blood was interpreted to indicate that destruction was random: 50% of the cells were estimated to have survived 29 days; their mean life-span was calculated to be 42 days and haemoglobin and erythrocyte production to be approximately 2.8 times the normal. No evidence was found of any failure in haemoglobin synthesis or erythrocyte formation. The last point was confirmed by James and Abbott (1955) in a similar but expanded study which included the estimation of [^{15}N]stercobilin. Their subject was a 21-year-old female (haemoglobin 6.0 g/dl, with 23% reticulocytes). Erythrocyte destruction was again found to be random: 50% of the cells were eliminated in 11 days and their mean life-span was 16 days. The erythrocyte turnover rate was calculated to be 6.3% per day and there was no evidence for more than one population. The stercobilin excretion curve paralleled the disappearance curve of labelled haem from the peripheral blood and there was no evidence of any excess initial labelling of stercobilin.

Weinstein and co-workers (1954) used ^{51}Cr to study the survival of the erythrocytes of a small number of patients in their own circulations. As expected, a major increase in cell destruction was found in Hb-SS disease (one patient gave a definitely two-component curve of elimination) and minor increases were found in Hb-SC disease and Hb-CC disease. The results were normal in individuals with the Hb-AS and Hb-AC traits.

Chernoff, Rucknagel and Jim (1955) transfused blood from Hb-SC disease patients into normal recipients with or without spleens. Using the Ashby technique, they found that the transfused cells were completely eliminated in 50–60 days irrespective of whether or not the spleen had been removed. These results were thought to indicate that the spleen played a comparatively small role in bringing about haemolysis. Chaplin, Keitel and Peterson (1956) also carried out some interesting experiments. They transfused three patients who had Hb-SS disease with normal Hb-AA blood so as to raise the level of haemoglobin to normal, and followed the rate at which the percentage of sickled cells in the circulation diminished following the transfusion (at a time when the rate of erythrocyte regeneration was low). Their data appeared to indicate that some of the patients' sickled cells had a very short life-span.

Sprague and Paterson (1958) published data on erythrocyte survival in Hb-SS and Hb-SC disease, and on the effect that splenectomy had on survival. Seven children with Hb-SS disease and splenomegaly were studied, six also after splenectomy: the mean ^{51}Cr T$_{50}$ before operation was 4.0 days; after operation it was 11.4 days (normal 30 ± 3 days). In seven older patients without splenomegaly (no splenectomy) the mean ^{51}Cr was 10 days, while in four out of five experiments in which blood from these patients was transfused to

normal recipients (with spleens) the survival was considerably less, i.e., the mean ^{51}Cr T$_{50}$ was 4.4 days compared with 9.2 days in the patients themselves. In seven patients with Hb-SC disease (three with splenomegaly) the mean ^{51}Cr T$_{50}$ was 15.7 days. This report emphasized that the spleen plays a significant role in the production of anaemia in children with Hb-SS disease (see also p. 28).

Further studies, using ^{51}Cr (and in some cases DF^{32}P, too), were reported by Erlandson, Schulman and Smith (1960), Malamos et al. (1963), Hathorn (1967), McCurdy (1969), Bensinger and Gillette (1974), McCurdy, Mahmoud and Sherman (1975) and McCurdy and Sherman (1978). The reported values for ^{51}Cr T$_{50}$ in the above series were: Hb-SS patients, 3.0–14.8 days; Hb-SC patients, 13.6–20.2 days, and Hb-S/β-thalassaemia patients, 10–18 days.

McCurdy (1969), McCurdy, Mahmoud and Sherman (1975) and McCurdy and Sherman (1978) used DF^{32}P as well as ^{51}Cr in their measurements and found that the results were concordant: e.g., ^{51}Cr T$_{50}$, 4.2–14.8 days (mean 9.52 days) in 22 Hb-SS patients; DF^{32}P, mean cell life-span (MCL) 7.8–23.9 days (mean 17.32 days) in 25 Hb-SS patients; mean ^{51}Cr T$_{50}$, 15.7 ± 2.7 days and DF^{32}P, MCL 28.9 ± 4.0 days in nine Hb-SC patients.

McCurdy and Sherman (1978) noted that 30% of those studied gave two-component survival curves and that there appeared to be a negative correlation between erythrocyte life-span and the numbers of irreversibly sickled cells present.

The question as to whether the binding of chromium to Hb S and the elution rates in vivo are the same as with Hb A had earlier been studied by Pearson (1963). His in-vitro data indicated that the site and strength of the binding of ^{51}Cr to Hb S, Hb C and Hb A were similar.

Bensinger and Gillette (1974) reviewed the published data on erythrocyte life-span in Hb-SS disease as determined by the Ashby, ^{51}Cr and DF^{32}P techniques, and presented data on 18 Hb-SS patients studied by CO excretion (see vol. 1, p. 50). Their results indicated a mean haem breakdown of 5–6 times the normal (range 3–14 times) and they concluded that their data implied a large reserve of bone-marrow erythropoietic activity in patients in a steady state.

COMPENSATORY ERYTHROPOIESIS IN SICKLE-CELL DISEASES

The early work of London and co-workers (1949) and James and Abbott (1955) using [^{15}N]glycine had failed to demonstrate any undue ineffective erythropoiesis in patients with Hb-SS anaemia, and the CO excretion data of Bensinger and Gillette (1974), referred to above, are in accord with this, as are the substantially raised reticulocyte counts of most patients. Studies using radioactive iron (^{59}Fe) have, too, generally demonstrated a fast turnover and a good utilization of iron in Hb-SS patients, with the findings in Hb-S/β-thalassaemia intermediate between those in Hb-SS anaemia and β-thalassaemia major (Malamos et al., 1963).

The data of Steinberg, Dreiling and Lovell (1977) on 10 patients indicated, however, a suboptimal response to their anaemia, with the iron turnover and erythrocyte production rate being only 2–3 times the normal. It was suggested that this may have been due to increased O_2 dissociation and an increase in cardiac output diminishing the hypoxic stimulus to erythropoiesis.

MECHANISM OF INCREASED HAEMOLYSIS IN SICKLE-CELL DISEASES

Several factors probably contribute to the diminished life-span of Hb-SS-containing erythrocytes. One is the abnormal rigidity of the cells, particularly of irreversibly sickled cells (ISCs), which would increase their sensitivity to lysis by mechanical forces [as demonstrated in vitro by the cells' increased mechanical fragility (p. 86)]. Another important factor is the unusual tendency of Hb-SS cells to adhere to, and to be phagocytosed by, macrophages.

Increased membrane rigidity

Factors which contribute to the cells' increased rigidity include the greatly increased viscosity of Hb S when deoxygenated and stiffening of the cell membrane. Amongst the causes of the stiffening are thought to be the binding of increased amount of $β^S$ chains (Bank et al., 1974) and of haemoglobin (Fischer et al., 1975) to the membrane (see also p. 83).

Instability of Hb S

Compared with Hb A, Hb S is unstable when exposed to mechanical forces. This, it has been suggested, may be responsible, at least in part, for the excessive amounts of denatured haemoglobin demonstrable in the membranes of Hb-SS cells.

According to Asakura et al. (1973), mechanical shaking causes oxyHb S in solution to undergo denaturation, with resultant turbidity, about 10 times as fast as Hb A. Haemoglobin from Hb-AS trait individuals denatures at an intermediate rate.

J. M. White (1974) compared the effect of mechanical shaking on newly synthesized Hb S and on Hb S that had been subjected in vivo to repeated sickling and unsickling. He found no difference in the rate of denaturation. In contrast to the effect of mechanical shaking on Hb S in dilute solution, no inclusions developed within intact erythrocytes in suspension when shaken for a similar period of time. He concluded that the unusual sensitivity of dilute solutions of Hb S to mechanical denaturation that is demonstrable in vitro has little pathogenetic significance.

Vella (1975) compared the stability of 22 different haemoglobins to mechanical trauma. Under the condition of his experiments, Hb S, with Hb Bucuresti, Köln, M Saskatoon, Shepherds Bush and Zürich, were the most unstable of the haemoglobins tested.

Bensinger and Beutler (1977) used the isopropanol precipitation test (see p. 352) to compare the stability of Hb S with that of Hb A. A precipitate was visible within 20 minutes using haemolysates derived from Hb-SS, Hb-AS or Hb-SC blood; in contrast, haemolysates from Hb-AC or Hb-AA blood took 40–60 minutes to precipitate. Bensinger and Beutler concluded that even fully oxygenated Hb S is relatively unstable.

Asakura and co-workers (1977) later reported that the amount of denatured haemoglobin demonstrable in Hb-S-containing cells was about 5 times that in normal cells. In contrast, erythrocytes from Hb-AA patients with reticulocytosis did not as a rule contain elevated amounts of denatured haemoglobin. Thus the amounts were normal or only very slightly raised in patients with hereditary spherocytosis or auto-immune haemolytic anaemia, irrespective of whether splenectomy had been carried out.

Intravascular haemolysis

The concept that a significant proportion of the increased haemolysis in Hb-SS disease (and probably also in Hb-SC disease and in Hb-S/β-thalassaemia) takes place intravascularly, as the result presumably of mechanical forces acting on cells abnormally sensitive to trauma, was supported by the observations of Crosby and Dameshek (1951) on the occurrence of haemoglobinaemia and haemosiderinuria in patients with various types of haemolytic anaemia. They found raised plasma-haemoglobin levels and also small amounts of urinary haemosiderin in sickle-cell anaemia but not in the sickle-cell trait.

Evidence that exercise plays a part in promoting the intravascular haemolysis has more recently been provided by Platt (1982). Following up the observation that a 21-year-old male Hb-SS patient developed haemoglobinuria after vigorous exercise, a rise in plasma-haemoglobin concentration (without haemoglobinuria) was demonstrated in four other patients who undertook a more moderate form of exercise — they simply walked up stairs wearing rubber-soled shoes. Platt concluded that the exercise-induced haemolysis was related to the mechanical lysis of dehydrated shear-sensitive cells and suggested that exercise might be a factor in the causation of the chronic haemolysis of Hb-SS disease.

Extravascular haemolysis: adhesion of Hb-SS cells to macrophages

Recently it has been realized that Hb-SS cells adhere more readily than do Hb-AA cells to macrophages in in-vitro systems, and it has been suggested that this abnormal tendency to adherence plays a significant part in the shortening of the life-span of Hb-SS erythrocytes. Possible reasons for the abnormal adherence include the redistribution of aminophosphatides in the outer leaflet of the erythrocyte membrane (see p. 208) and the presence on the erythrocyte surface of abnormal amounts of IgG. Both these phenomena are demonstrable, but to a lesser degree, in the case of normal erythocytes at the end of their life-span.

Miller and Hebbel (1981) reported that Hb-SS erythrocytes adhere to cultured unstimulated human bone-marrow macrophages more readily and persistently than do normal Hb-AA cells. An adherence ratio correlated positively with the ISC count and with other indicators of the rate of haemolysis. Hb-SS cells were ingested to a greater extent and more rapidly than were normal cells. Miller and Hebbel concluded that abnormal cell-to-cell interaction plays a part not only in vaso-occlusion but is also an important determinant of increased haemolysis.

Schwartz and co-workers (1983b, 1985) investigated the mechanism of the increased adherence of Hb-SS cells to macrophages. They used as test cells cultured human peripheral-blood monocytes and found that ISCs and deoxygenated reversibly sickled cells (RSCs) adhered more readily than did oxygenated Hb-SS and Hb-AA cells. ISCs were the most adherent, while re-oxygenation of RSCs diminished their adherence. Schwartz et al. showed that increased adherence was associated with an increased expression in the outer leaflet of the erythrocyte membrane of the aminophosphatides, phosphatidylserine (PS) and phosphatidylethanolamine; they enriched the erythrocyte membrane with a fluorescent analogue of PS and found that this caused increased adhesion, and they showed that enrichment with similar amounts of phosphatidylcholine failed to do this.

Preincubation of monocytes with PS liposomes caused an approximately 60% inhibition of adherence. Schwartz et al. suggested that PS on the surface of Hb-SS erythrocytes acted as a ligand that is recognized by monocytes and that its presence could play a significant role in bringing about a shortening of the erythrocyte life-span.

Hebbel and Miller (1984) reported further studies on the interaction of Hb-SS erythrocytes and cultured macrophages derived from human bone marrow. With their technique Hb-SS cells were ingested by 18.9% of the macrophages (mean value) while Hb-AA cells were ingested by only 3.1% of the macrophages (mean value). The difference was not related to the reticulocyte count but was strongly correlated with increased erythrocyte density. The interaction between cells and macrophages appeared to be partly immunological, caused by abnormal amounts of IgG on the erythrocyte surface, and partly due to chemical changes to the membrane brought about by dialdehyde products of excessive auto-oxidation. Hebbel and Miller suggested that malonyldialdehyde (MDA) enhances IgG binding either by causing the exposure of normally cryptic antigens or by leading to the formation of new antigens. They concluded that macrophages recognize Hb-SS cells abnormally readily not so much because the cells are abnormal as because they are 'senescent'.

Further evidence supporting the concept that shortening of the Hb-SS cell life-span may be brought about by an immunological mechanism was provided by Petz et al. (1984) who had used a sensitive complement-fixing antiglobulin test as a probe for abnormal amounts of IgG on the surface of erythrocytes of patients suffering from haemolytic anaemias not thought to be caused by an immune mechanism. Patients with hereditary spherocytosis, pyruvate-kinase deficiency or mechanical haemolytic anaemia were found to have less then 25 molecules of IgG on the surface of each cell; in contrast, 39 out of 62 Hb-SS patients (63%) had abnormally high numbers of molecules on each cell; the mean was 195 molecules, the maximum 890 molecules. None of the Hb-SS patients had been recently transfused. The orthodox direct antiglobulin test was positive in two; but in none of the patients could abnormal antibodies be demonstrated in their serum. However, eluates from the erythrocytes of six patients contained sufficient antibody against normal erythrocytes to be demonstrated by the indirect antiglobulin test. Petz et al. also obtained positive results in eight out of 14 Hb-SC, Hb-SD and Hb-S/β-thalassaemia patients, in seven out of 57 Hb-AS individuals and in five out of six patients with thalassaemia major.

Green, Rehn and Kaira (1985) separated Hb-SS blood into four fractions using a discontinuous Stractan gradient. Autologous IgG coating the erythrocytes was estimated by means of a ^{125}I-protein A (Staph. aureus) binding assay; in addition, the proportion of cells in each fraction that fluoresced when the cells were exposed to FITC-conjugated anti-human IgG was determined as well as the extent to which the cells reacted. The two most dense fractions of cells were found to bind on 2.7 and 1.8 times, respectively, as much IgG as the lightest (youngest) fraction. The fluorescence test also showed that the most dense cells tended to bind on the most IgG. Green, Rehn and Kaira concluded that some of the changes that affect the membrane of normal cells towards the end of their life-span (approximately 120 days) affect Hb-SS cells of a much younger (10–40 days) age; they suggested that the topography of the surface of Hb-SS cells is altered during the transformation of the cells to dense ISCs, with the result that cryptic antigenic sites are unmasked.

The more recent work of Galili, Clark and Shohet (1986) suggests that the antibody responsible for the observations of Petz et al. (1984) and probably, too, responsible for the enhanced phagocytosis of Hb-SS cells in vitro is the recently described normal antibody anti-Gal (anti-α-galactosyl IgG) (Galili et al., 1983, 1984).

Galili, Clark and Shohet (1986) employed as a probe a highly sensitive rosetting antiglobulin test, using K562 myeloid cells which bear a receptor for the FC portion of IgG molecules (Galili, Manny and Izak, 1981). Using a Stractan gradient, they separated blood into six fractions and found that 0.6% of the most dense fraction of Hb-AA cells, and approximately 40% of the most dense Hb-SS cells (mainly fractions IV–VI), had IgG bound to their membrane as indicated by the high proportion of rosettes formed. The IgG was found to be readily eluted by carbohydrates containing α-galactosyl residues and it seemed clear that the IgG was identical with anti-Gal, present in normal sera at high titre.

Affinity-purified anti-Gal interacted specifically with Hb-SS or Hb-AA cells depleted of bound antibody and similar results were obtained with a radio-labelled lectin with α-galactosyl specificity. In vitro, phagocytosis could be correlated with the presence of anti-Gal on the cells. Galili, Clark and Shohet concluded that the in-vivo binding of anti-Gal reflects, in the case of Hb-SS cells, an accelerated physiological ageing process involving the recognition of prematurely exposed α-galactosyl-bearing antigen sites and that this recognition contributes to the shortened life-span of Hb-SS erythrocytes.

Role of the spleen, liver and bone marrow

Spleen. As already referred to (p. 28), enlargement of the spleen in infancy and its subsequent shrinkage were early recognized as characteristic features of sickle-cell anaemia. Hahn and Gillespie (1927), in assigning to the spleen a secondary role in pathogenesis, stated that 'it merely performs its usual function in sickle cell anemia, that of capturing and destroying damaged or abnormal red blood corpuscles'. The initial splenomegaly is the consequence of the splenic pulp being engorged with blood; once there, cells become sickled as the result of anoxia, a relatively low pH and haemoconcentration, and they must find it difficult, because of their shape and rigidity, to leave the pulp and regain the general circulation. Weisman and co-workers (1953) provided experimental evidence that such cells become selectively trapped in the spleen, and Watson, Lichtman and Shapiro (1956) and Harris and co-workers (1956) reported that the proportion of ISCs in spleen-pulp blood is higher than in the peripheral circulation. Because the spleen pulp acts as a cul-de-sac, it is easy to understand how infarction eventually occurs and why the spleen shrinks to a small fibrotic organ in patients with Hb-SS disease whose erythrocytes sickle so readily. In Hb-SC disease and in the Hb-AS trait an added factor of generalized hypoxia, as in unpressurized aeroplane flights, seems to be required for infarction of the spleen to take place. The spleen in Hb-SS disease thus acts as an involuntary storehouse for sickled cells, and in doing so increases to some extent the rate at which sickled cells are destroyed. But as Hahn and Gillespie pointed out as long ago as 1927, 'in performing this office, it is damaged itself'.

Exceptionally, the spleen becomes massively

enlarged in Hb-SS disease as the result of becoming grossly engorged with blood, and the patient becomes markedly and dangerously anaemic (see p. 28). This can only happen in young people, before the spleen becomes fibrotic. Splenectomy in such cases can be life-saving; in more typical patients, on the other hand, it makes as a rule no great difference to their well-being (see p. 252).

The data obtained by in-vivo counting after labelling patients' erythrocytes with ^{51}Cr have supported the concept that the spleen plays a relatively minor role in the increased haemolysis of Hb-SS disease, despite the splenic sequestration of sickled cells. The eventual development of splenic fibrosis is no doubt the reason for this.

Lewis, Szur and Dacie (1960) studied four Hb-SS patients and one patient with Hb-SC disease. No excess ^{51}Cr counts were detected over the (impalpable) spleen of the Hb-SS patients, but there was a moderate excess in the case of the Hb-SC patient whose spleen was palpable. Excess counts were, however, detected over the liver in all five patients. Erlandson, Schulman and Smith's (1960) findings were similar. Hepatic sequestration was demonstrated in all eight Hb-SS patients and splenic sequestration in the two patients whose spleens could be palpated. The data of Hathorn (1967), who reported from Accra, were essentially the same: excess hepatic counts were demonstrated in seven out of nine patients, and excess splenic counts in all seven patients in whom the spleen was palpable. It is interesting to note that the [51]Cr T_{50} of the seven patients with splenomegaly was 3.4–5.2 days, whilst in the two patients in whom the spleen was impalpable it was longer, 9.2 and 9.4 days.

In contrast to Hb-SS disease, the spleen remains palpably enlarged throughout the life-time of patients suffering from Hb-SC disease or Hb-S/β-thalassaemia. This is presumably because the O_2 tension required for sickling is lower in these disorders. The spleen thus escapes infarction and fibrosis, and it normally contributes to the excess haemolysis throughout the life of the patient.

Liver. That the liver is involved to an important degree in the destruction of Hb-SS-containing erythrocytes is indicated by the in-vivo studies with [51]Cr (Vol. 1, p. 112) and by the histological findings in fatal cases. As already mentioned (p. 181), Edington (1955) found abundant evidence of erythrophagocytosis by Kupffer cells and of dilatation of the hepatic sinuses, and he and Walters (1958) emphasized that fibrin was deposited within the sinuses. It seems likely that sickling takes place to a marked degree within the liver in the slowly circulating deoxygenated portal blood.

Bone marrow. The bone-marrow sinuses would seem to be another site where the circulatory conditions are suitable for extensive sickling to take place and where sickled cells are destroyed. Indirect evidence for this is the frequency of bone pain and the occasional occurrence of objective evidence of the consequence of vascular obstruction, *i.e.*, necrosis of the bone marrow.

Mechanism of haemolysis within the spleen, liver and bone marrow. There seems little reason to doubt but that the slow circulation within the spleen, liver and bone marrow provides an ideal environment for the intimate erythrocyte and macrophage interaction described on page 224 to take place. This must be particularly true of the spleen, and it would be particularly interesting to know whether the serious complication of acute splenic sequestration is correlated with the presence of unusually large amounts of Hb-SS cell membrane IgG.

PATHOGENESIS OF THE CLINICAL MANIFESTATIONS AND INCREASED HAEMOLYSIS IN COMPOUND HETEROZYGOSITY FOR Hb S AND β-THALASSAEMIA OR ANOTHER VARIANT HAEMOGLOBIN

The factors that determine severity in the compound heterozygotes are in general the same as those that operate in homozygous Hb-SS disease. Their effect, however, is ameliorated by reduction in Hb-S concentration and would be, too, by Hb F, if present in high concentration. Hb-SC disease is, however, significantly, even surprisingly, severe taking into account that neither the presence of the Hb-AS nor Hb-AC trait lead as a rule to any clinical or haematological abnormality and that the concentration of Hb S in Hb-SC disease patients is usually only about 50% (see p. 156).

Hb-SC disease

Conley (1964), in studies of the crystallization of

haemoglobin in Hb-CC patients when their erythrocytes were suspended in hypertonic (3 g/dl) NaCl, found that crystals formed readily in Hb-SC erythrocytes despite the fact that the concentration of Hb C was less than 50%. He concluded that Hb C and Hb S interact with respect to crystal formation.

The relatively severe manifestation of Hb-SC disease presumably reflects an analogous interaction between Hb S and Hb C *in vivo* — namely, co-polymerization rather than co-crystallization under artificial conditions *in vitro*. According to Bunn *et al.* (1982), three factors are important: the proportion of Hb S is relatively high (higher than in the Hb-AS trait); the total haemoglobin concentration (MCHC) is unusually high in Hb-SC disease, and Hb C co-polymerizes with Hb S.

Bunn and his co-workers established that polymerization occurs about 15 times more rapidly in a 50:50 mixture of Hb C and Hb S (the usual finding in Hb-SC patients) compared with in a 60:40 mixture of Hb A and Hb S (the usual finding in the Hb-AS trait). Bunn *et al.* also reported that in density-separated fractions of Hb-SC blood the reticulocytes were more evenly distributed than in Hb-AA or Hb-AS blood, suggesting that Hb-SC cells when young have a high haemoglobin concentration; they concluded that the two factors that contribute to the increased sickling of Hb-SC cells, compared with Hb-AS cells, are the higher concentration of Hb S and the higher concentration of total (S+C) haemoglobin.

REFERENCES

ADACHI, K. & ASAKURA, T. (1982). Kinetics of the polymerization of hemoglobin in high and low phosphate buffers. *Blood Cells*, **8**, 213–224.

ADAMS, J. Q. (1957). Sodium and potassium alterations in red cells of patients with sicklemia. *J. Lab. clin. Med.*, **49**, 738–744.

ALLAN, D., LIMBRICK, A. R., THOMAS, P. & WESTERMAN, M. P. (1981). Microvesicles from sickle erythrocytes and their relation to irreversible sickling. *Brit. J. Haemat.*, **47**, 383–390.

ALLAN, D., LIMBRICK, A. R., THOMAS, P. & WESTERMAN, M. P. (1982). Release of spectrin-free spicules on reoxygenation of sickled erythrocytes. *Nature (Lond.)*, **295**, 612–613.

ALLISON, A. C. (1956). Observations on the sickling phenomenon and on the distribution of different haemoglobin types in erythrocyte populations. *Clin. Sci.*, **15**, 497–510.

ALLISON, A. C. (1957). Properties of sickle-cell haemoglobin. *Biochem. J.*, **65**, 212–219,

ANDERSON, I. S., YEUNG, K.-Y., HILLMAN, D. & LESSIN, L. S. (1975). Multiple myeloma in a patient with sickle cell anemia. Interacting effects on blood viscosity. *Amer. J. Med.*, **59**, 568–574.

ASAKURA, T., AGARWAL, P. L., RELMAN, D. A., McCRAY, J. A., CHANCE, B., SCHWARTZ, E., FRIEDMAN, S. & LUBIN, B. (1973). Mechanical instability of the oxy-form of sickle haemoglobin. *Nature (Lond.)*, **244**, 437–438.

ASAKURA, T. & MAYBERRY, J. (1984). Relationship between morphologic characteristics of sickle cells and method of deoxygenation. *J. Lab. clin. Med.*, **104**, 987–994.

ASAKURA, T., MINAKATA, K., ADACHI, K., RUSSELL, M. O. & SCHWARTZ, E. (1977). Denatured hemoglobin in sickle erythrocytes. *J. clin. Invest.*, **59**, 633–640.

ASCENZI, A. & SILVESTRONI, E. (1957). Étude anatomo-clinique d'un cas de maladie microdrépanocytique. *Acta haemat. (Basel)*, **18**, 205–218.

BAEZ, S., KAUL, D. K. & NAGEL, R. L. (1982). Microvascular determinants of blood flow behavior and HbSS erythrocyte plugging in microcirculation. *Blood Cells*, **8**, 127–137.

BAIRD, R. L., WEISS, D. L., FERGUSON, A. D., FRENCH, J. H. & SCOTT, R. B. (1964). Studies in sickle cell anemia. XXI. Clinico-pathological aspects of neurological manifestations. *Pediatrics*, **34**, 92–100.

BALLAS, S. K. & BURKA, E. R. (1980). Failure to demonstrate red cell membrane protein abnormalities in sickle cell anaemia. *Brit. J. Haemat.*, **46**, 627–629.

BANK, A., MEARS, G., WEISS, R., O'DONNELL, J. V. & NATTA, C. (1974). Preferential binding of β^S globin chains associated with stroma in sickle cell disorders. *J. clin. Invest.*, **54**, 805–809.

BARABINO, G. A., McINTIRE, L. V., ESKIN, S. G., SEARS, D. A. & UDDEN, M. M. (1985). Endothelial cell interactions with sickle cell, sickle trait, mechanically injured and normal erythrocytes. *Blood*, **66**, No. 5 (Suppl. 1), 55a (Abstract 108).

BARTLETT, G. R., HUGHES, L., BARNEY, C. & MARLOW, A. A. (1955). Erythrocyte metabolism in sickle cell anemia. *Proc. Soc. exp. Biol. Med.*, **88**, 288–289.

BAUER, J. (1940). Sickle cell disease: pathogenic,

clinical and therapeutic considerations. *Arch. Surg.*, **41**, 1344–1362.

BAUER, T. W., MOORE, G. W. & HUTCHINS, G. M. (1980). The liver in sickle cell disease. A clinicopathologic study of 70 patients. *Amer. J. Med.*, **69**, 833–837.

BENESCH, R. E., EDALJI, R., BENESCH, R. & KWONG, S. (1980). Solubilization of hemoglobin S by other hemoglobins. *Proc. natn. Acad. Sci. U.S.A.*, **77**, 5130–5134.

BENESCH, R. E., KWONG, S., BENESCH, R. & EDALJI, R. (1977). Location and bond type of intermolecular contacts in the polymerization of haemoglobin S. *Nature (Lond.)*, **269**, 772–775.

BENESCH, R. E., KWONG, S., EDALJI, R. & BENESCH, R. (1979). Alpha chain mutations with opposite effects on the gelation of Hb S. *J. biol. Chem.*, **254**, 8169–8172.

BENNETT, G. W. (1929a). Splenic atrophy with calcium and iron incrustations (nodular splenic atrophy). *Arch. Path.*, **7**, 71–77.

BENNETT, G. A. (1929b). Sickle cell anemia. Further investigation of a case of splenic atrophy with calcium and iron incrustations (nodular splenic atrophy). *Arch. Path.*, **7**, 801–803.

BENSINGER, T. W. & BEUTLER, E. (1977). Instability of the oxy form of sickle hemoglobin and of methemoglobin in isopropanol. *Amer. J. clin. Path.*, **67**, 180–183.

BENSINGER, T. W. & GILLETTE, P. N. (1974). Hemolysis in sickle cell disease. *Arch. intern. Med.*, **133**, 624–631.

BERETTA, L., GERLI, G. C., FERRARESI, R., AGOSTONI, A., GUALANDRI, V. & ORSINI, G. B. (1983). Antioxidant system in sickle red cells. *Acta haemat. (Basel)*, **70**, 194–197.

BERMAN, L. B. & TUBLIN, I. (1959). The nephropathies of sickle-cell disease. *Arch. intern. Med.*, **103**, 602–606.

BERNSTEIN, J. & WHITTEN, C. F. (1960). A histologic appraisal of the kidney in sickle cell anemia. *Arch. Path.*, **70**, 407–418.

BERTLES, J. F. (1974). Hemoglobin interaction and molecular basis of sickling. *Arch. intern. Med.*, **133**, 538–543.

BERTLES J. F. & DÖBLER, J. (1969). Reversible and irreversible sickling: a distinction by electron microscopy. *Blood*, **33**, 884–898.

BERTLES, J. F. & MILNER, P. F. A. (1968). Irreversibly sickled erythrocytes: a consequence of the heterogeneous distribution of hemoglobin types in sickle-cell anemia. *J. clin. Invest.*, **47**, 1731–1741.

BERTLES, J. F., RABINOWITZ, R. & DÖBLER, J. (1969). Relative exclusion of molecular species of hemoglobin during solid-phase formation in deoxygenated solutions of sickle hemoglobin (Hb S). *Blood*, **34**, 857 (Abstract 99).

BERTLES, J. F., RABINOWITZ, R. & DÖBLER, J. (1970). Hemoglobin interaction: modification of

solid phase composition in the sickling phenomenon. *Science*, **169**, 375–377.

BERTLES, J. F., ROTH, E. & ANKU, V. (1967). The hemoglobin of irreversibly sickled erythrocytes. *J. clin. Invest.*, **46**, 1037 (Abstract).

BESSIS, M., BRICKA, M. & BRETON-GORIUS, J. (1953). Différents aspects de la surface des erythrocytes falciformes observés au microscope électronique. *Rev. Hémat.*, **8**, 222–229.

BESSIS, M., BRICKA, M., BRETON-GORIUS, J. & TABUIS, J. (1954). New observations on sickle cells with special reference to their agglutinability. *Blood*, **9**, 39–45.

BESSIS, M. & DÖBLER, J. (1970). Discocytes et échinocytes dans l'anémie à cellules falciformes. II. Disposition des polymères d'hémoglobine. *Nouv. Rev. franç. Hémat.*, **10**, 793–800.

BESSIS, M., DÖBLER, K. & MANDON, P. (1970). Discocytes et échinocytes dans l'anémie à cellules falciformes. Examen au microscope électronique à balayage *Nouv. Rev. franç. Hémat.*, **10**, 63–74.

BESSIS, M., FEO, C. & JONES, E. (1982). Quantitation of red cell deformability during progressive deoxygenation and oxygenation in sickling disorders (the use of an automated ektacytometer). *Blood Cells*, **8**, 17–28.

BESSIS, M., NOMARSKI, G., THIÉRY, J. P. & BRETON-GORIUS, J. (1958). Études sur la falciformation des globules rouges au microscope polarisant et au microscope électronique. II. L'intérieur du globule. Comparaison avec les cristaux intraglobulaires. *Rev. Hémat.*, **13**, 249–270.

BEUTLER, E., GUINTO, E. & JOHNSON, C. (1976). Human red cell protein kinase in normal subjects with hereditary spherocytosis, sickle cell disease, and autoimmune hemolytic anemia. *Blood*, **48**, 887–898.

BILLETT, H. H., FABRY, M., BUCHANAN, I. & NAGEL, R. (1984). Evidence for the activation of platelets during the vaso-occlusive crisis of sickle cell disease. *Blood*, **64**, No. 5 (Suppl. 1), 46a (Abstract 96).

BOGOCH, A., CASSELMAN, W. G. B., MARGOLIES, M. P. & BOCKUS, H. L. (1955). Liver disease in sickle cell anemia. A correlation of clinical, biochemical, histologic and histochemical observations. *Amer. J. Med.*, **19**, 583–609.

BOOKCHIN, R. M., BALAZS, T. & LANDAU, L. C. (1976). Determinants of red cell sickling. Effects of varying pH and of increasing intracellular hemoglobin concentration by osmotic shrinkage. *J. Lab. clin. Med.*, **87**, 597–616.

BOOKCHIN, R. M., LEW, D. J., BALAZS, T., UEDA, Y. & LEW, V. L. (1984). Dehydration and delayed proton equilibria of red blood cells suspended in isosmotic phosphate buffers: implications for studies of sickled cells. *J. Lab. clin. Med.*, **104**, 855–866.

BOOKCHIN, R. M. & LEW, V. L. (1983). Red cell membrane abnormalities in sickle cell anemia. In: *Progress in Hematology*, Vol. XIII (ed. by E. B. Brown), pp. 1–23. Grune and Stratton, New York.

BOOKCHIN, R. M. & NAGEL, R. L. (1974). Interactions between human hemoglobins: sickling and related phenomena. *Seminars Hemat.*, **11**, 577–595.

BOOKCHIN, R. M., NAGEL, R. L. & RANNEY, H. M. (1967). Structure and properties of hemoglobin C$_{Harlem}$, a human hemoglobin variant with amino acid substitutions in 2 residues of the β-polypeptide chain. *J. biol. Chem.*, **242**, 248–255.

BOOKCHIN, R. M., NAGEL, R. L. & RANNEY, H. M. (1970). The effect of β^{73} ^{Asn} on the interactions of sickling hemoglobins. *Biochim. biophys. Acta*, **221**, 373–375.

BRADLOW, B. A. (1961). Liberation of material with platelet-like coagulant properties from intact red cells and particularly from reticulocytes. *Brit. J. Haemat.*, **7**, 476–495.

BREWER, G. J., WETTERSTROEM, N., WARTH, J. A., MITCHINSON, A., NEAR, K., BREWER, L. F. & HILL, G. M. (1983). The relationship of glutathione levels and Heinz body formation to irreversibly sickled cells in sickle cell anemia. *Blood*, **62**, No. 5 (Suppl. 1), 54a (Abstract 117).

BRIDGES, W. H. (1939). Cerebral vascular disease accompanying sickle cell anemia. *Amer. J. Path.*, **15**, 353–362.

BRIEHL, R. W. (1982). The effects of shear on the delay time for gelation. *Blood Cells*, **8**, 201–212.

BRITTENHAM, G. M., SCHECHTER, A. N. & NOGUCHI, C. T. (1985). Hemoglobin S polymerization: primary determinant of the hemolytic and clinical severity of the sickling syndromes. *Blood*, **65**, 183–189.

BROWN, C. H. III (1972). Bone marrow necrosis. A study of seventy cases. *Johns Hopk. med. J.*, **131**, 189–203.

BUCKALEW, V. M. JNR & SOMEREN, A. (1974). Renal manifestations of sickle cell disease. *Arch. intern. Med.*, **133**, 660–669.

BUNN, H. F., NOGUCHI, C. T., HOFRICHTER, J., SCHECHTER, G. P., SCHECHTER, A. N. & EATON, W. A. (1982). Molecular and cellular pathogenesis of hemoglobin SC disease. *Proc. natn. Acad. Sci. U.S.A.*, **79**, 7527–7531.

BURNS, E. R. (1985). Increased avidity of sickle erythrocytes for fibrinogen/fibrin: implications for vaso-occlusive crises. *Blood*, **66**, No. 5 (Suppl. 1), 56a (Abstract 112).

BURNS, E. R., WILKINSON, W. H. & NAGEL, R. L. (1983). Adherence properties of sickle erythrocytes in dynamic flow systems. *Blood*, **62**, No. 5 (Suppl. 1), 54a (Abstract 118).

BURNS, E. R., WILKINSON, W. H. & NAGEL, R. L. (1985). Adherence properties of sickle erythrocytes in dynamic flow systems. *J. Lab. clin. Med.*, **105**, 673–678.

CALLENDER, S. T. E., NICKEL, J. F., MOORE, C. V. & POWELL, E. O. (1949). Sickle cell disease: studied by measuring the survival of transfused red blood cells. *J. Lab. clin. Med.*, **34**, 90–104,

CAMPWALA, H. Q. & DESFORGES, J. (1982). Membrane-bound hemichrome in density-separated cohorts of normal (AA) and sickled (SS) cells. *J. Lab. clin. Med.*, **99**, 25–28.

CHAPLIN, H. JNR, KEITEL, H. G. & PETERSON, R. E. (1956). Hematologic observations on patients with sickle cell anaemia sustained at normal hemoglobin levels by multiple transfusions. *Blood*, **11**, 834–845.

CHARACHE, S. & CONLEY, C. L. (1964). Rate of sickling of red cells during deoxygenation of blood from persons with various sickling disorders. *Blood*, **24**, 25–48.

CHARACHE, S., DE LA MONTE, S. & MACDONALD, V. (1982). Increased blood viscosity in a patient with sickle cell anemia. *Blood Cells*, **8**, 103–109.

CHARACHE, S. & PAGE, D. L. (1987). Infarction of bone marrow in sickle cell disorders. *Ann. intern. Med.*, **67**, 1195–1200.

CHARACHE, S. & RICHARDSON, S. N. (1964). Prolonged survival of a patient with sickle cell anemia. *Arch. intern. Med.*, **113**, 884–849.

CHERNOFF, A. I., RUCKNAGEL, D. & JIM, R. (1955). Hemolytic mechanism in sickle cell-Hgb C disease. *Proc. Soc. exp. Biol. Med.*, **90**, 547–550.

CHIEN, S. (1977). Rheology of sickle cells and erythrocyte content. *Blood Cells*, **3**, 283–303.

CHIEN, S., KING, R. G., KAPERONIS, A. A. & USAMI, S. (1982). Viscoelastic properties of sickle cells and hemoglobin. *Blood Cells*, **8**, 53–64.

CHIEN, S., USAMI, S. & BERTLES, J. F. (1969). Abnormal rheology of oxygenated blood in sickle-cell anemia (Hb SS disease). *Blood*, **34**, 832 (Abstract 23).

CHIEN, S., USAMI, S. & BERTLES, J. F. (1970). Abnormal rheology of oxygenated blood in sickle cell anemia. *J. clin. Invest*, **49**, 623–634.

CHIU, D. & LUBIN, B. (1979). Abnormal vitamin E and glutathione peroxidase levels in sickle cell anemia. Evidence for increased susceptibility to lipid peroxidation in vivo. *J. Lab. clin. Med.*, **94**, 542–548.

CHIU, D., LUBIN, B., ROELOFSEN, B. & VAN DEENEN, L. L. M. (1981). Sickled erythrocytes accelerate clotting in vitro: an effect of abnormal membrane asymmetry. *Blood*, **55**, 398–401.

CHIU, D., LUBIN, B. & SHOHET, S. B. (1979). Erythrocyte membrane lipid reorganization during the sickling process. *Brit. J. Haemat.*, **41**, 223–234.

CLARK, L. J., CHAN, L. S., POWARS, D. R. & BAKER, R. F. (1981). Negative charge distribution and density on the surface of oxygenated normal and sickle red cells. *Blood*, **57**, 675–678.

CLARK, M. R., GUATELLI, J. C., MOHANDAS, N. & SHOHET, S. B. (1980). Influence of red cell water content on the morphology of sickling. *Blood*, **55**, 823–830.

CLARK, M. R., MOHANDAS, N., EMBURY, S. H. & LUBIN, B. H. (1982). A simple laboratory alternative to irreversibly sickled cell (ISC) counts. *Blood*, **60**, 659–662.

CLARK, M. R., MOHANDAS, N. & SHOHET, S. B. (1980). Deformability of oxygenated irreversibly sickled cells. *J. clin. Invest.*, **65**, 189–196.

CLARK, M. R., MORRISON, C. E. & SHOHET, S. B. (1978). Monovalent cation transport in irreversibly sickled cells. *J. clin. Invest.*, **62**, 329–337.

CLARK, M. R. & SHOHET, S. B. (1976). Hybrid erythrocytes for membrane studies in sickle cell disease. *Blood*, **47**, 121–131.

CLARK, M. R., UNGER, R. C. & SHOHET, S. B. (1978). Monovalent cation composition and ATP and lipid content of irreversibly sickled cells. *Blood*, **51**, 1169–1178.

CLARKSON, E. M. & MAIZELS, M. (1955). Sodium transfer in the erythrocyte of sickle-cell anaemia. *J. Physiol.*, **129**, 504–512.

CONLEY, C. L. (1964). Pathophysiological effects of some abnormal hemoglobins. *Medicine (Baltimore)*, **43**, 785–787.

CREPEAU, R. H., DYKES, G., GARRELL, R & EDELSTEIN, S. J. (1978). Diameter of haemoglobin S in fibres in sickled cells. *Nature (Lond.)*, **274**, 616–617.

CROSBY, W. H. & DAMESHEK, W. (1951). The significance of hemoglobinuria and associated hemosiderinuria, with particular reference to various types of hemolytic anemia. *J. Lab. clin. Med.*, **38**, 829–841.

DANISH, E. H. & HARRIS, J. W. (1983). Viscosity studies of deoxyhemoglobin S: evidence for formation of microaggregates during the lag phase. *J. Lab. clin. Med.*, **101**, 515–526.

DAS, S. K. & NAIR, R. C. (1980). Superoxide dismutase, glutathione peroxidase, catalase and lipid peroxidation of normal and sickled erythrocytes. *Brit. J. Haemat.*, **44**, 87–92.

DELAUNAY, J., GALAND, C. & BOIVIN, P. (1982). Erythrocyte membrane phosphorylation in sickle cell disease. *Nouv. Rev. franç. Hémat.*, **24**, 227–230.

DERVICHIAN, D. G., FOURNET, G., GUINIER, A. & PONDER, E. (1952). Structure submicroscopique des globules rouges contenant des hémoglobines anormales. *Rev. Hémat.*, **7**, 567–574.

DIGGS, L. W. (1932). The sickle cell phenomenon. I. Rate of sickling in moist preparations. *J. Lab. clin. Med.*, **17**, 913–920.

DIGGS, L. W. (1935). Siderofibrosis of the spleen in sickle cell anemia. *J. Amer. med. Ass.*, **104**, 538–541.

DIGGS, L. W. (1967). Bone and joint lesions in sickle-cell disease. *Clin. Orthop.*, **52**, 119–143.

DIGGS, L. W. (1969). Pulmonary lesions in sickle cell anemia. *Blood*, **34**, 734 (Abstract).

DIGGS, L. W. (1973). Anatomic lesions in sickle cell disease. In: *Sickle Cell Disease: Diagnosis, Management, Education and Research. A Symposium* (ed. by H. Abramson, J. F. Bertles and D. L. Wethers), pp. 189–229. C. V. Mosby, Saint Louis.

DIGGS, L. W., AHMANN, C. F. & BIBB, J. (1933). Incidence and significance of the sickle cell trait. *Ann. intern. Med.*, **7**, 769–778.

DIGGS, L. W. & BIBB, J. (1939). The erythrocyte in sickle cell anemia. Morphology, size, hemoglobin content, fragility and sedimentation rate. *J. Amer. med. Ass.*, **112**, 695–701.

DIGGS, L. W. & CHING, R. E. (1934). Pathology of sickle cell anemia. *Sth. med. J. (Bgham, Ala.)*, **27**, 839–845.

DINTENFASS, L. (1964). Rheology of packed red cells containing hemoglobins A-A, S-A, and S-S. *J. Lab. clin. Med.*, **64**, 594–600.

DIXON, E. & WINSLOW. R. M. (1981). The interaction between $(Ca^{2+} + Mg^{2+})$-ATPase and the soluble activator (calmodulin) in erythrocytes containing haemoglobin S. *Brit. J. Haemat.*, **47**, 391–401.

DÖBLER, J. & BERTLES, J. F. (1968), The physical state of hemoglobin in sickle-cell anemia erythrocytes in vivo. *J. exp. Med.*, **127**, 711–715.

DUROCHER, J. R., CONRAD, M. E. & PAYNE, R. C. (1974). Erythrocyte membrane proteins and sickle cell anemia. *Proc. Soc. exp. Biol. Med.*, **146**, 373–375.

DYKES, G., CREPEAU, R. H. & EDELSTEIN, S. J. (1978). Three dimensional reconstruction of the fibres of sickle cell haemoglobin. *Nature (Lond.)*, **272**, 506–510.

DYKES, G. W., CREPEAU, R. H. & EDELSTEIN, S. J. (1979). Three-dimensional reconstruction of the 14-filament fibers of hemoglobin S. *J. mol. Biol.*, **130**, 451–472.

EATON, J. W., BERGER, E., WHITE, J. G. & JACOB, H. S. (1978). Calcium-induced damage of haemoglobin SS and normal erythrocytes. *Brit. J. Haemat.*, **38**, 57–62.

EATON, J. W., JACOB, H. S. & WHITE, J. G. (1979). Membrane abnormalities of irreversibly sickled cells. *Seminars Hemat.*, **16**. 52–64.

EATON, J. W., SKELTON, T. D., SWOFFORD, H. S., KOLPIN, C. E. & JACOB, H. S. (1973). Elevated erythrocyte calcium in sickle cell disease. *Nature (Lond.)*, **246**, 105–106.

EATON, J. W., WHITE, J. G., JACOB, H. S. & BERGER, E. (1975). Ca^{2+} induced maintenance of sickling in Hb SS erythrocytes. *Blood*, **46**, 1051 (Abstract).

EATON, W. A., HOFRICHTER, J. & ROSS, P. D. (1976). Delay time of gelation: a possible determinant of clinical severity in sickle cell disease. *Blood*, **47**, 621–627.

EDINGTON, G. M. (1955). The pathology of sickle-cell disease in West Africa. *Trans. roy. Soc. trop. Med. Hyg.*, **49**, 253–267.

EMBURY, S. H., MICKOLS, W., KROOP, J., MAESTRE, M. F. & TINOCO, I. JNR (1985). Differential polarization imaging microscopy to detect the amount of and distribution of aligned polymer (AP) within individual sickle cells: effects of polymerization-modifying conditions and discovery of the homokentrocyte. *Blood*, **66**, No. 5 (Suppl. 1), 58a (Abstract 118).

EMMEL, V. E. (1917). A study of the erythrocytes in a case of severe anemia with elongated and sickle-shaped red blood corpuscles. *Arch. intern. Med.*, **20**, 586–598.

ERICKSON, B. N., WILLIAMS, H. H., HUMMEL, F. C., LEE, P. & MACY, I. G. (1937). The lipid and mineral distribution of the serum and erythrocytes in the hemolytic and hypochromic anemias of childhood. *J. biol. Chem.*, **118**, 569–598.

ERLANDSON, M. E., SCHULMAN, I. & SMITH, C. H. (1960). Studies on congenital hemolytic syndromes. III. Rates of destruction and production of erythrocytes in sickle cell anemia. *Pediatrics*, **25**, 629–644.

EVANS, E., MOHANDAS, N. & LEUNG, A. (1984). Static and dynamic rigidities of normal and sickle erythrocytes: major influence of cell hemoglobin concentration. *J. clin. Invest.*, **73**, 477–488.

FAIRBANKS, G., PALEK, J., DINO, J. & LIU, P. A. (1983). Protein kinase and membrane protein phosphorylation in normal and abnormal human erythrocytes: variation related to mean cell age. *Blood*, **61**, 850–857.

FINCH, J. T. (1978). Sickle-cell haemoglobin fibres. *Nature (Lond.)*, **272**, 496–497.

FINCH, J. T., PERUTZ, M. F., BERTLES, J. F. & DÖBLER, J. (1973). Structure of sickled erythrocytes and of sickle-cell hemoglobin fibers. *Proc. natn. Acad. Sci. U.S.A.*, **70**, 718–722.

FISCHER, S., NAGEL, R. L., BOOKCHIN, R. M., ROTH, E. F. JNR & TELLEZ-NAGEL, I. (1975). The binding of hemoglobin to membranes of normal and sickle erythrocytes. *Biochim. biophys. Acta*, **375**, 422–433.

GALILI, U., CLARK, M. R. & SHOHET, S. B. (1986). Excessive binding of natural anti-alpha-galactosyl immunoglobin [*sic*] G to sickle erythrocytes may contribute to extravascular cell destruction. *J. clin. Invest.*, **77**, 27–33.

GALILI, U., KORKESH, A., KAHANE, I. & RACHMILEWITZ, E. A. (1983). Demonstration of a natural anti-galactosyl IgG antibody on thalassemic red blood cells. *Blood*, **61**, 1258–1264.

GALILI, U., MANNY, N. & IZAK, G. (1981). EA rosette formation: a simple means to increase sensitivity of the antiglobulin test in patients with anti red cell antibodies. *Brit. J. Haemat.*, **47**, 227–233.

GALILI, U., RACHMILEWITZ, E. A., PELEG, A. & FLECHNER, I. (1984). A unique natural human IgG antibody with anti-α-galactosyl specificity. *J. exp. Med.*, **160**, 1519–1531.

GARRELL, R. L., CREPEAU, R. H. & EDELSTEIN, S. J. (1979). Cross-sectional views of hemoglobin S fibres by electron microscopy and computer modeling. *Proc. natn. Acad. Sci. U.S.A.*, **76**, 1140–1144.

GLADER, B. E., LUX, S. E., MULLER-SOYANO, A., PLATT, O. S., PROPPER, R. D. & NATHAN, D. G. (1978). Energy reserve and cation composition of irreversibly sickled cells. *Brit. J. Haemat.*, **40**, 527–532.

GLADER, B. E., LUX, S. E., MULLER, A., PROPPER, R. & NATHAN, D. G. (1976). Cation, water and ATP content of irreversibly sickled RBC's (ISC's) in vivo. *Clin. Res.*, **24**, 390A (Abstract).

GLADER, B. E. & MÜLLER, A. (1975). Irreversibly sickled cells (ISC's): a consequence of cellular dehydration. *Ped. Res.*, **9**, 321 (Abstract 389).

GLADER, B. E. & NATHAN, D. G. (1978). Cation permeability alterations during sickling: relationship to cation composition and cellular hydration of irreversibly sickled cells. *Blood*, **51**, 983–989.

GOPINATH, R. M. & VINCENZI, F. F. (1979). (Ca^{2+} + Mg^{2+})-ATPase activity of sickle membranes: decreased activation by red blood cell cytoplasmic activator. *Amer. J. Hemat.*, **7**, 303–312.

GORDON, E. M., KLEIN, B. L., BERMAN, B. W., STRANDJORD, S. E., SIMON, J. E. & COCCIA, P. F. (1983). The contact factors in sickle cell disease: evidence for chronic intravascular coagulation. *Blood*, **62**, No. 5 (Suppl. 1), 56a (Abstract 127).

GRAHAM, G. S. (1924). A case of sickle cell anemia with necropsy. *Arch. intern. Med.*, **34**, 778–800.

GRASSO, J. A., SULLIVAN, A. L. & SULLIVAN, L. W. (1975a). Ultrastructural studies of the bone marrow in sickle cell anaemia. I. The structure of sickled erythrocytes and reticulocytes and their phagocytic destruction. *Brit. J. Haemat.*, **31**, 135–148.

GRASSO, J. A., SULLIVAN, A. L. & SULLIVAN, L. W. (1975b). Ultrastructural studies of the bone marrow in sickle cell anaemia. II. The morphology of erythropoietic cells and their response to deoxygenation *in vitro*. *Brit. J. Haemat.*, **31**, 381–389.

GREEN, G. A., REHN, M. M. & KAIRA, V. K. (1985). Cell-bound autologous immunoglobulin in erythrocyte subpopulations from patients with sickle cell disease. *Blood*, **65**, 1127–1133.

GREEN, T. W., CONLEY, C. L. & BERTHRONG, M. (1953). The liver in sickle cell anemia. *Bull. Johns Hopk. Hosp.*, **92**, 99–127.

GREENBERG, M. S. & KASS, E. H. (1958). Studies on the destruction of red blood cells. XIII. Observations on the role of pH in the pathogenesis and treatment of painful crisis in sickle-cell disease. *Arch. intern. Med.*, **101**, 355–363.

GREENBERG, M. S., KASS, E. H. & CASTLE, W. B. (1957). Destruction of red blood cells. XII. Factors influencing the role of S hemoglobin in the pathologic physiology of sickle cell anemia and related disorders. *J. clin. Invest*, **36**, 833–843.

GRIGGS, R. C. & HARRIS, J. W. (1956). The biophysics of the variants of sickle-cell disease. *Arch. intern. Med.*, **97**, 315–326.

GULLEY, M. L., ROSS, D. W., FEO, C. & ORRINGER, E. P. (1982). The effect of cell hydration on the deformability of normal and sickle erythrocytes. *Amer. J. Hemat.*, **13**, 283–291.

GUY, R. B., GAVRILIS, P. K. & ROTHENBERG, S. P. (1973). In vitro and in vivo effect of hypotonic saline on the sickling phenomenon. *Amer. J. med. Sci.*, **266**, 267–277.

HAHN, E. V. & GILLESPIE, E. B. (1927). Sickle cell anemia. Report of a case greatly improved by splenectomy. Experimental study of sickle cell formation. *Arch. intern. Med.*, **39**, 233–254.

HAHN, J. A., MESSER, M. J. & BRADLEY, T. B. (1976). Ultrastructure of sickling and unsickling in time-lapse studies. *Brit. J. Haemat.*, **34**, 559–565.

HAM, T. H. & CASTLE, W. B. (1940). Relation of increased hypotonic fragility and of erythrostasis to the mechanism of hemolysis in certain anemias. *Trans. Ass. Amer. Phycns*, **55**, 127–131.

HAM, T. H., DUNN, R. F., SAYRE, R. W. & MURPHY, J. R. (1968). Physical properties of red cells as related to effects in vivo. I. Increased rigidity of erythrocytes as measured by viscosity of cells altered by chemical fixation, sickling and hypertonicity. *Blood*, **32**, 847–861.

HAM, T. H., SAYRE, R. W., DUNN, R. F. & MURPHY, J. R. (1968). Physical properties of red cells as related to effects in vivo. II. Effect of thermal treatment on rigidity of red cells, stroma and the sickle cell. *Blood*, **32**, 862–871.

HARRIS, J. W. (1950). Studies on the destruction of red blood cells. VIII. Molecular orientation in sickle cell hemoglobin solutions. *Proc. Soc. exp. Biol. Med.*, **75**, 197–201.

HARRIS, J. W. (1959). The role of physical and chemical factors in the sickling phenomenon. *Progr. Hemat.*, **2**, 47–109.

HARRIS, J. W. & BENSUSAN, H. B. (1975). The kinetics of the sol-gel transformation of deoxyhemoglobin S by continuous monitoring of viscosity. *J. Lab. clin. Med.*, **86**, 564–575.

HARRIS, J. W., BREWSTER, H. H., HAM, T. H. & CASTLE, W. B. (1956). Studies on the destruction of red blood cells. The biophysics and biology of sickle-cell disease. *Arch. intern. Med.*, **97**, 145–168.

HATHORN, M. (1967). Patterns of red cell destruction in sickle-cell anaemia. *Brit. J. Haemat.*, **13**, 746–751.

HAVELL, T. C., HILLMAN, D. & LESSIN, L. S. (1978). Deformability characteristics of sickle cells by microelastimetry. *Amer. J. Hemat.*, **4**, 9–16.

HEBBEL, R. P. (1985). Auto-oxidation and a membrane-associated 'Fenton reagent': a possible explanation for development of membrane lesions in sickle erythrocytes. *Clinics Haemat.*, **14**, 129–140.

HEBBEL, R. P. (1986). Erythrocyte antioxidants and membrane vulnerability. *J. Lab. clin. Med.*, **107**, 401–404.

HEBBEL, R. P., BOOGAERTS, M. A. C., EATON, J. W. & STEINBERG, M. H. (1980a). Erythrocyte adherence to endothelium and sickle-cell anemia: a possible determinant of disease severity. *New Engl. J. Med.*, **302**, 992–995.

HEBBEL, R. P., EATON, J. W., BALASINGAM, M. & STEINBERG, M. H. (1982). Spontaneous oxygen

radical generation by sickle erythrocytes. *J. clin. Invest.*, **70**, 1253–1259.

HEBBEL, R. P., EATON, J. W. & STEINBERG, (1981). Spontaneous oxygen radical generation by sickle erythrocytes. *Blood*, **58**, No. 5 (Suppl. 1), 60a (Abstract 150).

HEBBEL, R. P., EATON, J. W. & STEINBERG, M. H. (1982). Autooxidation and the membrane abnormalities of sickle RBC. *Blood*, **60**, No. 5 (Suppl. 1), 45a (Abstract 108).

HEBBEL, R. P., EATON, J. W., STEINBERG, M. H. & WHITE, J. G. (1982). Erythrocyte/endothelial interactions in the pathogenesis of sickle-cell disease: a "real logic" assessment. *Blood Cells*, **8**, 163–173.

HEBBEL, R. P. & MILLER, W. J. (1984). Phagocytosis of sickle erythrocytes: immunologic and oxidative determinants of hemolytic anemia. *Blood*, **64**, 733–741.

HEBBEL, R. P., MOLDOW, C. F. & STEINBERG, M. H. (1981). Modulation of erythrocyte endothelial interactions and the vasocclusive severity of sickling disorders. *Blood*, **58**, 947–952.

HEBBEL, R. P., SCHWARTZ, R. S. & MOHANDAS, N. (1985). The adhesive sickle erythrocyte: cause and consequence of abnormal interactions with endothelium, monocytes/macrophages and model membranes. *Clinics Haemat.*, **14**, 142–161.

HEBBEL, R. P. YAMADA, O., MOLDOW, C. F., JACOB, H. S., WHITE, J. G. & EATON, J. W. (1980b). Abnormal adherence of sickle erythrocytes to cultured vascular endothelium: possible mechanism for microvascular occlusion in sickle cell disease. *J. clin. Invest.*, **65**, 154–160.

HEBBEL, R. P., YAMADA, O., MOLDOW, C. F., WHITE, J. G. & EATON, J. W. (1978). Abnormal adherence of sickle erythrocytes. (HbS RBC) to vascular endothelium. *Blood*, **52**, No. 5 (Suppl. 1), 98 (Abstract 70).

HEIN, G. E., McCALLA, R. L. & THORNE, G. W. (1927). Sickle cell anemia. With report of a case with autopsy. *Amer. J. med. Sci.*, **173**, 763–772.

HELLERSTEIN, S. & BUNTHRARUNGROJ, T. (1974). Erythrocyte composition in sickle-cell anemia. *J. Lab. clin. Med.*, **83**, 611–624.

HOFRICHTER, J., ROSS, P. D. & EATON, W. A. (1974). Kinetics and mechanism of deoxyhemoglobin S gelation: a new approach to understanding sickle cell disease. *Proc. natn. Acad. Sci. U.S.A.*, **71**, 4864–4868.

HOFRICHTER, J., ROSS, P. D. & EATON, W. A. (1976). Supersaturation in sickle cell hemoglobin solutions. *Proc. natn. Acad. Sci. U.S.A.*, **73**, 3035–3039.

HOOVER, R., RUBIN, R., WISE, G. & WARREN, R. (1979). Adhesion of normal and sickle erythrocytes to endothelial monolayer cultures. *Blood*, **54**, 872–876.

HORNE, Mc. K. III (1981). Sickle cell anemia as a

rheologic disease. *Amer. J. Med.*, **70**, 288–297.

HOSEY, M. M. & TAO, M. (1976). Altered erythrocyte membrane phosphorylation in sickle cell disease. *Nature (Lond.)*, **263**, 424–425.

ITANO, H. A. (1953a). Human hemoglobin. *Science*, **117**, 89–94.

ITANO, H. A. (1953b). Solubilities of naturally occurring mixtures of human hemoglobin. *Arch. Biochem. Biophys.*, **47**, 148–159.

JAIN, S. K. & SHOHET, S. B. (1981). Calcium potentiates the peroxidation of erythrocyte membrane lipids. *Biochim. biophys. Acta*, **642**, 46–54.

JAIN, S. K. & SHOHET, S. B. (1984). A novel phospholipid in irreversibly sickled cells: evidence for in-vivo peroxidative membrane damage in sickle cell disease. *Blood*, **63**, 362–367.

JAMES, G. W. III & ABBOTT, L. D. JNR (1955). Erythrocyte destruction in sickle-cell anemia: simultaneous N^{15}-hemin and N^{15}-stercobilin studies. *Proc. Soc. exp. Biol. Med.*, **88**, 398–402.

JENSEN, M. & NATHAN, D. G. (1972). The relationship between the intracellular 2,3, DPG concentration and the sickling of hemoglobin S (Hb S) erythrocytes in vitro. *Blood*, **40**, 929 (Abstract).

JENSEN, M., SHOHET, S. B. & NATHAN, D. G. (1973) The role of red cell energy metabolism in the generation of irreversibly sickled cells in vitro. *Blood*, **42**, 835–842.

JENSEN, W. & LESSIN, L. (1970). Membrane alterations associated with the hemoglobinopathies. *Seminars Hemat.*, **7**, 409–426.

JENSEN, W. N. (1969). Fragmentation and the "freakish" poikilocyte. *Amer. J. med. Sci.*, **257**, 355–364.

JENSEN, W. N., BROMBERG, P. A. & BAREFIELD, K. (1969). Membrane deformation: a cause of irreversibly sickled cells (ISC). *Clin. Res.*, **17**, 464 (Abstract).

JENSEN, W. W., RUCKNAGEL, D. L. & TAYLOR, W. J. (1960). In vivo study of the sickle cell phenomenon. *J. Lab. clin. Med.*, **56**, 854–865.

KAPERONIS, A. A., BERTLES, J. F. & CHIEN, S. (1979). Variability of intracellular pH within individual populations of SS and AA erythrocytes. *Brit. J. Haemat.*, **43**, 391–400.

KAPERONIS, A. A., HANDLEY, D. A. & CHIEN, S. (1986). Fibers, crystals, and other forms of HbS polymers in deoxygenated sickle erythrocytes. *Amer. J. Hemat.*, **21**, 269–275.

KAUL, D. K., FABRY, M. E. & NAGEL, R. L. (1985). Vaso-occlusion by sickle cells: vascular tone and red cell density dependency of trapping. *Blood*, **66**, No. 5 (Suppl. 1), 60a (Abstract 128).

KAUL, D. K., FABRY, M. E., WINDISCH, P., BAEZ, S. & NAGEL, R. L. (1983). Erythrocytes in sickle cell anemia are heterogeneous in their rheological and hemodynamic characteristics. *J. clin. Invest.*, **72**, 22–31.

KENNY, M. W., MEAKIN, M. & STUART, J. (1981). Measurement of erythrocyte filterability using washed-erythrocyte and whole-blood methods. *Clin. Hemorheol.*, **1**, 135–146.

KENNY, M. W., MEAKIN, M., WORTHINGTON, D. J. & STUART, J. (1981). Erythrocyte deformability in sickle cell crisis. *Brit. J. Haemat.*, **49**, 103–109.

KIMMELSTIEL, P. (1948). Vascular occlusion and ischemic infarction in sickle cell disease. *Amer. J. med. Sci.*, **216**, 11–19.

KLIPSTEIN, F. A. & RANNEY, H. M. (1960). Electrophoretic components of the hemoglobin of red cell membranes. *J. clin. Invest.*, **39**, 1894–1899.

KLUG, P. P., KAYE, N. & JENSEN, W. N. (1982). Endothelial cell and vascular damage in the sickle cell disorders. *Blood Cells*, **8**, 175–184.

KLUG, P. P. & LESSIN, L. S. (1977). Microvascular blood flow of sickled erythrocyte: a dynamic morphologic study. *Blood Cells*, **3**, 263–272.

KLUG, P. P., LESSIN, L. S. & RADICE, P. (1974). Rheological aspects of sickle cell disease. *Arch. intern. Med.*, **133**, 577–590.

KONOTEY-AHULU, F. I. D., GALLO, E., LEHMANN, H. & RINGELHANN, B. (1968). Haemoglobin Korle-Bu (β73 aspartic acid → asparagine) showing one of the two amino acid substitutions. *J. med. Genet.*, **5**, 107–111.

KRAUS, L. M. MIYAJI, T., IUCHI, I. & KRAUS, A. P. (1966). Characterization of $\alpha^{23 \ \text{Glu NH}_2}$ in hemoglobin Memphis. Hemoglobin Memphis/S, a new variant of molecular disease. *Biochemistry*, **5**, 3701–3708.

LACELLE, P. L. (1977). Oxygen delivery to muscle cells during capillary occlusion by sickled erythrocytes. *Blood Cells*, **3**, 273–281.

LACHANT, N. A., DAVIDSON, W. D. & TANAKA, K. R. (1983). Impaired pentose phosphate shunt function in sickle cell disease: a potential mechanism for increased Heinz body formation and membrane lipid peroxidation. *Amer. J. Hemat.*, **15**, 1–13.

LAM, Y.-F., LIN, A. K.-L. C. & HO, C. (1979). A phosphorus-31 nuclear magnetic resonance investigation of intracellular environment of human normal and sickle cell blood. *Blood*, **54**, 196–209.

LANE, T. A., BALLAS, S. K. & BURKA, E. R. (1976). Lipid synthesis in human erythroid cells: the effect of sickling. *Blood*, **47**, 189–195.

LANGE, R. D., MINNICH, V. & MOORE, C. V. (1950). In vitro differences in behavior of sickle cell anemia and trait erythrocytes produced by variation in O_2 tension and pH. *J. Lab. clin. Med.*, **36**, 848 (Abstract).

LANGE, R. D., MINNICH, V. & MOORE C. V. (1951). Effect of oxygen tension and of pH on the sickling and mechanical fragility of erythroytes from patients with sickle cell anemia and the sickle cell trait. *J. Lab. clin. Med.*, **37**, 789–802.

LESSIN, L. S., JENSEN, W. N. & KLUG, P. (1972). Ultrastructure of the normal and hemoglobinopathic red blood cell membrane. Freeze-etching and stereoscan electron microscopic studies. *Arch. intern. Med.*, **129**, 306–332.

LESSIN, L. S. & WALLAS, C. (1973). Biochemical basis for membrane alterations in irreversibly sickled cells (ISC). *Blood*, **42**, 978 (Abstract 6).

LEWIS, S. M., SZUR, L. & DACIE, J. V. (1960). The pattern of erythrocyte destruction in haemolytic anaemia, as studied by radioactive chromium. *Brit. J. Haemat.*, **6**, 122–139.

LIN, C. Y., MORETTI, R., ADDIEGO, J., VICHINSKY, E., CHIU, D. & LUBIN, B. (1983). A vasoactive factor (VAF) may be a major determinant of vaso-occlusive crisis (VOC) in sickle cell disease (SCD). *Blood*, **62**, No. 5 (Suppl. 1), 57a (Abstract 129).

LIPOWSKY, H. H., USAMI, S. & CHIEN, S. (1982). Human SS red cell rheological behavior in the microcirculation of cremaster muscle. *Blood Cells*, **8**, 113–126.

LITOSCH, I. & LEE, K. S. (1980). Sickle red cell calcium metabolism: studies on Ca^{2+}-Mg^{2+} ATPase and Ca-binding properties of sickle red cell membranes. *Amer. J. Hemat.*, **8**, 377–397.

LIU, S. C., ZHAI, S. & PALEK, J. (1984). Free hemin pool in the cytosol of sickle erythrocytes. *Blood*, **64**, No. 5 (Suppl. 1), 50a (Abstract 112).

LONDON, I. M., SHEMIN, D., WEST, R. & RITTEMBERG, D. (1949). Heme synthesis and red blood cell dynamics in normal humans and in subjects with polycythemia vera, sickle-cell anemia, and pernicious anemia. *J. biol. Chem.*, **169**, 463–484.

LUBIN, B., CHIU, D., BASTACKY, J., ROELOFSEN, B. & VAN DEENEN, L. L. M. (1981a). Abnormalities in membrane phospholipid organization in sickled erythrocytes. *J. clin. Invest.*, **67**, 1643–1649.

LUBIN, B., CHIU, D., ROELOFSEN, B. & VAN DEENEN, L. L. M. (1981b). Abnormal membrane phospholipid asymmetry in sickle erythrocytes and its pathophysiologic significance. In: *Erythrocyte Membranes 2: Recent Clinical and Experimental Advances*, pp. 171–187. Alan R. Liss, New York.

LUCAS, G. S., CALDWELL, N. M. & STUART, J. (1985). Fluctuating deformity of oxygenated sickle erythrocytes in the asymptomatic state and in painful crisis. *Brit. J. Haemat.*, **59**, 363–368.

LUTHRA, M. G. & SEARS, D. A. (1982). Increased Ca^{++}, Mg^{++}, and $Na^+ + K^+$ ATPase activities in erythrocytes of sickle cell anemia. *Blood*, **60**, 1332–1336.

LUX, S. E. & JOHN, K. M. (1975). The membrane defect in irreversibly sickled red cells (ISCs). Irreversible deformation of the spectrin-actin lattice. *Blood*, **46**, 1051 (Abstract 154).

LUX, S. E., JOHN, K. M. & KARNOVSKY, M. J. (1976). Irreversible deformation of the spectrin-actin lattice in irreversibly sickled cells. *J. clin. Invest.*, **58**, 955–963.

McCoy, R. C. (1969). Ultrastructural alterations in the kidney of patients with sickle cell disease and the nephrotic syndrome. *Lab. Invest.*, **21**, 85–95.

McCURDY, P. R. (1969). ^{32}DFP and ^{51}Cr for measurement of red cell life span in abnormal hemoglobin syndromes. *Blood*, **33**, 214–224.

McCURDY, P. R., MAHMOUD, L. & SHERMAN, A. S. (1975). Red cell life span in sickle cell-hemoglobin C disease with a note about sickle cell-hemoglobin O_{ARAB}. *Blood*, **45**, 273–279.

McCURDY, P. R. & SHERMAN, A. S. (1978). Irreversibly sickled cells and red cell survival in sickle cell anemia. A study with both $DF^{32}P$ and ^{51}Cr. *Amer. J. Med.*, **64**, 253–258.

McKELLAR, M. & DACIE, J. V. (1958). Thromboplastic activity of the plasma in paroxysmal nocturnal haemoglobinuria. *Brit. J. Haemat.*, **4**, 404–415.

MAGDOFF-FAIRCHILD, B. & CHIU, C. C. (1979). X-ray diffraction studies of fibers and crystals of deoxygenated sickle cell hemoglobin. *Proc. natn. Acad. Sci. U.S.A.*, **76**, 223–226.

MAGDOFF-FAIRCHILD, B. M., POILLON, W. N., LI, TING-I & BERTLES, J. F. (1976). Thermodynamic studies of polymerization of deoxygenated sickle cell hemoglobin. *Proc. natn. Acad. Sci. U.S.A.*, **73**, 990–994.

MAGDOFF-FAIRCHILD, B. SWERDLOW, P. H. & BERTLES, J. F. (1972). Intermolecular organization of deoxygenated sickle haemoglobin determined by X-ray diffraction. *Nature (Lond.)*, **239**, 217–219.

MALAMOS, B., BELCHER, E. H., GYFTAKI, E. & BINOPOULOS, D. (1963). Simultaneous radioactive tracer studies of erythropoiesis and red-cell destruction in sickle-cell disease and sickle-cell haemoglobin/thalassaemia. *Brit. J. Haemat.*, **9**, 487–498.

MASYS, D. R., BROMBERG, P. A. & BALCERZAK, S. P. (1974). Red cells shrink during sickling. *Blood*, **44**, 885–889.

MAUGH, T. H. II (1981). A new understanding of sickle cell emerges. *Science*, **211**, 265–267.

MESSER, M. J. & HARRIS, J. W. (1970). Filtration characteristics of sickle cells: rates of alteration of filterability after deoxygenation and reoxygenation, and correlations with sickling and unsickling. *J. Lab. clin. Med.*, **76**, 537–547.

MILLER W. J. & HEBBEL. R. P. (1981). Macrophage/erythrocyte interactions and the anemia of sickle disease. *Clin. Res.*, **29**, 341a (Abstract).

MINTON, A. P. (1973). Models for the gelling behavior of binary mixtures of hemoglobin variants. *J. mol. Biol.*, **75**, 559–574.

MIZUKAMI, H., BARTNICKI, D. E., BURKE, S., BREWER, G. J. & MIZUKAMI, I. F. (1986). The effect of erythrocyte membrane on the birefringence formation of sickle cell hemoglobin. *Amer. J. Hemat.*, **21**, 233–241.

MOFFAT, K. (1974). Gelation of sickle cell hemoglobin: effects of hybrid tetramer formation in hemoglobin mixtures. *Science*, **185**, 274–277.

MOHANDAS, N. & EVANS, E. (1983). Increased adherence of sickle cells to endothelium: influence of both cellular and plasma factors. *Blood*, **62**, No. 5 (Suppl. 1), 58a (Abstract 133).

MOHANDAS, N. & EVANS, E. (1984). Adherence of sickle red cells to vascular endothelial cells: morphologic correlates and requirement for calcium and collagen-binding plasma proteins. *Blood*, **64**, No. 5 (Suppl. 1), 51a (Abstract 114).

MOHANDAS, N., EVANS, E. & KUKAN, B. (1984). Adherence of sickle erythrocytes to vascular endothelial cells: requirement for both cell membrane changes and plasma factors. *Blood*, **64**, 282–287.

MOHANDAS, N., EVANS, E., KUKAN, B. & LEUNG, A. (1985). Sickle erythrocyte adherence to vascular endothelium. Morphologic correlates and the requirement for divalent cations and collagen-binding plasma proteins. *J. clin. Invest.*, **76**, 1605–1612.

MOHANDAS, N., ROSSI, M. E. & CLARK, M. R. (1986). Association between morphologic distortion of sickle cells and deoxygenation-induced cation permeability increase. *Blood*, **68**, 450–454.

MURAYAMA, M. (1964). A molecular mechanism of sickled erythrocyte formation. *Nature (Lond.)*, **202**, 258–260.

MURAYAMA, M. (1965). Orientation of sickled erythrocytes in a magnetic field. *Nature (Lond.)*, **206**, 420–422.

MURAYAMA, M. (1966). Molecular mechanism of red cell "sickling". *Science*, **153**, 145–149.

MURAYAMA, M. (1967). Structure of sickle cell hemoglobin and molecular mechanism of the sickling phenomenon. *Clin. Chem.*, **14**, 578–588.

MURAYAMA, M., OLSON, R. A. & JENNINGS, W. H. (1965). Molecular orientation in horse hemoglobin crystals and sickled erythrocytes. *Biochim. biophys. Acta*, **94**, 194–199.

MURPHY, J. R., WENGARD, M. & BRERETON, W. (1976). Rheological studies of Hb SS blood: influence of hematocrit, hypertonicity, separation of cells, deoxygenation, and mixture with normal cells. *J. Lab. clin. Med.*, **87**, 475–486.

MURPHY, R. C. JNR & SHAPIRO, S. (1944). Sickle cell disease. I. Observations on behavior of erythrocytes in sickle cell disease. *Arch. intern. Med.*, **64**, 28–35.

MURPHY, R. C. JNR & SHAPIRO, S. (1945). The pathology of sickle cell disease. *Ann. intern. Med.*, **23**, 376–397.

NAGEL, R. L. & BOOKCHIN, R. M. (1974). The effect of 2,3 diphosphoglycerate on gelation of hemoglobin S and its molecular mechanism. *Clin. Res.*, **22**, 399A (Abstract).

NAGEL, R. L. & FABRY, M. E. (1985). The many pathophysiologies of sickle cell anemia. *Amer. J. Hemat.*, **20**, 195–199.

NAIR, C. R., MCCULLOUGH, M. S. & DAS, S. K.

(1977). Red cell membrane peroxidation and superoxide dismutase (EC.1.15.1.1) in sickle cell anemia. *Fed. Proc.*, **36**, 1067 (Abstract).

NASH, G. B., JOHNSON, C. S. & MEISELMAN, H. J. (1984). Mechanical properties of oxygenated red blood cells in sickle cell (HbSS) disease. *Blood*, **63**, 73–82.

NATTA, C., CREQUE, L. & NAVARRO, C. (1985). Compartmentalization of iron in sickle cell anemia — an autopsy study. *Amer. J. clin. Path.*, **83**, 76–77.

NATTA, C. L. & KREMZNER, L. T. (1982). Polyamines and membrane proteins in sickle cell disease. *Blood Cells*, **8**, 273–280.

NISHIO, I., TANAK, T., SUN, S.-T., IMANISHI, Y. & OHNISHI, S. T. (1983). Hemoglobin aggregation in single red blood cells of sickle cell anemia. *Science*, **220**, 1173–1175.

NOGUCHI, C. T. & SCHECHTER, A. N. (1981). The intracellular polymerization of sickle hemoglobin and its relevance to sickle cell disease. *Blood*, **58**, 1057–1068 (Review).

NOGUCHI, C. T., TORCHIA, D. A. & SCHECHTER, A. N. (1980). Determination of deoxyhemoglobin S polymer in sickle erythrocytes upon deoxygenation. *Proc. natn. Acad. Sci. U.S.A.*, **77**, 5487–5491.

NOGUCHI, C. T., TORCHIA, D. A. & SCHECHTER, A. N. (1982). Determination of sickle hemoglobin polymer in SS and AS erythrocytes. *Blood Cells*, **8**, 225–235.

O'BRIEN, R. T. (1978). Iron burden in sickle cell anemia. *J. Pediat.*, **92**, 579–582.

OHTSUKI, M., WHITE, S. L. ZEITLER, E., WELLEMS, T. E., FULLER, S. D., ZWICK, M., MACKINEN, M. W. & SIGLER, P. B. (1977). Electron microscopy of fibers and discs of hemoglobin S having sixfold symmetry. *Proc. natn. Acad. Sci. U.S.A.*, **74**, 5538–5542.

ORTIZ, O. E., LEW, V. L. & BOOKCHIN, R. M. (1986). Calcium accumulated by sickle cell anemia red cells does not affect their potassium ($^{86}Rb^+$) flux components. *Blood*, **67**, 710–715.

PADILLA, F., BROMBERG, P. A. & JENSEN, W. N. (1973). The sickle-unsickle cycle: a cause of cell fragmentation leading to permanently deformed cells. *Blood*, **41**, 653–660.

PALEK, J. (1973). Calcium accumulation during sickling of hemoglobin S (Hb SS) red cells. *Blood*, **42**, 988 (Abstract).

PALEK, J. (1977). Red cell membrane injury in sickle cell anaemia. *Brit. J. Haemat.*, **35**, 1–9 (Annotation).

PALEK, J. & LIU, S.-C. (1979). Dependence of spectrin organization in red blood cell membranes on cell metabolism: implications for control of red cell shape, deformability, and surface area. *Seminars Hemat.*, **16**, 75–93.

PALEK, J., THOMAE, M. & OZOG, D. (1977). Red cell calcium content and transmembrane calcium movements in sickle cell anemia. *J. Lab. clin. Med.*, **89**, 1365–1374.

PARFREY, N. A., MOORE, G. W. & HUTCHINS, G. M. (1985). Is pain crisis a cause of death in sickle cell disease? *Amer. J. clin. Path.*, **84**, 209–212.

PAULING, L., ITANO, H. A., SINGER, S. J. & WELLS, I. C. (1949). Sickle cell anemia, a molecular disease. *Science*, **110**, 543–548.

PEARSON, H. A. (1963). The binding of chromium^{51} to hemoglobin. I. In vitro studies. *Blood*, **22**, 218–230.

PERILLIE, P. E. & EPSTEIN, F. H. (1963). Sickling phenomenon produced by hypertonic solutions: a possible explanation for the hyposthenuria of sicklemia. *J. clin. Invest.*, **42**, 570–580.

PERUTZ, M. F., LIQUORI, A. M. & EIRICH, F. (1951). X-ray and solubility studies of the haemoglobin of sickle-cell anaemia patients. *Nature (Lond.)*, **167**, 929–931.

PERUTZ, M. F. & MITCHISON, J. M. (1950). State of haemoglobin in sickle-cell anaemia. *Nature (Lond.)*, **166**, 677–679.

PETZ, L. D., YAM, P., WILKINSON, L., GARRATTY, G., LUBIN, B. & MENTZER, W. (1984). Increased IgG molecules bound to the surface of red blood cells of patients with sickle cell anemia. *Blood*, **64**, 301–304.

PITCOCK, J. A., MUIRHEAD, E. E., HATCH, F. E., JOHNSON, J. G. KELLY, B. J. (1970). Early renal changes in sickle cell anemia. *Arch. Path.*, **90**, 403–410.

PLATT, O. S. (1982). Exercise-induced hemolysis in sickle cell anemia: shear sensitivity and erythrocyte dehydration. *Blood*, **59**, 1055–1060.

PLATT, O. S., FALCONE, J. F. & LUX, S. E. (1983). Abnormal spectrin-ankyrin interaction in hemoglobinopathies. *Blood*, **62**, No. 5 (Suppl. 1), 59a (Abstract 140).

PLATT, O. S., FALCONE, J. F. & LUX, S. E. (1985). Molecular defect in the sickle erythrocyte skeleton. Abnormal spectrin binding to sickle inside-out vesicles. *J. clin. Invest.*, **75**, 266–271.

PONDER, E. (1945). The sickling phenomenon and its bearing on the problem of red cell structure. *J. exp. Biol.*, **21**, 77–83.

PONDER, E. (1948). *Hemolysis and Related Phenomena*, pp. 145–153. Churchill, London, and Grune and Stratton, New York.

PONDER, E. (1958). Globules rouges normaux paracristallins et falciformes. *Rev. Hémat.*, **13**, 129–131 (Editorial).

PRANKERD, T. A. J. (1955). The uptake of radioactive phosphate and its distribution amongst esters in sickled cells. *Clin. Sci*, **14**, 381–386.

RAMPLING, M. W. (1975). Observations on the effect of CO_2 and temperature on the sickling phenomenon. *Europ. J. clin. Invest.*, **5**, 385–389.

RAMPLING, M. W. & SIRS, J. A. (1973). The rate of sickling of cells containing sickle-cell haemoglobin.

Clin. Sci. mol. Med., **45**, 655–664.

RANK, B. H., CARLSSON, J. & HEBBEL, R. P. (1985). Abnormal redox status of membrane-protein thiols in sickle erythrocytes. *J. clin. Invest.*, **75**, 1531–1537.

RANK, B., HEBBEL, R. P., JACOB, H. S. & CARLSSON, J. (1983). Abnormal redox status of RBC membrane protein thiols in sickle disease. *Blood*, **62**, No. 5 (Suppl. 1), 60a (Abstract 141).

REBUCK, J. W., STURROCK, R. M. & MONAGHAN, E. A. (1950). Sickling processes in anemia and trait erythrocytes with the electron microscopy of their incipient crystallization. *Fed. Proc.*, **9**, 340 (Abstract).

REBUCK, J. W., STURROCK, R. M. & MONTO, R. W. (1955). Sequential electron micrography of sickling. *Lab. Invest.*, **4**, 175–189.

RICH, A. R. (1928). The splenic lesion in sickle cell anemia. *Bull. Johns Hopk. Hosp.*, **43**, 398–399.

RIEBER, E. E., VELIZ, G. & POLLACK, S. (1977). Red cells in sickle cell crisis: observations on the pathophysiology of crisis. *Blood*, **49**, 967–979.

RIGGS, M. G. & INGRAM, V. M. (1975). Differences in erythrocyte membrane proteins and glycoproteins in sickle cell disease. *Biochem. biophys. Res. Commun.*, **74**, 191–198.

RODGERS, G. P., BONNER, R. F., NOGUCHI, C. T., NIENHUIS, A. W. & SCHECHTER, A. N. (1983). Evidence for abnormal peripheral vasomotor activity in patients with sickle cell disease. *Blood*, **62**, No. 5 (Suppl. 1), 60a (Abstract 143).

RODGERS, G. P., NOGUCHI, C. T. & SCHECHTER, A. N. (1984). A quantitative reappraisal of the "irreversible" sickled erythrocyte in sickle cell anemia. *Blood*, **64**. No. 5 (Suppl. 1), 52a (Abstract 119).

RODGERS, G. P., NOGUCHI, C. T. & SCHECHTER. A. N. (1985). Irreversibly sickled erythrocytes in sickle cell anemia: a quantitative reappraisal. *Amer. J. Hemat.*, **20**, 17–23.

RODGERS, G. P., SCHECHTER, A. N., NOGUCHI, C. T., KLEIN, H. G., NIENHUIS, A. W. & BONNER, R. F. (1984). Periodic microcirculatory flow in patients with sickle-cell disease. *New Engl. J. Med.*, **311**, 1534–1538.

ROSENBLATE, H. J., EISENSTEIN, R. & HOLMES. A. W. (1970). The liver in sickle cell anemia. A clinical-pathologic study. *Arch. Path.*, **90**, 235–245.

ROSSI, M. E., MOHANDAS, N. & CLARK, M. R. (1984). Is the cation leak of sickled cells caused by overstretching of the membrane? *Blood*, **64**, No. 5 (Suppl. 1), 52a (Abstract 120).

ROTH, E. F. JNR, NAGEL, R. L. & BOOKCHIN, R. M. (1981). pH dependency of potassium efflux from sickled red cells. *Amer. J. Hemat.*, **11**, 19–27.

RUBENSTEIN, E. (1961). Studies on the relationship of temperature to sickle cell anemia. *Amer. J. Med.*, **30**, 95–98.

SCHACTER, L. P., DELVILLANO, B. C., GORDON,

E. M. & KLEIN, B. L. (1985). Red cell superoxide dismutase and sickle cell anemia symptom severity. *Amer. J. Hemat.*, **19**, 137–144.

SCHMID-SCHÖNBEIN, H. (1982). Continuous viscous deformation of red blood cells in flow and their disturbance in sickle cell disease. *Blood Cells*, **8**, 29–51.

SCHMID-SCHÖNBEIN, H. & HEIDTMANN, H. (1982). Non-specific rheological abnormalities in sickle cell disease. *Blood Cells*, **8**, 89–101.

SCHNEIDER, R. G., TAKEDA, I., GUSTAVSON, L. P. & ALPERIN, J. B. (1972). Intraerythrocytic precipitations of haemoglobins S and C. *Nature new Biol.*, **235**, 88–90.

SCHRIER, S. L., BENSCH, K., JUNGA, I. & JOHNSON, M. (1975). Endocytosis and calcium (Ca) movements in sickle ghosts. *Clin. Res.*, **23**, 406A (Abstract).

SCHWARTZ, R. S., DÜZGÜNS, N., CHIU, D.T.-Y. & LUBIN, B. (1983a). Interaction of phosphatidylserine-phosphatidylcholine liposomes with sickle erythrocytes: evidence for altered membrane surface propeties. *J. clin. Invest*, **71**, 1570–1580.

SCHWARTZ, R. S., SCHROIT, A. J., TANAKA, Y., CHIU, D. & LUBIN, B. (1983b). Increased adherence of sickle erythrocytes to human peripheral monocytes is correlated with an increased content of outer leaflet aminophospholipids. *Blood*, **62**, No. 5 (Suppl. 1), 61a (Abstract 145).

SCHWARTZ, R. S., TANAKA, Y., FIDLER, I. J., CHIU, D. T.-Y., LUBIN, B. & SCHROIT, A. J. (1985). Increased adherence of sickled and phosphatidylserine-enriched human erythrocytes to cultured human peripheral blood monocytes. *J. clin. Invest.*, **75**, 1965–1972.

SCRIVER, J. B. & WAUGH, T. R. (1930). Studies on a case of sickle-cell anaemia. *Canad. med. Ass. J.*, **23**, 375–380.

SEARS, D. A. & LUTHRA, M. G. (1983). Membrane bound hemoglobin in the erythrocytes of sickle cell anemia. *J. Lab. clin. Med.*, **102**, 694–698.

SELF, F., McINTIRE, L. V. & ZANGER, B. (1977). Rheological evaluation of hemoglobin S and hemoglobin C hemoglobinopathies. *J. Lab. clin. Med.*, **89**, 488–497.

SERJEANT, G. R. (1970). Irreversibly sickled cells and splenomegaly in sickle-cell anaemia. *Brit. J. Haemat.*, **19**, 635–641.

SERJEANT, G. R. (1985). *Sickle Cell Disease.* 478 pp. Oxford University Press.

SERJEANT, G. R., PETCH, M. C. & SERJEANT, B. E. (1973). The in vivo sickle phenomenon: a reappraisal. *J. Lab. clin. Med.*, **81**, 850–856.

SERJEANT, G. R., SERJEANT, B. E., DESAI, P., MASON, K. P., SEWELL, A. & ENGLAND, J. M. (1978). The determinants of irreversibly sickled cells in homozygous sickle cell disease. *Brit. J. Haemat.*, **40**, 431–438.

SERJEANT, G. R., SERJEANT, B. E. & MILNER, P. F.

(1969). The irreversibly sickled cell: a determinant of haemolysis in sickle cell anemia. *Brit. J. Haemat.*, **17**, 527–533.

SHAKLAI, N., SHARMA, V. S. & RANNEY, H. M. (1981). Interaction of sickle cell hemoglobin with erythrocyte membranes. *Proc. natn. Acad. Sci. U.S.A.*, **78**, 65–68.

SHEN, S. C., CASTLE, W. B. & FLEMING, E. M. (1944). Experimental and clinical observations on increased mechanical fragility of erythrocytes. *Science*, **100**, 387–389.

SHEN, S. C., FLEMING, E. M. & CASTLE, W. B. (1949). Studies on the destruction of red blood cells. V. Irreversibly sickled erythrocytes: their experimental production in vitro. *Blood*, **4**, 498–504.

SHERMAN, I. T. (1940). The sickling phenomenon, with special reference to the differentiation of sickle cell anemia from the sickle cell trait. *Bull. Johns Hopk. Hosp.*, **67**, 309–324.

SHUNG, K. K., LEE, M. Y., REID, J. M. & FINCH, C. A. (1979). Effects of oxygen tension and pH on the ultrasonic absorption properties of sickle cells. *Blood*, **54**, 451–458.

SINGER, K. (1951). The pathogenesis of sickle cell anemia. A review. *Amer. J. clin. Path.*, **21**, 858–865.

SINGER, K. & CHERNOFF, A. I. (1952). Studies on abnormal hemoglobins. III. The interrelationship of type S (sickle cell) hemoglobin and type F (alkali resistant) hemoglobin in sickle cell anemia. *Blood*, **7**, 47–52.

SINGER, K. & FISHER, B. (1952). Studies on abnormal hemoglobins. V. The distribution of type S (sickle cell) hemoglobin and type F (alkali resistant) hemoglobin within the red cell population in sickle cell anemia. *Blood*, **7**. 1216–1226.

SINGER, K., ROBIN, S., KING, J. C. & JEFFERSON, R. N. (1948). The life span of the sickle cell and the pathogenesis of sickle cell anemia. *J. Lab. clin. Med.*, **33**, 975–984.

SINGER, K. & SINGER, L. (1953). Studies on abnormal hemoglobins. VIII. The gelling phenomenon of sickle cell hemoglobin: its biologic and diagnostic significance. *Blood*, **8**, 1008–1023.

SMITH, B. D. & LaCELLE, P. L. (1981). Erythrocyte-endothelial cell interactions in sickle cell anemia and diabetes mellitus. *Blood*, **58**, No. 5 (Suppl. 1), 64a (Abstract 166).

SMITH, C. M. II, KUETTNER, J. F., TUKEY, D. P., BURRIS, S. M. & WHITE, J. G. (1981). Variable deformability of irreversibly sickled erythrocytes. *Blood*, **58**, 71–77.

SMITH, J. E., MOHANDAS, N., CLARK, M. R., GREENQUIST, A. C. & SHOHET, S. B. (1980). Deformability and spectrin properties in three types of elongated red cells. *Amer. J. Hemat.* **8**, 1–13.

SONG, Y. S. (1955). Cirrhosis of the liver in sickle cell disease. Report of a case with a review of the literature. *Arch. Path.*, **60**, 235–239.

SONG, Y. S. (1957). Hepatic lesions in sickle cell anemia. *Amer. J. Path.*, **33**, 331–351.

SPECTOR, D., ZACHARY, J. B., STERIOFF, S. & MILLAN, J. (1978). Painful crises following renal transplantation in sickle cell anemia. *Amer. J. Med.*, **64**, 835–839.

SPRAGUE, C. C. & PATERSON, J. C. S. (1958). Role of the spleen and effect of splenectomy in sickle cell disease. *Blood*, **13**, 569–581.

STATIUS, VAN EPS, L. W., SCHOUTEN, H., SLOOFF, P. A. M. & VAN DELDEN, G. J. A. (1971). Sodium, potassium and calcium in erythrocytes in sickle-cell anemia. *Clin. chim. Acta*, **33**, 475–478.

STEINBERG, M. H., DREILING, B. J. & LOVELL, W. J. (1977). Sickle cell anemia: erythrokinetics, blood volumes, and a study of possible determinants of severity. *Amer. J. Hemat.*, **2**, 17–23.

STEINBERG, M. H., EATON, J. W., BERGER, E., COLEMAN, M. B. & OELSHLEGEL, F. J. (1978). Erythrocyte calcium abnormalities and the clinical severity of sickling disorders. *Brit. J. Haemat.*, **40**, 533–539.

STETSON, C. A. JNR (1966). The state of hemoglobin in sickled erythrocytes. *J. exp. Med.*, **123**, 341–346.

STOCKMAN, J. A., NIGRO, M. A., MISHKIN, M. M. & OSKI, F. A. (1972). Occlusion of large cerebral vessels in sickle cell anemia. *New Engl. J. Med.*, **287**, 846–849.

STUART, M. J. & SILLS, R. H. (1981). Deficiency of plasma prostacyclin or PGI_2 regenerating ability in sickle cell anaemia. *Brit. J. Haemat.*, **48**, 545–550.

SYDENSTRICKER, V. P. (1924). Further observations on sickle cell anemia. *J. Amer. med. Ass.*, **83**, 12–17.

SYDENSTRICKER, V. P., MULHERIN, W. A. & HOUSEAL, B. W. (1923). Sickle cell anemia: report of two cases in children, with necropsy in one case. *Amer. J. Dis. Child.*, **26**, 132–154.

THOMAS, A. N., PATTISON, C. & SERJEANT, G. R. (1982). Causes of death in sickle-cell disease in Jamaica. *Brit. med. J.*, **285**, 633–635.

TOMLINSON, W. J. (1945). A study of the circulation of the spleen in sicklemia and sickle cell anemia. *Amer. J. Path.*, **21**, 877–887.

TOSTESON, D. C. (1955). The effects of sickling on ion transport. II. The effect of sickling on sodium and cesium transport. *J. gen. Physiol.*, **39**, 55–67.

TOSTESON, D. C., CARLSEN, E. & DUNHAM, E. T. (1955). The effects of sickling on ion transport. I. Effect of sickling on potassium transport. *J. Gen. Physiol.*, **39**, 31–53.

TOSTESON, D. C., SHEA, E. & DARLING, R. C. (1952). Potassium and sodium of red blood cells in sickle cell anemia. *J. clin. Invest*, **31**, 406–411.

UEDA, Y. & BOOKCHIN, R. M. (1984). Effects of carbon dioxide and pH variations in vitro on blood respiratory functions, red blood cell volume, transmembrane pH gradients, and sickling in sickle cell anemia. *J. Lab. clin. Med.*, **104**, 146–159.

USAMI, S., CHIEN, S. & BERTLES, J. F. (1975). Deformability of sickle cells as studied by microsieving. *J. Lab. clin. Med.*, **86**, 274–279.

USAMI, S., CHIEN, S., SCHOLTZ, P. M. & BERTLES, J. F. (1975). Effect of deoxygenation on blood rheology in sickle cell disease. *Microvasc. Res.*, **9**, 324–334.

VANDEPITTE, J. M. & LOUIS, L. A. (1953). A new method for the differentiation of sickle-cell anaemia from the sickle-cell trait. *Lancet*, **ii**, 806–810.

VELLA, F. (1975). Mechanical stability of human haemoglobins. *Acta haemat. (Basel)*, **54**, 257–260.

WAGNER, G. M., SCHWARTZ, R. S., CHIU, D. T.-Y. & LUBIN, B. H. (1985). Membrane phospholipid organization and vesiculation of erthrocytes in sickle cell anaemia. *Clinics Haemat.*, **14**, 183–200.

WALKER, B. R., ALEXANDER, F., BIRDSALL, T. R. & WARREN, R. L. (1971). Glomerular lesions in sickle cell nephropathy. *J. Amer. med. Ass.*, **215**, 437–440.

WALTERS, J. H. (1958). Vascular occlusion in sickle-cell disease. *Proc. roy. Soc. Med.*, **51**, 646–648.

WATSON, J. (1948). A study of sickling of young erythrocytes in sickle cell anemia. *Blood*, **3**, 465–469.

WATSON, R. D. LICHTMAN, H. C. & SHAPIRO, H. D. (1956). Splenomegaly in sickle cell anemia. *Amer. J. Med.*, **20**, 196–206.

WAUTIER, J. L., GALACTEROS, F., WAUTIER, M. P., PINTIGNY, D. BEUZARD, Y., ROSA, J. & CAEN, J. P. (1985). Clinical manifestations and erythrocyte adhesion to endothelium in sickle cell syndrome. *Amer. J. Hemat.*, **19**, 121–130.

WAUTIER, J.-L., PINTIGNY, D., MACLOUF, J., WAUTIER, M.-P., CORVAZIER, E. & CAEN, J. (1986). Release of prostacyclin after erythrocyte adhesion to cultured vascular endothelium. *J. Lab. clin. Med.*, **107**, 210–215.

WAUTIER, J. L., PINTIGNY, D., WAUTIER, M. P., PATON, R. C., GALACTEROS, F., PASSA, P. & CAEN, J. P. (1983a). Fibrinogen, a modulator of erythrocyte adhesion to vascular endothelium. *J. Lab. clin. Med.*, **101**, 911–920.

WAUTIER, J. L., WAUTIER, M. P., PINTIGNY, F., GALACTEROS, F., COURILLON, A., PASSA, P. & CAEN, J. P. (1983b). Factors involved in cell adhesion to vascular endothelium. *Blood Cells*, **9**, 221–234.

WEED, R. I. & BESSIS, M. (1975). Measurement of ATP content in single erythrocytes: low levels in irreversible sickle cells. *Clin. Res.*, **23**, 442A (Abstract).

WEINBERG, A. G. & CURRARINO, G. (1972). Sickle cell dactylitis: histopathologic observations. *Amer. J. clin. Path.*, **58**, 518–523.

WEINSTEIN, I. M., SPURLING, C. L., KLEIN, H. & NECHELES, T. F. (1954). Radioactive sodium chromate for the study of survival of red blood cells. III. The abnormal hemoglobin syndromes. *Blood*, **9**, 1155–1164.

WEISMAN, R. JNR, HURLEY, T. H., HARRIS, J. W. & HAM, T. H. (1953). Studies of the function of the spleen in the hemolysis of red cells in hereditary spherocytosis and sickle cell disorders. *J. Lab. clin. Med.*, **42**, 965–966 (Abstract).

WENGER, G. D. & BALCERZAK, S. P. (1984). Viscometric and spectrophotometric measurements of hemoglobin S polymerization kinetics. *Blood*, **63**, 897–903.

WERTHAM, F., MITCHELL, N. & ANGRIST, A. (1942). The brain in sickle cell anemia. *Arch. Neurol.*, **47**, 752–767.

WESTERMAN, M. P. & ALLAN, D. (1983). Effects of valinomycin, A23187 and repetitive sickling on irreversible sickle cell formation. *Brit. J. Haemat.* **53**, 399–409.

WESTERMAN, M. P., DILOY-PURAY, M. & STRECZYN, M. (1979). Membrane components in the red cells of patients with sickle cell anemia: relationship to cell aging and to irreversibility of sickling. *Biochim. biophys. Acta*, **557**, 149–155.

WESTERMAN, M. P., PIERCE, L. E. & JENSEN, W. N. (1964). Erythrocyte and plasma lipids in sickle cell anemia. *Blood*, **23**, 200–205.

WETTERSTROEM, N. & BREWER, G. J. (1981). Sickle cell oxidant damage and its treatment. *Clin. Res.*, **29**, 721A (Abstract).

WETTERSTROEM, N., BREWER, G. J., WARTH, J. A., MITCHINSON, A. & DEAR, K. (1984). Relationship of glutathione levels and Heinz body formation to irreversibly sickled cells in sickle cell anemia. *J. Lab. clin. Med.*, **103**, 589–596.

WHITE, J. G. (1968). The fine structure of sickled hemoglobin in situ. *Blood*, **31**, 561–579.

WHITE, J. G. (1974). Ultrastructural features of erythrocyte and hemoglobin sickling. *Arch. intern. Med.*, **133**, 545–562.

WHITE, J. G. & HEAGAN, B. (1970a). The fine structure of cell-free sickled hemoglobin. *Amer. J. Path*, **58**, 1–17.

WHITE, J. G. & HEAGAN, B. (1970b). Gels of normal and sickled hemoglobin. Comparative study. *J. exp. Med.*, **131**, 1079–1092.

WHITE, J. M. (1974). Mechanical instability of sickle haemoglobin. Further evidence as to cause and clinical implications. *Biochim. biophys. Acta*, **336**, 505–508.

WILEY, J. S. & McCULLOCH, K. E. (1982). Calcium ions, drug action and the red cell membrane. *Pharmac. Ther.*, **18**, 271–292.

ZACHOWSKI, A., CRAESCU, C. T., GALACTEROS, F. & DEVAUX, P. F. (1985). Abnormality of phospholipid transverse diffusion in sickle erythrocytes. *J. clin. Invest.*, **75**, 1713–1717.

ZARKOWSKY, H S. & HOCHMUTH, R. M. (1975). Sickling times of individual erythrocytes at zero PO_2. *J. clin. Invest.*, **56**, 1023–1034.

ZARKOWSKY, H. S. & HOCHMUTH, R. M. (1977). Experimentally-induced alterations in the kinetics of erythocyte sickling. *Blood Cells*, **3**, 305–312.

ZIMMERMAN, C. P. & NATTA, C. (1981). Glutathione peroxidase activity of whole blood of patients with sickle cell anaemia. *Scand. J. Haemat.*, **26**, 177–181.

Sickle-cell disease V: treatment and antenatal diagnosis

The rapid development in recent years of the science of molecular biology, and the elaboration of the techniques of DNA analysis and gene cloning, suggest that gene substitution aimed at providing a cure for the sickle-cell diseases (and other serious genetically-determined diseases, too) will soon be more than a theoretical ideal. Time will no doubt reveal whether this form of radical therapy will ever prove to be practicable in the case of homozygous sickle-cell disease. In the meanwhile a good deal can be done to alleviate the worst consequences of harbouring Hb S. In this chapter an attempt has been made to summarize what has been achieved. The summaries refer primarily to the management of Hb-SS disease; but they apply, too, to Hb-SC disease and Hb-S/β-

thalassaemia, etc., in which the clinical problems are fortunately generally less serious. Good accounts of the early attempts at treatment are to be found in reviews by Margolies (1951) and Scott and Ferguson (1960) and by the WHO Scientific Group (1972); more recent accounts include those in Serjeant's (1974, 1985) monographs and in Huntsman and Lehmann's (1974), Milner's (1974), Sheehy and Plumb's (1977) Dean and Schechter's (1978) and Platt and Nathan's (1981) reviews.

Treatment will be considered under the following main headings: general health measures, including those designed to prevent painful crises; management of painful crises; symptomatic treatment of complications, other than the painful crisis; oxygen therapy; blood transfusion; splenectomy; use of anti-sickling chemicals and drugs; immunization against infections, and abortion based on prenatal diagnosis.

GENERAL HEALTH MEASURES

These include: regular attendance at a sickle-cell anaemia clinic with the aim of achieving a good rapport with the physician-in-charge and of ascertaining and recording each individual patient's clinical and haematological findings when in a steady state; instructing the patient (or his or her parents) as to the facts and problems of sickle-cell anaemia; the maintenance of as good a state of nutrition as possible, including the giving of vitamin supplements when indicated, particularly folic acid in pregnancy; the prompt diagnosis and effective treatment of infections and their prevention by appropriate immunization; the avoidance of dehydration and the avoidance of cold.

In tropical countries the prevention of malaria by chemotherapy is most important; and it is in Africa, particularly, where the benefit of better control of infections and infestations, and the improvement in nutrition and hygiene, have been shown most clearly to be of major benefit (Konetey-Ahulu, 1971, 1972), so much so that the expectation of life of an infant with Hb-SS disease is now many times better than it was even a few decades ago.

Folic acid supplementation

The possible value of adding folic acid to the daily diet of children was assessed in Jamaica by Rabb *et al.* (1983). A double-blind controlled trial was organized and the 117 participating children each received 5 mg of folic acid daily for 1 year. At the end of this time it was found that the folic acid supplement had made no significant difference to the incidence of major or minor infections, acute splenic sequestration or vaso-occlusive phenomena or to haemoglobin levels or growth-rate. However, the mean MCV of the patients receiving the folic acid was 4 fl less than that of the control patients, suggesting that some patients were mildly folate-deficient. Rabb *et al.* remarked that overt megaloblastic anaemia in Hb-SS children living in Jamaica at the time of the trial was rare — at one time it was probably less rare; and they concluded that it is now not essential to give Jamaican children daily supplements of folic acid. This does not mean that it is no longer important to give folic acid to pregnant women.

MANAGEMENT AND PREVENTION OF VASO-OCCLUSIVE CRISES

It is important to try to determine what has caused the crisis that has led the patient to seek treatment. As many crises are precipitated by infections, evidence of infection should be looked for carefully, and if found the infection must be treated promptly and effectively.

Control of pain. As already discussed (p. 22), vaso-occlusive crises lead to deep-seated pain in the affected organ or organs, which is often severe. In Jamaica, as described by Serjeant (1985, p. 204), most bone-pain crises have been controlled by the use of mild analgesics, such as paracetamol, and reassurance that the pain will subside without the necessity of admitting the patient to hospital. More potent analgesics may be necessary in some cases, but these have to be used with care, bearing in mind the possibility of addiction to a drug such as pethidine.

In an interesting letter to *The Lancet*, Brozovic and her colleagues (1986) summarized their experience of treating Hb-SS patients in painful crisis in London. Mild pain has generally been managed satisfactorily with the patient at home with the help of paracetamol, warmth, oral fluids and rest. For more severely affected patients, often with more than one organ affected, Brozovic *et al.* have found that opioids have generally been necessary, and they stress the paramount importance of the physician relieving the patient of his or her pain as promptly and effectively as possible. None of the 610 Hb-SS patients attending their clinics is known to be a drug addict.

Fluid replacement

It is important to prevent dehydration. Fluids should be given freely by mouth and intravenous therapy may be helpful: physiological saline, 50 g/l glucose or glucose saline have all been widely used intravenously, as well as intravenous sodium lactate or sodium bicarbonate. Whether one formula is better than another has not been clearly established. Platt and Nathan (1981) recommended that 2250 ml of fluid per m^2 should be given per 24 hours and that the serum electrolyte levels should be carefully checked and the rate of fluid administered adjusted accordingly. With the above rather conservative treatment most patients feel better within 48 hours.

The fact that most crises last only a few days (see p. 22) has made it difficult to assess the value of attempts at more specific treatment. A large number of different therapies have, nevertheless, been tried with the aim of alleviating existing crises and of shortening their duration or of preventing their occurrence. In general, the results have been indecisive and disappointing; and therapies that have reduced sickling *in vitro* have proved to be impracticable or unacceptably toxic *in vivo*. The little that has been achieved, despite much effort, is summarized in the following sections.

Alkalies

The knowledge that sickling *in vitro* is enhanced by a fall in pH has led to the expectation that therapy with alkalies might be beneficial. They have in fact been found to be of doubtful or, at the most, of limited value.

Torrance and Schnabel (1932), in a lengthy report on a male black aged 26, reported that he was 'promptly relieved of generalized bodily pains on two occasions after the exhibition of potassium sulphocyanate, potassium citrate and bicarbonate of sodium'.

Greenberg and Kass (1956, 1958) treated six patients in painful crisis with intravenous sodium bicarbonate; four responded promptly, two did not. Schwartz and McElfresh (1964), in 25 trials on 18 patients, concluded that the rapid intravenous infusion of sodium bicarbonate was not more effective than comparable infusions of saline and that, although acidosis *in vivo* and a lowered pH *in vitro* promoted sickling, alkalinization, as achieved in their study, was ineffective in the treatment of crises. The Cooperative Urea Trials Group (1974c) similarly found no differences in the number of remissions within 48 hours and in the duration of the crises between two groups of patients in crisis treated with intravenous sodium lactate (nine patients) or intravenous saline-dextrose solution (12 patients). However, their findings suggested that patients whose initial blood pH was low did better when treated with the alkali than with saline and dextrose.

The value of alkalies given by mouth is also controversial. Lehmann (1963) and Hugh-Jones, Lehmann and McAlister (1964), while doubting whether orally administered alkali was effective in the treatment of established crises, concluded that the regime was helpful, by increasing the alkali reserve, in preventing their onset. Barreras and Diggs (1971) concluded, however, that sodium citrate and water by mouth were as effective as intravenous sodium lactate in shortening the duration of crises and were superior to water alone by mouth.

Huntsman and Lehmann (1974) recommended the oral administration of sodium bicarbonate, in divided doses of up to 20 g daily, to increase the alkali reserve and to prevent acidosis, and also the intravenous administration of magnesium sulphate (see below).

Reduction in plasma osmolarity: hyponatraemia

The objective of therapy designed to induce hyponatraemia is to reduce the osmolarity of the plasma and hence the MCHC and in this way diminish sickling as the result of deoxygenation.

Guy, Gavrilis and Rothenberg (1973) described how suspending sickle-cell disease blood *in vitro* in phosphate-buffered saline solutions of diminishing salt content led to a decrease in the number of reversibly sickled cells when the suspension was deoxygenated; the percentage of ISCs, in contrast, was unchanged. No lysis took place unless the salt concentration was reduced below 0.4 g/dl. Saline solution at a concentration of 0.45 g/dl was administered at a rate of 5–10 ml/kg/hour to seven patients with sickle-cell disease in painful crisis (five Hb SS, two Hb SC). Seven of the patients appeared to respond favourably and the duration of the crises in three of them was substantially shorter than that of previous crises. Guy, Gavrilis and Rothenberg warned that the therapy should not be attempted if there was any evidence of renal disease or reduction in urinary output or in patients with any signs of cardiac failure.

Attempts have also been made to maintain hyponatraemia on a chronic basis by restricting the intake of salt. Several studies have shown that it is possible to achieve some benefit in this way, but the patients have found that the low salt diet and the necessary high fluid intake difficult to tolerate.

Rosa and co-workers (1980, 1982) reported that they had managed to induce sustained dilutional hyponatraemia in three Hb-SS patients by the use of DDAVP, an analogue of arginine vasopressin, combined with a high fluid intake and a low salt diet. The MCHC fell from 34–35.5% to 30–32.5% and the degree of sickling at low O_2 partial pressures was reduced. Serum Na^+ fell from 140 to 120–125 mM. The frequency of painful crises appeared to be reduced and acutely produced hyponatraemia was thought to have shortened the duration of crises. Rosa et al. considered these results to be encouraging. However, Leary and Abramson (1981), who had treated four patients, concluded that the regime was of little benefit and were concerned about its possible toxicity. Charache and Walker (1981) also concluded that the regime had little to offer and stressed that the four patients they studied found the necessary low salt intake and high water load difficult to tolerate for any length of time.

Charache, Moyer and Walker (1983), on the basis of a larger experience, concluded that, although it was possible to achieve a significant degree of hyponatraemia with or without the administration of DDAVP, the length of time patients so treated remained in hospital after admission for a painful crisis did not differ from that of patients who had received conventional treatment. Moreover, the regime required intensive laboratory surveillance. Further controlled trials, it was suggested, were not justified.

Magnesium salts

Reports of their possible value are conflicting. Hugh-Jones, Lehmann and McAlister (1964) treated six patients with oral magnesium glutamate and oral sodium bicarbonate and concluded

that they suffered from fewer crises subsequently and that their duration was shorter than formerly. The treatment had no effect on the haemoglobin level or erythrocyte life-span. Magnesium sulphate (1–2 ml of a 50% solution) given slowly intravenously appeared to relieve pain; this was attributed to its mild anticoagulant and vasodilatory effects. Basu and Woodruff (1966) studied 13 patients before and after treatment with oral acetazolamide and magnesium citrate. However, they appeared to derive no obvious clinical benefit, and the ^{51}Cr T_{50} was not significantly affected.

Oxygen

This has been administered many times to Hb-SS patients in acute crisis but the results have generally been disappointing. In theory, raising the arterial blood pO_2 would inhibit sickling and thus help to prevent the spread of vaso-occlusion; it could hardly be expected to restore the circulation within occluded capillaries. In patients suffering from the acute chest syndrome, irrespective of whether infection is present, the administration of oxygen can be helpful if the arterial-blood pO_2 is low. A theoretical objection to oxygen therapy continued for more than a day or so is depression of erythropoiesis, with consequent rapid increase in anaemia. This has been well documented (see below).

In early studies, Reinhard and co-workers (1943) tried the effect on three sickle-cell anaemia patients of breathing 80–100% oxygen. Continuing the treatment for 8–20 days did not, however, inhibit haemolysis and did not relieve pain. Moreover, not unexpectedly, compensatory erythropoiesis was markedly inhibited and the patients became more anaemic. More recently hyperbaric oxygen has been given a trial. Laszlo, Obenour and Saltzman (1969) exposed five patients (three Hb SS, one Hb SD and one Hb AS) to oxygen at 2 atmospheres for 20 minutes to 1 hour. The percentage of sickled cells in the peripheral blood fell and remained low for up to 24 hours, but the symptoms of a painful crisis were not alleviated and the renal concentrating ability was not improved. Haematuria in one patient, nevertheless, ceased. Reynolds (1971), however, reported a more encouraging experience; a 25-year-old female suffering from recurrent painful abdominal crises improved dramatically subjectively on three occasions after 90 minutes exposure to 2 atmospheres.

Solanki (1983) described the effect of treating a 24-year-old male suffering from sickle-cell anaemia and the acute chest syndrome by administering oxygen continuously for 4 days via a nasal catheter. This raised the arterial-blood pO_2 well above 100 mm Hg (13.3 kPa). The result was a fall in reticulocyte count from 10.6. to 1.4% and a fall in PCV from 26.5 to 17.5% (Fig. 15.1).

Embury and co-workers (1984) detailed the effect on three steady-state Hb-SS patients of the continuous administration of oxygen at a rate of 5 litres per minute over a 5-day period. Serum erythropoietin levels declined rapidly and were followed after 2 days by steep falls in the reticulocyte count. The ISC count fell considerably in all three patients from Day 1 onwards, only to rebound to higher than initial levels in two of the three patients when they no longer inhaled

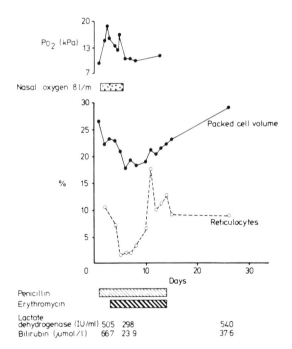

Fig. 15.1 Changes in haematological and respiratory data resulting from the treatment of a Hb-SS patient with oxygen.
PO_2 = arterial O_2 pressure (1 kPa ≡ 7.5 mm Hg).
[Reproduced by permission from Solanki (1983).]

oxygen; these two patients experienced painful crises 3–4 days later. Embury *et al.* concluded that, if oxygen therapy is to be given, it is best to administer the oxygen intermittently rather than continuously. Shulman (1984), in correspondence, stressed that the only role of oxygen therapy in Hb-SS disease is to improve arterial hypoxaemia caused by ventilation-perfusion imbalance in the acute chest syndrome; in such circumstances the oxygen should be given, in his opinion, continuously and when no longer required tapered off gradually to prevent any 'rebound' effect.

Vasodilator drugs: priscoline

Vasodilator drugs have been used from time to time, in an attempt presumably to unblock occluded capillaries. Priscoline was used by Smith, Rosenblatt and Bedo (1953) to treat seven children in crises. Their pain appeared to be relieved and the drug appeared to be useful in differential diagnosis. However, despite this favourable report vasodilator drugs do not seem to have been widely used. Presumably they have been found generally to be ineffective.

Dextran

The possibility that increasing the plasma volume would be effective in the treatment of Hb-SS patients in crisis, presumably by increasing the blood flow in areas affected by vaso-occlusion and by lowering of the PCV, was tested by Jenkins, Scott and Ferguson (1956) who treated nine children with an intravenous infusion of 6% dextran (mol. wt. 64 000) in 5% fructose. The symptoms of six of the nine improved, but their improvement did not necessarily parallel an increase in blood volume. The total mass of circulating haemoglobin increased in six patients and it was suggested that this was due to the mobilization, by expansion of the blood volume, of erythrocytes trapped in internal organs or peripheral capillaries. Watson-Williams (1963) and Garrett, Giles and Sage (1963), used Rheomacrodex and reported encouraging results in small numbers of patients. Oski and co-workers (1965), who treated a larger series, concluded, however, that dextran was no more beneficial than intravenous saline.

The experience of Barnes, Hendrickse and Watson-Williams (1965) was similar: they had treated 26 episodes of bone pain in 24 Nigerian children with Hb-SS disease with Rheomacrodex but found it no more effective than 50 g/l dextrose. Thus despite encouraging reports when first used, subsequent experience indicates that intravenously administered low molecular weight dextran is without clear benefit in the treatment of patients in vaso-occlusive crisis.

Fresh frozen plasma

This has also been used to treat Hb-SS patients in crisis, and there is some evidence that the treatment is beneficial. Huehns, Davies and Brozovic (1981) reported that they had treated 17 crises in 11 patients with fresh frozen plasma, giving 1 unit (c 500 ml) to children and 2 units to adults. Pain was relieved immediately in 15 of the crises (nine patients), and it was found in eight patients that their requirement for analgesics, given on demand, was less than that for previous crises. All the nine patients who responded left hospital within 4 days of admission. The apparent beneficial effect of the treatment was attributed to enhancement of blood flow from expansion of the plasma volume and to stimulation of PGI_2 (prostacyclin) production (leading to vasodilation and anti-platelet effects).

Anticoagulants

Oral anticoagulants have been administered to patients from time to time in an attempt to prevent the occurrence of vaso-occlusive crises. It is possible that they may help to do this but the possible complications consequent on their use would seem to outweigh any minor improvement achieved.

Griffiths (1955) described how tromexan had been given to a Hb-AS female who had developed a femoral thrombosis *post partum*. Whilst on the drug the sickling *in vitro* of a sealed blood preparation appeared to be markedly delayed. Rodman, Myerson and Pastor (1961) reported that a 32-year-old male had been virtually free from painful crises while receiving dicumarol. Salvaggio, Arnold and Banov (1963) treated 12 patients with warfarin for 12–34 months. The frequency of painful crises appeared to be reduced but there were seven episodes of bleeding, one being nearly fatal.

Heparin. Chaplin and co-workers (1984) reported that four patients had administered heparin to themselves at a minidosage (5000 units per 12 hours) for a period of 12 months. Compared with their experience of 12 months without heparin, two of the patients were markedly improved and two moderately improved. There had been an approximately 80% reduction in the time spent in hospital. There were no complications; in particular, no thrombocytopenia or evidence of osteoporosis.

Defibrination by arvin

The venom of the Malayan pit viper (*Agkistrodon rhodostoma*) contains a powerful defibrinating agent (arvin). Marketed under the name of Ancrod, the venom, although effective in reducing the plasma fibrinogen to very low levels, does not seem to have been of any practical value in the treatment of Hb-SS disease patients in crisis. Early results were encouraging (Gilles *et al.*, 1968), but they were not confirmed in a double-blind trial (Mann *et al.* 1972).

One of the difficulties about using arvin is the possibility of the eventual development of antibodies by the patient that neutralize its effect. Pitney (1968) had pointed out that this seemed to be less likely to develop if the venom was given intravenously rather than intramuscularly.

Steroid hormones

ACTH or adrenocorticosteroid therapy appears to have no place in the treatment of patients with Hb-SS disease. The same is probably true of sex hormones, for the potential dangers and undesirable sequelae of androgen or progesterone therapy would seem to outweigh any possible benefits (see below).

The results of the early use of ACTH were conflicting. Kass and co-workers (1951) treated two patients: the first patient underwent two crises after the start of treatment; the second patient had a mild crisis, then a rise in erythrocyte count. Sass (1952) reported dramatic symptomatic improvement in one patient without any significant change in blood count.

Sex hormones. Isaacs and Hayhoe (1967) reported that testosterone added to preparations of the bone marrow or peripheral blood of a Hb-AS subject inhibited sickling and that progesterone had a similar effect. They suggested that the hormones were acting on the erythrocyte membrane.

Lundh and Gardner (1970) treated 11 sickle-cell anaemia patients with testosterone for 3–16 weeks. In 10 of them (males and females) the erythrocyte mass increased by as much as 25–125%, but the cells' life-span appeared to be unaltered and Lundh and Gardner could demonstrate no effect on the sensitivity of the patients' erythrocytes to sickling *in vitro* at a range of O_2 tensions. All the patients gained weight and there were other undesirable effects. All the males suffered from priapism. However, the incidence of painful crises did not seem to be increased in the females despite the rise in PCV.

Raper, Black and Huntsman (1970) similarly found no change in in-vitro sickling in two male Hb-SS patients and four female Hb-AS individuals after the administration of testosterone and progesterone, respectively.

The results obtained by Isaacs, Effiong and Ayeni (1972) by the use of testosterone (in males) and progesterone (in females) were more encouraging. (They suggested that the dose of testosterone that Lundh and Gardner (1970) had been using was too high.) Forty-four patients in all were treated and 80% of those who received hormone treatment responded favourably, as assessed by a numerical scoring system, compared with control patients who had received injections of saline.

Zanger and co-workers (1974) treated 12 patients with Hb-SS disease with the oral androgen dromostanolone. The haemoglobin and PCV rose in eleven of them and in nine out of 10 an increase in erythrocyte iron turnover was demonstrated. However, there was no change in ^{51}Cr T_{50}, Hb-F or 2,3-DPG concentration or viscometric measurements. Side-effects were minimal and there were no upsets in liver function. However, three patients developed crises during the treatment. Zanger *et al.* concluded that dromostanolone was an effective stimulant of erythropoiesis in Hb-SS disease and that the increased erythrocyte mass might help to improve cardiac function; however, they concluded, too, that the rise in PCV might precipitate vaso-occlusive crises and also that the drug failed to affect favourably the abnormal physical and chemical character of the erythrocytes.

Alexanian and Nadell (1975) studied the effect of the administration of oxymetholone for at least 2 months to seven Hb-SS anaemia patients. Their erythrocyte mass increased by 17–75% but there was no change in erythrocyte life-span. One patient suffered from hepatic toxicity.

de Ceulaer and co-workers (1982) administered medroxyprogesterone acetate to 23 Hb-SS patients in a crossover trial. While receiving a placebo, their haematological indices remained unaltered; when given the drug, however, total haemoglobin and the erythrocyte count, erythrocyte mass and life-span, and the Hb-F percentage, all rose significantly; in contrast, the reticulocyte and ISC counts and total serum bilirubin fell. Painful crises were, too, less frequent, and de Ceulaer *et al.* concluded that medroxyprogesterone inhibits in-vivo sickling; their findings led them to suggest, too, that the injectable Depo-Provera might be the contraceptive of choice for Hb-SS women.

Serjeant, de Ceulaer and Maude (1985), in a similarly organized trial, administered stilboestrol to 11 Hb-SS men complaining of priapism and found that stilboestrol was better than the placebo in preventing attacks.

Conversion of haemoglobin S to methaemoglobin S or carboxyhaemoglobin S

Although the presence of methaemoglobin or carboxyhaemoglobin results in a left shift of the O_2-dissociation curve of Hb S, treatment of Hb-SS disease patients with methaemoglobin-producing drugs or with carbon monoxide (CO) can hardly be recommended as a practical form of therapy.

Methaemoglobin S. Beutler and Mikus (1961) administered sodium nitrite to Hb-SS patients so as to raise the methaemoglobin concentration to approximately 20%. Erythrocyte life-span was transiently increased, but this was followed eventually by the formation of Heinz bodies and an accelerated rate of erythrocyte destruction.

Carboxyhaemoglobin S. Sirs (1963) administered sufficient CO to a 29-year-old Hb-SS patient to produce about 4% Hb CO and reported a fall in the percentage of sickled cells in venous blood (fixed immediately after withdrawal) from 10.2 to 3.9. He suggested that oxygen containing 0.005% CO might be useful in the treatment of a patient during a crisis or before exposure to a lowered oxygen tension.

Purugganan and McElfresh (1964) failed to demonstrate in two Hb-SS boys a significant change in the percentage of sickled cells in peripheral capillary blood as the result of increasing the blood concentration of CO from 0% to 11.2% and 12.6%, respectively. The concentration of CO achieved was thought to be the highest that could be tolerated. In one patient the ^{51}Cr T_{50} fell from 8 days before the daily inhalation of CO to 5.5 days after 7 days of treatment. Beutler (1975), on the other hand, demonstrated an improvement in erythrocyte life-span in two patients following the administration of CO in sufficient amount to raise the HbCO concentration to 12% and 15%, respectively; he concluded, nevertheless, that the inhalation of CO was not a practicable method of treatment.

Franklin, Rosemeyer and Huehns (1983) studied in an in-vitro system the effect of liganded derivatives of haemoglobin (CO-Hb S and met-Hb S) on Hb-S polymerization and calculated that as much as 30% of CO-Hb S and as much as 60% of met-Hb S would have to be maintained to prevent sickling *in vivo*. Therapy with CO or with methaemoglobin-producing drugs was thus not practicable. They calculated, too, that for an anti-sickling reagent to be effective, it would have to be able to keep 30% of the Hb S in the fully oxy(R) form; they added that even 30% of the haemoglobin in the fully oxy form would be likely to compromise oxygen delivery to the tissues sufficiently to cause a counterproductive rise in haemoglobin.

SYMPTOMATIC TREATMENT OF PATIENTS SUFFERING FROM COMPLICATIONS OTHER THAN VASO-OCCLUSIVE CRISES

Sudden increase in anaemia. As already indicated, this may have several causes. An accurate diagnosis is essential. If due to folate deficiency, as is not rare in pregnancy, this can be corrected by oral folic acid; if due to an aplastic crisis, a transfusion of packed normal erythrocytes may be essential. If in a young child the result of a splenic sequestration crisis, transfusion may be urgently necessary and, if the crisis recurs, splenectomy should be considered (see p. 253). Increased anaemia due to an exacerbation of haemolysis is not common; it is likely that concurrent infection is the cause, with or without the presence of G6PD deficiency. How the patient is managed will depend upon the mechanism of the increased haemolysis. Blood transfusion may be necessary.

Complications requiring surgery. Patients with Hb-SS disease are not exempt from disorders that require surgical treatment; in addition, they suffer frequently from gallstones and cholecystitis, as do patients with other types of chronic haemolytic anaemia. The risk of surgery in a Hb-SS patient stems from the potentially harmful effects of anaesthesia and from the trauma of the operation itself; singly or in combination they can lead to vaso-occlusive crises. Particular care has to be taken to avoid anoxia and dehydration. If major surgery has to be undertaken, preparing the patient by an exchange-transfusion should certainly be considered.

Pregnancy. As discussed on page 44, the hazards of pregnancy and of the puerperium in patients with Hb-SS disease are now not nearly as serious as they were at one time. What is required is a high standard of antenatal and perinatal care.

The possible value of prophylactic blood transfusion is considered on page 249.

Leg ulceration. As already referred to (p. 26), leg ulcers quite commonly develop in Hb-SS patients. They are difficult to treat.

BLOOD TRANSFUSION

Transfusion with packed normal erythrocytes may be life-saving in Hb-SS patients who become severely anaemic; multiple transfusions, or preferably perhaps exchange-transfusion, may be an essential preliminary in any patient requiring major surgery. Transfusions should seldom be necessary or given to patients in a steady state, except, perhaps, in pregnancy when the harmful effect of severe anaemia on the mother and on the unborn child has to be considered.

In most Hb-SS patients in a steady state the haemoglobin is seldom lower than 6–7 g/dl; and at this level they often are able to lead almost normal lives. This is because the shift in the O_2-dissociation curve to the right and an increased cardiac output act together to ensure an almost normal delivery of oxygen to the tissues. For patients whose haemoglobin is higher than this, transfusion is likely to be unnecessary and unwise. Benefit at the most would be temporary: raising the haemoglobin depresses erythropoiesis so that in the presence of continuing increased haemolysis the haemoglobin will quickly fall to its pre-transfusion level. Also, transfusion, by raising the PCV, will increase the viscosity of the blood and even a small increase may precipitate a vaso-occlusive crisis in some patients. Details of the changes in blood picture resulting from multiple transfusions were given by Donegan, MacIlwaine and Leavell (1954) and Nadel and Spivack (1958). The results in some later series of patients are outlined below. The majority of the reports deal with attempts to assess the value of blood transfusion in the treatment of potentially serious complications of sickle-cell disease.

Transfusion in the treatment and prevention of vaso-occlusive phenomena

Anderson and co-workers (1963) reported on five

patients who had been treated by a partial exchange-transfusion at 5–6 week intervals over a period of up to 6 years, the aim being to have 15–40% of normal erythocytes in the circulation. Three of these patients were judged to have been markedly benefited and two moderately so. *In vitro*, adding normal Hb-AA cells to Hb-SS cells in the proportion of 3:7 was found not to reduce the percentage of Hb-SS cells which sickled at a given pH and degree of deoxygenation. However, the viscosity of the mixture was less than that of 100% Hb-SS cells.

Brody and co-workers (1970) described how limited exchange-transfusion had benefited eight patients suffering from painful vaso-occlusive crises. Their fever diminished and bone pain rapidly decreased, due it was considered to the treatment interrupting the cycle of hypoxia, vaso-occlusion and organ injury. The patients' average stay in hospital was 3 days, instead of an expected 7 days.

Sommer, Kontras and Craenen (1971) described how they had treated by a partial exchange-transfusion a 9-year-old boy, severely affected with sickle-cell anaemia, who had been admitted to hospital moribund in severe cardiac failure associated with multiple pulmonary emboli. He improved following a 1000-ml exchange and was subsequently partially exchanged at 8–12-week intervals. Additional simple transfusions were given as necessary in order to keep his haemoglobin at about 9 g/dl. On this regime he suffered from no further crises and his heart diminished markedly in size.

Seeler (1973) reported the resolution of priapism in five boys following transfusions of packed normal erythrocytes aimed at doubling the haematocrit value.

Charache (1974), in an interesting review, discussed the pros and cons, and difficulties and complications, of long-term transfusion therapy and illustrated his discussion with a description of a patient with Hb-SD disease who had been treated by partial exchange-transfusion every 3–4 weeks with the aim of reducing the proportion of patient's erythrocytes to less than 50%.

Green and co-workers (1975) described how two patients suffering from severe vaso-occlusive phenomena that failed to respond to conversative measures were treated successfully by means of large 6-litre exchange transfusions. One of the patients had Hb-S/β-thalassaemia and multiple skeletal pains; the other had Hb-SC disease and widespread pulmonary infarction. Green *et al.* cautioned, however, that large-scale exchange-transfusion should be considered only for patients who seemed likely to die.

Kernoff, Botha and Jacobs (1977) reported how they had successfully carried out an exchange-transfusion on a Hb-SS disease patient using a continuous-flow cell separator. A level of 90.8% Hb A was achieved.

Miller and co-workers (1980) studied the exercise capacity of 10 patients who had been partially exchange-transfused with normal blood with the aim of substantially reducing the proportion of Hb S present and at the same time keeping the haemoglobin and blood volume constant. The mean proportion of Hb A present rose to 55%. The exercise capacity of the patients improved and this was attributed to improved oxygen transport to the tissues secondary to the reduction in blood viscosity.

Sheehy, Law and Wade (1980) reported that they had successfully treated by exchange-transfusion a 21-year-old patient who was suffering from intrahepatic cholestasis, a serious and often fatal complication. They managed to reduce the concentration of Hb S to 3% by eight partial exchanges with packed cells and plasma; the patient's hepatic encephalopathy regressed and the serum bilirubin fell from the very high level of 146 mg/dl to 16 mg/dl.

Finch, Lee and Leonard (1982) described the interesting history of a female patient who had received approximately 600 transfusions prior to her death when aged 47. For the 13 years before she died she had received 2 units of packed erythrocytes every 3 weeks with the aim of keeping the haematocrit greater than 36%; the Hb-S proportion was usually less than 10%. During this whole period she experienced no further crises and an ankle ulcer healed. The reticulocyte count was as low as less than 1% and it was suggested that one effect of repeated transfusion is to lengthen the erythrocyte maturation time in the bone marrow, with the result that the Hb-S concentration within reticulocytes is unusually high. Finch, Lee and Leonard suggested that this would impede the passage of reticulocytes through the wall of the marrow sinuses.

Van de Pette, Pearson and Slater (1982) reported on five adult patients with sickle-cell disease suffering from life-threatening crises whom they had successfully treated by exchange-transfusion. Three of the patients had Hb-SC disease and in two of them the crisis had been precipitated by an aeroplane flight.

Transfusion in the prevention of strokes

Recent studies have indicated that, although regular transfusion helps to prevent further cerebral infarction, strokes are likely to occur again once transfusions are no longer given.

Russell and co-workers (1976) studied five Hb-SS children aged between 4 and 10 years who had suffered from strokes: three were transfused repeatedly to keep the Hb-S percentage less than 30; two were not transfused. Cerebral angiograms were abnormal in all five patients at the start of the study. One year later the angiograms in the patients who had not been transfused revealed progressive disease; those in the patients who had been transfused showed that the abnormalities had resolved in two of them and had partially resolved in one.

Lusher, Haghighat and Khalifa (1976) described the results of a prophylactic transfusion programme in a series of children all of whom had had one or more episodes of cerebral infarction. Of 15 children who had received buffy-coat-poor transfusions every 3 weeks for 9 months to $5\frac{3}{4}$ years none showed any progression of their neurological abnormalities and several had improved. One child, however, had developed hepatitis.

Wilimas and co-workers (1980) reported that they had transfused 12 children (11 Hb SS; one Hb SC), all of whom had previously suffered from strokes, with packed erythrocytes every 3–4 weeks so as to reduce the proportion of Hb S to less than 20%. The regime was halted after 1 year in 10 of the patients, and seven of them then suffered from a second stroke 5 weeks to 11 months later (median 3 months). Wilimas et al. concluded that short-term repeated transfusions will not prevent further strokes from developing after the treatment is stopped. In a commentary on their paper, Seeler and Royal (1980) stated that four out of 17 children under their own care, who had developed strokes, gave a history of surviving bacterial meningitis; they concluded that children with a history of stroke run a great risk of recurrence unless treated by a long-term transfusion regime and recommended that this be combined with chelation therapy, as used in thalassaemia major.

Kron and Cohen (1984) stressed that one way of preventing the accumulation of iron was to transfuse using a partial exchange-technique; they calculated that it would be possible to transfuse in this way for 30–40 years, keeping the proportion of Hb S present to between 10 and 30%, without iron overload developing, even without chelation.

Sarnaik and Lusher (1985) had transfused 49 sickle-cell anaemia patients on a regular basis for 2–10 years. The results were considered to be good in 40 patients who had had strokes and in six who had had developed splenic sequestration; three who had developed aseptic necrosis, however, derived no benefit. Cardiac function was normal in nine patients who had received more than 20 g of iron; in 15, however, there was biochemical and histochemical evidence of hepatic iron overload; one patient developed diabetes, and 21% formed anti-erythrocyte allo-antibodies.

Transfusion during pregnancy

The dangers to mother and infant of pregnancy in the sickle-cell disorders, and the improving prospect, have already been described (p. 44). Prophylactic transfusions appear to be helpful, but the most appropriate type of transfusion and their precise value is still somewhat uncertain.

When anaemia is very severe, as the result of poor nutrition and/or infection, transfusions can be life-saving. Fullerton and Turner (1962) in Nigeria, for instance, treated 115 severely anaemic pregnant patients by means of exchange-transfusion with only five deaths; 7% of this series of patients had a background of Hb-SS or Hb-SC disease. In a later report from Nigeria, Harrison, Ajabor and Lawson (1971) reported similarly successful results using exchange-transfusion in 46 severely anaemic pregnant women: only one mother and 12 fetuses were lost. They were, however, equally successful in a comparable series of 47 women whom they transfused slowly with 500 ml of packed cells to which 50 mg of ethacrynic acid (a rapidly-acting diuretic) had been added: in this series there were no maternal deaths, although 11 fetuses were lost.

Exchange-transfusion has also been used successfully in the United States in pregnant sickle-cell disease patients, not so often to treat severe anaemia as in an attempt to alleviate severe vaso-occlusive crises. Davey and co-workers (1978), for instance, reported that they had treated by means of a partial exchange-transfusion two pregnant Hb-SC patients who had serious respiratory complications thought to be secondary to infarction of the bone marrow and fat embolism.

Cunningham and co-workers (1979) reviewed the outcome of pregnancy in 37 patients (16 Hb SS, 19 Hb SC and two Hb-S/β-thalassaemia). They had been transfused throughout pregnancy with the aim of keeping the haematocrit above 25% and the Hb-S percentage below 60. There were no maternal deaths and maternal morbidity was described as minimal. Fetal deaths were fewer than anticipated on the basis of past experience but fetal morbidity was still excessive.

Morrison and co-workers (1980) reported on 75 patients (41 Hb SS, 25 Hb SC and nine Hb-S/β-thalassaemia), all of whom were treated by partial exchange-transfusion at 28 weeks and at 36–38 weeks. The effect on the patients' haemoglobin was to reduce the Hb-S percentage from 92 (mean value) before the exchange to 43 (mean value) afterwards. Again there were no maternal deaths and maternal morbidity was, too, considered to be significantly improved. The fetal perinatal death rate was 26 per 1000, which was considered an improvement, and there were fewer premature births and low birth-weight infants than expected.

COMPLICATIONS OF BLOOD TRANSFUSION

Patients suffering from sickle-cell disorders who are being treated by blood transfusion are prone, like all other recipients, to three main types of complication: the development of allo-antibodies against transfused blood-cell antigens which they themselves lack; overloading with iron; and infection, in particular by viruses such as those responsible for hepatitis and (recently) AIDS.

Allo-antibodies

Orlina, Unger and Koshy (1978) provided interesting data on the frequency with which allo-antibodies develop in Hb-SS patients who have received multiple transfusions. Fifty patients were investigated, 30 females and 20 males: 18 (36%) became immunized, of which 13 were female. Thirty-six antibodies were identified: 15 were anti-Rh, 12 anti-Lewis and five anti-K. The immunized patients had received more transfusions on the whole than the non-immunized, but there was some overlap and five non-immunized patients had received more than 15 transfusions. Orlina, Unger and Koshy concluded that, as the development of the antibodies was potentially important clinically, patients should be grouped for antigens of the ABO, Rhesus, Kell, Duffy and Kidd systems, at least, before commencing any programme of repeated blood transfusions.

Coles, Klein and Holland (1981) concluded, as a result of a review of patients transfused at the Clinical Center at the National Institutes of Health (NIH) and at the Johns Hopkins Hospital, that sickle-cell disease patients did not differ from thalassaemic patients in their propensity to form allo-antibodies when comparably transfused. The incidence of antibodies (23%) was approximately the same in both groups, and was similar to that of a previously reported series of multi-transfused patients who had undergone open-heart surgery at NIH. Coles, Klein and Holland stated that they did not feel that phenotypically matched blood was necessary for the routine transfusion of sickle-cell disease patients, but added that carefully matched blood would be required for patients who gave a history of a delayed transfusion reaction and for patients who appeared to be good antibody 'responders'.

Rosse and co-workers (1985) reported on the results of tests for allo-antibodies in 1856 Hb-SS patients of whom 72.2% had been transfused: 20.1% were found to be immunized against one or more erythrocyte antigens, a percentage considered to be greater than in most multi-transfused populations. More females had formed antibodies than males, and this did not seem to be accountable by pregnancy. A high proportion (70%) of the antibodies were directed against antigens, the incidence of which was lower in blacks than in Caucasians, e.g., the antigens E, C, K, Fy^a, Fy^b, Le^a and Le^b. The percentage of antibody-forming Hb-SC and Hb-S/β-thalassaemia patients was less than that of the Hb-SS patients, but fewer had been transfused.

Sarnaik, Schornack and Lusher (1986) reported on a similar investigation in which 245 Hb-SS children, all of whom had been transfused, were screened for allo-antibodies. In this group only 19 patients (7.75%) had developed antibodies: the median number of transfusions that they had received was 23, compared with three transfusions in the unsensitized patients. The most frequent antibody was anti-K (38%), the next most frequent anti-Le^a and anti-Le^b (24%, combined total); 14% of the antibodies were anti-Rh. Sarnaik, Schornack and Lusher considered that, as the incidence of antibodies consequent on multiple transfusions was low, phenotypically matched blood was probably not warranted for most Hb-SS patients who were receiving transfusions. [This opinion is contrary to that of Orlina, Unger and Koshy (1978) (see above) and that of Diamond et al. (1980) and Milner et al. (1985) (see below).]

Role of HLA group. Castro and co-workers (1983a) reported that eight out of 10 sickle-cell anaemia patients who had formed allo-antibodies were HLA-Bw35 positive, as compared with the normal incidence of 30% in blacks; they suggested that HLA antigen grouping may be useful in predicting which patients are likely to form allo-antibodies after transfusion.

Ofosu and her co-workers (1986) have studied the incidence of auto-antibodies in 80 sickle-cell disease patients and related the incidences to their HLA-A, -B,-C and -DR phenotypes; 73 of the patients had Hb-SS disease, four Hb-SC disease and three Hb-S/β-thalassaemia. The incidence of rheumatoid factor was significantly increased in both males and females; it was lower in highly transfused patients. The incidence of antinuclear factor (ANF) was significantly increased in males and that of anti-smooth muscle increased in females. A low incidence of ANF was associated with HLA-DR3 and an increased incidence of ANF was associated with HLA-A28 and HLA-B15.

Auto-transfusion. The presence of allo-antibodies may sometimes make it very difficult to find compatible normal blood: in such cases the patient's own blood may prove to be a valuable, if by no means an ideal, substitute when, for instance, the patient is faced with a surgical procedure in which haemorrhage is expected.

Castro (1980) and Castro and co-workers (1981) reported that Hb-SS erythrocytes, stored at 4°C in ACD or CPD preservative, behave very similarly to normal cells and that Hb-SS cells can be stored, when glycerolized, at −80–85°C for weeks or months and then used for auto-transfusion without loss of viability, although the post-thaw haemolysis is higher than normal.

Delayed transfusion reactions as a cause of crises. The importance of the presence of unsuspected allo-antibodies has been highlighted by reports of serious delayed transfusion reactions simulating crises in Hb-SS patients.

In a particularly interesting and detailed report, Chaplin and Cassell (1962) described how a 26-year-old male Hb-SS patient had received repeated transfusions for severe vaso-occlusive phenomena with blood which *in vitro* appeared to be entirely compatible. The transfused blood, nevertheless, was rapidly eliminated *in vivo*, and eventually anti-E and anti-K were demonstrated. Chaplin and Cassell recorded that 'A striking clinical observation was the regular onset of typical sickle cell "crisis" coincident with the rapid destruction of large volumes of donor erythrocytes'.

Solanki and McCurdy (1978) referred to delayed transfusion reactions as an 'often-missed entity'. They described how in eight patients transfusions were followed by unexplained falls in the haematocrit. Five of their patients had sickle-cell disease (one, Hb SC; four, Hb SS) and three of the Hb-SS patients developed a painful crisis following the transfusion. All five patients had formed multiple allo-antibodies.

Diamond and co-workers (1980) reported how three out of 18 patients receiving partial exchange-transfusion had become acutely ill 2–6 days after the transfusion with symptoms suggestive of a sickle-cell crisis. The basis of their illness was subsequently found to be haemolysis of a large proportion of the transfused erythrocytes; this was occasioned by anti-Jk[a] and anti-C and perhaps other allo-antibodies. Milner and co-workers (1985) described a further series of Hb-SS patients who had been similarly affected. The patients, of whom two died, became acutely ill within a few days of receiving blood transfusions. The illness of some of the patients mimicked vaso-occlusive crises associated with bone-marrow infarction; other patients developed signs and symptoms suggestive of biliary obstruction or renal insufficiency. Both Diamond *et al.* and Milner *et al.* emphasized the need for carefully matching recipient and donor erythrocyte antigens.

Iron overload

Cohen and Schwartz (1979) reported on the use of DFO (deferoxamine) as an iron chelator. The daily administration of 2.0 g of DFO, given by a 12-hour overnight subcutaneous infusion, resulted in the excretion of 13–39 mg of iron in the urine in a 24-hour period, and it was calculated that the amount excreted more than balanced the iron intake from the transfused blood in eight out of nine patients who were being transfused on a regular basis.

In a more recent report Wang *et al.* (1983) described how they had placed on a DFO regime six youths, aged between 10 and 17 years, who had received multiple transfusions for 5–8 years in an attempt to prevent the recurrence of strokes. After 1 year's treatment the serum-ferritin concentration was lowered in each case; there had, however, been no major improvement in liver function tests. As already referred to, Kron and Cohen (1984) recommended a partial exchange technique as a way of avoiding serious iron overload in patients for whom multiple transfusions were thought to be necessary.

Infection

Patients suffering from sickle-cell disease are at least as susceptible to infections transmitted by transfusions as are Hb-AA individuals. Camacho and co-workers (1983) referred to three repeatedly transfused Hb-SS patients who seemed likely to have developed a forme fruste of AIDS, while Gessain and co-workers (1984), reporting from Martinique where the incidence of HTLV-I antibodies in blood donors is relatively high (3.7%), described how they had found that the incidence of the antibodies in 57 Hb-SS patients was high (14%) compared with approximately 5% in 21 Hb-AS individuals.

SPLENECTOMY

This has been carried out on numerous occasions in patients suffering from sickle-cell disease. The results have often been disappointing. However, patients with hypersplenism are likely to derive considerable benefit and in patients who develop acute splenic sequestration splenectomy may be life-saving.

Early reports

Early reports of the results of splenectomy include those of Bell and co-workers (1927), Hahn and Gillespie (1927) and Stewart (1927). Shotton, Crockett and Leavell (1951) reviewed the results of the operation in 24 cases. The symptoms of 15 patients became less severe and there was some improvement in their erythrocyte count; of the others, four patients improved slightly and four did not benefit. The best results seem to have been obtained in patient who had the largest spleens. Dickstein and Koop (personal communication quoted by Margolies (1951)), for instance, described the effect of splenectomy in 16 children ranging from 14 months to 6 years of age and followed their progress for 1–4 years after the operation. Two of the children were not improved, but the other 14 did relatively well; their haemoglobins were maintained at slightly higher levels than before the operation and none had a major crisis following splenectomy.

As already referred to (p. 222), Sprague and Paterson (1958) reported that the ^{51}Cr half-times of tagged erythrocytes had more than doubled in six patients as a result of splenectomy. This was associated with a rise in the mean haemoglobin from 5.6 to 8.3 g/dl, and a reduction in the number of hospital admissions from 26 per 19.5 patient-years to two per 12.5 patient-years. A further seven Hb-SS patients were mentioned who had already been splenectomized and who after operation no longer needed transfusions.

Splenectomy for hypersplenism

As already mentioned (p. 28), patients (nearly always children) with Hb-SS disease occasionally develop, for reasons which are still not understood, exceptionally large spleens. In consequence they become unusually anaemic and sometimes dangerously so, with a haemoglobin sometimes less than 3.0 g/dl and with variable degrees, too, of thrombocytopenia. Splenectomy is then strongly indicated and may have to be carried out as an urgent procedure. Egdahl, Martin and Hilkovitz (1963) described five such patients. Before splenectomy their haemoglobin ranged from 1.6 to 3.8 g/dl; subsequently it stabilized at 6–10 g/dl and only one of the patients needed transfusing and this was on one occasion only.

Earlier, Watson, Lichtman and Shapiro (1956) had referred to six patients with particularly large spleens who needed frequent transfusions. In two of them it was possible to demonstrate that the survival of transfused normal erythrocytes was impaired, which suggested that an extravascular factor contributed to the haemolysis. Splenectomy in these two patients was of striking clinical benefit and this was associated with a return to normal of the survival of transfused normal cells.

Two interesting patients were described by Stevens (1970). Both were black Americans and gave long histories of anaemia and ill health. Haemoglobin electrophoresis revealed a single band of Hb S. Both patients had had a spleen which was massively enlarged on palpation. The first patient, a male, had been splenectomized when aged 12 and was followed up for 16 years subsequently. His spleen had weighed 970 g. Before splenectomy his haemoglobin had ranged between 4.0 and 7.6 g/dl, and he had been transfused on nine occasions: after splenectomy he needed no further transfusions and the minimum recorded haemoglobin was 7.7 g/dl. [It is interesting to note that this patient had been studied by Motulsky et al. (1958); they had estimated that 40% of his erythrocyte mass was trapped in his spleen.] The second patient was a female who was splenectomized when age $23\frac{1}{2}$ years. Her spleen weighed 1200 g, and after splenectomy her PCV stabilized at 26–28%. The ^{51}CR T_{50} was 4 days before splenectomy and 16 days subsequently. In a letter enclosed with a reprint, Stevens recorded that this patient had died after a 5-day illness 3 years after splenectomy and was found at necropsy to have developed massive pulmonary arterial thrombi with focal infarcts. She had been placed on oral contraceptives, and her death points to the danger of oestrogens in promoting thrombosis in splenectomized subjects, perhaps particularly, too, in patients with Hb-SS disease.

A further female patient splenectomized when an adult was described by Ballester and Warth (1979). Her spleen was palpable 6 cm below the left costal margin; it was tender on palpation and was the cause apparently of repeated attacks of left-sided abdominal pain. Her symptoms were completely relieved following splenectomy and cholecystectomy, carried out after an exchange-transfusion. Electrophoresis revealed Hb S, 3.1% Hb A_2 and 10% Hb F. The α:β globin-chain synthesis ratio was normal.

The reports referred to above show not only that splenectomy can be carried out in young children with Hb-SS disease without an unacceptable rate of complications, and also, too, in adults, but that considerable clinical and haematological benefit may also be expected if the spleen is large. Clearly, if a patient has to be maintained on transfusions and his or her spleen is palpable, particularly if the blood picture suggests chronic hypersplenism and the transfused blood appears to be surviving poorly, splenectomy should be seriously considered. The other important criterion for splenectomy is, in young children, a history of acute splenic sequestration (see below).

In older children and adults in whom the spleen has become fibrosed and is no longer palpable there would seem to be no case for contemplating splenectomy.

Splenectomy for acute splenic sequestration

Recently, Emond and co-workers (1984) reviewed the results of splenectomy, carried out between 1954 and 1982 on 60 Jamaican children and adolescents, aged between 9 months and 16 years, suffering from Hb-SS disease. There were three deaths, two possibly from post-splenectomy infection, and one from renal failure. In 14 patients the operation was carried out to prevent recurrence of acute splenic sequestration — it was seriously considered if the child had had two attacks; while in 14 patients the criterion for splenectomy was sustained hypersplenism — the spleen being palpable at least 4 cm below the costal margin, the haemoglobin being less than 6.5 g/dl, reticulocyte count greater than 15% and platelet count less than $200 \times 10^9/1$, on at least two occasions 6 months apart. In the hypersplenism cases, Edmond et al. documented a modest rise in haemoglobin and a striking rise in platelet count and more than a doubling of ISC count and erythrocyte survival. At the time of writing their review, they recommended giving patients benzyl penicillin pre-operatively and during the hospital admission, then depot benzathine penicillin monthly until the age of 7 years, as well as immunizing them pre-operatively with 14-valent pneumococcal vaccine and H. influenzae B vaccine.

Splenectomy has also been carried out in patients with Hb-SC disease or Hb-S/β-thalassaemia. Less is known about the results of the operation than in Hb-SS disease. It seems probable, however, that the benefit, if any, is slight.

CHEMICALS AND DRUGS THAT INHIBIT SICKLING *IN VITRO*; THEIR USE AND VALUE *IN VIVO*

A large number of chemicals and drugs are known which in appropriate doses inhibit to a greater or lesser extent the sickling *in vitro* of deoxygenated Hb-S-containing erythrocytes. The question has naturally been asked as to whether it is possible to use any of these substances *in vivo*, either as a short-term expedient to benefit a patient suffering from a painful vaso-occlusive crisis or on a long-term basis to prevent crises or other complications developing. A great deal of research has been undertaken in recent years in an attempt to find a drug or drugs that could be used safely for either purpose and the relevant literature is now extensive. The story is largely, although not quite entirely, of encouraging early reports and of a subsequent failure to confirm benefit — of hopes raised and dashed.

It is now realized that chemicals and drugs that inhibit sickling *in vitro* can do this in more than one way: for instance, some are known to disrupt or prevent the intermolecular bonding of Hb-S tetramers so that stacking of the molecules and the formation of fibres is interfered with; others act by shifting the O_2-dissociation curve of Hb S to the left, thus favouring the maintenance of the haemoglobin in its oxy conformation during its passage through the capillaries and veins. Other chemicals and drugs decrease the intracellular concentration of Hb S by interfering with the ionic equilibrium through the cell membrane and in this way increasing the cell's water content; others seem to act primarily on the membrane itself; still others act perhaps in more ways than one. Another altogether different approach has been to use drugs known to increase the formation of Hb F.

There is, of course, a vast difference between adding a chemical to a suspension of erythrocytes *in vitro* and observing a reduction in sickling, or inhibiting the gelation of Hb S in solution, and administering the same chemical to a patient orally or parenterally in a sufficient dosage to affect him favourably without exposing him to unwanted toxic side-effects. The chemical has first to penetrate the erythrocyte membrane. If it is able to do this, and perhaps inhibit to some extent the aggregation of Hb S, it has to do this without damaging other proteins in the body to a significant degree: to be more specific, it has to exert a favourable effect in a dosage that does not produce other unwanted effects — on, for instance, the nervous system. Then, if the chemical shifts the O_2-dissociation curve of the left — which would favour the maintenance of the haemoglobin in the oxy form at the partial pressure of oxygen in the peripheral vessels — it must not do this so effectively that the oxygen delivery to the tissues is impaired. Moreover, for a drug to be really valuable, it needs to be administered on a continuous basis, perhaps daily, in order to prevent crises or other complications developing — which is a much better form of therapy than attempting to alleviate a crisis or other event *after* it has occurred. Prevention implies life-long therapy and for this to be acceptable to the patient the regime of treatment has to be a simple one and one in which he or she has confidence; and the treatment must give rise to few, if possible no, undesirable side-effects. The

difficulty in finding such a drug can be readily understood.

One way of avoiding the toxic effects on the body as a whole of a drug known to inhibit sickling is to expose a portion of the patient's blood to the drug extracorporeally and then to reinfuse it back into the patient. This type of technique has in fact been quite widely used in an experimental fashion and good results have been obtained with several drugs (see below), *i.e.*, the blood after treatment has been shown to survive better in the patient than before it was exposed to the drug. However, the result of transfusing normal blood to the patient in what would amount to be a partial exchange-transfusion would ordinarily be even better — except for the possibility of the transmission of disease and the building up of antibodies against blood-cell antigens that the patient does not possess. Nevertheless, it is difficult to imagine that the extracorporeal drug-exposure technique will ever be widely used as a routine form of therapy.

Later in this Chapter the story of attempts at treating sickle-cell disease patients with a variety of chemicals and drugs will be summarized. No attempt, however, will be made to list all the chemicals and drugs which have been shown to affect sickling *in vitro*: the emphasis will be primarily on those which have also been given to Hb-SS patients in the course of clinical trials or have been administered for other reasons to patients not suffering from sickle-cell disease. Before, however, dealing with individual chemicals or drugs (in alphabetical order), reference will be made to some valuable reviews which have dealt in a general way with the problem of the use of chemicals and drugs in the treatment of the complications of sickle-cell disease or in their prevention.

Beutler (1974) discussed therapeutic strategy in an interesting short review. He pointed out that when an agent reduces sickling a relevant question is whether it does this by lowering the concentration of reduced haemoglobin at any given oxygen tension by a left shift in the O_2-dissociation curve — an effect common to many agents — or whether the agent has, perhaps in addition, a more direct effect. He concluded that all treatments which shift the O_2-dissociation curve to the left should be useful despite the consequent lowering of tissue pO_2; and he stressed that the main problem for the patient is not tissue hypoxia but impaired blood flow through the smallest blood vessels brought about by the sickling process.

Sunshine, Hofrichter and Eaton (1978) discussed the requirements for the therapeutic inhibition of the gelation of Hb S and the importance of the time between the initiation of gelling and the appearance of the polymer — the delay time. They stressed that this is sensitive to a wide range of physiological variables, *e.g.*, total haemoglobin concentration, pH, salt concentration and temperature, and also that it is extremely sensitive to the presence of other haemoglobins, such as Hb A or, particularly, Hb F. In mixtures of Hb S and Hb A, as found in Hb-S/β^+-thalassaemia with 15–30% Hb A, the delay time would be 10–100 times greater than with pure Hb S. They pointed out that for real therapeutic benefit an effect on the delay time of this order would be required — and would be difficult to achieve.

Dean and Schechter (1978) pointed out that it was widely appreciated at the time of writing their review that increasing the amount of non-gelling haemoglobin in Hb-SS disease patients would, or should, ameliorate their symptoms; the question was how to do this effectively and safely. In a useful Table they classified potential anti-sickling gelation inhibitors into those bringing about inhibition of haemoglobin intermolecular contacts (by non-co-valent or co-valent interactions) and those decreasing the amount of deoxy Hb S present (by increasing the O_2 affinity of Hb S or by decreasing its concentration). In addition, they referred to the agents which, by acting on the erythrocyte membrane, may inhibit sickling independently of any anti-gelling effect and also to the possibility of modifying the clinical consequences of sickling by agents which act on the microvascular entrapment of sickled cells. They discussed the many chemicals which affect gelling or sickling in one way or another and which had been, or were being, investigated, and they stressed the paramount importance of properly conducted clinical trials and of prior well-conducted toxicity tests on animals.

They stressed, too, the need for accurate techniques for measuring quantitatively the effect of drugs and chemicals on gelling and sickling.

Maugh (1981) emphasized at the time he wrote his review that 'the prospects for a successful therapy for sickle cell disease never looked better'. He based this rather optimistic view not on a 'medical miracle in the pipeline' but rather because of the greatly increased understanding of the molecular and atomic interactions that trigger the sickle-cell crisis and the availability of accurate techniques for assaying the effectiveness of new drugs *in vitro*; he also mentioned the improved possibilities of carrying out organized programmes to test in controlled trials the efficacy of new drugs. He suggested that combinations of drugs might be used in the future and stressed that for an agent to be effective it should be given prophylactically and that such an agent, given on a daily basis, must be very safe to use.

Klotz, Haney and King (1981), in a more detailed review of the many ways in which sickling can be affected, and the numerous chemicals and drugs that inhibit sickling or gelation of Hb S *in vitro*, referred in particular to aspirin, which acetylates haemoglobin weakly, and to the possibility of creating more effective acylsalicylates by chemical modification. The synthesis of double-headed aspirins was mentioned; 'dibromoaspirin' had, for instance, been found to be far more active in modifying haemoglobin than ordinary aspirin.

Chang and co-workers (1983) described how they had carried out a comparative in-vitro evaluation of 15 anti-sickling compounds, determining for each compound at two or three concentrations (2–100 mM) their effect on the solubility of deoxy Hb S, on sickling at various O_2 partial pressures, on the O_2 affinity of Hb S and of Hb-SS whole blood, and on erythrocyte morphology. Four of the drugs, urea, butylurea, L-phenylalanine and cetiedil citrate, were non-co-valent (characterized by the ease in which the drugs' effect could be removed by dialysis or washing); of these, butylurea was the most effective but it had to be present at a relatively high concentration (20–50 mM). Of the co-valent drugs tested, bis-(3,5 dibromosalicyl)-fumarate, nitrogen mustard and dimethyladipimidate, at 2–10 mM concentration, were the most potent inhibitors of gelation and/or sickling. Chang *et al.* stressed that all the compounds they had tested needed to be further developed before they could be considered for clinical use; none was an 'optimal agent'; some might have a practical application.

Rodgers, Noguchi and Schechter (1985) reviewed the possibilities available for the in-vivo assessment of the results of clinical trials of anti-sickling agents and pointed out that it was now possible to characterize regional organ perfusion and tissue biochemistry quantitatively by non-invasive techniques. They mentioned the use of bicycle ergometry to measure exercise tolerance, laser-Doppler velocimetry to measure cutaneous blood flow, positron emission tomography to measure, for instance, brain perfusion, magnetic resonance imaging for delineating physical and chemical variation in tissues, retinal fluorescein angiography, thermography and transcutaneous pO_2 measurement.

CHEMICALS AND DRUGS THAT HAVE BEEN USED: IN ALPHABETICAL ORDER

Acetazolamide (Diamox)

Tomlinson and Jacob (1945) stated that if erythrocytes capable of sickling were washed in normal saline and then resuspended in saline or plasma they would undergo sickling provided they had not been washed more than 5 times in the saline; and they suggested that prolonged washing removes a substance from the cells necessary for sickling and that this substance might be carbonic anhydrase.

Hilkovitz (1957) reported that the carbonic anhydrase inhibitor acetazolamide inhibits sickling *in vitro* and that when administered to an 8-month-old infant it diminished the number of sickled cells in the peripheral blood. Subsequent reports, however, have indicated that it is probably of no value, at least in doses that can be tolerated by the patient (Gailitis *et al.*, 1957; dos Santos and Lehmann, 1959; MacDougall and Jacob, 1959).

β-adrenergic blockers

Ohnishi and co-workers (1982) reported that in relatively high concentrations dichloroisoprotenol (DCI) and propanolol inhibit sickling *in vitro*; the drugs, too, were found to have some effect on the delay time of gelation of Hb S and on oxygen affinity. Sickling was reduced to approximately two-thirds of the non-drug level by 500 mM propanolol and to one-third by 5 mM DCI. Ohnishi *et al.* mentioned that these levels could not, however, be obtained safely *in vivo*.

Alkylureas

Elbaum and co-workers (1974, 1976) reported that alkylureas (methyl, ethyl, propyl and butyl) in 0.05–0.1 M concentration are able to inhibit the gelation of Hb S and sickling without denaturing the haemoglobin. Oxygen affinity is affected only minimally, as are osmotic fragility, GSH concentration and GSH reductase activity. Their effectiveness was found to increase with increase in the length of the alkyl chain, and their action was thought to substantiate the importance of hydrophobic interactions in the polymerization of Hb S. Harrington and Nagel (1977) reported on the effects of alkylureas and nitrogen mustards on the kinetics of sickling. Butylurea was found to lengthen the time required for sickling and to inhibit its extent; nitrogen mustard inhibited sickling without modifying the rate. Harrington and Nagel concluded that both types of chemical, if cautiously developed, might be clinically useful.

Amino acids

Rumen (1975) reported that L-homoserine, L-asparagine and L-glutamine inhibited sickling *in vitro* at 0.02 M concentrations. Noguchi and Schechter (1977) stated that phenylalanine was 2–5 times as effective on a molar basis as urea in inhibiting the gelation of Hb S.

Aspirin

Aspirin has been given to sickle-cell disease patients on many occasions. While some early results suggested that it was of value, controlled double-blind trials have not substantiated this.

According to Klotz and Tam (1973), incubation of Hb S (or Hb A) with aspirin leads to acetylation of haemoglobin and an increase in its O_2 affinity. They suggested in view of this that aspirin might ameliorate the severity of Hb-SS disease *in vivo*. de Furia and co-workers (1973), however, reported that aspirin makes no difference to the O_2 affinity of Hb S in intact erythrocytes either *in vitro* or *in vivo* and they concluded that there was no basis for thinking that aspirin might be useful in the treatment of Hb-SS disease patients. Walder and co-workers (1977), however, found that dibromosalicylic acid has a direct inhibiting effect on sickling as well as increasing the O_2 affinity of the acetylated haemoglobin.

Osamo, Photiades and Famodu (1981) reported quite marked improvement in a group of 50 Hb-SS patients in Benin, Nigeria, given 1.2 g of soluble aspirin daily in divided doses, compared with 50 patients not treated with the drug. [Both series of patients received paludrine and folic acid, too.] The mean haemoglobin, O_2 saturation and pO_2 of the capillary blood of the treated patients rose and there was a fall in erythrocyte 2,3-DPG, and they became less jaundiced. In three patients the mean erythrocyte life-span was reported to be more than doubled. Two subsequent trials (see below), however, have failed to show that aspirin therapy is of any benefit.

Greenberg and co-workers (1983) carried out a double-blind crossover study of the possible effectiveness of low doses of aspirin in 49 children and adolescents suffering from sickle-cell disease (40 Hb SS; eight Hb SC, and one Hb SO Arab). The patients were asked to take aspirin pills (81 mg, equivalent to 3–6 mg/kg) or placebo pills matched in appearance and taste, daily, morning and evening. During the 21 months of study, 70% of the patients had a maximum of two painful crises; 25% experienced four or more. Their frequency and severity did not appear to be influenced by taking aspirin, and Greenberg et al. concluded, because of the known influence of aspirin on platelet function, that platelets do not contribute to the initiation or progression of the vaso-occlusive process. Zago and co-workers (1984), too, failed to show that taking aspirin was of any value in a double-blind trial completed by 29 patients (25 Hb SS and four Hb-S/β^0-thalassaemia). The median daily dose of aspirin (31 mg/kg) was higher than in the trial of Greenberg et al. (1983), but no differences were noted in the two phases of the trial — aspirin or placebo — in the incidence of painful crises and infective episodes, in haemoglobin, PCV, reticulocyte count, Hb F and serum bilirubin, in ISC count, filterability and sickling of erythrocytes in vitro and in K^+ loss induced by hypoxia.

Bepridil

A preliminary report on bepridil, like cetiedil a membrane-acting agent, was given by Reilly and Asakura (1986). Like cetiedil, it causes the erythrocyte to swell and lowers the MCHC, and like cetiedil it inhibits the interaction of calmodulin with the cell membrane. It increases the intracellular Na^+ concentration and reduces that of K^+; it has no effect on the minimum gelling concentration of Hb S or on its O_2-dissociation curve. Bepridil is remarkable in that it inhibits sickling in vitro even when present at a molar ratio of drug to intracellular haemoglobin of less than 0.02. It causes 50% inhibition of sickling at 80 μM

concentration — this is half the concentration of cetiedil required for a similar degree of inhibition.

BW 12C (5-[2-formyl-3-hydroxyphenoxyl] pentanoic acid)

This aromatic aldehyde was shown by Kenny and Stuart (1983) to increase the deformability of Hb-SS erythrocytes at a concentration of 1.5 mM at all levels of deoxygenation below normal arterial pO_2, while at concentrations of 3.0 and 5.0 mM it completely prevented any reduction in deformity of cells exposed to a pO_2 level below that of normal venous blood. The chemical inhibits sickling in vitro and is known to bind to haemoglobin and stabilize it in the oxy comformation.

Keiden and co-workers (1986) described how they had given the drug to eight volunteers with Hb-SS disease or Hb-S/β-thalassaemia. The O_2-dissociation curve of their haemoglobin was shown to be shifted to the left when the drug was administered intravenously and at the highest dose given (20 mg/kg) up to 23% of the Hb S was calculated to have been modified to the high-affinity form. There was some evidence of a transient decrease in haemolysis. Keiden et al. pointed out that any reduction in oxygen delivery to the tissues might result in an increase in erythrocyte mass and whole-blood viscosity and that patients receiving BW 12C would need to be carefully watched to ensure that any rise in blood viscosity did not negate the benefit of increased erythrocyte deformability.

Cepharanthine

This is a bisbenzylisoquinoline alkaloid that has been used in Japan in the treatment of snake bite and has been found to produce few side-effects when given in large doses and over a long period of time. It was reported by Sato and Ohnishi (1982) to have an anti-sickling effect of the same order as that of chlorpromazine. The drug does not affect O_2 affinity or the delay time of the gelation of Hb S, and Sato and Ohnishi suggested that it exerted its effect through a membrane-linked reaction. Ohnishi (1983) found that cepharanthine at a 15 μM concentration inhibited by 50% the formation of ISCs created in vitro by submitting Hb-SS cells to repeated oxygenation-deoxygenation cycles.

Cetiedil

This drug, a smooth muscle relaxant, has been used to obtain symptomatic relief in intermittent claudication and Raynaud's phenomena. According to Asakura et al. (1980), Cabannes stated at the International Symposium on Vascular Disease held in Rome in February 1977 that cetiedil also inhibited sickling. This report led to the effect of the drug on erythrocytes being intensively studied. Benjamin, Kokkini and Peterson (1980) found that the drug inhibits sickling *in vitro* and improves the filterability of Hb-SS erythrocytes in a dose-dependent manner, the optimum concentration being 20–200 μM. No adverse effect on the survival of drug-treated erythrocytes was found in dogs and in four human patients with Hb-SS disease, in three of whom a slight increase in the ^{51}Cr T_{50} was noted. The drug did not appear to have an effect on the gelation of Hb S or affect its oxygen affinity, and it was suggested that it affected sickling through an action on the erythrocyte membrane.

Asakura and co-workers (1980) independently reached the same conclusions. They found that in a 140 μM concentration cetiedil causes 50% inhibition of sickling irrespective of whether the drug is added before or after sickling had occurred. The O_2-dissociation curve did not seem to be significantly altered and the minimum gelling concentration of Hb S was found to be increased by less than 10% in the presence of 218 μM cetiedil. Asakura *et al*. noted that erythrocytes treated with high concentrations of the drug became swollen and spheroidal and they concluded that it might be affecting the cells' membrane.

The mode of action of cetiedil has been studied in further detail by several groups of workers. Its failure to affect the oxygen affinity and gelation of Hb S has been confirmed, and it has been shown to act by causing an increase in intracellular cation concentration and a consequent gain in cell water. The haemoglobin concentration is thus reduced. Preliminary clinical trials have indicated that *in vivo* the drug can have a favourable effect on the course of vaso-occlusive crises (see below).

Berkowitz and Orringer (1981, 1982) concluded that cetiedil inhibits the specific increase in K^+ permeability that follows a rise in cytoplasmic Ca^{2+} and that it causes, too, a rise in passive Na^+ movement, *i.e.* in Na^+ influx, both changes tending to lower the concentration of Hb S.

Schmidt, Asakura and Schwartz (1982a,b) emphasized the importance of ATP. With fresh cells, cetiedil in a concentration exceeding 100 μM was found to cause the movement of Na^+ and K^+ to increase considerably, with the cell swelling due to gain in Na^+ exceeding loss of K^+; when ouabain was added to the system, Na^+ gain and K^+ loss, and net gain in water, were all increased. External Ca^{2+} inhibited the cetiedil-induced changes, and with cells depleted of ATP cetiedil was found to inhibit the K^+ loss occasioned by the presence of external Ca^{2+}. Schmidt, Asakura and Schwartz concluded that the changes induced by cetiedil are complex and that their data supported the hypothesis that its anti-sickling effect *in vitro* results from dilution of the Hb S secondary to net intracellular gain in cation and water.

Berkowitz and Orringer (1984) investigated the part played by calcium in the ionic and water changes which take place when erythroytes are exposed to cetiedil. They concluded that the drug inhibits the Gardos phenomenon — the accelerated transmembrane movement of K^+ and Cl^- following a rise in intracellular Ca^{2+}. Their studies indicated that cetiedil does not prevent the accumulation of Ca^{2+} by Hb-S-containing erythrocytes; it acts, they concluded, by 'the opening of the K-specific gate in the erythrocyte membrane'. The effect appeared to be irreversible as it could not be reversed by repeatedly washing the cells.

Benjamin and co-workers (1983, 1986) have described the results of a carefully conducted double-blind randomized trial of cetiedil given in an attempt· to alleviate the severity of vaso-occlusive crises. Sixty-seven patients with sickle-cell disease (87% Hb SS) giving a history of vaso-occlusive crises of 4–24 hours' duration were treated with cetiedil at a concentration of 0.2, 0.3 or 0.4 mg/kg (or given a placebo) by means of a 30-minute intravenous infusion every 8 hours for 4 days. The effect of the treatment (or placebo) on the number of painful sites, on pain intensity scores and on the duration of the crises was carefully recorded. The results were considered to be 'excellent or good' in 85% of the patients who had recieved the largest (0.4 mg/kg) dose of cetiedil compared with 25% of the patients who had received the placebo. Possible side-effects — headache, nausea and vomiting and a dry mouth — were noted in all four groups, but they were not serious. Benjamin *et al*. concluded that cetiedil could be given safely and that its use had resulted in a measurable improvement; they stressed, however, the need for more trials, with objective criteria of effect rigorously adhered to, before cetiedil should be made generally available to practising physicians.

Cyanate

Kilmartin and Rossi-Bernardi (1971) showed that cyanate at 0.01–0.1 M concentration caused the progressive carbamylation of terminal NH_2 groups of horse haemoglobin and increased its oxygen affinity. Cerami and Manning (1971) reported that potassium cyanate (KCNO) irreversibly inhibited the sickling of Hb-S-containing erythrocytes and that the concentration of cyanate necessary to achieve this (0.01–0.1 M) was much less than the required concentration of urea (1M). A concentration of KCNO as little as 5 mM was also found to cause detectable inhibition of the gelling of Hb S, and carbamylation of the terminal valine residues was considered to be responsible for this. Cerami and Manning concluded that KCNO might be used to prevent sickling *in vivo*, and they established that the presence of several carbamyl groups on the haemoglobin molecule, although inhibiting sickling, does not affect the molecule's ability to bind and release oxygen and transport carbon dioxide.

It was soon established that cyanate affected sickling by increasing the affinity of the haemoglobin molecule for oxygen, so that at any partial pressure of oxygen more of the haemoglobin would be in the oxy form and less in the deoxy form of Hb S than normal (Diederich *et al.*, 1971; Diederich and Milam, 1972). Sickling at tissue oxygen tensions would thus be significantly reduced (May *et al.*, 1972).

The metabolism of cyanate-treated erythrocytes was studied by de Furia *et al.* (1972): glycolysis, ATP and 2,3-DPG concentration, and osmotic fragility and rate of autohaemolysis, were not affected; K^+ loss was less than that of untreated cells; PK activity was decreased by approximately 25%, but the activity of all other enzymes studied appeared not to be affected. The Bohr effect was unaltered and the pH was not changed. Glader and Conrad (1972), however, observed irreversible inactivation of G6PD, and a fall in GSH concentration when erythrocytes were exposed to 10–50 mM cyanate.

Gillette, Manning and Cerami (1971) reported the interesting finding that cyanate-treated Hb-SS erythrocytes, carbamylated *in vitro*, would survive much better *in vivo* after such treatment than before. In seven subjects the mean ^{51}Cr T_{50} increased from 9.9 to 20.7 days, indicating that the anti-sickling effect produced by cyanate *in vitro* was retained even if the treated cells were returned to the circulation. This, in their view, provided a rationale for the possible therapeutic use of cyanate.

The work summarized above gave rise to much experimental work in man and in animals, mainly directed to the possible therapeutic value of cyanate and to the way in which it interferes with sickling [see reviews of Cerami (1972), Gillette, Lu and Peterson (1973), Peterson and Cerami (1974) and Harkness and Roth (1975)]. It soon became clear, however, that cyanate forms firm co-valent bonds with functional groups of a variety of proteins. Thus Crist and co-workers (1972), in experiments with rats, showed that cyanate and carbamyl phosphate caused the carbamylation of brain and liver proteins to a varying extent, in addition to haemoglobin. The effects of the administration of cyanate *in vivo*, in doses large enough to have a significant action on haemoglobin, on this evidence thus seemed unlikely to be confined to haemoglobin, and this has in fact been found to be so, particularly in relation to the nervous system (see later).

Life-span of cyanate-treated erythrocytes

The relatively much improved survival *in vivo* of erythrocytes treated with cyanate *in vitro* that was reported by Gillette, Manning and Cerami (1971) was soon confirmed (Alter, Kan and Nathan, 1972; May *et al.*, 1972; Milner and Charache, 1973).

Alter, Kan and Nathan (1972) followed the survival of two 50-ml samples of the blood of two Hb-SS patients. One sample from each patient was labelled (via the reticulocytes) with [^{14}C] leucine and the other with [^3H] leucine, and one sample from each was carbamylated with cyanate (CNO) before both samples were reinfused into the donors. The T_{50} of the carbamylated cells was approximately trebled, but remained below normal — 14 days, increased to 50 days (with CNO) in one patient; 10 days, increased to 28 days (with CNO) in the other. [This technique has the advantage that the comparisons are carried out simultaneously (and not sequentially as in ^{51}Cr studies) and it avoids any error caused by carbamylation possibly affecting the rate of chromium elution.]

Milner and Charache (1973) carried out similar studies: they avoided ^{51}Cr and used instead DFP labelled in three ways, with ^{3}H, ^{14}C and [32]P. They established that the increase in life-span following carbamylation is proportional to the concentration of cyanate; also that the carbamylation exerts its best effect on young (relatively undamaged) erythrocytes, and that, in contrast, the life-span of (already severely damaged) ISCs is not affected. Milner and Charache concluded from their data that at the levels of carbamylation likely to be achieved by taking cyanate orally only a modest improvement in life-span could be expected.

Castro and co-workers (1973b), in a discussion of the possible value of assessing the survival of human erythrocytes after transfusion to rats (with artificially reduced RE-cell function and complement activity), stated that the survival of Hb-S-containing erythrocytes was improved by carbamylation with cyanate. This did not, however, prevent their accelerated removal in hypoxic animals.

The above-quoted studies indicated that carbamylation *in vitro* at the concentrations of cyanate used, and at the temperature of exposure, did not affect adversely (at least in a major way) the life-span of the treated cells after reinfusion into human subjects. [If there were any adverse effects their consequences were being submerged by the beneficial effect of inhibiting sickling.] In rabbits, the experiments of Lane and Burka (1976) indicated that, as expected, any damage due to cyanate is dose-dependent. Thus when erythrocytes were exposed to 30–50 mM cyanate their life-span was reduced by 40–65% while the life-span of cells exposed to 15 mM cyanate for 30 minutes at 4°C was unaltered.

Effect of cyanate on erythrocyte deformability and morphology

Durocher and co-workers (1974) reported that carbamylation decreased the filtration time of both Hb-SS cells and Hb-AA cells through 3 μm polycarbonate filters and postulated that this was brought about by cyanate binding to, and carbamylating, cell membrane proteins as well as haemoglobin. They suggested that the improved life-span *in vivo* of cyanate-treated erythrocytes might be related to improvement in their rheological properties apart from an effect on haemoglobin.

According to Wagner *et al.* (1975), the morphology of normal and carbamylated Hb-SS cells is the same over a wide range of oxygen tensions. They found, too, that the filterability of cyanate-treated erythrocytes was improved over a wide range of oxygen tensions, *i.e.* from 10 to 50% O_2 saturation. They suggested that carbamylation results in more haemoglobin molecules being 'relaxed' at a given oxygen tension and/or that carbamylation interferes with the apposition of the binding sites required for polymerization.

Results of treating Hb-SS patients with cyanate. Gillette and co-workers (1972, 1974) and Peterson and co-workers (1973) gave an account of their early results when sodium cyanate was administered orally. Thirty-one patients, 7–49 years of age, were treated at a dose range of 10–35 mg/kg daily over a 6–18-month period. At first the results of treatment seemed promising; and the drug appeared to cause no substantial toxic effects, except occasionally to produce gastro-intestinal symptoms or drowsiness. However, in a footnote to Gillette and co-workers' (1974) paper it was stated that six out of the 14 patients who had received 35 mg/kg daily (a high dose), or more, had developed a neuropathy and had lost weight (see later). Before the possible development of a neuropathy was appreciated, it looked as if the treatment had no great effect on the clinical state of the patients. It seemed, however, that the frequency of crises might have been reduced, particularly in those receiving high doses of cyanate. The haemoglobin of the 16 patients on a low-dose regime was unaffected, but in those receiving a high dose there was a small rise: before treatment their mean haemoglobin was 8.2 g/dl, after treatment 9.3 g/dl, and one patient achieved a haemoglobin within the normal range. Gillette *et al.* (1972) had reported a fall in serum bilirubin.

The reports quoted above suggested that to achieve any worthwhile result with orally administered cyanate high doses would have to be given; and the development of neuropathy was a severe blow to the hope that cyanate taken orally would prove to be of real practical value.

Peterson and co-workers (1974) and Peterson and Cerami (1974) described the results of a detailed neurophysiological study on 27 patients. Of those who had received high doses of cyanate (mean 38 mg/kg/day for a mean duration of 478 days), 16 were found to have nerve conduction defects; in contrast, no such defects were demonstrable in the remaining 11 patients who had received smaller doses for shorter periods (mean 33 mg/kg/day for a mean duration of 278 days). Those on the higher doses, too, lost 9% of their pretreatment weight. Clinically, the neuropathy led to weakness, paraesthesiae, numbness and impaired sensation; histological examination revealed demyelination. Details of two patients were given whose neuropathy improved when the cyanate treatment was stopped.

The potentially toxic effects of cyanate were underlined by a study carried out on rats by Alter, Kan and Nathan (1974b). The animals lost weight, and they became lethargic and developed diarrhoea and spasticity, particularly of their hind limbs. The neuromuscular system appeared to be more sensitive than the haemopoietic, as the animals were able to respond to the carbamylation-induced increase in haemoglobin oxygen affinity. *In vitro*, however, cyanate could be shown to inhibit haemoglobin synthesis (Alter, Kan and Nathan, 1974a).

A further blow to the clinical use of cyanate was the report by Nicholson *et al.* (1976) of the development of cataracts in two relatively young patients. The first, who suffered from Hb-S/β-thalassaemia, developed visual symptoms 4 months after the start of a second course of cyanate treatment; the second, who had Hb-SS disease, developed lesions after about 15 months of treatment.

Extracorporeal treatment of Hb-SS erythrocytes with cyanate. The manifest dangers of the oral administration of cyanate led to the idea that it might, nevertheless, be worthwhile exposing *in vitro* part of a patient's erythrocyte mass periodically to cyanate and then reinfusing it, thereby, hopefully, sparing the patients from the general toxic effects of the chemical.

Diederich, Gill and Lawson (1974) and Diederich and co-workers (1976) treated 10 patients in this way. The results were promising. Approximately 20% of the erythrocyte mass was exposed to cyanate each week throughout a 2-year period. Referring to eight patients who had been treated in this way for more than 2 years, Diederich *et al.* (1976) reported that after about 3 months 35–50% of the circulating erythrocytes were carbamylated. The patients' mean whole-blood $p_{50}O_2$ fell from 33 to 26 mm Hg; their mean haemoglobin rose

from 6.4 g/dl to 9.13 g/dl, and the absolute reticulocyte and ISC counts fell by 58 and 63%, respectively. The mean erythrocyte life-span increased from 13.0 to 21.6 days. There were no toxic effects and the frequency of painful crises appeared to be substantially reduced (by about 80%). The incidence of crises seemingly provoked by infections decreased by approximately 50% while that of those of unexplained origin fell almost to zero.

Langer and co-workers (1976) subjected four patients to a similar, although not identical, regime. Every 4–6 weeks the patients underwent a series of venesections of about one-tenth of their blood volume; the venesected erythrocytes were carbamylated and reinfused the following day. The venesections were carried out in clusters, *i.e.*, daily until the $p_{50}O_2$ had fallen to approximately 20 mm Hg. The patient was then observed until the $p_{50}O_2$ had risen to 24–26 mm Hg when the series of venesections was repeated. This regime led to the patients having a population of cells with a high oxygen affinity and with a life-span which was only slightly reduced (MCL 38 days). Their mean haemoglobin increased over a 6-month period by 24%, but the serum bilirubin concentration did not fall, and the degree of sickling at any given concentration of oxygen was not altered. The patients stated that they felt that the treatment was of benefit; their painful crises, however, continued. An attempt to assess their frequency and severity by a severity-frequency index indicated a 23% improvement.

A more recent development has been continuous extracorporeal carbamylation carried out at intervals over long periods. Lee and co-workers (1982) and Balcerzak and co-workers (1982) described their preliminary results. Lee *et al.* treated two patients for 4–6 hours every 2 weeks on 15 and 17 occasions, respectively. Their haemoglobin rose slowly, the $p_{50}O_2$ fell significantly and the ^{51}Cr T_{50} increased. The amount of cyanate returned to the patient was small and the nervous system and eyes appeared to be unaffected. Before each treatment 40–60% of the erythrocytes were not carbamylated and Lee *et al.* concluded that to obtain a higher degree of carbamylation more frequent treatments would be necessary. Balzerzak *et al.* (1982) treated four patients similarly, exposing their blood extracorporeally to cyanate for up to 6 hours and achieving, as had Lee *et al.*, carbamylation levels of 1–2 mol per mol of haemoglobin tetramer. The treatment was persisted with for more than 1 year in three of the patients with a rise in haemoglobin and a fall in reticulocyte count and $p_{50}O_2$, and possibly with some benefit in a fourth patient. All four patients suffered from headaches, and severe headache, with nausea and vomiting, led to the withdrawal of one of them from the trial. There was no evidence of damage to the nervous system or eyes; on the other hand, the patients did not seem to have derived any clinical benefit from the procedure. Both groups demonstrated the feasibility and safety of continuous extracorporeal carbamylation but did not establish its clinical importance — this was not their aim.

A further elaborate procedure of uncertain clinical relevance was described by Castro, Rana and Poillon (1986) who investigated the possibility of bleeding sickle-cell anaemia patients when in a steady state, carbamylating the withdrawn blood and then cryopreserving it with glycerol and storing it at $-80°C$. Their aim was to create a stockpile of blood that could be used later in an exchange-transfusion to treat the donor in a vaso-occlusive or other crisis. The carbamylated and frozen blood of four patients (three Hb SS and one Hb-S/β-thalassaemia) was stored for periods of 62–153 days and, although about 25% of the erythrocytes were lost during storage, the survival of the remaining cells was found to be almost twice as long as that of fresh cells before carbamylation and storage. At the high concentration of cyanate used, the $p_{50}O_2$ was as low as 13.3 mm Hg (mean) and gelation at zero pO_2 was markedly inhibited, too. Castro, Rana and Poillon pointed out that the success of an exchange-transfusion, in the treatment of a vaso-occlusive crisis, would depend on how the increased blood flow consequent on decreased sickling would compensate for the low unloading of oxygen at tissue O_2 levels.

DBA

Ekong and co-workers (1975) reported that the substance DBA (3,4-dihydro-2,2-dimethyl-2H-l-benzopyran-6-butyric acid), derived via xanthoxylol from a small tree (*Fagara xanthoxyloides*), common in coastal areas of West Africa, prevents sickling and the gelation of Hb S. According to Poillon and Bertles (1977), DBA (and ethanol) increase the solubility of deoxyHb S. Together the two chemicals increase its solubility in an additive fashion. Isaacs-Sodeye and co-workers (1975) administered *Fagara xanthoxyloides* root extract to four Hb-SS patients over a 3-month period and concluded that the treatment, assessed by a 'pain score', gave them grounds for cautious optimism. The potential value of DBA as a therapeutic agent, however, was rendered doubtful by the failure of Honig, Vida and Ferenc (1978) to demonstrate that DBA at a 10 mM concentration had any effect on sickling *in vitro*; it did, however, increase the $p_{50}O_2$ of sickled cells, but only by 3 mm Hg.

Abu, Anyaibe and Headings (1981) reported that chromatographic fractionation of root bark from *Fagara xanthoxyloides* yielded five fractions capable of reversing metabisulphite-induced sickling of Hb-SS erythrocytes *in vitro*.

DMA (dimethyl adipimidate)

Lubin and co-workers (1975) reported that prior treatment of Hb-SS erythrocytes with 5 mM DMA (a bifunctional imidoester) would completely prevent sickling on deoxygenation; they found, too, that the oxygen affinity of the treated cells was increased. According to Pennathur-Das et al. (1978, 1982, 1984), DMA, at pH 7.4, increases the solubility of deoxyHb S and its O_2 affinity, causes inter- as well as intra-tetrameric cross-linking, decreases K^+ leak from hypoxic cells and inhibits the gelation of deoxyHb S in solution. It was found to cause no change in cellular deformability.

Guis and co-workers (1984) described how the in-vitro exposure of the erythrocytes of five Hb-SS patients to dimethyl adipimidate (DMA) greatly improved the survival of the cells when they were transfused back into the donors: the ^{51}Cr T_{50} was normal in four of the patients and only a little reduced (T_{50} 20 days) in the fifth. The experiment was repeated in three of the patients 3–6 months later and in each case the cells' survival was found then to be markedly shortened. This was shown to be the result of the development of an antibody against the DMA-treated cells (Fig. 15.2). The marked improvement in survival in the first series of experiments was superior, according to Guis et al., to that previously achieved by treating Hb-SS erythrocytes *in vitro* with cyanate, urea, zinc, cetiedil, methyl acetimidate or nitrogen mustard.

Ethacrynic acid

This chemical was shown by Castro et al. (1985) to prolong the life-span of Hb-SS erythrocytes transfused into rats. The mean T_{50} of survival was 3.9 hours compared with 2.6 hours when the cells were untreated. Ethacrynic acid was, however, considered not to be suitable for in-vivo use in man because of its diuretic properties. The possibility was raised of using it as an extracorporeal agent.

Glyceraldehyde

Nigen and Manning (1977), reported that DL-glyceraldehyde at 5–10 mM concentrations would reduce the sickling of Hb-SS erythrocytes even in the complete absence of oxygen. Inhibition was time- and concentration-dependent and not reversed by washing the cells with buffer. Incubation of Hb-SS cells with the chemical resulted in a small increase in O_2 affinity, a moderate reduction in the Hill coefficient and a substantial increase in the minimum concentration of deoxyHb S required for gelling. Nigen and Manning concluded that the main effect of DL-glyceraldehyde was a reduction in the ability of deoxyHb S to polymerize — they

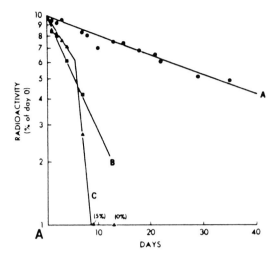

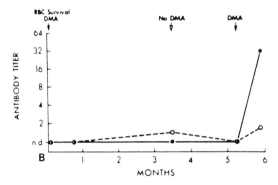

Fig. 15.2 Survival of ^{51}Cr-labelled autologous erythrocytes in an adult Hb-SS patient.

Upper chart: A: DMA-treated cells (first exposure); B: Control, untreated cells; C: DMA-treated cells (second exposure).

Lower chart: development of antibodies to DMA-treated erythrocytes. Continuous line: antiglobulin test. Interrupted line: low ionic strength saline test (37°).

[Reproduced by permission from Guis *et al.* (1984).]

had demonstrated modification of up to two lysine residues per molecule of haemoglobin. They pointed out, too, that the chemical had been used in animals as an anti-tumour agent and speculated that it might be of therapeutic use in man in Hb-SS disease. In a later paper, Nigen and Manning (1978), however, concluded that it was premature to consider clinical studies. They reported that the D and L isomers of glyceraldehyde were equally effective in inhibiting sickling *in vitro*, but found that neither could reverse the sickling of cells already sickled as the result of deoxygenation. The viscosity of cells treated with 5–20 mM DL-glycer-

aldehyde was shown to be reduced and their filterability improved.

Benjamin and Manning (1986) demonstrated an improvement in the survival *in vivo* of Hb-SS erythrocytes exposed *in vitro* to glyceraldehyde at a 10 or 20 mM concentration: the mean ^{51}Cr T_{50} of the treated cells of five patients was 9.0 ± 1.4 days compared with 5.8 ± 1.6 days, in the case of the untreated cells. Benjamin and Manning stressed the need for extensive toxicity trials before contemplating treating Hb-SS patients with glyceraldehyde by the oral or parenteral route.

Methyl acetimidate (MAI)

This compound inhibits the sickling of Hb-SS erythrocytes even when completely deoxygenated (Chao, Berenfeld and Gabuzda, 1976). Gabuzda and co-workers (1980) later reported on the effect on the survival *in vivo* of Hb-SS erythrocytes that had been exposed to the drug *in vitro*. The ^{51}Cr T_{50} was substantially increased in 10 out of 13 patients, the mean T_{50} being prolonged from 8.4 ± 1.1 days to 24.4 ± 4.6 days. However, five of the patients developed antibodies against the MAI-treated cells, which reduced the survival times of treated cells in later studies. [See above for a similar immune response to DMA-treated cells.]

Nitrogen mustard (HN$_2$) and nor-nitrogen mustard (nor-HN$_2$)

HN$_2$ inhibits sickling *in vitro* and in increasing concentration causes a progressive rise in the minimum concentration of Hb S in solution required for gelling on deoxygenation (Roth, 1972). The chemical was thought to interfere with the polymerization of Hb-S molecules but to have little effect on O$_2$ affinity or haem-to-haem interaction. Roth and co-workers (1975) investigated the effect *in vitro* of HN$_2$ and nor-HN$_2$ on the metabolism of rabbit erythrocytes. Nor-HN$_2$ at 10 mg/ml concentration did not appear to affect the metabolism or the function of the erythrocytes: HN$_2$, on the other hand, inhibited GSH reductase and alkylated GSH, and the in-vivo survival of rabbit erythrocytes so treated was impaired. The O$_2$ affinity of haemoglobin did not appear to be altered by either compound. It was concluded that nor-HN$_2$ might be used to treat Hb-SS erythrocytes extracorporeally.

Charache and co-workers (1976) experimented with dog erythrocytes and found that the survival of nor-HN$_2$-treated cells was reduced by about one-half. They suggested that if alkylation of Hb-SS cells was attempted *in vitro* the blood should be rendered lymphocyte-free so as to avoid the possibility of transfusing back alkylated and potentially mutated (but still viable) lymphocytes.

Oligopeptides

Yang (1975) suggested that oligopeptides which mimicked portions of the amino-acid sequence of the β^S-globin chain might conceivably be used therapeutically by competing for binding sites between Hb-S molecules so as to interfere with the gelation of Hb S when deoxygenated. Kubota and Young (1977) reported that several oligopeptide amides which mimicked the NH_2 terminus of the β^S chain did in fact increase the minimum concentration of Hb S required for gelling. How to get the oligopeptides across the membrane of the Hb-S-containing erythrocyte remained to be solved and the possibility was raised of obtaining and using carriers for trans-membrane passage.

Voltano, Gorecki and Rich (1977) reported that a number of tri- and tetrapeptides could be used in this way to inhibit the aggregation and gelation of Hb S *in vitro*. In searching for a therapeutically successful compound, it was stressed: (1) that the chemical must bind sufficiently to the Hb-S molecule to prevent its aggregation, yet not to interfere with the loading and unloading of oxygen, (2) that the chemical must be able to penetrate the cell membrane, and (3) that it must be non-toxic.

Perfluorocarbon compounds

A variety of perfluorocarbon compounds have been developed; all dissolve relatively large amounts of oxygen, and the possibility of using them as blood substitutes has been explored. They appear, too, to have a beneficial effect on the rheological properties of Hb-S-containing erythrocytes (Smith *et al.*, 1983).

Reindorf and co-workers (1985) showed that Fluosol-43 reduced the percentage of Hb-S-containing erythrocytes which sickled when deoxygenated, reduced the viscosity of deoxygenated sickled cells at low shear rates, and increased their deformability as measured by filtration through Nucleopore filters. Both Smith *et al.* (1983) and Reindorf *et al.* (1985) suggested that perfluorocarbon compounds might be of benefit in the treatment of severe vaso-occlusive crises.

Phenothiazines

Bounameaux (1961) reported that the anti-malarial drug Nivaquine and various antihistaminics, *e.g.*, Phenergan, Lactargil, Antistine and Pyribenzamine, were able to inhibit sickling *in vitro*.

This lead was followed up by Lewis (1964) who stated that in-vitro sickling was retarded in six African patients (four Hb SS, two Hb SC) who had been given 100–300 mg of promazine daily; while Hathorn and Lewis (1966) reported that the life-span of the erythrocytes of 11 patients was slightly increased following the administration of the drug in a similar dosage.

Lewis and Gyang (1965) had reported that they had screened 53 phenothiazine derivatives for their ability to inhibit sickling *in vitro* and also to inhibit the enzyme G6PD. Desmethylchlorpromazine was noted to be particularly effective and some correlation was found between the capacity of the drugs to inhibit sickling and their ability to inhibit G6PD. These actions were not, however, correlated with the drugs' tranquillizing action.

Later work, however, has failed to confirm that phenothiazines are of any clinical value — except as inducers of somnolence — or that the life-span of Hb-SS erythrocytes is favourably affected (Pearson and Noyes, 1966; Knight, Woodruff and Pettitt, 1968; Oski, Call and Lessen, 1968; Mahmood, 1969).

More recently, renewed interest has, however, been taken in the anti-sickling effect of anti-psychotic drugs. Ohnishi and co-workers (1981) and Ohnishi (1982b), experimenting with phenothiazine derivatives, including chlorpromazine, demonstrated a linear relationship between their anti-sickling action and inhibition of calmodulin-stimulated phosphodiesterase activity. They suggested that the drugs act on the erythrocyte membrane and that the polymerization of deoxygenated Hb S is influenced by this. The compounds were found to cause the erythrocytes to assume a cup-shaped form at the concentrations they inhibit the sickling of Hb-SS cells.

Piracetam (2-oxo-pyrrolidine acetamide)

Piracetam has been reported to inhibit the sickling of deoxygenated Hb-SS erythrocytes *in vitro* and it has been suggested that, *in vivo*, it may help to alleviate vaso-occlusive crises (de Melo, 1976; de Araujo and Nero, 1977). Costa, Zago and Bottura (1979), however, failed to demonstrate any significant anti-sickling effect. Nalbandian and co-workers (1981, 1983), nevertheless, found that the adherence of Hb-SS cells to cultured rat or human endothelium was diminished in the presence of the drug and suggested, in view of this, and of other evidence, that clinical trials should be carried out.

Asakura and co-workers (1981) reported that Piracetam caused 50% inhibition of sickling, and prolongation of the delay time, at 300 mM concentration; the O_2-equilibrium curve was shifted to the right and there was, too, an anti-gelling effect. Asakura *et al.* drew attention to the relatively high dose of the drug likely to be required for a worthwhile anti-sickling effect *in vivo*.

Procaine hydrochloride

Baker, Powars and Haywood (1974) reported that procaine hydrochloride, a cationic anaesthetic, is able to diminish the rigidity of the membrane of ISCs and that ISCs once formed *in vitro* can be rendered more deformable by procaine. Displacement of membrane-bound calcium was suggested as a possible mechanism of its action.

Pyridoxal and pyridoxine

Pyridoxal-5-phosphate interacts with the amino terminus of the β^S chain and, with this in mind, Beutler, Paniker and West (1972) administered 400 mg of pyridoxine daily to two patients with Hb-SS disease without, however, any discernible effect on their haemoglobin concentration, the ^{51}Cr T_{50} or the $p_{50}O_2$, or on the frequency of painful crises.

Laboratory data on the effect on pyridoxal compounds on the haemoglobin molecule were reported by Benesch, Benesch and Yung (1977) and Benesch et al. (1977). The compounds inhibit gelation by increasing the solubility of Hb S, and 5'-deoxypyridoxal increases the O_2 affinity of haemoglobin. Kark and co-workers (1978) reported that pyridoxal (but not pyridoxine) substantially reduces sickling and considered that this was due to its effect on O_2 affinity, which was equivalent to that of glyceraldehyde. Kark et al. (1982) concluded that exposing erythrocytes to pyridoxal or pyridoxal 5'-phosphate did not cause any severe impairment of the cells' metabolism. Kuranstin-Mills and Lessin (1982) reported that pyridoxine and pyridoxal improved the deformability of Hb-S-containing erythrocytes and reduced the formation of intracellular fibrils when the cells were deoxygenated.

Natta and Reynolds (1983) found that the pyridoxal phosphate (PLP) level in the plasma of 16 Hb-SS patients was subnormal, while that in the erythrocytes was greater than in controls — this was thought to be due perhaps to PLP having a greater affinity for β^S-globin chains than β^A chains. Natta and Reynolds administered 50 mg of pyridoxine twice daily for 1 month to six Hb-SS patients. This resulted in an increase in plasma and erythrocyte pyridoxal-phosphate concentration and a slight rise in haematocrit. It was suggested that pyridoxine given orally to Hb-SS patients might be of benefit.

Ticlopidine

This is an amphiphilic molecule that has been used as a platelet antiaggregant. According to Sablayrolles et al. (1985), it had been shown in a double-blind trial conducted by Cabannes et al. (1981) in the Ivory Coast to protect against the vaso-occlusive crises of sickle-cell disease. The in-vitro studies of Sablayrolles et al. suggest, however, that the drug is unlikely to affect sickling favourably in the concentrations that have been achieved in vivo. The drug binds strongly to the erythocyte membrane and acts, they suggested, as a membrane expander, with the haemoglobin concentration being lowered in consequence of this.

Trental

This is a xanthine derivative (pentoxifylline). According to Ambrus et al. (1985), it was able to prevent vascular occlusion in monkeys transfused with human Hb-SS cells and given air to breathe containing oxygen at a low tension. Ambrus et al. mentioned, too, that a human patient treated with Trental over a 3-year period appeared to have benefited. Trental is thought to inhibit the aggregation of platelets, increase the fluidity of the erythrocyte membrane and release tissue activators of plasminogen and of prostacyclin (PgI$_2$) from the vessel wall.

Urea

The use of urea as an anti-sickling agent was described by Nalbandian et al. in a series of publications in 1971 (e.g., Nalbandian and Evans, 1971; Nalbandian et al., 1971,a,b,c). [In these publications reference was also made to descriptions of the use of urea in Army Medical Research Laboratory Reports published in 1970.] It was already known that in vitro urea in moderately high concentrations (e.g., 0.1–1.0 M) would reduce or abolish the increase in viscosity of solutions of Hb S on deoxygenation by apparently interfering with the aggregation which takes place between molecules of deoxy Hb S.

Nalbandian and co-workers' preliminary reports indicated that sickling in vitro could be blocked and reversed by urea, as illustrated by scanning electron micrographs (Nalbandian et al., 1971b). Equally striking appeared to be the clinical success in terminating crises, which followed the rapid intravenous injection of urea in invert sugar solution, the aim being to achieve a blood urea nitrogen (BUN) level of 1.5–2.0 g/l (Nalbandian et al., 1971c). It was admitted, however, that the diuresis provoked by the treatment needed to be countered by increasing the fluid intake appropriately. Nalbandian and co-workers (1971a) reported on the results of long-term oral therapy given with the aim of preventing the occurence of crises. In 80 patients managed in this way it was stated that the 'frequency of sickle cell crisis has been eliminated', and it was stressed that less urea was required to prevent sickling than to reverse it once it had occurred; hence oral prophylactic treatment was to be preferred to attempts to treat established crises by intravenously administered urea.

These early apparent successes with urea therapy seemed to be confirmed by a preliminary report from McCurdy and Mahmood (1971): 40–320 g of urea in 10% invert sugar were given 24 times to 14 patients in painful crises; 17 of the crises appeared to be terminated. Diuresis was, however, an important consequence, and the BUN levels attained were similar in those who had apparently responded to the treatment as in those who did not improve. McCurdy and Mahmood warned against the real risk of dehydration and advised against treating children; and they stressed that urea therapy could only be regarded as experimental.

Opio and Barnes (1972) treated 23 patients in Africa suffering from bone-pain crises with intravenous 10% invert sugar to which in 12 of them 16% urea had been added. The addition of the urea to the solution of invert sugar appeared not to make any difference to the clinical outcome. Opio and Barnes pointed out, however, that they had achieved lower levels of BUN than had Nalbandian and co-workers and that most of their patients had been in crisis for a relatively long time (mean 59 hours), and also that in seven of the patients receiving urea there was evidence of overt infection.

Segel and co-workers (1972), in a comparative study of the effects of urea and cyanate on sickling *in vitro*, concluded that, although they could demonstrate an inhibiting effect of urea on sickling *in vitro*, the necessary concentration required to bring this about was higher than could possibly be achieved *in vivo*.

Subsequent controlled clinical trials have, too, failed to demonstrate that urea therapy is in fact of any clear value in the treatment or prevention of vaso-occlusive crises — which shows how difficult it is to form accurate judgements of the value of 'new' treatments when attempting to manage patients who develop crises of uncertain duration and in whom assessment of success in treatment is largely subjective. Thus Lubin and Oski (1973) treated 11 children with Hb-SS disease with oral urea for periods of 7 days to 16 months (average 7.8 months) without any clear effect on the incidence of painful crises or frequency of hospital admissions.

Kraus (1973) reported that intravenously administered 100 g/l invert sugar, 50 g/l dextrose in saline,

sodium bicarbonate solution or 0.166 M lactate were just as good as 100–150 g/l urea in the invert sugar solution in the control of vaso-occlusive crises. All the results were, however, considered to be 'less than satisfactory'. Similar results, *i.e.*, that neither urea nor alkali was superior to invert sugar alone in combating painful vaso-occlusive crises were reported by the Cooperative Urea Trials Group (1974a,b). Similarly, the results were negative in a more recent double-blind trial designed to see whether low-dose urea given orally would prevent the onset of crises. In this trial, reported by Gail *et al.* (1982), low-dose urea was compared with high-dose urea and a similarly tasting control. Seventy-nine patients were entered into the trial; the average follow-up time was 13.7 months, and 33 of the patients suffered from one or more crises during the period of the trial. Their haemoglobin and bilirubin and weight, and the time of onset of crises, appeared to be independent of the therapy they were receiving.

The haematological effects of urea treatment have naturally been studied. Bensinger and co-workers (1971) found an increase in CO production as the result of the intravenous infusion of 80–90 g of urea in invert sugar and attributed this to the destruction of sickled cells or to an increase in the turnover of early-labelled haem. Bensinger and co-workers (1972) and Lipp, Rudders and Pisciotta (1972) failed, however, to demonstrate any significant effect on erythrocyte life-span by the ^{51}Cr and DF^{32}P techniques.

May and Huehns (1975) in an in-vitro study of the effect of urea on sickling, in concentrations up to 1M, found that it increased the O_2 affinity of Hb-SS cells (and Hb-AA cells) and deduced that this was the result of the polymerization of Hb-SS molecules being inhibited. However, at the concentrations of urea recommended for treatment the effect was slight. May and Huehns concluded that unless urea in the recommended doses affected sickling by a mechanism other than by an action on haemoglobin, *e.g.*, by an effect perhaps on the erythrocyte membrane, it could be of little use in treatment.

The story of urea therapy is thus one of disappointment. However, although it failed to establish itself as a useful and practical measure, its introduction did lead to consideration of the possible value of cyanate, a contaminant (degradation product) of urea preparations. [According to Cerami and Manning (1971) a solution of 1M urea will contain in equilibrium at 37°C and pH 7.4 cyanate at 5 mM concentration.]

Vitamin E (α-tocopherol)

Chiu and Lubin (1979) and Natta and Machlin (1979) have reported that the vitamin-E concentration in the plasma of Hb-SS patients tends to be low, and with this in mind, Natta, Machlin and Brin (1980) treated six

Hb-SS patients with a daily dose of 450 i.u. of vitamin E (as α-tocopherol) given orally for 6–35 weeks. The plasma level of the vitamin increased and the percentage of circulating ISCs fell from 25 ± 3 to 11 ± 1, and the percentage of ISCs remained below pretreatment levels as long as the vitamin therapy was continued. Natta, Machlin and Brin commented that the practical value of the therapy remained to be determined.

Zinc

The possibility that patients with Hb-SS disease might be deficient in zinc (Serjeant, Galloway and Gueri, 1970; Oelshlegel et al., 1973; Schoomaker et al., 1973; Prasad et al., 1975), and the known ability of zinc to act as an antagonist of calcium, has led to studies of zinc as a possible therapeutic agent in Hb-SS disease. Its practical value remains, however, doubtful at the time of writing. Its possible use has been the subject of several reviews (Brewer, 1976, 1980, 1981).

Serjeant, Galloway and Gueri (1970) reported that they had treated with oral zinc sulphate 17 patients with Hb-SS disease who had leg ulcers and found that healing, although slow, was faster than in a control series of 17 patients who had received a placebo instead of the zinc. Of the treated patients, 13 improved and in six healing was complete compared with eight improved and complete healing in three of the control series. The basis of this treatment was that previous reports had indicated that oral zinc sulphate would accelerate the healing of wounds. Serjeant, Galloway and Gueri also reported that their patients' serum zinc levels were significantly subnormal before treatment; they mentioned, however, that low serum levels had earlier been reported in thalassaemia, pernicious anaemia, malignant disease and chronic infections.

Schoomaker and co-workers (1973) stated that deficiency of zinc causes delayed puberty, a short stature, hypogonadism and delayed healing of chronic leg ulcers and postulated that many of the growth and healing disturbances in Hb-SS diseases were due to deficiency of zinc. They reported that the mean concentrations of zinc in the erythrocytes, plasma and hair were subnormal in 27 adult Hb-SS patients, compared with 22 normal black adults, and that the urinary excretion of zinc was greater in the patients (749 ±

206 μg/day) than in the normal controls (643 ± 198 μg/day).

Prasad and co-workers (1976) estimated erythrocyte and plasma levels of zinc, copper and magnesium in 84 adult Hb-SS patients and confirmed their previous findings; namely, that the erythrocyte and plasma zinc levels tended to be low and that the urinary excretion of zinc was abnormally high. The copper and magnesium levels were probably normal. Prasad et al. reiterated their view that zinc deficiency might be responsible for retardation of growth and hypogonadism in Hb-SS disease. Similar findings, namely, that the plasma zinc concentration is low and the urinary excretion of zinc is high, were reported by Niell, Leach and Kraus (1979) in a series of 34 Hb-SS patients in a steady state and in six patients in a crisis.

Interaction between zinc and calcium. Brewer and Oelshlegel (1974) showed that added zinc improved the filterability of Hb-SS erythrocytes at intermediate O_2 tensions and suggested that this was being brought about by an antagonizing effect on calcium.

Kruckeberg and co-workers (1975) reported that zinc had an effect on the morphology of sickle-cell ghosts — which became 'flat, thin and amorphous', and it was suggested that this was the consequence of the displacement of calcium in the membrane by the zinc. Experimentally, Schoomaker, Brewer and Oelshlegel (1976) were able to show that pretreating rats with zinc improved the survival of human Hb-SS erythrocytes in animals breathing 15–16% oxygen, and also that exposure in vitro of Hb-SS cells to zinc resulted in an increase in their O_2 affinity and an improvement in their survival when injected into rats.

Brewer (1980) discussed the role of the calcium-binding protein calmodulin, and its interaction with spectrin and actin, in the regulation of erythrocyte membrane expansion and contraction and suggested that the beneficial effect of zinc on the sickling of Hb-SS-containing cells was through its inhibiting effect on calcium-activated calmodulin.

Effect of zinc therapy in Hb-SS disease. Brewer, Brewer and Prasad (1975) stated that orally administered zinc reduced the incidence of crises and improved the blood picture and reported that the ISC count fell significantly in three out of five patients after several weeks of therapy. Prasad and co-workers (1975) reported that they had treated seven men and two women with Hb-SS disease with 600 mg of zinc sulphate daily. All but one of the patients gained weight, two 17-year-olds gained in height, five males experienced increased growth of hair, and leg ulcers healed in one patient and were improved in two others. Brewer, Brewer and Prasad (1977) stated that the mean ISC count of 12 patients, treated over a 3–18-month period, fell from 28.0 to 18.6%.

Prasad, Rabbani and Warth (1979) reported that the plasma ammonia level is above normal in Hb-SS disease patients and that this could be lowered by treatment with zinc; and Prasad and co-workers (1981) stated that the administration of zinc is followed by a rise in the serum testosterone level (as well as by an increase in neutrophil zinc and alkaline phosphatase activity). Brewer (1981) suggested that low plasma zinc levels, when present in Hb-SS disease patients, were due to excessive loss of zinc in the urine; he recommended that the giving of daily supplements of zinc to Hb-SS disease children should be seriously considered, not so much to influence the frequency of crises but to improve their growth and development.

TREATMENT DESIGNED TO RAISE HB-F LEVELS

If it were possible to reactivate the γ-globin gene so that the production of Hb F was permanently increased, this would probably be of considerable benefit to a Hb-SS patient. Adamson (1984), in an Editorial, reviewed the background to attempts to achieve this desirable switch from Hb A to Hb F. Azacytidine and hydroxyurea have in fact been administered experimentally to fully informed, severely affected Hb-SS patients in an attempt to raise their Hb-F levels sufficiently to alleviate their symptoms. The results have been moderately encouraging (see below), but whether the benefit will outweigh the drugs' toxicity and carcinogenic potentiality remains to be determined.

5-azacytidine (5-aza)

DeSimone and co-workers (1982) reported that they had administered 5-aza to baboons that had been made anaemic by bleeding to see whether the drug would stimulate the synthesis of Hb F. They

argued that a drug known to inhibit methylation of sequences in DNA might act in this way. They found in fact that the administration of the 5-aza resulted in increases in Hb-F synthesis so that the peak levels of Hb F in the peripheral blood were 6–30 times higher than those achieved by bleeding alone. The main effect was an increase in the amount of Hb F per F cell. Following this observation, Charache and co-workers (1982) administered the drug to a severely affected Hb-SS patient. No clinical or haematological signs of toxicity were detected after three 3-day courses of 90 mg/m^2/day given intravenously in 4 hours on Days 0, 30 and 40. However, the Hb-F percentage in the peripheral blood and the percentage of F-containing cells and the amount of Hb F per cell all substantially increased and there were, too, rises in MCV and MCH and an increase in erythrocyte life-span. Methylation of DNA in nucleated cells retrieved from the peripheral blood was shown to be decreased. Charache et al. suggested that more intensive therapy might raise the Hb-F percentage to a level which could lessen clinical severity.

Ley and co-workers (1983) treated two patients with Hb-SS disease and two with β$^+$-thalassaemia with 5-aza at a dosage of 2 mg/kg/day for 7 days. There was no apparent toxicity and γ:β globin-chain synthesis was shown to increase 4–6-fold as the result of the treatment and to remain elevated for 7–14 days subsequently. The Hb-F percentage increased from 6 to 13.7 and from 1.6 to 8.9, respectively, in the two Hb-SS patients, and Stractan gradient separation revealed a marked decrease in the proportion of very dense cells present. In a postcript, Ley et al. reported that they had treated four additional patients and that all of them had increased the production of Hb F. Mild to moderate nausea was attributed to the drug being infused too rapidly.

Dover, Charache and Vogelsang (1983) and Dover and co-workers (1985) reported that they had administered 5-aza by subcutaneous injection (or orally with tetrahydrouridine) to four adult Hb-SS patients for periods of 30–300 days; they gave the drug daily or on alternate days or on three consecutive days each week. No marrow toxicity was detected and the total reticulocyte count was unaltered. However, the percentage of Hb-F-containing reticulocytes increased 2–5-fold within 5 days of the start of treatment. Charache and co-workers (1983) reported on one patient who had been given four courses of therapy which had resulted in an increase in Hb-F percentage from 1.8 to 8.9 and increases in the percentage of Hb-F-containing reticulocytes and erythrocytes. They were able to demonstrate that the treatment had resulted in the hypomethylation of DNA at two of 15 restriction sites around the γ-δ-β-globin gene complex. Dover et al. (1985) pointed out that, although all the patients increased the synthesis of Hb F in response to treatment, the rapidity with which they responded varied considerably; they also pointed out that the long-term effects of the treatment were unknown and that little information was available as to the drug's carcinogenicity in man.

Hydroxyurea

Nathan and co-workers (1983) and Letvin and co-workers (1984) reported that hydroxyurea (Hu), a widely used cytotoxic/cytostatic chemical, increased the production of Hb F when administered to monkeys. They had bled two young Cynomolgus monkeys and noted that after bleeding the percentage of Hb-F-containing erythrocytes (F cells) rose to 13 and 20, and the percentage of Hb F from zero to 3 and 5, respectively. Subsequently, 5-Hu given at a dosage of 50 mg/kg for 5 days produced a small and transient increase in F-cell and Hb-F percentages; 2 weeks, later, however, a similar course at a dosage of 100 mg/kg resulted in a prompt and dramatic increase in the percentage of F cells and Hb F. This work had been undertaken as a follow-up to the observation that a severely affected Hb-SS patient suffering from a chronic bone crisis appeared to have responded to the administration of Hu at a dose of 50 mg/kg/day, given in an attempt to limit the formation of sickle cells, by increasing the formation of Hb F. The Hb-F percentage in this patient had increased from less than 1 to 30%, only to return to the base-line when the treatment was discontinued. Further details of the responses of human patients were given by Platt et al. (1984). Two adult females had been given four 5-day courses of Hu at a dose-rate of 50 mg/kg/day. The Hb-F percentage in the peripheral blood increased from 7.9 to 12.3 in one patient and from 5.3 to 7.4 in the other. The total haemoglobin increased, too. The percentage of Hb-F-containing reticulocytes increased within 48 hours, reached a peak in 7–11 days and fell back in 18–21 days. Additional single-day doses of the drug maintained a raised Hb-F percentage. The lowest total granulocyte count recorded was 1.6 × 10^9/1. Platt et al. concluded that Hu might

prove to be useful in the treatment of severely affected Hb-SS patients but warned against its potential toxicity.

Charache, Dover and Nora (1985) reported that they had treated two Hb-SS patients for 2 years with Hu. The percentage of Hb F in the peripheral blood, and the percentage of Hb-F-containing reticulocytes and Hb-F cells, increased considerably and both patients suffered from fewer crises; one patient developed folate deficiency and the other disseminated herpes zoster. Charache, Dover and Nora concluded that Hu might prove to be an effective and safe means of treating patients who are resistant to more conventional treatment despite a slow response and the unknown risk of cancer, and the necessity to adjust the treatment regime to each patient's requirement.

Dover and co-workers (1986), in a fuller report from the Johns Hopkins Hospital and the National Institutes of Health, described how they had treated with Hu four Hb-SS patients who had previously been treated with 5-azathioprine (5-aza) and four additional patients who were given Hu only. The drug was administered at a dose-rate of 50 mg/kg/day for 3 or 5 days. Hu, in contrast to 5-aza, was found to lead to early suppression of the reticulocyte count and in some of the patients to decreased CFU-E colony growth in bone-marrow cultures. The patients' ability to increase Hb-F production was found to be variable and was best in the patients in whom CFU-E formation was least suppressed. Dover et al. concluded that neither 5-aza nor Hu was likely to be of real therapeutic benefit in Hb-SS disease and that in any case controlled trials would have to be carried out; moreover, the carcinogenicity of the drugs was uncertain. They concluded that Hu was more difficult to use then 5-aza, because the dose required for increased Hb-F production was close to that which is cytotoxic.

EVALUATION OF ANTI-SICKLING DRUGS: A SUMMARY

One of the clinical features of sickle-cell disease is the unpredictability of its clinical consequences in any individual patient. This makes it difficult to assess the value of any drug given as treatment, whether to alleviate and shorten acute episodes or to prevent their occurrence. Ultimately, however, the success or failure of any form of treatment can only be judged by the patient's reaction to it — how he or she feels and whether he or she wishes to persevere with the treatment — and by the severity of the side-effects (if any) it produces.

Changes, such as a rise in haemoglobin, fall in reticulocyte count, ISC percentage and serum bilirubin, and improvement in erythrocyte life-span, are useful indicators of response but are irrelevant if the patient finds the treatment intolerable. As the descriptions in the preceding pages indicate, finding a drug that is really effective in the treatment of acute episodes of Hb-SS disease or in their prevention, and that can be safely administered on a long-term basis, has proved to be a most difficult task.

While assessment *in vivo* in man of the effect of an experimental drug has to be the final test, a great deal can be learnt from laboratory studies. These studies have been directed particularly to the effect of the drug on the occurrence of sickling under conditons of reduced oxygen tension or on the filterability of Hb-S-containing erythocytes. Alternatively, the effect of the drug on the increase in viscosity of Hb-S solutions when exposed to reduced O_2 tension or on the concentration of Hb S required for gelation has been studied. The techniques used have become increasingly sophisticated and automated.

Paniker, Ben-Bassat and Beutler (1972) assessed the viscosity of Hb-S solutions by a falling ball technique, and Ohnishi (1982a) employed automated instruments to establish the relationship between pO_2 and blood viscosity and between pO_2 and erythrocyte filterability.

Johnson and co-workers (1985) used an ektacytometer to measure the flexibility of intact erythrocytes under conditons in which the pO_2 could be varied over a wide range of tensions. The curves obtained were considered to indicate whether the compound tested affected O_2 affinity or increased the solubility of deoxyHb. Johnson *et al.* stressed that their technique measures the deformability of cells containing deoxyHb rather than their shape and that some compounds that are effective in preventing sickling do not necessarily restore cell deformability. They suggested that the results obtained with their technique bridged the gap between measurements on isolated haemoglobin solutions and studies *in vivo*.

ANTENATAL DIAGNOSIS OF SICKLE-CELL DISEASES: THERAPEUTIC ABORTION

Since the early 1970s considerable attention has been directed to the possibility of diagnosing the sickle-cell diseases (and the thalassaemias) in the unborn child. The subject is of great importance, for the possibility of diagnosing accurately homozygous Hb-SS disease (or β-thalassaemia major) at an early stage of fetal life raises the question of the desirability of a therapeutic abortion.

In this Chapter will be summarized what has been achieved in relation to the diagnosis of sickle-cell disease. The development of the techniques by which samples of fetal blood or chorionic villi can be obtained, and the ways in which a judgement as to the genotype of the fetus can be arrived at from the samples, are dealt with in more detail in Chapter 20 (pp. 536–541) when the antenatal diagnosis of thalassaemia is discussed.

The successful demonstration of β^S globin-chain synthesis in fetal blood stems from the reports of Kan *et al.* (1972), Kazazian and Woodhead (1974), Alter *et al.* (1976 a,b) Kan, Golbus and Trecartin (1976) and Kan *et al.* (1977).

The earliest work in the field was briefly reviewed by Kazazian (1972); and the scientific principles behind the diagnostic procedures, and their important social and ethical implications, have been dealt with in numerous reviews, including those of Alter *et al.* (1974), Nathan and Alter (1975), Nathan, Alter and Frigoletto (1975), Kan (1977) and Alter (1979). The results obtained in 21 centres throughout the world practising the antenatal diagnosis of haemoglobinopathies from July 1974 to March 1981 were summarized by Alter (1981): she reported that more than 1900 diagnostic procedures had by then been carried out, 92% for thalassaemia and 8% for sickle-cell diseases, with an overall fetal loss of 5.6% and a small error rate (0.9%, mostly false negatives).

At first the procedures consisted essentially of obtaining fetal red cells by fetoscopy (or transplacental puncture) and of testing their ability, in the case of suspected Hb S, to synthesize β^A and β^S

chains, using radioisotope techniques. In Hb-SS disease, no β^A chains would be demonstrable, as in the first successful antenatal diagnoses reported by Alter *et al.* (1976a,b) and Kan, Golbus and Trecartin (1976); in the Hb-AS trait, both β^A and β^S chains would be present (Kan *et al.*, 1972).

An important step forward was the determination of the genotype by analysis of fetal DNA by molecular-biological techniques, the DNA being obtained by amniocentesis, a safer procedure than fetal blood sampling. Using this technique, Kan and Dozy (1978) were able to demonstrate that DNA cultured from a fetus produced both 7.6 kb and 13.0 kb β-globin gene fragments when subjected to restriction enzyme analysis. As it was known that the family in which the fetus was conceived carried the Hb-S gene in the 13.0 kb fragment, Kan and Dozy were able to diagnose that the fetus had the Hb-AS trait, a conclusion which was confirmed by a globin-chain synthesis study carried out on the blood of the fetus. Phillips and his co-workers (1979), using similar techniques, were able to diagnose successfully the fetal genotype in two families: the genotype of one fetus was *AS* and that of the other *S/O* Arab.

One disadvantage of the above approach is the need for family analysis. Geever and co-workers (1981) reported that, using the restriction endonuclease *Dde* I, it was possible to carry out direct analysis. This is because the presence of the altered codon associated with the Hb-S allele would result in the elimination of a restriction site for *Dde* I and the production of a large (376 bp) fragment.

Chang and Kan (1981) reported that they had used the *Dde* I enzyme successfully. Its disadvantage was, however, that it produced relatively small DNA fragments, so that sufficient DNA for analysis could only be obtained if the amniotic cells were cultured. Chang, Golbus and Kan (1982) and Chang and Kan (1982) described how, using the enzyme *Mst* II, they had developed a assay which was sufficiently sensitive to be used on uncultured cells. The enzyme yields a 1.15-kb fragment with normal DNA and a 1.35-kb fragment with Hb-S DNA. Chang and Kan mentioned that they had used the assay on four fetuses: by the direct analysis of 20 ml of amniotic fluid they had been able to diagnose one as having

the *AA* genotype, two the *AS* genotype and one the *SS* genotype. The fetus whose genotype was thought to be *SS* was aborted and the diagnosis was found to be correct. Orkin and co-workers (1982) similarly used the *Mst* II enzyme successfully: six fetuses at risk were investigated and definitive diagnoses were arrived at in each case.

Boehm and co-workers (1983) reported an experience based on the analysis of fetal DNA from 95 conceptions, 57 of the fetuses being at risk of sickle-cell disease. The DNA was obtained by amniocentesis and digested with one to five restriction endonucleases, including *Dde* I and *Mst* II, each of which was capable of detecting one or more restriction-site polymorphisms. Prenatal diagnosis was found to be correct in all cases available for confirmation (up to the time the report was written).

A further molecular-biological technique capable of being applied to the antenatal diagnosis of sickle-cell disease was introduced by Connor and her co-workers (1983). They had synthesized two 19-base oligonucleotides, one complementary to the normal β^A-globin gene, the other complementary to the β^S-globin gene. These were used as probes in DNA hybridization after they had been radioactively labelled. DNA from normal (Hb-AA) individuals was found to hybridize only with the β^A-specific probe and that from Hb-SS individuals to hybridize only with the β^S-specific probe; DNA from $\beta^A\beta^S$ heterozygotes hybridized with both probes.

A further important advance was reported by Williamson and his co-workers in 1981. They demonstrated that it is possible to obtain sufficient DNA for analysis by biopsy of fetal chorionic tissue without disturbing the fetus. The great advantage of this method of obtaining fetal DNA is that a sample can be obtained relatively early in pregnancy, even before the 10th week. This is substantially earlier than fetal blood can be sampled or amniocentesis carried out (see p. 537). Goosens and co-workers (1983) applied this technique to eight pregnancies in which the fetus was at risk of sickle-cell disease and managed to analyse the DNA so obtained satisfactorily: two fetuses were diagnosed as being genotypically *SS*; the others, *AA* or *AS*.

The implications of the availability of practical

and accurate means of diagnosing sickle-cell disease in the unborn fetus at an early age — a striking example of how high technology can be applied to important medical and human problems — are indeed important. In the Third World, however, as pointed out by Konotey-Ahulu (1982), selective abortion could not possibly be applied on a significant scale. With 1 million births every 4 months in West Africa alone, 140 000 amniocenteses would be required to screen for sickle-cell disease and up to 35 000 abortions. Moreover, whether abortion should be proceeded with when homozygous Hb-SS disease is diagnosed in the unborn fetus is a matter on which opinions can and do differ. As already discussed (p. 19), Hb-SS disease is sometimes a relatively mild affliction which is compatible with a long life; and as Konetey-Ahulu (1977) pointed out some Hb-SS sufferers have managed to lead highly successful and productive lives.

BONE-MARROW TRANSPLANTATION

Transplantation of bone marrow from a (Hb-AS) sibling to a patient with Hb-SS disease offers a wonderful way of restoring the patient to full health. Unfortunately, the complications of allogeneic transplantation, even using a well-matched donor, are still sufficiently menacing (and potentially lethal) as virtually to preclude its use. At the time of writing, for the above reasons, transplantation remains a dream rather than a reality. The situation differs markedly from that in leukaemia where transplantation has been established to be a useful form of treatment which, despite its dangers, offers in many cases the best chance of cure (and in some types of leukaemia the only chance of cure). As compared with leukaemia, Hb-SS disease is not necessarily lethal and in some cases it is not a great impediment to the patient leading an almost normal life; it is for these reasons, and because of the danger to the patient associated with the procedure, that transplantation cannot be recommended as a practical form of therapy at the present time. An account of a patient who was successfully transplanted is summarized below. The transplantation was, however, carried out primarily because the patient had developed leukaemia.

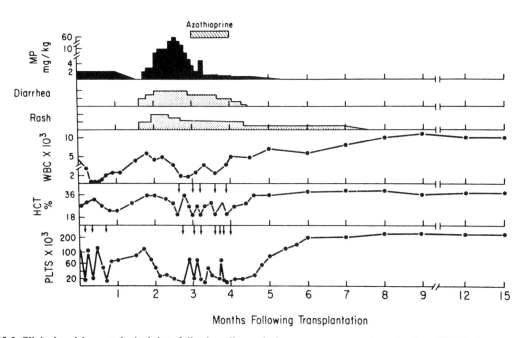

Fig. 15.3 Clinical and haematological data following allogeneic bone-marrow transplantation in a Hb-SS girl suffering from acute myeloblastic leukaemia.

MP denotes methylprednisolone; the arrows refer to transfusion of packed erythrocytes or platelets. [Reproduced by permission from Johnson et al. (1984).]

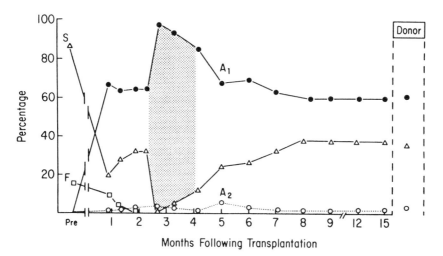

Fig. 15.4 Haemoglobin electrophoresis pattern before and after the bone-marrow transplantation.
Same patient as in Figure 15.3. The shaded area indicates acute graft-versus-host disease for which blood transfusions were required. [Reproduced by permission from Johnson et al. (1984).]

Johnson and co-workers' (1984) patient, an 8-year-old female, had been diagnosed as suffering from Hb-SS disease when she was 2 years old. When she was aged 8 she developed acute M2 myeloblastic leukaemia. Chemotherapy resulted in remission and as she had a sibling (who had the Hb-AS trait) who was ABO compatible, with a complete match also at the A, B and D loci of the major histocompatibility complex, she was transplanted with the marrow of this sibling (a boy aged 4 years). The transplant was accepted and the patient eventually went into a complete re-mission, after surviving a stormy post-transplant course, which included severe acute and then chronic GVH disease, as well as aseptic necrosis of the right femoral head and streptococcal septi-caemia and pneumonia. The patient's karyotype became XY and the blood-group antigens became those of the donor; the haematocrit stabilized at approximately 36% and the platelet and leucocyte counts rose to within the normal range. The Hb-S percentage stabilized at 35 and that of Hb A rose to 62, almost exactly the same relative proportions as in the donor's blood (Figs. 15.3 and 15.4).

REFERENCES

ABU, S., ANYAIBE, S. & HEADINGS, V. (1981). Chromatographic fractionation of anti-sickling agents in *Fagara xanthoxyloides*. *Acta haemat. (Basel)*, **66**, 19–12.

ADAMSON, J. W. (1984). Hemoglobin — from F to A, and back. *New Engl. J. Med.*, **310**, 917–918 (Editorial).

ALEXANIAN, R. & NADELL, J. (1975). Oxymetholone treatment for sickle cell anemia. *Blood*, **45**, 769–777.

ALTER, B. P. (1979). Prenatal diagnosis of hemoglobinopathies and other hematologic diseases. *J. Pediat.*, **95**, 501–513.

ALTER, B. P. (1981). Prenatal diagnosis of haemoglobinopathies: a status report. *Lancet*, **ii**, 1152–1155.

ALTER, B. P., FRIEDMAN, S., HOBBINS, J. C., MAHONEY, M. J., SHERMAN, A. S., McSWEENEY, J. F., SCHWARTZ, E. & NATHAN D. G. (1976a). Prenatal diagnosis of sickle-cell anemia and alpha G-Philadelphia. *New Engl. J. Med.*, **294**, 1040–1041.

ALTER, B. P., KAN, Y. W., FRIGOLETTO, F. D. & NATHAN, D. G. (1974). The antenatal diagnosis of the haemoglobinopathies. *Clinics Haemat.*, **3**, 509–526.

ALTER, B. P., KAN, Y. W. & NATHAN, D. G. (1972). Reticulocyte survival in sickle cell anemia: effect of cyanate. *Blood*, **40**, 733–739.

ALTER, B. P., KAN, Y. W. & NATHAN, D. G. (1974a). Inhibition of hemoglobin synthesis by cyanate in vitro. *Blood*, **43**, 57–68.

ALTER, B. P., KAN, Y. W. & NATHAN, D. G.

(1974b). Toxic effects of high-dose cyanate administration in rodents. *Blood*, **43**, 69–77.

ALTER, B. P., MODELL, C. B., FAIRWEATHER, D., HOBBINS, J. C., MAHONEY, M. J., FRIGOLETTO, F. D., SHERMAN, A. S. & NATHAN, D. G. (1976b). Prenatal diagnosis of hemoglobinopathies: a review of 15 cases. *New Engl. J. Med.*, **295**, 1437–1443.

AMBRUS, C. M., AMBRUS, J. L., SILLS, R., BANNERMAN, R., LOGUE, G., BETTIGOLE, R. & BAHSIN, A. (1985). Vaso-occlusive crisis of sickle cell disease, effects of Trental. *Blood*, **66**, No. 5 (Suppl. 1), 55a (Abstract 106).

ANDERSON, R., CASSELL, M., MULLINAX, G. L. & CHAPLIN, H. JNR (1963). Effect of normal cells on viscosity of sickle-cell blood: in vitro studies and report of six years' experience with a prophylactic program of "partial exchange transfusion". *Arch. intern. Med.*, **111**, 286–294.

ASAKURA, T., OHNISHI, S. T., ADACHI, K., OZGUC, M., HASHIMOTO, K., DEVLIN, M. T. & SCHWARTZ, E. (1981). Effect of piracetam on sickle erythrocytes and sickle hemoglobin. *Biochim. biophys. Acta*, **668**, 397–405.

ASAKURA, T., OHNISHI, S. T., ADACHI, K., OZGUC, M., HASHIMOTO, K., SINGER, M., RUSSELL, M. O. & SCHWARTZ, E. (1980). Effect of cetiedil on erythrocyte sickling: new type of antisickling agent that may affect erythrocyte membranes. *Proc. natn. Acad. Sci. U.S.A.*, **77**, 2955–2959.

BAKER, R., POWARS, D. & HAYWOOD, L. J. (1974). Restoration of the deformability of "irreversibly" sickled cells by procaine hydrochloride. *Biochem. biophys. Res. Commun.*, **59**, 548–556.

BALCERZAK, S. P., GREVER, M. R., SING, D.R., BISHOP, J. N. & SEGAL, M. L. (1982). Preliminary studies of continuous extracorporeal carbamylation in the treatment of sickle cell anemia. *J. Lab. clin. Med.*, **100**, 345–355.

BALLESTER, O. F. & WARTH, J. (1979). Sickle cell anemia: recurrent splenic pain relieved by splenectomy. *Ann. intern. Med.*, **90**, 349–350.

BARNES, P. M., HENDRICKSE, R. G. & WATSON-WILLIAMS, E. J. (1965). Low-molecular-weight dextran in treatment of bone-pain crises in sickle-cell disease. A double-blind trial. *Lancet*, **ii**, 1271–1273.

BARRERAS, L. & DIGGS, L. W. (1971). Sodium citrate orally for painful sickle cell crises. *J. Amer. med. Ass.*, **215**, 762–768.

BASU, A. K. & WOODRUFF, A. W. (1966). Effect of acetazolamide and magnesium therapy on erythrocyte survival in sickle-cell anaemia and sickle-cell-haemoglobin-C disease. *Trans. roy. Soc. trop. Med. Hyg.*, **60**, 64–69.

BELL, A. J., KOTTE, R. H., MITCHELL, A. G., COOLEY, T. B. & LEE, P. (1927). Sickle cell anemia. Reports of two cases in young children, in which splenectomy was performed. *Amer. J. Dis. Child.*, **34**, 923–933.

BENESCH, E., BENESCH, R. E., EDALJI, R. & SUZUKI, T. (1977). 5'-Deoxypyridoxal as a potential antisickling agent. *Proc. natn. Acad. Sci. U.S.A.*, **74**, 1721–1723.

BENESCH, R., BENESCH, R. E. & YUNG, S. (1977). Chemical modifications that inhibit gelation of sickle hemoglobin. *Proc. natn. Acad. Sci. U.S.A.*, **71**, 1504–1505.

BENJAMIN, L. J., BERKOWITZ, L. R., ORRINGER, E., MANKAD, V. N., PRASAD, A. S., LEWKOW, L. M., CHILLAR, R. K. & PETERSON, C. M. (1986). A collaborative, double-blind randomized study of cetiedil citrate in sickle cell crisis. *Blood*, **67**, 1442–1447.

BENJAMIN, L. J., KOKKINI, G. & PETERSON, C. M. (1980). Cetiedil: its potential usefulness in sickle cell disease. *Blood*, **55**, 265–270.

BENJAMIN, L. J. & MANNING, J. M. (1986). Enhanced survival of sickle erythrocytes upon treatment with glyceraldehye. *Blood*, **67**, 544–546.

BENJAMIN, L. J., PETERSON, C. M., ORRINGER, E. P., BERKOWITZ, L. R., KREISBERG, R. A., MANKAD, V. N., PRASAD, A. S., LEWKOW, L. M. & CHILLAR, R. K. (1983). Effects of cetiedil in acute sickle cell crisis. *Blood*, **62**, No. 5 (Suppl. 1), 53a (Abstract 113).

BENSINGER, T. A., MAHMOOD, L., CONRAD, M. E. & McCURDY, P. (1972). The effect of oral urea administration on red cell survival in sickle cell disease. *Amer. J. med. Sci.*, **264**, 283–287.

BENSINGER, T. A., MAISELS, M. J., MAHMOOD, L., McCURDY, P. & CONRAD, M. E. (1971). Effect of intravenous urea in invert sugar on heme catobolism in sickle-cell anemia. *New Engl. J. Med.*, **285**, 995–997.

BERKOWITZ, L. R. & ORRINGER, E. P. (1981). Effect of cetiedil, an in vitro antisickling agent, on erythrocyte membrane cation permeability. *J. clin. Invest.*, **68**, 1215–1220.

BERKOWITZ, L. R. & ORRINGER, E. P. (1982). Effects of cetiedil on monovalent cation permeability in the erythrocyte. An explanation for the efficiency of cetiedil in the treatment of sickle cell anemia. *Blood Cells*, **8**, 283–288.

BERKOWITZ, L. R. & ORRINGER, E. P. (1984). An analysis of the mechanism by which cetiedil inhibits the Gardos phenomenon. *Amer. J. Hemat.*, **17**, 217–223.

BEUTLER, E. (1974). Hypothesis: changes in the O_2 dissociation curve and sickling: a general formulation and therapeutic strategy. *Blood*, **43**, 297–300.

BEUTLER, E. (1975). The effect of carbon monoxide on red cell life span in sickle cell disease. *Blood*, **46**, 253–259.

BEUTLER, E. & MIKUS, B. J. (1961). Effect of methemoglobin formation in sickle cell disease. *J. clin. Invest.*, **40**, 1856–1871.

BEUTLER, E. PANIKER, N. V. & WEST, C. J. (1972).

Pyridoxine administration in sickle cell disease: an unsuccessful attempt to influence the properties of sickle hemoglobin. *Biochem. Med.*, **6**, 139–143.

BOEHM, C. D., ANTONARAKIS, S. E., PHILLIPS, J. A. III, STETTIN, G. & KAZAZIAN, H. H. JNR (1983). Prenatal diagnosis using DNA polymorphisms. Report on 95 pregnancies at risk for sickle-cell disease or β-thalassemia. *New Engl. J. Med.*, **308**, 1054–1058.

BOUNAMEAUX, Y. (1961). Action inhibitrice de la nivaquire et de divers antihistaminiques sur la formation d'hématies en faucilles dans l'anémie drépanocytaire *C.R. Soc. Biol. (Paris)*, **155**, 425–426.

BREWER, G. J. (1976). A view of the current status of antisickling therapy. *Amer. J. Hemat.*, **1**, 121–128.

BREWER, G. J. (1980). Calmodulin, zinc and calcium in cellular and membrane regulation: an interpretive review. *Amer. J. Hemat.*, **8**, 231–248.

BREWER, G. (1981). Zinc supplementation treatment of growth retardation and hypogonadism in sickle cell patients. *Amer. J. Hemat.*, **10**, 195–198 (Editorial).

BREWER, G. J., BREWER, L. F. & PRASAD, A. S. (1975). Zinc therapy suppression of erythrocyte morphological abnormalities in sickle cell anemia (SCA). *Clin. Res.*, **23**, 522A (Abstract).

BREWER, G. J., BREWER, L. F. & PRASAD, A. S. (1977). Suppression of irreversibly sickled erythrocytes by zinc therapy in sickle cell anemia. *J. Lab. clin. Med.*, **90**, 549–554.

BREWER, G. J. & OELSHLEGEL, F. J. JNR (1974). Antisickling effects of zinc. *Biochem. biophys. Res. Commun.*, **58**, 854–861.

BRODY, J. I., GOLDSMITH, M. H., PARK, S. K. & SOLTYS, H. D. (1970). Symptomatic crises of sickle cell anemia treated by limited exchange transfusion. *Ann. intern. Med.*, **72**, 327–335.

BROZOVIC, M., DAVIES, S. C., YARDUMIAN, A., BELLINGHAM, A., MARSH, G. & STEPHENS, A. D. (1986). Pain relief in sickle cell crises. *Lancet*, **ii**, 624–625 (Letter).

CAMACHO, F. J., MOLL, B., NOEL, B. E., BECKER, N. H., SPIGLAND, I., EMESON, E. E., GREENWALD, E. S. & WIERNIK, P. H. (1983). Lymphadenopathy and immunodeficiency in patients with sickle cell disease. *Blood*, **62**, No. 5 (Suppl. 1), 54a (Abstract 119).

CASTRO, O. (1980). Viability and function of stored sickle erythrocytes. *Transfusion*, **20**, 696–703.

CASTRO, O., ALARIF, L., OFOSU, M. & SCOTT, R. B. (1983a). HLA-Bw35 is associated with red cell alloimmunization in sickle cell disease. *Blood*, **62**, No. 5 (Suppl. 1), 233a (Abstract 838).

CASTRO, O., HARDY, K. P., WINTER, W. P., HORNBLOWER, M & MERYMAN, H. T. (1981). Freeze preservation of sickle erythrocytes. *Amer. J. Hemat.*, **10**, 297–304.

CASTRO, O., ORLIN, J., ROSEN, M. W. & FINCH, S. C. (1973b). Survival of human sickle-cell erythrocytes in heterologous species: response to variation in oxygen tension. *Proc. natn. Acad. Sci. U.S.A.*, **70**, 2356–2359.

CASTRO, O., RAINEY, D., INASI, B., MITCHELL, K. & ABRAHAM, D. (1985). Ethacrynic acid improves the intravascular recovery and survival of human sickle cells in rats. *Blood*, **66**, No. 5 (Suppl. 1), 57a (Abstract 114).

CASTRO, O., RANA, S. R. & POILLON, W. N. (1986). Autologous survival of cyanate-treated cryopreserved sickle erythrocytes. *Amer. J. Hemat.*, **21**, 409–413.

CERAMI, A. (1972). Cyanate as an inhibitor of red-cell sickling. *New Engl. J. Med.*, **287**, 807–812.

CERAMI, A. & MANNING, J. M. (1971). Potassium cyanate as an inhibitor of the sickling of erythrocytes in vitro. *Proc. natn. Acad. Sci. U.S.A.*, **68**, 1180–1183.

CHANG, H., EWERT, S. M., BOOKCHIN, R. M. & NAGEL, R. L. (1983). Comparative evaluation of fifteen anti-sickling agents. *Blood*, **61**, 693–704.

CHANG, J. C., GOLBUS, M. S. & KAN, Y. K. (1982). Antenatal diagnosis of sickle cell anaemia by sensitive DNA assay. *Lancet*, **i**, 1463.

CHANG, J. C. & KAN, Y. W. (1981). Antenatal diagnosis of sickle cell anaemia by direct analysis of the sickle mutation. *Lancet*, **ii**, 1127–1129.

CHANG, J. C. & KAN, Y. W. (1982). A sensitive new prenatal test for sickle-cell anemia. *New Engl. J. Med.*, **307**, 30–32.

CHAO, T. L., BERENFELD, M. R. & GABUZDA, T. G. (1976). Inhibition of sickling by methyl acetimidate. *FEBS Lett.*, **62**, 57–59.

CHAPLIN, H. JNR & CASSELL, M. (1962). The occasional fallibility of *in vitro* compatibility tests. *Transfusion*, **2**, 375–384.

CHAPLIN, H., MONROE, M. C., MALECEK, A. C. & MURPHY, W. A. (1984). Preliminary trial of minidose heparin prophylaxis for sickle cell pain crisis. *Blood*, **64**, No. 5 (Suppl. 1), 47a (Abstract 97).

CHARACHE, S. (1974). The treatment of sickle cell anemia. *Arch. intern. Med.*, **133**, 698–705.

CHARACHE, S., DOVER, G. & NORA, R. (1985). Treatment of sickle cell anemia with hydroxyurea (HU): two years experience. *Blood*, **66**, No. 5 (Suppl. 1), 57a (Abstract 115).

CHARACHE, S., DOVER, G. J., SMITH, K. D. & TALBOT, C. C. (1982). Treatment of sickle cell anemia with azacytidine. *Blood*, **60**, No. 5 (Suppl. 1), 44a (Abstract 102).

CHARACHE, S., DOVER, G., SMITH, K., TALBOT, C. C., MOYER, M. & BOYER, S. (1983). Treatment of sickle cell anemia with 5-azacytidine results in increased fetal hemoglobin production and is associated with nonrandom hypomethylation of DNA around the γ-δ-β-globin gene complex. *Proc. natn. Acad. Sci. U.S.A.*, **80**, 4842–4846.

CHARACHE, S., DREYER, R., ZIMMERMAN, I. & HSU,

C.-K. (1976). Evaluation of extracorporeal alkylation of red cells as a potential treatment for sickle cell anemia. *Blood*, **47**, 481–488.

CHARACHE, S., MOYER, M. A. & WALKER, W. G. (1983). Treatment of acute sickle cell crisis with a vasopressin analogue. *Amer. J. Hemat.*, **15**, 315–319.

CHARACHE, S. & WALKER, W. G. (1981). Failure of desmopressin to lower serum sodium or prevent crisis in patients with sickle cell anemia. *Blood*, **58**, 892–896.

CHIU, D. & LUBIN, B. (1979). Abnormal vitamin E and glutathione peroxidase levels in sickle cell anemia. Evidence for increased susceptibility to lipid peroxidation in vivo. *J. Lab. clin. Med.*, **94**, 542–548.

COHEN, A. & SCHWARTZ, E. (1979). Iron chelation therapy in sickle cell anemia. *Amer. J. Hemat.*, **7** 69–76.

COLES, S. M., KLEIN, H. G. & HOLLAND P. V. (1981). Alloimmunization in two multitransfused patient populations. *Transfusion*, **21**, 462–466.

CONNOR, B. J., REYES, A. A., MORIN, C., ITAKURA, K., TEPLITZ, R. L. & WALLACE, R. B. (1983). Detection of sickle cell β^S-globin allele by hybridization with synthetic oligonucleotides. *Proc. natn. Acad. Sci. U.S.A.*, **80**, 278–282.

COOPERATIVE UREA TRIALS GROUP (1974a). Clinical trials of therapy for sickle cell vaso-occlusive crises. *J. Amer. med. Ass.*, **228**, 1120–1124.

COOPERATIVE UREA TRIALS GROUP (1974b). Treatment of sickle cell crisis with urea in invert sugar. A controlled trial. *J. Amer. med. Ass.*, **288**, 1125–1128.

COOPERATIVE UREA TRIALS GROUP (1974c). Therapy for sickle cell vaso-occlusive crises. Controlled clinical trials and cooperative study of intravenously administered alkali. *J. Amer. med. Ass.*, **228**, 1129–1131.

COSTA, F. F., ZAGO, M. A. & BOTTURA. C. (1979). Effects of piracetam and iodoacetate on erythrocyte sickling. *Lancet*, **ii**, 1302.

CRIST, R., GRISOLIA, S., BETTIS, C. & DIEDERICH, A. (1972). In vivo carbamylation of brain, blood and liver proteins by carbamyl phosphate (CP) and cyanate. *Fed. Proc.*, **31**, 231 (Abstract).

CUNNINGHAM, F. G., PRITCHARD, J. A., MASON, R. & CHASE, G. (1979). Prophylactic transfusions of normal red blood cells during pregnancies complicated by sickle cell hemoglobinopathies. *Amer. J. Obstet. Gynec.*, **135**, 994–1003.

DAVEY, R. J., ESPOSITO, D. J., JACOBSON, R. J. & CORN, M. (1978). Partial exchange transfusion as treatment for hemoglobin SC disease in pregnancy. *Arch. intern. Med.*, **138**, 937–939.

DE ARAUJO, J. T. & NERO, G. S. (1977). Piracetam and acetamide in sickle-cell disease. *Lancet*, **ii**, 411 (Letter).

DE CEULAER, K., HAYES, R., GRUBER, C. &

SERJEANT, G. R. (1982). Medroxyprogesterone acetate in homozygous sickle-cell disease. *Lancet*, **ii**, 229–231.

DE FURIA, F. G., CERAMI, A., BUNN, H. F., LU, Y. S. & PETERSON, C. M. (1973). The effect of aspirin on sickling and oxygen affinity of erythrocytes. *Proc. natn. Acad. Sci. U.S.A.*, **70**, 3707–3710.

DE FURIA, F. G., MILLER, D. R., CERAMI, A. & MANNING, J. M. (1972). The effects of cyanate in vitro on red blood cell metabolism and function in sickle cell anemia. *J. clin. Invest.*, **51**, 566–574.

DE MELO, G. O. S. (1976). Piracetam in sickle-cell anaemia. *Lancet*, **ii**, 1139–1140 (Letter).

DEAN, J. & SCHECHTER, A. N. (1978). Sickle-cell anemia: molecular and cellular bases of therapeutic approaches. *New Engl. J. Med.*, **299**, 752–763, 804–811, 863–870.

DESIMONE, J., HELLER, P., HALL, L & ZWIERS, D. (1982). 5-Azacytidine stimulates fetal hemoglobin synthesis in anemic baboons. *Proc. natn. Acad. Sci. U.S.A.*, **79**, 4428–4431.

DIAMOND, W. J., BROWN, F. L. JNR, BITTERMAN, P., KLEIN, H. G., DAVEY, R. J. & WINSLOW, R. M. (1980). Delayed hemolytic transfusion reaction presenting as sickle-cell crisis. *Ann. intern. Med.*, **93**, 231–233.

DIEDERICH, D., CARRERAS, J., TRUEWORTHY, R., GRISOLIA, S. & LOWMAN, J. T. (1971). Carbamylation induced alterations in red cell function. *Blood*, **38**, 795 (Abstract).

DIEDERICH, D., GILL, P. & LAWSON, B. (1974). In vitro red cell carbamylation in the management of sickle anemia. *Clin. Res.*, **22**, 387A (Abstract).

DIEDERICH, D. & MILAM, L. (1972). Relationship between the oxygen affinity and *in vitro* sickling propensity of carbamylated sickle erythrocytes. *Biochem. biophys. Res., Commun.*, **46**, 1255–1261.

DIEDERICH, D. A., TRUEWORTHY, R. C., GILL, P., CADER, A. M., LARSEN, W. E., LAWSON, B., ODENBAUGH, A., CURRAN, M. & DIEDERICH, A. (1976). Hematologic and clinical responses in patients with sickle cell anemia after chronic extracorporeal red cell carbamylation. *J. clin. Invest.*, **58**, 642–653.

DONEGAN, C. C. JNR, MACILWAINE, W. A. & LEAVELL, B. S. (1954). Hematologic studies on patients with sickle cell anemia following multiple transfusions. *Amer. J. Med.*, **17**, 29–35.

DOS SANTOS, W. D. & LEHMANN, H. (1959). Acetazolamide in sickle-cell anaemia. *Brit. med. J.*, **ii**, 139–140.

DOVER, G. J., CHARACHE, S., BOYER, S. H., VOGELSANG, G. & MOYER, M. (1985). 5-Azacytidine increases HbF production and reduces anemia in sickle cell disease: dose-response analysis of subcutaneous and oral dosage regimens. *Blood*, **66**, 527–532.

DOVER, G., CHARACHE, S. & VOGELSANG G. (1983). 5-

Azacytidine increases HbF production in sickle cell anemia: results of 300 days of therapy. *Blood*, **62**, No. 5 (Suppl. 1), 55a (Abstract 122).

DOVER, G. J., HUMPHRIES, R. K., MOORE, J. G., LEY, T. J., YOUNG, N. S., CHARACHE, S. & NIENHUIS, A. W. (1986). Hydroxyurea induction of hemoglobin F production in sickle cell disease: relationship between cytotoxicity and F cell production. *Blood*, **67**, 735–738.

DUROCHER, J. R., GLADER, B. E., GAINES, L. T. & CONRAD, M. E. (1974). Effect of cyanate on erythrocyte deformability. *Blood*, **43**, 277–280.

EGDAHL, R. H., MARTIN, W. W. & HILKOVITZ, G. (1963). Splenectomy for hypersplenism in sickle cell anemia. *J. Amer. med. Ass.*, **186**, 745–746.

EKONG, D. E. U., OKUGUN, J. I., ENYENIHI, V. U., BALOGH-NAIR, V., NAKANISHI, K. & NATTA, C. (1975). New antisickling agent, 3,4-dihydro-2,2-dimethyl-2H-1 benzopyran-6-butyric acid. *Nature (Lond.)*, **258**, 743–746.

ELBAUM, D., NAGEL, R. L., BOOKCHIN, R. M. & HERSKOVITS, T. T. (1974). Effect of alkylureas on the polymerization of hemoglobin S. *Proc. natn. Acad. Sci. U.S.A.*, **71**, 4718–4722.

ELBAUM, D., ROTH, E. F. JNR, NEUMANN, G., JAFFE, E. R., BOOKCHIN, R. M. & NAGEL, R. L. (1976). Molecular and cellular effects of antisickling concentrations of alkylureas. *Blood*, **48**, 273–282.

EMBURY, S. H., GARCIA, J. F., MOHANDAS, N., PENNATHUR-DAS, R. & CLARK, M. R. (1984). Effects of oxygen inhalation on endogenous erythropoietin kinetics, erythropoiesis, and properties of blood cells in sickle-cell anemia. *New Engl. J. Med.*, **311**, 291–295.

EMOND, A. M., MORAIS, P., VENUGOPAL, S., CARPENTER, R. G. & SERJEANT, G. R. (1984). Role of splenectomy in homozygous sickle cell disease in childhood. *Lancet*, i, 88–91.

FINCH, C. A., LEE, M. Y. & LEONARD, J. M. (1982). Continuous RBC transfusions in a patient with sickle cell disease. *Arch. intern. Med.*, **142**, 279–282.

FRANKLIN, I. M., ROSEMEYER, M. A. & HUEHNS, E. R. (1983). Sickle cell disease: the proportion of liganded haemoglobin needed to prevent crises. *Brit. J. Haemat.*, **54**, 579–587.

FULLERTON, W. T. & TURNER, A. G. (1962). Exchange transfusion in treatment of severe anaemia in pregnancy. *Lancet*, i, 75–78.

GABUZDA, T. G., CHAO, T. L., BERENFELD, M. R. & GELBART, T. (1980). In vivo survival studies of ^{51}Cr-labelled methyl acetimidate treated erythrocytes in patients with sickle cell disease. *Blood*, **56**, 1041–1047.

GAIL, M., BEACH, J., DARK, A., LEWIS, R. & MORROW, H. (1982). A double-blind randomized trial of low-dose oral urea to prevent sickle cell crises. *J. chr. Dis.*, **35**, 151–161.

GAILITIS, J., ALEGRE, J. A., MOTOLA, B. & HOLOGGITAS, J. (1957). Acetazoleamide (Diamox) in

sickle cell disease. *Rhode Island Med. J.*, **40**, 679–680.

GARRETT, J. V., GILES, H. McC. & SAGE, R. H. (1963). Crisis in sickle cell anaemia treated with rheomacrodex. *Lancet*, i, 1431 (Letter).

GEEVER, R. F., WILSON, L. B., NALLASETH, F. S., MILNER, P. F., BITTNER, M. & WILSON, J. T. (1981). Direct identification of sickle cell anemia by blot hybridization. *Proc. natn. Acad. Sci. U.S.A.*, **78**, 5081–5085.

GESSAIN, A., GAZZOLO, L., YOYO, M., FORTIER, L., ROBERT-GUROFF, M. & DE-THÉ, G. (1984). Sickle-cell-anaemia patients from Martinique have an increased prevalence of HTLV-1 antibodies. *Lancet*, ii, 1155–1156 (Letter).

GILLES, H. M., REID, H. A., ODUTOLA, A., RANSOME KUTI, O., LESI, F. & RANSOME-KUTI, S. (1968). Arvin treatment for sickle-cell crisis. *Lancet*, ii 542–543.

GILLETTE, P. N., LU, Y. S. & PETERSON, C. M. (1973). The pharmacology of cyanate with a summary of its initial usage in sickle cell disease. In: *Progress in Hematology*, Vol. VIII (ed. by E.B.Brown), pp. 181–190. Grune and Stratton, New York.

GILLETTE, P. N., MANNING, J. M. & CERAMI, A. (1971). Increased survival of sickle-cell erythrocytes after treatment *in vitro* with sodium cyanate. *Proc. natn. Acad. Sci. U.S.A.*, **68**, 2791–2793.

GILLETTE, P. N., PETERSON, C. M., LU, Y. S. & CERAMI, A. (1974). Sodium cyanate as a potential treatment for sickle-cell disease. *New Engl. J. Med.*, **290**, 654–660.

GILLETTE, P. N., PETERSON, C. M., MANNING, J. M. & CERAMI, A. (1972). Decrease in the hemolytic anemia of sickle cell disease after administration of sodium cyanate. *J. clin. Invest.*, **51**, 36a (Abstract).

GLADER, B. E. & CONRAD, M. E. (1972). Cyanate inhibition of erythrocyte glucose-6-phosphate dehydrogenase. *Nature (Lond.)*, **237**, 336–338.

GOOSENS, M., DUMEZ, Y., KAPLAN, L., LUPKER, M., CHABRET, C., HENRION, R. & ROSA, J. (1983). Prenatal diagnosis of sickle-cell anemia in the first trimester of pregnancy. *New Engl. J. Med.*, **309**, 831–833.

GREEN, M., HALL, R. J., HUNTSMAN, R. G., LAWSON, A., PEARSON, T. C. & WHEELER, P. C. (1975). Sickle cell crisis treated by exchange transfusions: treatment of two patients with heterozygous sickle cell syndrome. *J. Amer. med. Ass.*, **231**, 948–950.

GREENBERG, J., OHENE-FREMPONG, K., HALUS, J., WAY, C. & SCHWARTZ, E. (1983). Trial of low doses of aspirin as prophylaxis in sickle cell disease. *J. Pediat.*, **102**, 781–784.

GREENBERG, M. S. & KASS, E. H. (1956). Alkali in the treatment of painful crises in patients with sickle cell anemia. *J. clin. Invest.*, **35**, 707–708 (Abstract).

GREENBERG, M. S. & KASS, E. H. (1958). Studies on

the destruction of red blood cells. VIII. Observations on the role of pH in the pathogenesis and treatment of painful crisis in sickle-cell disease. *Arch. intern. Med.*, **101**, 355–363.

GRIFFITHS, F. E. D. (1955). Ethyl biscoumacetate as an inhibitor of sickling. *Lancet*, **ii**, 20–21.

GUIS, M. S., LANDO, W. M., MOHANDAS, N., PENNATHUR-DAS, R., PREISLER, H., LUBIN, B. H., MENTZER, W. C. & HOLMES, M. A. (1984). Prolongation of sickle cell survival by dimethyl adipimidate is compromised by immune sensitization. *Blood*, **64**, 161–165.

GUY, R. B., GAVRILIS, P. K. & ROTHENBERG, S. P. (1973). In vitro and in vivo effect of hypotonic saline on the sickling phenomenon. *Amer. J. med. Sci.*, **266**, 267–277.

HAHN, E. V. & GILLESPIE, E. B. (1927). Sickle cell anemia. Report of a case improved by splenectomy. *Arch. intern. Med.*, **39**, 233–254.

HARKNESS, D. R. & ROTH, S. (1975). Clinical evaluation of cyanate in sickle cell anemia. In: *Progress in Hematology*, Vol. IX (ed. by E. L. Brown), pp. 157–184. Grune and Stratton, New York.

HARRINGTON, J. P. & NAGEL, R. L. (1977). The effects of alkylureas and nitrogen mustards on the kinetics of red cell sickling. *J. Lab. clin. Med.*, **90**, 863–872.

HARRISON, K. A., AJABOR, L. N. & LAWSON, J. B. (1971). Ethacrynic acid and packed-blood-cell transfusion in treatment of severe anaemia in pregnancy. *Lancet*, **i**, 11–14.

HATHORN, M. & LEWIS, R. A. (1966). Inhibition of sickling by phenothiazines. Effect on red-cell survival. *Brit. J. Haemat.*, **12**, 195–201.

HILKOVITZ, G. (1957). Sickle-cell disease: new method of treatment. Preliminary Report. *Brit. med. J.*, **ii**, 266–269.

HONIG, G. R., VIDA, L. N. & FERENC, C. (1978). Effects *in vitro* of the proposed antisickling agent DBA. *Nature (Lond.)*, **272**, 833–834.

HUEHNS, E. R., DAVIES, S. C. & BROZOVIC, M. (1981). Fresh frozen plasma for vaso-occlusive crises in sickle cell disease. *Lancet*, **i**, 1310–1311 (Letter).

HUGH-JONES, K., LEHMANN, H. & McALISTER, J. M. (1964). Some experiences in managing sickle-cell anaemia in children and young adults, using alkalis and magnesium. *Brit. med. J.*, **ii**, 226–229.

HUNTSMAN, R. G. & LEHMANN, H. (1974). Treatment of sickle-cell disease. *Brit. J. Haemat.*, **28**, 437–443 (Annotation).

ISAACS, W. A., EFFIONG, C. E. & AYENI, O. (1972). Steroid treatment in the prevention of painful episodes in sickle-cell disease. *Lancet*, **i**, 570–571.

ISAACS, W. A. & HAYHOE, F. G. J. (1967). Steroid hormones in sickle-cell disease. *Nature (Lond.)*, **215**, 1139–1142.

ISAACS-SODEYE, W. A., SOFOWORA, E. A., WILLIAMS, A. O., MARQUIS, V. O., ADEKUNLE, A. &

ANDERSON, C. O. (1975). Extract of *Fagara xanthoxyloides* root in sickle cell anaemia. Toxicology and preliminary clinical trials. *Acta haemat. (Basel)*, **53**, 158–164.

JENKINS, M. E., SCOTT, R. B. & FERGUSON, A. D. (1956). Studies in sickle cell anemia. VII. Blood volume relationships and the use of a plasma extender in sickle cell disease in childhood: a preliminary report. *Pediatrics*, **18**, 239–248.

JOHNSON, F. L., LOOK, A. T., GOCKERMAN, J., RUGGIERO, M. R., DALLA-POZZA, L. & BILLINGS, F. T. III (1984). Bone-marrow transplantation in a patient with sickle-cell anemia. *New Engl. J. Med.*, **311**, 780–783.

JOHNSON, R. M., FÉO, C. J., NOSSAL, M. & DOBO, I. (1985). Evaluation of covalent antisickling compounds by PO_2 scan ektacytometry. *Blood*, **66**, 432–438.

KAN, Y. K. (1977). Prenatal diagnosis of hemoglobin disorders. In: *Progress in Hematology*, Vol. X (ed. by E. B. Brown), pp. 91–104. Grune and Stratton, New York.

KAN, Y. W. & DOZY, A. M. (1978). Antenatal diagnosis of sickle-cell anaemia by D.N.A. analysis of amniotic-fluid cells. *Lancet*, **ii**, 910–912.

KAN, Y. W., DOZY, A. M., ALTER, B. P., FRIGOLETTO, F. D. & NATHAN, D. G. (1972). Detection of the sickle gene in the human fetus. Potential for intrauterine diagnosis of sickle cell anemia. *New Engl. J. Med.*, **287**, 1–5.

KAN Y. W., GOLBUS, M. S. & TRECARTIN, R. (1976). Prenatal diagnosis of sickle-cell anemia. *New Engl. J. Med.*, **294**, 1039–1040.

KAN, Y. W., GOLBUS, M. S., TRECARTIN, R. F. & FILLY, R. A. (1977). Prenatal diagnosis of β-thalassaemia and sickle-cell anaemia: experience with 24 cases. *Lancet*, **i**, 269–271.

KARK, J. A., BONGIOVANNI, R., HICKS, C. H., TARASSOFF, P. G., HANNAH, J. S. & YOSHIDA. G. Y. (1982). Modification of intracellular hemoglobin with pyridoxal and pyridoxal 5′-phosphate. *Blood Cells*, **8**, 299–314.

KARK, J. A., KALE, M. P., TARASSOFF, P. G., WOODS, M. & LESSIN, L. S. (1978). Inhibition of erythrocyte sickling in vitro by pyridoxal. *J. clin. Invest.*, **62**, 888–891.

KASS, E. H., INGBAR, S. H. HARRIS, J. W. & LEY, A. B. (1951). Chemical abnormalities in the erythrocytes of sickle cell anemia, their relationship to sulfhydryl metabolism and the effects of ACTH. *J. clin. Invest.*, **30**, 652–653 (Abstract).

KAZAZIAN, H. H. (1972). Antenatal detection of sickle-cell anemia. *New Engl. J. Med.*, **287**, 41–42 (Annotation).

KAZAZIAN, H. H. JNR & WOODHEAD, A. P. (1974). Adult hemoglobin synthesis in the human fetus. *Ann. N.Y. Acad. Sci.*, **241**, 691–698.

KEIDEN, A. J., FRANKLIN, I. M., WHITE, R. D., JOY, M., HUEHNS, E. R. & STUART, J. (1986). Effect of

BW12C on oxygen affinity of haemoglobin in sickle-cell disease. *Lancet*, **i**, 831–834.

KENNY, M. W. & STUART, J. (1983). Preservation of deformability (filterability) of sickle cells by BW12C during progressive deoxygenation. *Brit. J. Haemat.*, **55**, 465–571.

KERNOFF, L. M., BOTHA, M. C. & JACOBS, P. (1977). Exchange transfusion in sickle cell disease using a continuous-flow blood cell separator. *Transfusion*, **17**, 269–271.

KILMARTIN, J. V. & ROSSI-BERNARDI, L. (1971). The binding of carbon dioxide by horse haemoglobin. *Biochem. J.*, **124**, 31–45.

KLOTZ, I. M., HANEY, D. N. & KING, L. C. (1981). Rational approaches to therapy: anti-sickling agents. *Science*, **213**, 724–731.

KLOTZ, I. M. & TAM, J. W. O. (1973). Acetylation of sickle cell hemoglobin by aspirin. *Proc. natn. Acad. Sci. U.S.A.*, **70**, 1313–1315.

KNIGHT, R., WOODRUFF, A. W. & PETTITT, L. E. (1968). Some applications of radiochromium ^{51}Cr in assessing the value of therapeutic regimes and the effects of crises in haemoglobinopathic states. *Trans. roy. Soc. trop. Med. Hyg.*, **62**, 92–104.

KONOTEY-AHULU, F. I. D. (1971). Treatment and prevention of sickle-cell crisis. *Lancet*, **ii**, 1255 (Letter).

KONOTEY-AHULU, F. I. D. (1972). Management of patients with sickle-cell disease. *Lancet*, **ii**, 772 (Letter).

KONOTEY-AHULU, F. I. D. (1977). Antenatal diagnosis of haemoglobinopathies. *Lancet*, **i**, 597–598 (Letter).

KONOTEY-AHULU, F. I. D. (1982). Ethics of amniocentesis and selective abortion for sickle cell disease. *Lancet*; **i**, 38–39 (Letter).

KRAUS, A. P. (1973). Clinical trials of therapy for sickle cell vaso-occlusive crises. *Blood*, **42**, 979 (Abstract).

KRON, E. & COHEN, A. (1984). Improved transfusion program for prevention of recurrent stroke in sickle cell anemia. *Blood*, **64**, No. 5 (Suppl. 1), 49a (Abstract 108).

KRUCKEBERG, W. C., OELSHLEGEL, F. J. JNR, SHORE, S. H. & BREWER, G. J. (1975). Effects of zinc on the morphology of sickle RBC ghosts as observed by scanning electron microscopy (SEM). *Clin. Res.*, **23**, 262 (Abstract).

KUBOTA, S. & YOUNG, J. T. (1977). Oligopeptides as potential antiaggregation agents for deoxyhemoglobin S. *Proc. natn. Acad. Sci. U.S.A.*, **74**, 5431–5434.

KURANSTIN-MILLS, J. & LESSIN, L. S. (1982). Rheological assessment of antisickling effects of pyridoxine and pyridoxal. *Blood Cells*, **8**, 315–328.

LANE, T. A. & BURKA, E. R. (1976). Decreased life span and membrane damage of carbamylated erythrocytes in vitro. *Blood*, **47**, 909–917.

LANGER, E. E., STAMATOYANNOPOULOS, G., HLASTALA, M. P., ADAMSON, J. W., FIGLEY, M.,

LABBE, R. F., DETTER, J. C. & FINCH, C. A. (1976). Extracorporeal treatment with cyanate in sickle cell disease: preliminary observations in four patients. *J. Lab. clin. Med.*, **87**, 462–474.

LASZLO, J., OBENOUR, W. JNR & SALTZMAN, H. A. (1969). Effects of hyperbaric oxygenation on sickle syndromes. *Sth. med. J. (Bgham, Ala.)*, **62**, 453–457.

LEARY, M. & ABRAMSON, N. (1981). Induced hyponatremia for sickle-cell crisis. *New Engl. J. Med.*, **304**, 844–845 (Letter).

LEE, M. Y., UVELLI, D. A., AGODOA, L. C. Y., SCRIBNER, B. H., FINCH, C. A. & BABB, A. L. (1982). Clinical studies of a continuous extracorporeal cyanate treatment system for patients with sickle cell disease. *J. Lab. clin. Med.*, **100**, 334–344.

LEHMANN, H. (1963). Treatment of sickle-cell anaemia. *Brit. med. J.*, **i**, 1158–1159 (Letter).

LETVIN, N. L., LINCH, D. C., BEARDSLEY, G. P., McINTYRE, K. W. & NATHAN, D. G. (1984). Augmentation of fetal-hemoglobin production in anemic monkeys by hydroxyurea. *New Engl. J. Med.*, **310**, 869–874.

LEWIS, R. A. (1964). Inhibition of sickling by phenothiazines: effect of promazine. *Ghana med. J.*, **3**, 3–8.

LEWIS, R. A. & GYANG, F. N. (1965). Inhibition of sickling by phenothiazines: comparison of derivatives. *Arch. int. Pharmacodyn.*, **158**, 158–171.

LEY, T. J., DeSIMONE, J., NOGUCHI, C. T., TURNER, P. H., SCHECHTER, A. N., HELLER, P. & NIENHUIS, A. W. (1983). 5-Azacytidine increases γ-globin synthesis and reduces the proportion of dense cells in patients with sickle cell anemia. *Blood*, **62**, 370–380.

LIPP, E. C., RUDDERS, R. A. & PISCIOTTA, A. V. (1972). Oral urea therapy in sickle-cell anemia. A preliminary report. *Ann. intern. Med.*, **76**, 765–768.

LUBIN, B. H. & OSKI, F. A. (1973). Oral urea therapy in children with sickle cell anemia. *J. Pediat.*, **82**, 311–313.

LUBIN, B. H., PENA, V., MENTZER, W. C. & BYMUN, E. (1975). Dimethyl adipimidate: a new antisickling agent. *Proc. natn. Acad. Sci. U.S.A.*, **72**, 43–46.

LUNDH, B. & GARDNER, F. H. (1970). The haematological response to androgens in sickle cell anaemia. *Scand. J. Haemat.*, **7**, 389–397.

LUSHER, J. M., HAGHIGHAT. H. & KHALIFA, A. S. (1976). A prophylactic transfusion program for children with sickle cell anemia complicated by CNS infarction. *Amer. J. Hemat.*, **1**, 265–273.

McCURDY, P. R. & MAHMOOD, L. (1971). Intravenous urea treatment of the painful crisis of sickle-cell disease. A preliminary report. *New Engl. J. Med.*, **285**, 992–994.

MacDOUGALL, L. G. & JACOB, G. (1959). Acetazolamide in the treatment of sickle-cell anaemia. *Brit. med. J.*, **ii**, 141.

MAHMOOD, A. (1969). A double-blind trial of a phenothiazine compound in the treatment of clinical crisis of sickle cell anaemia. *Brit. J. Haemat.*, **16**, 181–184.

MANN, J. R., DEEBLE, T. J., BREEZE, G. R. & STUART, J. (1972). Ancrod in sickle-cell crisis. *Lancet*, **i**, 934-937.

MARGOLIES, M. P. (1951). Sickle cell anemia. A composite study and survey. *Medicine (Baltimore)*, **30**, 357–443.

MAUGH, T. H. II (1981). Sickle cell (II): many agents near trials. *Science*, **211**, 468–470.

MAY, A., BELLINGHAM, A. J., HUEHNS, E. R. & BEAVAN, G. H. (1972). Effect of cyanate on sickling. *Lancet*, **i**, 658–661.

MAY, A. & HUEHNS, E. R. (1975). The effect of urea on sickling. *Brit. J. Haemat.*, **30**, 21–29.

MILLER, D. M., WINSLOW, R. M., KLEIN, H. G., WILSON, K. C., BROWN, F. L. & STATHAM, N. J. (1980). Improved exercise performance after exchange transfusion in subjects with sickle cell anemia. *Blood*, **56**, 1127–1131.

MILNER, P. F. (1974). The sickling disorders. *Seminars Hemat.*, **3**, 289–331.

MILNER, P. F. & CHARACHE, S. (1973). Life span of carbamylated red cells in sickle cell anemia. *J. clin. Invest.*, **52**, 3161–3171.

MILNER, P. F., SQUIRES, J. E., LARISON, P. J., CHARLES, W. T. & KRAUSS, J. S. (1985). Posttransfusion crises in sickle cell anemia: role of delayed hemolytic reactions to transfusion. *Sth. med. J. (Bgham, Ala.)*, **78**, 1462–1469.

MORRISON, J. C., SCHNEIDER, J. M., WHYBREW, W. D., BUCOVAZ, E. T. & MEIZEL, D. M. (1980). Prophylactic transfusions in pregnant patients with sickle haemoglobinopathies: benefit versus risk. *Obstet. and Gynec.*, **56**, 274–280.

MOTULSKY, A. G., CASSERD, F., GIBLETT, E. R., BROUN, G. O. JNR, & FINCH, C. A. (1958). Anaemia and the spleen. *New Engl. J. Med.*, **259**, 1164–1169, 1215–1219.

NADEL, J. A. & SPIVACK, A. P. (1958). Surgical management of sickle cell anemia: the use of packed red blood cell transfusions. *Ann. intern. Med.*, **48**, 399–406.

NALBANDIAN, R. M., ANDERSON, J. W., LUSHER, J. M., AGUSTSSON, A. & HENRY, R. L. (1971a). Oral urea and the prophylactic treatment of sickle cell disease — a preliminary report. *Amer. J. med. Sci*, **261**, 325–334.

NALBANDIAN, R. M. & EVANS, T. N. (1971). Sickle cell anemia: a molecular approach to pathogenesis, diagnosis and treatment. *Mich. Med.*, **70**, 411–417.

NALBANDIAN, R. M., HENRY, R. L. BARNHART, M. I., NICHOLS, B. M., CAMP, J. R. JNR, & WOLF, P. L. (1971b). Sickling reversed and blocked by urea in invert sugar: optical and electron microscopic evidence. *Amer. J. Path.*, **64**, 405–422.

NALBANDIAN, R. M., HENRY, R. L., BUREK, L. & DIGLIO, C. A. (1981). Diminished adherence of sickle erythrocytes to rat and human vascular endothelium by piracetam. *Blood*, **58**, No. 5 (Suppl. 1), 63a (Abstract 161).

NALBANDIAN, R. M., HENRY, R. L., BUREK, C. L., DIGLIO, C. A., GOLDMAN, A. I., TAYLOR, G. W. & HOFFMAN, W. H. (1983). Diminished adherence of sickle erythrocytes to cultured vascular endothelium by piracetam. *Amer. J. Hemat.*, **15**, 147–151.

NALBANDIAN, R. M., SHULTZ, G., LUSHER, J. M., ANDERSON, J. W. & HENRY, R. L. (1971c). Sickle cell crisis terminated by intravenous urea in sugar solutions — a preliminary report. *Amer. J. med. Sci*, **261**, 309–324.

NATHAN, D. G. & ALTER, B. P. (1975). Antenatal diagnosis of the haemoglobinopathies. *Brit. J. Haemat.*, **31**, (Suppl), 143–154.

NATHAN, D. G., ALTER, B. P. & FRIGOLETTO, F. D. (1975). Antenatal diagnosis of hemoglobinopathies: social and technical considerations. *Seminars Hemat.*, **12**, 305–321.

NATHAN, D. G., LINCH, D., BEARDSLEY, P., PLATT, O. & LETVIN, N. (1983). Fetal hemoglobin (HbF) production is enhanced by hydroxyurea. *Blood*, **62**, No. 5 (Suppl. 1), 74a (Abstract 199).

NATTA, C. L. & MACHLIN, L. J. (1979). Plasma levels of tocopherol in sickle cell anemia subjects. *Amer. J. clin. Nutr.*, **32**, 1359–1362.

NATTA, C. L., MACHLIN, L. J. & BRIN, M. (1980). A decrease in irreversibly sickled erythrocytes in sickle cell anemia patients given vitamin E. *Amer. J. clin. Nutr.*, **33**, 968–971.

NATTA, C. L. & REYNOLDS, R. D. (1983). Low plasma pyridoxal phosphate in sickle cell anemia. Response to pyridoxine. *Blood*, **62**, No. 5 (Suppl. 1), 59a (Abstract 137).

NICHOLSON, D. H., HARKNESS, D. R., BENSON, W. E. & PETERSON, C. M. (1976). Cyanate-induced cataracts in patients with sickle-cell hemoglobinopathies. *Arch. Ophthal. (Chicago)*, **94**, 927–930.

NIELL, H. B., LEACH, B. E. & KRAUS, A. P. (1979). Zinc metabolism in sickle cell anemia. *J. Amer. med. Ass.*, **242**, 2686–2687.

NIGEN, A. M. & MANNING, J. M. (1977). Inhibition of erythrocyte sickling in vitro by DL-glyceraldehyde. *Proc. natn. Acad. Sci. U.S.A.*, **74**, 367–371.

NIGEN, A. M. & MANNING, J. M. (1978). Effects of glyceraldehyde on the structural and functional properties of sickle erythrocytes. *J. clin. Invest.*, **61**, 11–19.

NOGUCHI, C. T. & SCHECHTER, A. N. (1977). Effects of amino acids on gelation kinetics and solubility of sickle hemoglobin. *Biochem. biophys. Res. Commun.*, **74**, 637–642.

OELSHLEGEL, F. J. JNR, BREWER, G. J., PRASAD, A. S., KNUTSEN, C. & SCHOOMAKER, E. B. (1973).

Effect of zinc on increasing oxygen affinity of sickle and normal red blood cells. *Biochem. biophys. Res. Commun.*, 53, 560–566.

OFOSU, M. D., SAUNDERS, D. A., DUNSTON, G. M., CASTRO, O. & ALARIF, L. (1986). Association of HLA and autoantibody in transfused sickle cell disease patients. *Amer. J. Hemat.*, 22, 27–33.

OHNISHI, S. T. (1982a). Viscosity and filtrability measurements of sickle-cell suspensions in the development of anti-sickling drugs. *Blood Cells*, 8, 79–87.

OHNISHI, S. T. (1982b). Antisickling effects of membrane-interacting compounds. *Blood Cells*, 8, 337–343.

OHNISHI, S. T. (1983). Inhibition of the *in vitro* formation of irreversibly sickled cells by cepharanthine. *Brit. J. Haemat.*, 55, 665–671.

OHNISHI, S. T., DEVLIN, M. T., SATO, T., HASHIMOTO, K. & SINGER, M. (1981). Possible use of non-neuroleptic isomers of anti-pyschotics in anti-sickling therapy. *Europ. J. Pharm.*, 75, 121–125.

OHNISHI, S. T., HASHIMOTO, K., SATO, T., DEVLIN, M. T. & SINGER, M. (1982). Effect of β-adrenergic blockers on the sickling phenomenon. *Canad. J. Physiol. Pharm.*, 60, 148–153.

OPIO, E. & BARNES, P. M. (1972). Intravenous urea in treatment of bone-pain crises of sickle-cell disease. A double-blind trial. *Lancet*, ii, 160–162.

ORKIN, S. H., LITTLE, P. F. R., KAZAZIAN, H. H. JNR & BOEHM, C. D. (1982). Improved detection of the sickle mutation by DNA analysis. Application to prenatal diagnosis. *New Engl. J. Med.*, 307, 32–36.

ORLINA, A. R., UNGER, P. J. & KOSHY, M. (1978). Post-transfusion alloimmunization in patients with sickle cell disease. *Amer. J. Hemat.*, 5, 101–106.

OSAMO, N. O., PHOTIADES, D. P. & FAMODU, A. A. (1981). Therapeutic effect of aspirin in sickle cell anaemia. *Acta haemat. (Basel)*, 66, 102–107.

OSKI, F., CALL, F. L. II & LESSEN, L. (1968). Failure of promazine HCl to prevent the painful episodes in sickle cell anemia. *J. Pediat.*, 73, 265–266.

OSKI, F. A., VINER, E. D., PURUGGANAN, H. & McELFRESH, A. E. (1965). Low molecular weight dextran in sickle-cell crisis. *J. Amer. med. Ass.*, 191, 43.

PANIKER, N. V., BEN-BASSAT, I. & BEUTLER, E. (1972). Evaluation of sickle hemoglobin and desickling agents by falling ball viscometry. *J. Lab. clin. Med.*, 80, 282–290.

PEARSON, H. A. & NOYES, W. D. (1966). Failure of phenothiazines in sickle cell anemia. *J. Amer. med. Ass.*, 199, 33–34.

PENNATHUR-DAS, R., HEATH, R. H., MENTZER, W. C. & LUBIN, B. H. (1982). Modification of hemoglobin S with dimethyl adipimidate. Contribution of inter-tetrameric cross-linking to

changes in properties. *Biochim. biophys. Acta*, 706, 80–85.

PENNATHUR-DAS, R., LANDE, W. M., MENTZER, W. C. & LUBIN, B. H. (1978). Effect of dimethyl adipimidate (DMA) on red blood cell (RBC) deformability and hemoglobin (Hb)-S gelation. *Biophys. J.*, 21, 51a (Abstract).

PENNATHUR-DAS, R., LANDE, W. M., MENTZER, W. C., MOHANDAS, N., PREISLER, H., KLEMAN, K. M., HEATH, R. H. & LUBIN, B. H. (1984). Influence of pH on the rheologic and antisickling effects of dimethyl adipimidate. *J. Lab. clin. Med.*, 104, 718–729.

PETERSON, C. M. & CERAMI, A. (1974). Therapy of sickle disease: an approach with sodium cyanate. *Seminars Hemat.*, 11, 569–595.

PETERSON, C. M., LU, Y. S., MANNING, J. M. & GILLETTE, P. N. (1973). Studies with oral cyanate in sickle-cell disease. *J. Clin. Invest.*, 52, 64a (Abstract).

PETERSON, C. M., TSAIRIS, P., OHNISHI, A., LU, Y. S., GRADY, R., CERAMI, A. & DYCK, P. J. (1974). Sodium cyanate induced polyneuropathy in patients with sickle-cell disease. *Ann. intern. Med.*, 81, 152–158.

PHILLIPS, J. A. III, SCOTT, A. F., KAZAZIAN, H. H. JNR, SMITH, K. D., STETTEN, G. & THOMAS, G. H. (1979). Prenatal diagnosis of hemoglobinopathies by restriction endonuclease analysis: pregnancies at risk for sickle cell anemia and S–O^{Arab} disease. *Johns Hopk. med. J.*, 145, 57–60.

PITNEY, W. R. (1968). Arvin treatment for sickle-cell crisis. *Lancet*, iii, 682 (Letter).

PLATT, O. & NATHAN, D. G. (1981). Sickle cell disease. In: *Hematology of Infancy and Childhood*, 2nd edn (ed. by D. G. Nathan and F. A. Oski), pp. 687–725. W. B. Saunders, Philadelphia.

PLATT, O. S., ORKIN, S. H., DOVER, G., BEARDSLEY, G. P., MILLER, B. & NATHAN, D. G. (1984). Hydroxyurea enhances fetal hemoglobin production in sickle cell anemia. *J. clin. Invest*, 74, 652–656.

POILLON, W. N. & BERTLES, J. F. (1977). Effects of ethanol and 3,4-dihydro-2,2-dimethyl-2H-l-benzopyran-6-butyric acid on the solubility of sickle hemoglobin. *Biochem. biophys. Res. Commun.*, 75, 636–642.

PRASAD, A. S., ABBASI, A. A., RABBANI, P. & DUMOUCHELLE, E. (1981). Effect of zinc supplementation on serum testosterone level in adult male sickle cell anemia subjects. *Amer. J. Hemat.*, 10, 119–127.

PRASAD, A. S., ORTEGA, J., BREWER, G. J., OBERLEAS, D. & SCHOOMAKER, E. B. (1976). Trace elements in sickle cell disease. *J. Amer. med. Ass.*, 235, 2396–2398.

PRASAD, A. S., RABBANI, P. & WARTH, J. A. (1979). Effect of zinc on hyperammonemia in sickle cell anemia subjects. *Amer. J. Hemat.*, 7, 325–327.

PRASAD, A. S., SCHOOMAKER, E. B., ORTEGA, J.,

BREWER, G. J., OBERLEAS, D. & OELSHELGEL, F. J. JNR (1975). Zinc deficiency in sickle cell disease. *Clin. Chem.*, **21**, 582–587.

PURUGGANAN, H. B. & McELFRESH, A. E. (1964). Failure of carbonmonoxy sickle-cell haemoglobin to alter the sickle state. *Lancet*, i, 79–80.

RABB, L. M., GRANDISON, Y., MASON, K., HAYES, R. J., SERJEANT, B. & SERJEANT, G. R. (1983). A trial of folate supplementation in children with homozygous sickle cell disease. *Brit. J. Haemat.*, **54**, 589–594.

RAPER, A. B., BLACK, A. J. & HUNTSMAN, R. G. (1970). Sickling and steroid hormones. *Trans. roy. Soc. trop. Med. Hyg.*, **64**, 293–295.

REILLY, M. P. & ASAKURA, T. (1986). Antisickling effect of bepridil. *Lancet*, i, 848 (Letter).

REINDORF, C. A., KURANTSIN-MILLS, J., ALLOTEY, J. B. & CASTRO, O. (1985). Perfluorocarbon compounds: effects on the rheological properties of sickle erythrocytes in vitro. *Amer. J. Hemat.*, **19**, 229–236.

REINHARD, E. H. MOORE, C. V., DUBACH, R. & WADE, L. J. (1943). The effect of breathing 80 to 100% oxygen on the erythrocyte equilibrium in patients with sickle cell anemia. *J. Amer. med. Ass.*, **121**, 1245 (Abstract).

REYNOLDS, J. D. H. (1971). Painful sickle cell crisis. Successful treatment with hyperbaric oxygen therapy. *J. Amer. med. Ass.*, **216**, 1977–1978.

RODGERS, G. P., NOGUCHI, C. T. & SCHECHTER, A. N. (1985). Noninvasive techniques to evaluate the vaso-occlusive manifestations of sickle cell disease. *Amer. J. pediat. Hemat./Oncol.*, 7, 245–253.

RODMAN, T., MYERSON, R. M. & PASTOR, B. H. (1961). Prevention of the painful crises of sickle cell anemia with prothrombinopenic anticoagulants: report of a case. *Amer. J. med. Sci.*, **242**, 707–711.

ROSA, R. M., BIERER, B. E., BUNN, F. & EPSTEIN, F. H. (1982). The treatment of sickle cell anemia. with induced hyponatremia. *Blood Cells*, **8**, 329–335.

ROSA, R. M., BIERER, B. E., THOMAS, R., STOFF, J. S., KRUSKALL, M., ROBINSON, S., BUNN, H. F. & EPSTEIN, F. H. (1980). A study of induced hyponatraemia in the prevention and treatment of sickle-cell crisis. *New Engl. J. Med.*, **303**, 1138–1143.

ROSS, P. D. & SUBRAMANIAN, S. (1977). Inhibition of sickle cell hemoglobin gelation by some aromatic compounds. *Biochem. biophys. Res. Commun.*, **77**, 1217–1223.

ROSSE, W. F., GALLAGHER, D., ALTMAN, N., CASTRO, O., DOSIK, H., KINNEY, T. R., JNR, WANG, W. & GIBBONS, P. (1985). Alloimmunization to red blood cells antigen in patients with sickle cell disease. *Blood*, **66**, No. 5 (Suppl. 1), 65a (Abstract 146).

ROTH, E. F. JNR (1972). Nitrogen mustard: an "in vitro" inhibitor of erythrocyte sickling. *Biochem. biophys. Res. Commun.*, **48**, 612–618.

ROTH, E. F. JNR, NAGEL, R. L., NEUMAN, G.,

VANDERHOFF, G., KAPLAN, B. H. & JAFFÉ, E. R. (1975). Metabolic effects of antisickling amounts of nitrogen and nor-nitrogen mustard on rabbit and human erythrocytes. *Blood*, **45**, 779–788.

RUMEN, N. M. (1975). Inhibition of sickling in erythroytes by amino acids. *Blood*, **45**, 45–48.

RUSSELL, M. O., GOLDBERG, H. I., REIS, L., FRIEDMAN, S., SLATER, R., REIVICH, M. & SCHWARTZ, E. (1976). Transfusion therapy for cerebrovascular abnormalities in sickle cell disease. *J. Pediat.*, **88**, 382–387.

SABLAYROLLES, M., WAJCMAN, H., CASTAIGNE, J.-P. & LABIE, D. (1985). Membrane expansion as a mechanism explaining the antisickling action of ticlopidine observed in vitro. *Amer. J. Hemat.*, **18**, 121–130.

SALVAGGIO, J. E., ARNOLD, C. A. & BANOV, G. H. (1963). Long-term anticoagulation in sickle-cell disease: a clinical study. *New Engl. J. Med.*, **269**, 182–186.

SARNAIK, S. & LUSHER, J. M. (1985). Effects of long-term transfusion on patients with sickle cell anemia. *Blood*, **66**, No. 5 (Suppl. 1), 65a (Abstract 148).

SARNAIK, S., SCHORNACK, J. & LUSHER, J. M. (1986). The incidence of the development of irregular red cell antibodies in patients with sickle cell anemia. *Transfusion*, **26**, 249–252.

SASS, M. (1952). ACTH and cortisone in the treatment of sickle-cell anemia. Report of a case. *New Engl. J. Med.*, **246**, 583–584.

SATO, T. & OHNISHI, S. T. (1982). In vitro anti-sickling effect of cepharanthine. *Europ. J. Pharm.*, **83**, 91–95.

SCHMIDT, W. F. III, ASAKURA, T. & SCHWARTZ, E. (1982a). Effect of cetiedil on cation and water movements in erythrocytes. *J. clin. Invest.*, **69**, 589–594.

SCHMIDT, W. F., ASAKURA, T. & SCHWARTZ, E. (1982b). The effect of cetiedil on red cell membrane permeability. *Blood Cells*, **8**, 289–298.

SCHOOMAKER, E. B., BREWER, G. J. & OELSHLEGEL, F. J. JNR (1976). Zinc in the treatment of homozygous sickle cell anemia: studies in an animal model. *Amer. J. Hemat.*, **1**, 45–57.

SCHOOMAKER, E. B., PRASAD, A., OELSHLEGEL, F. J. JNR, ORTEGA, J. & BREWER, G. J. (1973). Role of zinc in sickle cell disease. I. Zinc deficiency through hemolysis. *Clin. Res.*, **21**, 834 (Abstract).

SCHWARTZ, E. & McELFRESH, A. E. (1964). Treatment of painful crises of sickle cell disease. A double blind study. *J. Pediat.*, **64**, 132–133.

SCOTT, R. B. & FERGUSON, A. D. (1960). Studies in sickle-cell anemia. XIV. Management of the child with sickle-cell anemia. *Amer. J. Dis. Child.*, **100**, 85–93.

SEELER, R. A. (1973). Intensive transfusion therapy for priapism in boys with sickle cell anemia. *J. Urol.*, **100**, 360–361.

SEELER, R. A. & ROYAL, J. E. (1980). Commentary:

sickle cell anemia, stroke, and transfusion. *J. Pediat.*, **96**, 243–244.

SEGEL, G. B., FEIG, S. A., MENTZER, W. C., McCAFFREY, R. P., WELLS, R., BUNN, H. F., SHOHET, S. B. & NATHAN, D. (1972). Effects of urea and cyanate on sickling in vitro. *New Engl. J. Med.*, **287**, 59–64.

SERJEANT, G. R. (1974). *The Clinical Features of Sickle Cell Disease.* 357 pp. North-Holland Publishing Co., Amsterdam, Oxford.

SERJEANT, G. R. (1985). *Sickle Cell Disease.* 474 pp. Oxford University Press.

SERJEANT, G. R., DE CEULAER, K. & MAUDE, G. H. (1985). Stilboestrol and stuttering priapism in homozygous sickle-cell disease. *Lancet*, ii, 1274–1276.

SERJEANT, G. R., GALLOWAY, R. E. & GUERI, M. C. (1970). Oral zinc sulphate in sickle-cell ulcers. *Lancet*, ii, 891–892.

SHEEHY, T. W., LAW, D. E. & WADE, B. H. (1980). Exchange transfusion for sickle cell intrahepatic cholestasis. *Arch. intern. Med.*, **140**, 1364–1366.

SHEEHY, T. W. & PLUMB, V. J. (1977). Treatment of sickle cell disease. *Arch. intern. Med.*, **137**, 779–782.

SHOTTON, D., CROCKETT, J. L. JNR & LEAVELL, B. S. (1951). Splenectomy in sickle cell anemia: report of a case and review of the literature. *Blood*, **6**, 365–371.

SHULMAN, L. L. (1984). Oxygen therapy in sickle-cell anemia. *New Engl. J. Med.*, **311**, 1319–1320 (Letter).

SIRS, J. A. (1963). The use of carbon monoxide to prevent sickle-cell formation. *Lancet*, i, 971–972.

SMITH, C. M. II, BUTZ, M., TUKEY, D. P., BURRIS, S. M., CLAWSON, C. C., HEBBEL, R. P., WHITE, J. G. & VERCELLOTTI, G. M. (1983). The deformation and adhesion of oxygenated sickle erythrocytes are improved by a perflurochemical blood substitute. *Blood*, **62**, No. 5 (Suppl. 1), 61a (Abstract 146).

SMITH, E., ROSENBLATT, P. & BEDO, A. V. (1953). Sickle-cell anemia crisis: report on seven patients treated with Priscoline. *J. Pediat.*, **43**, 655–660.

SOLANKI, D. L. (1983). Sickle cell anaemia, oxygen treatment, and anaemic crisis. *Brit. med. J.*, **287**, 725–726.

SOLANKI, D. & McCURDY, P. R. (1978). Delayed hemolytic transfusion reactions: an often missed entity. *J. Amer. med. Ass.*, **239**, 729–731.

SOMMER, A., KONTRAS, S. B. & CRAENEN, J. M. (1971). Partial exchange transfusion in sickle cell anemia complicated by heart disease. *J. Amer. med. Ass.*, **215**, 483–484.

SPRAGUE, C. C. & PATERSON, J. C. S. (1958). Role of the spleen and effect of splenectomy in sickle cell disease. *Blood*, **13**, 569–581.

STEVENS, A. R. (1970). Splenectomy in sickle cell anemia. *Arch. intern. Med.*, **125**, 883–884.

STEWART, W. B. (1927). Sickle cell anemia. Report of

case with splenectomy. *Amer. J. Dis. Child.*, **34**, 72–80.

SUNSHINE, H. R., HOFRICHTER, J. & EATON, W. A. (1978). Requirements for therapeutic inhibition of sickle haemoglobin gelation. *Nature (Lond.)*, **275**, 238–240.

TOMLINSON, W. J. & JACOB, J. E. (1945). Studies of sickle-cell formation in normal saline, plasma, and sera with carbonic anhydrase inhibitors. *J. Lab. clin. Med.*, **30**, 107–111.

TORRANCE, E. G. & SCHNABEL, T. G. (1932). Potassium sulphocyanate: a note on its use for the painful crises in sickle cell anemia. *Ann. intern. Med.*, **6**, 782–788.

VAN DE PETTE, J. E. W., PEARSON, T. C. & SLATER, N. G. P. (1982). Exchange transfusion in life-threatening sickling crises. *J. roy. Soc. Med.*, **75**, 777–780.

VOLTANO, J. R., GORECKI, M. & RICH, A. (1977). Sickle hemoglobin aggregation: a new class of inhibitors. *Science*, **196**, 1216–1219.

WAGNER, S. M., BISHOP, J., BROMBERG, P. A. & BALCERZAK, S. P. (1975). Enhancement of filterability of sickle cells by cyanate: an effect independent of oxygen saturation. *J. Lab. clin. Med.*, **85**, 445–450.

WALDER, J. A., ZAUGG, R. H., IWAOKA, R. S., WATKIN, W. G. & KLOTZ, I. M. (1977). Alternative aspirins as antisickling agents: acetyl-3,5-dibromosalicylic acid. *Proc. natn. Acad. Sci. U.S.A.*, **74**, 5499–5503.

WANG, W., BIRDWELL, N., HANNA, M., PRESBURY, G., ZEE, P., PARVEY, L. & WILIMAS, J. (1983). Iron chelation in chronically transfused sickle cell patients. *Blood*, **62**, No. 5 (Suppl. 1), 62a (Abstract 149).

WATSON, R. J., LICHTMAN, H. C. & SHAPIRO, H. D. (1956). Splenomegaly in sickle cell anemia. *Amer. J. Med.*, **20**, 196–206.

WATSON-WILLIAMS, E. J. (1963). Sickle-cell crisis treated with rheomacrodex. *Lancet*, i, 1053 (Letter).

WHO SCIENTIFIC GROUP (1972). Report on treatment of haemoglobinopathies and allied disorders. *Wld Hlth Org. tech. Rep. Ser.*, No. 509, 83 pp.

WILIMAS, J., GOFF, J. R., ANDERSON, H. R. JNR, LANGSTON, J. W. & THOMPSON, E. (1980). Efficacy of transfusion therapy for one to two years in patients with sickle cell disease and cerebrovascular accidents. *J. Pediat.*, **96**, 205–208.

WILLIAMSON, R., ESKDALE, J., COLEMAN, D. V., NIAZI, M., LOEFFLER, F. E. & MODELL, B. M. (1981). Direct gene analysis of chorionic villi: a possible technique for first-trimester antenatal diagnosis of haemoglobinopathies. *Lancet*, ii, 1125–1127.

YANG, J. T. (1975). Intermolecular contacts of deoxyhemoglobin S: a hypothesis and search for possible anti-sickling agents. *Biochem. biophys. Res. Commun.*, **63**, 232–238.

ZAGO, M. A., COSTA, F. F., ISMAEL, S. J., TONE, L. G. & BOTTURA, C. (1984). Treatment of sickle cell diseases with aspirin. *Acta haemat. (Basel)*, **72**, 61–64.

ZANGER, B., ALFREY, C. P., McINTIRE, L. V. & LEVERETT, L. B. (1974). The effects of dromostanolone in sickle cell anemia. *J. Lab. clin. Med.*, **84**, 889–901.

Haemoglobin C, haemoglobin C Harlem, haemoglobin D, haemoglobin E and haemoglobin O: effect of the combination of these haemoglobins with another abnormal haemoglobin or thalassaemia

HAEMOGLOBIN C: DISCOVERY AND GEOGRAPHICAL DISTRIBUTION

Haemoglobin C (Hb C) was first described by Itano and Neel (1950) as 'hemoglobin III', and its presence in black Americans was reported by Kaplan, Zuelzer and Neel in 1951. It was soon recognized to be an allele of Hb A and Hb S (Ranney, 1954) and, as already described (p. 146), compound heterozygosity for Hb S and Hb C leads to a mild form of sickle-cell disease. A single gene for Hb C has no clinical effect (the Hb-AC trait) but homozygosity gives rise to a rather characteristic mild haemolytic syndrome (Hb-CC disease). Hb C does not cause the erythrocytes to sickle.

Edington and Lehmann (1954) were the first to report the presence of Hb C outside the United States, finding in a survey of blood samples from 200 Africans in Ghana an incidence of 12%; and it soon became clear that the main focus for Hb C is in West Africa (Allison, 1956a,b; Neel et al., 1956) (Fig. 16.1).

Edington and Lehmann (1956), who compared the relative frequency of carriers of Hb C and Hb S in North and South Ghana, made the point that while the total population carrying an abnormal haemoglobin was similar in the two populations Hb C was much more frequent in the north. Neel (1957) reported a frequency of 20% in the north of the country. Presumably the gene arose there and subsequently became strongly established, probably by reason of being selected for by malaria (see below). In American blacks Hb C is much less common than in Ghana, most surveys reporting an incidence of 2–3% for the Hb-AC trait (Smith and Conley, 1953; Schneider, 1954, 1956). On this basis one in about 6000 black Americans would be expected to be homozygous for Hb C.

Although clearly a black-African characteristic, a small number of cases of Hb-AC trait or Hb-CC disease have been reported in other racial groups: e.g., in a white family of Dutch and German origin living in Curacao (Huisman, van der Schaaf and van der Sar, 1955); in Algeria, where Hb C appears to be the most common type of abnormal haemoglobin (Cabannes et al., 1956), and in an Italian family (Diggs et al., 1954).

Although not nearly as lethal as Hb S when homozygous, Hb-C homozygotes are probably at some disadvantage compared with normal individuals. If so, the same problem arises as with Hb S: how is it that the gene has been maintained at a high concentration in certain populations, and have Hb-AC heterozygotes some advantage over other genotypes? In relation to the attractive possibility that the possession of Hb C might protect against malaria, the evidence appears to be less strong than with Hb S. Edington and Laing (1957) reported that they had failed to find evidence in favour of any protection. However, Thompson (1962, 1963) later reported that the intensity of infection with *Pl. falciparum* (the parasite density) was significantly lower in affected children whose haemoglobin genotype was *AC* than in those in which it was *AA*.

A recent study by Olson and Nagel (1986) has shown that cultured *Pl. falciparum* parasites do not grow in Hb-CC cells, apparently because the abnormal osmotic response of the parasitized cells interferes with the erythrocyte rupture required for the liberation of merozoites. Hb-AC cells were, on the other hand, found to be able to support the growth of the parasites. Olson and Nagel, nevertheless, suggested that this did not negate the possibility that the parasites conferred by some other mechanism an advantage to their possessors in malarious regions.

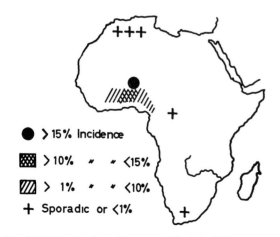

Fig. 16.1 Distribution of haemoglobin C in Africa.
[Redrawn and reproduced by permission from Lehmann (1959).]

Nature of Hb C

This is now known to be the result of lysine being substituted for glutamic acid in the β6 (A3) position (Hunt and Ingram, 1958, 1960). Hb C is thus $\alpha_2\beta_2^{6\ \text{Glu} \rightarrow \text{Lys}}$. This substitution is responsible for the haemoglobin's relatively high positive charge and for its clear separation on electrophoresis at pH 8.6 from Hb A and Hb S. According to Reiss, Ranney and Shaklai (1982), its high positive charge probably explains, too, the much greater affinity that Hb C has for the erythrocyte membrane compared with that of Hb A (or Hb S).

HAEMOGLOBIN-AC TRAIT

As already mentioned, the presence of the Hb-AC trait is not normally accompanied by any clinical symptoms or signs. For example, Smith and Krevans (1959) reported that of 240 Hb-AC subjects only one of them had experienced unexplained haematuria.

Blood picture

The patients are normally not anaemic. However, an excess of target cells in stained blood films is characteristic, although not diagnostic (Fig. 16.2): the number present, however, is variable, some films showing very few, if any; others as many as 40% (Kaplan, Zuelzer and Neel, 1953; Smith and Conley, 1953; Watson, 1956). There is no undue anisocytosis and poikilocytosis, and the MCV and MCH and reticulocyte count are normal. Steinberg (1975) gave the following data for haemoglobin, MCV and MCH based on the study of 35 Hb-AC heterozygotes: haemoglobin 14.8 ± 1.4 g/dl, MCV 86.2 ± 6.5 fl and MCH 29.4 ± 2.3 pg.

Osmotic resistance is increased (Booth and Mead, 1983). The serum bilirubin is typically normal and the mean erythrocyte life-span is normal or very slightly subnormal.

Prindle and McCurdy (1970), using ^{51}Cr and DF^{32}P, found in six patients that the mean ^{51}Cr T$_{50}$ was 25.8 days (range 22.7–31.5 days) and the mean life-span calculated from the DF^{32}P data was 86.8 days (range

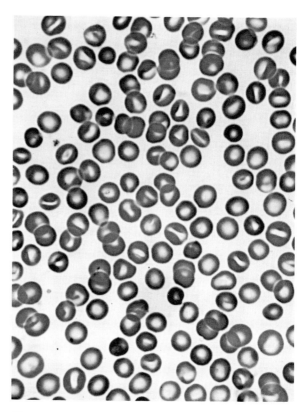

Fig. 16.2 Photomicrograph of a blood film, Hb-AC trait.
Shows slight anisocytosis, target cells and a few contracted cells. × 750.

77.4–102.6 days). Prindle and McCurdy also reported that the erythrocyte mass tended to be low, the mean in eight patients being 17.8 ± 1.8 ml/kg and concluded that, in addition to a slight reduction in life-span, erythrocyte production is subnormal; they suggested that this might be the consequence of a shift in the O$_2$-dissociation curve to the right so that oxygen becomes available to the tissues unusually easily (but produced no data in support of this suggestion).

Electrophoresis of haemoglobin

According to early observations, 25–39% of the haemoglobin separates on electrophoresis as Hb C, the remainder as Hb A (Schneider, 1954; Zuelzer, Neel and Robinson, 1956). Smith and Krevans (1959) gave the mean percentage of Hb C as 33%. Steinberg (1975), however, has reported higher percentages, the mean in 35 individuals being 42.1 ± 3.2%. Hb F and Hb A$_2$ are present in normal amounts. At birth Hb C is present in only small amounts in the cord blood of Hb-AC heterozygotes; it can, however, be demonstrated by refined methods of analysis.

An important factor in the rather wide range of Hb-C percentages in Hb-AC heterozygotes is the presence of the gene (or genes) for α-thalassaemia in the population. Huisman's (1977) data illustrate this. The percentage of Hb C (plus Hb A_2) in Hb-AC heterozygotes according to their α-globin genotypes was: αα/αα, 43.8 ± 1.5; −α/αα, 37.5 ± 1.4; and −α/−α, 32.2 ± 0.8. In a more recent study, Cameron, Smith and Cody (1984) reported on 318 Hb-AC heterozygotes. The mean Hb-C (plus Hb-A_2) percentage was 41.2 ± 3.8, with a range of 28.8–49.3. The pattern of distribution was skewed to the left, a finding considered to be consistent with the incidence of the α-thalassaemia gene in the population. If 2.5%, the likely mean percentage of Hb A_2, was subtracted from the mean Hb-C plus Hb-A_2 percentage, the resultant 38.7% was almost exactly the same as that of the mean percentage of Hb S in Hb AS heterozygotes, suggesting that both abnormal haemoglobins have a similar affinity for α chains.

According to Abraham et al. (1984), Hb C and Hb A are glycosylated in vivo to approximately the same extent in Hb-AC heterozygotes, with or without diabetes.

HOMOZYGOUS HAEMOGLOBIN-C (Hb-CC) DISEASE

Homozygosity for Hb C leads to a mild haemolytic syndrome, with a rather characteristic blood picture.

Clinical findings

Spaet, Alway and Ward (1953) were the first to describe a patient, a black child aged 4 years, who was a homozygote for Hb C. Other reports soon followed and the rather distinct clinical syndrome was quickly recognized.

Most of the early descriptions referred to black Americans [Levin et al., 1953; Ranney, Larson and McCormack, 1953; Schneider, 1954; Singer et al., 1954a; Terry, Motulsky and Rath, 1954; Hartz and Schwartz, 1955; Lange and Hagen, 1955 (identical twins)]. Most of these patients were discovered in the course of surveys of the incidence of abnormal haemoglobins or as a result of their entering into hospital for some reason other than anaemia. Subsequently, a small number of cases have been reported in which the

patients have belonged to other racial groups and in whom the origin of the Hb C has been uncertain. Thus, Lewis, Anderson and Baskind (1957) described Hb-CC disease in a white South African of Dutch parentage, Albahary et al. (1958) in a South-Vietnamese; Galbraith and Green (1960) in a man of English and Irish forebears, Scott, Dworatzek and Crookston (1963) in a Sicilian-Canadian patient and Marti et al. (1965) in a South Italian (who possibly had Hb-C/thalassaemia) and Mulla and Chrobak (1973) in Jordanian and Kuwaiti families.

Most patients lead almost normal lives. However, they are usually mildly anaemic and they may complain of intermittent jaundice or abdominal discomfort. Joint pains, too, have occasionally been complained of, but crises similar to those of Hb-SS disease do not seem to be experienced. Ulceration of the leg does not usually occur, nor does haematuria, although this has been reported (Lewis, Anderson and Baskind, 1957). X-ray of the skeleton typically reveals nothing abnormal.

The spleen is usually palpable but it is seldom markedly enlarged. However, spleens extending 17, 8 and 8 cm, respectively, below the costal margin were reported in three adult females by Tanaka and Clifford (1958) and a spleen reaching 15 cm below the costal margin was recorded by Marti et al. (1965) in an adult male.

Smith and Krevans (1959) reviewed the clinical manifestations of 35 patients with Hb-CC disease, including nine whom they had personally studied. Their symptoms were variable but they included abdominal pain (nine of the patients), joint pains, headache, haemorrhagic phenomena and jaundice. None of the patients complained of their eyes. The spleen was palpable in 34 of them. There were nine uncomplicated pregnancies; one patient, however, developed a superimposed severe megaloblastic anaemia.

Hb-CC disease seems to be compatible with normal life expectancy and Ransone and Lange (1957) referred to a patient, suffering from gout, whose haemoglobinopathy was first diagnosed when he was 79.

Blood picture

Anaemia is variable but the haemoglobin is usually above 10 g/dl and it may be normal (Table 16.1).

Table 16.1 Haematological findings in certain haemoglobinopathies associated with increased haemolysis.

Disease	Haemoglobin (g/dl)	Erythrocyte count (× 10^{12}/l)	MCV (fl)	MCH (pg)	MCHC (g/dl)	Reticulocyte count (%)	Target cells (%)
Hb-CC	10.0–14.5	4.0–5.5	60–90	20–32	34–40	1.5–7	20–80
Hb-C/β-thal	7.0–12.7	4.6–6.0	50–67	15–22	22–34	2–7	20–60
Hb-C/HPFH	12–14	3.8–5.8	80–90	25–27		<1–4	2–20
Hb-DD	9.5–15	5.5–6.5	67–80	23–27	32–35	1–4	50–80
Hb-D/β-thal	7.5–14	5.2–7.0	50–70	16–21		<1–3.5	'Many'
Hb EE	9.0–16	4.0–8.0	55–90	19–30	33–34	<1–1.5	5–45
Hb-E/β-thal	3.0–12	1.5–3.5	70–100	16–30	25–33	2–6	5–25
Hb E/HPFH	12.5–13.3	4.8–6.3	64–77	21–26		1–2	'Present'
Hb-OO	7.0–12	2.5–?		29–30		1–5	'Few'
Hb-O/β-thal	6.0–13	2.0–4.0				3.5–8	40–90

The figures quoted are believed to represent the findings in the majority of patients in each category. In the rare syndromes only very approximate figures can be quoted. The findings are affected by the age of the patient, as well as by the α-globin genotype, and to a small extent probably by sex.

The erythrocytes are normocytic or slightly microcytic and there is, as a rule, little anisocytosis and poikilocytosis. However, some shrunken cells resembling microspherocytes, as a rule without

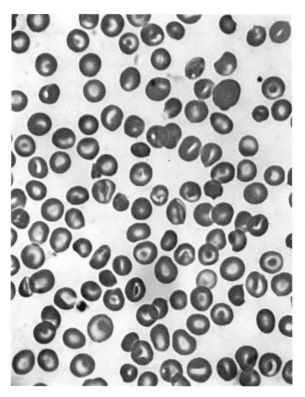

Fig. 16.3 Photomicrograph of a blood film, Hb-CC disease.
Shows anisocytosis, target cells and some contracted microcytes. × 750.

perfectly rounded contours, are usually present (Fig. 16.3). Target cells are characteristically present in large numbers: almost invariably more than 20%, and sometimes almost 100%, of the cells are affected. In dried films some cells may appear to have folded over in the long axis of the cell so as to produce 'boat-shaped' (Terry, Motulsky and Rath, 1954) or 'folded' forms (Smith and Krevans, 1959).

Charache and co-workers (1967) gave the following figures for the haemoglobin and erythrocyte count of 12 patients: haemoglobin 10.6–14.5 g/dl; erythrocytes 3.07–5.77 × 10^{12}/l. Murphy's (1968) data, based on the study of nine patients, were very similar: haemoglobin 10.7–15.0 g/dl, mean 12.4 g/dl; erythrocytes 3.94–5.50 × 10^{12}/l, mean 4.57 × 10^{12}/l.

An interesting phenomenon is the occurrence of crystals of haemoglobin within erythrocytes (Fig. 16.4). This was first reported by Diggs *et al.* (1954) in an Italian youth who had undergone splenectomy 2 years previously. About 2% of the erythrocytes contained single crystals 6–10 μm in length and 2–3μm in width. The crystals appeared to be six-sided and had blunt or pointed ends. A further instance of the same phenomenon was reported by Wheby, Thorup and Leavell (1956), also in a splenectomized patient. Rod-shaped erythrocytes, possibly containing crystals, were present in small numbers in the peripheral blood of five of Smith and Krevans's (1959)

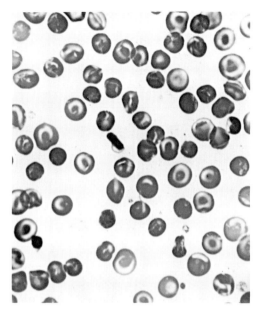

Fig. 16.4 Photomicrograph of a blood film, Hb-CC disease after splenectomy.
Shows anisocytosis, target cells and quite large numbers of contracted microcytes, and one crystal of haemoglobin.
× 700. (Film provided by courtesy of Dr Adrian Stephens.)

patients, and they were present in large numbers in the blood of one of their patients after splenectomy.

These early observations firmly linked the presence of relatively large numbers of erythrocytes containing a large crystal of haemoglobin with splenectomy. Wheby, Thorup and Leavell (1956) reported, however, that they had been unable to find any crystals within erythrocytes in imprints of the spleen of one of their two patients after its removal or in preparations of bone marrow made prior to splenectomy, in contrast to their presence in preparations made after splenectomy. They did not suggest an explanation for this except to state that: 'This finding would suggest that the spleen plays some role in the production of crystals.' A possible explanation is that crystals form after splenectomy because the erythrocytes then survive longer in the circulation. The longer-surviving cells continue to lose water with the result that the haemoglobin undergoes crystallization in some of the oldest cells while they are still circulating (see also p. 294).

Krauss and Diggs (1956) observed that intra-erythrocytic crystals developed when citrated blood from patients with Hb-SC disease or Hb-C/thalassaemia, in whom the proportion of Hb C exceeded 58%, was allowed to dry slowly *in vitro*. Crystallization of haemoglobin within normal erythrocytes did not occur under

these circumstances, nor within the cells of subjects with the Hb-AC trait in whom the percentage of Hb C was less than 44. Ager and Lehmann (1957), however, in a similar study found that erythrocytes containing several different types of haemoglobin would undergo crystallization when blood to which 2% sodium metabisulphite had been added was kept *in vitro* in a medium of increasing osmolarity, as might be produced by slow drying. Under these circumstances Hb C did not crystallize more readily than did the others.

Scott, Dworatzek and Crookston (1963) found that if an unstained 'wet' preparation of Hb-CC blood was left, partially sealed, at room temperature for 1–3 hours, rhomboidal crystals, usually 3–4 μm in length, but occasionally rod-like extending to 7–10 μm, would form in many of the cells. They noted, too, that in cells in which crystals had formed, the cytoplasm surrounding the crystals was clear and colourless. Freshly-drawn blood appeared to be devoid of crystals.

Conley (1964) and Conley and Charache (1967), too, provided clear evidence that Hb C has an abnormal tendency to crystallize. He found, when Hb-CC cells were suspended in a hyperosmotic medium, *e.g.*, 3 g/dl NaCl, that a 'large and beautiful' crystal developed in almost every cell and that this did not happen with Hb-AA or Hb-SS cells (Fig. 16.5). Conley (1964) had been

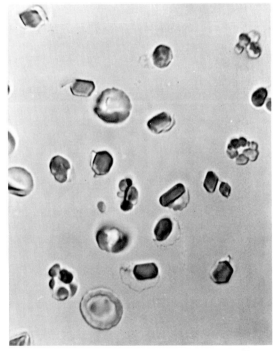

Fig. 16.5 Photomicrograph of Hb-CC erythrocytes suspended in 3.0 g/dl NaCl.
Shows the formation of intracellular crystals of haemoglobin. [Reproduced by permission from Conley (1964).]

able to find only a few such crystals in the films of the fresh blood of four out of 10 Hb-CC patients (who had not been splenectomized); at the most only 1–2 crystal-containing cells per film could be found. He concluded that crystal development was a reflection of the intracellular concentration of Hb C. Charache and co-workers (1967) carried out some quantitative studies and showed that a higher salt concentration in the suspending medium was required for crystals to form in reticulocytes than in older cells; they also found that in haemolysates crystallization took place with haemoglobin concentrations exceeding 35 g/dl while in intact erythrocytes a concentration as high as 45 g/dl was necessary. Lessin, Jensen and Padilla (1968) found that when Hb-CC cells were suspended in 3 g/dl NaCl about 25% of the cells contained birefringent crystals after 12 hours.

Additional observations on the mechanism and significance of the crystallization of Hb C have more recently been reported. Fabry and co-workers (1981) submitted the blood of a splenectomized Hb-CC patient and three patients with a spleen *in situ* to Percoll-Renograffin continuous density gradient separation. A heavy distinct crystal-containing band of erythrocytes was present in the splenectomized patient but was not found in preparations from the other three patients. Fabry *et al.* deduced from this that in patients with an intact spleen crystal-containing cells are effectively removed. They concluded by means of ^{31}P nuclear magnetic resonance and by measuring changes in viscosity that intracellular aggregation of Hb C takes place on deoxygenation even when no crystals form (see also p. 294).

The results of further interesting studies were reported by Hirsch *et al.* (1985). They fractionated the blood of two splenectomized Hb-CC patients on Percoll-Stractan gradients and found that crystals obtained from the densest fraction melted on deoxygenation. It thus seems that the crystals of Hb C that form in Hb-CC erythrocytes are in the oxygenated state. Hirsch *et al.* noted, too, that when the crystals melted the cells containing them underwent a spherocytic transformation (Fig. 16.6).

Absolute values

The MCV and MCH tend to be low and the MCHC tends to be high but the values overlap with the normal (Table 16.1). Charache and co-workers (1967) reported the following figures based on the study of 12 patients: MCV 55–94 fl, MCH 20–34 pg and MCHC 34–39 g/dl. Murphy's

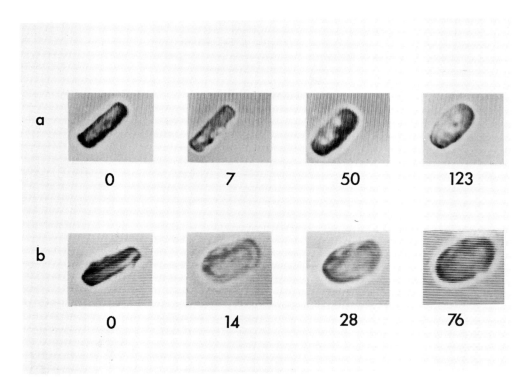

Fig. 16.6 Time-sequence video recordings of oxyHb C crystals after exposure to iso-osmotic sodium dithionite.
There are two sequences of pictures, **a** and **b**, that illustrate the change in form of two crystals exposed for different times to deoxygenation. The figures represent times in seconds. [Reproduced by permission from Hirsch *et al.* (1985).]

(1968) data, obtained from nine patients, were similar: MCV 65–83 fl, mean 71.6 fl; MCH 20.2–31.0 pg, mean 26.9 pg; MCHC 35.2–41.1 g/dl, mean 38.0 g/dl.

Other laboratory findings

Oxygen affinity. According to Murphy (1976), the mean p_{50} O_2 was 29.5 mm Hg when the measurement was made on the whole blood of 10 Hb-CC patients compared with the whole blood of six Hb-AA individuals who gave a mean value of 26.5 mm Hg, *i.e.*, the O_2 affinity of Hb-CC cells is slightly reduced. Murphy also reported that the intracellular pH and total cation content of Hb-CC cells were lower than normal; the concentration of 2,3-DPG was normal.

Reticulocyte count. This is usually raised but it may be normal. Smith and Krevans (1959) reported that the count exceeded 1.5% in 20 of 32 patients and was greater than 6% in five of them. Murphy (1968) gave a range of 1.9–5.0% in nine patients, with a mean of 3.6%.

Osmotic fragility. This is markedly diminished (Booth and Mead, 1983), and the increased resistance is even more marked after incubation for 24 hours at 37°C (Lewis, Anderson and Baskind, 1957).

Autohaemolysis. This has been reported as being less than normal, with added glucose failing to diminish the rate of haemolysis further (Lewis, Anderson and Baskind, 1957; Dedman, Emanueli and Trobaugh, 1959).

Erythrocyte sedimentation rate. Using the Wintrobe method, Abel and Beier (1961) reported that they had observed unexpectedly low sedimentation rates in six patients with Hb-CC disease. In five, there was no visible sedimentation in 1 hour; and this was true also of three out of eight patients with Hb-SC disease. In contrast, the results obtained with Hb-SS, Hb-AC and Hb-AS blood showed no definite trends and, after correction for anaemia, were usually normal. No explanation was offered for the curious behaviour of the Hb-CC blood.

Leucocyte and platelet counts. These have mostly been reported as normal (in patients in a steady state and in the absence of intercurrent illness). Singer and co-workers (1954a), however,

mentioned that one of their patients had thrombocytopenia (perhaps due to hypersplenism) and Smith and Krevans (1959) stated that eight patients had been recorded as having had thrombocytopenia.

Serum bilirubin. This is normal or slightly raised.

Erythrocyte life-span

This is slightly to moderately reduced.

The earliest studies were carried out by the Ashby method, the patients' cells being eliminated from the circulation of normal recipients in 40–55 days (Spaet, Alway and Ward, 1953; Singer *et al.*, 1954a; Terry, Motulsky and Rath, 1954). Later studies using ^{51}Cr by Ransone and Lange (1957), Tanaka and Clifford (1958), Dedman, Emanueli and Trobaugh (1959) and Galbraith and Green (1960) gave ^{51}Cr T_{50} values of 18–24 days in five patients. Prindle and McCurdy (1970) used both ^{51}Cr and DF^{32}P in studies on four patients. The results were: ^{51}Cr T_{50}, 18.7–19.5 days; DF^{32}P mean cell life-span, 35–40 days (excluding the findings in one patient who had concurrent acute leukaemia).

Ferrokinetic studies

Thomas, Motulsky and Walters (1955) calculated that in the patient they had studied haemoglobin production was only 1.7 times the normal despite a subnormal haemoglobin level (9.4 g/dl), and Jensen, Schoefield and Agner (1957), in reviewing the published accounts of Hb-CC disease, pointed out that the erythrocyte renewal rate, usually about twice normal, seemed to be an inadequate response to the haemolysis. Movitt and co-workers (1964), who studied two patients in a steady state, estimated that haemoglobin production was 3 and 2.5 times the normal, respectively, while erythrocyte destruction was about 4 times the normal. These inadequate responses seem likely to be due to a shift to the right in the oxygen-dissociation curve of Hb-CC cells facilitating the delivery of oxygen to the tissues and thereby reducing the stimulus for erythropoiesis [see Murphy (1976) and Vol. 1, p. 18].

Bone marrow

A moderate degree of normoblastic hyperplasia, commensurate with the reticulocyte count, is present. Megaloblastic erythropoiesis is unusual but has been reported, *e.g.*, by Smith and Krevans (1959) in a pregnant patient.

Electrophoresis of haemoglobin

Almost 100% of the haemoglobin is Hb C and this

Table 16.2 Haemoglobin percentages in certain haemoglobin genotypes associated with increased haemolysis.

Haemoglobin genotype	Hb A	Hb A_2	Hb F	Hb C	Hb D	Hb E	Hb O
CC	0	2–3.5	2.5–4	94–96			
C/β-thal	0–25		<1–5.5	75–93			
C/HPFH			6–35	60–70			
DD	0	2–3.5	<1–2.5		96–98		
D/β-thal		3.5–6	1–6		93–94		
EE	0	2–3.5	<1–6			90–98	
E/β-thal	0–30		6–35			55–85	
OO	0	2–3.5	1–2				95–97
O/β-thal	0–?	4	6				90

The figures quoted are believed to represent the findings in the majority of patients in each category. In the rare syndromes only very approximate figures can be quoted. The findings are affected by the age of the patient, as well as by the α-globin genotype.

produces a band, at pH 8.6, very close to where Hb A_2 is to be found, which is nearer to the cathode and line of origin than Hb S. Hb A is absent in Hb-CC patients, and Hb F is only present in small amounts, e.g., 2.4–3.7% (Lange and Hagen, 1955; Thomas, Motulsky and Walters, 1955; Watson, 1956) (Table 16.2).

Abraham and co-workers (1984) reported that the percentage of glycosylated haemoglobin (Hb C_{1C}) in Hb-CC patients and Hb-SC patients was higher than that previously reported in Hb-SS patients.

PATHOLOGY OF HOMOZYGOUS HAEMOGLOBIN-C DISEASE

Reports are available on the histopathology of several spleens removed from Hb-CC patients at operation (Diggs et al., 1954; Singer et al., 1954a; Wheby, Thorup and Leavell, 1956; Smith and Krevans, 1959) or necropsy (Jensen, Schoefield and Agner, 1957). Increased congestion of the sinuses and spleen pulp is the main feature, and the capsule, trabeculae and inter-sinusoidal reticulum have been reported to be thickened. Jensen, Schoefield and Agner found multiple ante-mortem thrombi within the pulmonary arteries in one patient. The relationship, if any, between these thrombi and the presence of Hb C was uncertain. The spleen of this patient weighed 575 g and that of Wheby, Thorup and Leavell's patient 1000 g, which is unusually massive for Hb-CC disease.

Steinberg, Gatling and Tavassoli (1983) described the presence of multiple nodules of haemangiosarcoma in a 830-g spleen surgically removed from a 54-year-old Hb-CC patient. Signs of hyposplenism in peripheral-blood films were thought to reflect 'splenic decompen-sation' due to the partial replacement of normal splenic tissue by tumour.

PATHOGENESIS OF HOMOZYGOUS HAEMOGLOBIN-C DISEASE

The slight to moderate reduction of erythrocyte life-span in Hb-CC disease has already been mentioned (p. 292), and also the apparent failure of erythropoiesis to compensate for this sufficiently to restore the haemoglobin level to within the normal range, a failure which is probably the consequence of a shift in the O_2-dissociation curve of the Hb-CC cells to the right (Murphy, 1976) (see p. 292).

The increased haemolysis seems to be linked, at least in part, with the enlargement of the spleen which is such a regular feature of the disease. It seems likely that an important factor leading to the splenomegaly is the raised viscosity of the blood and the decreased deformability of Hb-CC cells (Charache et al., 1967; Conley and Charache, 1967; Murphy, 1968). Charache and co-workers (1967) attributed the decreased deformability to the intracellular haemoglobin being in a precrystalline state in which crystallization does not occur despite the MCHC exceeding the solubility of the haemoglobin in haemolysates; they suggested that the decreased deformability led to fragmentation with the formation of exceptionally rigid microspherocytes.

Bunn, Forget and Ranney (1977) also concluded that the shortened life-span of Hb-CC erythrocytes probably resulted from their increased rigidity causing the cells to traverse capillaries less readily than normal cells.

As already mentioned, the main histopathological finding in the enlarged spleen of Hb-CC disease is congestion, *i.e.* erythrocyte sequestration, presumably because the unusual rigidity of the erythrocytes prevents their easy passage from the spleen pulp to the venous sinuses. Murphy (1967, 1968) attributed the abnormal rheological property of intracellular Hb C to an increase in the proportion of intracellular water bound to Hb C and a proportional decrease in the water available for osmotic equilibrium. As already noted (p. 291), the MCHC of Hb-CC cells tends to be unusually high.

Lawrence, Jensen and Ponder (1969) reported on the ultrastructural changes which Hb-CC cells undergo when suspended in hypertonic saline. Their findings indicate that the haemoglobin molecules aggregate as water is lost and that the molecules eventually polymerize and form crystals. They attributed the increased rigidity of Hb-CC cells to the aggregation of haemoglobin molecules adjacent to the cell membrane and the development of microspherocytes *in vivo* to loss of membrane and water.

An important clinical difference between Hb-CC disease and Hb-SS disease is that in the former vaso-occlusive crises do not occur despite the increased viscosity of Hb-CC blood. According to Fabry *et al.* (1981), Hb-CC patients escape 'micro-circulatory impairment' because the increased viscosity of their blood is offset by the small diameter and size of the erythrocytes. They reported that in perfusion experiments using the rat mesoappendix as a test system they had failed to find any abnormal resistance to the flow of Hb-CC cells, irrespective of whether the cells were oxygenated or deoxygenated. The oxygenated cells from a splenectomized patient behaved normally, too; but when deoxygenated the flow through the system was moderately but significantly impaired.

Hirsch and her co-workers (1985) suggested that a change in the ligand state of Hb C (from oxy to deoxy), leading to the melting of intracellular crystals, might help to prevent the occurrence of vaso-occlusion. As already referred to (p. 291), Hirsch *et al.* found that when crystals of Hb C melt under deoxygenated conditions the cells containing them become spherocytic. This observations may explain why crystal-containing cells are not found (or at least difficult to find) in spleen-pulp blood (Wheby, Thorup and Leavell, 1956). It seems likely that cells in which crystals have formed are, nevertheless, sequestered in the spleen because of their rigidity and spherocytic shape.

Brugnara and co-workers (1985) discussed the mechanism by which the intracellular cation and water content of Hb-CC cells becomes subnormal, as reported by Murphy (1967, 1968). They demonstrated that the cells regulate their volume by a ouabain- and bumetanide-insensitive pathway which is stimulated by increased cell volume and which is sensitive to pH. Their data did not support the hypothesis that the Ca^{2+}-dependent pathway for K^+ transport is the mechanism that is responsible for the low K^+ content of Hb-CC cells.

Summary. There seems little doubt but that the increased haemolysis in Hb-CC disease is the direct consequence of the increased rigidity of the erythrocytes and that the contracted spherocyte-like cells seen in blood films are erythrocytes at the end of their life-span. The characteristic splenomegaly of Hb-CC disease is probably the result of the sequestration of these cells within the spleen pulp. The cause and mechanism of the target-cell shape of the erythrocytes, which is so characteristic of Hb-CC disease, remains an interesting mystery.

TREATMENT OF HOMOZYGOUS HAEMOGLOBIN-C DISEASE

The presence of splenomegaly in almost all Hb-CC patients, and the histological evidence of congestion with erythrocytes, suggest that splenectomy should be beneficial. The operation has, in fact, been carried out in a small number of patients. The results have been variable. The haemoglobin has risen in some of the patients (Wheby, Thorup and Leavell, 1956), but in others there has been no change (Singer *et al.*, 1954a). In view of the apparently inconsistent results of splenectomy, and because the degree of increased haemolysis is usually not marked, it would seem best not to consider splenectomy except in exceptional circumstances, *e.g.*, when the spleen is markedly large and the cause of abdominal symptoms, or when anaemia is unusually severe.

COMBINATION OF HOMOZYGOUS HAEMOGLOBIN-C DISEASE WITH α-THALASSAEMIA

Steinberg (1975) described a 13-year-old black female whose parents each had the Hb-AC trait. Her father, however, in addition appeared to be carrying a gene for α-thalassaemia. She was mildly anaemic but not iron-deficient: haemoglobin 11.8 g/dl, MCV 74 fl, MCH 26.1 pg, with 2.1% reticulocytes. Electrophoresis of her haemoglobin revealed 77.3% Hb C (including Hb A_2) and 22.7% Hb F. Hb A was absent. The distribution of Hb F in her erythrocytes was heterogeneous. The α: non-α globin-chain synthesis ratio was markedly subnormal in the propositus and in her father, 0.63 and 0.66, respectively; the ratio in her (Hb-AC) mother was normal (0.99).

COMBINATION OF HAEMOGLOBIN C WITH β-THALASSAEMIA

This combination (Hb-C/β-thalassaemia) was first described in American blacks by Singer *et al.* (1954b) and Zuelzer and Kaplan (1954). It was subsequently reported in two white siblings of Italian origin living in the United States by Erlandson, Smith and Schulman (1956) and by Smith and Krevans (1959) in a black boy. Perosa, Manganelli and Dalfino (1960) reported its occurrence in an Italian resident in Italy and Coquelet and co-workers (1970) described it in a Sicilian family.

Blood picture

The patients have been mildly or moderately anaemic, with relatively high erythrocyte counts, moderately raised reticulocyte counts (2.0–7.0%) and marked microcytosis (50–67 fl) (Table 16.1). The spleen is usually palpable.

The erythrocytes are markedly pleomorphic and as a rule many target cells (20–60%) and microspherocytes [approximately 25% in the patient of Smith and Krevans (1959)], as well as hypo-

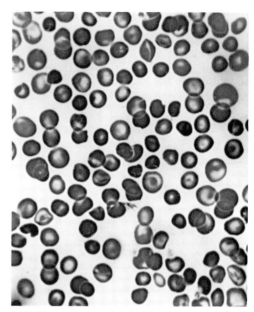

Fig. 16.7 Photomicrograph of a blood film, Hb-C/β-thalassaemia.
Shows anisocytosis, target cells and quite large numbers of microcytes. × 700. (Film provided by courtesy of Dr Adrian Stephens.)

chromic poikilocytes and cell fragments, can be seen in stained films (Fig. 16.7). An increased osmotic fragility span has been reported [in Zuelzer and Kaplan's (1954) patient, 0.66–0.12 g/dl NaCl].

Electrophoresis of haemoglobin

An Hb-C plus Hb-A plus Hb-F pattern is found, but the proportions of the haemoglobin have varied widely from case to case, no doubt reflecting the heterogeneity of the thalassaemia gene (Table 16.2).

Singer and co-workers (1954b) reported that the haemoglobin in both of their patients consisted of approximately 75% Hb C, the remainder being Hb A with a small amount of Hb F (2.4–2.7%). The haemoglobin of Zuelzer and Kaplan's (1954) patient contained, on the other hand, far less Hb C (29%); the remainder was Hb A, and there was less than 2% Hb F. The two children reported by Erlandson, Smith and Schulman (1956) were remarkable for the high concentration of Hb C, 90 and 93%, respectively, and only small amounts of Hb F were present (1.4 and 0.4%). Smith and Krevans's (1959) patient had 15% Hb A and 2% Hb F; the remainder was Hb C. The patient of Coquelet *et al.* (1970) had 12% Hb A, 82.5% Hb C and 5.5% Hb F.

Diagnosis of Hb-C/β-thalassaemia

This has to be based on the electrophoretic findings — a variable Hb-C plus Hb-A plus Hb-F pattern, the blood count findings, the appearance of the blood film and a family history in which Hb C is present in one side of the family and a type of β-thalassaemia in the other.

COMBINATION OF HAEMOGLOBIN C WITH HEREDITARY PERSISTENCE OF FETAL HAEMOGLOBIN

The rare combination of the gene for Hb C and that for a type of HPFH was reported by McCormick and Humphreys (1960), Kraus, Koch and Burckett (1961) and Schneider, Levin and Everett (1961) in patients in the United States and by Thompson and Lehmann (1962) in a family in Ghana. Excess haemolysis seems to have been slight at the most in these patients, and it is clear that the combination of the genes for Hb C and HPFH is of less clinical importance than is the Hb-C and β-thalassaemia gene combination. Anaemia is absent or minimal (Table 16.1).

McCormick and Humphreys's (1960) patient was a 64-year-old black female who was suffering from severe renal failure (from which she died) and which no doubt was responsible, at least in part, for her severe anaemia. Her haemoglobin was 5.8 g/dl and blood films showed anisopoikilocytosis, microcytes and target cells; the spleen was not palpable. Electrophoresis of her haemoglobin revealed 60% Hb C, 13.3% Hb A and 26.7% Hb F. HPFH was demonstrable in the mother's side of her family.

The propositus in the family studied by Kraus, Koch and Burckett (1961) was a 48-year-old black female who had complained of arthritis for 4 years. Her liver and spleen (4 cm) were palpable. She was mildly anaemic but not jaundiced: haemoglobin 11.3 g/dl, MCV 83 fl, reticulocyte count 1.3%, bilirubin 0.5 mg/dl, serum iron 92 μg/dl; 27% of the erythrocytes in stained films were target cells. Electrophoresis of her haemoglobin revealed 69% Hb C and 31% Hb F. Three other members of her family had the same combination with 34–39% Hb F and possibly traces of Hb A (up to 4.5%); the rest of the haemoglobin was Hb C. None was anaemic, but two had raised reticulocyte counts, 4.1 and 4.2%, respectively. Their serum bilirubin was normal.

The patient described by Schneider, Levin and Everett (1961), a black female aged 31, was not anaemic and her spleen was not palpable. The erythrocyte count was 5.4×10^{12}/l, haemoglobin 13.8 g/dl and reticulocyte count 0.3%. Only a few target cells were present in stained blood films. On electrophoresis, 62% of her haemoglobin was Hb C and 6–13% Hb F, the remainder was Hb A. [In this family the Hb-A/HPFH heterozygotes had only 7–13% Hb F.]

The Ghanaian patient, a girl aged 7, referred to by Thompson and Lehmann (1962) had a haemoglobin of 13.4 g/dl of which 26.9% was Hb F. She had had episodes of fever and abdominal pain, but clinical examination revealed no abnormalities and the spleen was not palpable. Her blood film was characterized by numerous target cells.

COMBINATION OF HAEMOGLOBIN C WITH NON-REACTING β-CHAIN VARIANTS

Hb K Woolwich. Ringelhann and co-workers (1971) referred to a Ghanaian who was a heterozygote for both Hb C and Hb K Woolwich ($\alpha_2\beta_2^{132 \; Lys \to Gln}$). The patient was clinically normal and apparently not anaemic.

Hb N Baltimore. Heterozygosity for both Hb C and Hb N Baltimore ($\alpha_2 \; \beta_2^{95 \; Lys \to Glu}$) was described by Johnson, Powars and Schroeder (1976). Their patient had a mild hypochromic microcytic anaemia with target cells in stained films. He had had, however, a peptic ulcer and there was no evidence for a haemolytic component to his anaemia.

Hb P Galveston. The combination of Hb C plus Hb P Galveston was reported in members of a black family by Huisman (1978). Their haematological values were, however, normal.

COMBINATION OF HAEMOGLOBIN C WITH α-CHAIN VARIANTS

Hb G Philadelphia. This haemoglobin ($\alpha_2^{68Asn \to Lys}\beta_2$) appears to be the commonest α-chain variant met with in the American black population. However, its presence with Hb C is usually not accompanied by appreciable anaemia or symptoms attributable to the haemoglobinopathy. A 1-year-old black child with this combination was described by Raper et al. (1960). The child was iron-deficient and target cells were present in blood films. His father had the same haemoglobin genotype but was not anaemic. Four haemoglobins were demonstrable on electrophoresis: Hb C, Hb A, Hb G Bristol (= G Philadelphia) and a hybrid (Hb-C/Hb-G Bristol).

McCurdy, Pearson and Gerald (1961) described a further patient with the same combination. He was a 47-year-old black American who 2 years previously had undergone splenectomy following an accident. The PCV was 38%, MCV 72 fl and reticulocyte count 1.8%. The ^{51}Cr T_{50} was 16 days. Films showed target cells, folded cells, microspherocytes and cells containing elongated crystals. Electrophoresis showed four components: Hb C 44%, 'Hb D' (= Hb G Philadelphia) 14%, Hb A (or Hb F) 18% and a slow-running hybrid haemoglobin Hb-C/'Hb-D' 24%. There was 6.5% Hb F by alkali denaturation.

Further examples of the same genotype were described by Weatherall, Sigler and Baglioni (1962) in three brothers. Their haemoglobins, too, separated into four components on electrophoresis. They were not anaemic, or only very slightly so (haemoglobin 12.3–15.0 g/dl), and they had reticulocyte counts of 0.9–1.8%. Blood films were reported to show anisocytosis, hypochromia, target cells and some spherocytes. Additional patients with Hb C and Hb G Philadelphia were referred to by McCurdy et al. (1975): in three of them the PCV was 36.8–38.4%, MCV 72–86 fl and reticulocyte count 1.2–1.8%. The ^{51}Cr T_{50} was 30.5 days in one patient and 16 days in a second patient who had had a gastrectomy.

HAEMOGLOBIN C HARLEM

Haemoglobin C Harlem is particularly interesting for two reasons: the haemoglobin stems from a double mutation affecting the β-globin gene, and it causes erythrocytes bearing it to sickle on deoxygenation. [One of the mutations is in fact identical with that of haemoglobin S.] The variant was first reported under the tentative label 'hemoglobin C Georgetown'. [Either designation, C Harlem or C Georgetown, is unfortunate as the haemoglobin is not related to haemoglobin C: the use of the letter C stemmed from the haemoglobin's property of running in almost exactly the same position as genuine haemoglobin C on electrophoresis at pH 8.6.]

Haemoglobin C Georgetown. In 1963, Pierce, Rath and McCoy described what they believed to be a new variant haemoglobin in the blood of four members of three generations of a black American family. The new variant was remarkable in that, although associated with pronounced sickling when blood containing it was deoxygenated by being sealed under a cover-slip or by the addition of sodium metabisulphite, the haemoglobin ran on electrophoresis at pH 8.6 not as Hb S but close to the position expected of Hb C. None of those who carried the trait was significantly anaemic. Later, Gerald and Rath (1966) reported that the variant, which they had tentatively referred to as 'hemoglobin C Georgetown', appeared to be associated with two different mutations affecting the same gene.

Haemoglobin C Harlem. Bookchin, Davis and Ranney reported in 1968 a more complete study of a variant haemoglobin having similar properties to 'hemoglobin C Georgetown'. They were able to establish that their 'new' sickling haemoglobin, which they referred to as 'hemoglobin C Harlem' (Hb C_H), was the product of a double mutation affecting the β-globin gene, namely, $\beta^{6\ \text{Glu} \rightarrow \text{Val}}$ (as in Hb S) plus $\beta^{73\ \text{Asp} \rightarrow \text{Asn}}$ (see also p. 6). The propositus in the family they had studied was a male aged 45; he had 11.9–13.4 g/dl haemoglobin, 0.2–0.8% reticulocytes, 40% Hb C_H and 2.4% Hb F. The variant was present in six other family members, too, all being heterozygous for the new haemoglobin: none was significantly anaemic, although a son of the propositus had 3.0% reticulocytes, with 11.0 g/dl haemoglobin. Their blood films were normal except for occasional target cells. None of the seven affected members in the family had suffered from any clinical symptoms attributable to the abnormal haemoglobin, but in all seven there was evidence of impaired renal concentration (as in Hb-AS heterozygotes). Purified Hb C_H was found to require a much higher concentration than Hb S for gelling to take place when deoxygenated. Both Hb C_H and Hb S were found to interact similarly with Hb A.

Compound heterozygosity for haemoglobin C and haemoglobin C Harlem

Wong and co-workers (1969) described a patient of genotype Hb C/C Harlem. He was a 39-year-old black who was admitted into hospital with painless gross haematuria. He gave no history of past illness except for symptoms suggestive of pyelonephritis 4 years previously. He was found to have 10 g/dl haemoglobin, and many target cells and occasional sickled cells were present in blood films. The spleen was palpable 5 cm below the left costal margin. Electrophoresis revealed a combination of Hb C and Hb C Harlem, the latter migrating cathodally to Hb C. His blood underwent typical sickling when deoxygenated.

The haematuria subsided spontaneously; it was attributed to the presence of the abnormal sickling haemoglobin.

HAEMOGLOBIN D

As already referred to (p. 5), haemoglobin D (Hb D) was first described by Itano in 1951 in three members of a white American family suspected of having sickle-cell anaemia. Further reports of the occurrence of 'Hb D' in other racial groups soon followed, e.g., in Sikhs, Punjabi and Gujerati Indians in India (Bird, Lehmann and Mourant, 1955; Bird and Lehmann, 1956a,b) and in Uganda (Jacob, Lehmann and Raper, 1956), in Algerians (Cabannes, Sendra and Dalaut, 1955), in Turks and Persians (Aksoy and Lehmann, 1956; Hynes and Lehmann, 1956; Göksel and Tartaroglu, 1960), in Congolese (Vandepitte and Catrysse, 1957), in Filipinos (Vella, 1958), in black Americans (Chernoff and Farr, 1956; Marder and Conley, 1959), in Chinese (rarely) (Vella, 1960) and in Thais (Wasi et al., 1968b).

Additional reports in European families include those of Dacie (1954), Konigsberg et al. (1965) and Vella and Lehmann (1974) (British), Arends, Layrisse and Rincon (1959) (Portuguese), Deliyannis, Ballas and Christakis (1969) and Gouttas et al. (1960a) (Greek), Martin et al. (1960) (German), Ramot et al. (1969) (Bulgarian), Ungar et al. (1973) (Australian English), Lischka et al. (1984) (Austrian) and Husquinet et al. (1986) (Belgian).

Konigsberg and co-workers (1965) pointed out that the occurrence of Hb D Punjab in the United Kingdom, France and Portugal was a reflection of the bonds that existed between these countries and India in the 17–20th centuries, e.g. by the marriage of British soldiers in India to Indian women. Hb D too, is now known to be not very rare in black Americans. Thus Chernoff and Farr (1956) found four Hb-AD heterozygotes in 1000 blood samples from hospital patients in Saint Louis. The maximum incidence of Hb D seems, however, to be in Sikhs [five cases in 279 blood samples, according to Bird and Lehmann (1956b)] and in Gujeratis [1%, according to Jacob, Lehmann and Raper (1956)]. Vella and Lehmann (1974) gave a comprehensive account of the global distribution of Hb D. Lehmann and Huntsman (1966, p. 199) had earlier pointed out that the area in which it is found in highest concentration in Asia is the region which was invaded by the Mongols, implying a possible origin from further north-east.

Nature of Hb D. There are in fact several 'Hb Ds', all of which migrate on electrophoresis at alkaline pH in an identical way to Hb S (Benzer, Ingram and Lehmann, 1958). But most can be separated from Hb S at an acid pH (6.0–6.5). Almost all the Hb Ds described above in the different racial groups, however, have proved to be identical — namely, to have glutamine (Gln) substituted for glutamic acid (Glu) at the β 121 residue (Baglioni, 1962). This Hb D is Hb D Punjab (or Hb D Los Angeles). The solubility of Hb D Punjab is similar to that of Hb A and its presence does not result in sickling on deoxygenation.

Hb-AD heterozygotes suffer from no clinical or haematological ill-effects and Hb-DD homozygotes have at the worst a mild, easily compensated haemolytic anaemia. Compound heterozygotes for Hb D and β-thalassaemia suffer from a mild to moderately severe thalassaemia-like syndrome (see below), while most Hb-SD patients have a rather mild form of sickle-cell disease (see p. 160).

The other β-chain Hb-D variants, e.g. Hb D Ibadan ($\alpha_2\beta_2^{87\ Thr\ \rightarrow\ Lys}$), appear to be harmless. Thus, Watson Williams and co-workers (1965) described a Yoruba Nigerian, a compound heterozygote for Hb S and Hb D Ibadan, who had no symptoms and normal haematological values. As in the Hb-AS trait, however, his erythrocytes sickled *in vitro*.

Haemoglobin-AD trait

As referred to above, Hb-AD trait carriers are clinically and haematologically normal. On electrophoresis 34–40% of the haemoglobin is Hb D (Wasi *et al.*, 1968b; Ungar *et al.*, 1973). Hb F is not present (in adults) in significant amounts.

HOMOZYGOUS HAEMOGLOBIN-D (Hb-DD) DISEASE

A 25-year-old Sikh, thought to have homozygous Hb-DD disease, was described briefly by Bird and Lehmann (1956a,b). He had complained of no symptoms attributable to his abnormal haemoglobin and his spleen was not palpable. He was, however, slightly anaemic: haemoglobin 12.8 g/dl, erythrocytes $7.1 \times 10^{12}/l$, MCV 63 fl, MCH 18 pg, reticulocytes 0.7% and serum bilirubin 0.3 mg/dl. Numerous target cells and some contracted cells could be seen in stained blood films. The mean erythrocyte diameter was normal (7.6 μm) and the mean cell thickness was diminished (1.4 μm): osmotic fragility was markedly reduced. [According to Bird (personal communication to the author), this patient was eventually shown to be suffering from Hb-D/β-thalassaemia.]

Chernoff and Farr (1956) and Chernoff (1958) described as being homozygous for Hb D a 40-year-old black female. She had three sisters all of whom had the Hb-D trait. Her own haemoglobin was almost all Hb D, there being no increase in Hb F. Her father, who had American-Indian relatives and her mother who had English relatives, had both died before her abnormal haemoglobin had been detected. She was diagnosed as being anaemic when aged 26. The haemoglobin was 12–13 g/dl and erythrocyte count $5.5–6.5 \times 10^{12}/l$; the MCV was 67 fl and MCH 23 pg. There were 1.0–1.5% reticulocytes, and 50–80% of the erythrocytes were target cells. The osmotic fragility curve was shifted symmetrically towards increased resistance, and the ^{51}Cr T_{50} was slightly subnormal (21 days).

A small number of other genuine Hb-D homozygotes have subsequently been described, *e.g.*, by Stout, Holland and Bird (1964), Özsoylu (1970) and Politis-Tsegos *et al.* (1975).

Stout, Holland and Bird's (1964) two patients were slightly anaemic; their haemoglobin was 10.1 and 9.4 g/dl, respectively, and they had slightly raised reticulocyte counts (2.3% and 4.0%).

Özsoylu's (1970) patient, a male aged 52, was not anaemic: his haemoglobin was 14.7 g/dl, erythrocyte count $5.6 \times 10^{12}/l$, MCV 77 fl, MCH 26 pg and reticulocyte count $63 \times 10^{9}/l$ (normal). He was also G6PD-deficient, but he had had no crises attributable to this.

Politis-Tsegos and her co-workers' (1975) patient was an Indian blood donor who was found to be homozygous for Hb D Punjab in the course of a screening programme. He was, however, not anaemic: haemoglobin 15 g/dl, erythrocytes $5.59 \times 10^{12}/l$, MCV 79 fl, MCH 27 pg, MCHC 34 g/dl and reticulocytes 1.4%. Blood films were characterized by slight anisocytosis and a few target cells. Electrophoresis of his haemoglobin revealed a single band in the region of Hb S. His blood did not sickle and the band was identified as being that of Hb D. There was 0.2% Hb F and 3.3% Hb A_2. The oxygen affinity of his haemoglobin was slightly increased and α: β globin-chain synthesis was found to be balanced. Osmotic fragility was decreased. Autohaemolysis was increased: 7% at 48 hours, reduced to 0.55% by added glucose.

Hb-DD disease, as judged from the small number of cases that have been described, is thus a mild and clinically unimportant condition. A moderate degree of microcytosis and hypochromia seem to be regular features as are the target cells to be seen in stained blood films (except in Özsoylu's case). Anaemia is slight or absent (Table 16.1).

Haemoglobin electrophoresis. At pH 8.6 a single band is formed in the same position as would be occupied by Hb S. Small amounts only of Hb F (< 2.4%) have been demonstrated by alkali denaturation.

HAEMOGLOBIN-D/β-THALASSAEMIA

Hb-D/β-thalassaemia has been more frequently described than homozygous Hb-DD disease. It is associated with rather more anaemia, and blood films show a greater degree of anisopoikilocytosis; the erythrocyte count tends to be high and the

MCV is lower (Table 16.1). On electrophoresis a single band of Hb D is a characteristic finding, as in genuine Hb-DD disease, and family studies, in particular the absence of Hb D in one parent, may be required to establish the diagnosis beyond doubt.

Case reports that have been published include those of Hynes and Lehmann (1956), Sukumaran, Sanghvi and Nazreth (1960), Marengo-Rowe, McCracken and Flanagan (1968), Ramot *et al.* (1969), Jain, Andleigh and Mehta (1970), Jain (1971), Oldrini, Salmini and Maiocio (1973), Tsistrakis *et al.* (1975), Rieder (1976), Wong and Ali (1980), Uva, Fernandes and Pilar (1983), Trent *et al.* (1984) and Worthington and Lehmann (1985).

Hynes and Lehmann's (1956) patient was a Persian girl aged 18: her haemoglobin was 11.3 g/dl, erythrocyte count 5.4×10^{12}/l, MCV 65 fl and MCH 20.9 pg.

Sukumaran, Sanghvi and Nazreth's (1960) four Hb-D/β-thalassaemia patients were members of two Indian families. Their haemoglobin ranged between 7.2 and 13.3 g/dl, erythrocyte count $5.21–6.48 \times 10^{12}$/l, MCV 50–70 fl and reticulocyte count 2.0–3.4%. The findings in Marengo-Rowe, McCracken and Flanagan's (1968) patient, an Indian girl aged 18, were very similar. Ramot and co-workers' (1969) patient was a Bulgarian boy aged 3 years; his haemoglobin was 9.5 g/dl and there were 6% reticulocytes; his spleen was palpable 6 cm below the left costal margin. The two patients of Tsistrakis *et al.* (1975) were adult Greek males: they were mildly jaundiced and had a palpable spleen; their haemoglobin was 11.2 and 13.9 g/dl, respectively, and MCV 70–71 fl.

Wong and Ali's (1980) patients belonged to two Canadian families: one patient was of East-Indian origin and had Hb-D/β$^+$-thalassaemia, the other was of Italian origin and had Hb-D/β^0-thalassaemia.

Uva, Fernandes and Pilar (1983) reported that three members of a Portuguese family had Hb-D/β^0-thalassaemia. They had high erythrocyte counts, $6.14–6.8 \times 10^{12}$/l; their haemoglobin was 10.6–11.8 g/dl, MCV 53–55 fl and MCH 16.0–18.2 pg. There was 93–93.7% Hb D and 4.8–5.7% Hb A$_2$. [The blood picture was similar to that of other members of the family who were Hb-A/β^0-thalassaemia heterozygotes.] Erythrocyte osmotic resistance was markedly increased in the three Hb-D/β^0-thalassaemia heterozygotes; it was normal in a Hb-AD heterozygote.

Worthington and Lehmann (1985) gave a detailed description of a large English family in which one member was found (by accident) to be a compound heterozygote for Hb D Punjab and β^0-thalassaemia.

This finding led to the discovery that the proband's brother and his mother (and 20 of her relatives) had hitherto unsuspected β^0-thalassaemia minor. Her ancestors had lived in the Midlands since at least the 18th century. The proband's father carried the Hb-AD trait; his ancestors had come to the Midlands from Monmouthshire in the 19th century.

The Hb-F percentages have been variable in the above-quoted cases. *e.g.*, from 0 to 6.0 in the adults. The Hb-A$_2$ percentages have similarly been variable, exceeding 3.7 in 12 patients and being 3.0 in four patients.

HAEMOGLOBIN-D/α-THALASSAEMIA

The combination of Hb D and α-thalassaemia has seldom been reported. A possible example was, however, described by Çavdar and Arcasoy (1974) in a Turkish family.

More recently, Trent and co-workers (1984) reported that four members of an Afghan family were compound heterozygotes for Hb D Punjab and α-thalassaemia. Their α genotype was established by restriction enzyme analysis: three were of the $-\alpha/\alpha\alpha$ genotype and one (the proposita) was of the $-\alpha/-\alpha$ genotype. The proposita had a significant degree of microcytosis (MCV 67 fl) and was possibly slightly anaemic (Hb 12.9 g/dl). An interesting finding was that the percentage of Hb D (30) was lowest in the Hb AD patient who was of the $-\alpha/-\alpha$ genotype; it was 35–37 in the patients of $-\alpha/\alpha\alpha$ genotype. This finding was considered to support the concept that the fewer α chains that are available the more likely is their association with normal β chains rather than with a variant haemoglobin's β chains for which their affinity is less.

COMPOUND HETEROZYGOSITY FOR HAEMOGLOBIN D AND HAEMOGLOBIN O INDONESIA

Hb O Indonesia is an α-chain variant (α_2^{116} $_{\text{Glu} \rightarrow \text{Lys}}$ β$_2$). The boy described by Rahbar, Nowzari and Poosti (1975) was mildly anaemic, but it was not clear whether or not his haemoglobinopathy was responsible for this as he had a hydronephrosis. On electrophoresis his haemoglobin separated into four components, namely, Hb A, Hb D, Hb O Indonesia and a Hb-O/Hb-D hybrid, $\alpha_2^O \beta^D_2$.

HAEMOGLOBIN E

Haemoglobin E (Hb E) was first described as the fourth abnormal human haemoglobin by Itano, Bergren and Sturgeon (1954) in an American family of partly Indian origin and by Chernoff, Minnich and Chongchareonsuk (1954) in the blood of eight Thai subjects. It was next identified in Veddas living in Ceylon by Graff *et al.* (1955). It was not long, however, before Hb E was found to be widespread in the Far East. Its incidence is highest in the indigenous populations of Burma (Lehmann, Story and Thein, 1956), Thailand (Na-Nakorn *et al.*, 1956; Na-Nakorn, 1959; Wasi, Na-Nakorn and Suingdumrong, 1967; Wasi, 1981), Kampuchea (Cambodia) (Brumpt *et al.*,

1958) and Laos (Sicard, Kaplan and Labie, 1978). It is, however, also quite common in Malaysia (Lehmann and Singh, 1956), Indonesia (Lie Injo, 1955, 1956, 1959, 1964, 1969; Lie-Injo and Oey, 1957), India (Chatterjea *et al.*, 1957) and in the Philippines (Stransky and Campos, 1957; Stransky, 1958) (Fig. 16.8).

Hb E appears to be rare in China — it was not found in any of 213 Chinese tested by Na-Nakorn *et al.* (1956). It is rare, too, in the Japanese; it was, however, reported in two families by Shibata, Iuchi and Hamilton (1964) and Miyaji *et al.* (1973). It is not uncommon in Eti-Turks (Aksoy and Lehmann, 1957; Aksoy and Tanrikulu, 1960)

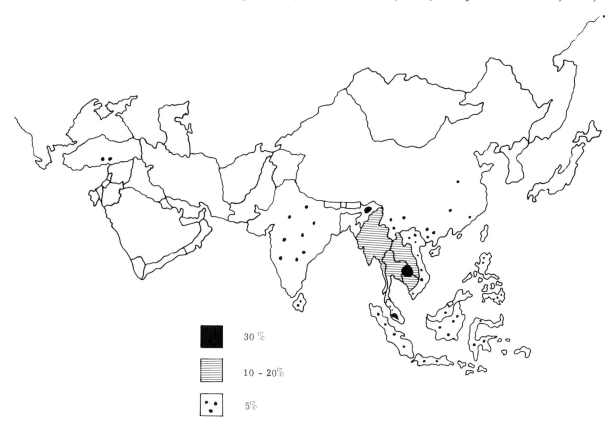

30 %

10 - 20%

5%

Distribution of haemoglobin E. At the three foci, namely Assam, the Laos-Cambodia-Thailand junction, and Malaysia (among aborigine groups) the frequencies are as high as 50 per cent or more.

Fig. 16.8 Distribution of haemoglobin E in Asia.
[Reproduced by permission from Wasi (1981).]

and it has been reported, too, in Greeks (Gouttas *et al.*, 1960b; Aksoy, 1962) and Egyptians (Hoerman *et al.*, 1961) and in a Saudi family (Hardy and Ragbeer, 1985). Vella and co-workers (1973) mentioned that three unrelated Canadians of European origin had the Hb-AE trait.

The distribution of Hb E in the Far East has naturally raised the question as to whether its high incidence in certain areas is connected with the past prevalence of malaria. This would imply that the presence of Hb E in some way increased an individual's resistance to the infection. This idea, first advanced by Na-Nakorn *et al.* (1956), has been difficult to prove, but on balance the evidence from distribution studies seems to suggest that the hypothesis of protection by malaria is correct (Flatz, Pik and Sundharagiati, 1964; Flatz, 1967). Flatz (1967) pointed out that homozygotes for Hb E or β-thalassaemia or compound heterozygotes for Hb E and thalassaemia were at a definite disadvantage, so that the maintenance of the high frequencies of the genes had to depend upon some advantage possessed by the heterozygotes and that this advantage might be mediated by protection against *Pl. falciparum* malaria. It should be noted, however, that Chatterjea (1964) had stated that of 11 patients with Hb-E/thalassaemia only two could be infected with *Pl. vivax*, compared with 13 out of 14 controls, and that this resistance was not seen with induced infection with *Pl. falciparum*.

Origin of the β^E-globin gene

As is the case with Hb S, there is now evidence that Hb E has had more than one origin. Antonarakis and his co-workers (1982) determined the haplotypes at three polymorphic restriction sites in the β-globin gene to predict the framework of 23 β^E-globin genes, derived from unselected Cambodians. Their data suggested that the β^E-globin gene (resulting from a GAG → AAG mutation at codon 26) was present in two different frameworks. Further studies, including an investigation of two European families, have indicated that the same mutation has arisen in five different haplotypes in the β-globin gene cluster, three in South-East Asians and two in Europeans (Kazazian *et al.*, 1984).

CLINICAL AND HAEMATOLOGICAL CONSEQUENCES OF THE PRESENCE OF HAEMOGLOBIN E

The consequences of the presence of Hb E are quite similar to those produced by Hb C. Individuals who have the Hb-AE trait are not anaemic and have no symptoms attributable to their abnormal haemoglobin. Hb-EE homozygotes are usually not anaemic (except sometimes in the presence of infections) and typically do not present with any haemoglobinopathy-produced symptoms. Individuals who are heterozygous for both Hb E and β-thalassaemia suffer, however, from a thalassaemia-like syndrome which is sometimes severe. Compound heterozygosity for Hb E and Hb S is very much less common, and the few patients that have been reported have had haemolytic anaemia of mild to moderate severity but few symptoms (see p. 163).

Haemoglobin-E trait

As already stated, individuals carrying the haemoglobin-E (Hb-AE) trait do not suffer any clinical disability and they are not normally anaemic. However, their erythrocytes tend to be microcytic and hypochromic and some target cells, and occasional cells showing punctate basophilia, may be seen in stained blood films (Fig. 16.9). Osmotic

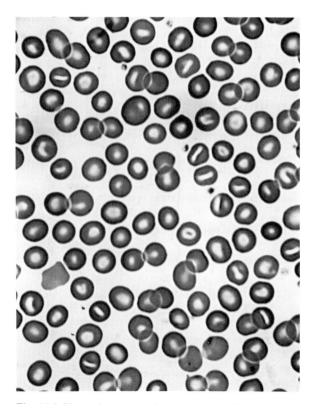

Fig. 16.9 Photomicrograph of a blood film, Hb-AE trait.
Shows slight anisocytosis and some target cells. × 750.

resistance is slightly increased (Chernoff *et al.*, 1956; Lie-Injo and Oey, 1957) and autohaemolysis similarly tends to be increased (Swarup, Ghosh and Chatterjea, 1960c).

Hb E is not present at birth in appreciable quantities, but it can be detected by the time an infant is 2 months old (Lie-Injo, 1956). In adults more than 20% but well less than 50% of the haemoglobin is Hb E; usually there is about 30%. Almost all the remainder is Hb A; Hb F is not increased in amount.

Fairbanks and co-workers (1979) studied in detail the blood picture in 21 Hb-AE trait subjects who were resident in the United States and stressed its similarity with that of thalassaemia minor. Their haemoglobin ranged from 11.6 to 16.6 g/dl, erythrocyte count 4.96–7.07 × 10^{12}/l, MCV 59–75 fl, MCH 17.1–26.9 pg, MCHC 27.6–36.0 g/dl, Hb E (including Hb A_2) 19.4–33.9% (median 30%) and Hb F 0.4–4.6%.

Microcytes, target cells and a few poikilocytes could be seen in blood films. The possibility of β-thalassaemia and/or iron deficiency could not be excluded in some of the cases but the association between Hb E and microcytosis seemed to be highly significant. The erythrocyte count was abnormally high in half the cases. Instability of Hb E could be demonstrated by the isopropanol and 2,6-dichlorphenolindophenol tests (see p. 352).

HOMOZYGOUS HAEMOGLOBIN-E (Hb-EE) DISEASE

Homozygotes for Hb E were recognized soon after Hb E was discovered. As already mentioned, they suffer from little or no disability attributable to their haemoglobinopathy, and anaemia, if present at all, is generally slight. The spleen is usually not palpable and there is no evidence of overt increased haemolysis. Brumpt and co-workers (1958), referring to cases described in Kampuchea (Cambodia) where the incidence of Hb E is very high, described the homozygous state not as a disease but as a 'terain hématique fragile' on which malnutrition, parasites and above all thalassaemia lead to severe anaemia. Lie-Injo (1969) emphasized the role of intercurrent infections, even mild ones, in the causation of anaemia.

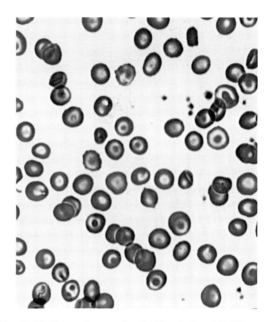

Fig. 16.10 Photomicrograph of a blood film, Hb-EE disease.
Shows anisocytosis, microcytosis and target cells. × 700. (Film provided by courtesy of Dr Wanchai Wanachiwanawin.)

The erythrocyte count is often high and the MCV and MCH are typically lower than normal; the MCHC is usually within the normal range (Table 16.1). Osmotic resistance is markedly increased and autohaemolysis usually moderately increased (Swarup, Ghosh and Chatterjea (1960c). Stained films show a moderate amount of aniso-cytosis and microcytosis but rather little poikilo-cytosis (Fig. 16.10); the target-cell percentage is variable but may reach 60 (Chernoff *et al.*, 1956; Lehmann, Story and Thein, 1956; Na-Nakorn *et al.*, 1956; Lie-Injo and Oey, 1957; Na-Nakorn and Minnich, 1957).

Electrophoresis of haemoglobin yields a single band, Hb E accounting for 90–98% of the total haemoglobin. The amount of Hb F is normal in adult patients or may be slightly increased (Table 16.2).

The two Burmese patients reported by Lehmann, Story and Thein (1956) were fit and normally active and their spleen was not palpable. Their haemoglobin ranged from 13.6 g/dl to 16.3 g/dl; the erythrocyte counts were unusually high, 7.47–8.44 × 10^{12}/l, with correspondingly low MCVs (59 and 55 fl) and MCHs (18.2 and 19.3 pg). There were 0.6% and 1.5% reticulocytes and 5% and 9% target cells, respectively, in stained films. Osmotic resistance was markedly increased. There was no increase in Hb F.

The six Thai patients described by Chernoff et al. (1956) were considered to be of rather small stature and some of them gave a history of tiredness and arthralgia and possible jaundice. The spleen was palpable in one and the liver in another. Their haemoglobin ranged from 8.8 to 13.2 g/dl, erythrocyte counts 3.97–5.55 × 10^{12}/l, MCVs 65–72 fl and MCHCs 29–34 g/l. There were 0.4–1.4% reticulocytes and 11–48% of the erythrocytes were target cells.

Their bone marrow was judged to show minimal hyperplasia. Electrophoresis of their haemoglobin demonstrated a single band of Hb E and there was up to 6.4% Hb F.

Further cases of Hb-EE disease were reported by Na-Nakorn and Minnich (1957) in Thais, by Lie-Injo and Oey (1957) in Indonesians, and by Swarup, Ghosh and Chatterjea (1960a) and Chatterjea (1965) in Indians from Calcutta. Na-Nakorn and Minnich (1957) made the point that it may be difficult to distinguish Hb-EE disease from mild cases of Hb-E/thalassaemia. Chatterjea (1965) gave details of seven patients: they were in fact slightly anaemic, their haemoglobin being 9.2–10.4 g/dl, but the reticulocyte count was normal, 0.6–1.5%. There was [unusually] no significant degree of microcytosis or hypochromia, the MCV (80–95 fl) and MCH (29–31 pg) being normal. The rate of autohaemolysis was normal or slightly increased — 1.6–12.5%, mean 6.2% at 48 hours without added glucose.

Ong (1975) described how pregnancy is well tolerated in Hb-EE disease (and in the Hb-AE trait).

More recently, Fairbanks and co-workers (1980) reported detailed studies on two patients (one from Thailand, the other from Vietnam) living in the United States. They made the point that mild chronic increased haemolysis is not a feature of Hb-EE disease — in one of their patients the ^{51}Cr T_{50} was 28 days; they stressed, too, that if such a patient is anaemic this should not necessarily be attributed to the haemoglobinopathy. The O_2-dissociation curve of their patients' haemoglobin was displaced slightly to the right (p_{50} 32 mm Hg) and the α:non-α chain synthesis was increased (as in β-thalassaemia trait).

Nature of haemoglobin E

Hb E results from the substitution of lysine for glutamic acid at the β26 (B8) position of the β chain (Hunt and Ingram, 1961). Its constitution is thus $\alpha_2\beta_2^{26\ Glu\to Lys}$. On electrophoresis at an alkaline pH Hb E runs with Hb C and Hb A_2.

Hb E is relatively unstable. Frischer and Bowman (1975) observed that haemolysates of blood samples from the Far East (containing Hb E) developed turbidity in the presence of the dye 2,6-dichlorphenolindophenol (DCPI). Fairbanks and co-workers (1979), too, reported that Hb E was unusually easily precipitated by isopropanol and DCPI. Ali, Quinlan and Wong (1980) found that all 13 samples of Hb E they tested were precipitated by isopropanol, compared to 16 samples of Hb C, none of which underwent precipitation.

Hb E is also abnormally sensitive to oxidant stress. Macdonald and Charache (1983) compared the sensitivity of Hb E, Hb S, Hb A and Hb F to oxidation by menadione and acetylphenylhydrazine. Hb E was the most reactive: the rate of oxidation was only slightly increased, but Hb E produced much more haemichrome than the other haemoglobins. The order of precipitation was Hb E > Hb S > Hb A > Hb F. Swarup, Ghosh and Chatterjea (1960b) had earlier found that GSH was unstable in 12 out of 20 cases of Hb-E/thalassaemia, despite high levels of G6PD. Swarup, Ghosh and Chatterjea (1966) concluded that this was brought about by an unexplained deficiency of NADP.

Globin-chain synthesis. Feldman and Rieder (1973) found in haemoglobin synthesis studies that the specific activity of β^E chains in Hb-AE heterozygotes was greater than that of β^A chains despite a Hb-A:Hb-E ratio of 3:1 in the peripheral blood. This was interpreted as indicating instability of Hb E and its preferential destruction.

The α:non-α globin-synthesis ratio has also been measured. Abnormally high ratios were reported by Fairbanks et al. (1980) in two Hb-EE patients and by Bird et al. (1984) in six out of eight patients (six Hb-AE, one Hb-E/β-thalassaemia and one Hb EE, the latter two patients giving the most abnormal results (see also p. 309).

Oxygen affinity. The whole-blood O_2-dissociation curve in Hb-EE patients is shifted slightly to the right (Bellingham and Huehns, 1968; Fairbanks et al., 1980). According to Gacon, Wajcman and Labie (1974) and May and Huehns (1977), this can be explained by an increased erythrocyte content of 2,3,DPG. The O_2 affinity of purified Hb E is normal (Bunn et al., 1972).

Pathogenesis of Hb-EE disease

As already referred to (p. 302), patients with Hb-EE disease show no evidence of overt increased haemolysis. In fact, the few studies on erythrocyte life-span that have been carried out have given just subnormal or normal results, e.g., ^{51}Cr T_{50} 23 days (Na-Nakorn and Minnich, 1957) and 28 days (Fairbanks et al., 1980). To what extent the slight instability of Hb E contributes to any reduction in life-span is uncertain; it does not seem to have any clinical importance although it may be responsible, at least in part, for the low MCH (and MCV).

The benign nature of Hb-EE disease is somewhat surprising, bearing in mind that the presence of a single Hb-E gene in combination with that for β-thalassaemia leads generally to a disorder often comparable in severity to that of homozygous β-thalassaemia. Excess α-globin chains do not seem, however, to be as damaging in Hb-EE disease as they are in homozygous thalassaemia.

As with Hb C, the way in which the presence of Hb E leads to target-cell formation remains obscure.

Treatment of Hb-EE disease

No treatment seems indicated, but as in β-thalassaemia minor, the long-continued administration of iron, in an attempt to raise the MCH, is contraindicated. As already mentioned, if a patient shown to have Hb-EE disease is anaemic, a cause for anaemia other than the haemoglobinopathy should be sought.

COMPOUND HETEROZYGOSITY FOR HAEMOGLOBIN E AND β-THALASSAEMIA (Hb-E/β-THALASSAEMIA)

Hb-E/β-thalassaemia is an important and not uncommon cause of ill health in the Far East. In 1954 a series of patients were described in Thailand by Minnich et al. as suffering from Mediterranean anaemia; on reinvestigation, however, five of them were found to have Hb-E/thalassaemia (Chernoff, Minnich and Chongchareonsuk, 1954;

Chernoff et al., 1956) Further cases in other Asiatic racial groups were soon reported, e.g. by Sturgeon, Itano and Bergren (1955) (in a Hindu), by Lie-Injo et al. (1956), van Gool, Punt and de Vries (1956) and Punt and van Gool (1957) in Indonesians and Indonesian-Dutch, by Chatterjea et al. (1957) and Chatterjea (1965) in Bengalees, by Nagaratnam et al. (1958) in a Ceylonese family and by Klefstad-Sillonville et al. (1962) in Cambodians.

A severe familial haemolytic anaemia (Stransky and Regala's anaemia), rather similar to, but not identical with, thalassaemia major, had been recognized in the Far East well before Hb E had been discovered. Stransky (1952), in an interesting Newsletter dealing with the occurrence of anaemia in the Philippines (based on his experiences there since 1939), wrote as follows: 'We have observed an interesting form of familial hemolytic anemia, possibly related to Cooley's anemia, but not identical with it. Symptoms appear in early childhood or even later in life. There is stunting of growth, severe anemia, marked jaundice and splenomegaly. Hemoglobin of the fetal type is found in only a few cases and in moderate amounts. Splenectomy is unsuccessful.' As a succinct description of Hb-E/β-thalassaemia this could hardly be bettered and there seems little doubt but that this was the diagnosis in some at least of Stransky's patients. Accounts of their illness make interesting reading (Stransky and Regala, 1946; Stransky, 1951).

Clinical expression. The clinical findings and course of Hb-E/β-thalassaemia are very similar to those of β-thalassaemia major. The symptoms vary rather widely, but anaemia is often severe (Table 16.1). According to Wasi et al. (1969), whose experience was then based on more than 400 patients, the clinical severity of the disease in Thailand lies between that of Hb-H disease and typical homozygous β-thalassaemia.

The patients' facies resemble that of β-thalassaemia major (Figs. 16.11 and 16.12), and growth and sexual development are usually retarded. The abdomen may eventually become greatly enlarged. This is mainly the result of splenomegaly but the liver may be massively enlarged, too. Bone, joint and muscle pains are typically not complained of. Ulcers of the leg may occur but are not common. Pregnancy may be hazardous, with increase in anaemia and premature delivery (Lie-Injo, Hoo and Kho, 1959).

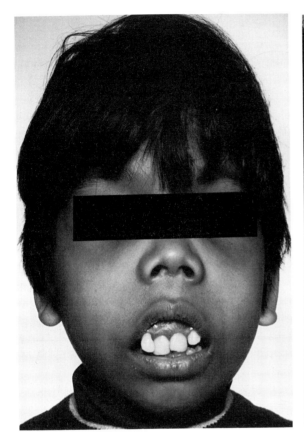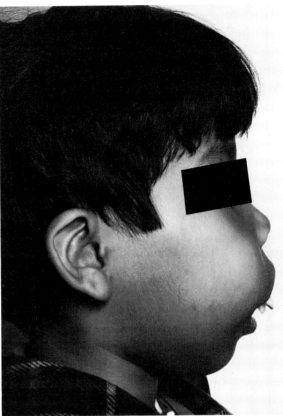

Fig. 16.11 Haemoglobin-E/β-thalassaemia.
  Shows facial distortion due to expansion of the facial bones caused by hyperplasia of the bone marrow. Front and side views, patient aged 10. (Reproduced by courtesy of Dr J. van der Pette.)

Of the 32 patients referred to by Chernoff *et al.* (1956), 28 were judged to be severely and four moderately severely affected. The disorder was usually discernible in the 1st year of life and in only four of the patients were major symptoms postponed until after the 10th year. Most of the children had presented with an enlarged spleen (from 5 cm below the left costal margin to the brim of the pelvis), pallor and intermittent jaundice. Some had had crises characterized by pyrexia and darkening of the urine.

Aksoy and co-workers (1963) described three unusual patients. One had severe pancytopenia associated with massive splenomegaly. Following the removal of a 2090-g spleen the haemoglobin rose from 3.8 to 8.8 g/dl, the total leucocyte count from 2.2 to 14.2 × 10⁹/l and the platelet count from 50 to 440 × 10⁹/l. The other two patients were male twins aged 26; their blood pictures were closely similar and the results of haemoglobin electrophoresis were almost identical: Hb E 87% and 87.5%; Hb F 10% and 9.2%, and Hb A 3.0% and 3.3%.

Flatz, Pik and Sringam (1965), in a paper describing regional differences in the distribution of Hb E in Thai-land, stressed that Hb-E/β-thalassaemia patients had a poor life expectancy and a low fertility; they also pointed out that Hb E and β-thalassaemia are distributed in Thailand in a reciprocal fashion.

Mehta and co-workers (1980) referred to 16 patients, from five different areas of India: 10 had a disorder clinically equivalent to thalassaemia intermedia; five were severely affected and required blood transfusion from early childhood. Fourteen of the patients were of the Hb-E/ β⁺-thalassaemia variety; only one had Hb-E/ β⁰-thalassaemia. One patient had Hb-E/δβ-thalassaemia.

Tumour-like masses of bone marrow

As in thalassaemia intermedia (see p. 427), adult patients with Hb-E/β-thalassaemia occasionally develop tumour-like extramedullary masses of bone marrow. These sometimes give rise to serious consequences.

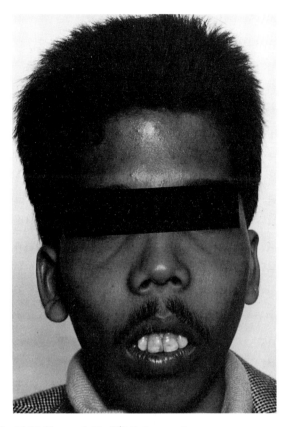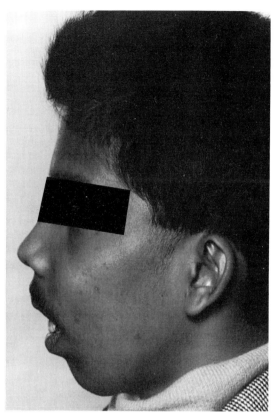

Fig. 16.12 Haemoglobin-E/β-thalassaemia.
Same patient as shown in Figure 16.11. Shows encouraging improvement in facial distortion. Patient aged 24. (Reproduced by courtesy of Dr J. van der Pette.)

Da Costa, Loh and Hanam (1974) described a 55-year-old female who presented with cough and dyspnoea. X-ray examination revealed very large mediastinal masses and the diagnosis was not cleared up until biopsy was undertaken. Dhechakaisaya, Shuang-shoti and Susakares [1979, quoted by Fucharoen et al. (1981)] described a patient with extramedullary haemopoiesis within the cranial dura mater and choroid plexus that was associated with terminal convulsions. Fucharoen and co-workers (1981) themselves reported the occurrence in a 27-year-old female, who died of respiratory failure, cerebral anoxia and cardiac arrest, of an intracranial mass, 10 × 9 × 1.2 cm in size, that was attached to the dura and falx cerebri; it had extended over the central part of both hemispheres and had led to atrophy of the underlying brain tissue. [This patient had had, too, an auto-immune haemolytic anaemia for which she had undergone splenectomy; she also had developed spinal-cord compression as the result of having extramedullary masses for which she had received deep X-ray therapy.]
Issaragrisil, Piankijagum and Wasi (1981) described

12 patients, aged between 17 and 40 years, with Hb-E/β[0]-thalassaemia, all of whom had developed symptoms and signs of spinal-cord compression. This was proved by surgery in two of the patients and by myelography in six. In the remaining patients a prompt response to deep X-ray therapy (1500–3500 rads) substantiated the diagnosis of cord compression by haemopoietic tissue. Recovery or improvement in the neurological symptoms and signs followed blood transfusion in some of the patients, but the responses were slow and uncertain compared to that resulting from radiotherapy. Issaragrisil et al. pointed out that they had not seen the syndrome in Hb-H disease patients in Thailand despite its prevalence; they emphasized, however, that Hb-H disease is generally a less severe disorder than is Hb-E/-thalassaemia.

Blood picture

This resembles that of β-thalassaemia major: anisopoikilocytosis, microcytosis and hypochromia are usually conspicuous and there may be punctate basophilia; target cells are present in variable numbers and usually, too, small numbers of contracted spherocyte-like cells (Fig. 16.13). Normoblasts are typically present and after splenectomy they are often responsible for a high proportion of the total nucleated cell count. Macrocytes, too, are conspicuous after splenectomy, many being target cells (Fig. 16.14). Osmotic resistance is markedly increased.

The haematological findings in the 32 patients described by Chernoff *et al.* (1956) were as follows: haemoglobin 3.0–7.0 g/dl, erythrocyte count 1.5–3.5 $\times 10^{12}$/l, MCV 65–75 fl, MCHC 27–29 g/dl, reticulocyte count 4–6%, target cells 5–25%, spherocytes 6–9%, osmotic fragility 90% lysis in 0.16–0.20 g/dl NaCl. Chatterjea's (1965) data were based on a vast experience gained in Calcutta (545 cases): haemoglobin 2.9–12.9 (mean 6.0) g/dl, erythrocyte count 0.97–3.9 (mean 2.47) $\times 10^{12}$/l, reticulocyte count 2.2–35 (mean 8.5)%, MCV 68–112 (mean 84) fl, MCH 16–34 (mean 24.3) pg, MCHC 24–35 (mean 27.7) g/dl, serum bilirubin 0.2–5.3 (mean 1.3) mg/dl, autohaemolysis (48 hours at 37°C) without added glucose 4.6–15%, with added glucose 0.5–13%.

Bunyaratrej and co-workers (1985) used a scanning electron microscope to study erythrocyte morphology in 79 patients with Hb-E/β-thalassaemia who had not been transfused for at least 2 months. The many abnormal cells present were categorized into *torocytes* (thin cells with a thickened rim), *codocytes* (target cells), *dacryocytes* (tear-drop cells), *keratocytes* (burr or spur cells), *schizocytes* (fragments) and *echinocytes* (crenated cells). Splenectomy, a large spleen and severe anaemia were each associated with a diminished number of normal cells (*discocytes*); splenectomy, too, led to increased percentages of target cells and echinocytes. Large spleens were associated with increased evidence of fragmentation; splenectomy, on the other hand, led to a notable reduction — an observation linking fragmentation with the presence of a spleen.

Haemoglobin electrophoresis

Hb E (usually 55–85%) and Hb F are always demonstrable; Hb A may be absent or a small or moderate proportion may be present (Table 16.2). The amount of Hb F naturally depends to some extent on the patient's age: *e.g.*, Chernoff *et al.* (1956) reported 5.5–85%, Chatterjea *et al.* (1957) 5.8–49% (with 39% in one patient aged 20 years), Chatterjea (1965) 7–58% (mean 28%). Hb A varied from O to 28.3% in the 20 patients described by Chatterjea *et al.* (1957).

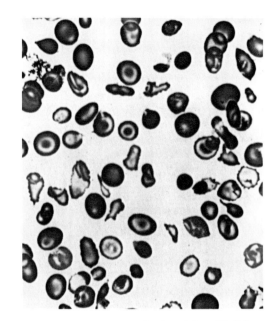

Fig. 16.13 Photomicrograph of a blood film, Hb-E/β-thalassaemia.
Shows marked anisocytosis, poikilocytosis and anisochromasia; also target cells and contracted spherocyte-like cells. × 700. (Film provided by courtesy of Dr Wanchai Wanachiwanawin.)

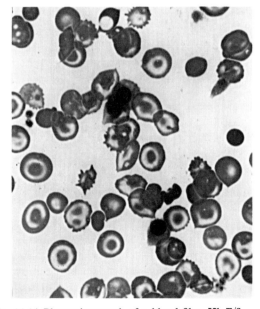

Fig. 16.14 Photomicrograph of a blood film, Hb-E/β-thalassaemia after splenectomy.
Shows marked anisocytosis and macrocytosis; also echinocytosis, many target cells and a few spherocyte-like cells. Three normoblasts are present. × 700.

Wasi and co-workers (1969) gave details of their findings in a large number of Thai patients. Ten of them, from four unrelated families, formed Hb A: the mean values for Hb E were 55%, Hb F 16% and Hb A 29%. A much greater number of patients failed to form Hb A, *i.e.*, had Hb-E/β^0-thalassaemia, than in the Indian patients of Chatterjea *et al.* (1957). Four patients in one family in which Hb A_2 was not elevated in family members with thalassaemia trait were considered to have Hb-E/$\delta\beta$-thalassaemia.

Erythrocyte life-span

This is shortened and undoubtedly contributes to the severity of the patients' anaemia.

Hosain and co-workers (1962) studied five patients and concluded that the pattern of elimination of ^{51}Cr-labelled erythrocytes fitted a double exponential curve: the mean cell life (MCL) in the five cases ranged from 4 to 21 days, with a fast component (MCL 1 day) and a slow component (MCL 22–24 days). The extent of the fast component was directly correlated with the reticulocyte count but it was not clear whether it was the reticulocytes that were actually being rapidly eliminated from the circulation.

PATHOLOGY OF HAEMOGLOBIN-E/β-THALASSAEMIA

Bhamarapravati and co-workers (1967) published details of 20 necropsies. The main findings were as follows: widespread siderosis of reticulo-endothelial and parenchyma cells, *e.g.* in liver and kidney; hyperplasia of haemopoietic tissue; in some cases monolobular or septal hepatic cirrhosis, and in other patients proliferative lesions of the renal glomeruli.

The occurrence in some patients of tumour-like masses of haemopoietic tissue has already been referred to (p. 306).

PATHOGENESIS OF HAEMOGLOBIN-E/β-THALASSAEMIA

Three factors contribute to the anaemia of Hb-E/β-thalassaemia: ineffective erythropoiesis,

reduction in erythrocyte life-span and enlargement of the spleen. These factors are the same as operate in homozygous β-thalassaemia. In summary, unbalanced globin-chain production (i.e. reduced β^E and β^A globin-chain production and thus relatively excessive α-chain production), and possibly, too, the instability of Hb E, lead to ineffective erythropoiesis. The consequent failure to form haemoglobin results in the microcytosis and hypochromia (and the anisocytosis and poikilocytosis and fragmentation). The poorly produced and deformed erythrocytes have a reduced life-span. The splenomegaly results from the sequestration of abnormal erythrocytes; it is also a work hypertrophy phenomenon, secondary to the diminished erythrocyte life-span, to which it itself may contribute by virtue of its enlargement.

Ineffective erythropoiesis

The nature and mechanism of ineffective erythropoiesis in Hb-E/β-thalassaemia has been repeatedly studied, and it has been shown that the synthesis of Hb E is impaired because β^E mRNA is unstable (see below).

Early work using ^{59}Fe showed that despite a rapid plasma iron clearance the utilization of iron by erythrocyte precursors is much less than normal. Swarup and co-workers (1961) found in four Hb-E/β-thalassaemia patients that only approximately 20% of the administered iron appeared in the peripheral blood, compared with an expected percentage of about 80.

Ruymann, Popejoy and Brouillard (1978) studied a Thai girl aged 13 years. The α:β^E+γ chain ratio was 1.26 in bone-marrow reticulocytes and 1.90 in peripheral-blood reticulocytes. The γ:β^E chain ratio was 0.36 using reticulocytes from both sources. Despite this, the ratio of Hb E to Hb F in the peripheral blood was 49:51. No β^A chains were demonstrable. The circulating erythrocyte haem turnover rate was calculated to be about 6 times the normal, indicating markedly ineffective erythropoiesis. Splenectomy was carried out, and the ^{51}Cr T_{50} rose from 22.7 days to 32.8 days after the operation. Heinz-body-like inclusions (excess α chains) could be found in the peripheral blood after splenectomy; none had been seen before the operation.

According to Testa *et al.* (1980), an important mechanism leading to the high levels of Hb F in the peripheral blood is the increased survival of cells containing most Hb F.

Later studies have shown clearly that the β^E globin chain is inefficiently synthesized (Testa *et al.*, 1980; Benz *et al.*, 1981; Wasi *et al.*, 1982). According to Traeger *et al.* (1980), who studied Hb-AE heterozygotes and Hb-EE homozygotes, and Benz *et al.* (1981) who studied Hb-E/β-thalassaemia compound heterozygotes, this is due to an abnormally low production of β^E mRNA. This results apparently from β^E mRNA being unstable (Traeger, Winichagoon and Wood, 1982).

Wickramasinghe and his co-workers (1981) reported on an electron-microscope study of erythroblasts in the peripheral blood of two Hb-E/β-thalassaemia patients who had not undergone splenectomy and of three patients whose spleen had been removed. Intracellular precipitates (probably of α-globin chains), and other mild dyserythropoietic changes, were found to be present in early and late polychromatic erythroblasts, and in reticulocytes, too. Bone-marrow macrophages had phagocytosed erythroblasts. The changes were similar to those seen in homozygous β-thalassaemia.

Dorléac and co-workers (1984) emphasized that the presence of the β^E gene leads to thalassaemia-like features; they cited how the erythrocyte indices in Hb-EE homozygotes mimic those in β-thalassaemia minor and the extent to which β^E-globin synthesis is impaired. They themselves demonstrated in the membrane of Hb-AE erythrocytes a kinetic abnormality of neutral phosphatase similar to that which they had previously found in various types of β-thalassaemia; they also demonstrated increased binding of Hb E (and Hb A) to Hb-AE erythrocyte ghosts.

ANTENATAL DIAGNOSIS OF HAEMOGLOBIN-E/β-THALASSAEMIA

The clinical severity of Hb-E/β-thalassaemia, and its frequency in Asia, have stimulated research into the possibility of detecting the mutations antenatally. Thein and co-workers (1986) have reported success in detecting Hb E specifically and directly in DNA obtained by chorion biopsy using a synthetic oligonucleotide probe. They concluded that using the β^E probe in combination with oligonucleotide probes for the common types of β-thalassaemia would make it possible to detect a large proportion of affected fetuses in the first trimester.

TREATMENT OF HAEMOGLOBIN-E/β-THALASSAEMIA

The problem is the same as in homozygous β-thal-assaemia. Transfusions should be avoided, if possible, but cannot be withheld from a seriously anaemic patient. If many are needed, then the dangerous consequences of iron overload have to be faced up to and treatment with iron chelators considered.

Splenectomy

As in homozygous β-thalassaemia, little benefit can be expected from splenectomy except when there are special circumstances.

Chatterjea and co-workers (1961) reported on 34 Hb-E/β-thalassaemia patients aged from 1 to 10 years, who had been submitted to splenectomy. The mean haemoglobin level rose only a little from 5.7 to 7.5 g/dl, but there were major rises in mean reticulocyte, leucocyte and platelet counts and in the mean number of circulating normoblasts (from 2384 to 46 046 per μl). Ten of the patients had died after splenectomy, two of post-operative complications and eight of infections. Chatterjea *et al.* concluded that the operation should not be undertaken unless the spleen is massively enlarged and/or there are signs of hypersplenism or there is a history of repeated crises or evidence of the rapid destruction of donor erythrocytes associated with splenic sequestration.

Wasi and co-workers (1969) reported that the haemoglobin of 143 patients submitted to splenectomy rose only in those who had presented with signs of hypersplenism — presumably patients with massive splenomegaly, unusually low haemoglobin levels and neutropenia and thrombocytopenia.

Bunyaratrej and co-workers (1985), as part of their detailed survey of erythrocyte morphology in Hb-E/β-thalassaemia, compared the blood picture of 49 patients with their spleen *in situ* with that of 30 patients who had undergone splenectomy. They found that there were no significant differences in haemoglobin, PCV, erythrocyte count, MCH and MCHC; the MCV was, however, significantly higher in the splenectomized patients, mean 82.9 ± 1.8 fl compared with 69.2 ± 0.7 fl before the operation. There were, however, major differences in erythrocyte morphology (see p. 308 and Figs. 16.13 and 16.14).

HAEMOGLOBIN-E/α-THALASSAEMIA

The combination of two α-thalassaemia genes in the same patient in addition to Hb E was described by Tuchinda *et al.* (1964). Five Thai families had been studied and children forming

Hb E and Hb Bart's or Hb H identified. These were considered to possess two α-thalassaemia genes in addition to a single gene for Hb E. Three groups were distinguished with respect to the amount of Hb E formed: those with 10–16% Hb E were considered to possess two α genes; those with 22–28% Hb E three α genes; those with 30–34% Hb E to possess normal α genes, *i.e.* to be simple HE heterozygotes. It was suggested that the presence of α-thalassaemia genes decreases the amount of β^E polypeptide chains formed relative to those of β^A, as well as the number of α chains formed relative to non-α chains.

A fuller description of Hb-E/α-thalassaemia was given by Wasi *et al.* (1967). Clinically, the syndrome could not be distinguished from homozygous β-thalassaemia, Hb-E/β-thalassaemia and Hb-H disease, all prevalent in Thailand. The 21 patients they described ranged in age from 5 to 38 years. They were all anaemic (haemoglobin 3.2–9.8 g/dl) and almost all were jaundiced, and the liver and spleen were palpable in nearly all of them. The blood picture was strikingly abnormal, with marked anisochromasia, anisopoikilocytosis and fragmentation, and target cells were present in variable numbers. A characteristic feature was the presence of inclusions (thought to be of Hb H) which stained with methylene blue in 'wet' preparations. In contrast to Hb-H disease, however, relatively few erythrocytes contained these inclusion bodies. Haemoglobin electrophoresis revealed: Hb E 12.2–18.9%, Hb Bart's 3.4.–18%, Hb F 1.5–5.2%; the remainder was Hb A, with a small amount of an unidentified fraction, thought probably to be Hb δ_4 or Hb β_4^E. Occasionally a faint band was seen in the position of Hb H. Splenectomy was carried out in six of the patients; the anaemia of two of them was improved — one had hypersplenism.

The percentage of haemoglobin that was Hb E in the above-described patients was noted by Wasi *et al.* (1967) to be much less than in simple Hb-AE heterozygotes, as had earlier been found in the patients reported by Tuchinda *et al.* in 1964. Tuchinda, Beale and Lehmann (1967) suggested that this stemmed from β^A chains being more successful than β^E chains in competing for the limited number of α chains being synthesized. Fessas (1968) attributed it to instability of the β^E chains making more β^A chains available.

Wong and Ali (1982), in a more recent study of nine members of two South-East Asian families, were able to contrast the blood picture and the α:non-α globin synthesis ratio in four different Hb-E syndromes: they demonstrated a progressive decrease in the ratio from Hb EE (1.43–1.60), Hb AE (1.15–1.02), Hb-AE/α-thal-2 (0.83) to Hb-AE/Hb-H disease (0.54).

Winichagoon and co-workers (1985) studied by means of restriction endonuclease DNA mapping the α-thal-

assaemia genotype in 42 Thai patients suffering from Hb-E/β⁰-thalassaemia. Seven of them were found to have the α-thal-2 haplotype: in five this was of the rightward or 3.7 kb type and in two the leftward or 4.2 kb type. All seven patients with α-thalassaemia had a haemoglobin above 7.4 g/dl and attended the anaemia clinic only occasionally: those without α-thalassaemia had a haemoglobin above or below 7.4 g/dl and attended the clinic regularly. Winichagoon *et al.* concluded that the concomitant presence of α-thalassaemia can alleviate the severity of Hb-E/β⁰-thalassaemia.

COMBINATION OF HAEMOGLOBIN E WITH HEREDITARY PERSISTENCE OF FETAL HAEMOGLOBIN (HPFH)

Wasi, Pootrakul and Na-Nakorn (1968a) reported the occurrence of the above association in a Thai family. The Hb-A/HPFH heterozygotes were healthy and had 21–22% Hb F, with low Hb-A_2 levels. Three members of the family were Hb-E/HPFH heterozygotes; they, too, were healthy and were not considered to be anaemic: their haemoglobin was 12.5–13.3 g/dl, erythrocyte count 4.78–6.27 $\times$ 10^{12}/l, MCV 64–77 fl, MCH 21–26 pg, and reticulocyte counts 1.2–2.0%. Target cells could be seen in stained blood films. Electrophoresis revealed that Hb A was absent: there was 34–41% Hb E; the remaining haemoglobin was Hb F.

COMBINATION OF HAEMOGLOBIN E, α-THALASSAEMIA AND HAEMOGLOBIN CONSTANT SPRING

Ganesan and co-workers (1977) described the presence of Hb E, α-thalassaemia and Hb Constant Spring in a Malaysian family. The propositus was a 20-year-old female who was thought to be a heterozygote for Hb E and Hb Constant Spring and to also carry a gene for α-thalassaemia. She had a haemoglobin of 8.7 g/dl and her spleen was palpable 2 cm below the left costal margin. She had a markedly abnormal blood picture, with hypochromia and marked anisopoikilocytosis. A few of the erythrocytes contained Hb-H-like inclusions demonstrable in wet preparations. The MCV was 72 fl and MCH 19 pg, and there were 4.2% reticulocytes; the serum bilirubin was 1.4 mg/dl. Haemoglobin electrophoresis revealed, in addition to Hb A, 16% Hb E, 1.9% Hb Bart's and 1% Hb Constant Spring. There was 1.7% Hb F. The brother of the propositus had typical Hb-H disease as well as Hb Constant Spring.

COMBINATION OF HAEMOGLOBIN E WITH HAEMOGLOBIN NEW YORK

Pootrakul and co-workers (1971) described the

occurrence in a Thai family of Hb E and Hb New York ($\alpha_2\beta_2^{113 \ Val \rightarrow Glu}$). Two male sibs were compound heterozygotes: neither was significantly anaemic and the erythrocyte morphology was normal.

HAEMOGLOBIN E AND SOUTH-EAST ASIAN HEREDITARY OVALOCYTOSIS (SEAHO)

Lie-Injo and co-workers (1972) observed Hb E plus elliptocytosis in 61 out of 1384 Malaysians. The combination did not, however, appear to be associated with symptoms or haematological abnormalities (other than the elliptocytosis). Four were Hb-E homozygotes (as well as having SEAHO); they had a slight increase in Hb F and their blood films were considered to show slightly more anisopoikilocytosis than was usually found in heterozygous Hb-E/SEAHO or in either trait separately, or in homozygous Hb E. The Hb E and SEAHO were inherited independently.

HAEMOGLOBIN O

'Hb-O' was first described as a 'new' haemoglobin by Lie-Injo and Sadono (1958). Six Hb-AO heterozygotes were found amongst 455 Buginesi living in Sulawasi (Celebes) and five similar individuals were discovered in three other tribes. The haemoglobin was originally referred to as Hb Buginese, and there was no evidence of any haematological abnormality in the Hb-AO heterozygotes. Subsequently, further examples of 'Hb O' were found in an Arab family in Israel in which two members, a boy and a girl, were shown to be compound heterozygotes for 'Hb O' and Hb S; both were anaemic (Ramot et al., 1960) (p. 163). Next, Baglioni and Lehmann (1962) showed that the Indonesian and Arab varieties of 'Hb O' were different: i.e., Hb O Indonesia is an α-chain variant ($\alpha_2^{116 \ Glu \rightarrow Lys} \beta_2$) and Hb O Arab a β-chain variant ($\alpha_2\beta_2^{121 \ Glu \rightarrow Lys}$), which has a motility at alkaline pH closely similar to that of Hb C. Recently, Hb O Arab has been found in a Sicilian family (Sciarratta et al., 1985).

HOMOZYGOUS HAEMOGLOBIN-O (Hb-OO) DISEASE

A small number of patients homozygous for Hb O have been described. They seem to have suffered from mildly to moderately increased haemolysis (Table 16.1).

Kantchev and co-workers (1975), in describing the syndrome associated with compound heterozygosity for Hb O Arab and β-thalassaemia (see below), stated in an added note that they had identified a 5-year-old girl, living in East Thrace, who appeared to be homozygous for Hb O. She had the facies of an individual with a haemoglobinopathy; her spleen was palpable 2 cm below the left costal margin, and she was mildly jaundiced and appeared to be anaemic. The haemoglobin was 7.0 g/dl and erythrocyte count 2.5×10^{12}/l. Haemoglobin electrophoresis revealed that almost all the haemoglobin was Hb O; Hb A could not be demonstrated and there was 2% of Hb F.

A similar case was described by Efremov et al. (1977) in a gipsy family living in Yugoslavia. The propositus was a young female who appeared to have been mildly chronically anaemic since childhood, and to have had episodes of acute haemolysis. Splenectomy had been carried out when she was 14. When studied aged 18, the haemoglobin was 11.2–12.0 g/dl, MCH 29–30 pg, reticulocyte count 0.9–4.9% and bilirubin 3.6 mg/dl. Her blood film was described as showing anisopoikilocytosis and target cells. The ^{51}Cr T$_{50}$ was 25 days. Electrophoresis of haemoglobin revealed a single band of Hb O Arab. There was 1.2–1.6% Hb F. Hb O Arab was identified in members of the family in three generations. The Hb-AO heterozygotes (38–43% Hb O) had no symptoms attributable to their abnormal haemoglobin, but their blood films were reported to show slight anisopoikilocytosis and hypochromia, and a few target cells, and osmotic fragility was decreased.

COMPOUND HETEROZYGOSITY FOR HAEMOGLOBIN O ARAB AND β-THALASSAEMIA

A small number of patients heterozygous for both Hb O Arab and β-thalassaemia have been reported, most of whom have been moderately severely anaemia (Table 16.1).

Kantchev, Tcholakov and Baglioni (1965) described how they had observed several examples of a severe hypochromic, apparently haemolytic, anaemia in unrelated adults living in the Burgas region of Bulgaria, adjacent to Turkey. The patients were slightly jaundiced and their spleen was palpable. Osmotic resistance was increased and 40–90% of their erythrocytes were target cells. Haemoglobin electrophoresis revealed that Hb A was absent and that a single band of a more slowly moving haemoglobin, identified as Hb O Arab, was present. Four family trees were illustrated: in three of them one parent of the propositus had Hb AO and the other parent β-thalassaemia trait (not uncommon in this formerly malarious region of Bulgaria). In the fourth family the data were insufficient to exclude the possibility that the propositus was homozygous for Hb O.

Further data on 16 compound heterozygotes for Hb O Arab and β-thalassaemia were given by Kantchev et al. (1975). They were slightly to moderately severely anaemic: the haemoglobin ranged between 6 and 13 g/dl, erythrocyte count 2.0–4.0 × 10^{12}/l and reticulocyte count 3.5–8.2%: the maximum serum bilirubin recorded was 6 mg/dl. Blood films showed hypochromia and anisopoikilocytosis, with microcytes and macrocytes and 40–90% of target cells. Haemoglobin electrophoresis revealed a complete absence of Hb A. The general condition of the patients (aged 1–73 years) was good between attacks of increased haemolysis, which were usually precipitated by infections.

Kantchev and co-workers (1975) concluded that the combination of Hb O and β-thalassaemia results in a syndrome that is more severe than β-thalassaemia minor (Hb A plus β-thalassaemia); they judged its severity to be similar to that of Hb-E/β-thalassaemia. They drew attention, however, to the fact that the black West-Indian patient referred to by Milner et al. (1970) as having Hb-O Arab/β-thalassaemia (and who formed some Hb A) was free from symptoms attributable to the haemoglobinopathy.

A further patient, a 29-year-old pregnant Hungarian female, with splenomegaly and moderate anaemia, was described by Horányi et al. (1980) as suffering from Hb O Arab/β-thalassaemia. The PCV was 32%. Haemoglobin electrophoresis revealed 90% Hb O Arab, 5.9% Hb F and 3.9% Hb A_2.

DOUBLE HETEROZYGOSITY FOR HAEMOGLOBIN O ARAB AND α-THALASSAEMIA

El-Hazmi and Lehmann (1980) reported the occurrence of this combination in a 38-year-old Saudi-Arabian female. She had a microcytic hypochromic anaemia unresponsive to treatment with iron. The haemoglobin was 8.3 g/dl and erythrocyte count 4.2 × 10^{12}/l, with 5% reticulocytes. There was marked anisopoikilocytosis and occasional target cells were present. The spleen was enlarged and splenectomy was carried out.

Study of her haemoglobin revealed that she was heterozygous for Hb O Arab. However, in addition, globin-chain synthesis studies revealed, in both haemin-free and haemin-containing media, that the synthesis of α chains was markedly decreased compared to that of non-α chains. This led to the diagnosis of α-thalassaemia. Her family, unfortunately, could not be investigated.

REFERENCES

ABEL, C. C. & BEIER, L. (1961). Erythrocyte sedimentation rate in various hemoglobinopathies. *Amer. J. med. Sci.*, **242**, 463–467.

ABRAHAM, E. C., CAMERON, B. F., ABRAHAM, A. & STALLINGS, M. (1984). Glycosylated hemoglobins in heterozygotes and homozygotes for hemoglobin C with or without diabetes. *J. Lab. clin. Med.*, **104**, 602–609.

AGER, J. A. M. & LEHMANN, H. (1957). Intra-erythrocytic haemoglobin crystals. *J. clin. Path.*, **10**, 336–338.

AKSOY, M. (1962). Haemoglobins S and E in Turkish people. *Nature (Lond.)*, **193**, 786–787.

AKSOY, M., ÇETINGIL, A. I., KOCABALKAN, N., ŞESTAKOF, D., ALARDAĞ, T., SEÇER, G. & BOSTANCI, N. (1963). Thalassemia-hemoglobin E disease in Turkey, with hypersplenism in one case. *Amer. J. Med.*, **34**, 851–855.

AKSOY, M. & LEHMANN, H. (1956). A further example of haemoglobin D — in a Turkish family. *Trans. roy. Soc. trop. Med. Hyg.*, **50**, 179–180.

AKSOY, M. & LEHMANN, H. (1957). The first observation of sickle-cell haemoglobin E disease. *Nature (Lond.)*, **179**, 1248–1249.

AKSOY, M. & TANRIKULU, K. (1960). The hemoglobin E syndromes. I. Hemoglobin E in Eti-Turks. *Blood*, **15**, 606–609.

ALBAHARY, C., DREYFUS, J. C., LABIE, D., SCHAPIRA, G. & TRAM, L. (1958). Hémoglobines anormales au Sud-Vietnam (Hémoglobinose C homozygote. Trait E. Hémoglobine nouvelle). *Rev. Hémat.*, **13**, 163–170.

ALI, M. A. M., QUINLAN, A. & WONG, S. C. (1980). Indentification of hemoglobin E by the isopropanol solubility test. *Clin. Biochem.*, **13**, 146–148.

ALLISON, A. C. (1956a). Sickle-cell anaemia and haemoglobin C. *Trans. roy. Soc. trop. Med. Hyg.*, **50**, 185–203.

ALLISON, A. C. (1956b). The sickle-cell and haemoglobin C genes in some African populations.

Ann. hum. Genet., **21**, 67–89.

ANTONARAKIS, S. E., ORKIN, S. H., KAZAZIAN, H. H. JNR, GOFF, S. C., BOEHM, C. D., WABER, P. G., SEXTON, J. P., OSTRER, H., FAIRBANKS, V. F. & CHAKRAVATI, A. (1982). Evidence for multiple origins of the β^E-globin gene in Southeast Asia. *Proc. natn. Acad. Sci. U.S.A.*, **79**, 6608–6611.

ARENDS, T., LAYRISSE, M. & RINCON, A. R. (1959). Sickle cell-haemoglobin D disease in a Portuguese child. *Acta haemat. (Basel)*, **22**, 128–126.

BAGLIONI, C. (1962). Abnormal human haemoglobins. VIII. Chemical studies on haemoglobin D. *Biochim. biophys. Acta*, **59**, 437–449.

BAGLIONI, C. & LEHMANN, H. (1962). Chemical heterogeneity of haemoglobin O. *Nature (Lond.)*, **196**, 229–232.

BELLINGHAM, A. J. & HUEHNS, E. R. (1968). Compensation in haemolytic anaemias caused by abnormal haemoglobins. *Nature (Lond.)*, **218**, 924–926.

BENZ, E. J., BERMAN, B. W., TONKONOW, B. L., COUPAL, E., COATES, T., BOXER, L. A., ALTMAN, A. & ADAMS, J. G. III (1981). Molecular analysis of the β-thalassemia phenotype associated with inheritance of hemoglobin E ($\alpha_2\beta_2^{26}$ Glu→Lys). *J. clin. Invest.*, **68**, 118–126.

BENZER, S., INGRAM, V. M. & LEHMANN, H. (1958). Three varieties of human haemoglobin D. *Nature (Lond.)*, **182**, 852–854.

BHAMARAPRAVATI, N., NA-NAKORN, S., WASI, P. & TUCHINDA, S. (1967). Pathology of abnormal hemoglobin diseases seen in Thailand. 1. Pathology of β-thalassaemia hemoglobin E disease. *Amer. J. clin. Path.*, **47**, 745–758.

BIRD, A. R., WOOD, K., LEISEGANG, F., MATTHEW, C. G., ELLIS, P., HARTLEY, P. S. & KARABUS, C. D. (1984). Haemoglobin E variants: a clinical, haematological and biosynthetic study of 4 South African families. *Acta haemat. (Basel)*, **72**, 135–137.

BIRD, G. W. G. & LEHMANN, H. (1956a). The finding of haemoglobin D in a Sikh. *Man*, **56**, 1–2.

BIRD, G. W. G. & LEHMANN, H. (1956b). Haemoglobin D in India. *Brit. med. J.*, **i**, 514 (Letter).

BIRD, G. W. G., LEHMANN, H. & MOURANT, A. E. (1955). A third example of haemoglobin D. *Trans. roy. Soc. trop. Med. Hyg.*, **49**, 399–400 (Letter).

BOOKCHIN, R. M., DAVIS, R. P. & RANNEY, H. M. (1968). Clinical features of hemoglobin C$_{Harlem}$, a new sickling hemoglobin. *Ann. intern. Med.*, **68**, 8–18.

BOOTH, F. & MEAD, S. V. (1983). Resistance to lysis of erythrocytes containing haemoglobin C — detected in a differential white cell counting system. *J. clin. Path.*, **36**, 816–818.

BRUGNARA, C., KOPIN, A. S., BUNN, H. F. & TOSTESON, D. C. (1985). Regulation of cation content and cell volume in hemoglobin [sic] erythrocytes from patients with homozygous

hemoglobin C disease. *J. clin. Invest.*, **75**, 1608–1617.

BRUMPT, L., BRUMPT, V., COQUELET, M. L. & TRAVERSE, P. M. DE (1958). La détection de l'hémoglobine E (Étude des populations Cambodgiennes). *Rev. Hémat.*, **13**, 21–30.

BUNN, H. F., FORGET, B. G. & RANNEY, H. M. (1977). *Human Hemoglobins*, p. 224. Saunders, Philadelphia, London, Toronto.

BUNN, H. F., MERIWETHER, W. D., BALCERZAK, S. P. & RUCKNAGEL, D. L. (1972). Oxygen equilibrium of hemoglobin E. *J. clin. Invest.*, **51**, 2984–2987.

BUNYARATREJ, A., SAHAPHONG, S., BHAMARAPRAVATI, N. & WASI, P. (1985). Quantitative changes in red blood cell shapes in relation to clinical features in β-thalassemia/Hb E disease. *Amer. J. clin. Path*, **83**, 555–559.

CABANNES, R., DUZER, A., PORTIER, A., MASSONAT, J., SENDRA, L. & BUHR, J. L. (1956). Hémoglobines anormales chez l'Algérien musulman. *Sang*, **27**, 580–585.

CABANNES, R., SENDRA, L. & DALAUT (1955). Hémoglobinose D. Anomalie hémoglobinique héréditaire retrouvée chez l'Algérien Musulman. Observations de deux familles. *Algérie méd.*, **59**, 387–395.

CAMERON, B. F., SMITH, D. B. & CODY, B. (1984). Hemoglobin C in heterozygote carriers. *Amer. J. Hemat.*, **17**, 437–438.

CAVDAR, A. O. & ARCASOY, A. (1974). Hb D Punjab–alpha thalassemia combination in a Turkish family. *Scand. J. Haemat.*, **13**, 313–319.

CHARACHE, S., CONLEY, C. L., WAUGH, D. F., UGORETZ, R. J., SPURRELL, J. R. & GAYLE, E. (1967). Pathogenesis of hemolytic anemia in homozygous hemoglobin C disease. *J. clin. Invest.*, **46**, 1795–1811.

CHATTERJEA, J. B. (1959). Haemoglobinopathy in India. In: *Abnormal Haemoglobins. A Symposium* (ed. by J. H. P. Jonxis and J. F. Delafresnaye), pp. 322–339. Blackwell Scientific Publications, Oxford.

CHATTERJEA, J. B. (1964). Malaria and haemoglobin E. *Lancet*, **ii**, 1185.

CHATTERJEA, J. B. (1965). Some aspects of haemoglobin E and its genetic interaction with thalassemia. *Ind. J. med. Res.*, **53**, 377–398.

CHATTERJEA, J. B., RAY, R. N., SWARUP, S. & GHOSH, S. K. (1961). Observations on splenectomy in thalassaemia syndrome. *J. Indian med. Ass.*, **37**, 1–7.

CHATTERJEA, J. B., SAHA, A. K., RAY, R. N. & GHOSH, S. K. (1957). Hemoglobin E-thalassemia disease. *Ind. J. med. Sci.*, **11**, 553–564.

CHERNOFF, A. I. (1958). The hemoglobin D syndromes. *Blood*, **13**, 116–127.

CHERNOFF, A. I. & FARR, P. C. (1956). On the prevalence of hemoglobin D in the American

Negro. *Blood*, **11**, 907–909.

CHERNOFF, A. I., MINNICH, V. & CHONGCHAREONSUK, S. (1954). Hemoglobin E, a hereditary abnormality of human hemoglobin. *Science*, **120**, 605–606.

CHERNOFF, A. I., MINNICH, V., NA-NAKORN, S., TUCHINDA, S., KASHEMSANT, C. & CHERNOFF, R. R. (1956). Studies on hemoglobin E. 1. The clinical, hematologic, and genetic characteristics of the hemoglobin E syndromes. *J. Lab. clin. Med.*, **47**, 455–489.

CONLEY, C. L. (1964). Pathophysiological effects of some abnormal hemoglobins. *Medicine (Baltimore)*, **43**, 785–787.

CONLEY, C. L. & CHARACHE, S. (1967). Mechanisms by which some abnormal hemoglobins produce clinical manifestations. *Seminars Hemat.*, **4**, 53–71.

COQUELET, M. L., DE TRAVERSE, P. M., ISRAEL, J., PELLETIER, P. & BLATRIX, C. (1970). La double hétérozygotie hémoglobinose C-thalassémie chez les européens. Étude d'une famille sicilienne. *Nouv. Rev. franç. Hémat.*, **10**, 461–475.

DA COSTA, J. L., LOH, Y. S. & HANAM, E. (1974). Extramedullary hemopoiesis with multiple tumor-simulating mediastinal masses in hemoglobin-E thalassemia disease. *Chest.*, **65**, 210–212.

DACIE, J. V. (1954). *The Haemolytic Anaemias: Congenital and Acquired*, p. 146. Churchill, London.

DEDMAN, R. E., EMANUELI, A. & TROBAUGH, F. E. JNR (1959). Hemolytic studies in homozygous hemoglobin C disease. *Amer. J. clin. Path.*, **31**, 487–495.

DELIYANNIS, G. A., BALLAS, A. & CHRISTAKIS, I. (1969). Haemoglobin D in a Greek family. *Acta haemat. (Basel)*, **41**, 121–125.

DHECHAKAISAYA, S., SHUANGSHOTI, S. & SUSAKARES, A. (1979). Extramedullary hematopoiesis of cranial dura mater and choroid plexus and terminal convulsions in a patient with thalassemia hemoglobin E disease. *J. med. Ass. Thailand*, **62**, 503. [Quoted by Fucharoen *et al.* (1981).]

DIGGS, L. W., KRAUS, A. P., MORRISON, D. B. & RUDNICKI, R. P. T. (1954). Intraerythrocytic crystals in a white patient with hemoglobin C in the absence of other types of hemoglobin. *Blood*, **9**, 1172–1184.

DORLÉAC, E., MORLÉ, L., GENTILHOMME, O., JACCOUD, P., BAUDONNET, C. & DELAUNEY, J. (1984). Thalassemia-like abnormalities of the red cell membrane in hemoglobin E trait and disease. *Amer. J. Hemat.*, **16**, 207–217.

EDINGTON, G. M. & LAING, W. N. (1957). Relationship between haemoglobin C and S and malaria in Ghana. *Brit. med. J.*, **ii**, 143–145.

EDINGTON, G. M. & LEHMANN, H. (1954). A case of sickle cell-haemoglobin C disease and a survey of haemoglobin C incidence in West Africa. *Trans. roy. Soc. trop. Med. Hyg.*, **48**, 332–335.

EDINGTON, G. M. & LEHMANN, H. (1956). The distribution of haemoglobin C in West Africa. *Man*, **56**, 34–36.

EFREMOV, G. D., SADIKARIO, A., STOJANCOV, A., DOJCINOV, D. & HUISMAN, T. H. J. (1977). Homozygous hemoglobin O Arab in a gypsy family in Yugoslavia. *Hemoglobin*, **1**, 389–394.

EL-HAZMI, M. A. F. & LEHMANN, H. (1980). Human haemoglobins and haemoglobinopathies in Arabia: Hb O Arab in Saudi Arabia. *Acta haemat. (Basel)*, **63**, 268–273.

ERLANDSON, M., SMITH, C. H. & SCHULMAN, I. (1956). Thalassemia-hemoglobin C disease in White siblings. *Pediatrics*, **17**, 740–746.

FABRY, M. E., KAUL, D. K., RAVENTOS, C., BAEZ, S., RIEDER, R. & NAGEL, R. L. (1981). Some aspects of the pathophysiology of homozygous Hb CC erythrocytes. *J. clin. Invest.*, **67**, 1284–1291.

FAIRBANKS, V. F., GILCHRIST, G. S., BRIMHALL, B., JEREB, J. A. & GOLDSTON, E. C. (1979). Hemoglobin E trait reexamined: a cause of microcytosis and erythrocytosis. *Blood*, **53**, 109–115.

FAIRBANKS, V. F., OLIVEROS, R., BRANDABUR, J. H., WILLIS, R. R. & FIESTER, R. F. (1980). Homozygous hemoglobin E mimics β-thalassaemia minor without anemia or hemolysis: hematologic, functional, and biosynthetic studies of first North American cases. *Amer. J. Hemat.*, **8**, 109–121.

FELDMAN, R. & RIEDER, R. F. (1973). The interaction of hemoglobin E with beta thalassemia: a study of hemoglobin synthesis in a family of mixed Burmese and Iranian origin. *Blood*, **42**, 783–791.

FESSAS, P. (1968). Haemoglobin E and α-thalassaemia. *Brit. med. J.*, **i**, 764–765.

FLATZ, G. (1967). Hemoglobin E: distribution and population dynamics. *Humangenetik*, **3**, 189–234.

FLATZ, G., PIK, C. & SRINGAM, S. (1965). Haemoglobin E and β-thalassaemia: their distribution in Thailand. *Ann. hum. Genet.*, **29**, 151–170.

FLATZ, G., PIK, C. & SUNDHARAGIATI, B. (1964). Malaria and haemoglobin E in Thailand. *Lancet*, **ii**, 385–387.

FRISCHER, H. & BOWMAN, J. (1975). Hemoglobin E, an oxidatively unstable mutation. *J. Lab. clin. Med.*, **85**, 531–539.

FUCHAROEN, S., TUNTHANAVATANA, C., SONAKUL, D. & WASI, P. (1981). Intracranial extramedullary hematopoiesis in β⁰-thalassemia/hemoglobin E disease. *Amer. J. Haemat.*, **10**, 75–78.

GACON, G., WAJCMAN, H. & LABIE, D. (1974). Hemoglobin E: its oxygen affinity in relation with the ionic environment. *FEBS Lett.*, **41**, 147–150.

GALBRAITH, P. A. & GREEN, P. T. (1960). Hemoglobin C disease in an Anglo-Saxon family. *Amer. J. Med.*, **28**, 969–972.

GANESAN, J., LIE-INJO, L. E., NG, T. S. & GEORGE, R. (1977). Interaction of haemoglobin E with α-thalassaemia and haemoglobin Constant Spring. *Acta haemat. (Basel)*, **57**, 109–115.

GELPI, A. P. (1970). Sickle cell disease in Saudi Arabs. *Acta haemat. (Basel)*, **43**, 89–99.

GERALD, P. S. & RATH, C. E. (1966). Hemoglobin C$_{Georgetown}$; first abnormal hemoglobin due to two different mutations in the same gene. *J. clin. Invest.*, **45**, 1012 (Abstract).

GÖKSEL, V. & TARTAROGLU, N. (1960). Hemoglobin D. *Blut*, **6**, 213–217.

GOUTTAS, A., TSEVRENIS, H., PAPASPYROU, A., POUGOURAS, P., FERTAKIS, A. & VOVIAS, — . (1960a). L'hémoglobinose D en Grèce. *Sang*, **31**, 303–306.

GOUTTAS, A., TSEVRENIS, H., ROMBOS, C., PAPASPYROU, A. & GARIDI, M. (1960b). L'hémoglobinose E en Grèce. *Sang*, **31**, 1–5.

GRAFF, J. A. E., IKIN, E. W., LEHMANN, H., MOURANT, A.E., PARKIN, D. M. & WICKREMASINGHE, R. L. (1955). Haemoglobin E and blood groups in the Veddas. *J. Physiol.*, **127**, 41P (Abstract).

HARDY, M. J. & RAGBEER, M. S. (1985). Homozygous HbE and HbSE in a Saudi family. *Hemoglobin*, **9**, 47–52.

HARTZ, W. H. JNR & SCHWARTZ, S. O. (1955). Hemoglobin C disease. Report of four cases. *Blood*. **10**, 235–246.

HIRSCH, R. E., RAVENTOS-SUAREZ, C., OLSON, J. & NAGEL, R. L. (1985). Ligand state of intraerythrocytic circulating HbC crystals in homozygote CC patients. *Blood*, **66**, 775–777.

HOERMAN, C. K., KAMEL, K. & ANONY, A. Y. (1961). Haemoglobin E in Egypt. *Nature (Lond.)*, **189**, 69–70.

HORÁNYI, M., SZELÉNYI, J., RONA, G., LANG, A., LEHMANN, H. & HOLLÁN, S. R. (1980). Haemoglobin O Arab, beta-thalassaemia and glucose-6-phosphate dehydrogenase deficiency in a Hungarian family. *Folia haemat. (Lpz.)*, **107**, 654–660.

HOSAIN, F., HOSAIN, P., SWARUP, S. S. & CHATTERJEA, J. B. (1962). Double exponential nature in chromium-51 red blood cell survival curves in haemoglobin E thalassaemia and relation with reticulocytes. *Nature (Lond.)*, **196**, 76–77.

HUISMAN, T. H. J. (1977). Trimodality in the percentages of β chain variants in heterozygotes: the effect of the number of active Hb$_a$ structural loci. *Hemoglobin*, **1**, 349–382.

HUISMAN, T. H. J. (1978). The hemoglobin P-Galveston–Hb-C condition in members of a black family from South Carolina. *FEBS Lett.*, **94**, 68–72.

HUISMAN, T. H. J., VAN DER SCHAAF, P. C. & VAN DER SAR, A. (1955). Some characteristic properties of hemoglobin C. *Blood*, **10**, 1079–1091.

HUNT, J. A. & INGRAM, V. M. (1958). Allelomorphism and chemical differences of the human haemoglobins A, S and C. *Nature (Lond.)*, **181**, 1062–1063.

HUNT, J. A. & INGRAM, V. M. (1960). Abnormal human haemoglobins. IV. The chemical difference between normal human haemoglobin and haemoglobin C. *Biochim. biophys. Acta*, **42**, 409–421.

HUNT, J. A. & INGRAM, V. M. (1961). Abnormal human haemoglobins. VI. The chemical difference between haemoglobins A and E. *Biochim. biophys. Acta*, **49**, 520–536.

HUSQUINET, H., PARENT, M. T., SCHOOS-BARBETTE, S., DODINVAL-VERSIE, J., LAMBOTTE, C. & GALACTEROS, F. (1986). Hemoglobin D-Los Angeles [β121 (GH4) GLU→GLN] in the province of Liege, Belgium. *Hemoglobin*, **10**, 587–592.

HYNES, M. & LEHMANN, H. (1956). Haemoglobin D in a Persian girl: presumably the first case of haemoglobin-D-thalassaemia. *Brit. med. J.*, ii, 923–925.

ISSARAGRISIL, S., PIANKIJAGUM, A. & WASI, P. (1981). Spinal cord compression in thalassemia. Report of 12 cases and recommendations for treatment. *Arch. intern. Med.*, **141**, 1033–1036.

ITANO, H. A. (1951). A third abnormal hemoglobin associated with hereditary hemolytic anemia. *Proc. natn. Acad. Sci. U.S.A.*, **37**, 775–784.

ITANO, H. A., BERGREN, W. R. & STURGEON, P. (1954). Identification of a fourth abnormal human hemoglobin. *J. Amer. chem. Soc.*, **76**, 2278 (Letter).

ITANO, H. A. & NEEL, J. V. (1950). A new inherited abnormality of human hemoglobin. *Proc. natn. Acad. Sci. U.S.A.*, **36**, 613–617.

JACOB, G. F., LEHMANN, H. & RAPER, A. B. (1956). Haemoglobin D in Indians of Gujerati origin in Uganda. *E. Afr. med. J.*, **33**, 135–138.

JAIN, R. C. (1971). Hemoglobin D disease. Report of a case. *Amer. J. clin. Path.*, **56**, 40–42.

JAIN, R. C., ANDLEIGH, H. S. & MEHTA, J. B. (1970). Haemoglobin D-thalassemia. A case report. *Acta haemat. (Basel)*, **44**, 124–127.

JENSEN, W. N., SCHOEFIELD, R. A. & AGNER, R. (1957). Clinical and necropsy findings in hemoglobin C disease. *Blood*, **12**, 74–83.

JOHNSON, C., POWARS, D. & SCHROEDER, W. A. (1976). A case with both hemoglobins C and N-Baltimore. *Acta haemat. (Basel)*, **56**, 183–188.

KANTCHEV, K. N., TCHOLAKOV, B. & BAGLIONI, C. (1965). Haemoglobin O Arab in Bulgaria. *Nature (Lond.)*, **205**, 187–188.

KANTCHEV, K. N., TCHOLAKOW, B. N., CASEY, R., LEHMANN, H. & EL HAZMI, M. (1975). Twelve families with Hb O Arab in the Burgas district of Bulgaria. Observations on sixteen examples of Hb O Arab-β⁰ thalassaemia. *Humangenetik*, **26**, 93–97.

KAPLAN, E., ZUELZER, W. W. & NEEL, J. V. (1951). A new inherited abnormality of hemoglobin and its interaction with sickle cell hemoglobin. *Blood*, **6**, 1240–1259.

KAPLAN, E., ZUELZER, W. W. & NEEL, J. V. (1953). Further studies on hemoglobin C. II. The hematologic effects of hemoglobin C alone and in combination with sickle cell hemoglobin. *Blood*, **8**, 735–746.

KAZAZIAN, H. H. JNR, WABER, P. G., BOEHM, C. D., LEE, J. I., ANTONARAKIS, S. E. & FAIRBANKS, V. F. (1984). Hemoglobin E in Europeans: further evidence for multiple origins of the β^E-globin gene. *Amer. J. hum. Genet.*, **36**, 212–217.

KLEFSTAD-SILLONVILLE, F., LABÉGORRE, J., RANC, A. & UNG-POLENG. (1962). Six cas d'association thalassémie-hémoglobinose E observés au Cambodge. *Presse méd.*, **70**, 433–436.

KONIGSBERG, W., HUNTSMAN, R. G., WADIA, F. & LEHMANN, H. (1965). Haemoglobin D$_{\beta \text{ Punjab}}$ in an East Anglian family. *J. roy. anthropol. Inst.*, **95**, 295–306.

KRAUS, A. P. & DIGGS, L. W. (1956). In vitro crystallization of hemoglobin occurring in citrated blood from patients with hemoglobin C. *J. Lab. clin. Med.*, **47**, 700–705.

KRAUS, A. P., KOCH, B. & BURCKETT, L. (1961). Two families showing interaction of haemoglobin C or thalassaemia with high foetal haemoglobin in adults. *Brit. med. J.*, **i**, 1434–1436.

LANGE, R. D. & HAGEN, P. S. (1955). Hemoglobin C disease in identical twins. *Amer. J. med. Sci.*, **229**, 655–660.

LAWRENCE, S. L., JENSEN, W. N. & PONDER, E. (1969). Molecular mechanism of hemolytic anemia in homozygous hemoglobin C disease. Electron microscopic study by the freeze-etching technique. *J. exp. Med.*, **130**, 443–466.

LEHMANN, H. (1959). Distribution of variations in human haemoglobin synthesis. In: *Abnormal Haemoglobins. A Symposium* (ed. by J. H. P. Jonxis and J. F. Delafresnaye), pp. 202–215. Blackwell Scientific Publications, Oxford.

LEHMANN, H. & HUNTSMAN, R. A. (1966). *Man's Haemoglobins, including the Haemoglobinopathies and their Investigation*. 331 pp. North-Holland Publishing Co., Amsterdam.

LEHMANN, H. & SINGH, R. B. (1956). Haemoglobin E in Malaya. *Nature (Lond.)*, **178**, 695–696.

LEHMANN, H., STORY, P. & THEIN, H. (1956). Haemoglobin E in Burmese. Two cases of haemoglobin E disease. *Brit. med. J.*, **i**, 544–547.

LESSIN, L. S., JENSEN, W. N. & PADILLA, F. (1968). Molecular rearrangement in intraerythrocytic crystallization in hemoglobin C disease. *Clin. Res.*, **16**, 307 (Abstract).

LEVIN, W. C., SCHNEIDER, R. G., CUDD, J. A. & JOHNSON, J. E. JNR (1953). A family with homozygous hemoglobin C and sickle cell union: a clinical, hematological and electrophoretic study. *J. Lab. clin. Med.*, **42**, 918–919 (Abstract).

LEWIS, S. M., ANDERSON, C. G. & BASKIND, E. (1957). Homozygous haemoglobin-C disease in a white family with special reference to blood autolysis studies. *Brit. J. Haemat.*, **3**, 68–76.

LIE-INJO, L. E. (1955). Haemoglobin E in Indonesia. *Nature (Lond.)*, **176**, 469–470.

LIE-INJO, L. E. (1956). Post natal formation of haemoglobin E. *Nature (Lond.)*, **178**, 1056.

LIE-INJO, L. E. (1959). Pathological haemoglobins in Indonesia. In: *Abnormal Haemoglobins. A Symposium* (ed. by J. P. H. Jonxis and J. F. Delafresnaye), pp 368–384. Blackwell Scientific Publications, Oxford.

LIE-INJO, L. E. (1964). Haemoglobinopathies in East Asia. *Ann. hum. Genet.*, **28**, 101–111.

LIE-INJO, L. E. (1969). Distribution of genetic red cell defects in Southeast Asia. *Trans. roy. Soc. trop. Med. Hyg.*, **63**, 664–674.

LIE-INJO, L. E., FIX, A., BOLTON, J. M. & GILMAN, R. H. (1972). Haemoglobin E-hereditary elliptocytosis in Malayan aborigines. *Acta haemat. (Basel)*, **47**, 210–216.

LIE-INJO, L. E., HOO, S. T. & KHO, L. K. (1959). A case of haemoglobin E-thalassaemia disease complicated by pregnancy. *Acta haemat. (Basel)*, **22**, 194–200.

LIE-INJO, L. E., MURSADIK, LIOE, L. D. & ODANG, U. (1956). Haemoglobin E-thalassaemia disease in Indonesia. *Docum. Med. geogr. trop. (Amst.)*, **8**, 135–143.

LIE-INJO, L. E. & OEY, H. G. (1957). Homozygous haemoglobin-E disease in Indonesia. *Lancet*, **i**, 20–23.

LIE-INJO, L. E. & SADONO (1958). Haemoglobin O (Buginese X) in Sulawesi. *Brit. med. J.*, **i**, 1461–1462.

LISCHKA, A., POLLAK, A., BAUER, K., ASCHAUER, H. & BRAUNITZER, G. (1984). Hemoglobin D "Los Angeles" in an Austrian family: biochemical identification, clinical aspects and kindred study. *Hemoglobin*, **8**, 353–361.

McCORMICK, W. F. & HUMPHREYS, E. W. (1960). High fetal-hemoglobin C disease: a new syndrome. *Blood*, **16**, 1736–1744.

McCURDY, P. R., PEARSON, H. & GERALD, P. S. (1961). A new hemoglobinopathy of unusual genetic significance. *J. Lab. clin. Med.*, **58**, 86–94.

McCURDY, P. R., SHERMAN, A. S., KAMUZORA, H. & LEHMANN, H. (1975). Globin synthesis in subjects doubly heterozygous for hemoglobin G-Philadelphia and hemoglobin S or C. *J. Lab. clin. Med.*, **85**, 891–897.

MacDONALD, V. W. & CHARACHE, S. (1983). Differences in the reaction sequences associated with drug-induced oxidation of hemoglobins E, S, A, and F. *J. Lab. clin. Med.*, **102**, 762–772.

MARDER, V. J. & CONLEY, C. L. (1959). Electrophoresis of hemoglobin on agar gels. Frequency of hemoglobin D in a negro population. *Bull. Johns Hopk. Hosp.*, **105**, 77–88.

MARENGO-ROWE, A. J., McCRACKEN, A. W. &

FLANAGAN, P. (1968). Complete suppression of haemoglobin A synthesis in haemoglobin D Los Angeles-beta thalassaemia. *J. clin. Path.*, **21**, 508–510.

MARTI, H. R., LEHMANN, H., KEISER, G. & SIEGENTHALER, W. (1965). Hämoglobin C bei Europäern: ein neuer, wahrscheinlich homozygoter und 3 heterozygote Träger der Anomalie. *Blut*, **11**, 321–325.

MARTIN, H., HEUPKE, G., PFLEIDERER, G. & WÖRNER, W. (1960). Hämoglobin D in einer Frankfurter Familie. *Folia haemat. (Frankfurt)*, **4**, 233–241.

MAY, A. & HUEHNS, E. R. (1977). The oxygen affinity of haemoglobin E. *Brit. J. Haemat.*, **30**, 177–184.

MEHTA, B. C., AGARWAL, M. B., VARANDANI, D. G., JOSHI, R. H. & BHARGAVA, A. B. (1980). Hemoglobin E-thalassemia: a study of 16 cases. *Acta haemat. (Basel)*, **64**, 201–204.

MILNER, P. F., MILLER, C., GREY, R., SEAKINS, M., DEJONG, W. W. & WENT, L. N. (1970). Hemoglobin O Arab in four negro families and its interaction with hemoglobin S and hemoglobin C. *New Engl. J. Med.*, **283**, 1417–1425.

MINNICH, V., NA-NAKORN, S., CHONGCHAREONSUK, S. & KOCHASENI, S. (1954). Mediterranean anemia. A study of thirty-two cases in Thailand. *Blood*, **9**, 1–23.

MIYAJI, T., MATSUMOTO, K., UEDA, S., IUCHI, I. & SHIBATA, S. (1973). The second Japanese family of Hb E found in Otsu, Shiga Prefecture. *Acta haemat. jap.*, **36**, 25–31.

MOVITT, E. R., POLLYCOVE, J. F., MANGUM, J. F. & PORTER, W. R. (1964). Hemoglobin C disease: quantitative determination of iron kinetics and hemoglobin synthesis. *Amer. J. med. Sci.*, **247**, 558–564.

MULLA, N. & CHROBAK, L. (1973). Haemoglobin C in Arabs in Kuwait. *Acta haemat. (Basel)*, **50**, 112–115.

MURPHY, J. R. (1967). Hb CC disease: an abnormality in cell water. *J. clin. Invest.*, **46**, 1099 (Abstract).

MURPHY, J. R. (1968). Hemoglobin CC disease: rheological properties of erythrocytes and abnormalities in cell water. *J. clin. Invest.*, **47**, 1483–1495.

MURPHY, J. R. (1976). Hemoglobin CC erythrocytes: decreased intracellular pH and decreased O_2 affinity — anemia. *Seminars Hemat.*, **13**, 177–180.

NAGARATNAM, N., WICKREMASINGHE, R. L., JAYAWICKREME, U. S., & MAHESON, V. S. (1958). Haemoglobin E syndromes in a Ceylonese family. *Brit. med. J.*, **i**, 866–868.

NA-NAKORN, S. (1959). Haemoglobinopathies in Thailand. In: *Abnormal Haemoglobins. A Symposium* (ed. by J. H. P. Jonxis and J. F. Delafresnaye),

pp. 357–367. Blackwell Scientific Publications, Oxford.

NA-NAKORN, S. & MINNICH, V. (1957). Studies on hemoglobin E. III. Homozygous hemoglobin E and variants of thalassemia and hemoglobin E. A family study. *Blood*, **12**, 529–538.

NA-NAKORN, S., MINNICH, V., CHERNOFF, A. I., QUAGQUI-PUAG, S. & CHAVALEKVIRAJ, K. (1956). Studies on hemoglobin E. II. The incidence of hemoglobin E in Thailand. *J. Lab. clin. Med.*, **47**, 490–498.

NEEL, J. V. (1957). Human hemoglobin types. Their epidemiologic implications. *New Engl. J. Med.*, **256**, 161–171.

NEEL, J. V., HIERNAUX, J., LINHARD, J., ROBINSON, A. R., ZUELZER, W. W. & LIVINGSTONE, F. R. (1956). Data on the occurrence of hemoglobin C and other abnormal hemoglobins in some African populations. *Amer. J. hum. Genet.*, **8**, 138–150.

OLDRINI, R., SALMINI, G. & MAIOIO, A. T. (1973). Studio di un case di associazione Hb D-β microcitemia. *Haematologica*, **58**, 515–521.

OLSON, J. A. & NAGEL, R. L. (1986). Synchronized cultures of *P falciparum* in abnormal red cells: the mechanism of the inhibition of growth in HbCC cells. *Blood*, **67**, 997–1001.

ONG, H. C. (1975). Maternal and fetal outcome associated with hemoglobin E trait and hemoglobin E disease. *Obstet. and Gynec.*, **45**, 672–674.

ÖZSOYLU, S. (1970). Homozygous hemoglobin D Punjab. *Acta haemat. (Basel)*, **43**, 353–359.

PAPAYANNOPOULOU, TH., LIM, G., McGUIRE, T. C., AHERN, V., NUTE, P. E. & STAMATOYANNOPOULOS, G. (1977). Use of specific fluorescent antibodies for the identification of hemoglobin C in erythrocytes. *Amer. J. Hemat.*, **2**, 105–112.

PEROSA, L., MANGANELLI, G. & DALFINO, G. (1960). Primo caso di HB C-talassemia in Italia. *Boll. Soc. Ital. Biol. sper.*, **36**, 93–96.

PIERCE, L. E., RATH, C. E. & McCOY, K. (1963). New hemoglobin variant with sickling properties. *New Engl. J. Med.*, **268**, 862–866.

POLITIS-TSEGOS, C., KYNOCH, P., LANG, A., LEHMANN, H., LORKIN, P. A., STATHOPOULOU, R. & WAKEFIELD, G. (1975). *J. med. Genet.*, **12**, 269–274.

POOTRAKUL, S.-N., WASI, P., NA-NAKORN, S. & DIXON, G. H. (1971). Double heterozygosity for hemoglobin E and hemoglobin New York in a Thai family. *J. med. Ass. Thailand*, **54**, 688–697.

PRINDLE, K. H. JNR & McCURDY, P. R. (1970). Red cell lifespan in hemoglobin C disorders (with special reference to hemoglobin C trait). *Blood*, **36**, 14–19.

PUNT, K. & GOOL, J. VAN (1957). Thalassaemia-haemoglobin E-disease in two Indo-European boys. *Acta haemat. (Basel)*, **17**, 305–314.

RAHBAR, S., NOWZARI, G. & POOSTI, M. (1975). A double heterozygous hemoglobin: hemoglobin

O$_{Indonesia}$ and hemoglobin D$_{Punjab}$ in an individual. *Amer. J. clin. Path.*, **64**, 416–420.

RAMOT, B., FISHER, S., REMEZ, D., SCHNEERSON, R., KAHANE, D., AGER, J. A. M. & LEHMANN, H. (1960). Haemoglobin O in an Arab family. Sickle-cell haemoglobin O trait. *Brit. med. J.*, **ii**, 1262–1264.

RAMOT, B., ROTEM, J., RAHBAR, S., JACOBS, A. S., UDEM, L. & RANNEY, H. M. (1969). Hemoglobin D$_{Punjab}$ in a Bulgarian Jewish family. *Israel J. med. Sci.*, **5**, 1066–1070.

RANNEY, H. M. (1954). Observations on the inheritance of sickle-cell hemoglobin and hemoglobin C. *J. clin. Invest.*, **33**, 1634–1641.

RANNEY, H. M., LARSON, D. L. & McCORMACK, G. H. JNR (1953). Some clinical, biochemical and genetic observations on hemoglobin C. *J. clin. Invest.*, **32**, 1277–1284.

RANSONE, J. W. & LANGE, R. D. (1957). Homozygous hemoglobin C disease in a 79 year old man with gout. *Ann. intern, Med.*, **46**, 420–424.

RAPER, A. B., GAMMACK, D. B., HUEHNS, E. R. & SHOOTER, E. M. (1960). Four haemoglobins in one individual. A study of the genetic interaction of Hb-G and Hb-C. *Brit. med. J.*, **ii**, 1257–1261.

REISS, G. H., RANNEY, H. M. & SHAKLAI, N. (1982). Association of hemoglobin C with erythrocyte ghosts. *J. clin. Invest.*, **70**, 946–952.

RIEDER, R. F. (1976). Globin chain synthesis in Hb D (Punjab)-β-thalassemia. *Blood*, **47**, 113–120.

RINGELHANN, B., KONOTEY-AHULU, F. I. D., TALAPATRA, N. C., NKRUMAH, F. H., WILTSHIRE, B. G. & LEHMANN, H. (1971). Hemoglobin K Woolwich ($\alpha_2\beta_2$ 132 lysine → glutamine) in Ghana. *Acta haemat. (Basel)*, **45**, 250–258.

RUYMANN, F. B., POPEJOY, L. A. & BROUILLARD, R. B. (1978). Splenic sequestration and ineffective erythropoiesis in hemoglobin E-β-thalassemia disease. *Pediat. Res.*, **12**, 1020–1023.

SCHNEIDER, R. G. (1954). Incidence of hemoglobin C trait in 505 normal negroes. A family with homozygous hemoglobin C and sickle-cell trait union. *J. Lab. clin. Med.*, **44**, 133–144.

SCHNEIDER, R. G. (1956). Incidence of electrophoretically distinct abnormalities of hemoglobin in 1550 Negro hospital patients. *Amer. J. clin. Path.*, **26**, 1270–1276.

SCHNEIDER, R. G., LEVIN, W. C. & EVERETT, C. (1961). A family with S and C hemoglobins and the hereditary persistence of F hemoglobin. A comparison of C thalassemia disease with the CF syndrome. *New Engl. J. Med.*, **265**, 1278–1283.

SCIARRATTA, C. V., IVALDI, G., SANSONE, G. & DI PIETRO, P. (1985). Hb O-Arab [β121 (GH4) GLU→LYS] in Italy. *Hemoglobin*, **9**, 513–515.

SCOTT, J. G., DWORATZEK, J. & CROOKSTON, J. H. (1963). Hemoglobin C disease in a Sicilian-Canadian family. *Canad. med. Ass. J.*, **89**, 1239–1241.

SHIBATA, S., IUCHI, I. & HAMILTON, H. B. (1964).

The first instance of hemoglobin E in a Japanese family. *Proc. Jap. Acad.*, **40**, 846–851.

SICARD, D., KAPLAN, J.-C. & LABIE, D. (1978). Haemoglobinopathies and G.-6-P.D. deficiency in Laos. *Lancet*, **ii**, 571–572 (Letter).

SINGER, K., CHAPMAN, A. Z., GOLDBERG, S. R., RUBINSTEIN, H. M. & ROSENBLUM, S. A. (1954a). Studies on abnormal hemoglobins. IX. Pure (homozygous) hemoglobin C disease. *Blood*, **9**, 1023–1031.

SINGER, K., KRAUS, A. P., SINGER, L., RUBINSTEIN, H. M. & GOLDBERG, S. R. (1954b). Studies on abnormal hemoglobins. X. A new syndrome: hemoglobin C-thalassemia disease. *Blood*, **9**, 1032–1046.

SMITH, E. W. & CONLEY, C. L. (1953). Filter paper electrophoresis of human hemoglobins with special reference to the incidence and clinical significance of hemoglobin C. *Bull. Johns Hopk. Hosp.*, **93**, 94–106.

SMITH, E. W. & KREVANS, J. R. (1959). Clinical manifestations of hemoglobin C disorders. *Bull. Johns Hopk. Hosp.*, **104**, 17–43.

SPAET, T. H., ALWAY, R. H. & WARD, G. (1953). Homozygous Type "C" hemoglobin. *Pediatrics*, **12**, 483–490.

STEINBERG, M. H. (1975). Haemoglobin C/α thalassemia: haematological and biosynthetic studies. *Brit. J. Haemat.*, **30**, 337–342.

STEINBERG, M. H., GATLING, R. R. & TAVASSOLI, M. (1983). Evidence of hyposplenism in the presence of splenomegaly. *Scand. J. Haemat.*, **31**, 437–439.

STOUT, C., HOLLAND, C. K. & BIRD, R. M. (1964). Hemoglobin D in an Oklahoma family. *Arch. intern. Med.*, **114**, 296–300.

STRANSKY, E. (1951). A peculiar familial hemolytic anemia in the tropics. Its differential diagnosis from thalassemia (Mediterranean anemia). *Acta haemat. (Basel)*, **6**, 193–207.

STRANSKY, E. (1952). Foreign newsletter — Philippine Islands. *Blood*, **7**, 574–575.

STRANSKY, E. (1958). On hemoglobin E-disease in the Philippines. *Acta haemat. jap.*, **21**, Suppl. I (Congress Number), 218–220.

STRANSKY, E. & CAMPOS, P. I. (1957). On hemoglobin E in the Philippines (hemolytic anemia, Stransky-Regala type). *J. Philipp. med. Ass.*, **33**, 731–739.

STRANSKY, E. & REGALA, A. C. (1946). New type of familial congenital chronic hemolytic anemia. *Amer. J. Dis. Child.*, **71**, 492–505.

STURGEON, P., ITANO, H. A. & BERGREN, W. R. (1955). Clinical manifestations of inherited abnormal hemoglobins. I. The interaction of hemoglobin-S with hemoglobin-D. *Blood*, **10**, 389–404.

SUKUMARAN, P. K., SANGHVI, L. D. & NAZRETH, F. A. (1960. Haemoglobin D-thalassemia. A report of two families. *Acta haemat. (Basel)*, **23**, 309–319.

SWARUP, S., CHATTERJEA, R. B., HOSAIN, P. & HOSAIN, F. (1961). A comparative study on iron turnovers with special reference of Hb. E-thalassaemia using small doses of Fe^{59}. *Indian J. med. Res.*, **49**, 256–261.

SWARUP, S., GHOSH, S. K. & CHATTERJEA, J. B. (1960a). Haemoglobin E disease in Bengalees. *J. Indian med. Ass.*, **35**, 13–15.

SWARUP, S., GHOSH, S. K. & CHATTERJEA, J. B. (1960b). Glutathione stability test in haemoglobin *E* –thalassaemia disease. *Nature (Lond.)*, **188**, 153.

SWARUP, S., GHOSH, S. K. & CHATTERJEA, J. B. (1960c). Observations on autohaemolysis in thalassaemia syndrome. *Proc. natn. Inst. Sci. India*, 26 B (Suppl.), 158–164.

SWARUP, S., GHOSH, S. K. & CHATTERJEA, J. B. (1966). Stability of erythrocyte reduced glutathione and nicotinadenine dinucleotide phosphate in HbE-thalassaemia disease. *Experientia*, **22**, 580–581.

TANAKA, K. R. & CLIFFORD, G. O. (1958). Homozygous hemoglobin C disease: report of three cases. *Ann. intern. Med.*, **49**, 30–42.

TERRY, D. W., MOTULSKY, A. & RATH, C. (1954). Homozygous hemoglobin C. A new hereditary hemolytic disease. *New Engl. J. Med.*, **251**, 365–373.

TESTA, U., DUBART, A., HINARD, N., GALACTEROS, F., VAINCHENKER, W., ROUYER-FESSARD, P., BEUZARD, Y. & ROSA, J. (1980). Beta^0-thalassemia/Hb E association. Hemoglobin synthesis in blood reticulocytes and bone marrow cells fractionated by density gradient and in blood erythroid colonies in culture. *Acta haemat. (Basel)*, **64**, 42–52.

THEIN, S. L., LYNCH, J. R., WEATHERALL, D. J. & WALLACE, R. B. (1986). Direct detection of haemoglobin E with synthetic oligonucleotides. *Lancet*, **i**, 93 (Letter).

THOMAS, E. D., MOTULSKY, A. G. & WALTERS, D. H. (1955). Homozygous hemoglobin C disease. Report of a case with studies on the pathophysiology and neonatal formation of hemoglobin C. *Amer. J. Med.*, **18**, 832–838.

THOMPSON, G. R. (1962). Significance of haemoglobins S and C in Ghana. *Brit. med. J.*, **i**, 682–685.

THOMPSON, G. R. (1963). Malaria and stress in relation to haemoglobins. *Brit. med. J.*, **ii**, 976–978.

THOMPSON, G. R. & LEHMANN, H. (1962). Combinations of high levels of haemoglobin F with haemoglobins A, S and C in Ghana. *Brit. med. J.*, **i**, 1521–1523.

TRAEGER, J., WINICHAGOON, P. & WOOD, W. G. (1982). Instability of β^E-messenger RNA during erythroid cell maturation in hemoglobin E homozygotes. *J. clin. Invest.*, **69**, 1050–1053.

TRAEGER, J., WOOD, W. G., CLEGG, J. B., WEATHERALL, D. J. & WASI, P. (1980). Defective synthesis of HbE is due to reduced levels of

β^E mRNA. *Nature (Lond.)*, **288**, 497–499.

TRENT, R. J., HARRIS, M. G., FLEMING, P. J., WYATT, K., HUGHES, W. G. & KRONENBERG, H. (1984). Haemoglobin D Punjab. Interaction with α thalassaemia and diagnosis by gene mapping. *Scand. J. Haemat.*, **32**, 275–282.

TSISTRAKIS, G. A., SCAMPARDONIS, G. J., CLONIZAKIS, J. P. & CONCOURIS, L. L. (1975). Haemoglobin D and D thalassaemia. A family report, comprising 18 members. *Acta haemat. (Basel)*, **54**, 172–179.

TUCHINDA, S., BEALE, D. & LEHMANN, H. (1967). The suppression of haemoglobin E synthesis when haemoglobin H disease and haemoglobin E trait occur together. *Humangenetik*, **3**, 312–318.

TUCHINDA, S., RUCKNAGEL, D. L., MINNICH, V., BOONYAPRAKOB, U., BALANKURA, K. & SUVATTEE, V. (1964). The coexistence of the genes for hemoglobin E and α thalassaemia in Thais, with resultant suppression of hemoglobin E synthesis. *Amer. J. hum. Genet.*, **16**, 311–335.

UNGAR, B., SYMONS, H. S., ANDERSON, G. R., STUBBS, A. E., WILTSHIRE, B. G. & LEHMANN, H. (1973). Haemoglobin D Punjab in a European family in Australia. *Med. J. Aust.*, **1**, 354–356.

UVA, L. S., FERNANDES, A. & PILAR, M. (1983). Double hétérozygotie hémoglobine D/β^{0}thalassémie. Communication de trois cas dans une famille portugaise. *Nouv. Rev. Franç. Hémat.*, **25**, 387–390.

VAN GOOL, J., PUNT, K. & DE VRIES, S. I. (1956). Thalassemie-Hb.E-ziekte bij twee Indonesische jongens. *Ned. T. Geneesk*, **100**, 3582–3585.

VANDEPITTE, J. & CATRYSSE, R. (1957). Hemoglobine D dans une famille Congolaise. *Ann. Soc. belge Méd. trop.*, **37**, 697–702.

VELLA, F. (1958). Haemoglobin D trait in a Filipino family. *Med. J. Malaya*, **12**, 602–604.

VELLA, F. (1960). Abnormal haemoglobin variants in 10,441 Chinese subjects. *Acta haemat. (Basel)*, **23**, 393–397.

VELLA, F., LABOSSIERE, A., WILTSHIRE, B., LEHMANN, H., SHOJANIA, A. M. & HILL, J. R. (1973). The occurrence of hemoglobins E and E$_{Saskatoon}$ in Central Canada. *Amer. J. clin. Path.*, **60**, 314–318.

VELLA, F. & LEHMANN, H. (1974). Haemoglobin D Punjab (D Los Angeles). *J. Med. Genet.*, **11**, 341–348.

WASI, P. (1981). Haemoglobinopathies including thalassaemia. Part I: tropical Asia. *Clinics Haemat.*, **10**, 707–726.

WASI, P., NA-NAKORN, S., POOTRAKUL, SA-NGA, SOOKANEK, M., DISTHASONGCHAN, P., PORNPATKUL, M. & PANICH, V. (1969). Alpha- and beta-thalassaemia in Thailand. *Ann. N.Y. Acad. Sci.*, **165**, 60–82.

WASI, P., NA-NAKORN, S. & SUINGDUMRONG, A. (1967). Studies on the distribution of haemoglobin E, thalassaemias and glucose-6-phosphate dehydrogenase deficiency in North-Eastern Thailand. *Nature (Lond.)*, **214**, 501–502.

WASI, P., POOTRAKUL, S. & NA-NAKORN, S. (1968a). Hereditary persistence of foetal haemoglobin in a Thai family: the first instance in the mongol race and in association with haemoglobin E. *Brit. J. Haemat.*, **14**, 501–506.

WASI, P., POOTRAKUL, S., NA-NAKORN, S., BEALE, D. & LEHMANN, H. (1968b). Haemoglobin D β Los Angeles (D Punjab, $\alpha_2\beta_2$ 121 Glu NH$_2$) in a Thai family. *Acta haemat. (Basel)*, **39**, 151–158.

WASI, P., SOOKANEK, M., POOTRAKUL, S., NA-NAKORN, S. & SUINGDUMRONG, A. (1967). Haemoglobin E and α-thalassaemia. *Brit. med. J.*, **iv**, 29–32.

WASI, P., WINICHAGOON, P., BARAMEE, T. & FUCHAROEN, S. (1982). Globin chain synthesis in heterozygous and homozygous hemoglobin E. *Hemoglobin*, **6**, 75–78.

WATSON, R. J. (1956). Hemoglobins and disease. *Advanc. intern. Med.*, **8**, 305–335.

WATSON-WILLIAMS, E. J., BEALE, D., IRVINE, D. & LEHMANN, H. (1965). A new haemoglobin, D Ibadan (β-87 threonine → lysine), producing no sickle-cell haemoglobin D disease with haemoglobin S. *Nature (Lond.)*, **205**, 1273–1276.

WEATHERALL, D. J., SIGLER, A. T. & BAGLIONI, C. (1962). Four hemoglobins in each of three brothers. Genetic and biochemical significance. *Bull. Johns Hopk. Hosp.*, **111**, 143–156.

WHEBY, M. S., THORUP, O. A. & LEAVELL, B. S. (1956). Homozygous hemoglobin C disease in siblings: further comment on intraerythrocytic crystals. *Blood*, **11**, 266–272.

WICKRAMASINGHE, S. N., HUGHES, M., WASI, P., FUCHAROEN, S. & MODELL, B. (1981). Ineffective erythropoiesis in haemoglobin Eβ-thalassaemia: an electron microscope study. *Brit. J. Haemat.*, **48**, 451–457.

WINICHAGOON, P., FUCHAROEN, S., WEATHERALL, D. & WASI, P. (1985). Concomitant inheritance of α-thalassemia in β⁰-thalassemia/Hb E disease. *Amer. J. Hemat.*, **20**, 217–222.

WONG, S. C. & ALI M. A. M. (1980). Haemoglobin D Los Angeles, D-β⁺- thalassaemia, and D-β⁰-thalassaemia. A report of two Canadian families. *Acta haemat. (Basel)*, **63**, 151–155.

WONG, S. C. & ALI, M. A. M. (1982). Hemoglobin E diseases: hematological, analytical, and biosynthetic studies in homozygotes and double heterozygotes for α-thalassaemia. *Amer. J. Hemat.*, **13**, 15–21.

WONG, Y. S., TANAKA, K. R., GREENBERG, L. H. & OKADA, T. (1969). Hematuria associated with hemoglobin C$_{Harlem}$: a sickling hemoglobin variant. *J. Urol.*, **102**, 762–764.

WORTHINGTON, S. & LEHMANN, H. (1985). The first observation of Hb D Punjab β⁰thalassaemia in an English family with 22 cases of unsuspected β⁰thalassaemia minor amongst its members. *J. med. Genet.*, **22**, 377–381.

ZUELZER, W. & KAPLAN, E. (1954). Thalassemia-hemoglobin C disease. A new syndrome presumably due to the combination of the genes for thalassemia and hemoglobin C. *Blood*, **9**, 1047–1054.

ZUELZER, W. W., NEEL, J. V. & ROBINSON, A. R. (1956). Abnormal hemoglobins. *Prog. Hemat.*, **1**, 91–137. Grune and Stratton, New York.

The unstable haemoglobin haemolytic anaemias

Synonyms

Idiopathic Heinz body anaemia (Cathie, 1952); hereditary Heinz-body anaemia (Dacie et al., 1964); unstable haemoglobin haemolytic anaemias (Carrell and Lehmann, 1969); unstable hemoglobin disease (Wrightstone, 1984).

HISTORY

In June 1952, Cathie described in the *Great Ormond Street Journal* under the title 'Apparent idiopathic Heinz body anaemia' the history of a patient who had a congenital haemolytic anaemia of uncertain type. In June 1948, a male child aged 16 months had been admitted to the Hospital for Sick Children, London, for the investigation of pallor and jaundice. His spleen was palpable, the haemoglobin was 7 g/dl and there were 37% reticulocytes. Both his parents, and other relatives, appeared to be healthy. Congenital haemolytic jaundice was diagnosed. The child was transfused and splenectomy carried out. Anaemia, however, recurred and laparotomy was undertaken to exclude the presence of an accessory spleen. None was found. In January 1950, the present author, who had been asked to see the child, found that the majority of his erythrocytes contained large inclusions which were considered to be Heinz bodies. Reinvestigation many years later, at University College Hospital, London, established that the patient was forming an unstable haemoglobin which was referred to as Hb Bristol (Steadman, Yates and Huehns, 1970).

In the late 1950s and early 1960s, before the pathogenesis of the unstable haemoglobin haemolytic anaemias (UHbHAs) had been established, a small number of rather similar case reports were published under a variety of titles* [Allison, 1957 (a very brief report); Lange and Akeroyd, 1958; Schmid, Williams and Clemens, 1958; Fiorio, 1959; Schmid, Brecher and Clemens, 1959; Scott et al., 1960; Lelong et al., 1961; Mozziconacci et

al., 1961; Worms et al., 1961; Shibata et al., 1963; André, Dreyfus and le Bulloc'h-Combrisson, 1964; Braunsteiner et al., 1964; Goudemand et al., 1964; Gregoratos, Vennes and Moser 1964 — the same patient was previously reported by Lange and Akeroyd; Sheehy, 1964; Miwa et al., 1965; Sansone and Pik, 1965; Seringe et al., 1965]. With the publication of these accounts it became clear that a rare but remarkable and important type of congenital haemolytic anaemia existed which had previously not been recognized.

A characteristic finding in all of the above-described patients was the presence in a large proportion of their erythrocytes of large inclusions which most of the authors considered to be similar to, if not identical with, Heinz bodies. An additional feature also common to the patients is that they had all undergone splenectomy (as had Cathie's patient). A point made by some authors, *e.g.* Lange and Akeroyd (1958), against identifying the inclusions as Heinz bodies was that they could be seen in Romanowsky-stained fixed blood films. (Genuine Heinz bodies were thought not to stain under these circumstances.) The present author pointed out, when shown the films of Lange and Akeroyd's patient, that he had seen the same appearances in a splenectomized human patient suffering from acetylphenylhydrazine poisoning and also in Cathie's case (Fig. 17.1).

In most instances the patient's haemoglobin had been submitted to electrophoresis. In some of the patients no abnormal bands were seen — there were, however, in some instances small rises in the percentage of Hb F and Hb A_2 (Lange and Akeroyd, 1958; Schmid, Brecher and Clemens, 1959; Mozziconacci et al., 1961; Worms et al. 1961; Miwa et al., 1965). In other patients an abnormal band (or bands), usually slow moving, had been found, the nature of which could not at the time be established (Scott et al., 1960; Shibata et al., 1963; André, Dreyfus and le Bulloc'h-Combrisson, 1964; Goudemand et al., 1964; Sheehy, 1964; Sansone and Pik, 1965). No tests for the heat stability of the patients' haemoglobin were carried out.

Common to most of these early accounts was the description of the passing by the patient of abnormally dark brown or even blackish urine, and this was reflected in the way the disorder was

---

* The severely affected infant described by Lelong et al. (1961) seems unlikely to have had an UHbHA. Splenectomy carried out at 17 months resulted in immediate and lasting benefit and after splenectomy Heinz bodies were noted to be present in only 2–3% of erythrocytes.

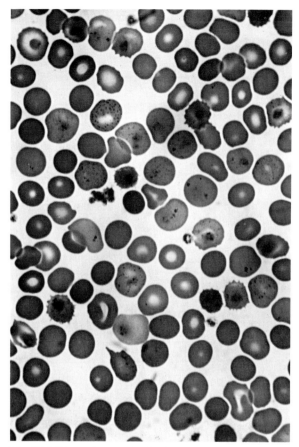

Fig. 17.1 Photomicrograph of a blood film. The film was made in 1950 from the original patient described by Cathie (1952) (Hb Bristol). After splenectomy.
Shows much punctuate basophilia, Pappenheimer bodies and dimly visible Heinz bodies, mostly in crenated and contracted cells. Romanowsky stain. × 750.

referred to. Thus 'abnormal pigment metabolism' (Lange and Akeroyd; Scott *et al.*, Miwa *et al.*), 'defect in pigment metabolism' (Schmid, Brecher and Clemens), 'urines noires' (French authors), 'mesobilifuscinurie' (Braunsteiner *et al.*), 'pigmenturia' (Sheehy) and 'bilifuscinuria' (Sansone and Pik) appear in the titles of some of the papers referred to above. The nature of the pigment(s) causing the darkening of the urine is considered on page 366.

Another important feature illustrated in these early papers is that the disorder could be a familial one. Thus more than one generation was affected in the case reports of Schmid, Brecher and Clemens (1959), Goudemand *et al.* (1964), André *et al.* (1964) and Sansone and Pik (1965).

It is interesting to consider how the patients' illness was viewed by the authors at the time their descriptions were published. Cathie (1952) concluded that the presence of the Heinz bodies was a developmental rather than a toxic phenomenon; Lange and Akeroyd (1958) and Schmid, Brecher and Clemens (1959) thought that the disorder was the consequence of an erythrocyte metabolic defect. Scott and co-workers (1960) wrote 'a likely hypothesis would be that the patient's cells contain an unstable hemoglobin, analogous to hemoglobin H, which somehow results in shortening of erythrocyte survival'. Shibata and co-workers (1963), who also demonstrated the presence of an abnormal haemoglobin, attributed its production to a congenital enzymatic defect in the erythrocytes. Goudemand and co-workers (1964) concluded that the disorder was a new type of haemoglobinopathy with spontaneous precipitation of an abnormal haemoglobin as the erythrocytes aged, leading to the appearance of abnormal inclusions and determining the destruction of the erythrocytes at a 'precocious age'.

Thus, before the nature of the unstable haemoglobin haemolytic anaemias was really understood there were strong indications that the disorder could stem from the presence of an abnormal haemoglobin. It was Grimes and Meisler (1962) who showed conclusively that this supposition was true by demonstrating by means of a simple laboratory test that an abnormal haemoglobin in the patient they studied was indubitably unstable. They had available to them the blood of a 10-year-old girl who had been referred to the present author for investigation. She had been splenectomized as an infant for a severe congenital haemolytic anaemia, but had continued to be anaemic and jaundiced and to pass dark urine. Almost all her erythrocytes contained Heinz bodies.

Grimes and Meisler were able to show that erythrocyte metabolism was essentially normal. The HMP shunt functioned adequately: the concentration of GSH was normal and exposure to acetylphenylhydrazine resulted in only a slight fall; the enzymes in the HMP shunt were very active, in excess of those in the EM pathway. Catalase activity was normal. It seemed, therefore, most unlikely that the presence of the Heinz bodies could be the result of an erythrocyte metabolic defect. Submitting the haemoglobin to a raised temperature revealed, however, a striking and convincing abnormality. When a stroma-free haemolysate was heated for a few minutes at 50°C a red-brown precipitate formed which increased in amount with time so that eventually about 20% of the haemoglobin precipitated. Precipitation (denaturation) also took place when a solution of purified patient's haemoglobin in phosphate buffered saline at pH 6.5 was similarly heated. Haemolysates of normal blood, reticulocyte-rich blood or cord blood did not form significant precipitates at 50°C within the same time limits. Some methaemoglobin was formed as the result of the heating and if the haemoglobin was converted to methaemoglobin beforehand the precipitate formed more quickly. On the other hand, the presence of sodium dithionite suppressed precipitate formation and it was concluded that it was necessary for methaemoglobin to be present for precipitation to take place. The haem : globin ratio in the precipitate was found to be lower than in normal haemoglobin. Grimes and Meisler 'concluded tentatively that in congenital Heinz-body anaemia the formation of Heinz bodies *in vivo* is the end-result of the presence in the red cells of an unstable haemoglobin fraction, the instability of which can be demonstrated *in vitro* by heat treatment of solutions of the haemoglobin'. Further details of the patient whose blood Grimes and Meisler had studied were given by Grimes, Meisler and Dacie (1964); her unstable haemoglobin was eventually identified and named Hb Hammersmith (see p. 329).

Grimes and Meisler's short paper has proved to be an important landmark in the history of the unstable haemoglobin haemolytic anaemias, for it has provided, alongside subsequently devised alternative simple tests of haemoglobin denaturation (see p. 352), a reliable way of making the diagnosis, particularly in patients who have not undergone splenectomy and whose erythrocytes in consequence do not contain Heinz bodies (see p. 346).

Parallel with the early work on Hb Hammersmith referred to above, two other distinct and unusual haemoglobins were being investigated at about the same time. Both were unstable: one was

Hb Zürich (Hitzig et al., 1960); the other was Hb Köln (Pribilla, 1962).

Haemoglobin Zürich

Under the title 'Hämoglobin Zürich: eine neue Hämoglobinanomalie mit sulfonamidinduzierter Innenkörperanämie' Hitzig and co-workers (1960) described the occurrence of a 'new' haemoglobin in 15 members in four generations of a large Swiss family. The abnormal haemoglobin was discovered following the occurrence of severe acute haemolytic episodes in two members of the family who had been given therapeutic doses of a sulphonamide drug.

The propositus (Case 1) was a female infant who, when aged 7 months, had become anaemic and jaundiced following the administration of Elkosin for otitis media. A similar but more severe episode followed the administration of a sulphonamide for a febrile illness when she was aged 2 years and 9 months. Blood films at that time showed erythrocyte fragments and 'egg-shell' forms and about 84% of the cells could be seen to contain large inclusions when stained supravitally with brilliant cresyl blue. The child's father (Case 2) suffered a similar but not so severe episode when he was treated for cystitis with a sulphonamide. Approximately 99% of his erythrocytes, including reticulocytes, contained inclusions, and his peripheral-blood picture was similar to that of his daughter. The haemolytic episodes were accompanied by a substantial leucocytosis, with a shift to the left in neutrophil segmentation, and were followed by a reticulocytosis. Both patients recovered well from their acute episodes, the intra-erythrocytic inclusions disappearing within a few days. G6PD activity, measured after the patients had recovered from their acute crises, was normal. ^{51}Cr erythrocyte survival studies were carried out on the child's father (Case 2). During the episodes of acute haemolysis the T_{50} was 1.5 days; when he was free of symptoms 5 months later it was still subnormal at 13 days. His haemoglobin was then 13.7 g/dl and the reticulocyte count 7.9%, *i.e.*, there was evidence of moderately increased haemolysis. Family studies showed that Hb Zürich could be found in both sexes and that it was transmitted by a dominant gene. All the positive individuals, including Cases 1 and 2, were heterozygotes.

Electrophoresis on starch block at pH 8.6 of haemolysates derived from both patients demonstrated the presence of a substantial amount of an abnormal haemoglobin component which ran more slowly than Hb A but faster than Hb S, and was clearly separated from Hb A. In the haemolysate from Case 1 the abnormal haemoglobin amounted to approximately 22% of the total haemoglobin and in Case 2 to about 28%. The abnormal haemoglobin was as alkali-sensitive as was Hb A; it was, however, more sensitive than Hb A to denaturation by heat, the rate of denaturation at 70°C of the cyanhaemoglobin derivative being recorded as 25 times faster.

Fingerprints of digests of the haemoglobin and of its separated β chains revealed multiple differences from those derived from Hb A; fingerprints prepared from α chains appeared, on the other hand, to be identical. Although the molecular abnormality of Hb Zürich could not be established at the time their paper was completed, Hitzig and his co-workers considered that they were dealing with a haemoglobin that had not been observed previously and they stressed that the association of a haemoglobinopathy with a drug-induced inclusion-body anaemia without any demonstrable enzyme defect was a new entity.

The description of Hb Zürich by Hitzig et al. (1960) was soon followed by several further publications based on studies carried out on the same Swiss family. Thus the clinical and haematological findings were described again in detail by Frick, Hitzig and Stauffer (1961) and Frick, Hitzig and Betke (1962). Frick, Hitzig and Betke (1962) described how ^{51}Cr-tagged erythrocytes from the patient described as Case 2 had been transfused to normal recipients who were then given test doses of several drugs. All the sulphonamides they tested, as well as primaquine, promptly caused the destruction of the test cells. Frick, Hitzig and Betke considered that the disorder affecting their patients could be distinguished from 'inclusion-body anaemia' as described by Lange and Akeroyd (1958); they stressed in particular that in inclusion-body anaemia lysis is unremitting and that drug therapy is not necessary for the inclusions to be present. Some of their conclusions can be challenged in the light of present knowledge of the unstable haemoglobins and their clinical effects, but there is no doubt that Hb Zürich is a remarkable abnormal haemoglobin and that its discovery, too, was an important landmark in the history of the unstable haemoglobin haemolytic anaemias.

Stauffer (1961), who dealt with the genetical aspects of Hb Zürich, reported that 15 heterozygotes were detected in four successive generations amongst 65 individuals studied. In addition to the two patients originally described, who had had

severe episodes of haemolysis, a further individual gave a history of jaundice following sulphonamide therapy or infection. The remaining heterozygotes appeared to be in good health. Hb Zürich comprised 13–29% of their total haemoglobin.

Further details of the physicochemical properties of the abnormal haemoglobin were given by Huisman et al. (1961) and Bachmann and Marti (1962). Muller and Kingma (1961), working with blood supplied by Drs Marti and Hitzig, showed that histidine (β63) was replaced by arginine.

Some more recent studies on Hb Zürich are referred to on page 369.

Haemoglobin Köln

The story of Hb Köln starts with a short communication given to a Haemoglobin Colloquium held in Vienna. Pribilla (1962) reported that an abnormal haemoglobin component had been found in a middle-Rhenish family suffering from a thalassaemia-like condition. They had no obvious Mediterranean, African or Asiatic connections. This component, which on electrophoresis formed a minor band between Hb A and Hb A$_2$ and comprised about 5% of the total haemoglobin, appeared to be a 'new' haemoglobin and was named Hb Köln. A fuller description of the family and its haemoglobin was given by Pribilla and co-workers (1965) under the title 'Hämoglobin-Köln-Krankheit: familiäre hypochrome hämolytische Anämie mit Hämoglobinanomalie'. Five certain, and four possible, cases were found in four generations. The patients were moderately anaemic: haemoglobin 10.5–13.5 g/dl, reticulocytes 190–270 × 10^9/l, MCH 26–28 pg, MCV 96–122 fl, bilirubin 1.0–2.5 mg/dl; and there was anisocytosis, microcytosis and punctate basophilia. Osmotic fragility was slightly diminished. Their spleen was palpable. Physicochemical studies led to the conclusion that the anomalous haemoglobin was characterized by an abnormality in its β-globin chain between residues 83 to 120. Later it was shown by Carrell, Lehmann and Pribilla (1967) in Cambridge that the German Hb Köln had the same abnormality (methionine for valine in the β 98 position) as had earlier been found in two families in Great Britain (see below).

Dacie and co-workers (1964) described in detail

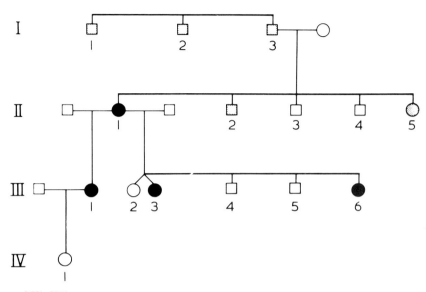

Fig. 17.2 Inheritance of Hb Köln.
Filled symbols denote affected patients; shaded symbols denote probably affected patients. [From Dacie *et al.* (1964).]

the clinical and haematological findings in a British family resident in London* in which four members suffered from a mild to moderately severe compensated haemolytic anaemia and six other members probably did so. Inheritance of the anaemia clearly followed an autosomal dominant pattern (Fig. 17.2). One of the patients had undergone splenectomy and 55–62% of her erythrocytes contained large, usually single, inclusions, considered to be Heinz bodies, which readily stained with methyl violet. The other affected members of the family had not had their spleen removed and their erythrocytes appeared to be free of Heinz bodies. However, if their blood was incubated at 37°C under sterile conditions for 48 hours and then exposed to methyl violet Heinz bodies could be seen in many of the cells.

At first sight the morphology of the erythrocytes of the affected patients whose spleens had not been removed appeared unremarkable, slight anisochromasia and polychromasia being the most obvious features. Closer inspection, however, revealed the presence of occasional relatively densely staining contracted cells with irregular

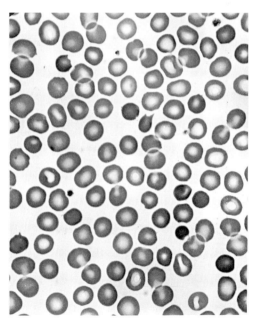

Fig. 17.3 Photomicrograph of a blood film of a patient with Hb Köln, with spleen *in situ*. Patient II-1 of Figure 17.2, a married woman aged 39.
A few contracted erythrocytes with an irregular contour are present. × 700.

* A brief description of the patient in this family who had undergone splenectomy (A. F.) was given by Dacie (1960, p. 196).

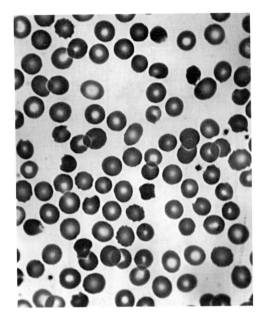

Fig. 17.4 Photomicrograph of a blood film of a patient with Hb Köln, with spleen *in situ*. Patient III-3 of Figure 17.2, one of two dissimilar twins, a girl aged 14.
The morphological changes are similar but more pronounced than those of her mother (Fig. 17.3). × 700.

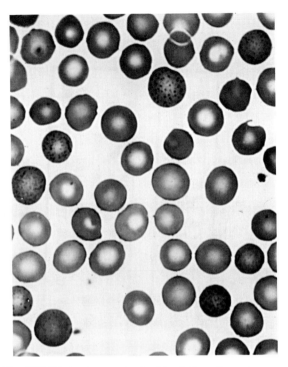

Fig. 17.5 Photomicrograph of a blood film of a patient with Hb Köln. From the same patient whose blood film is illustrated in Figure 17.4.
In this film punctuate basophilia is conspicuous. × 1200.

outlines (Figs. 17.3 and 17.4) as well as punctate basophilia. The degree of abnormality varied from patient to patient; in one patient cells showing punctate basophilia were strikingly frequent, approximately 10% being affected (Fig. 17.5).

Haemolysates prepared from the erythrocytes of the affected patients contained an unstable component which readily precipitated if the haemolysates were heated at 50°C (Fig. 17.6). Electrophoresis in various media showed trailing behind Hb A stretching to beyond Hb A_2, in which three abnormal peaks could be discerned (Fig. 17.7).

Hutchison and co-workers (1964) were at the same time investigating a Scottish family (resident in Glasgow but with remote German connections) with a similar mild to moderate haemolytic anaemia. Ten members in three generations were known to be affected and there were four deceased members who had probably been affected. An abnormal slow-running minor haemoglobin component could be demonstrated by paper electrophoresis and the existence of a heat-precipitable fraction became obvious if haemolysates were

heated at 50°C. Studies of the haemoglobin demonstrated an abnormal fingerprint, the findings being identical with that derived from a blood sample obtained from one of Professor Pribilla's patients. It was concluded that the β chain was abnormal and that the abnormality was located somewhere between residues 83 and 120. Later, Carrell, Lehmann and Hutchison (1966) were able to show that the abnormal haemoglobin was characterized by methionine being substituted for valine in the β 98 position. As has already been referred to, the same abnormality was demonstrated subsequently in haemoglobin samples from the German and London families.

Haemoglobin 'Ube-I'

In 1963 Shibata and co-workers had described the clinical history and haematological findings in a Japanese girl aged 15 years who had been found to be anaemic and to have a palpable spleen as a young child. Splenectomy had been carried for

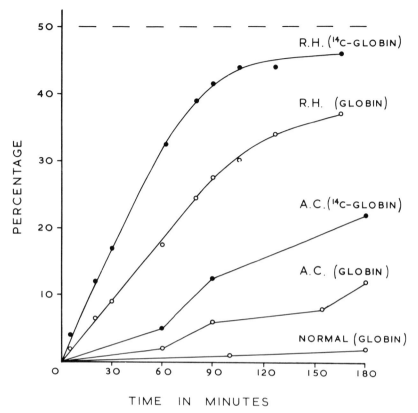

Fig. 17.6 Chart illustrating the result of heating at 50°C haemolysates prepared from two patients with an unstable haemoglobin. R.H. has Hb Hammersmith: A.C. has Hb Köln [patient III-1 (Fig. 17.2)] and had undergone splenectomy.
The closed circles represents the percentage of globin precipitated when the haemolysates were prepared from Heinz-body-free whole blood. The open circles represent the amount of radioactivity in the precipitated material expressed as a percentage of the total amount of radioactivity in haemolysates prepared from whole blood previously labelled with [^{14}C]leucine. [From Dacie *et al.* (1964).]

'hypersplenism'. Electrophoresis demonstrated a slow-running haemoglobin component, and many of the erythrocytes contained single large Heinz bodies. Physicochemical studies of the abnormal haemoglobin, which was named 'Hb Ube-I' revealed blocking of the SH groups of the cysteine residue in the β 98 position. It was not, however, possible to demonstrate at the time an amino-acid substitution. Subsequently, however, one was demonstrated and was shown to be identical with that of Hb Köln, namely, methionine for valine in the β 98 position (Ohba, Miyaji and Shibata, 1973). 'Hb Ube-I' is thus the same as Hb Köln.

Hb Köln appears to be the commonest of the abnormal haemoglobins giving rise to UHbHA and the disorder has by now quite a large literature.

Haemoglobin Hammersmith

Dacie (1960, p. 196) referred to a child suffering from 'congenital Heinz-body anaemia', then under study at Hammersmith Hospital, who was thought to be suffering from a disorder similar to that of Cathie's (1952) patient. She had undergone splenectomy as an infant and her strikingly abnormal Romanowsky-stained blood film was illustrated as Figure 81. Nearly every erythrocyte showed some degree of basophilic stippling, crenation was also conspicuous and some of the smaller crenated erythrocytes contained pale basophilic inclusions the size of Heinz bodies (Fig. 17.8). In wet methyl-violet-stained preparations many of the cells could, in fact, be seen to contain single large Heinz bodies.

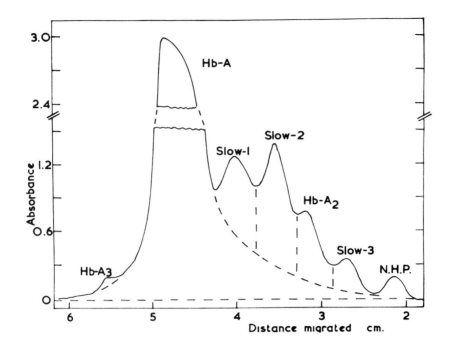

Fig. 17.7 Electrophoresis on starch gel at pH 8.6 of the blood of a patient with Hb Köln, illustrating the presence of three abnormal slow-running peaks.
[From Dacie *et al.* (1964).]

A fuller description of this patient was given by Grimes, Meisler and Dacie (1964). She had been born in 1951 and as an infant was known to have been jaundiced when 2 weeks of age. At 18 months she was noticed to be pale and to be passing dark urine. The haemoglobin was found to be 6.0 g/dl and there were about 70% reticulocytes. Stained blood films showed marked polychomasia and occasional erythrocytes exhibited punctate basophilia. A few small cells with moderately smooth outlines were present. Heinz bodies were not visible (in stained films) and it is not known whether any were present in fresh blood before splenectomy. This was carried out in September 1953 when she was 2 years and 4 months of age. The spleen weighed 158 g. Increased haemolysis, nevertheless, persisted and peripheral-blood films took on the appearances described above (Fig. 17.8). The child received transfusions at approximately 3-monthly intervals for the next 9 months. Subsequently, however, she managed to maintain a reasonably constant haemoglobin level and to lead an almost normal life. Between 1954 and 1957 she was transfused only 3 times.

Between 1960 and 1963 her haemoglobin varied between 6.1 and 8.3 g/dl, with 22–47% reticulocytes. Approximately 80% of the erythrocytes contained Heinz bodies. The leucocyte count ranged between 5.0 and 14.0 × 10⁹/l and the platelet count between 230 and 825 × 10⁹/l. Osmotic fragility was increased, lysis commencing in 0.6% NaCl, but it was incomplete in 0.2% NaCl. Autohaemolysis was markedly increased: 16–24% at 48 hours, reduced by only a small amount by the addition of glucose. The urine was dark reddish-brown: it contained excess urobilin and unidentified pigments.

Electrophoresis of haemoglobin on paper at pH 8.6 revealed no clear abnormalities; there was 3.2% Hb A_2. On starch gel a weak trail could be discerned behind Hb A; and with stored haemolysates several haem-containing bands could be seen between Hb A and the starting position. There was 3–7% Hb F. 1–2% of methaemoglobin was present in haemolysates of fresh cells, and this increased to the high figure of 11% when whole blood was incubated at 37°C for 48 hours.

Approximately 30% of the haemoglobin precipitated when stroma-free, Heinz-body-free haemolysates were

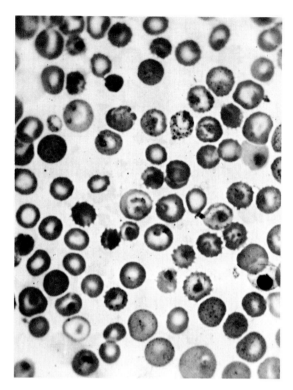

Fig. 17.8 Photomicrograph of a blood film of a patient (R.H.) with Hb Hammersmith. After splenectomy.
Contracted and crenated erythrocytes are conspicuous and Heinz bodies can be seen in some of the cells. Macrocytosis is conspicuous, too. Punctate basophilia is a striking feature. Romanowsky stain. × 700.

heated at 50°C. The precipitate was red-brown in colour. When [U-^{14}C]leucine was used to label globin in reticulocytes, almost one-half of the radioactivity was found in the heat-labile fraction (Fig. 17.6).

Glucose consumption by erythrocytes was increased; the ATP concentration was less than 50% normal and that of ADP was in the low normal range. The concentration of GSH was slightly low. The activity of the HMP shunt was strikingly high, being well in excess of that of the EM pathway.

Attempts to demonstrate the nature of the haemoglobin abnormality leading to its thermolability were at first unsuccessful. The experiments using [U-^{14}C]leucine suggested that about half the haemoglobin the patient was synthesizing was abnormal and heat-precipitable, and it was concluded that the Heinz bodies seen in post-splenectomy blood were the end products of the abnormal haemoglobin's degradation *in vivo*.

The patient's parents are normal; their first child was stillborn and there are two other children who are also normal.

The nature of Hb Hammersmith was finally determined at the MRC Abnormal Haemoglobin Unit at Cambridge as the substitution of serine for phenylalanine at the 42nd position in the β chain, *i.e.* Hb Hammersmith is β 42 (GD1) Phe → Ser (Dacie *et al.*, 1967). This identification of the abnormality in Hb Hammersmith was based on studies on the haemoglobin of the Hammersmith patient and on studies of the haemoglobin of a similar patient investigated at Coventry (Shinton, Thursby-Pelham and Williams, 1969). The two patients were unrelated, and in both instances it appears as if the abnormal haemoglobin had been formed in consequence of a new mutation.

RECENT OBSERVATIONS

The observations summarized in the foregoing sketch of the history of the UHbHAs provided the foundation on which much future work and progress in understanding have been based. In a remarkably short time a large number of unstable haemoglobins were described, differing one from the other in the molecular abnormality responsible for their instability (Tables 17.1–17.3), and it is now clear that the associated haemolytic syndrome is not as rare as it at one time appeared to be. It is remarkable that it remained unrecognized for so long. With some of the molecular variants in which instability can be demonstrated *in vitro*, this does not seem to be associated with any discernible increased haemolysis.

In the remainder of this Chapter, the clinical, haematological and molecular features of the syndrome are discussed and its pathogenesis and treatment considered. Reviews already published include those of Carrell and Lehmann (1969), Fairbanks, Opfell and Burgert (1969), Huehns and Bellingham (1969), Lehmann and Carrell (1969), Necheles and Allen (1969), Huehns (1970, 1974, 1982), White and Dacie (1971), Koler *et al.*, (1973), Rieder (1974), White (1974), Shibata (1975), Bunn, Forget and Ranney (1977), Carrell and Winterbourn (1981), Beutler (1983), Niazi and Shibata (1983a,b, 1984a,b) and Bunn and Forget (1986).

Table 17.1 β-chain amino-acid substitutions giving rise to unstable haemoglobins associated with increased haemolysis.

Name of variant (alphabetical order)	Amino acid involved: position in molecule	Amino acid substituted	Oxygen affinity: normal (N), increased (↑) or decreased (↓)	Increased haemolysis: severe, moderate or mild	Family history: positive or negative. Racial origin of patients	Key references
Abraham Lincoln = Perth = Köbe	Leucine β32 (B14)	Proline	N	Severe	Neg Afro-American	Honig et al. (1973) Ohba et al. (1980)
Altdorf	Alanine β135 (H13)	Proline	↑	Moderate	Pos Italian-Swiss	Marti et al. (1976)
Atlanta	Leucine β75 (E19)	Proline		Mild	Pos —	Hubbard et al. (1975)
Baylor	Leucine β81 (EF5)	Arginine	↑	Mild	Neg —	Schneider et al. (1976b)
Belfast	Tryptophan β15 (A12)	Arginine	↑ ? Absent	Mild	Pos Caucasian	Kennedy et al (1974) Gacon et al. (1976)
Bicêtre	Histidine β63 (E7)	Proline	N	Severe	Neg — Neg — — Caucasian	Wajcman, Gacon and Labie (1975) Allard et al. (1976) Miller et al. (1986)
Borås	Leucine β88 (F4)	Arginine		Mild	Pos Swedish	Svensson and Strand (1967)★ Hollender et al. (1969)
Bristol	Valine β67 (E11)	Aspartic acid	↓	Severe Severe	Neg British — Japanese	Cathie (1952)★ Steadman, Yates and Huehns (1970) Ohba et al. (1980, 1985c)
= Niigata						
Bryn Mawr	Phenylalanine β85 (F1)	Serine	↑	Moderate	Neg Caucasian	Bradley et al. (1972)
Bucureşti = Louisville	Phenylalanine β42 (CD1)	Leucine	↓	Moderate	Pos Roumanian	Bratu et al. (1971)
Buenos Aires = Bryn Mawr	Phenylalanine β85 (F1)	Serine	↑	Moderate	Pos Argentinian	de Weinstein et al. (1973)
Burke	Glycine β107 (G9)	Arginine	↓	Mild or moderate	Pos Japanese	Kobayashi et al. (1986)
Bushwick	Glycine β74 (E18)	Valine		Mild Moderate	Pos Italian-American — Japanese	Rieder et al (1975) Ohba et al (1985d)
Caspar = Southampton	Leucine β106 (G8)	Proline	↑	Moderate	Neg —	Jones et al. (1972) Koler et al. (1973)
Castilla	Leucine β32 (B14)	Arginine	↓	Severe	Neg Spanish	Garel et al. (1975) Thillet et al. (1980)
Chiba = Hammersmith	Phenylalanine β42 (CD1)	Serine	↓	Severe	Neg Japanese	Ohba et al. (1975a)

Table 17.1 (*cont'd*)

Name of variant (alphabetical order)	Amino acid involved: position in molecule	Amino acid substituted	Oxygen affinity: normal (N), increased (↑) or decreased (↓)	Increased haemolysis: severe, moderate or mild	Family history: positive or negative. Racial origin of patients	Key references
Christchurch	Phenylalanine β71 (E15)	Serine	↓	Moderate	— —	Carrell and Owen (1971); Carrell and Winterbourn (1981)
			N	Moderate	Neg Japanese	Ohba *et al.* (1985a)
Collingwood	Valine β60 (E4)	Alanine	N	Mild	— Greek	Williamson *et al.* (1983)
Cranston	Tyrosine β145 (HC2) and histidine β146 (HC3)	Chain elongated; β145 and 146 replaced by 13 residues making 157 residues in all, including isoleucine as β146	↑	Mild	Pos Italian-American	Bunn *et al.* (1975a, b)
Duarte	Alanine β62 (E6)	Proline	↑	Moderate	Pos German	Beutler, Lang and Lehmann (1974)
Genova	Leucine β28 (B10)	Proline	↑	Moderate	Pos Italian	Sansone and Centa (1964)★ Sansone and Pik (1965)★ Sansone, Carrell and Lehmann (1967)
					Pos Breton	Labie *et al.* (1977)
					Pos Kenyan	Kendall *et al.* (1979)
					Pos Cuban	Martinez, Carnot and Hernández (1983)
= Hyogo					— Japanese	Ohba *et al.* (1980)
Guantanamo	Alanine β128 (H6)	Aspartic acid		Mild	Pos Afro-Cuban	Martinez, Lima and Colombo (1977)
Hammersmith	Phenylalanine β42 (CD1)	Serine	↓	Severe	Neg British	Grimes, Meisler and Dacie (1964)★ Dacie *et al.* (1967)
= Chiba						Ohba *et al.* (1980)
Indianapolis	Cysteine β112 (G14)	Arginine		Severe	Pos Caucasian	Adams *et al.* (1979)
				Mild	Pos Spanish	Baiget *et al.* (1986)
Istanbul	Histidine β92 (F8)	Glutamine	↑	Moderate	Neg —	Aksoy *et al.* (1972)
= Saint Etienne					— —	Aksoy and Erdem (1979)
I Toulouse	Lysine β66 (E10)	Glutamic acid	N	Mild	— French	Rosa *et al.* (1969) Labie *et al.* (1971)

(*cont'd*)

Table 17.1 (*cont'd*)

Name of variant (alphabetical order)	Amino acid involved: position in molecule	Amino acid substituted	Oxygen affinity: normal (N), increased (↑) or decreased (↓)	Increased haemolysis: severe, moderate or mild	Family history: positive or negative. Racial origin of patients	Key references
Köln	Valine β98 (FG5)	Methionine	↑	Moderate	Pos German	Pribilla (1962)★ Pribilla *et al.* (1965) Carrell, Lehmann and Hutchison (1966)
					Pos Malaysian	Lie-Injo *et al.* (1972)
					Pos Jewish	Hällen, Charlesworth and Lehmann (1972) Kolski and Miller (1976)
Louisville = Bucureşti	Phenylalanine β42 (CD1)	Leucine	↓	Moderate	Pos English-Irish-American Indian	Keeling *et al.* (1972)
				Moderate	Neg Canadian	Smiley *et al.* (1978)
Lufkin	Glycine β29 (B4)	Aspartic acid	↑	Mild	— Afro-American	Schmidt *et al.* (1977)
Madrid	Alanine β115 (G17)	Proline		Moderate	Neg Spanish	Outeirino *et al.* (1974)
Mizuho	Leucine β68 (E12)	Proline	↑	Severe	— Japanese	Ohba *et al.* (1977)
Moscva	Glycine β24 (B6)	Aspartic acid	↓		— Russian	Idelson *et al.* (1974a)
Mozhaisk	Histidine β92 (F8)	Arginine	↑	Severe	— Russian	Spivak *et al.* (1982)
Nagoya	Histidine β97 (FG4)	Proline	↑	Mild	Pos Japanese	Ohba *et al.* (1985b)
Newcastle	Histidine β92 (F8)	Proline		Moderate	Pos —	Finney *et al.* (1975)
Nottingham	Valine β98 (FG5)	Glycine	↑	Severe	Neg English	Gordon-Smith *et al.* (1973)
Okaloosa	Leucine β48 (CD7)	Arginine	↓	Mild	Pos Caucasian	Charache *et al.* (1973)
Olmsted	Leucine β141 (H19)	Arginine		Severe	Neg Caucasian	Fairbanks, Opfell and Burgert (1969)★ Lorkin, Lehmann and Fairbanks (1975)
Pasedena	Leucine β75 (E19)	Arginine	↑	Mild	— French	Johnson *et al.* (1980)
Perth = Abraham Lincoln	Leucine β32 (B14)	Proline	N	Moderate	Neg —	Jackson, Yates and Huehns (1973)
Peterborough	Valine β111 (G13)	Phenylalanine	↓	Mild	Pos Italian	King *et al.* (1972)
Philly	Tyrosine β35 (C1)	Phenylalanine	↑	Moderate	Pos Italian-German-French	Rieder, Oski and Clegg (1969)

Table 17.1 (*cont'd*)

Name of variant (alphabetical order)	Amino acid involved: position in molecule	Amino acid substituted	Oxygen affinity: normal (N), increased ($\uparrow$) or decreased ($\downarrow$)	Increased haemolysis: severe, moderate or mild	Family history: positive or negative. Racial origin of patients	Key references
Riverdale-Bronx	Glycine β24 (B6)	Arginine	$\uparrow$	Moderate	— Jewish-German	Ranney *et al.* (1968)
Rush	Glutamic acid β101 (G3)	Glutamine	N	Mild	Pos Afro-American	Adams *et al.* (1972b, 1974)
Sabine	Leucine β91 (F7)	Proline		Severe	Neg English-Scottish-Irish	Mills, Levin and Alperin (1968)★ Schneider *et al.* (1969)
				Moderate	Neg Yugoslavian	Bogoevski *et al.* (1983)
Saint-Etienne = Istanbul	Histidine β92 (F8)	Glutamine	$\uparrow$	Mild	Neg Caucasian	Beuzard *et al.* (1972) Rosa *et al.* (1972) Cohen Solal *et al.* (1972)
Saint Louis	Leucine β28 (B10)	Glutamine	$\uparrow$	Severe; cyanosis	Neg French	Cohen-Solal *et al.* (1973) Thillet *et al.* (1976)
Saitama	Histidine β117 (G19)	Proline	$\downarrow$	Severe	Neg Japanese	Ohba *et al.* (1983)
Santa Ana	Leucine β88 (F4)	Proline		Moderate	Pos French	Goudemand *et al.* (1964)★ Opfell, Lorkin and Lehmann (1968) Biserte *et al.* (1970)
				Moderate	Neg Caucasian	Tanaka *et al.* (1985)
Savannah	Glycine β24 (B6)	Valine	$\uparrow$	Severe	Neg Caucasian	Huisman *et al.* (1971)
Seattle	Alanine β70 (E14)	Aspartic acid	$\downarrow$	Mild	Pos Caucasian	Huehns (1965)★ Huehns and Shooter (1965)★ Huehns *et al.* (1970) Kurachi *et al.* (1973)
Sendagi	Phenylalanine β42 (CD1)	Valine	$\downarrow$	Moderate	Pos Japanese	Ogata *et al.* (1986)
Shelby	Glutamine β131 (H9)	Lysine	$\uparrow$	Mild	Pos Afro-American	Moo-Penn *et al.* (1976) Moo-Penn *et al.* (1984)
Shepherds Bush	Glycine β74 (E18)	Aspartic acid	$\uparrow$	Mild; severe after sulphonamide	Pos British South African	White *et al.* (1970)
				Mild	Pos Sicilian	Sansone *et al.* (1977)
Southampton = Caspar	Leucine β106 (G8)	Proline	$\uparrow$	Severe	Neg English	Hyde *et al.* (1972)

(*cont'd*)

Table 17.1 (*cont'd*)

Name of variant (alphabetical order)	Amino acid involved: position in molecule	Amino acid substituted	Oxygen affinity: normal (N), increased (↑) or decreased (↓)	Increased haemolysis: severe, moderate or mild	Family history: positive or negative. Racial origin of patients	Key references
Sydney	Valine β67 (E11)	Alanine		Mild	Pos German	Raik, Hunter and Lindsay (1967) Carrell *et al.* (1967)
Toyoake	Alanine β142 (H20)	Proline	↑	Mild	Neg Japanese	Hirano *et al.* (1981)
Tübingen	Leucine β106 (G8)	Glutamine	↑	Mild; also cyanosis	Pos German	Kleihauer *et al.* (1971) Kohne *et al.* (1976)
Ube-I = Köln, Sendai, Keio, Sapporo	Valine β98 (FG5)	Methionine	↑		— Japanese	Shibata *et al.* (1963)★ Ohba, Miyaji and Shibata (1973) Ohba *et al.* (1980)
Vaasa	Glutamine β39 (C5)	Glutamic acid		Mild	Pos Finnish	Kendall *et al.* (1977)
Volga	Alanine β27 (B9)	Aspartic acid		Severe	Neg Russian	Idelson *et al.* (1975)
				Severe	Pos Dutch	Kuis-Reerink *et al.* (1976)
				Moderate	Pos Italian	Sciarratta *et al.* (1985)
Wien	Tyrosine β130 (H8)	Aspartic acid		Moderate	Pos —	Braunsteiner *et al.* (1964)★ Lorkin *et al.* (1974)
Yokahama	Leucine β31 (B13)	Proline	↑	Severe	Pos Japanese	Nakatsuji *et al.* (1981a).
Zürich	Histidine β63 (E7)	Arginine	↑	Mild; severe after sulphonamide therapy	Pos —	Hitzig *et al.* (1960)★ Muller and Kingma (1961) Winterhalter *et al.* (1969)

References marked with an asterisk★ are to papers published before the unstable haemoglobin had been identified. The tabulations of Lehmann and Kynoch (1976) and of the International Hemoglobin Information Center (1986) are valuable sources of information.

Table 17.2 β-chain amino-acid deletions giving rise to unstable haemoglobins.

Name of variant (alphabetical order)	Amino acid involved: position in molecule	Oxygen affinity: normal (N), increased (↑) or decreased (↓)	Increased haemolysis: severe, moderate, mild or not apparent (N.A.)	Family history: positive or negative. Racial origin of patients	Key refeences
Freiburg	Valine β23 (B5)	↑	Mild or N.A.; also cyanosis	Pos —	Betke and Kleihauer (1962) Jones et al. (1966)
Gun Hill	Leucine, histidine, cysteine, aspartic acid and lysine β91–95 (F7-FG2)	↑	Mild	Pos German-English Neg Afro-American	Bradley and Rieder (1965)★ Bradley, Wohl and Rieder (1967) Murari et al. (1977)
Leiden	Glutamic acid β6 (A3)	↑	Mild; also crisis after infection	Pos Dutch Pos Zulu — Yugoslavian	de Jong, Went and Bernini (1968) Rieder and James (1974) Perlman et al. (1981) Jurićić et al. (1983)
Lyons	Lysine β17 (A14)	↑	N.A.	Pos Spanish and N. African	Cohen-Solal et al. (1974)
Niteroi	Phenylalanine β42 (CD1)	↓	Mild, with crises associated with drugs and infections	— Brazilian	International Hemoglobin Information Center (1986)
Saint Antoine	Glycine β74 (E18)	N	Mild	— French	Wajcman, Labie and Schapira (1973)
Tochigi	Glycine β56–59 (D7–E3)		Moderate	Pos Japanese	Shibata et al. (1970)
Tours	Threonine β98 (F3)	↑	? Severe	— French	Wajcman, Labie and Schapira (1973)

Reference marked with an asterisk★ is to a paper published before the unstable haemoglobin had been identified.

Table 17.3 α-chain amino-acid substitutions giving rise to unstable haemoglobins associated with increased hacmolysis.

Name of variant (alphabetical order)	Amino acid involved: position in molecule	Amino acid substituted	Oxygen affinity: normal (N), increased (↑) or decreased (↓)	Increased haemolysis: severe, moderate, mild or not apparent (N.A.)	Family history: positive or negative. Racial origin of patients	Key references
Ann Arbor	Leucine α80 (F1)	Arginine		Mild or N.A.	Pos Caucasian	Rucknagel, Spencer and Brandt (1968)
Bibba	Leucine α136 (H19)	Proline		Severe	— —	Kleihauer et al. (1968)
Dakar	Histidine α112 (G19)	Glutamine	↑	Mild	Pos —	Rosa et al. (1968)
Hasharon = Sinai	Aspartic acid α47 (CD5)	Histidine		Mild or N.A.	Pos Askenazi Jewish	Halbrecht et al. (1967) Charache and Montdzac (1967) Charache et al. (1969) Levine et al. (1975) Giglioni et al. (1980)
Hirosaki	Phenylalanine α43 (CD1)	Leucine		Mild or moderate	Pos Japanese	Ohba et al. (1975b)
L. Ferrara	Aspartic acid α47 (CD5)	Histidine		Mild or N.A.	Pos Jewish	Bianco et al. (1963) Nagel et al. (1969)
Moabit	Leucine α86 (F7)	Arginine	↓	Mild	— Turkish	Knuth et al. (1979)
Petah Tikva	Alanine α110 (G17)	Aspartic acid		Mild	Pos Iraqi Jewish	Honig et al. (1981)
Port Phillip	Leucine α91 (FG3)	Proline		Mild	— Chinese	Brennan et al. (1977b)
Setif	Asparagine α94 (G1)	Tyrosine	↓	Mild or N.A.	— Iranian	Nozari et al. (1977)
Suan-Dok	Leucine α109 (G16)	Arginine		Mild	Pos Thai	Sanguansermsri et al. (1979)
Torino	Phenylalanine α43 (CD1)	Valine		Mild; crisis after receiving sulphonamide	— Italian	Beretta et al. (1968)
Tottori	Glycine α59 (E8)	Valine		Moderate	Pos Japanese	Nakatsuji et al. (1981b)

CLINICAL FEATURES

Genetics

It seems as if all the patients so far recorded as suffering from UHbHA have been heterozygous for the gene determining their unstable haemoglobin with the exception of a few patients who have been compound heterozygotes for two different unstable haemoglobins (Casey et al., 1978; Brennan et al., 1983). Other patients have been compound heterozygotes for an unstable haemoglobin and another type of haemoglobinopathy (Table 17.4).

The fact that patients homozygous for an un-stable haemoglobin do not seem to have been described can be most likely attributed to the rarity of this type of abnormal haemoglobin. Moreover, should a fetus inherit a gene for a markedly unstable haemoglobin from both parents it seems likely that this would result in death *in utero* if the abnormal haemoglobin was an α-chain variant or death within the first few months of post-natal life if the β chain was abnormal.

In the majority of cases of UHbHA a positive family history of the disease has been established (Tables 17.1–17.3), the inheritance pattern being

Table 17.4 Unstable haemoglobins associated with another abnormal haemoglobin or thalassaemia in compound heterozygotes.

Unstable haemoglobin (alphabetical order)	Associated abnormal haemoglobin or thalassaemia	Severity of increased haemolysis or anaemia	References
Atlanta*	Coventry*	Severe (in infancy)	Brennan et al. (1983)
Caribbean	Hb S	No evidence of increased haemolysis	Ahern et al. (1976)
Coventry	α-thalassaemia	Mild to moderate	Nozari, Rahbar and Lehmann (1978)
Duarte	β-thalassaemia	Mild	Beutler, Lang and Lehmann (1974)
Hofu	β°-thalassaemia	Moderate	Arends et al. (1985)
Hope	Hb S	Mild	Steinberg et al. (1974).
Leiden	β°-thalassaemia	Severe	Lie-Injo et al. (1977)
Leslie	β°-thalassaemia, Hb S, Hb C	Mild to moderate	Lutcher and Huisman (1975) Lutcher et al. (1976)
North Shore-Caracas	Hb S, Hb C	Mild anaemia; ? increased haemolysis	Arends et al. (1977)
Petah Tikva	α-thalassaemia	Similar to mild Hb-H disease	Honig et al. (1981)
Peterborough	Hb Lepore	Moderate	King et al. (1972)
Saint Etienne	Swiss type of HPFH		Testa et al. (1979)
Saki	Hb S	Slight anaemia, no clinical effect	Beuzard et al. (1975)
Saki	β-thalassaemia	Moderate	Milner et al. (1976)
Shelby	β°-thalassaemia	Moderate	Moo-Penn et al. (1984)
Sydney	Hb Coventry (β141 deleted)	Mild	Casey et al. (1976, 1978) Lehmann (1978)

*Subsequent work (Brennan et al., 1986) has indicated that this patient, and two of his children, were forming, in addition to Hb A and Hb Atlanta, a variant, Hb Atlanta-Coventry, resulting from two mutations in the same β-globin chain (β75 Leu → Pro plus β141 Leu deleted).

clearly that of a dominant autosomal gene, with both sexes being affected equally. In a significant proportion of cases, however, both parents and other relatives of the propositus have been shown not to be forming the abnormal haemoglobin. In such circumstances the unstable haemoglobin appears to have arisen as the result of a new mutation. Of the early reports, this was so in Cathie's (1952) patient (Hb Bristol) and also true of the patients forming Hb Hammersmith. With the patients forming Hb Zürich and Hb Koln, respectively, there were, however, clear-cut positive family histories. The presence or absence of a positive family history is noted with respect to the unstable haemoglobins listed in Tables 17.1–17.3. Stamatoyannopoulos, Nute and Miller (1981) reported that they had been able to amass from the literature or from personal communications, a total of 35 unstable haemoglobins arising apparently from de-novo mutations: included in the 35 were 24 different variants. By 1984, Stamatoyannopoulos and Nute had traced 42 examples of unstable haemoglobins arising from de-novo mutations, as well as 15 cases of Hb M. They used this information to calculate mutation rates per nucleotide.

The expression of the abnormal gene within individual members of an affected family, as judged by the proportion of unstable haemoglobin present in their peripheral-blood erythrocytes and their clinical state, has been fairly constant. Thus in four members of the family described by de Jong, Went and Bernini (1968) Hb Leiden comprised approximately one-third of the total haemoglobin and a similar proportion (32–36%) of Hb Okaloosa was present in five members of the family described by Charache et al. (1973). With Hb Zürich, however, the proportion of abnormal haemoglobin was recorded by Stauffer (1961) as varying more widely — between 13% and 29%: the majority of the 15 affected members were in good health and only three of them had developed haemolytic crises (two severe, one less severe), on each occasion following the administration of a sulphonamide drug. In the case of Hb Koln, on the other hand, affected members of a family usually suffer from continuous mild to moderately increased haemolysis irrespective of exposure to any drug, as in the family reported by

Dacie et al. (1964). Other patients have suffered from continuous haemolysis of far greater severity, as did, for example, the young girl and her father described by Adams et al. (1979) (Hb Indianapolis).

The differences in severity to which different families are affected are no doubt a reflection of the nature of the haemoglobin abnormality and its effect on the haemoglobin molecules' stability (see p. 358).

Severity

As indicated above, the clinical effects of the presence of an unstable haemoglobin vary widely. Some patients have a severe haemolytic anaemia manifest in the neonatal period as jaundice and producing within the first year of life a severe grade of anaemia requiring repeated transfusions, e.g., the patients with Hb Bristol, Hb Hammersmith, Hb Bicêtre (Allard et al., 1976), and Hb Perth (Grové et al., 1977); others have mild to moderate compensated but continuous haemolytic anaemia as with Hb Koln. Still other patients have no apparent disturbance of health: there is little or no increased haemolysis, except perhaps following oxidant drug therapy, as with Hb Zurich, or following an acute infection (see p. 342). Finally, there are slightly unstable variants (compared with Hb A) that appear to be completely innocuous, as with Hb Sogn (Monn and Bjark, 1970), or cause increased haemolysis in perhaps one individual only out of several affected members of a family carrying the unstable haemoglobin or cause increased haemolysis in some families carrying the abnormal haemoglobin but not in others carrying the same haemoglobin, as in the case of Hb Hasharon (Halbrecht et al., 1967; Charache et al., 1969).

Race

Although UHbHA was originally described in patients from Northern Europe, i.e., of British, German and Swiss origin, it is now clear that the disorders are not confined to any particular race. Thus cases have been reported, too, in Japanese (Shibata et al., 1963; Ohba et al., 1980), Ashkenazi Jews (Halbrecht et al., 1967), black Afro-Americans (Sathiapalan and Robinson, 1968), Sicilians (Sansone et al., 1977), Malays (Lie-Injo *et al.*, 1972), European Jews (Hällén, Charlesworth and Lehmann, 1972), a Nama child from Namidia (Grové *et al.*, 1977), Chinese (Lie-Injo *et al.*, 1977), Arabs (Ben-Bassat *et al.*, 1969), a Turkish patient (Knuth *et al.*, 1979), in an (East) Indian (Wong *et al.*, 1980) and in Zulus (Perlman *et al.*, 1981) as well as in Europeans of Dutch, French, Hungarian, Italian, Roumanian, Russian, Swedish and Ukrainian origin.

It is of great interest that identical mutations leading to the formation of some abnormal haemoglobins have occurred in widely separated ethnically different racial groups where there seems to have been no possibility of genetic contact. Thus Hb Köln has been identified in Japanese and Malaysian families as well as in European families and Hb Hammersmith in Japanese and Sudanese families in addition to two unconnected British families [see Table 17.1 and also Ohba *et al.* (1980)].

Age at presentation

In the majority of cases the disorder has been recognized in infancy, or at least early in childhood, but when increased haemolysis is not greatly increased the patient may have reached adult life before it is realized that he or she had a chronic haemolytic anaemia. This was true for instance of the patients described by Prato *et al.* (1970) (Hb Torino), Adams *et al.* (1974) (Hb Rush) and Beutler, Lang and Lehmann (1974) (Hb Duarte).

As has been mentioned, some individuals never develop significant symptoms and in such cases diagnosis has been made following a routine blood examination or as the result of screening for the presence of a haemoglobinopathy or in the course of studying a family in which one member has been found to have a haemolytic anaemia, as with Hb Sogn (Monn, Gaffney and Lehmann, 1968), Hb Etobicoke (Crookston *et al.*, 1969) and Hb Okaloosa (Charache *et al.*, 1973).

When a diagnosis of haemolytic anaemia has been made in infancy, this has usually not been made until the infant has reached the age of 9 months to 1 year, when for the first time he or she has been recognized to be unnaturally pale. An unusual degree of neonatal jaundice has, never-

theless, been recorded in a few instances, *e.g.*, by Cathie (1952) (Hb Bristol), Grimes, Meisler and Dacie (1964) and Shinton, Thursby-Pelham and Williams (1969) (Hb Hammersmith) and Yamada *et al.* (1971) (Hb Tochigi). The patient described by Ohba *et al.* (1975a) was sufficiently jaundiced to require an exchange transfusion; she had 'Hb Chiba', later shown to be identical with Hb Hammersmith. These severe cases are clearly exceptional, and it is no doubt because most unstable haemoglobins stem from abnormalities in the β chain of haemoglobin (relatively unimportant at birth and in early post-natal life), and also because in many instances the effect of the mutant haemoglobin on the molecules' stability is not too serious, that the infant is usually spared an important degree of increased haemolysis during the first few months of life.

Drugs as a cause of haemolytic crises

The important role of sulphonamide drugs in precipitating haemolytic crises in patients with Hb Zurich has already been referred to (p. 325). With most unstable haemoglobins, however, oxidant drug therapy seems not to have caused haemolytic episodes. There have, however, been exceptions. Thus transient increased haemolysis was recorded following the administration of a sulphonamide to patients with Hb Torino by Beretta *et al.* (1968), Prato *et al.* (1970) and Sansone *et al.* (1976), with Hb Shepherds Bush by White *et al.* (1970), with Hb M Saskatoon by Stavem *et al.* (1972) and with Hb Leiden by Rieder and James (1974). Exacerbation of haemolysis following sulphonamide therapy has also been reported in patients belonging to the two American families with Hb Zurich described by Rieder, Zinkham and Holtzman (1965) and Dickerman, Holtzman and Zinkham (1973). Virshup and co-workers (1983) have more recently reported a severe episode of haemolysis in a Hb-Zurich patient who had been treated with phenoazopyridine (Pyridium), and they were able to show, too, that the erythrocytes of three affected but asymptomatic patients were extremely sensitive to this drug *in vitro*, as judged by methaemoglobin and Heinz-body formation and loss of GSH.

Patients with Hb Köln probably do not suffer from increased haemolysis following the administration of oxidant drugs in therapeutic doses. Thus although Vaughan Jones and co-workers (1967) recorded a haemolytic episode, with haemoglobinuria, 10 days after the onset of a febrile illness for which aspirin, phenacetin and codeine had been given, Miller and co-workers (1971) were unable to demonstrate any adverse effect on the survival of ^{51}Cr-labelled Hb-Köln blood transfused to a normal subject when the recipient was given test doses of sulphisoxazole or primaquine.

Infections as a cause of haemolytic crises

There are many reports of crises of haemolysis following the occurrence of infections, bacterial or viral, that have occurred in the absence of the administration of any potentially haemolytic drug. They have, for example, been recorded with Hb Zürich (Rieder, Zinkham and Holtzman, 1965; Zinkham et al., 1979b), Hb Leiden (de Jong, Went and Bernini, 1968; Perlman et al., 1981), Hb Buenos Aires (de Weinstein et al., 1973), Hb Abraham Lincoln (Honig et al., 1973), Hb Bushwick (Rieder et al., 1975; Ohba et al., 1985d), Hb Perth (Grové et al., 1977) and Hb Shuangfeng (Chihchaun et al., 1981). It is probable that some degree of increased haemolysis is a regular accompaniment of infections, even quite minor ones, as it is in other types of haemolytic anaemia.

The mechanism of the increased haemolysis associated with infections in patients forming unstable haemoglobins has been the subject of some interesting studies. Zinkham and co-workers (1979b) noted that a 16-year-old male patient, heterozygous for Hb Zürich, became more anaemic, and his spleen enlarged, when he experienced an infection which caused his temperature to rise to 40–41°C. (No antipyretics were taken.) Heinz bodies were then found in 18% of his erythrocytes. On recovery, the percentage dropped to zero, the usual finding in this patient. In vitro, it was found that the concentration of GSH decreased and Heinz bodies appeared in erythrocytes when his blood was incubated at 41°C for 3–6 hours. (With normal blood Heinz bodies did

not appear until after 12–24 hours' incubation at this temperature.)

Winterbourn and co-workers (1981) have confirmed and extended the above observations. They experimented with Hbs Christchurch, Volga and Köln and showed with each haemoglobin that raising the temperature from 37°C to 40°C increased significantly the rate of oxidation of haemoglobin and speed of Heinz-body formation both in suspensions of intact erythrocytes and in solutions of haemoglobin. They also found that incubating an unstable haemoglobin (or Hb A) with neutrophils activated by phorbol myristate acetate resulted in accelerated methaemoglobin and Heinz-body formation. They suggested (on the basis of their in-vitro experiments) that a rise in temperature from 37°C to 40°C in vivo would increase Heinz-body formation significantly, and also the rate of haemolysis, and that pyrexia per se was more important than the cause of the pyrexia. The primary oxidation product of neutrophil activation was thought to be superoxide, the presence of which would give rise to H_2O_2. While the unstable haemoglobins were oxidized to methaemoglobin no more rapidly than was Hb A in the presence of the neutrophils, the methaemoglobin derived from the unstable haemoglobin was found to be more unstable than that formed from Hb A and to denature more quickly.

Aplastic crises

A small number of UHbHA patients have experienced aplastic crises that have developed apparently in consequence of an infection. This was so with the children described, respectively, by Schmid, Brecher and Clemens (1959), Sathiapalan and Robinson (1968) and Jackson, Yates and Huehns (1973).

SYMPTOMS

Patients who have an UHbHA complain of the usual symptoms of anaemia: e.g., pallor, exhaustion, palpitations and shortness of breath. They also may complain of jaundice and of abdominal pain from time to time, particularly over an enlarged spleen or in association with pigment gallstones. The passage of abnormally dark urine is, as already mentioned, a rather special symptom which should alert the physician, in a patient with a hereditary haemolytic anaemia, to the possibility that an unstable haemoglobin is the cause. As already stressed, all the patients' symptoms, and signs of increased haemolysis, too, tend to increase in severity in association with infections.

Another possible complaint is of a dusky hue to the skin. This is cyanosis, and it has been noticed particularly in severely affected patients, *e.g.*, in the patient with Hb Hammersmith described by Grimes, Meisler and Dacie (1964); but a dusky icteric tinge to the skin has also been obvious in patients whose haemolysis is less severe, as in the patients described by Raik, Hunter and Lindsay (1967) (Hb Sydney). The cyanosis probably results from an increased content in the blood of methaemoglobin or to increased deoxygenation of the blood in patients whose haemoglobin has a reduced O_2 affinity, or to both mechanisms acting in combination.

Growth and development

Most affected patients have grown and developed normally. Remarkably, too, many severely affected patients, as judged by the level of their haemoglobin — often in the 6–8 g/dl range — have lived almost normal lives. These are patients whose abnormal haemoglobin has a reduced oxygen affinity, with the result that the passage of oxygen to the tissues from the blood at capillary oxygen tensions is facilitated (see p. 361). The original patient with Hb Hammersmith enjoyed dancing, even swimming, without undue fatigue or dyspnoea despite a haemoglobin of 7–8 g/dl (White and Dacie, 1971) (see Fig. 17.17, p. 362).

Pregnancy

Many patients with an UHbHA have become pregnant and have been delivered of a healthy child or a child apparently healthy at birth who has developed the symptoms and signs of a haemolytic anaemia later. Pregnancy does not seem to be associated with any especial hazard to the mother.

Urine

As has been mentioned, abnormally dark urine is commonly passed by patients with an UHbHA, and this was early recognized as an important component of the inclusion-body haemolytic anaemia syndrome. The degree of darkening parallels the severity of the increased haemolysis and in some mildly affected patients, *e.g.*, those with Hb Köln, the urine colour may be normal or at least not different from that of patients with other types of haemolytic anaemia of comparable severity. The abnormal brown to black pigments excreted seem to be dipyrrols which have been referred to as mesobilifuscins. Their origin — anabolic or catabolic — is considered on page 366.

Splenomegaly

Enlargement of the spleen seems to be a constant feature of an UHbHA. The spleen is easily palpated as a rule, *i.e.*, it can be felt usually 2–5 cm below the left costal margin. Some very large spleens have, however, been reported. That of the patient described by Mozziconacci *et al.* (1961) extended to 22 cm below the costal margin of an 11-year-old female, and that of the male patient aged 21 described by Opfell, Lorkin and Lehmann (1968) (Hb Santa Ana) extended to the iliac crest and weighed 1920 g, while that of this patient's daughter aged 10 years weighed 552 g. The 8-year-old patient with Hb Caspar described by Koler *et al.* (1973) had a spleen which weighed 750 g.

Hypersplenism. A small number of patients with an UHbHA and an unusually large spleen have been diagnosed as suffering from hypersplenism. This was so with the patient of Shibata *et al.* (1963) (Hb 'Ube-I') and in the case of the patient, a 17-year-old male, with Hb Köln and thrombocytopenia (67×10^9/l platelets), described by Pedersen *et al.* (1973) the spleen weighed 840 g. The enlarged spleen of the 49-year-old male (who also had Hb Köln) described by Egan and Fairbanks (1973) stretched to below the umbilicus and weighed 1660 g. This patient's platelet count was 55×10^9/l and his leucocyte count 4×10^9/l. Splenectomy was followed by an erythrocytosis accompanied by a rise in haemoglobin to 19.2 g/dl.

The histological findings in the enlarged spleen of UHbHA are discussed on page 354.

Liver

The liver has often been reported as slightly enlarged in severe grades of UHbHA, particularly if the patient is a child. Possible pathological changes are considered on page 355.

Gallstones

Pigment gallstones commonly form in UHbHA: they may be a cause of pain and they may lead, too, to cholecystitis. Cholecystectomy has quite frequently been carried out, usually when the patient has become an adult.

As in other types of haemolytic anaemia, the investigation of a patient admitted to hospital for cholecystectomy has occasionally led to the diagnosis of an UHbHA, e.g., the 43-year-old female patient of Adams et al. (1974) with Hb Rush.

Ulceration of the leg

This has rarely occurred, in contrast to the frequency of ulceration in HS and Hb-SS disease. The patient described by Jackson, Yates and Huehns (1973), when aged 20, injured a leg and subsequently developed an indolent ulcer associated with superficial thrombophlebitis affecting his legs and arms. He had undergone splenectomy as a child.

BLOOD PICTURE

The remarkable appearance of the erythrocytes in stained dried blood films of some of the patients with an UHbHA has been repeatedly remarked on. The early descriptions were based almost entirely on films from severely affected patients who had undergone splenectomy.

Cathie (1952) referred to marked polychromasia and anisocytosis, with 'many bizarre forms'. Lange and Akeroyd (1958) described the post-splenectomy appearances as 'extreme anisocytosis and poikilocytosis, polychromatophilia, basophilic stippling, spherocytosis, target cells, Howell-Jolly bodies and bizarre inclusion bodies'. Dacie (1960, p. 196), in referring to the blood film of the patient later shown to have Hb Hammersmith, stated that 'nearly every cell showed some degree

of punctate basophilia and small contracted crenated cells, in which outlines of Heinz bodies could be easily seen, were conspicuous'. These abnormalities are well illustrated in Figure 17.8. Punctate basophilia is indeed most conspicuous: some of the basophilic granules, staining generally intensely, are Pappenheimer bodies, i.e., siderotic granules; the other granules that are diffusely and more or less evenly spread throughout the cell cytoplasm do not stain for iron and have the appearance of 'classical' punctate basophilia.

Less severely affected patients have correspondingly less abnormal films, both before and after splenectomy. In Figures 17.3 and 17.4 are illustrated films from two members of the mildly affected Hb-Köln family described by Grimes, Meisler and Dacie (1964). The patients had not undergone splenectomy. There is slight anisocytosis, but the most abnormal feature is the presence of moderate numbers of contracted relatively deeply staining cells with irregular outlines. These probably represent cells from which Heinz bodies have been removed during the cells' passage through the spleen, with resultant damage to the cell membrane. Punctate basophilia is not obvious in these photographs but it was a marked feature in the film of one of the patients made on another occasion (Fig. 17.5). Figure 17.9 is a photograph of the film of the one member of this family who had had splenectomy. Although abnormal, the film is nothing like as abnormal as those of the severely affected patients, with Hb Bristol and Hb Hammersmith, respectively, illustrated in Figures 17.1 and 17.8. There is some anisocytosis and considerable post-splenectomy crenation, and large inclusion bodies with pale centres can be seen in many of the cells. Staining with methyl violet showed that the majority of the cells contained Heinz bodies. Figure 17.10 is a photograph of a post-splenectomy blood film of a patient with Hb Nottingham. The changes are of intermediate severity.

Absolute values

MCV. Severely affected patients tend to have a high MCV. That of the patient with Hb Hammersmith averaged 135 fl. In less severely affected patients the recorded values for the MCV have been lower, e.g., mean 108 fl, range

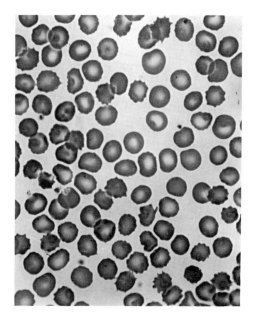

Fig. 17.9 Photomicrograph of a blood film of a patient (A.C.) with Hb Köln. After splenectomy.
Contracted and crenated erythrocytes are quite conspicuous, and Heinz bodies can be seen in many of the cells. Punctate basophilia is not evident in the photograph and the film as a whole is much less abnormal than that of R.H., with Hb Hammersmith, illustrated in Figure 17.8. Romanowsky stain. × 700.

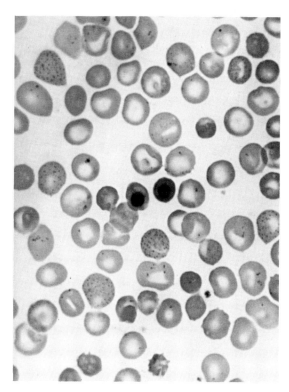

Fig. 17.10 Photomicrograph of a blood film of a patient (S.E.) with Hb Nottingham. After splenectomy.
Some contracted and crenated erythrocytes are present and Heinz bodies can be seen in some of the cells. Punctate basophilia is conspicuous and some macrocytes are present. The changes are intermediate in severity between those shown in Figures 17.8 and 17.9. Romanowsky stain. × 700.

99–109 fl, in four patients with Hb Köln (Dacie *et al.*, 1964). The macrocytosis is a reflection of a young erythrocyte population and also probably is an effect of splenectomy (when this has been carried out).

MCH and MCHC. Both values tend to be subnormal. This is due to loss of some of the abnormal haemoglobin as Heinz bodies and also, in some cases at least, to impaired synthesis of the abnormal haemoglobin. Exceptionally, the result of loss of the abnormal haemoglobin in consequence of its extreme lability has been such as to cause the blood picture to mimic that of severe thalassaemia. This was, for instance, the case in the family forming Hb Indianapolis (Adams *et al.*, 1979). In two affected members the MCV was 72–75 fl and the MCH 22.7–26.2 pg. Lower values still (MCV 71.9 fl and MCH 22.1 pg) were found in the propositus in the family described as forming Hb Suan-Dok (Sanguansermsri *et al.*, 1979) who also had α-thalassaemia (see also p. 433).

Reticulocytes

High reticulocyte counts are the typical finding in cases of UHbHA and, as in other chronic haemolytic anaemias, the highest counts tend to be found in the most anaemic and severely affected patients, particularly if splenectomy has been carried out. In the patient, for instance, with Hb Hammersmith described by Grimes, Meisler and Dacie (1964), the count ranged over a number of years between 22% and 47%, and similar high counts have been recorded in other severely affected patients, *e.g.*, in the patient with Hb Abraham Lincoln described by Honig *et al.* (1973).

It may be difficult to distinguish reticulocytes with very small amounts of reticulo-filamentous material from cells containing other types of small inclusions that stain basophilically, *e.g.*, sidero-cytes. [This can lead to error in both directions — undercounting and overcounting reticulocytes. Heinz bodies, which stain less intensely, should not be a cause of confusion.] Koler and co-workers (1973) made an interesting observation: they found in two splenectomized patients with Hb Caspar that estimation of erythrocyte RNA indicated that the recorded reticulocyte counts, based on New methylene blue staining, were higher than they should be. [Normally, the RNA content and reticulocyte count are closely corre-lated.] They suggested that inclusions were devel-oping and staining as the result of the exposure of the unstable haemoglobin to the New meth-ylene blue and that cells containing these inclu-sions were being scored as reticulocytes (see p. 352).

Heinz bodies

It is a characteristic feature of patients with an UHbHA that Heinz bodies can be readily seen in vitally stained preparations of their blood if splen-ectomy has been carried out. Typically from about 50 to 90%, or even more, of the erythro-cytes can then be seen to contain a single, large, slightly irregularly-shaped inclusion. These stain pale blue with brilliant cresyl blue (Fig. 17.11), slightly darker blue with New methylene blue and violet to black with methyl violet (Fig. 3.33, vol. 1, p. 86). It is equally characteristic that Heinz bodies cannot usually be seen if blood taken before splenectomy is examined in the same way. This is because the developing Heinz bodies are removed from the erythrocytes during their passage through the spleen. Nevertheless, Heinz bodies have been recorded in a large proportion of the erythrocytes of patients (before splen-ectomy) whose unstable haemoglobin is particularly sensitive to the oxidant effect of drugs, for example in patients with Hb Zürich (Frick, Hitzig and Stauffer, 1961) and Hb Torino (Prato *et al.*, 1970) after the administration of sulphonamides in normal therapeutic doses. There are, too, a small number of reports of Heinz-body-containing erythrocytes being noted in patients before splen-ectomy, who had not been taking drugs thought to be potentially harmful (*e.g.*, as reported by

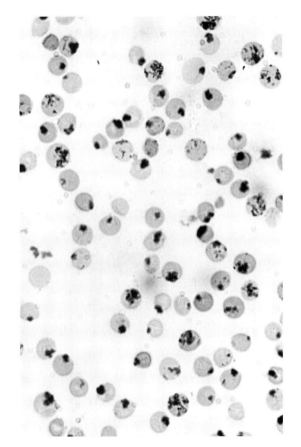

Fig. 17.11 Photomicrograph of the blood of a patient with Hb Hammersmith (R.H.) stained with brilliant creysl blue.
Shows Heinz bodies in almost all the erythrocytes, as well as reticulo-filamentous material in reticulocytes.

Vaughan Jones *et al.*, 1967; Hollán *et al.*, 1970; Nowicki and Martin, 1971, 1972; and Knuth *et al.*, 1979). The significance of these unusual reports is uncertain. Possible causal mechanisms include an unusually unstable haemoglobin, rela-tive hyposplenism, the presence of an infection or that the inclusions observed were not Heinz bodies.

In post-splenectomy blood films of mildly affected patients, stained by Romanowsky dyes, the Heinz bodies can usually be recognized in some of the erythrocytes, at least, as rings of material (globin) staining darkly with the eosin component of the stain (Fig. 17.9).

In severely affected patients with high reticulo-cyte counts and much punctate basophilia Heinz bodies appear as pale lilac-blue staining inclusions in films stained by Romanowsky dyes in the usual way, and it seems that this appearance is due to the staining of basophilic material, derived from the cytoplasm of juvenile cells, which has been adsorbed to the surface of, or incorporated into, the Heinz body (Fig. 17.1 and 17.8). Lange and Akeroyd had as far back as 1958 described the inclusions as staining a light blue-grey in Leishman-Giemsa preparations and had pointed out that a faint ring of tiny granules could be seen around the periphery of some of the inclusions and that the Prussian-blue reaction accentuated the ring.

If blood from patients with an UHbHA, initially free from Heinz bodies, is incubated at 37°C Heinz bodies readily develop if the incubation is prolonged. In the case of the four unsplenectomized patients with Hb Köln described by Dacie et al. (1964) Heinz bodies could be seen in their blood after 48 hours' incubation in significantly greater size and number than in control normal blood in which very small Heinz bodies were possibly visible. Subsequently, this phenomenon has been reported after 24–48 hours' incubation of the blood of patients belonging to other families with Hb Köln (Miller et al., 1971; Lie-Injo et al., 1972) and of the blood of patients with other types of unstable haemoglobin [Raik, Hunter and Lindsay, 1967 (Hb Sydney); Sathiapalan and Robinson, 1968 (Hb Kings County); Hollán et al., 1970 (Hb Santa Ana); Huehns et al., 1970 (Hb Seattle); Hyde et al., 1972 (Hb Southampton); Kennedy et al., 1974 (Hb Belfast), etc.] The simple procedure of incubating for 24–48 hours at 37°C blood from a patient, with a spleen in situ, suspected of having an UHbHA and then examining it for Heinz bodies is in fact a useful way of making a tentative diagnosis.

Leucocytes

As in other types of haemolytic anaemia, very high leucocyte counts have been recorded in association with haemolytic crises. Thus in the original patient with Hb Zürich, a girl 2 years and 9 months of age, the leucocyte count rose to $52 \times 10^9/l$ as the haemoglobin fell precipitously to 3.4 g/dl. The response of the 2-year-old female

child with Hb Nottingham who was admitted to hospital with a gastro-intestinal infection was notable, too, although less dramatic: she had a haemoglobin of 5.0 g/dl, 49% reticulocytes, $5 \times 10^9/l$ erythroblasts and a leucocyte count $18.3 \times 10^9/l$, with a marked shift to the left (Gordon-Smith et al., 1973).

Patients who have had their spleen removed tend to have permanently a moderately high leucocyte count, as in patients with other types of haemolytic anaemia after splenectomy (McBride, Dacie and Shapley, 1968). For example, the patient with Hb Perth reported by Jackson, Yates and Huehns (1973) had a leucocyte count of 11–18 $\times 10^9/l$ over a 12-year period. The haemoglobin ranged between 7 and 14 g/dl (usually 10–12 g) and there were 17–75% reticulocytes.

Platelets

Before splenectomy, the platelet count is usually normal; it is probably seldom if ever raised. Some moderately low counts have, on the other hand, been occasionally reported, e.g., by Hutchison et al., (1964) and Rieder and Bradley (1968). Some but not all of these low counts have been recorded in patients who have had a greatly enlarged spleen, as in the patient described by Opfell, Lorkin and Lehmann (1968).

After splenectomy, the platelet count is usually substantially and permanently raised and may exceed $500 \times 10^9/l$, as in patients who have undergone splenectomy for other types of haemolytic anaemia in whom increased haemolysis, nevertheless, has persisted (Hirsh and Dacie, 1966). Patients with UHbHA whose post-splenectomy platelet count exceeded $500 \times 10^9/l$ include those reported by Svensson and Strand (1967) ('Hb Borås'), Allard et al. (1976) (Hb Bicêtre) and Lie-Injo et al. (1977) (Hb Leiden/β^0-thalassaemia combination).

Post-splenectomy erythrocytosis

Following splenectomy, the erythrocyte count and haemoglobin may occasionally rise to above the normal range, as in the patients (both with Hb Köln, a high O_2-affinity haemoglobin) described by Jackson, Way and Woodliff (1967) and Egan and Fairbanks (1973). The latter suggested that splenectomy had reduced the rate of haemolysis sufficiently for erythrocytosis to develop as compensation for a left-shifted O_2-dissociation curve.

Osmotic fragility

Erythrocyte osmotic fragility has been recorded in most of the reports of UHbHA. A frequent finding has been a small tail of fragile cells and a larger population of unusually resistant cells, i.e. a prolonged span of lysis. Particularly is this so after splenectomy. After incubation of blood for 24 hours at 37°C these changes are often exaggerated. The findings with fresh or incubated blood are, however, in no way diagnostic or suggestive of UHbHA, except in as much as the incubated blood may assume a brownish tinge due to methaemoglobin formation (see below).

Autohaemolysis

Before the true nature of their illness was appreciated, the patients belonging to the P family, later shown to have Hb Koln, had been regarded tentatively as suffering from Type-I hereditary non-spherocytic haemolytic anaemia on the basis of the autohaemolysis test (Dacie, 1960; Cases 6–8, p. 182). Similar results were obtained by Hutchison et al. (1964) and Vaughan Jones et al. (1967) with members of the Glasgow Hb-Koln family. With the blood of more severely affected patients, higher percentages of lysis have been recorded, usually with a substantial reduction of lysis in the presence of added glucose (Scott et al., 1960; Goudemand et al., 1964; Ben-Bassat et al., 1969; Rieder, Oski and Clegg, 1969, etc.)

Exceptionally, more lysis has been observed in the presence of added glucose than in its absence (Miwa et al., 1965; Mills, Levin and Alperin, 1968). As with measurement of osmotic lysis, the autohaemolysis percentages are no help in diagnosis (and not distinguishable from those seen in HS), except in as much as UHbHA blood kept at 37°C for 48 hours is very likely to assume a brownish tinge due to the formation of methaemoglobin.

Methaemoglobinaemia

Small but significantly greater than normal amounts of methaemoglobin (usually <5%) have been found in the fresh blood of many patients with an UHbHA when it has been carefully looked for. Occasionally the amount present has been sufficient to give the skin of the patient a dusky hue, as in the original patient with Hb Hammersmith and in the patients with Hb Freiberg who were producing as much as 10% methaemoglobin (Betke and Kleihauer, 1962; Jones et al. 1966). A level as high as 12.3% was, too, recorded by Kleihauer et al. (1968) in a patient with Hb Bibba and as much as 15% by Thillet et al. (1976) in a patient with Hb Saint Louis.

In contrast, in a minority of patients methaemoglobin levels have been apparently normal (<1%), e.g., in the patients described by Miller et al. (1971) (Hb Koln), Hyde et al. (1972) (Hb Southampton) and Honig et al. (1973) (Hb Abraham Lincoln). Even so, the level generally rises substantially after incubation. Blood from the patient described by Jackson, Yates and Huehns (1973) (Hb Perth) behaved exceptionally, for less than 1% methaemoglobin had formed after 24 hours at 37°C.

As already mentioned, incubation at 37°C of UHbHA blood typically results in the formation of so much methaemoglobin that the blood becomes brownish to the naked eye. In the case of Hb Köln, Hutchison and co-workers (1964) recorded 17.3% methaemoglobin after 18 hours' incubation, Jackson, Way and Woodliff (1967) 11% after 24 hours and Vaughan Jones and co-workers (1967) 12–22% after 48 hours, reduced to 4–12% in the presence of added glucose. With Hb Seattle, Huehns and co-workers (1970) reported a methaemoglobin level of 23% after 24 hours' incubation at 37°C.

The differences in the rates of formation of methaemoglobin between the various unstable haemoglobins no doubt reflect subtle differences between the nature of the abnormal haemoglobins and differences, too, between the erythrocyte reducing power of the individual patient.

Haptoglobin and haemopexin

Extensive data on serum haptoglobin and haemopexin levels in a variety of types of haemolytic anaemia were reported by Zinkham et al. (1979a) as a background to studies on 14 patients belonging to an American family with Hb Zurich. In contrast to HS patients before splenectomy, of whom only one out of 18 had haemopexin levels below the normal range, all but two of the Hb-Zürich patients had subnormal levels; in eight of them haemopexin was absent and in two nearly so. The amount of haptoglobin was normal in two patients and slightly subnormal in one; it was absent in 10 and almost absent in two. The low haemopexin levels were thought to reflect the continuous loss of haem from unstable haemoglobin molecules.

HAEMOGLOBIN ELECTROPHORESIS

One reason why it took so long to recognize that the UHbHAs were haemoglobinopathies was the fact that the abnormal haemoglobin frequently failed to separate from Hb A when haemolysates were submitted to standard methods of electrophoresis. A reason for failure to separate is that, even when the amino-acid substitution results in a charge change, the change might be neutralized by an alteration in the tertiary structure of the haemoglobin molecule. In cases where the electrophoretic pattern has been clearly abnormal, the most frequently reported abnormality has been an additional band running behind Hb A and in front of the position occupied by Hb S if it was present. Two other features (which were initially confusing) that have quite often been reported are weak bands migrating just to the anodal side of Hb A, representing probably haem-depleted unstable haemoglobin, and free α chains forming a band at the cathodal side of the origin.

The first clear descriptions of an electrophoretic abnormality indicating the presence of an abnormal haemoglobin were provided by Scott et al. (1960), who reported that starch-block electrophoresis of their patient's blood revealed an abnormal band, equivalent to about 10% of the total haemoglobin, between Hb A and Hb A₂, and by Hitzig et al. (1960), who, in their description of Hb Zürich, described an abnormal band running between the position of Hb A and Hb S.

Other relatively early reports of abnormal bands include those of Dacie et al. (1964), Goudemand et al. (1964), Pribilla et al. (1965), Sansone and Pik (1965) and Carrell, Lehmann and Hutchison (1966) (Hb Köln), Raik, Hunter and Lindsay (1967) (Hb Sydney) and Opfell, Lorkin and Lehmann (1968) (Hb Santa Ana).

Sheehy (1964) and Huehns and co-workers (1970) (Hb Seattle) described rapidly migrating abnormal components, Bradley and Rieder (1965) and Bradley, Wohl and Rieder (1967) an abnormal band in the region of Hb A₂ or Hb C (Hb Gun Hill), de Jong, Went and Bernini (1968) a band migrating like Hb S (Hb Leiden) and Sansone, Carrell and Lehmann (1967) a normal pattern except for the presence of slowly moving α chains (Hb Genova).

Free α chains

As already mentioned, electrophoretically slow moving weak bands occupying the position expected of free α chains have been observed with a number of β-chain variant unstable haemoglobins. In some instances these bands have been the sole abnormality demonstrable by routine methods of electrophoresis. This was so with Hb Christchurch (Carrell and Owen, 1971), Hb Madrid (Outeirino et al., 1974) and Hb Genova (Kendall et al., 1979).

Haemoglobin A₂

An increased percentage of Hb A₂ has been frequently reported in β-chain variants.

Values greater than 2.5% were reported by Stauffer (1961) (Hb Zürich), Dacie et al. (1964) (Hb Köln), Bratu et al. (1971) (Hb Bucureşti), King et al. (1972) (Hb Peterborough), de Weinstein et al. (1973) (Hb Buenos Aires), Honig et al. (1973) (Hb Abraham Lincoln), Outeirino et al. (1974) (Hb Madrid), Grové et al. (1977) (Hb Perth), Kendall et al. (1979) (Hb Genova) and Perlman et al. (1981) (Hb Leiden).

Haemoglobin F

Small rises in Hb F have been frequently reported in children and adults with UHbHA.

Lange and Akeroyd (1958) reported 2.8–3.4% and Scott et al. (1960) 2.3–3.2%. Less commonly the increases have been substantial. For instance, 12–13% was recorded by Mills, Levin and Alperin (1968) and by Schneider et al. (1969) in a girl aged 12 with Hb Sabine, 12% by Cohen Solal and Labie (1973) in a boy aged 10 with Hb Genova, 12.8% by Outeirino et al. (1974) in a 16-year-old Spanish boy with Hb Madrid, 19% by Godeau et al (1976) in an 8-year-old boy with Hb Saint Etienne and 11.7% by Grové et al. (1977) in a 13-year-old Nama boy with Hb Perth.

The cause of these high Hb-F levels is uncertain. A response to 'haematological stress' was suggested by Godeau *et al.* (1976) in relation to their patient. In a later report this patient was, however, described as a compound heterozygote for Hb Saint Etienne and the Swiss type of hereditary persistence of fetal haemoglobin (HPFH) (Testa *et al.*, 1979). Godeau and co-workers (1976) referred to Hb Istanbul and Hb Saint Etienne as having the same amino-acid substitution ($\alpha_2\beta_2^{92 \ (F8) \ His \ Gln}$) and yet having apparently widely different clinical effects — Hb Instanbul being associated with a severe haemolytic anaemia and Hb Saint Etienne with a much milder disorder. This difference, it was suggested, could be explained by the Hb-F percentage being high (and protective) in the case of Hb Saint Etienne and within the normal range with Hb Istanbul.

HAEMOGLOBIN INSTABILITY

Heat lability

As has already been referred to, the demonstration by Grimes and Meisler (1962) that a haemolysate from a patient with a severe form of congenital haemolytic anaemia contained a heat-labile component was an important milestone in the understanding of the disorder then referred to as congenital Heinz-body anaemia. Grimes and Meisler's test was soon widely employed and found to be reliable, and its use led to the introduction of the descriptive term 'unstable haemoglobin haemolytic anaemia'. The temperature initially selected to test for heat lability was 50°C and in the patient studied, who was later shown to have Hb Hammersmith, a visible precipitate developed within a few minutes. The amount of the precipitate increased steeply over 60 minutes or so and then more slowly, and it reached a maximum of about 30% of the total haemoglobin in 2–3 hours. Grimes and Meisler also tested haemolysates from four patients with relatively mild hereditary non-spherocytic haemolytic anaemia, one of whom had had her spleen removed and many of whose erythrocytes contained Heinz bodies. All these haemolysates contained a heat-labile component, although in small proportion, 4–12% (Grimes, Meisler and Dacie, 1964). [These patients were later shown to be forming Hb Köln.]

Later reports have indicated that the amount of heat-labile haemoglobin that can be demonstrated varies widely from patient to patient. This depends upon the rate at which the abnormal haemoglobin is being synthesized relative to Hb A and the rate at which it undergoes denaturation (see p. 367).

Modifications of Grimes and Meisler's test have been introduced, chiefly with respect to the temperature to which the haemolysates are exposed. Clearly, the higher the temperature the faster will the haemoglobin precipitate. Normal Hb A will, of course, undergo denaturation if the temperature is sufficiently high and the time of exposure sufficiently prolonged (Fig. 17.12). Even so, unstable haemoglobins denature faster than Hb A at any selected temperature. Thus Betke and co-workers (1960) described how Hb H denatured faster than Hb A at 65° and 69°C over a 3-minute period and Bachmann and Marti (1962) reported that Hb Zürich was destroyed 3 times as fast as Hb A at 70°C.

The original temperature selected by Grimes and Meisler (50°C) is, however, one at which the precipitability of the great majority of unstable haemoglobins can be clearly distinguished from that of Hb A. Schneiderman, Junga and Fawley (1970) carried out the test using a 1% solution of haemoglobin in various buffers and found that precipitation occurred earlier in tris and barbital buffers than in sodium phosphate buffer.

The colour of the precipitate varies from red-brown as in Hb Hammersmith (globin with most of its haems still attached) to almost white (globin with most of its haems detached) as in Hb Santa Ana (Opfell, Lorkin and Lehmann, 1968). Bratu and co-workers (1971) reported in studies on Hb Bucuresti the interesting observation that the precipitate developing at 50°C, which was red at 1 hour and contained only a little free globin, contained a higher proportion of free globin after 2 hours.

Ueda and co-workers (1970) recommended carrying out heat lability tests in glass capillary tubes. Precipitation exceeding 4% after 1 hour at 50°C was taken as indicating an unstable haemoglobin.

Some selected and interesting findings, illustrative of the heat sensitivity of individual abnormal haemoglobins at various temperatures, are summarized below.

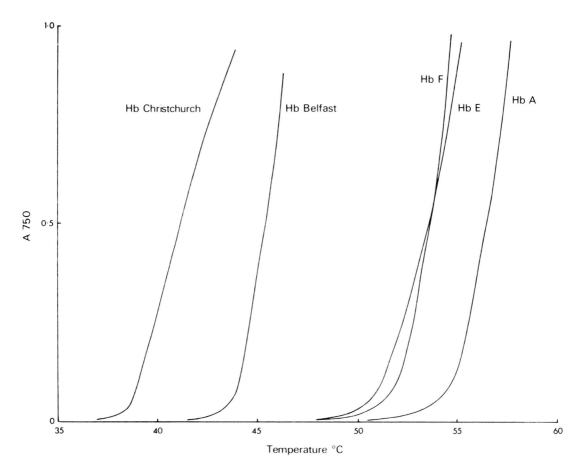

Fig. 17.12 Illustrates the contrasting heat sensitivity of two unstable haemoglobins, Hb Christchurch and Hb Belfast, compared to that of Hb A, Hb F and Hb E.
(Reproduced by courtesy of Professor R. W. Carrell.)

Hb Sinai. Not precipitated at 55°C but precipitated more rapidly than Hb AS and Hb AC at 60° and 65°C; 16–19% precipitated (Charache and Mondzac, 1967).

Hb Sogn. Slight precipitation at 58°C after 5 minutes (nil with Hb A); 17% precipitated at 58°C after 15 minutes (8% with Hb A) (Monn, Gaffney and Lehmann, 1968).

Hb Philly. 26–30% precipitated at 50°C, but 12–24 hours were required for full precipitation (Rieder, Oski and Clegg, 1969).

Hb Seattle. 50% precipitated at 72°C for 2 minutes. Hb A did not precipitate in this time until the temperature was raised to 80°C (Huehns et al., 1970).

Hb Savannah. 30% precipitated at 65°C for 8–10 minutes (Huisman et al., 1971).

Hb Tochigi. 20–24% precipitated at 50°C in three members of the family (Yamada et al., 1971).

Hb Köln. 20% precipitated at 65°C within 10 minutes

(3% Hb A precipitated in this time) (Pedersen et al., 1973).

Hb Toyoake. Precipitated at 50°C, but precipitation incomplete at 4 hours; at 60°C, 28.5% precipitated rapidly (Hirano et al., 1981).

The following two contrasting reports are of unusual interest:

Hb Leslie. As much as 96% of the haemoglobin precipitated at 62°C after 20 minutes. The propositus was a compound heterozygote for Hb Leslie and β^0-thalassaemia and was not forming any Hb A (Lutcher et al., 1976)!

Hb Indianapolis. No unstable haemoglobin could be demonstrated by simple tests. It seemed that the β-chain variant that was being produced was extremely labile, so much so that it could not be detected in the peripheral blood! The patient's blood picture resembled severe thalassaemia (Adams et al., 1979).

Precipitation by isopropanol

In 1972 Carrell and Kay described how adding haemolysates to buffered isopropanol at 38°C could be used to detect unstable haemoglobins. Haemolysates from 200 normal blood samples yielded no precipitate within 30 minutes; in contrast, haemolysates from six patients with UHbHA developed precipitates within 5 minutes which became flocculent by 20 minutes, the amount of precipitate varying between 13% (Hb Köln) and 21% (Hbs Sydney and Niteroi). Brosious, Morrison and Schmidt (1976) considered the possibility of false positive results in the isopropanol test arising from storage and high levels of Hb F; they recommended keeping the blood at 4°C, if it had to be stored, and adding 2% KCN to convert methaemoglobin to the cyan derivative as an additional precaution.

Johnson and co-workers (1980) stated that, although a heat precipitation test was clearly positive with a haemolysate containing Hb Pasadena, no precipitate formed in the presence of isopropanol. The patient, a 27-year-old male, had had clinically obvious haemolytic anaemia as a child, but when studied the Hb was 16.1 g/dl. There were, however, 10% reticulocytes.

The amounts of precipitate produced by the heating and isopropanol methods, and the relative sensitivity of both methods, are probably usually very similar, although there seems to be little comparative quantitative data. Most reports have simply indicated that both tests were positive. Knuth and co-workers (1979), however, reported that 12% of Hb Moabit was precipitated by isopropanol while 21% was precipitated by heating.

Haemoglobins precipitated by heating or isopropanol seem generally to be mechanically unstable as well, e.g. Hb Köln (Asakura et al., 1975). Vella (1975) reported, however, one exception: this was Hb Riverdale Bronx, which was found to be unstable on heating and in the isopropanol test but not abnormally unstable on shaking.

Precipitation by zinc acetate

Carrell and Lehmann (1981a,b) reported that solutions of zinc acetate buffered to a pH 7.0, will precipitate unstable haemoglobins from haemolysates at 37°C, and at 50°C, within 30 minutes, while not, in similar concentrations, precipitating Hb A. The result was negative, too, with blood containing up to 20% F or 3% methaemoglobin.

Precipitation by brilliant cresyl blue (BCB)

Heinz bodies rapidly stain pale blue if exposed to BCB at the concentrations used to stain reticulocytes in blood suspensions. If incubation is prolonged, multiple pale-blue-staining inclusions will develop in erythrocytes originally free from Heinz bodies, as in blood from UHbHA patients prior to splenectomy, i.e., the unstable haemoglobin is denatured in time by the dye and precipitates.

Precipitation by BCB was recorded by Bradley and Rieder (1965) with Hb Gun Hill and by Rieder, Zinkham and Holtzman (1965) with Hb Zürich. Rieder and Bradley (1968) gave some details as to how long it took for the inclusions to develop. With the blood of their Hb-Gun-Hill patient (who had not undergone splenectomy), no inclusions could at first be seen, but at 1 hour they were just discernible and they could be easily seen at 3 hours. (With normal erythrocytes none could be seen even after 24 hours' incubation.) Precipitation and staining was also obtained with New methylene blue (a redox dye) but not with methyl violet (not a redox dye, but capable of staining preformed Heinz bodies deeply). Rieder, Oski and Clegg (1969) reported similar results with Hb Philly, i.e., inclusions were visible after 1 hour and prominent in 2 hours. More recent reports of precipitates developing after BCB incubation include those of King et al. (1972) (Hb Peterborough), Kennedy et al. (1974) (Hb Belfast), Outeirino et al. (1974) (Hb Madrid) and Perlman et al. (1981) (Hb Leiden). Incubation of suspensions of patients' erythrocytes in BCB solution, if prolonged for 2 or more hours, would seem to provide a useful screening test for an UHbHA, as does the incubation of whole blood for longer periods of time (24–48 hours) without the addition of a redox dye.

ERYTHROCYTE LIFE-SPAN

Many of the case reports of UHbHA include data on erythrocyte life-span, almost all obtained with the use of ^{51}Cr. The possible unreliability of such data was considered by White and Dacie (1971) who pointed out that in a series of patients the ^{51}Cr T$_{50}$ figures were poorly correlated with haemoglobin levels. Amongst possible reasons for this were abnormal binding of ^{51}Cr by unstable haemoglobins and unusual susceptibility of unstable haemoglobins to damage by chromium. Experiments with Hb Köln, Hb Hammersmith and Hb Shepherds Bush had demonstrated in each case more binding of ^{51}Cr to the unstable haemoglobin than to Hb A. Hb Köln, for instance, bound 2–3 times more chromium and this was almost entirely bound to the abnormal β chain. Whether this increased binding affected the rate of elution of ^{51}Cr was uncertain. However, it was pointed out that loss of erythrocyte radioactivity would inevitably reflect loss of unstable β chains (as Heinz bodies) in patients before splenectomy, as well as loss of whole erythrocytes, and that this would result in falsely low ^{51}Cr values.

Pedersen and co-workers (1973) reported some interesting data. In a male aged 17 with Hb Köln the ^{51}Cr T_{50} was 7.3 days, while the mean erythrocyte life-span deduced from DF^{32}P data was 30.6 days. The ^{51}Cr elution rate, calculated from the difference between the loss of circulating radioactivity due to ^{51}Cr and that due to ^{32}P, was 5.6% per day before splenectomy and 1.9% after splenectomy, a difference presumably the result of the continuous loss of ^{51}Cr bound to Heinz bodies which were being removed from circulation by the spleen when *in situ*. In a similar study, Bentley, Lewis and White (1974) found, however, in two patients with Hb Köln that the mean erythrocyte life-span, calculated from ^{51}Cr and DF^{32}P data, was almost the same: DF^{32}P 21.3 days, ^{51}Cr 26.1 days in a patient before splenectomy; DF^{32}P 34.8 days, ^{51}Cr 32.4 days in another patient after splenectomy. In a patient with Hb Hammersmith the findings were similar: mean erythrocyte life-span, DF^{32}P 5.8 days, ^{51}Cr 6.6 days. The unexpected close similarity between the DF^{32}P and ^{51}Cr data of Bentley, Lewis and White (1974) in the patient (before splenectomy) could be due to loss of ^{51}Cr bound to Heinz bodies being paralleled by loss of DF^{32}P attached to cell membrane (lost in the spleen during the process of Heinz-body extraction).

Some of the more interesting earlier published data on erythrocyte life-span in cases of UHbHA are summarized below. (It may be assumed that mean life-spans calculated from ^{51}Cr T_{50} figures obtained on patients with their spleen *in situ* are underestimates.)

Schmid, Brecher and Clemens (1959) reported that the ^{51}Cr T_{50} of their propositus was 4 days and that of

his son 6 days. Erythrocytes from 1000 ml of the blood of the propositus (who had been splenectomized) were transfused to a normal recipient. A febrile episode with chills, malaise and splenic tenderness resulted that was most severe 2–5 days after the transfusion. For the first 3 days the recipient's urine was brown in colour. The transfused erythrocytes disappeared from his circulation at the same rate as in the patient (T_{50} approximately 5 days) but all the transfused inclusions (Heinz bodies) had disappeared within 3 days and siderotic granules within 5 days, *i.e.* they had a shorter survival (no doubt due to splenic removal) than had the erythrocytes themselves.

Scott and co-workers (1960), whose patient had also been splenectomized, reported a ^{51}Cr T_{50} of 8 days. However, a sample of his blood transfused to a normal recipient, with spleen *in situ*, survived much less well, the T_{50} being 2 days. Studies similar to the above were carried out by Frick, Hitzig and Betke (1962) in a patient with Hb Zürich (their Case 2, in clinical remission, 5 and 12 months, respectively, after a drug-induced haemolytic episode): the ^{51}Cr T_{50} was 13 days and 11 days on the two occasions. Each time, too, a sample of the patient's erythrocytes was transfused to two normal recipients: the ^{51}Cr T_{50s} were slightly less, 9 days and 12 days, without, apparently, significant uptake of radioactivity by the spleen. Normal recipients, transfused with samples of the patient's (Hb Zürich) erythrocytes, were also given test doses of a variety of drugs: all sulphonamides tested as well as primaquine induced prompt haemolysis.

Sheehy (1964) also showed that his patient's erythrocytes survived less well in a normal recipient with a spleen *in situ* (^{51}Cr T_{50} 4 days) than in the patient himself (^{51}Cr T_{50} 11 days).

Goudemand and co-workers (1964) similarly transfused patient's blood into a normal recipient: 500 ml of blood (taken from the patient after splenectomy) were transfused; inclusions were not demonstrated in the recipient's blood subsequently, but dark urine was passed for the next 48 hours. [The same experiment carried out with the patient's blood taken before splenectomy did not produce any 'pigmenturia'.]

André, Dreyfus and le Bolloc'h-Combrisson (1964) obtained evidence for a double population of erythrocytes in a patient studied after splenectomy, the ^{51}Cr T_{50s} being 3–5 days and 24 days, respectively.

Honig and co-workers (1973) used both ^{51}Cr and [^{14}C]leucine to study erythrocyte life-span in a severely affected 26-year-old female with Hb Abraham Lincoln. The ^{51}Cr T_{50} was 2.4 days and the T_{50} of leucine-labelled reticulocytes 7.2 days. In contrast, Charache and co-workers (1973) used DF^{32}P in an individual with Hb Okaloosa. She was asymptomatic and gave no history of anaemia or jaundice, and her spleen could not be palpated. The mean erythrocyte life-span was calculated to be 47.8 days (that of a normal control was 79.5 days).

In summary, the survival studies described above, and others in literature not referred to, indicate that erythrocyte life-span is variably but sometimes very severely shortened in UHbHA. It seems likely, however, that T_{50} values obtained with ^{51}Cr are falsely low in patients with a spleen *in situ*. Erythrocytes taken from splenectomized patients and transfused to normal recipients have been shown to be rapidly eliminated, a finding which illustrates the importance of the spleen as a haemolytic organ in UHbHA (see also p. 371). Heinz bodies present in transfused erythrocytes are removed even faster than the erythrocytes themselves in recipients with a functioning spleen.

ERYTHROKINETICS

Few studies seem to have been undertaken. Where, however, globin-chain synthesis is impaired some evidence of ineffective erythropoiesis is to be expected. Adams and co-workers (1979) reported some pertinent findings in a patient with Hb Indianapolis in whom synthesis of the abnormal globin chain was impaired to a degree similar to that seen in severe β-thalassaemia. Thus the plasma iron turnover was several times the normal, erythrocyte iron turnover was approximately twice normal and the percentage of iron utilized at 14 days was less than half normal.

PATHOLOGY

Spleen

As already referred to, the spleen is usually easily palpable in patients with UHbHA. On excision, the organ has often been found to be surprisingly large. For instance, Egan and Fairbanks (1973) recorded that the spleen of a 63-year-old male (with Hb Köln) weighed 1660 g, Goudemand and co-workers (1964) that the spleen of a 30-year-old male weighed 800 g and Miwa *et al.* (1965) that the spleen of a girl aged 11 years weighed 600 g. Opfell, Lorkin and Lehmann (1968) reported that the spleen of a 22-year-old male with Hb Santa Ana weighed 1920 g, Ben-Bassat and co-workers (1969) that the spleen of an 11-year-old male weighed 650 g and Huisman *et al.* (1971) that the

spleen of a 19-month-old infant with Hb Savannah weighed 175 g.

When cut into the spleen has usually been described as dark red in colour. Microscopically, the Malpighian bodies have been reported as normal in size and structure but widely separated by an expanded pulp engorged with blood, in which there is a variable degree of reticulo-endothelial cell hyperplasia. The amount of iron demonstrable by Perls's reaction has been variable too, no doubt depending upon the extent to which the patient has been transfused prior to splenectomy. A striking feature, described and illustrated by Dacie *et al.* (1964) in the spleen of one of their Hb-Köln patients — and one which may be characteristic of a Heinz-body anaemia — is the presence of iron-negative granules, 1–2 μm in size, in the cytoplasm of the littoral cells of the sinuses (Fig. 17.13). The granules stain blue-black with Giemsa's stain and in unstained sections they are golden-brown in colour. They appear to be Heinz bodies removed from erythrocytes at the time of their passage into the splenic sinuses via the gaps which exist between the littoral cells. Granules conforming to the

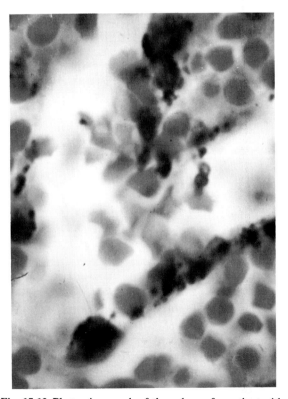

Fig. 17.13 Photomicrograph of the spleen of a patient with Hb Köln (A.C.), showing many dark-staining Heinz bodies within the littoral cells of the splenic sinuses
Giemsa stain. × 1200. [From Dacie *et al.* (1964).]

above description were recorded, too, in spleens from cases of UHbHA by Goudemand *et al.* (1964) and Miwa *et al.* (1965).

Liver

Schmid, Brecher and Clemens (1959) reported that examination of necropsy material showed a large amount of granular pigment within Kupffer cells which gave a negative Prussian-blue reaction. Gregoratos, Vennes and Moser (1964) also recorded post-mortem findings. Their patient was the one originally described by Lange and Akeroyd in 1958. She had died aged 18 following a blood transfusion. There was minimal portal fibrosis, acute centrolobular cell necrosis, and iron pigment, bile pigment and a third unidentified pigment within hepatocytes, principally in the centrolobular area.

Granules that failed to stain positively for iron were reported in liver-biopsy sections in hepatocytes by Goudemand *et al.* (1964) and by Miwa *et al.* (1965) in Kupffer cells, and were considered by these authors to be similar to the granules (presumably Heinz bodies) seen by them in sections of the spleen.

Bone marrow

The bone marrow is typically hyperplastic, with increased erythropoiesis commensurate with the increase in reticulocyte count. Erythroblastopenia resulting in an aplastic crisis is a rare event and marked megaloblastic change does not seem to have been noted.

Frisch and co-workers (1974) reported on an ultrastructural study carried out on marrow-biopsy material from two UHbHA patients, one with Hb Hammersmith, the other with Hb Nottingham. Multiple abnormalities indicative of dyserythropoiesis were noted, particularly in the case of Hb Nottingham. These included bi- and multi-nucleated erythroblasts, cytoplasmic bridges, microtubules, abnormalities of the nuclear envelope, widened nuclear pores, alteration in the density of chromatin, abundant iron-laden mitochondria and a variety of nuclear and cytoplasmic inclusions, including structures thought to be Heinz bodies, and membraneous material presumed to be endoplasmic reticulum. None of the findings was considered to be specific for, or diagnostic of, UHbHA.

MOLECULAR PATHOLOGY OF THE UNSTABLE HAEMOGLOBIN HAEMOLYTIC ANAEMIAS

As already indicated, Hb Zürich was the first unstable haemoglobin to be identified in terms of its molecular abnormality. This was accomplished by Muller and Kingma in 1961, who, working with a blood sample obtained from Drs Marti and Hitzig, identified the molecular abnormality as the substitution of arginine for histidine, the 63rd amino acid in the β-globin chain.

The next series of advances stemmed from the Medical Research Council Abnormal Haemoglobin Unit, Biochemistry Department, University of Cambridge (Director, Professor H. Lehmann) where the amino-acid substitutions of no less than four unstable haemoglobins associated with cases of chronic (not drug-precipitated) UHbHA were identified and published in 1966 and 1967 [Carrell, Lehmann and Hutchison, 1966 (Hb Köln); Sansone, Carrell and Lehmann, 1967 (Hb Genova); Carrell *et al.*, 1967 (Hb Sydney); Dacie *et al.*, 1967 (Hb Hammersmith)]. All these substitutions, and that of Hb Zürich, involved the β-globin chain. In 1967, too, was published the first account of an actual deletion, not a substitution, of amino acids, five in the β chain being deleted in Hb Gun Hill (Bradley, Wohl and Rieder). In 1968 appeared the first account of an α-chain deletion, Hb Bibba (Kleihauer *et al.*).

These early pioneer reports have been followed by an astonishingly large number of descriptions of additional substitutions of amino acids affecting the α or β chain, but particularly the β chain, as well as further examples of amino-acid deletions, all of which have been shown to have led to the formation of unstable haemoglobins. In addition, there have been reports of a small number of cases in which an amino acid has been replaced not by another amino acid but by the imino acid proline.

The names of many of the variant haemoglobins, the chain involved, the substitution or deletion, and a summary of the associated clinical manifestations and key references, are listed in Tables 17.1–17.3. At the time of writing 'new'

unstable haemoglobins continue to be described. The International Hemoglobin Information Center listed in its 1986 alphabetical variant list the names of 124 haemoglobins labelled as slightly unstable, unstable or, in the case of Hb Indianapolis, very unstable. Niazi and Shibata (1984b), in Part IV of their review, had listed 17 unstable variants that were the cause of uncompensated

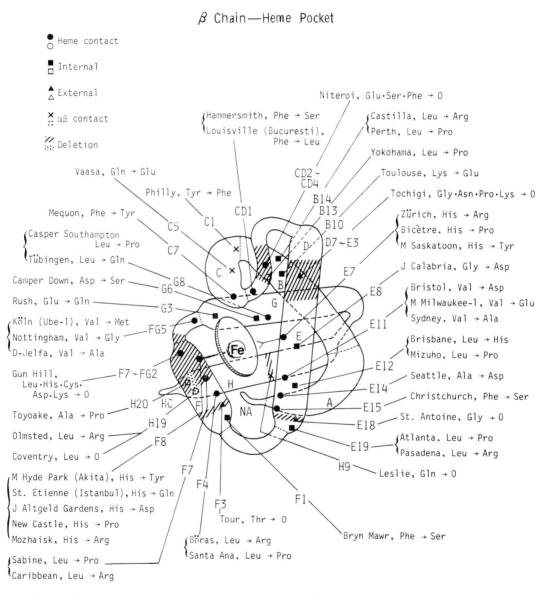

Fig. 17.14 Diagram illustrating the location within the β-globin chain of amino-acid substitutions or deletions giving rise to unstable haemoglobins. Substitutions in the vicinity of the haem pocket.
[Reproduced by permission from Niazi and Shibata (1983a).]

severe haemolytic anaemia, 17 variants that caused moderate haemolytic anaemia which could become compensated for after splenectomy, 36 variants that led to mild haemolytic anaemia except during a crisis (which in certain cases might follow an infection or the taking of a drug) and 33 variants in which the haemoglobin molecule could be shown to be mildly or moderately unstable but in which its instability did not appear to be associated with any clinical manifestations.

Figure 17.14–17.16, reproduced (by permission) from Niazi and Shibata's (1983a,b, 1984a,b) review, illustrate the very large number of variants known (up to 1984) and the distribution of the variants within the β- and α-globin chains.

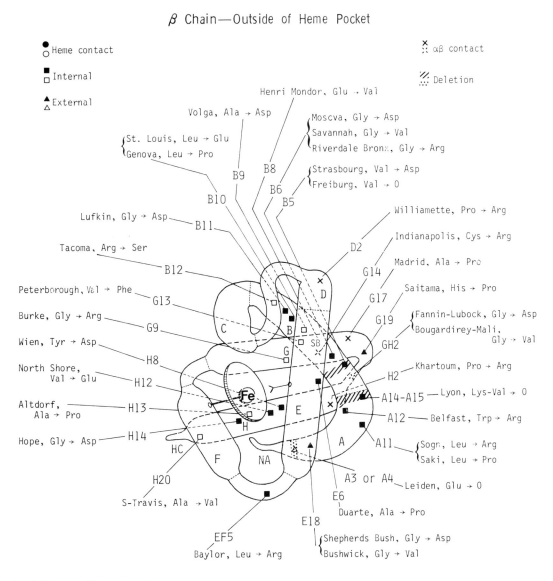

Fig. 17.15 Diagram illustrating the location within the β-globin chain of amino-acid substitutions or deletions giving rise to unstable haemoglobins. Substitutions not in the vicinity of the haem pocket.

[Reproduced by permission from Niazi and Shibata (1983a).]

α Chain

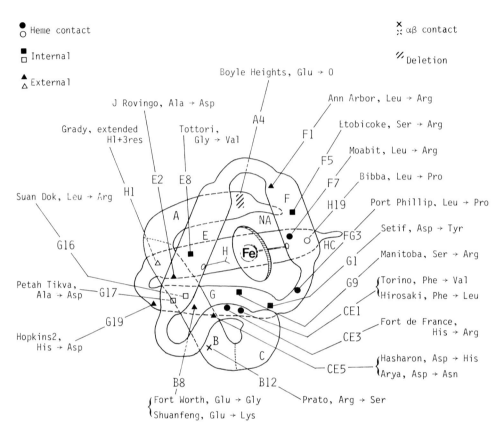

Fig. 17.16 Diagram illustrating the location within the α-globin chain of amino-acid substitutions or deletions giving rise to unstable haemoglobins.
[Reproduced by permission from Niazi and Shibata (1983a).]

MECHANISM OF HAEMOGLOBIN INSTABILITY

All the abnormal haemoglobins considered in this Chapter have one feature in common — an instability of the molecule that is greater than that of normal Hb A. It is an interesting fact that the discovery of the unstable human haemoglobins in the early 1960s coincided in time with a great surge of interest in, and the undertaking of much basic research into, the molecular structure of the haemoglobin molecule. The realization that a variety of clinical syndromes, especially haemolytic anaemias and cyanosis due to methaemoglobinaemia, could be brought about by the presence of a variant haemoglobin, and that the molecule's stability and respiratory function might be jeopardized by the replacement of a single amino acid by another, as the result of a mutation, provided a great stimulus to this work.

In 1968 Perutz and Lehmann, in their classic paper on the molecular pathology of human haemoglobin, concluded that the haemoglobin molecule is in fact 'insensitive to replacements of most of the amino-acid residues on its surface, but extremely sensitive to even quite small alterations of internal non-polar contacts, especially those near the haems', and that 'replacements at the contacts between α and β subunits affect respiratory function'. In support of these conclusions they tabulated the unstable haemoglobins that had been described up to the time they wrote their paper and analysed the effect of the amino-acid replacement on the molecule's structure and function, and, in a further table, they listed the larger number of mutants involving external replacements, then known to them, that had no clinical effect in the heterozygous state.

A detailed consideration of the way in which the stability of the normal haemoglobin tetramer is thought to be maintained is beyond the scope of this book. The following, however, is a brief summary.

The globin molecules are highly ordered structures and native globin is soluble because the amino-acid side chains that are hydrophilic are arranged externally and can interact with water. The side chains that are hydrophobic are arranged internally and form bonding van der Waals forces with each other and exclude water from the interior of the molecule. These interactions are one of the forces that help to maintain the stability of the molecule. Another important stabilizing force is interaction between the haem molecule and its globin chain by means of hydrophobic bonds with certain internal side chains. A further stabilizing force is provided by the interaction between the four subunits of the molecule, particularly the $\alpha\beta$ dimer contacts. As is illustrated below, the molecule's stability may be seriously affected by interference with any of the forces that normally stabilize it. The 'experiments of nature' that lead to haemoglobin instability and to the UHbHAs show how this can be brought about by the replacement by a new mutant amino acid of an amino acid that normally plays a key role in the stabilizing process by virtue of its position in the molecule, or by the deletion of an amino acid or a series of amino acids.

It is possible to classify the unstable haemoglobins into categories according to the position and function in the molecule of the amino acid that is substituted or deleted (see White and Dacie, 1971):

1. Substitutions of a haem-contact amino acid resulting in a molecule with a tendency to lose haem from the abnormal haemoglobin chain.

2. Substitutions of a non-polar amino acid in the interior of the molecule by a polar (charged) amino acid, a haem-contact amino acid not being involved.

3. Substitutions of an amino acid that forms critical hydrophobic stabilizing contacts with amino acids of another helix of the same chain or of another chain.

4. Deletions of an amino acid or sequence of amino acids resulting in an interruption to the continuity of a helical segment and a weakening of the internal arrangement of the non-polar amino acids.

Representative examples of well-known haemoglobins of each category are listed below. (References to descriptions of the haemoglobins referred to are given in Tables 17.1–17.3.)

Haem-contact amino-acid substitutions: β chain

Hb Bristol. Aspartic acid, a polar amino acid, is substituted for valine $\beta67$ (E11); the short side chain of aspartic acid is placed internally and is neutralized, probably by histidine $\beta63$, resulting in a severe alteration of the E helix. This results in marked instability.

Hb Hammersmith. Serine is substituted for phenylalanine $\beta42$ (CD1). The side chain of serine is too short to make contact with haem, leaving a gap at the surface of the haem pocket; its polar OH group allows a water molecule to enter the pocket. This results in marked instability.

Hb Köln. Methionine is substituted for valine $\beta98$ (FG5). Methionine is a larger molecule and its insertion into the FG segment, a tight corner, results in severe distortion of the segment and weakening of haem binding. A moderate degree of instability results.

Hb Santa Ana. The imino acid proline is substituted for leucine $\beta88$ (F4). Proline is unable to make the haem contacts normally made by leucine, leaving a space in the haem pocket into which water can enter. Moderately severe instability is the result.

Hb Sydney. Alanine is substituted for valine $\beta67$ (E11). Alanine is too short to make a haem contact and loosens the haem group. The effect on the molecule's stability is, however, slight.

Hb Zürich. Arginine is substituted for histidine $\beta63$ (E7). The side chain of arginine, a polar amino acid, cannot be accommodated in the haem pocket site; it protrudes on the surface and leaves a cavity at the ligand side of the iron atom. The resultant instability is, however, slight, except in the presence of oxidant drugs.

Haem-contact amino-acid substitutions: α chain

Hb Bibba. The amino acid proline is substituted for leucine $\alpha136$ (H19). The presence of proline breaks a haem contact and leads to unfolding of amino acids $\alpha136$–138 of the H helix. Severe instability results.

Hb Torino. Valine is substituted for phenylalanine α43 (CD1). As compared with Hb Hammersmith, the substitution of valine for phenylalanine is less serious. Valine is non-polar and does not introduce water into the haem pocket. However, a haem contact is removed and the CD segment is distorted.

Substitutions of a non-polar amino acid in the interior of the molecule by a polar amino acid not involved in a haem contact

Hb Riverdale-Bronx. Arginine is substituted for glycine β24 (B6), an internal non-polar amino acid. The guanidinium group of arginine is probably on the surface; its presence may distort that part of the E helix which forms part of the haem pocket. This results in moderately severe instability.

Hb Seattle. Aspartic acid is substituted for alanine β70 (E14) an external amino acid. Glutamic acid probably interacts with histidine β77 (EF1) and distorts the E helix. A moderate degree of instability is the result.

Hb Shepherds Bush. Aspartic acid is substituted for glycine β74 (E18), an internal non-polar amino acid. The aspartic acid side chain is probably at the surface and bonded to histidine β77 (EF1). The resultant distortion weakens part of the haem pocket. Moderately severe instability results.

Hb Sogn. Arginine is substituted for leucine β14 (A11), which normally makes contact with several amino acids that help to stabilize the A and H helices and the GH segment. The side chain of arginine, on the molecule's surface, would break these contacts. This, however, causes little instability.

Substitutions of amino acids that form critical hydrophobic stabilizing contacts

Hb Philly. Phenylalanine is substituted for tyrosine β35 (C1). Phenylalanine removes the hydrogen bond between tyrosine β35 (C1) and aspartic acid α126 (H9), weakening the $\alpha_1\beta_1$ contact. Hb Philly readily dissociates into subunits. Moderate instability results.

Deletions of an amino acid or a sequence of amino acids

Hb Freiburg. Valine β23 (B5) is deleted. Its absence results in glutamine β22 (B4) being drawn below the surface and the AB segment being distorted. The effect on the molecule's stability is, however, slight.

Hb Gun Hill. Five amino acids β91–95 (F7–FG2) are deleted, so that a large part of the FG segment is missing. The result is loss of some haem contacts and part of the $\alpha_1\beta_1$ contact as well. Despite this major lesion there is but slight instability.

Hb Leiden. Glutamine β6 or β7 (A3 or A4) is deleted, with disruption of the A helix. The molecule is but slightly unstable.

It is fascinating to compare the result on the haemoglobin molecule's stability, and the clinical effects on the patient, of a single amino acid being replaced by one or other of several different substituents. A striking example is valine β67 (E11) which may be replaced by alanine, glutamic acid or aspartic acid resulting, respectively, in Hb Sydney, associated with a mild UHbHA, Hb M-Milwaukee, associated with a type of hereditary methaemoglobinaemia, and Hb Bristol, giving rise to a

Table 17.5 Effect of the substitution of valine [β67 (E11)] by one of three amino acids.

Amino acid in β67 position	Chemical formula	Role in molecule and effect of substitution	Clinical presentation
Valine (non-polar)	H_2N CH_3 / CH–CH / HOOC CH_3	Makes a normal contact through CH_3 groups	Hb A: normal
Alanine (non-polar)	H_2N / CH–CH_3 / HOOC	Fails to make haem contact; side chain too short	Hb Sydney: mild haemolytic anaemia
Glutamic acid (polar)	H_2N / CH–CH_2–CH_2–COOH / HOOC	Reaches Fe^{2+} of haem and oxidizes it to Fe^{3+}; side chain charged and long	Hb M Milwaukee: methaemoglobinaemia
Aspartic acid (polar)	H_2N / CH–CH_2–COOH / HOOC	E helix grossly distorted; side chain charged but too short to reach surface; neutralized internally	Hb Bristol: severe haemolytic anaemia

Adapted from White and Dacie (1971).

very severe haemolytic anaemia (see Steadman, Yates and Huehns, 1970). The way in which these differences in clinical expression can be explained by the difference in the length and charge of a side chain of the substituted amino acid is illustrated in Table 17.5.

Elongation of a globin chain

In at least one instance haemoglobin instability has resulted from the elongation of the β chain. In the case of Hb Cranston the abnormal β chain is composed of 157 amino acids with iso-leucine as residue 146 (Bunn et al., 1975a,b). A woman and her son each had a compensated haemolytic anaemia. Hb Cranston comprised about 25% of the total haemoglobin; its O_2 affinity was markedly increased.

A γ-chain substitution

Lee-Potter and co-workers (1975) described as a new cause for haemolytic anaemia in the newborn the occurrence of an unstable variant of Hb F, referred to by them as Hb Poole. Glycine was shown to be substituted for tryptophan at position 130.

The affected infant, one of two dissimilar twins delivered at 36 weeks, became jaundiced between the 3rd–7th days and the urine was noticed to be dark on the 11th day. The haemoglobin was then 13.1 g/dl and a few contracted erythrocytes were seen in blood films. The infant could not be followed up beyond 10 weeks. It was then clinically well, with haemoglobin 12.4 g/dl and 1.4% reticulocytes. The heat and propanol precipitation tests were positive, as well as the ascorbate-cyanide and acetylphenylhydrazine tests. This report is believed to be the first description of an unstable γ-chain variant. The severity of increased haemolysis, if any, is uncertain.

OXYGEN AFFINITY OF UNSTABLE HAEMOGLOBINS

One of the consequences of an amino-acid substitution or deletion leading to haemoglobin instability is that the interaction of the altered molecule with oxygen may be affected, either by an increase or a reduction in O_2 affinity or by an alteration in haem-haem interactions. Such alterations may powerfully affect a patient's response to his disorder. A reduced O_2 affinity allows him or her to tolerate low haemoglobin levels, often without symptoms of anaemia, because of the unusual ease in which oxyhaemoglobin gives up oxygen at capillary O_2 tensions. In contrast, a higher than normal affinity diminishes the transfer of oxygen from oxyhaemoglobin to tissues and leads to the occurrence of symptoms at relatively high haemoglobin levels and may reduce seriously the capacity of the patient to respond to an increased oxygen demand as, for instance, that which results from exercise, despite increased compensatory erythropoiesis brought about by the erythropoietin mechanism. The result of having an unstable haemoglobin with a high oxygen affinity (e.g. Hb Köln) is that the patient has a relatively high haemoglobin level and perhaps may be not anaemic at all despite a considerably increased rate of haemolysis; while a patient with a similar degree of increased haemolysis but having an unstable haemoglobin with a low oxygen affinity (e.g. Hb Hammersmith) is usually moderately severely anaemic but relatively free from symptoms.

The early work on the clinical affect of alterations in the O_2 affinity of haemoglobin has already been summarized (Vol. 1, p. 18). Interest in the role of haemoglobin, as opposed, for instance, to the role of 2,3-DPG in controlling O_2 affinity, stemmed from the observations of Bellingham and Huehns (1968), Bunn (1969) and Stamatoyannopoulos, Parer and Finch (1969).

Stamatoyannopoulos, Parer and Finch (1969) had investigated three patients, a 33-year-old female and her two sons, 40–44% of whose haemoglobin was Hb Seattle. They were moderately anaemic (haematocrit 24–33%), yet the urine erythropoietin excretion was low. Oxygen delivery to the tissues thus appeared to be adequate. An erythrokinetic study demonstrated a subnormal response to anaemia. The $p_{50}O_2$ of whole blood was found to be high (41–44 mm Hg) denoting decreased O_2 affinity, and study of isolated haemoglobin fractions confirmed that this was due to the presence of Hb Seattle.

Morimoto and co-workers (1971), in an important review based on the O_2-affinity findings in 16 different variant haemoglobins, considered from the stereochemical point of view how the amino-acid replacements could bring about increased or decreased O_2 affinity. [In an earlier paper Perutz and Lehmann (1968) had reported that, while the haemoglobin molecule was insensitive to replacements of most of the amino acids on its surface (although extremely sensitive to quite small alterations of internal non-polar contacts), replacements near the haems or at the contacts between the α and β subunits affected its respiratory function.] Morimoto et al. concluded that the equilibrium between the oxy and deoxy forms of haemoglobin could be altered in a number of ways. They instanced destabiliz-ation of one of the forms because the mutation led to the production of an amino-acid side chain which was a misfit in one form but not in the other, or because the mutation resulted in a concentration of groups of equal charge which repelled each other in one but not in the other form, or because it led to the loss of a hydrogen bond that stabilized one or other of the quaternary structures; they emphasized that the equilibrium between the two allosteric forms of haemoglobin is so sensitively balanced that the loss or gain of a single pair of hydrogen bonds has a major effect on the O_2-dissociation curve.

A considerable number of laboratory studies have, too, been carried out with the aim of defining as precisely as possible the O_2 affinity of the abnormal haemoglobin and the relative roles played by the abnormal haemoglobin and other factors such as 2,3-DPG concentration in deter-mining the O_2 affinity of intact erythrocytes (see below).

Data on the O_2 affinity of individual unstable haemoglobins are included in Tables 17.1–17.3. According to the International Hemoglobin Infor-

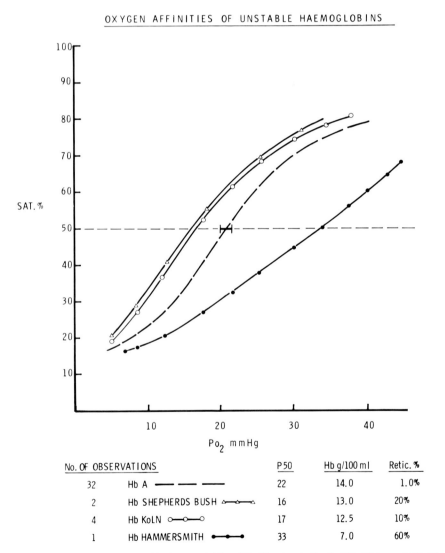

OXYGEN AFFINITIES OF UNSTABLE HAEMOGLOBINS

No. OF OBSERVATIONS		P 50	Hb g/100 ml	Retic. %
32	Hb A ▬ ▬ ▬	22	14.0	1.0%
2	Hb SHEPHERDS BUSH △—△—△	16	13.0	20%
4	Hb KoLN ○—○—○	17	12.5	10%
1	Hb HAMMERSMITH ●—●—●	33	7.0	60%

Fig. 17.17 O_2-affinity curves of three unstable haemoglobins, Hb Shepherds Bush, Hb Köln and Hb Hammersmith, compared with that of Hb A.
The O_2 affinity of Hb Hammersmith is strikingly reduced; that of Hb Shepherds Bush and Hb Köln is increased. (Reproduced by courtesy of Professor J. M. White.)

mation Center (1986) list, the majority of unstable haemoglobins have an increased O_2 affinity. Early data on Hbs Seattle, Köln, Shepherds Bush and Hammersmith are summarized below (see also Fig. 17.17).

de Furia and Miller (1972) studied a 14-year-old girl with Hb Köln 2 years after splenectomy, at a time when her haemolytic anaemia was well compensated and the erythrocyte mass was normal, *i.e.* 26 ml/kg. The $p_{50}O_2$ was low at 17.6 mm Hg, the concentration of 2,3-DPG was raised, that of ATP was lowered and erythrocyte pH was normal. Isolated Hb Köln was found to have a high O_2 affinity and the Hill number (n) was decreased, but 2,3-DPG reactivity was normal.

Woodson, Heywood and Lenfant (1974) studied O_2 transport in two slightly anaemic patients who were similarly heterozygous for Hb Koln. Cardiac output and O_2 consumption were found to be normal, but the reserve capacity of the O_2 transport system was reduced.

May and Huehns (1972) studied Hb Shepherds Bush. Their patient, a 30-year-old woman, had a well-compensated haemolytic anaemia, her haemoglobin being 13 g/dl with 5–8% reticulocytes. The O_2 affinity of her erythrocytes (containing 25% Hb Shepherds Bush and 75% Hb A), as well as that of purified Hb Shepherds Bush, was increased under all experimental conditions. This appeared to be one-third due to the intrinsic increased O_2 affinity of the abnormal haemoglobin and two-thirds due to a diminished response to 2,3-DPG. There was no evidence of interaction between Hb Shepherds Bush and Hb A. May and Huehns (1975) reported on similar studies which they had carried out on Hb Hammersmith obtained from the original patient (Grimes, Meisler and Dacie, 1964). She had a low haemoglobin (6–8 g/dl) and a high reticulocyte count. The O_2 affinity of her intact erythrocytes was found to be decreased. Part of this was shown to be due to an increased concentration of 2,3-DPG but most appeared to be the result of the reduced O_2 affinity of the abnormal haemoglobin. Haem-haem interaction was reduced and the Bohr (pH) effect was abnormal, causing a further decrease in O_2 affinity at physiological pH. The O_2 affinity of lysates containing 30–32% of the abnormal haemoglobin was found to be low, the Bohr effect normal and haem-haem interaction only slightly decreased; interaction with 2,3-DPG was normal.

MECHANISM OF FORMATION OF HEINZ BODIES

It is widely accepted that Heinz bodies represent insoluble denatured globin chains and result from the breaking up of unstable haemoglobin mol-ecules. The exact sequence of events leading to their formation is of considerable interest.

Experimental studies using normal erythrocytes and oxidative chemicals, such as acetylphenylhydrazine, indicated that the formation of methaemoglobin is an early stage in the denaturation process (Harley and Mauer, 1960; Jandl, Engle and Allen, 1960), but it is less certain that this is true of the spontaneous degradation of unstable haemoglobin molecules. The formation of methaemoglobin is in fact probably not an essential first step. However, as already referred to (p. 348), with some unstable haemoglobins quite large amounts of methaemoglobin may be present in freshly withdrawn blood while in other cases the amount present, normal or barely raised in fresh blood, increases markedly if the blood is kept at 37°C. Subtle differences in the molecular pathology of individual unstable haemoglobins seem likely to be responsible for these differences in behaviour.

Winterhalter and Jacob (1969), Jacob (1970) and Jacob and Winterhalter (1970a,b), working with Hbs Hammersmith, Köln and Zürich, derived from patients with haemolytic anaemias of severe, moderate and mild degrees, respectively, concluded that it was the loss of haem from the abnormal β chains that was the crucial event that led to molecular degradation of these particular haemoglobins. They envisaged, and obtained evidence for, the following sequence. The unstable molecules lose haem, then split into haem-containing (soluble) α chains and haem-depleted (insoluble) β chains, the latter forming the bulk of Heinz-body material. The denaturing chains attach to cytoplasmic GSH and membrane thiols (SH groups) in mixed disulphide linkages, the latter interaction being responsible for the attachment of the Heinz bodies to the cells' membrane. Experimentally, an intermediate compound formed by adding half-stoichiometric amounts of haem to globin, behaved *in vitro* (at 50°C) exactly as did the naturally-occurring unstable haemoglobins.

In studies on Hb Köln, Wajcman and co-workers (1971a,b) reached a similar conclusion, namely, that after the spontaneous loss of haem the remainder of the molecule behaves like an experimentally made semihaemoglobin. Amongst the consequences noted were: the O_2-dissociation curve becomes hyperbolic with an interaction coefficient of 1.0; 2,3-DPG binds but does not modify O_2 affinity; the dissociation equilibrium is displaced to that of the dimeric form.

In the case of Hbs Hammersmith, Köln and Zürich, Jacob and Winterhalter (1970a,b), recalling that the responsible mutations affect amino acids situated close

β - Chain Mutations in Heinz-Body
Forming Hemoglobins

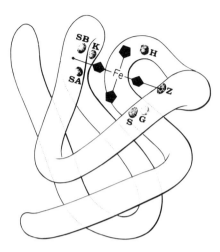

K = KÖLN; β^{98} *Valine* ⟶ *Methionine*
H = HAMMERSMITH; β^{42} *Phenylalanine* ⟶ *Serine*
Z = ZURICH; β^{63} *Histidine* ⟶ *Arginine*
G = GENOVA; β^{28} *Leucine* ⟶ *Proline*
S = SYDNEY; β^{67} *Valine* ⟶ *Alanine*
SA = SANTA ANA; β^{88} *Leucine* ⟶ *Proline*
SB = SABINE; β^{91} *Leucine* ⟶ *Proline*

Fig. 17.18 Diagram illustrating the proximity to the haem pocket of amino-acid substitutions in the β-globin chain giving rise to unstable haemoglobins.

[Reproduced by permission from Jacob and Winterhalter (1970a).]

to the haem pocket, emphasized that it was this close proximity that was responsible for the loss of haem (Fig. 17.18). Jacob (1970), however, pointed out that haem loss was not the only mechanism leading to the break-up of the haemoglobin molecule. He mentioned Hb Philly and Hb Riverdale Bronx as examples of unstable haemoglobins where the responsible mutation is at the α and β chain contact region and not near the haem pocket. In this position substitution would impair the linkage between subunits and lead the break-up of the molecule into unstable α and β chain monomers. Jacob pointed out that Heinz bodies produced by Hbs Philly and Riverdale Bronx are reddish in colour, *i.e.* haem-replete, rather than whitish (haem-depleted).

Winterbourn and Carrell (1972) studied the same problem, particularly in relation to Hb Christchurch in which serine is substituted for phenylalanine, an internal haem-contact amino acid, at the β71 (E15) position. The replacement leads to haemolytic anaemia of moderate severity. They found that Heinz bodies obtained from the patient they studied contained α and β chains, derived solely from the abnormal molecules,

in approximately equal amounts and also that heat-derived precipitates from Hb Christchurch, as well as from Hbs Hammersmith, Köln and Sydney, were composed of β chains with apparently, too, equal amounts of co-precipitated normal α chains. With Hbs Christchurch and Sydney, they obtained evidence for four haem molecules per globin tetramer in precipitated material and they noted that erythrocyte ghosts containing Heinz bodies obtained from these haemoglobins were brown in colour. Winterbourn and Carrell (1972) concluded that, although with some types of abnormal haemoglobin the abnormal chains alone precipitate, having first lost their haem groups, this was unlikely to be a general mechanism of Heinz-body formation.

Rachmilewitz and Harari (1971), Rachmilewitz and White (1973) and Rachmilewitz (1974) reported that when haemolysates of Hb Köln were oxidized with potassium ferricyanide the change in absorption spectrum indicated that haemichromes were being formed, *i.e.*, the Hb Köln was being dissociated into free haem-containing α and β subunits. A similar change had previously been demonstrated with Hbs Freiberg and Riverdale Bronx. They suggested that the dissociation of the haemoglobin tetramer into haem-containing α and β subunits was a common mechanism in the break-up of unstable haemoglobins.

Winterbourn and Carrell (1973) had studied the attachment of Heinz bodies to the membranes of Hb Christchurch erythrocytes as well as the binding on of normal erythrocyte ghosts to heat-precipitated Hb A. Using SDS PAGE, no protein bands corresponding to haemoglobin co-valently bound to a ghost protein were detected and SH-reducing and blocking agents appeared not to affect the attachment of the insoluble haemoglobin to the ghosts. Winterbourn and Carrell concluded, contrary to the views summarized by Jacob (1970) (working with Hb Köln, in particular), that covalent bonding, particularly SH bonding, is not implicated in the attachment of Heinz bodies to the erythrocyte membrane. Hydrophobic bonding, involving numerous van der Waal bonds was suggested as the likely alternative.

Winterbourn and Carrell (1974), in a further study of the subsequent changes occurring during the precipitation of Hbs Christchurch and Sydney, and of Hb A, as the result of mild heating, found that all three haemoglobins precipitated with a full haem complement. Hb Köln, on the other hand, appeared to become half-haem depleted and β chains were present in the precipitate in slight excess. In all cases the spectrum of the precipitated material conformed to that of haemichrome. There appeared to be no evidence that SH oxidation contributed to the precipitation process and GSH did not seem to be able to protect the haemoglobins from precipitation. Mixed disulphide formation between the haemoglobin and GSH was insignificant and blockage of β93 cysteine could not be demonstrated. Winterbourn and Carrell mentioned that the colours of the precipitates resulting from heating differed from haemoglobin to haemoglobin — visibly dark with Hbs Christchurch and Sydney (containing close to four haems per globin molecule) and much paler in the case of Hb Köln (with two or fewer haems per globin molecule). They concluded that their results generally favoured the concept of precipitation of both chains rather than dissociation and precipitation of unstable β chains followed by α chains, a conclusion with differs considerably from that of Jacob and Winterhalter (see above) who, working with Hbs Hammersmith, Köln and Zürich, had stressed the crucial role of haem loss in initiating the precipitation of β chains and that the normal α chains did not co-precipitate in significant amounts.

Winterbourn, McGrath and Carrell (1976) reported on the reactions between superoxide (O_2^-) ions and normal and unstable haemoglobins. Superoxide was found to be released on auto-oxidation of Hbs Christchurch, Belfast and Köln faster than from Hb A. The reactions of Hbs Christchurch and Belfast with the O_2^- ions, were, however, identical with that of Hb A and occurred at the same rate; that of Hb Köln differed in that the thiol groups of the β93 cysteines reacted with the O_2^- ions as well as the haem groups. Haemichrome formation occurred very rapidly with Hbs Christchurch and Belfast as compared with Hb A, quite independently of O_2^- production or utilization. Winterbourn, McGrath and Carrell concluded, in relation to the relative importance of haemichrome formation and precipitation of protein and the production of O_2 radicals as promoters of haemolysis in the UHbHAs, that the increased ease of haemichrome formation with resultant protein precipitation seemed likely to be the major cause under normal circumstances. However, the O_2 radical mechanism was thought likely to be of great importance under conditions of oxidant stress, as the additional reduction requirements of UHbHA erythrocytes compared to normal cells would make them abnormally sensitive to oxidant injury.

In their 1981 review Carrell and Winterbourn ably summarized the available evidence as to the mechanism of haemoglobin denaturation, with particular reference to methaemoglobin and haemichrome formation. They stressed that it is the rapid conversion of methaemoglobin to haemichrome that is the critical step in the precipitation of the unstable haemoglobins.

lactate formation, is substantially increased. In the UHbHAs this is particularly true of metabolism via the HM shunt (Grimes, Meisler and Dacie, 1964). The activity of individual glycolytic enzymes is normal, or more usually increased. On the other hand, the concentration of ATP has generally been reported to be normal or low and the same is true of that of GSH; the stability of GSH, however, to acetylphenylhydrazine *in vitro* is normal. 2,3-DPG concentrations are, too, usually normal. All these changes can be looked upon as secondary responses to the presence of a denaturing abnormal haemoglobin.

Low ATP levels were reported by Grimes, Meisler and Dacie (1964), Miller et al. (1971) and Wajcman et al. (1971b) in Hb Köln patients from different families and by Miwa et al. (1965), Mills, Levin and Alperin (1968), Hollán et al. (1970) and Yamada et al. (1971) in patients with other types of UHbHA. The low levels have generally been presumed to be the result of increased utilization rather than of defective production.

The concentration of 2,3-DPG was reported to be increased by de Furia and Miller (1972) and by Rosa et al. (1972). In contrast, Wajcman and co-workers (1971b) reported a lower than normal level in a patient with Hb Köln UHbHA.

Reductions in GSH concentrations (in most instances small) were described by Miwa et al. (1965), Hollán et al. (1970), Yamada et al. (1971) and Allard et al. (1976). The reduction in GSH level, when present, has been attributed to its forming mixed disulphides with SH groups, *e.g.* with β93 cysteines on denaturing globin. According to Jacob, Brain and Dacie (1967), 7 times as much $G^{35}SH$ bound to Hb Köln as to Hb A. This increased GSH binding is probably responsible for the heightened level of HM shunt metabolism that has been observed in some instances (Jacob, Brain and Dacie, 1968).

EFFECT OF AN UNSTABLE HAEMOGLOBIN ON ERYTHROCYTE METABOLISM

As in other types of haemolytic anaemia associated with an increased reticulocyte response, the rate of glycolysis within the EM pathway and the HM shunt, as indicated by glucose utilization and

EFFECT OF AN UNSTABLE HAEMOGLOBIN ON THE ERYTHROCYTE MEMBRANE

As already mentioned, the Heinz bodies that are spontaneously produced in the UHbHAs generally coalesce (at least in patients after splenectomy)

and attach themselves to the erythrocyte membrane, and they adhere to erythrocyte ghosts when these are prepared from intact Heinz-body containing cells. It seems highly likely that this attachment has a deleterious effect on membrane integrity and function and that this plays an important part in the premature demise of the cells.

The work of Jacob and his co-workers (Jacob, Brain and Dacie, 1967, 1968; Jacob et al., 1968; Jacob, 1970) suggested that with Hb Köln, at least, the Heinz bodies are attached to the cell membranes by S-S linkages between the abnormal β-globin chains and membrane SH groups and that membrane permeability is increased in the vicinity of these attachments and that this leads to the destruction of the affected cells in organs rich in reticulo-endothelial cells such as the spleen. According to Jacob, Brain and Dacie (1967), blockading the β93 SH groups of Hb A with paramercuribenzoate (PMB) leads to excessive haem loss and an increase in heat precipitability. Hb-Köln erythrocytes were found to be even more susceptible than normal Hb-A-containing cells to the effects of PMB, as assessed by cation leakage, increase in osmotic fragility and rate of autohaemolysis. This increased susceptibility is probably due to the depletion of membrane SH groups as the result of their reaction with Heinz bodies, as can be demonstrated by titration with DTNB [5,5′dithiobis (2-nitrobenzoic acid)]. The role of SH groups in the binding of Heinz bodies to erythrocyte membranes is well illustrated by the fact that mercaptoethanol is able to release the bodies from their attachment.

The increased susceptibility of unstable haemoglobins to the effects of SH blocking reagents such as PMB has been utilized as a means of demonstrating haemoglobin instability and of selectively separating the pathological chain (André et al., 1970; Huisman et al., 1971; Cohen Solal and Labie, 1973; Wrightstone et al., 1973; Allard et al., 1976, etc.).

Carrell, Winterbourn and Rachmilewitz (1975), in discussing the role of activated oxygen and haemolysis, had concluded that, as a consequence of the molecular instability leading to the formation of haemichromes and Heinz bodies and an increased turnover of methaemoglobin, the conse-quent increased formation of superoxide would lead to membrane damage.

Another possible mechanism leading to decreased erythrocyte survival is the occurrence within the cell membrane of high molecular weight polypeptide aggregates capable of causing decreased membrane deformability. Treating normal erythrocytes with the cross-linking agent malonyldialdehyde leads to the formation of such aggregates. Allen and co-workers (1984) reported that similar aggregates were present in untreated Hb-Köln erythrocyte membranes derived from splenectomized patients.

'DIPYRROLURIA'

As mentioned on page 324, one of the features of the UHbHAs that was well recognized and commented on in early descriptions, even before the disorders were recognized to be haemoglobinopathies, was the passage of dark, even almost blackish, urine. The exact reason for, and the nature of, the dark colouration, nevertheless, proved difficult to establish. The pigment, or more probably pigments, have, however, generally been regarded as degradation products of haem, dipyrrols (dipyrrylmethenes) or mesobilifuscins, derived from haem molecules which have partly broken down after separation from globin. Whether the pigments are correctly viewed as catabolic products of haem after separation from fully formed haemoglobin molecules or as byproducts of the synthesis of haem, i.e. degradation products of haem molecules not utilized and never incorporated into abnormal globin chains, has been debated.

The view that dipyrrylmethenes (mesobilifuscins) are mainly, if not normally entirely, anabolic pigments received strong support from the [^{15}N]glycine studies carried out on human subjects by Gilbertson et al. (1959). Three of their test subjects were anaemic (one had a haemolytic anaemia, but not an UHbHA); one was a normal volunteer. Mesobilifuscin excretion was found not to be related to stercobilin excretion, which could be greatly elevated without the former being appreciably altered. The early ^{15}N peak of mesobilifuscin excretion, too, often preceded that of early-appearing stercobilin. These results were reasonably held to support the view that mesobilifuscin pigments were derived from a pigment pool synthesized in excess of requirements. It does not follow, however, that the same explanation holds good for the UHbHAs in which the excretion of apparently similar (but perhaps not identical) pigments is very greatly increased. There is in fact some evidence that suggests that part at least of the pigments is catabolic in origin.

Schmid, Brecher and Clemens (1959) transfused the erythrocytes derived from 1000 ml of blood of one of their patients to a normal recipient. The latter experienced febrile episodes, chills, malaise and splenic tenderness over the subsequent 5 days and excreted for the first 3 days brown-coloured urine. The ^{51}Cr T_{50} of the transfused blood was 5 days, so there is no doubt that the transfused blood was destroyed rapidly, and it seemed highly likely that it was the source of the brown pigment that had been excreted in the first few days. Schmid, Brecher and Clemens also recorded, however, that the son of the donor, who was also affected, when in an aplastic crisis, passed urine that was virtually free from dark pigments, an observation compatible with the pigment having an anabolic origin!

Goudemand and co-workers (1964) undertook a similar transfusion experiment and obtained the same result: 500 ml of their patient's blood (taken after splenectomy) was transfused to a normal recipient who then passed dark urine for the next 48 hours. Before splenectomy, when the donor's erythrocytes were free from Heinz bodies, a similar experiment had been carried out. The recipient was the same, but on this occasion no 'pigmenturia' resulted.

Kreimer-Birnbaum and co-workers (1966) described how in a patient with severe thalassaemia intermedia they had found in the urine a dipyrrol pigment which they considered to be closely similar to that excreted by the Glasgow Hb-Köln patients. A [^{14}C]glycine study indicated in the thalassaemia patient that the pigment was indeed a product of ineffective erythropoiesis. Fairbanks and Burgert (1967) had studied five UHbHA patients: they concluded that mesobilifuscin was a minor urinary pigment which contributed little to its mahogany-brown colour; the colouration was, in their opinion, primarily due to the presence of a water-soluble pigment of approximately 1500 mol. wt., possibly a polypeptide-polypyrrole complex. Mesobilifuscin was stated to have a mol. wt. of about 500 and to be a tetrapyrrole rather than a dipyrrole (Fairbanks, Opfell and Burgert, 1969).

Kreimer-Birnbaum, Pinkerton and Bannerman (1968) carried out a metabolic study on a patient with Hb Köln and a mild UHbHA. [2-^{14}C]glycine was used to label Hb A and Hb Köln; the two haemoglobins were subsequently separated and their radioactivity assessed, and the dipyrrolic fraction of the urine was also counted. The radioactivity curves suggested very early destruction of Hb Köln and the urine dipyrrol fraction was highly radioactive for the first 2 days after the labelling,

its radioactivity being maximal 6 hours after the administration of the isotope. Clearly, this interesting study does not differentiate between an anabolic or catabolic origin of the dipyrrols; however, if catabolic, the detachment of the haems must have occurred at an early stage in haemoglobin formation.

RATE OF SYNTHESIS OF UNSTABLE HAEMOGLOBINS

Quite soon after the presence of an unstable haemoglobin was recognized as a cause of certain hereditary haemolytic anaemias it was realized that in patients heterozygous for the unstable haemoglobin the proportion of the abnormal haemoglobin, compared to that of Hb A, in haemolysates prepared from the patients' peripheral blood was always less, and sometimes very much less, than 50%. This observation posed the question as to whether the low proportion of the unstable haemoglobin was due to defective synthesis of the abnormal globin chain or to the post-synthetic removal of denaturing haemoglobin from erythrocytes in the form of Heinz bodies. Careful studies have indicated that both mechanisms operate. With some haemoglobins loss by one mechanism or the other is so great that little if any abnormal haemoglobin can be demonstrated in the peripheral blood. The blood picture may then be that of a hypochromic anaemia and confusion with thalassaemia possible (see below).

In theory, the synthesis of an abnormal haemoglobin can be impaired either by defective synthesis of the abnormal chain (by perhaps defective initiation, slow assembly time or defective termination) or by defective association of the abnormal α or β chain with its normal β and α chain partner (White, 1971). The following section summarizes some of the studies that have been carried out on the synthesis of *unstable* haemoglobins.

In the case of Hb Köln, White and Brain (1968, 1970) studied three patients in whom 10–20% of the haemoglobin in peripheral-blood erythrocytes was abnormal. Using [^{14}C]leucine, they found that $\beta^{Köln}$ chains were synthesized more slowly than β^A chains and that the net synthesis of Hb Köln was less than that of Hb A. Charache and co-workers (1969) similarly concluded that Hb

Hasharon was synthesized more slowly than Hb A and pointed out that the decreased synthesis of an abnormal haemoglobin could be protective. Charache and Ostertag (1970) made the same point when describing another 'low-output' haemoglobin (Hb Hopkins-2). Heterozygotes for the haemoglobin, combined with Hb A or Hb S, were not anaemic, although the reticulocyte count might be slightly elevated.

The findings of White and Dacie (1970), working with Hb Hammersmith, were different: the $\beta^{Hammersmith}$ chains appeared to be synthesized at approximately the same rate as were β^A chains and it seemed therefore that the abnormality in this haemoglobin did not affect the assembly of the abnormal haemoglobin. It appeared, too, as if the different severities of Hb Köln (relatively mild haemolysis) and Hb Hammersmith (severe haemolysis) could be correlated with the differences in the amounts of unstable haemoglobin synthesized (about 3 times as much Hb Hammersmith as Hb Köln) and in the intracellular concentration of the abnormal haemoglobin (35–40% of the total haemoglobin in the case of Hb Hammersmith and only 10–15% in the case of Hb Köln).

White (1971), in a review, discussed the data then available as to the proportion of unstable haemoglobin present in the peripheral-blood haemoglobin of affected patients. In the α-chain variants this was invariably less than 15% of the total; in the β-chain variants it was generally higher, being greater than 25% in all but four haemoglobins (Köln, Borås, Santa Ana and Sabine). In the case of Hb Köln it appeared that part at least of the apparent failure to synthesize the abnormal chain could be explained by some chains being so unstable that they were broken down almost immediately they were assembled so that they were never able to form tetramers with α chains (Huehns and Steadman, 1970). With Hb Borås, the experimental data indicated a marked deficiency in synthesis and not early precipitation of the abnormal chain (White, 1971). Rieder (1971) described experiments that he had carried out on Hb Gun Hill, the exceptionally interesting unstable haemoglobin associated with deletion of five amino acids in the β chain. When reticulocytes were incubated with [^{14}C]leucine the incorporation of radioactivity into Hb Gun Hill was found to be 2–3 times that into Hb A. His studies also demonstrated that lack of strong haem binding to globin did not hinder the synthesis of the abnormal chains.

Rucknagel, Brandt and Spencer (1971) discussed the possible reasons why the proportion of the α-chain variant haemoglobin in heterozygotes is characteristically low and included in their argument the findings in the unstable variant Hb Ann Arbor ($\alpha_2^{80\ Leu \rightarrow Arg}\beta_2$), in which the percentage of the abnormal haemoglobin had been found to vary from 2 to 13. They concluded that the α chain is more sensitive than is the β chain to amino-acid substitutions. In the case of Hb Ann Arbor, it was suggested that the abnormal molecule might be degraded more rapidly than Hb A in hetero-

zygotes or that the abnormal amino acid was being encoded by a degenerate codon resulting in reduced synthesis of the polypeptide chain.

Adams and co-workers (1972a) also studied Hb Ann Arbor, labelling reticulocytes with [^{3}H] and [^{14}C]leucine. Their studies suggested that the low proportion of the unstable haemoglobin (14% in the patient they studied) was the result of the preferential destruction of the variant α chains and also that the reduced concentration of α chains resulted, by feed-back regulation, in a decreased synthesis of normal β chains.

Cohen Solal and Labie (1973) worked with Hb Genova and concluded that the abnormal β chain was synthesized normally and that the relatively low proportion of the abnormal haemoglobin in the peripheral blood (about 20%) was the result of a defect in the association of the subunits which led to their precipitation.

Rieder and James (1974) investigated the balance of α- and β-globin synthesis in two patients with the β-chain variant Hb Leiden. A significant excess of α-chain synthesis was demonstrated, the $\beta:\alpha$ ratio being 0.47–0.63 with peripheral-blood reticulocytes and 0.82 with marrow cells, findings resembling those of heterozygous β-thalassaemia. The incubation studies indicated, too, preferential destruction of β^{Leiden} chains.

Honig and co-workers (1974) studied Hb Abraham Lincoln and concluded that the low level of this β-chain variant haemoglobin in the peripheral blood resulted from the early degradation of a fraction of the newly synthesized abnormal β chains plus a less than normal rate of synthesis.

Cohen-Solal, Lebeau and Rosa (1974) experimented with the unstable β-chain variant Hb Saint Louis. As with Hb Genova (with a substitution at the same site, $\beta28$), synthesis of the abnormal chain appeared to be normal. The state of haem iron, ferric or ferrous, did not appear to affect the rate of synthesis.

Rieder and co-workers (1975) studied the β-chain variant Hb Bushwick, present in an Italian-American family. [^{3}H]leucine studies showed that although the $\beta^{Bushwick}$ and β^A chains were synthesized initially in approximately similar amounts, the $\beta^A:\beta^{Bushwick}$ ratio increased markedly after 50–120 minutes' incubation, indicating early post-synthetic loss of the abnormal chain. The peripheral-blood erythrocytes of the propositus were, however, not hypochromic (MCH 30.1 pg), indicating apparently an increased synthesis of β^A chains in response to the excess of α chains present.

Despite the finding in Hb Bushwick, mentioned above, with certain unstable haemoglobins the post-synthetic destruction of the abnormal globin chain may take place so quickly (or failure of synthesis may be so nearly complete) that the patient presents with a hypochromic blood picture simulating in many respects that of thalassaemia.

Schneider and co-workers (1971), in describing the α-chain variant Hb Fort Worth, reported that the propositus, a 29-year-old black female, and her son, had a haemoglobin of 11.3–12.1 g/dl and an MCH of 23.3–22.8 pg, with normal serum-iron levels. Only 5% of abnormal haemoglobin could be demonstrated in haemolysates. Adams and co-workers (1979) described two Caucasian patients, a girl aged 9 years and her father, who were much more severely affected. Both were heterozygous for Hb Indianapolis; they had been severely anaemic since childhood and had needed transfusions. Splenectomy had been carried out and Heinz bodies were found in erythrocytes subsequently. The MCH was 26.2 and 22.7 pg, respectively, and erythrokinetic studies indicated ineffective erythropoiesis as in severe β-thalassaemia. Biosynthetic studies indicated that the abnormal $\beta^{Indianapolis}$ chains were being destroyed so rapidly that their net synthesis was essentially zero, the half-life of the abnormal chains being calculated to be only 7 minutes. They could not be demonstrated in peripheral-blood haemolysates.

HAEMOGLOBIN F AS A PROTECTIVE FACTOR

The proportion of Hb F present in patients with a β-chain UHbHA has an important influence on the severity of the patient's haemolytic anaemia. Clearly the more $\alpha_2^A \gamma_2$ chain (Hb F) combinations formed the smaller is the amount of abnormal haemoglobin ($\alpha_2^A \beta_2^{unstable\ Hb}$) that can be formed and the better off the patient is likely to be. (The same is true of Hb-SS disease, see p. 48).

Godeau and co-workers (1976) studied the blood of an 8-year-old girl with Hb Saint Etienne that contained 19% Hb F. They found that the Hb F was heterogeneously distributed amongst the erythrocytes and that two populations could be distinguished, one with high Hb F and low i antigen content, and the other with high Hb Saint Etienne and high i antigen content.

Aksoy and Erdem (1979) compared the clinical histories and laboratory findings in two patients with UHbHAs associated with Hb Istanbul and Hb Saint Etienne, respectively. [Both these haemoglobins result from the same amino-acid substitution, β92 (F8), histidine replaced by glutamine.] The patient with Hb Istanbul had a moderately severe haemolytic anaemia with overt signs of increased haemolysis, ameliorated to some extent by splenectomy; 2% adult-type Hb F was

present. The patient with Hb Saint Etienne (a boy aged 11 years) (Rosa et al., 1972) had a much milder illness: 19% of Hb F was present, and this was of the fetal type.

EFFECT OF CYANIDE AND CARBON MONOXIDE ON HAEMOGLOBIN INSTABILITY

Jacob, Brain and Dacie (1967, 1968) showed that cyanide (CN) and carbon monoxide (CO) could prevent haem from being detached from Hb Köln and retarded Heinz-body development and heat precipitability. Rieder (1970), working with Hb Philly, demonstrated the importance of CN in stabilizing the molecule: CN decreased precipitation at 50°C and prevented the development of inclusions when erythrocytes containing Hb Philly were exposed to the redox dye New methylene blue. Stabilization by CN was demonstrated to require the binding of the ligand to one haem only of an αβ dimer. Thus Hb Gun Hill, with haem groups only on α chains, was heat stable in the presence of CN.

More recently, Zinkham and his co-workers (Zinkham, Houtchens and Caughey, 1980, 1983; Virshup et al., 1983) showed that there is a clear link between the clinical severity of the UHbHA associated with Hb Zürich and CO levels in the patients' peripheral blood, i.e. with the smoking habit of the patient. [Previously it had been shown that the affinity of Hb Zürich for CO was at least as high as that of Hb A (Tucker et al., 1978).] Fifteen asymptomatic subjects with Hb Zürich were studied from two unrelated American families: nine did not smoke and had 3.9–6.7% HbCO in their blood; six smokers had 9.8–19.7%. The rates of haemolysis, as indicated by PCV and reticulocyte counts and by haptoglobin and haemopexin levels, were less in the smokers than in the non-smokers. The rates of Heinz-body formation at 41°C and the amount of haemoglobin precipitated from haemolysates by isopropanol were similarly less in the smokers. Smoking was, however, not recommended as a practical therapeutic measure for the following reasons: patients who smoked would, of course, suffer from the same general health risks as do smokers in general; moreover, the presence of HbCO shifts the O_2-dissociation curve to the left.

Virshup and co-workers (1983), in the course of investigating a Hb-Zürich patient who had developed a severe haemolytic anaemia following the taking of therapeutic doses of phenazopyridine (PAP), found that CO was able to inhibit the powerful oxidant effect of PAP on Hb-Zürich erythrocytes *in vitro*, as indicated by Heinz-body and methaemoglobin formation. This was brought about, it was suggested, by the CO preventing superoxide and hydrogen peroxide formation.

ROLE OF THE SPLEEN

The finding of Heinz bodies in the erythrocytes of patients with an UHbHA after removal of the spleen where none could be seen before the operation, as well as the rapid removal of Heinz bodies from erythrocytes taken from splenectomized patients and transfused experimentally to recipients with a spleen *in situ*, demonstrate the importance of the spleen in the pathogenesis of the UHbHAs. Aside from removing insoluble Heinz bodies by the pitting process, the spleen is an important site of erythrocyte destruction. Damage to the cell membrane, resulting in increased rigidity and heightened permeability, by leading to entrapment of the cell, is the likely cause of its premature destruction (Jacob, 1970). The spleen's enlargement — it is almost always palpable in patients with an UHbHA — is a reflection of its involvement in the increased haemolysis, as also is the modest to marked accumulation of radio-activity within the spleen demonstrable in patients in whom in-vivo counting has been carried out after labelling erythrocytes with ^{51}Cr (Sansone and Pik, 1965; Raik, Hunter and Lindsay, 1967; Knuth *et al.*, 1979, etc.).

DIAGNOSIS OF AN UNSTABLE HAEMOGLOBIN HAEMOLYTIC ANAEMIA

The clinical and laboratory features of a case of UHbHA present as a rule an unmistakable picture. They have been dealt with at length in the preceding pages of this Chapter and are summarized below.

Clinical history

Typically, the patient is chronically anaemic and is jaundiced and has a palpable spleen. In severity, however, his/her illness ranges from an anaemia manifest in the first year of life, which requires transfusion, to a barely perceptible illness not diagnosed until the patient is an adult. Two features that may be present (not necessarily together) are highly suggestive of an UHbHA, as opposed to another type of hereditary haemolytic anaemia. They are cyanosis, usually continuous and of mild to moderate degree, and the passage of dark brown or almost black urine. A history of a similar disorder in a family member other than the propositus may or may not be obtainable. If positive, evidence of parent to child transmission supports a diagnosis of an UHbHA.

Blood picture

Before splenectomy, the picture is of a non-spherocytic haemolytic anaemia. Two features are suggestive of an UHbHA: the presence of some distorted and contracted cells and punctate baso-philia. Heinz bodies should be demonstrable in untreated blood incubated at 37°C for 24 hours and in about 2 hours if the blood is incubated in the presence of a redox dye such as brilliant cresyl blue.

After splenectomy, the blood picture is usually much more characteristic: Heinz bodies may be recognizable in Romanowsky-stained films and punctate basophilia is often very conspicuous. Heinz bodies should be demonstrable in the majority of erythrocytes in wet preparations of fresh blood stained with dyes such as methyl violet.

Haemoglobin studies

An abnormal component can usually, but not always, be demonstrated by electrophoresis carried out by standard methods. Almost by definition, however, haemoglobin instability will be demonstrable. This can be simply tested for by exposing a haemolysate of the patient's blood to heat, e.g. 50°C, or above, or to isopropanol. In each case the haemoglobin, if unstable, denatures and precipitates faster than does Hb A.

TREATMENT OF AN UNSTABLE HAEMOGLOBIN HAEMOLYTIC ANAEMIA

No specific treatment, i.e. one directed to correcting the genetically determined defect, is at present available. According to Fairbanks and Normanbhoy (1969), the ingestion of 5 mg of riboflavin daily, in an attempt to increase GSH reductase activity, by three patients forming Hbs Köln, H and Olmsted, respectively, failed to influence the rate of haemolysis.

Preventive and palliative treatments are, however, available. These will be considered under four headings: avoidance of harm (avoidance of drugs); prompt recognition and treatment of infections; blood transfusion, and splenectomy.

Avoidance of drugs

The harmful effect of oxidant drugs, e.g., sulphonamides in normal therapeutic doses, has already been discussed in relation to Hb Zürich and certain other unstable haemoglobins (p. 325), and it would clearly be wise to use such drugs cautiously in all patients known to be forming an unstable haemoglobin. It seems probable, however, that oxidant drugs are much more harmful to certain unstable haemoglobins than to others and in practice exacerbations unequivocally associated with drug-taking have seldom been reported.

Prompt recognition and treatment of infections

Increases in anaemia and jaundice associated with infections have repeatedly been reported and have often led to blood transfusions being given, especially to small children. There is good reason, therefore, to watch carefully for infections and to diagnose them at an early stage, and to treat them promptly and effectively, using an antibiotic, if appropriate, rather than a sulphonamide. The giving of penicillin as a prophylactic to a child who has undergone splenectomy and immunizing against, for instance, pneumococcal antigens, have been discussed in an earlier chapter of this book (Vol. 1, p. 119). Either or both prophylactics should be considered in the case of a child splenectomized for an UHbHA.

Blood transfusion

As with other hereditary haemolytic anaemias, blood transfusion may be necessary in the worst affected patients, particularly in small children when anaemia and jaundice have been exacerbated in association with infections. They should not be withheld for the fear of iron overload, although this can be a problem. However, if repeated transfusions appear to be necessary, splenectomy should certainly be considered (see below).

Splenectomy

Most of the patients who have had an UHbHA of moderate to serious grade have had their spleen removed and most of them appear to have derived some benefit, their haemoglobin being maintained as a rule at a level a few grams per dl higher than before splenectomy. Few patients have, however, been followed in detail and erythrocyte life-span has seldom been measured before and after splenectomy. However, when a splenectomized patient's erythrocytes have been transfused to a recipient with spleen in situ, they have been rapidly eliminated.

In view of the enlargement of the spleen and its

Table 17.6 Effect of splenectomy in unstable haemoglobin haemolytic anaemia.

Name of unstable haemoglobin (alphabetical order)	Age of patient at time of splenectomy	Result of splenectomy	References
Abraham Lincoln	5 years	? Not improved	Honig et al. (1973)
Atlanta (and Coventry)	4 years	Greatly improved	Brennan et al. (1983)
Bibba	'Infancy'	? Improved	Kleihauer et al. (1968)
Bicêtre	10 months	Improved	Allard et al. (1976) Miller et al. (1986)
Bristol	16 months	? Not improved	Cathie (1952)★ Steadman, Yates and Huehns (1970)
Bucureşti	19 years	? Improved	Bratu et al. (1971)
Caspar	(1) 8 years (2) 4 years	Improved ? Improved	Koler et al. (1973)
Duarte	Two older sisters of propositus	Both died of thrombo-embolic complications within 1 years of splenectomy	Beutler et al. (1974)
'Frankfurt'	(1) ? 25 years (2) ? 2½ years	? Improved	Nowicki and Martin (1971, 1972)
Genova	16 years 4 years (for rupture)	Not improved ? Improved Improved Improved	Sansone and Pik (1965) Wrightstone et al. (1973) Kendall et al. (1979) Martinez, Carnot and Hernández (1983)
Hammersmith	2 years 2 years	? Not improved ? Improved	Grimes, Meisler and Dacie (1964)★ Shinton, Thursby-Pelham and Williams (1969)
Hirosaki	(1) 10 years (2) 10 years	? Not improved, One of the children died 5 years later in a severe haemolytic crisis associated with a 'common cold'	Ohba et al. (1975b)
Indianapolis	9 years	? Not improved	Adams et al. (1979)
Istanbul	29 years	Improved	Aksoy et al. (1972)
Köln	24 years	Improved	Hutchison et al. (1964)
	12 years 6 years	Improved Improved; Hb 17.8 g/dl after splenectomy	Vaughan Jones et al. (1967) Jackson, Way and Woodliff (1967)
	18 years 17 years	? Improved Improved	Wajcman et al. (1971b) Pedersen et al. (1973)
Mizuho	4 years	Improved	Ohba et al. (1977)
Perth	6 years 11 years	? Improved Not improved	Jackson et al. (1973) Grové et al. (1977)
Sabine	18 months	Not improved	Schneider et al. (1969)
Santa Ana	(1) 22 years (2) 10 years	Improved	Opfell, Lorkin and Lehmann (1968)
Savannah	19 months	? Improved	Huisman et al. (1971)
Ube I (= Köln)	10 years	Improved	Shibata et al. (1963)
Wein	16 years	Improved	Braunsteiner et al. (1964)★

References marked with an asterisk★ are to reports published before the unstable haemoglobin had been identified.

involvement in haemolysis, it is likely that its removal will always be followed by some increase in erythrocyte life-span, but where the abnormal haemoglobin is markedly unstable and erythrocyte life-span is in consequence markedly shortened a modest improvement is unlikely to be of much clinical benefit. The same is probably true of patients in whom erythrocyte life-span is but slightly shortened. Between these two extremes are patients with haemolytic anaemia of moderate intensity that they are not fully able to compensate for: these are the patients who probably derive most benefit from splenectomy.

In coming to a decision as to the advisability of splenectomy, the same considerations apply as in other types of hereditary haemolytic anaemia in which a partial reduction in the rate of haemolysis is the best that can be hoped for. In particular, the following points have to be taken into account: the age of the patient; the severity of haemolysis and how the patient tolerates the increased haemolysis — the oxygen affinity of the abnormal haemoglobin being an important factor; the patient's transfusion requirements, if any, and whether he or she has symptoms in consequence of pigment gallstones. To be weighed against some decrease in the rate of haemolysis as the result of splenectomy are the small but not negligible immediate surgical risk of the operation, the long-term risk (especially in small children) of serious sepsis subsequently, and the risk of post-splenectomy thrombocytosis and thrombo-embolism. [These risks have been discussed at length in Vol. 1, pp. 116–122.] In patients in whom a moderate degree of increased haemolysis has been associated with an unstable haemoglobin having an increased oxygen affinity, a lessening of haemolysis has been followed by undesirable persistent polycythaemia and supranormal haemoglobin levels in a few patients.

The results of splenectomy in patients with an UHbHA, as far as the writer has been able to judge from the information recorded in the literature, are summarized in Table 17.6.

HAEMOGLOBIN M AND INCREASED HAEMOLYSIS

The haemoglobin Ms comprise an interesting group of variant haemoglobins, the presence of which leads to hereditary cyanosis caused by methaemoglobinaemia. The condition was first recognized in Germany by Hörlein and Weber (1948) who were able to show that the methaemoglobinaemia was associated with an abnormality in the globin moiety of haemoglobin. Not unexpectedly, perhaps, it is now realized that several different types of Hb M exist which differ one from the other in the causal amino-acid substitution.

The Hb Ms are mentioned briefly in the present Chapter because they are to a variable extent unstable haemoglobins and in some affected families at least the presence of a Hb M has been associated with minor degrees of increased haemolysis. The instability is brought about by a disturbance to the bonding of the haem group consequent on the replacment of a haem-linked histidine in either the α chain (α58 or α87) or β chain (β63 or β92).

Except in the case of Hb Iwata, the affected histidine is replaced by tyrosine, the phenolic group of which forms a stable complex with the haem iron, blocking it permanently in the ferric state (Niazi and Shibata, 1984a).

Most of the reports that have indicated haemoglobin instability and/or have provided evidence suggestive of slightly increased haemolysis have been concerned with patients suffering from either Hb M Hyde Park = M Akita (β92 His→Tyr) or Hb M Saskatoon (β63 His→Tyr). In the case of Hb Hyde Park = Hb Akita the reports include those of Becroft, Carrell and Lehmann (1968), Hayashi et al. (1968), Stamatoyannopoulos et al. (1976), Heller (1969), Shibata et al. (1969), Efremov et al. (1974) and Shibata et al. (1976). Reports dealing with Hb M Saskatoon include those of Josephson et al. (1962), Hobolth (1965), Stavem et al. (1972), Efremov et al. (1974), Baine et al. (1980) and Blouquit et al. (1985). In the case of the patient of Stavem et al., slight constant haemolysis was markedly increased following the taking of a sulphonamide.

As has already been referred to (p. 348), minor degrees of methaemoglobinaemia, as well as accelerated methaemoglobin formation *in vitro*, have been observed with other unstable haemoglobins,

not labelled as a Hb M. With these haemoglobins increased haemolysis has been the dominant clinical phenomenon. In some cases, however, in-vivo methaemoglobinaemia has been sufficient for cyanosis to be an obvious feature of the patient's clinical history.

REFERENCES

ADAMS, J. G. III, BOXER, L. A., BAEHNER, R. L., FORGET, B. G., TSISTRAKIS, G. A. & STEINBERG, M. H. (1979). Hemoglobin Indianapolis (β122 [G14] arginine). An unstable β-chain variant producing the phenotype of severe β-thalassemia. *J. clin. Invest.*, **63**, 931–938.

ADAMS, J. G. III, WINTER, W. P., RUCKNAGEL, D. L. & SPENCER, H. H. (1972a). Biosynthesis of hemoglobin Ann Arbor: evidence for catabolic and feedback regulation. *Science*, **176**, 1427–1429.

ADAMS, J. G., WINTER, W. P., TAUSK, K. & HELLER, P. (1972b). Hemoglobin Rush [β-101 (G-3) Glu → Gln]: a new unstable hemoglobin. *Blood*, **40**, 947 (Abstract).

ADAMS, J. G. III, WINTER, W. P., TAUSK, K. & HELLER, P. (1974). Hemoglobin Rush [β101 (G3) glutamine]: a new unstable hemoglobin causing mild hemolytic anemia. *Blood*, **43**, 261–269.

AHERN, E., AHERN, V., HILTON, T., SERJEANT, G. R., SERJEANT, B. E., SEAKINS, M., LANG, A., MIDDLETON, A. & LEHMANN, H. (1976). Haemoglobin Caribbean β91 (F7) Leu → Arg: a mildly unstable haemoglobin with low oxygen affinity. *FEBS Lett.*, **69**, 99–102.

AKSOY, M. & ERDEM, S. (1979). Differences between individuals with hemoglobins Istanbul and Saint-Etienne (α2β2 92F8 His-Gln). *Acta haemat. (Basel)*, **61**, 295–297.

AKSOY, M., ERDEM, S., EFREMOV, G. D., WILSON, J. B., HUISMAN, T. H. J., SCHROEDER, W. A., SHELTON, J. R., SHELTON, J. B., ULITIN, O. N. & MÜFTÜOĞLU, A. (1972). Hemoglobin Istanbul: substitution of glutamine for histidine in a proximal histidine (F8 (92) β). *J. clin. Invest.*, **51**, 2380–2387.

ALBERTI, R., MARIUZZI, G. M., ARTIBANI, L., BRUNI, E. & TENTORI, L. (1974). A new haemoglobin variant: J Rovigo α53 (E-2) alanine → aspartic acid. *Biochim. biophys. Acta*, **342**, 1–4.

ALLARD, C., MOHANDAS, N., WACJMAN, H. & KRISNNAMOORTHY, R. (1976). Un cas d'instabilité majeure de l'hémoglobine: l'hémoglobine Bicêtre. *Nouv. Rev. franç Hémat.*, **16**, 23–35.

ALLEN, D. W., BURGOYNE, C. F., GROAT, J. D., SMITH, C. M. II & WHITE J. G. (1984). Comparison of hemoglobin Köln erythrocyte membranes with malonyldialdehyde-reacted normal

erythrocyte membranes. *Blood*, **64**, 1263–1269.

ALLISON, A. C. (1956). Observations on the sickling phenomenon and on the distribution of different haemoglobin types in erythrocyte populations. *Clin. Sci.*, **15**, 497–510.

ALLISON, A. C. (1957). Acute haemolytic anaemia with distortion and fragmentation of erythrocytes in children. *Brit. J. Haemat.*, **3**, 1–17.

ANDRÉ, R., DREYFUS, B. & LE BOLLOC'H-COMBRISSON, A. (1964). Anémie hémolytique familiale avec inclusions intra-érythrocytaires et urines noires. *Bull. Soc. méd. Hôp. Paris*, **115**, 475–482.

ANDRÉ, R., DUHAMEL, G. & NAJMAN, A. (1970). Les anémies hémolytiques congénitales avec inclusions intra-érythrocytaires. *Ann. Méd. interne*, **121**, 389–398.

ARENDS, T., GARLIN, G., GUEVARA J. M. I., AMESTY, C., PÉREZ-BÁNDEZ, O., LORKIN, P. A., LEHMANN, H. & CASTILLO, O. (1985). Hemoglobin Hofu associated with β°-thalassemia. *Acta haemat. (Basel)*, **73**, 51–54.

ARENDS, T., LEHMANN, H., PLOWMAN, D. & STATHOPOULOU, R. (1977). Haemoglobin North Shore-Caracas β134 (H12) Valine → Glutamic acid. *FEBS Lett.*, **80**, 261–265.

ASAKURA, T., ADACHI, K., SHAPIRO, M., FRIEDMAN, S. & SCHWARTZ, E. (1975). Mechanical precipitation of hemoglobin Köln. *Biochim. biophys. Acta*, **412**, 197–201.

BACHMANN, F. & MARTI, H. R. (1962). Hemoglobin Zürich. II. Physiochemical properties of the abnormal hemoglobin. *Blood*, **20**, 272–286.

BAIGET, M., GOMEZ PEREIRA, C., JUE, D. L., JOHNSON, M. H., McGUFFEY, J. E. & MOO-PENN, W. F. (1986). A case of hemoglobin Indianapolis [β112 (G14) Cys → Arg] in an individual from Cordoba, Spain. *Hemoglobin*, **10**, 483–494.

BAINE, R. M., WRIGHT, J. M., JOHNSON, M. H. & CADENA, C. L. (1980). Biosynthetic evidence for instability of Hb M Saskatoon. *Hemoglobin*, **4**, 201–207.

BAUR, E. W. & MOTULSKY, A. G. (1965). Hemoglobin Tacoma — a β-chain variant associated with increased Hb A2. *Humangenetik*, **1**, 621–634.

BECROFT, D. M. O., CARRELL, R. W. & LEHMANN, H. (1968). Haemoglobin M^Hyde Park: a hereditary methaemoglobinaemia in a Caucasian child. *N.Z.*

med. J., **68**, 72–76.

BELLINGHAM, A. J. & HUEHNS, E. R. (1968). Compensation in haemolytic anaemias caused by abnormal haemoglobins. *Nature (Lond.)*, **218**, 924–926.

BEN-BASSAT, I., BROK-SIMONI, F., BENYAMINOV, M., DANON, D. & RAMOT, (1969). Congenital inclusion body hemolytic anaemia. Study of a family. *Israel J. med. Sci.*, **5**, 383–394.

BENTLEY, S. A., LEWIS, S. M. & WHITE, J. M. (1974). Red cell survival studies in patients with unstable haemoglobin disorders. *Brit. J. Haemat.*, **26**, 85–92.

BERETTA, A., PRATO, V., GALLO, E. & LEHMANN, H. (1968). Haemoglobin Torino-α43 (CD1) phenylalanine → valine. *Nature (Lond.)* **217**, 1016–1018.

BETKE, K. & KLEIHAUER, E. (1962). Hämoglobinanomalien in der deutschen Bevölkerung. *Schweiz. med. Wschr.*, **42**, 1316–1318.

BETKE, K., MARTI, H. R., KLEIHAUER, E. & BUTIKOFER, E. (1960). Hitzelabilität und Säurestabilitat von Hämoglobin H. *Klin. Wschr.*, **38**, 529–532.

BEUTLER, E. (1983). Hemoglobinopathies associated with unstable hemoglobin. In: *Hematology*, 3rd edn (ed. by W. J. Williams, E. Beutler, A. J. Erslev and M. A. Lichtman), pp. 609–617. McGraw-Hill Book Company, New York.

BEUTLER, E., LANG, A. & LEHMANN, H. (1974). Hemoglobin Duarte: ($\alpha_2\beta_2^{62\ (E6)\ Ala \rightarrow Pro}$): a new unstable hemoglobin with increased oxygen affinity. *Blood*, **43**, 527–535.

BEUZARD, Y., BASSET, P., BRACONNIER, F., EL GAMMEL, H., MARTIN, L., OUDARD, J. L. & THILLET, J. (1975). Haemoglobin Saki $\alpha_2\beta_2^{14\ Leu \rightarrow Pro\ (A_{11})}$ structure and function. *Biochim. biophys. Acta*, **393**, 182–187.

BEUZARD, Y., COURVALIN, J. CL., COHEN SOLAL, M., GAREL, M. C. & ROSA. J. (1972). Structural studies of hemoglobin Saint-Etienne β92 (F8) His → Gln: a new abnormal hemoglobin with loss of β proximal histidine and absence of heme on the β chains. *FEBS Lett.* **27**, 76–80.

BIANCO, J., MODIANO, G., BOTTINI, E. & LUCCI, R. (1963). Alteration in the α-chain of haemoglobin L Ferrara. *Nature (Lond.)*, **198**, 395–396.

BISERTE, G., GOUDEMAND, M., VOISIN, D., CHARLESWORTH, D., LORKIN, P. A., & LEHMANN, H. (1970). Hémoglobine instable au cours d'une anémie hémolytique à inclusions érythrocytaires et urines noires. Hémoglobine trouvée à Lille, analogue à l'hémoglobine Santa Ana β88 (F4) Leucine → Proline. *Nouv. Rev. franç. Hémat.*, **10**, 201–208.

BLOUQUIT, Y., AROUS, N., DELANOE-GARIN, J., RIOU, J., LACOMBE, C., ROSA, J. & GALACTEROS, F. (1985). Hemoglobin M Saskatoon ($\alpha_2\beta_2$63 (E7) His → Tyr) in an Algerian family. *Hemoglobin*, **9**,

509–511.

BOGOEVSKI, P., EFREMOV, G. D., KEZIC, J., LAM, H., WILSON, J. B. & HUISMAN, T. H. J. (1983). Hb Sabine or $\alpha_2\beta_2$91 (F7) Leu → Pro in a Yugoslavian boy. *Hemoglobin*, **7**, 195–200.

BRADLEY, T. B. JNR & RIEDER, R. F. (1965). Hemoglobin$_{\text{Gun Hill}}$, a β chain abnormality associated with a haemolytic state. *Blood*, **28**, 975–976 (Abstract).

BRADLEY, T. B., WOHL, R. C., MURPHY, S. B., OSKI, F. A. & BUNN, H. F. (1972). Properties of hemoglobin Bryn Mawr, $\beta^{85\ Phe \rightarrow Ser}$, a new spontaneous mutation producing an unstable hemoglobin with high oxygen affinity. *Blood*, **40**, 947 (Abstract).

BRADLEY, T. B. JNR, WOHL, R. C. & RIEDER, R. F. (1967). Hemoglobin Gun Hill: deletion of five amino acid residues and impaired heme-globin binding. *Science*, **157**, 1581–1583.

BRATU, V., LORKIN, P. A., LEHMANN, H. & PREDESCU, C. (1971). Haemoglobin Bucureşti β42 (CD1) Phe → Leu, a cause of unstable haemoglobin haemolytic anaemia. *Biochim. biophys. Acta*, **251**, 1–6.

BRAUNSTEINER, H., DIENSTL, F., SAILER, S. & SANDHOFER, F. (1964). Angeborene hämolytische Anämie mit Mesobilifuscinurie und Innenkörperbildung nach Splenectomie. *Acta haemat. (Basel)*, **32**, 314–320.

BRENNAN, S. O., JONES, K. O. A., CRETHAR, L., ARNOLD, B. J., FLEMING, P. J. & WINTERBOURN, C. C. (1977a). Haemoglobin North Shore, β134 Val → Glu, a new unstable haemoglobin. *Biochim. biophys. Acta*, **494**, 403–407.

BRENNAN, S. O., TAURO, G. P., MELROSE, W. & CARRELL, R. W. (1977b). Haemoglobin Port Phillip α91 (FG3) Leu → Pro. A new unstable haemoglobin. *FEBS Lett.*, **81**, 115–117.

BRENNAN. S. O., WILLIAMSON, D., SYMMANS, W. A. & CARRELL, R. W. (1983). Two unstable haemoglobins in one individual: Hb Atlanta (β75 Leu → Pro) and Hb Coventry (β141 Leu deleted). *Hemoglobin*, **7**, 303–312.

BRENNAN, S. O., WILLIAMSON, D., SYMMANS, W. A. & CARRELL, R. W. (1986). Two de novo mutations in one β globin chain: hemoglobin Atlanta-Coventry, β75 Leu → Pro and β141 Leu deleted. *Hemoglobin*, **10**, 225–237.

BRIMHALL, B., JONES, R. T., BAUER, E. W. & MOTULSKY, A. G. (1969). Structural characterization of hemoglobin Tacoma. *Biochemistry*, **8**, 2125–2129.

BROSIOUS, E. M., MORRISON, B. Y. & SCHMIDT, R. M. (1976). Effects of hemoglobin F levels, KCN, and storage on the isopropanol precipitation test for unstable hemoglobins. *Amer. J. clin. Path.*, **66**, 878–882.

BUNN, H. F. (1969). Subunit dissociation of certain abnormal human hemoglobins. *J. clin. Invest.*, **48**, 126–138.

BUNN, H. F. & FORGET, B. G. (1986). *Hemoglobin: Molecular, Genetic and Clinical Aspects*, pp. 565–594. W. B. Saunders, Philadelphia.

BUNN, H. F., FORGET, B. G. & RANNEY, H. M. (1977). *Human Hemoglobins*, pp. 282–311. W. B. Saunders, Philadelphia.

BUNN, H. F., SCHMIDT, G. J., HANEY, D. N. & DLUHY, R. G. (1975a). Hemoglobin Cranston, an unstable variant having an elongated β chain due to nonhomologous crossover between two normal β chain genes. *Proc. natn. Acad. Sci. U.S.A.*, **72**, 3609–3613.

BUNN, H. F., SCHMIDT, G.J., MUSS, H. & DLUHY, R. G. (1975b). Hemoglobin Cranston, an unstable variant having an elongated β-chain due to unequal crossover between two normal genes. *Clin Res.*, **23**, 401A (Abstract).

BURKERT, L. B., SHARMA, V. S., PISCIOTTA, A. W., RANNEY, M. & BRUCKHEIMER, S. (1976). Hemoglobin Mequon β41(C7) phenylalanine → tyrosine. *Blood*, **48**, 645–651.

CARRELL, R. W. & KAY, R. (1972). A simple method for the detection of unstable haemoglobins. *Brit. J. Haemat.*, **23**, 615–619.

CARRELL, R. W. & LEHMANN, H. (1969). The unstable haemoglobin haemolytic anaemias. *Seminars Hemat.*, **6**, 116–132.

CARRELL, R. W. & LEHMANN, H. (1981a). Zinc acetate as a precipitant of unstable haemoglobins. *J. clin. Path.*, **34**, 796–799.

CARRELL, R. W. & LEHMANN, H. (1981b). Precipitation of hemoglobin by zinc: the detection and isolation of unstable hemoglobins and the concentration of dilute hemoglobin solutions. In: *The Red Cell: Fifth Ann Arbor Conference*, pp. 3–14. Alan R. Liss, New York.

CARRELL, R. W., LEHMANN, H. & HUTCHISON, H. E. (1966). Haemoglobin Köln (β-98 valine → methionine): an unstable protein causing inclusion-body anaemia. *Nature (Lond.)*, **210**, 915–916.

CARRELL, R. W., LEHMANN, H., LORKIN, P. A., RAIK, E. & HUNTER, E. (1967). Haemoglobin Sydney: β67 (Ell) valine → alanine: an emerging pattern of unstable haemoglobins. *Nature (Lond.)*, **215**, 626–628.

CARRELL, R. W., LEHMANN, H. & PRIBILLA, W. (1967). Strukturanalyse des Hämoglobin Köln. *Klin. Wschr.*, **45**, 1189–1193.

CARRELL, R. W. & OWEN, M. C. (1971). A new approach to haemoglobin variant identification. Haemoglobin Christchurch β71 (E15) phenylalanine → serine. *Biochim. biophys. Acta*, **236**, 507–511.

CARRELL, R. W. & WINTERBOURN, C. C. (1981). The unstable hemoglobins. In: *Human Hemoglobins and Hemoglobinopathies: a Review to 1981* (ed. by R. G. Schneider, S. Charache and W. A. Schroeder). *Texas Rep. Biol. Med.*, **40**, 431–445.

CARRELL, R. W., WINTERBOURN, C. C. & RACHMILEWITZ, E. A. (1975). Activated oxygen and haemolysis. *Brit. J. Haemat.*, **30**, 259–264 (Annotation).

CASEY, P., KYNOCH, P. A. M., LANG, A., LEHMANN, H., NOZARI, G. & SHINTON, N. K. (1978). Double heterozygosity for two unstable haemoglobins: Hb Sydney (β67 [E 11] Val → Ala) and Hb Coventry (β141 [H19] Leu deleted). *Brit. J. Haemat.*, **38**, 195–209.

CASEY, R., LANG, A., LEHMANN, H. & SHINTON, N. K. (1976). Double heterozygosity for two unstable haemoglobins: Hb Sydney (β67 E 11 (Val → Ala) and Hb Coventry (β141 (H19) Leu deleted). *Brit. J. Haemat.*, **33**, 143–144 (Abstract).

CATHIE, I. A. B. (1952). Apparent idiopathic Heinz body anaemia. *Gt. Ormond St. J.*, No. 3, 43–48.

CHARACHE, S., BRIMHALL, B., MILNER, P. & COBB, L. (1973). Hemoglobin Okaloosa (β48 (CD7) leucine → arginine). An unstable variant with low oxygen affinity. *J. clin. Invest.*, **52**, 2858–2864.

CHARACHE, S. & MONDZAC, A. M. (1967). Hemoglobin Sinai ($\alpha_2^{47\ his}\ \beta_2$): an unstable hemoglobin causing occult hemolysis. *Blood*, **30**, 879 (Abstract No. 54).

CHARACHE, S., MONDZAC, A. M., GESSNER, U. & GAYLE, E. E. (1969). Hemoglobin Hasharon ($\alpha_2^{47\ his}$ (CD5)β_2): a hemoglobin found in low concentration. *J. clin. Invest.*, **48**, 834–847.

CHARACHE, S. & OSTERTAG, W. (1970). Hemoglobin Hopkins-2 ((α112 Asp)$_2\beta_2$): "low-output" protects from potentially harmful effects. *Blood*, **36**, 852 (Abstract).

CHARACHE, S., OSTERTAG, W. & VON EHRENSTEIN, G. (1972). Clinical studies and physiological properties of Hopkins-2 haemoglobin. *Nature new Biol.*, **237**, 88–90

CHEN-MAROTEL, J., BRACONNIER, F., BLOQUIT, Y., MARTIN-CABURI, J., KAMMERER, J. & ROSA, J. (1979). Hemoglobin Bougardirey-Mali β119(GH2) gly → val. An electrophoretically silent variant migrating in isoelectrofocusing as Hb F. *Hemoglobin*, **3**, 253–262.

CHIHCHUAN, L., HAINAN, T., HWEIYUEN, L., SHANGZHI, H., RUIYOU, L. & BAUSENG, W. (1981). Hemoglobin Shuangfeng (α27(B8) glu → lys): a new unstable hemoglobin variant. *Hemoglobin*, **5**, 691–700.

COHEN SOLAL, M., BLOUQUIT, Y., GAREL, M. C., THILLET, J., GAILLARD, L., CREYSSEL, R., GIBAUD, A. & ROSA, J. (1974). Haemoglobin Lyon (β17–18 (A14–15) Lys → Val → O): determination by sequenator analysis. *Biochim. biophys. Acta*, **351**, 306–316.

COHEN SOLAL, M. & LABIE, D. (1973). A new case of hemoglobin Genova $\alpha_2\beta_2^{28\ (B10)\ Leu\text{-}Pro}$. Further studies on the mechanism of instability and defective synthesis. *Biochim. biophys. Acta*, **295**, 67–76.

COHEN-SOLAL, M., LEBEAU, M. & ROSA, J. (1974). "In vitro" normal biosynthesis of an unstable ferrihemoglobin: hemoglobin Saint Louis B10 (β28) leu → glu. *Nouv. Rev. franç. Hémat.*, **14**, 621–626.

COHEN-SOLAL, M., SELIGMANN, M., THILLET, J. & ROSA, J. (1973). Haemoglobin Saint Louis β28 (B10) leucine → glutamine. A new unstable haemoglobin only present in a ferri form. *FEBS Lett.*, **33**, 37–41.

COHEN SOLAL, M., THILLET, J., GAILLARDON, J. & ROSA, J. (1972). Functional properties of hemoglobin Saint-Etienne: a variant carrying heme only on α chains. *Rev. Europ. Etudes clin. biol.*, **17**, 988–993

CROOKSTON, J. H., FARQUHARSON, H. A., BEALE, D. & LEHMANN, H. (1969). Hemoglobin Etobicoke: α84 (F5) serine replaced by arginine. *Canad. J. Biochem.* **47**, 143–146.

DACIE, J. V. (1960). *The Haemolytic Anaemias: Congenital and Acquired. Part I — The Congenital Anaemias.* Churchill, London.

DACIE, J. V., GRIMES, A. J., MEISLER, A., STEINGOLD, L., HEMSTED, E. H., BEAVEN, G. H. & WHITE, J. C. (1964). Hereditary Heinz-body anaemia: a report of studies on five patients with mild anaemia. *Brit. J. Haemat.*, **10**, 388–402.

DACIE, J. V., SHINTON, N. K., GAFFNEY, P. J. JNR, CARRELL, R. W. & LEHMANN, H. (1967). Haemoglobin Hammersmith (β42 (CD1) Phe → Ser). *Nature (Lond.)*, **216**, 663–665.

DE FURIA, F. G. & MILLER, D. R. (1972). Oxygen affinity in hemoglobin Köln disease. *Blood*, **39**, 398–406.

DE JONG, W. W. W., WENT, L. N. & BERNINI, L. F. (1968). Hemoglobin Leiden: deletion of β6 or 7 glutamic acid. *Nature (Lond.)* **220**, 788–790.

DE WEINSTEIN, B. I., WHITE, J. M., WILTSHIRE, B. G. & LEHMANN, H. (1973). A new unstable haemoglobin: Hb Buenos Aires β85 (F1) Phe → Ser. *Acta haemat. (Basel)*, **50**, 357–363.

DICKERMAN, J. D., HOLTZMAN, N. A. & ZINKHAM, W. H. (1973). Hemoglobin Zürich. A third family presenting with hemolytic reactions to sulfonamides. *Amer. J. Med.*, **55**, 638–642.

EFREMOV, C. D., HUISMAN, T. H. J., STANULOVIC, M., ZUROVEC, M., DUMA, H., WILSON, J. B. & JEREMIC, V. (1974). Hemoglobin M Saskatoon and hemoglobin M Hyde Park in two Yugoslavian families. *Scand. J. Haemat.*, **13**, 48–60.

EGAN, E. L. & FAIRBANKS, V. F. (1973). Postsplenectomy erythrocytosis in hemoglobin Köln disease. *New Engl. J. Med.*, **288**, 929–931.

FAIRBANKS, V. F. & BURGERT, E. O. JNR (1967). Mesobilifuscin in urine. *Brit. med. J.*, **i**, 430 (Letter).

FAIRBANKS, V. F. & NOMANBHOY, Y. T. (1969). Failure of riboflavin ingestion to modify the anemia and glutathione reductase activity of erythrocytes in three unstable hemoglobin disorders (Köln, H, Olmsted). *Programme of Meeting of American Society of Hematology, Cleveland, 1969. Abstract. No. 237.*

FAIRBANKS, V. F., OPFELL, R. W. & BURGERT, E. O. JNR (1969). Three families with unstable hemoglobinopathies (Köln, Olmsted and Santa Ana) causing hemolytic anemia with inclusion bodies and pigmenturia. *Amer. J. Med.* **46**, 344–359.

FINNEY, R., CASEY, R., LEHMANN, H. & WALKER, W. (1975). Hb Newcastle: β92 (F8) His → Pro. *FEBS Lett.*, **60**, 435–437.

FIORIO, G. (1959). Considerazioni sui rapporti fra corpi di Heinz e iperemolisi nel quadro di forme particolari di ittero emolitico. *Riv. clin. Pediat.*, **64**, 101–113.

FRICK, P. G., HITZIG, W. H. & BETKE, K. (1962). Hemoglobin Zürich. I. A new hemoglobin anomaly associated with acute hemolytic episodes with inclusion bodies after sulfonamide therapy. *Blood*, **20**, 261–271.

FRICK, P. G., HITZIG, W. H. & STAUFFER, U. (1961). Das Hämoglobin-Zürich-Syndrom. *Schweiz. med. Wschr.*, **91**, 1203–1205.

FRISCH, B., LEWIS, S. M., SHERMAN, D., WHITE, J. M. & GORDON-SMITH, E. C. (1974). The ultrastructure of erythropoiesis in two haemoglobinopathies. *Brit. J. Haemat.*, **28**, 109–117.

GACON, G., WAJCMAN, H., LABIE, D. & COSSON, A. (1975). A new unstable hemoglobin mutated in β96 (FG5) Val → Ala: Hb Djelfa. *FEBS Lett.*, **58**, 238–240.

GACON, G., WAJCMAN, H., LABIE, D., VARET, B. & CHRISTOFOROV, B. (1976). A second case of haemoglobin Belfast (β15 [A12] Trp → Arg) observed in a French patient. *Acta haemat. (Basel)*, **55**, 313–319.

GAREL, M. C., BLOUQUIT, Y., ROSA, J., AROUS, N. & GARCIA, C. R. (1975). Hemoglobin Castilla β32 (B14) Leu-Arg; a new unstable variant producing severe hemolytic disease. *FEBS Lett.*, **58**, 145–148.

GIGLIONI, B., COMI, P., TARAMELLI, R., OTTOLENGHI, S., CIOCCA-VASINO, M. A., ANÈ, C., CAPPELLINI, M. D. & GIANNI, A. M. (1980). Organization of α-globin genes in Hb Hasharon (α47 asp → his) carriers. *Blood*, **56**, 1145–1149.

GILBERTSEN, A. S., LOWRY, P. T., HAWKINSON, V. & WATSON, C. J. (1959). Studies of the dipyrrylmethene ("fuscin") pigments. I. The anabolic significance of the fecal mesobilifuscin. *J. clin. Invest.*, **38**, 1166–1174.

GODEAU, J. F., BEUZARD, Y. G., CACHELEUX, J., BRIZARD, C. P., GIBAUD, A. & ROSA, J. (1976). Association of hemoglobin Saint Etienne ($\alpha_2\beta_2^{92F8}_{His-Gln}$) with hemoglobins A and F. Synthesis and subunit exchange *in vitro*. *J. biol. Chem.*, **251**, 4346–4354.

GORDON-SMITH, E. C., DACIE, J. V., BLECHER, T. E., FRENCH, E. A., WILTSHIRE, B. G. & LEHMANN, H. (1973). Hemoglobin Nottingham, βFG5 (98) Val → Gly: a new unstable haemoglobin producing severe haemolysis. *Proc. roy. Soc. Med.*, **66**, 507–508.

GOUDEMAND, M., BISERTE, G., HABAY, D. & VOISIN, D. (1964). Hémoglobine anormale et anémie hémolytique familiale avec inclusions érythrocytaires et urines noires. *Nouv. Rev. franç. Hémat.*, **4**, 487–504.

GREGORATOS, G., VENNES, G. J. & MOSER, R. H. (1964). Congenital inclusion body hemolytic anemia associated with epilepsy and disordered pyridoxine metabolism. *Blood*, **24**, 164–177.

GRIMES, A. J. & MEISLER, A. (1962). Possible cause of Heinz bodies in congenital Heinz-body anaemia. *Nature (Lond.)*, **194**, 190–191.

GRIMES, A. J., MEISLER, A. & DACIE, J. V. (1964). Congenital Heinz-body anaemia: further evidence on the cause of Heinz-body production in red cells. *Brit. J. Haemat.*, **10**, 281–290.

GROVÉ, S. S., JENKINS, T., KAMUZORA, H. L. & LEHMANN, H. (1977). Congenital Heinz body haemolytic anaemia due to haemoglobin Perth in a Nama child seemingly aggravated by the high nitrate content of the water supply. *Acta haemat. (Basel)*, **57**, 143–151.

HALBRECHT, I., ISAACS, W. A., LEHMANN, H. & BEN-PORAT, F. (1967). Hemoglobin Hasharon (α47 aspartic acid → histidine). *Israel J. med. Sci.*, **3**, 827–831.

HÄLLÉN, J., CHARLESWORTH, D. & LEHMANN, H. (1972). Haemoglobin Köln in a Jewish family. *Acta med. scand.*, **191**, 177–180.

HARANO, T., HARANO, K., SHIBATA, S., VEDA, S., NAKASHIMA, Y., IMAI, K. & SEKI, M. (1982). Hemoglobin variant with slight instability and increased oxygen affinity, Hb Etobicoke [α84 (F5) Ser → Arg]: the first case detected in Japan. *Hemoglobin*, **6**, 613–617.

HARLEY, J. D. & MAUER, A. M. (1960). Studies on the formation of Heinz bodies. I. Methemoglobin production and oxyhemoglobin destruction. *Blood*, **16**, 1722–1735.

HAYASHI, A., SUZUKI, T., SHIMIZU, A., IMAI, K., MORIMOTO, H., MIYAJI, T. & SHIBATA, S. (1968). Some observation on the physiochemical properties of hemoglobin M_Hyde Park *Arch. Biochem. Biophys.*, **125**, 895–901.

HAYASHI, A., SUZUKI, T. & STAMATOYANNOPOULOS, G. (1974). Electrophoretic and functional abnormalities in hemoglobin Tacoma, β30 (B12) Arg → Ser. *Biochim. biophys. Acta*, **351**, 453–456.

HELLER, P. (1969). Hemoglobin M — an early chapter in the saga of molecular pathology. *Ann. intern. Med.*, **70**, 1038–1041.

HIRANO, M. OHBA, Y., IMAI, K., INO, T., MORISHITA, Y., MATSUI, T., SHIMIZU, S., SUMI, H., YAMAMOTO, K. & MIYAJI, T. (1981). Hb Toyoake: β142 (H20) Ala → Pro. A new unstable hemoglobin with high oxygen affinity. *Blood*, **57**, 697–704.

HIRSH, J. & DACIE, J. V. (1966). Persistent post-splenectomy thrombocytosis and thrombo-embolism: a consequence of continuing anaemia. *Brit. J. Haemat.*, **12**, 44–53.

HITZIG, N. H., FRICK, P. G., BETKE, K. & HUSMAN, T. H. J. (1960). Hämoglobin Zürich: eine neue Hämoglobinanomalie mit sulfonamidinduzierter Innernkörperanämie. *Helvet. paediat. Acta*, **15**, 141–155.

HOBOLTH, N. (1965). Haemoglobin M_Arthus. I. Clinical family study. *Acta paediat. scand.*, **54**, 357–362.

HOLLÁN, S. R., SZELÉNYI, J. G., MILTENYI, M., CHARLESWORTH, D., LORKIN, P. A. & LEHMANN, H. (1970). Unstable haemoglobin disease caused by Hb Santa Ana-β88 (F4) Leu → Pro. *Haematologia*, **4**, 141–155.

HOLLENDER, A., LORKIN, P. A., LEHMANN, H. & SVENSSON, B. (1969). New unstable haemoglobin Borås: β88 (F4) leucine → arginine. *Nature (Lond.)*, **22**, 953–955.

HONIG, G. R., GREEN, D., SHAMSUDDIN, M., VIDA, L. N., MASON, R. G., GNARRA, D. J. & MAURER, H. S. (1973). Hemoglobin Abraham Lincoln β32 (B14) leucine → proline. An unstable variant producing severe hemolytic disease. *J. clin. Invest.*, **52**, 1746–1755.

HONIG, G. R., MASON, R. G., VIDA, L. N. & SHAMSUDDIN, M. (1974). Synthesis of hemoglobin Abraham Lincoln (β32 leu → pro). *Blood*, **43**, 657–664.

HONIG, G. R., SHAMSUDDIN, M., ZAIZOV, R., STEINHERZ, M., SOLAR, I. & KIRSCHMANN, (1981). Hemoglobin Petah Tikva (α100 Ala → Asp): a new unstable variant with α-thalassemia-like expression. *Blood*, **57**, 705–711.

HÖRLEIN, H. & WEBER, G. (1948). Über chronische familiäre Methämoglobinämie und eine neue Modifikation des Methämoglobins. *Dtsch. med. Wschr.*, **73**, 476–478.

HUBBARD, M., WINTON, E. F., LINDEMAN, J. G., DESSAUER, P. L., WILSON, J. B., WRIGHTSTONE, R. N. & HUISMAN, T. H. J. (1975). Hemoglobin Atlanta or $\alpha_2\beta_2^{75\,Leu\;Pro\,(E19)}$; an unstable variant found in several members of a Caucasian family. *Biochim. biophys. Acta*, **386**, 538–541.

HUEHNS, E. R. (1965). Abnormal haemoglobins causing haemolytic anaemia. *Proc. roy. Soc. Med.*, **58**, 514–516.

HUEHNS, E. R. (1970). Diseases due to abnormalities of hemoglobin structure. *Ann. Rev. Med.*, **21**, 157–178.

HUEHNS, E. R. (1974). The unstable haemoglobins. In: *Blood and its Disorders* (ed. by R. M. Hardisty and D. J. Weatherall), pp 596–609. Blackwell Scientific Publications, Oxford.

HUEHNS, E. R. (1982). The structure and function of haemoglobin: clinical disorders due to abnormal haemoglobin structure. In: *Blood and its Disorders*, 2nd edn (ed. by R. M. Hardisty and D. J. Weatherall), pp. 323–400. Blackwell Scientific

Publications, Oxford.

HUEHNS, E. R. & BELLINGHAM, A. J. (1969). Diseases of function and stability of haemoglobin. *Brit. J. Haemat.*, 17, 1–10 (Annotation).

HUEHNS, E. R., HECHT, F., YOSHIDA, A., STOMATOYANNOPOULOS, G., HARTMAN. J. & MOTULSKY, A. G. (1970). Hemoglobin-Seattle ($\alpha_2{}^A\beta_2{}^{76\ Glu}$): an unstable hemoglobin causing chronic hemolytic anaemia. *Blood*, 36, 209–218.

HUEHNS, E. R. & SHOOTER, E. M. (1965). Human haemoglobins. *J. med. Genet.*, 2, 48–90 (Review).

HUEHNS, E. R. & STEADMAN, J. H. (1970). Peptide chain synthesis in unstable haemoglobin diseases. *Proc. XIII Congr. int. Soc. Hemat.*, p. 7. Lehmann-Verlag, Munich (Abstract).

HUISMAN, T. H. J., BROWN, A. K., EFREMOV, G. D., WILSON, J. B., REYNOLDS, C. A., UY, R. & SMITH, L. L. (1971). Hemoglobin Savannah (B6 (24) β-glycine → valine): an unstable variant causing anemia with inclusion bodies. *J. clin. Invest.*, 50, 650–659.

HUISMAN, T. H. J., HORTON, B., BRIDGES, M. T., BETKE, K. & HITZIG, W. H. (1961). A new abnormal human haemoglobin: Hb-Zürich. *Clin. chim. Acta*, 6, 347–355.

HUTCHISON, H. E., PINKERTON, P. H., WATERS, P., DOUGLAS, A. S., LEHMANN, H. & BEALE, D. (1964). Hereditary Heinz-body anaemia, thrombocytopenia, and haemoglobinopathy (Hb Köln) in a Glasgow family. *Brit. med. J.*, ii, 1099–1103.

HYDE, R. D., HALL, M. D., WILTSHIRE, B. G., & LEHMANN, H. (1972). Haemoglobin Southampton β106 (G8) Leu → Pro: an unstable variant producing severe haemolysis. *Lancet*, ii, 1170–1172.

IDELSON, L. I., DIDKOWSKY, N. A., CASEY, R., LORKIN, P. A., & LEHMANN, H. (1974a). New unstable haemoglobin (Hb MOSCVA, β24 (B4) Gly → Asp) found in the USSR. *Nature (Lond.)*, 249, 768–770.

IDELSON, L. I., DIDKOWSKY, A., CASEY, R., LORKIN, P. A. & LEHMANN, H. (1974b). Structure and function of haemoglobin Tacoma (β30ᐧArg → Ser) found in a second family. *Acta haemat. (Basel)*, 52, 303–311.

IDELSON, L. I., DIDKOVSKY, N. A., FILIPPOVA, A. V., CASEY, R., KYNOCH, P. A. M. & LEYMAN [sic], H. (1975). Haemoglobin Volga, β27 (B9) Ala → Asp, a new highly unstable haemoglobin with a suppressed charge. *FEBS Lett.*, 58, 122–125.

INTERNATIONAL HEMOGLOBIN INFORMATION CENTER (1986). Alphabetical hemoglobin variant list. *Hemoglobin*, 10, 329–351.

JACKSON, J. M., WAY, B. J. & WOODLIFF, H. J. (1967). A west Australian family with a haemolytic disorder associated with haemoglobin Köln. *Brit. J. Haemat.*, 13, 474–481.

JACKSON, J. M., YATES, A. & HUEHNS, E. R. (1973). Haemoglobin Perth: β32 (B14) Leu → Pro, an unstable haemglobin causing haemolysis. *Brit. J. Haemat.*, 25, 607–610.

JACOB, H. S. (1970). Mechanisms of Heinz body formation and attachment to red cell membrane. *Seminars Hemat.*, 7, 341–354.

JACOB, H. S., BRAIN, M. C. & DACIE, J. V. (1967). Blockade of membrane and globin thiols in the pathogenesis of congenital Heinz body hemolytic anemia (CHBHA) with dipyrroluria. *J. clin. Invest.*, 46, 1073–1074 (Abstract).

JACOB, H. S., BRAIN, M. C. & DACIE, J. V. (1968). Altered sulfhydryl reactivity of hemoglobins and red blood cell membranes in congenital Heinz body hemolytic anemia. *J. clin. Invest.*, 47, 2664–2677.

JACOB, H. S., BRAIN, M. C., DACIE, J. V., CARRELL, R. W. & LEHMANN, H. (1968). Abnormal haem binding and globin SH group blockade in unstable haemoglobins. *Nature*, 218, 1214–1217.

JACOB, H. & WINTERHALTER, K. (1970a). Unstable hemoglobins: the role of heme loss in Heinz body formation. *Proc. natn. Acad. Sci. U.S.A.*, 65, 697–701.

JACOB, H. S. & WINTERHALTER, K. H. (1970b). The role of hemoglobin heme loss in Heinz body formation: studies with a partially heme-deficient hemoglobin and with genetically unstable hemoglobins. *J. clin. Invest.*, 49, 2008–2016.

JANDL, J. H., ENGLE, L. K. & ALLEN, D. W. (1960). Oxidative hemolysis and precipitation of hemoglobin. I. Heinz body anemias as an acceleration of red cell aging. *J. clin. Invest*, 39, 1818–1836.

JOHNSON, C. C., MOYES, D., SCHROEDER, W. A., SHELTON, J. B., SHELTON, J. R. & BEUTLER, E. (1980). Hemoglobin Pasadena, $\alpha_2\beta_2 75$ (E19) Leu → Arg: identification by high performance liquid chromatography of a new unstable variant with increased oxygen affinity. *Biochim. biophys. Acta*, 623, 360–367.

JONES, R. T., BRIMHALL, B., HUISMAN, T. H. J., KLEIHAUER, E. & BETKE, K. (1966). Hemoglobin Freiburg: abnormal hemoglobin due to deletion of a single amino acid residue. *Science*, 154, 1024–1027.

JONES, R. T., KOLER, R. D., DUERST, M. & STOCKLEN, Z. (1972). Hemoglobin Casper G8 β106 Leu → Pro: further evidence that hemoglobin mutations are not random. *Adv. exp. Med. Biol.*, 28, 79–98.

JOSEPHSON, A. M., WEINSTEIN, H. G., YAKULIS, B. S., SINGER, L. & HELLER, P. (1962). A new variant of hemoglobin M disease: hemoglobin $M_{Chicago}$. *J. Lab. clin. Med.*, 59, 918–925.

JURIĆIĆ, D., RUZDIĆ, I., BEER, Z., EFREMOV, G. D., CASEY, R. & LEHMANN, H. (1983). Hemoglobin Leiden [β6 or 7 (A3 or A4) Glu → O] in a Yugoslavian woman arisen by a new mutation. *Hemoglobin*, 7, 271–277.

KEELING, M. M., OGDEN, L. L., WRIGHTSTONE, R. N., WILSON, J. B., REYNOLDS, C. A.,

KITCHENS, J. L. & HUISMAN, T. H. J. (1972). Hemoglobin Louisville (β42 (CD1) Phe → Leu): an unstable variant causing mild hemolytic anemia. *J. clin. Invest.*, 50, 2395–3402.

KENDALL, A. G., TEN-PAS, A., WILSON, J. B., COPE, N., BOLCH, K. & HUISMAN, T. H. J. (1977). Hb Vaasa or $\alpha_2\beta_2$ (39(C5) gln → glu). A mildly unstable variant found in a Finnish family. *Hemoglobin*, 1, 292–295.

KENDALL, A., YOUNG, S., OUNE, N., WILTSHIRE, B. & LEHMANN, H. (1979). The unstable Hb Genova (β28 Leu → Pro) in an East African family. Family study and the effect of splenectomy. *Acta haemat. (Basel)*, 61, 278–282.

KENNEDY, C. C., BLUNDELL, G., LORKIN, P. A., LANG, A. & LEHMANN, H. (1974). Haemoglobin Belfast 15 [sic] (A12) Tryptophan → Arginine: A new unstable haemoglobin variant. *Brit. med. J.*, iv, 324–326.

KING, M. A. R., WILTSHIRE, B. G., LEHMANN, H. & MORIMOTO, H. (1972). An unstable haemoglobin with reduced oxygen affinity: haemoglobin Peterborough, β111 (G13) valine → phenylalanine, its interaction with normal haemoglobin and with haemoglobin Lepore. *Brit. J. Haemat.*, 22, 125–134.

KLEIHAUER, E. F., REYNOLDS, C. A., DOZY, A. M., WILSON, J. B., MOORES, R. R., BERENSON, M. P., WRIGHT, C.-S. & HUISMAN, T. H. J. (1968). Hemoglobin$_{Bibba}$ or $\beta_2{}^{136\ Pro}\beta_2$, an unstable α-chain abnormal hemoglobin. *Biochim. biophys. Acta*, 154, 220–222.

KLEIHAUER, E., WALLER, H. D., BENÖHR, H. C., KOHNE, E. & GELINSKY, P. (1971). Hb Tübingen. Eine neue β-Kettenvariante (βTp10–12) mit erhöhter Spotanoxydation. *Klin. Wschr.*, 49, 651–658.

KNUTH, A., PRIBILLA, W., MARTI, H. R. & WINTERHALTER, K. H. (1979). Hemoglobin Moabit: alpha 86 (F7) Leu → Arg. A new unstable abnormal hemoglobin. *Acta haemat. (Basel)*, 61, 121–124.

KOBAYASHI, S., NARA, T., NAKANO, Y., FUKAZAWA, H., KAWAMURA, G., KITAJIMA, H., SUGITA, M., JOH, K., OHBA, Y., HATTORI, Y. & MIYAJI, T. (1986). Hemoglobin Burke: an unstable hemoglobin rarely associated with hemolytic episodes. *Hemoglobin*, 10, 661–666.

KOHNE, E., KLEY, H. P., KLEIHAUER, E., VERSMOLD, H., BENÖHR, H. C. & BRAUNITZER, G. (1976). Structural and functional characteristics of Hb Tübingen: β106 (G8) Leu → Gln. *FEBS Lett.*, 64, 443–447.

KOLER, R. D., JONES, R. T., BIGLEY, R. H., LITT, M., LOVREIN, E., BROOKS, R., LAHEY, M. E. & FOWLER, R. (1973). Hemoglobin Caspar: β106 (G8) Leu → Pro. A contemporary mutation. *Amer. J. Med.*, 55, 549–558.

KOLSKI, G. B. & MILLER, D. R. (1976). Heme synthesis in hereditary hemolytic anemias: decreased δ-amino levulinic acid synthetase in hemoglobin Köln disease. *Pediat. Res.*, 10, 702–706.

KREIMER-BIRNBAUM, M., PINKERTON, P. H. & BANNERMAN, R. M. (1968). Metabolism of haemoglobin Köln, an unstable haemoglobin. *Nature (Lond.)*, 219, 494–495.

KREIMER-BIRNBAUM, M., PINKERTON, P. H., BANNERMAN, R. M. & HUTCHISON, H. E. (1966). Dipyrrolic urinary pigments in congenital Heinz-body anaemia due to Hb Köln and in thalassaemia. *Brit. med. J.*, ii, 396

KUIS-REERINK, J. D., JONXIS, J. H. P., NIAZI, G. A., WILSON, J. B., BOLCH, K. C., GRAVELY, M. & HUISMAN, T. H. J. (1976). Hb Volga or $\alpha_2\beta_2{}^{27\ (B9)}{}_{Ala–Asp}$: an unstable hemoglobin variant in three generations of a Dutch family. *Biochim. biophys. Acta*, 439, 63–69.

KURACHI, S., HERMANDSON, M., HORNUNG, S. & STAMATOYANNOPOULOS, G. (1973). Structure of haemoglobin Seattle. *Nature new Biol.*, 243, 275–276.

LABIE, D., BERNADOU, A., WAJEMAN, H. & BILSQUI-PASQUIER, G. (1977). Observation familiale d'une hémoglobine Genova β28 (B10) Leu → Pro. Étude clinique, hématologique, génétique et biochimique d'une famille française. *Nouv. Rev. franç. Hémat.*, 12, 502–506.

LABIE, D., ROSA, J., BELKHODJA, O. & BIERME, R. (1971). Hemoglobin Toulouse $\alpha_2\beta_2{}^{66\ (E10)\ Lys\ →\ Glu}$; structure and consequence in molecular pathology. *Biochim. biophys. Acta*, 236, 201–207.

LANGE, R. D. & AKEROYD, J. H. (1958). Congenital hemolytic anemia with abnormal pigment metabolism and red cell inclusion bodies: a new clinical syndrome. *Blood*, 13, 950–958.

LEE-POTTER, J. P., DEACON-SMITH, R. A., SIMKISS, M. J., KAMUZORA, H. & LEHMANN, H. (1975). A new cause of haemolytic anaemia in the newborn: a description of an unstable fetal haemoglobin: F Poole, $\alpha_2{}^{G}\gamma_2$130 tryptophan → glycine. *J. clin. Path.*, 28, 317–320.

LEHMANN, H. (1978). Hemoglobin Coventry, a βδ chain? In: *The Red Cell*, pp. 81–89. Alan R. Liss, New York.

LEHMANN, H. & CARRELL, R. W. (1969). Variations in the structure of human haemoglobin: with particular reference to the unstable haemoglobins. *Brit. med. Bull.*, 25, 14–19.

LEHMANN, H. & KYNOCH, P. A. M. (1976). *Human Haemoglobin Variants and their Characteristics*. 241 pp. North-Holland Publishing Company, Amsterdam.

LELONG, M., FLEURY, J., ALAGILLE, D., MALASSENET, R., LORTHOLARY, P. & PARA, M. (1961). L'anémie hémolytique constitutionnelle non sphérocytaire avec pigmenturie. Un cas avec étude enzymatique. *Nouv. Rev. franç. Hémat.*, 1, 819–831.

LEVINE, R. L., LINCOLN, D. R., BUCHHOLZ, W. M., GRIBBLE, T. J. & SCHWARTZ, H. C. (1975). Hemoglobin Hasharon in a premature infant with hemolytic anemia. *Pediat. Res.*, 9, 7–11.

LIE-INJO, L. E., GANESAN, J., RANDHAWA, Z. I., PETERSON, D. & KANE, J. P. (1977). Hb Leiden $-\beta^0$ thalassemia in a Chinese with severe hemolytic anemia. *Amer. J. Hemat.*, **2**, 335–342.

LIE-INJO, L. E., LOPEZ, C. G., EAPEN, J. S., ERAVELLY, J., WILTSHIRE, B. G. & LEHMANN, H. (1972). Unstable haemoglobin Köln disease in members of a Malay family. *J. med. Genet.*, **9**, 340–343.

LORKIN, P. A., LEHMANN, H. & FAIRBANKS, V. F., (1975). The amino acid substitution in Hb Olmsted: β141 (H19) leucine → arginine. *Biochim. biophys. Acta*, **386**, 256–259.

LORKIN, P. A., PIETSCHMANN, H., BRAUNSTEINER, H. & LEHMANN, H. (1974). Structure of haemglobin Wien β130 (H8) tyrosine-aspartic acid: an unstable haemoglobin variant. *Acta haemat. (Basel)*, **51**, 351–361.

LUTCHER, C. L. & HUISMAN, T. H. J. (1975). Hb-Leslie, an unstable variant due to a deletion of Glu β131 occurring in combination with β^0-thalassemia, Hb-S, and Hb-C. *Clin. Res.*, **23**, 278A.

LUTCHER, C. L., WILSON, J. B., GRAVELY, M. E., STEVENS, P. D., CHEN, C. J., LINDEMAN, J. G., WONG, S. C., MILLER, A., GOTTLEIB, M. & HUISMAN, T. H. J. (1976). Hb Leslie, an unstable hemoglobin due to deletion of glutaminyl residue β131 (H9) occurring in association with β^0-thalassemia, HbC, and HbS. *Blood*, **47**, 99–112.

McBRIDE, J. A., DACIE, J. V. & SHAPLEY, R. (1968). The effect of splenectomy on the leucocyte count. *Brit. J. Haemat.*, **14**, 225–231.

MARINUCCI, M., MALVILIO, F., FONTANAROSA, P. P., TENTORI, L. & BRANCATI, C. (1979). Studies on a family with Hb J Calabria [$\alpha_2\beta_2$64 (E8) Gly → Asp]. *Hemoglobin*, **3**, 327–340.

MARTI, H. R., WINTERHALTER, K. J., DI IORIO, E. E., LORKIN, P. A. & LEHMANN, H. (1976). Hb Altdorf $\alpha_2\beta_2$135 (H13) Ala → Pro: a new electrophoretically silent unstable haemoglobin variant from Switzerland. *FEBS Lett.*, **63**, 193–196.

MARTINEZ, G., CARNOT, J. & HERNÁNDEZ, P. (1983). Hb Genova in a Cuban family, clinical differences between families. *Hemoglobin*, **7**, 591–594.

MARTINEZ, G., LIMA, F. & COLOMBO, B. (1977). Haemoglobin J Guantanamo ($\alpha_2\beta_2$128 (H6) Ala → Asp): a new fast haemoglobin found in a Cuban family. *Biochim. biophys. Acta*, **491**, 1–6.

MAY, A. & HUEHNS, E. R. (1972). The control of oxygen affinity of red cells with Hb-Shepherds Bush. *Brit. J. Haemat.*, **22**, 599–607.

MAY, A. & HUEHNS, E. R. (1975). The oxygen affinity of haemoglobin Hammersmith. *Brit. J. Haemat.*, **30**, 185–195.

MILLER, D. R., WEED, R. I., STAMATOYANNOPOULOS, G. & YOSHIDA, A. (1971). Hemoglobin Köln disease occurring as a fresh mutation: erythrocyte metabolism and survival. *Blood*, **38**, 715–729.

MILLER, D. R., WILSON, J. B., KUTLAR, A. &

HUISMAN, T. H. J. (1986). Hb Bicêtre or $\alpha_2\beta_2$63 (E7) His → Pro in a white male: clinical observations over a period of 25 years. *Amer. J. Hemat.*, **21**, 209–214.

MILLS, G. C., LEVIN, W. C. & ALPERIN, J. B. (1968). Hemolytic anemia associated with low erythrocyte ATP. *Blood*, **32**, 15–32.

MILNER, P. F., CORLEY, C. C., POMEROY, W. L., WILSON, J. B., GRAVELY, M. & HUISMAN, T. H. J. (1976). Thalassemia intermedia caused by heterozygosity for both β-thalassemia and hemoglobin Saki [β14 (A11) Leu-Pro]. *Amer. J. Hemat.*, **1**, 283–292.

MIWA, S., KATO, H., SAITO, M., CHIBA, A., IRISAWA, K & OHYAMA, H. (1965). Congenital hemolytic anemia with abnormal pigment metabolism and red cell inclusion bodies. Report of a case and review of literature. *Acta haemat. jap.*, **28**, 593–608.

MONN, E., & BJARK, P. (1970). Hb Sogn (β14 arginine). Haematological and genetical studies. *Scand. J. Haemat.*, **7**, 455–459.

MONN, E., GAFFNEY, P. J. JNR & LEHMANN, H. (1968). Haemoglobin Sogn (β_{14} arginine). A new haemoglobin variant. *Scand. J. Haemat.*, **5**, 353–360.

MOO-PENN, W. F., JOHNSON, M. H., McGUFFEY, J. E. & JUE, D. L. (1984). Hemoglobin Shelby [β131 (H9) Gln → Lys]: a correction to the structure of hemoglobin Deaconess and hemoglobin Leslie. *Hemoglobin*, **8**, 583–593.

MOO-PENN, W. F., JUE, D. L., BECHTEL, K. C., JOHNSON, M. H., BEMIS, E., BROSIOUS, E. & SCHMIDT, R. M. (1976). Hemoglobin Deaconess. A new deletion mutant β131 (H9) glutamine deleted. *Biochem. biophys. Res. Commun.*, **65**, 8–15.

MORIMOTO, H., LEHMANN, H. & PERUTZ, M. F. (1971). Molecular pathology of human haemoglobin: stereochemical interpretation of abnormal oxygen affinities. *Nature (Lond.)*, **232**, 408–413.

MOZZICONACCI, P., ATTAL, C., PHAM-HUU-TRUNG, MALASSENET, R. & BESSIS, M. (1961). Nouveau cas d'anémie hémolytique congénitale avec inclusions intra-érythrocytaires et urines noires. Importance de la splénectomie dans l'apparition de ces inclusions. *Nouv. Rev. franç. Hémat.*, **1**, 832–846.

MULLER, C. J. & KINGMA, S. (1961). Haemoglobin Zürich: $\alpha_2^A\beta_2^{63 \text{ Arg}}$. *Biochim. biophys. Acta*, **50**, 595.

MURARI, T., SMITH, L. L., WILSON, J. B., SCHNEIDER, R. G., & HUISMAN, T. H. J. (1977). Some properties of hemoglobin Gun Hill. *Hemoglobin*, **1**, 267–282.

NAGEL, R. L., RANNEY, H. M., BRADLEY, T. B., JACOBS, A. & UDEM, L. (1969). Hemoglobin L Ferrara in a Jewish family associated with a haemolytic state in the propositus. *Blood*, **34**, 157–165.

NAKATSUJI, T., MIWA, S., OHBA, Y., HATTORI, Y., MIYAJI, T., HINO, S. & MATSUMOTO, N. (1981a).

A new unstable hemoglobin, Hb Yokahama β31 (B13) Leu → Pro, causing hemolytic anemia. *Hemoglobin*, 5, 667–678.

NAKATSUJI, T., MIWA, S., OHBA, Y., MIYA, I. T., MATSUMOTO, N. & MATSUOKA, I. (1981b). Hemoglobin Tottori (α59 [E8] glycine → valine). A new unstable hemoglobin. *Hemoglobin*, 5, 427–439.

NECHELES, T. F. & ALLEN, D. M. (1969). Heinz-body anaemias. *New Engl. J. Med.*, 280, 203–206.

NIAZI, G. A. & SHIBATA, S. (1983a). Instability of hemoglobin molecule — a review. Part I. *Kawasaki med. J.*, 9, 205–208.

NIAZI, G. A. & SHIBATA, S. (1983b). Instability of hemoglobin molecule: unstable hemoglobins with substitution at the heme contacts — a review. Part II. *Kawasaki med. J.*, 9, 209–218.

NIAZI, G. A. & SHIBATA, S. (1984a). Instability of hemoglobin molecule: unstable hemoglobins with substitutions at $\alpha_1\beta_1$ and $\alpha_1\beta_2$ contacts, in central cavity, at external surface or with deletions. — A review. Part III. *Kawasaki med. J.*, 10, 1–16.

NIAZI, G. A. & SHIBATA, S. (1984b). Instability of hemoglobin molecule: clinical and laboratory manifestations. — A review. Part IV. *Kawasaki med. J.*, 10, 17–20.

NOWICKI, L. & MARTIN, H. (1971). Hb Frankfurt: ein neues instabiles Hämoglobin als Ursache einer Heinzkörperanämie in einer deutschen Sippe. *Klin. Wschr.*, 49, 1115–1120.

NOWICKI, L. & MARTIN, H. (1972). Hb Frankfurt: ein neues instabiles Hämoglobin. II. Versuche zur Aufklärung der Strukturanomalie. *Klin. Wschr.* 50, 454–461.

NOZARI, G., RAHBAR, S., DARBRE, P. & LEHMANN, H. (1977). Hemoglobin Setif (α94 (G1) Asp → Tyr) in Iran: a report of 9 cases. *Hemoglobin*, 1, 289–292.

NOZARI, G., RAHBAR, S. & LEHMANN, H. (1978). Haemoglobin Coventry (β41 deleted) in Iran. *FEBS Lett.*, 95, 88–90.

OGATA, K., ITO, T., OKAZAKI, T., DAN, K., NOMURA, T., NOZAWA, Y. & KAJITA, A. (1986). Hemoglobin Sendagi (β42 PHE → VAL): a new unstable hemoglobin variant having an amino acid substitution at CD1 of the β-chain. *Hemoglobin*, 10, 469–481.

OHBA, Y., HASEGAWA, Y., AMINO, H., MIWA, S., NAKATSUJI, T., HATTORI, Y. & MIYAJI, T. (1983). Hemoglobin Saitama or β117 (G19) His → Pro, a new variant causing hemolytic disease. *Hemoglobin*, 7, 47–56.

OHBA, Y., HATTORI, Y., MIYAJI, T., TAKAHASHI, K., MORISAKI, T., FUJII, H., MIWA, S. & WATANABE, O. (1985a). An example of Hb Christchurch in Japan. Identification by high-performance liquid chromatography. *Hemoglobin*, 9, 483–488

OHBA, Y., IMANAKA, M., MATSUOKA, M., HATTORI, Y., MIYAJI, T., FUNAKI, C., SHIBATA, K., SHIMOKATA, H., KUZUYA, F. & MIWA, S. (1985b).

A new unstable, high oxygen affinity hemoglobin: Hb Nagoya or 97 (FG4) His → Pro. *Hemoglobin*, 9, 11–24.

OHBA, Y., MATSUOKA, M., FUYUNO, K., YAMAMOTO, K., NISHIJIMA, S, & MIYAJI, T. (1981). Further studies on hemoglobin Hofu, β126 (H4) Val → Glu, with special reference to its stability. *Hemoglobin*, 5, 89–95.

OHBA, Y., MATSUOKA, M., MIYAJI, T., SHIBUYA, T. & SAKURAGAWA, M. (1985c). Hemoglobin Bristol or β67 (E11) Val → Asp in Japan. *Hemoglobin*, 9, 79–85.

OHBA, Y., MIYAJI, T., HATTORI, Y., FUYUNO, K. & MATSUOKA, M. (1980). Unstable hemoglobins in Japan. *Hemoglobin*, 4, 307–312.

OHBA, Y., MIYAJI, T., IHZUMI, T. & SHIBATA, A. (1985d). Hb Bushwick, an unstable hemoglobin with tendency to lose heme. *Hemoglobin*, 9, 517–523.

OHBA, Y., MIYAJI, T., MATSUOKA, M., SUGIYAMA, K., SUZUKI, T. & SUGIURA, A. (1977). Hemoglobin Mizuho or beta 68 (E12) leucine → proline, a new unstable variant associated with severe hemolytic anemia. *Hemoglobin*, 1, 467–477.

OHBA, Y., MIYAJI, T., MATSUOKA, M., YAMAGUCHI, K., YONEMITSU, H., ISHII, T., & SHIBATA, S. (1975a). Hemoglobin Chiba: Hb Hammersmith in a Japanese girl. *Acta haemat. jap.*, 38, 53–58.

OHBA, Y., MIYAJI, T., MATSUOKA, M., YOKOYAMA, M., NUMAKURA, H., NAGATA, K., TAKEBE, Y. IZUMI, Y. & SHIBATA, S. (1975b). Hemoglobin Hirosaki (α43 [CE1] Phe → Leu), a new unstable variant. *Biochim. biophys. Acta*, 405, 155–160.

OHBA, Y., MIYAJI, T. & SHIBATA, S. (1973). Identical substitution in Hb Ube-1 and Hb Köln. *Nature new Biol.*, 243, 205–207.

OPFELL, R. W., LORKIN, P. A. & LEHMANN, H. (1968). Hereditary non-spherocytic haemolytic anaemia with post-splenectomy inclusion bodies and pigmenturia caused by an unstable haemoglobin Santa Ana-β88 (F4) leucine → proline. *J. med Genet.*, 5, 292–297.

OUTEIRINO, J., CASEY, R., WHITE, J. M. & LEHMANN, H. (1974). Haemoglobin Madrid β-115 (G17) alanine → proline: an unstable variant associated with haemolytic anaemia. *Acta haemat. (Basel)*, 52, 53–60.

PEDERSEN, P. R., McCURDY, P. R., WRIGHTSTONE, R. N., WILSON, J. B., SMITH, L. L. & HUISMAN, T. H. J. (1973). Hemoglobin Köln in a black: pre- and post-splenectomy red cell survival ($DF^{32}P$ and ^{51}Cr) and the pathogenesis of hemoglobin instability. *Blood*, 42, 771–781.

PERLMAN, M. M., WILTSHIRE, B. G., STEVENS, K., CASSEL, R. & LEHMANN, H. (1981). Haemoglobin Leiden in a South African negro. A case report. *S. Afr. med. J.*, 59, 537–540.

PERUTZ, M. F. & LEHMANN, H. (1968). Molecular pathology of human haemoglobin. *Nature (Lond.)*,

219, 902–909.

PRATO, V., GALLO, E., RICCO, G., MAZZA, U., BIANCO, C. & LEHMANN, H. (1970). Haemolytic anaemia due to haemoglobin Torino. *Brit. J. Haemat.*, **19**, 105–115.

PRIBILLA, W. (1962). Thalassämia-ähnliche Erkrankung mit neuem Minor-Hämoglobin (Hb Köln). In: Hämoglobin Colloquium Wien 31.8.1961, pp. 73–74. Georg Thieme, Stuttgart.

PRIBILLA, W., KLESSE, P., BETKE, K., LEHMANN, H. & BEALE, D. (1965). Hämoglobin-Köln-Krankheit: familiare hypochrome hämolytische Anämie mit Hämoglobinanomalie. *Klin. Wschr.*, **43** 1049–1053.

RACHMILEWITZ, E. A. (1974). Denaturation of the normal and abnormal hemoglobin molecule. *Seminars Hemat.*, **11**, 441–462.

RACHMILEWITZ, E. A. & HARARI, E. (1971). Intermediate hemichrome formation after oxidation of three unstable hemoglobins (Freiburg, Riverdale-Bronx and Köln). *Hämat. Bluttransf.*, **10**, 241–250.

RACHMILEWITZ, E. A. & WHITE, J. M. (1973). Haemichrome formation during the *in vitro* oxidation of Hb Köln. *Nature new Biol.*, **241**, 115–117.

RAIK, E., HUNTER, E. G. & LINDSAY, D. A. (1967). Compensated hereditary haemolytic disease resulting from an unstable haemoglobin fraction. *Med. J. Aust.*, **1**, 955–958.

RANNEY, H. M., JACOBS, A. S., UDEM, L. & ZALUSKY, R. (1968). Hemoglobin Riverdale-Bronx an unstable hemoglobin resulting from the substitution of arginine for glycine at helical residue B6 of the β polypeptide chain. *Biochem. biophys. Res. Commun.*, **33**, 1004–1011.

RIEDER, R. F. (1970). Hemoglobin stability. Observations on the denaturation of normal and abnormal hemoglobins by oxidant dyes, heat and alkali. *J. clin. Invest.*, **49**, 2369–2376.

RIEDER, R. F. (1971). Synthesis of hemoglobin Gun Hill: increased synthesis of the heme-free β^{GH} globin chain and subunit exchange with a free α-chain pool. *J. clin. Invest.*, **50**, 388–400.

RIEDER, R. F. (1974). Human hemoglobin stability and instability: molecular mechanisms and some clinical correlations. *Seminars Hemat.*, **11**, 423–440.

RIEDER, R. F. & BRADLEY, T. B. JNR (1968). Hemoglobin Gun Hill: an unstable protein associated with chronic hemolysis. *Blood*, **32**, 355–369.

RIEDER, R. F. & JAMES, G. W. III (1974). Inbalance in α and β globin synthesis associated with a hemoglobinopathy. *J. clin. Invest.*, **54,** 948–956.

RIEDER, R. F., OSKI, F. A. & CLEGG, J. B. (1969). Hemoglobin Philly (β35 tyrosine → phenylalanine): studies in the molecular pathology of hemoglobin. *J. clin. Invest.*, **48**, 1627–1642.

RIEDER, F. R., WOLF, D. J., CLEGG, J. B. & LEE, S. L. (1975). Rapid postsynthetic destruction of unstable hemoglobin Bushwick. *Nature (Lond.)*,

254, 725–727.

RIEDER, R. F., ZINKHAM, W. H. & HOLTZMAN, N. A. (1965). Hemoglobin Zürich Clinical, chemical and kinetic studies. *Amer. J. Med.*, **39**, 4–20.

ROSA, J., BRIZARD, C. P., GIBAUD, A., BEUZARD, Y., COURVALIN, J. CL., COHEN-SOLAL, M., GAREL, M. C. & THILLET, J. (1972). L'hémoglobine Saint-Etienne: $\alpha^A\beta_2$ 92 His → Gln (F8), une nouvelle variété d'hémoglobine instable avec absence d'hème sur les chaînes β. *Nouv. Rev. franç. Hémat.*, **12**, 691–700.

ROSA, J., LABIE, D., WAJCMAN, H., BOIGNE, J. M., CABANNES, R., BIERME, R. & RUFFIE, J. (1969). Haemoglobin I Toulouse: β66 (E10) lys → glu: a new abnormal haemoglobin with a mutation localized on the E10 porphyrin surrounding zone. *Nature (Lond.)*, **223**, 190–191.

ROSA, J., OUDART, J. L., PAGNIER, J., BELKHODJA, O., BOIGNÉ, J. M. & LABIE, D. (1968). A new hemoglobin: $\alpha_2^{112 \text{ His-Gln}}\beta_2$: Hb Dakar. *XII Congr. int. Soc. Hemat., New York*. Abstracts of the Simultaneous Sessions T-6, p. 72.

RUCKNAGEL, D. L., BRANDT, N. J. & SPENCER, H. H. (1971). α-chain mutants of human hemoglobin contributing to the genetics of the α-locus. *Proc. 1st Inter-American Symp. Hemoglobins, Caracas 1969. Genetical, Functional and Physical Studies of Hemoglobins*, pp. 53–54. Karger, Basel.

RUCKNAGEL, D. L., SPENCER, H. H. & BRANDT, N. J. (1968). Hemoglobin Ann. Abor, a complex alpha chain abnormality. *Proc. XII Congr. int. Soc. Hemat.*, p. 56 (Abstract K-11).

SANGUANSERMSRI T., MATRAGOON, S., CHANGLOAH, L. & FLATZ, G. (1979). Hemoglobin Suan-Dok $(\alpha_2^{109 \text{ (G16) leu-arg}}\beta_2)$: an unstable variant associated with α-thalassemia. *Hemoglobin*, **3**, 161–174.

SANSONE, G., CARRELL, R. W. & LEHMANN, H. (1967). Haemoglobin Genova: β28 (B10) leucine → proline. *Nature (Lond.)*, **214**, 877–879.

SANSONE, G. & CENTA, A. (1964). Una nouva emoglobina: l'emoglobina Galliera Genova, in un caso familiare di anaemia emolitica non sferocitaria con mesobilifuscinuria e corpi inclusi endoeritrocitari. *Accad. med.*, **79**, 167–171.

SANSONE, G. & PIK, C. (1965). Familial haemolytic anaemia with erythrocyte inclusion bodies, bilifuscinuria and abnormal haemoglobin (haemoglobin Galliera Genova). *Brit. J. Haemat.*, **11**, 511–517.

SANSONE, G., SCIARRATTA, G. V., GENOVA, R., DARBRE, P. D. & LEHMANN, H. (1977). Haemoglobin Shepherds Bush (β74 [E18] Gly → Asp) in an Italian family. *Acta haemat. (Basel)*, **57**, 102–108.

SANSONE, G., SCIARRATTA, G. V., LANG, A., LORKIN, P. A. & LEHMANN, H. (1976). A drug-induced haemolytic anaemia due to Hb Torino (α43(CD1) Phe → Val). Second finding in an Italian family.

Acta haemat. (Basel), **56**, 225–233.

SATHIAPALAN, R. & ROBINSON, M. G. (1968). Hereditary haemolytic anaemia due to an abnormal haemoglobin (haemoglobin Kings County). *Brit. J. Haemat.*, **15**, 579–587.

SCHMID, R., BRECHER, G. & CLEMENS, T. (1959). Familial hemolytic anemia with erythrocyte inclusion bodies and a defect in pigment metabolism. *Blood*, **14**, 991–1007.

SCHMID, R., WILLIAMS, G. Z. & CLEMENS, T. JNR (1958). Familial hemolytic anemia with spontaneous erythrocyte inclusion bodies. *Proc. Sixth Congr. int. Soc. Hemat.*, Boston, Aug. 2 — Sept. 1, 1956, p. 742. Grune and Stratton, New York.

SCHMIDT, R. M., BECHTEL, K. C., JOHNSON, M. H., THERREL, B. L. JNR & MOO-PENN, W. F. (1977). Hemoglobin Lufkin: β29 (B11) Gly → Asp. An unstable variant involving an internal amino acid residue. *Hemoglobin*, **1**, 799–814.

SCHNEIDER, R. G., BERKMAN, N. L., BRIMHALL, B. & JONES, R. T. (1976a). Hemoglobin Fannin-Lubbock [$α_2β_2$119 (GH2) Gly → Asp]; a slightly unstable mutant. *Biochim. biophys. Acta*, **453**, 478–483.

SCHNEIDER, R. G., BRIMHALL, B., JONES, R. T., BRYANT, R., MITCHELL, C. B. & GOLDBERG, A. I. (1971). Hb Ft. Worth: α 27 Glu → Gly (B8): a variant present in unusually low concentration. *Biochim. biophys. Acta*, **243**, 164–169.

SCHNEIDER, R. G., HETTIG, R. A., BILUNOS, M. & BRIMHALL, B. (1976b). Hemoglobin Baylor ($α_2β_2$81 (EF5) Leu → Arg) — an unstable mutant with high oxygen affinity. *Hemoglobin*, **1**, 85–96.

SCHNEIDER, R. G., UEDA, S., ALPERIN, J. B., BRIMHALL, B. & JONES, R. T. (1968). Hemoglobin Sealy ($α_2^{47\ His}β_2$): a new variant in a Jewish family. *Amer. J. human Gen.*, **20**, 151–156.

SCHNEIDER, R. G., UEDA, S., ALPERIN, J. B., BRIMHALL, B. & JONES, R. T. (1969). Hemoglobin Sabine beta 91 (F7) Leu → Pro. An unstable variant causing severe anaemia with inclusion bodies. *New Engl. J. Med*, **280**, 739–745.

SCHNEIDERMAN, L. J., JUNGA, I. G. & FAWLEY, D. E. (1970). Effect of phosphate and non-phosphate buffers on thermolability of unstable haemoglobins. *Nature (Lond.)*, **225**, 1041–1042.

SCIARRATTA, C. V., IVALDI, G., SANSONE, G., WILSON, J. B., WEBBER, B. B. & HUISMAN, T. H. J. (1985). Hb Volga or $α_2β_2$ 27 (B9) ALA → ASP in an Italian family. *Hemoglobin*. **9**, 91–93.

SCOTT, J. L., HAUT, A., CARTWRIGHT, G. E. & WINTROBE, M. M. (1960). Congenital hemolytic disease associated with red cell inclusion bodies, abnormal pigment metabolism and a electrophoretic hemoglobin abnormality. *Blood*, **16**, 1239–1252.

SERINGE, PH., ROSA, J., COMBRISSON, A., HALLEZ, J., GOROUBEN, J.-CL & DESPRÉS, P. (1965). Maladie hémolytique congénitale avec hémoglobine anormale, inclusions intra-érythrocytaires et urine noires. *Presse Méd.*, **73**, 3051–3056.

SHEEHY, T. W. (1964). Inclusion body anemia with pigmenturia. *Arch. intern. Med.*, **114**, 83–88.

SHIBATA, S. (1975). Unstable abnormal hemoglobins in Japan. In: *Abnormal Haemoglobins and Thalassaemia. Diagnostic Aspects*, pp. 161–183. Academic Press, New York.

SHIBATA, S., IUCHI, I., MIYAJI, T., UEDA, S. & TAKEDA, I. (1963). Hemolytic disease associated with the production of abnormal hemoglobin and intraerythrocytic Heinz bodies. *Acta haemat. jap.*, **26**, 164–173.

SHIBATA, S., MIYAJI, T., UEDA, S., MATSUOKA. M, IUCHI, I., YAMADA, K. & SHINKAI, N. (1970). Hemoglobin Tochigi (β56–59 deleted). A new unstable hemoglobin discovered in a Japanese family. *Proc. Japan Acad.*, **46**, 440–445.

SHIBATA, S., YAMAMOTO, K., OHBA, Y., MIYAJI, T., KARITA, K. & IUCHI, I. (1969). Hemoglobin M Akita disease. *Acta haemat. jap.*, **32**, 149–167.

SHIBATA, S., YAWATA, Y., YAMADA, O., KORESAWA, S. & UEDA, S. (1976). Altered erythropoiesis and increased hemolysis in hemoglobin M Akita (M Hyde Park β 92 His → Tyr) disease. *Hemoglobin*, **1**, 111–124.

SHINTON, N. K., THURSBY-PELHAM, D. C. & WILLIAMS, H. P. (1969) Congenital Heinz-body haemolytic anaemia due to haemoglobin Hammersmith. *Postgrad. med. J.*, **45**, 629–632.

SMILEY, R. K., GRAVELY, M. E., WILSON, J. B. & HUISMAN, T. H. J. (1978). Hemoglobin Louisville (β42 (CD1) Phe → Leu) occurring as a fresh mutation in a Canadian woman. *Hemoglobin*, **2**, 89–90.

SPIVAK, V. A., MOLCHANOVA, T. P., POSTNIKOV, Y. U., ASEEVA, E. A., LUTSENKO, I. N. & TODAREV, Y. U. (1982). A new abnormal hemoglobin: Hb Mozhaisk β92 (F8) His → Arg. *Hemoglobin*, **6**, 169–181.

STAMATOYANNOPOULOS, G. & NUTE, P. E. (1984). Cases of unstable hemoglobin and methemoglobin produced by de novo mutation. *Hemoglobin*, **8**, 85–95.

STAMATOYANNOPOULOS, G., NUTE, P. E., GIBLETT, E., DETTER, J. & CHARD, R. (1976). Haemoglobin M Hyde Park occurring as a fresh mutation: diagnostic, structural, and genetic considerations. *J. mol. Genet.*, **13**, 142–147.

STAMATOYANNOPOULOS, G., NUTE, P. E. & MILLER, M. (1981). De novo mutations producing unstable haemoglobins or hemoglobin M. 1. Establishment of a depository and use of data to test for an association of de novo mutation with advanced parental age. *Human Genet.*, **58**, 396–404.

STAMATOYANNOPOULOS, G., PARER, J. T. & FINCH, C. A. (1969). Physiologic implications of a hemoglobin with decreased oxygen affinity (hemoglobin Seattle). *New Engl. J. Med.*, **281**, 915–919.

STAUFFER, U. G. (1961). Familienuntersuchung der

Hämoglobin-Zürich-Sippe. *Helv. paediat. Acta*, **16**, 226–243.

STAVEM, P., STRÖMME, J., LORKIN, P. A. & LEHMANN, H. (1972). Haemoglobin M Saskatoon with slight constant haemolysis, markedly increased by sulphonamides. *Scand. J. Haemat.*, **9**, 566–571.

STEADMAN, J. H., YATES, A. & HUEHNS, E. R. (1970). Idiopathic Heinz body anaemia: Hb-Bristol (β67 (E11) Val → Asp). *Brit. J. Haemat.*, **18**, 435–446.

STEINBERG, M. H., ADAMS, J. G., THIGPEN, J. T., MORRISON, F. S. & DREILING, B. J. (1974). Hemoglobin Hope ($\alpha_2\beta_2^{136\text{-gly-ash}}$) — S disease: clinical and biochemical studies. *J. Lab. clin. Med.*, **84**, 632–642.

SVENSSON, B. & STRAND, L. (1967). A Swedish family with haemolytic anaemia, Heinz bodies and an abnormal haemoglobin. *Scand. J. Haemat.*, **4**, 241–248.

TANAKA, Y., KELLEHER, J. F., SCHWARTZ, E. & ASAKARA, T. (1985). Oxygen binding and stability properties of Hb Santa Ana (β88 Leu → Pro). *Hemoglobin*, **9**, 157–169.

TESTA, U., BEUZARD, Y., VAINCHENKER, W., GOOSSENS, M., DUBART, A., MONPLAISIR, N., BRIZARD, C. P., PAPAYANNOPOULOU, TH. & ROSA, J. (1979). Elevated HbF associated with an unstable hemoglobin, hemoglobin Saint Etienne; Hb synthesis in blood BFUe in culture. *Blood*, **54**, 334–343.

THILLET, J., COHEN-SOLAL, M., SELIGMANN, M. & ROSA, J. (1976). Functional and physicochemical studies of hemoglobin St. Louis β28 (B10) Leu → Gln. *J. clin. Invest.*, **58**, 1098–1106.

THILLET, J., GAREL, M. C., BIERME, R. & ROSA, J. (1980). Oxidation properties of two hemoglobin variants with their mutation localized in the heme pocket: Hb Castilla β32 (B14) Leu → Arg and Hb Toulouse β66 (E10) Lys → Glu, and abnormal functional properties of Hb Castilla. *Biochim. biophys. Acta*, **624**, 293–303.

TUCKER, P. W., PHILLIPS, S. E. V., PERUTZ, M. F., HOUTCHENS, R. & CAUGHEY, W. S. (1978). Structure of hemoglobins Zürich [His E7 (63) β → Arg] and Sydney [Val E11(67) β → Ala] and the role of the distal residues in ligand binding. *Proc. natn. Acad. Sci. U.S.A.*, **75**, 1076–1080.

UEDA, S., MATSUOUKA, M., MIYAJI, T., UEDA, N., AOKI, K., IZAWA, M. & SHIBATA, S. (1970). Heat denaturation test for unstable hemoglobin, with a note on its application to hemoglobin survey in Japan. *Acta haemat. jap.*, **33**, 281–290.

VAUGHAN JONES, R., GRIMES, A. J., CARRELL, R. W. & LEHMANN, H. (1967). Köln haemoglobinopathy. Further data and a comparison with other hereditary Heinz body anaemias. *Brit. J. Haemat.*, **13**, 394–408.

VELLA, F. (1975). Mechanical stability of human haemoglobins. *Acta haemat. (Basel)*, **54**, 257–260.

VIRSHUP, D. M., ZINKHAM, W. H., SIROTA, R. L. & CAUGHEY, W. S. (1983). Unique sensitivity of Hb Zürich to oxidative injury by phenoazopyridine: reversal of the effects by elevating carboxyhemoglobin levels in vivo and in vitro. *Amer. J. Haemat.*, **14**, 315–324.

WAJCMAN, H., BÝCKOVA, V., HAIDAS, S. & LABIE, D. (1971a). Consequences of heme loss in unstable hemoglobins; a study of hemoglobin Köln. *FEBS Lett.*, **13**, 145–148.

WAJCMAN, H., GACON, F. & LABIE, D. (1975). A new haemoglobin variant involving the distal histidine: Hb Bicetre β63 (E7) His → Pro. *3rd Meeting Europ. African Div. int. Soc. Haemat., London*. Abstract 30: 01.

WAJCMAN, H., LABIE, D. & SCHAPIRA, G. (1973). Two new hemoglobin variants with deletion. Hemoglobin Tours: Thr β87 (F3) deleted and hemoglobin St. Antoine: gly → leu β74–75 (E18–19) deleted. Consequences for oxygen affinity and protein stability. *Biochim. biophys. Acta*, **295**, 495–504.

WAJCMAN, H., PAGNIER, J., LABIE, D. & BOIVIN, P. (1971b). Hémoglobine Köln; physiopathologie d'une hémoglobine perdant spontanément son hème. *Nouv. Rev. franç. Hémat.*, **11**, 317–330.

WHITE, J. M. (1971). The synthesis of abnormal haemoglobins. *Series haemat.*, **4**, 116–132.

WHITE, J. M. (1974). The unstable haemoglobin disorders. *Clinics Haemat.*, **3**, 333–356.

WHITE, J. M. & BRAIN, M. C (1968). Haemoglobin Köln: relative synthesis of α^A,β^A and $\beta^{K\ddot{o}ln}$ chains. *XII Congr. int. Soc. Hemat. New York*. Abstract M-9, p. 65.

WHITE, J. M. & BRAIN, M. C. (1970). Defective synthesis of an unstable haemoglobin: haemoglobin Köln (β^{98} Val-Met). *Brit. J. Haemat.*, **18**, 195–209.

WHITE, J. M., BRAIN, M. C., LORKIN, P. A., LEHMANN, H. & SMITH, M. (1970). Mild "unstable haemoglobin haemolytic anaemia" caused by haemoglobin Shepherds Bush (B74 (E18) Gly → Asp). *Nature (Lond.)*, **225**, 939–941.

WHITE, J. M. & DACIE, J. V. (1970). *In vitro* synthesis of Hb Hammersmith (CD1 Phe → Ser). *Nature (Lond.)*, **225**, 860–861.

WHITE, J. M. & DACIE, J. V. (1971). The unstable haemoglobins: molecular and clinical features. In: *Progress in Hematology*, Vol. VI (ed. by Elmer B. Brown and Carl V. Moore), pp. 69–109. Grune and Stratton, New York and London.

WILLIAMSON, D., BRENNAN, S. O., MUIR, H. & CARRELL, R. W. (1983). Hemoglobin Collingwood β60(E4) Val → Ala — a new unstable hemoglobin. *Hemoglobin*, **7**, 511–519.

WINTERBOURN, C. C. & CARRELL, R. W. (1972). Characterization of Heinz bodies in unstable haemoglobin haemolytic anaemia. *Nature (Lond.)* **240**, 150–152.

WINTERBOURN, C. C. & CARRELL, R. W. (1973). The

attachment of Heinz bodies to the red cell membrane. *Brit. J. Haemat.*, **25**, 585–592.

WINTERBOURN, C. C. & CARRELL, R. W. (1974). Studies of hemoglobin denaturation and Heinz body formation in the unstable hemoglobins. *J. clin. Invest.*, **54**, 678–689.

WINTERBOURN, C. C., McGRATH, B. M. & CARRELL, R. W. (1976). Reactions involving superoxide and normal and unstable haemoglobins. *Biochem. J.*, **155**, 493–502.

WINTERBOURN, C. C., WILLIAMSON, D., VISSERS, M. C. M. & CARRELL, R. W. (1981). Unstable haemoglobin haemolytic crises: contribution of pyrexia and neutrophil oxidants. *Brit. J. Haemat.*, **49**, 111–116.

WINTERHALTER, K. H., ANDERSON, N. M., AMICONI, G., ANTONINI, E. & BRUNORI, M. (1969). Functional properties of hemoglobin Zürich. *Europ. J. Biochem.*, **11**, 435–440.

WINTERHALTER, K. & JACOB, H. (1969). Heme deficiency of beta chains a cause of hemoglobin precipitation in congenital Heinz body hemolytic anemia (CHBHA). *J. clin. Invest.*, **48**, 89a–90a.

WONG, S. C., ALI, M. A. A., PAI, M. & BARR, R. D. (1980). A new case of unstable haemoglobin Genova $(\alpha_2\beta_2^{28(\beta 10)\ \text{Leu} \rightarrow \text{Pro}})$ in Canada: as a result of a sporadic mutation and causing Heinz body haemolytic anaemia. *Acta haemat. (Basel)*, **63**, 222–225.

WOODSON, R. D., HEYWOOD, J. D. & LENFANT, C. (1974). Oxygen transport in hemoglobin Köln. Effect of increased oxygen affinity in absence of compensatory erythrocytosis. *Arch. intern. Med.*, **134**, 711–715.

WORMS, R., BERNARD, J., BESSIS, M. & MALASSENET, R. (1961). Anémie hémolytique congénitale avec inclusions intra-érythrocytaires et urines noires. Rapport d'un nouveau cas avec étude de microscopie électronique. *Nouv. Rev. franç. Hémat.*, **1**, 805–818.

WRIGHTSTONE, R. N. (1984). Unstable hemoglobins. *Sphere* (Medical College of Georgia Comprehensive Sickle Cell Center), **9**, No. 4.

WRIGHTSTONE, R. N., WILSON, J. B., REYNOLDS, C. A. & HUISMAN, T. H. J. (1973). Hb-Genova $(\alpha_2\beta_2^{28(B10)\ \text{Leu} \rightarrow \text{Pro}})$; methods for detection and analysis of unstable hemoglobins. *Clin. chim. Acta*, **44**, 217–227.

YAMADA, K. SHINKAI, N., NAKAZAWA, S., YAMADA, Z., SAITO, K., MIWA, S., MIYAJI, T. SHIBATA, S. (1971). Hemoglobin Tochigi disease, a new unstable hemoglobin hemolytic anemia found in a Japanese family. *Acta haemat. jap.*, **34**, 484–497.

ZINKHAM, W. H., HOUTCHENS, R. A. & CAUGHEY, W. S. (1980). Carboxyhemoglobin levels in an unstable hemoglobin disorder (Hb Zürich): effect on phenotypic expression. *Science*, **209**, 406–408.

ZINKHAM, W. H., HOUTCHENS, R. A. & CAUGHEY, W. S. (1983). Relation between variations in the phenotypic expression of an unstable hemoglobin disorder (hemoglobin Zürich) and carboxyhemoglobin levels. *Amer. J. Med.*, **74**, 23–29.

ZINKHAM, W. H., LILJESTRAND, J. D., DIXON, S. M. & HUTCHISON, J. L. (1979b). Observations on the rate and mechanism of hemolysis in individuals with Hb Zürich [His E7 (63) β → Arg]: II. Thermal denaturation as a cause of anemia during fever. *Johns Hopk. med. J.*, **144**, 109–116.

ZINKHAM, W. H., VANGROV, J. S., DIXON, S. M. & HUTCHISON, J. L. (1979a). Observations on the rate and mechanism of hemolysis in individuals with Hb Zürich [His E7 (63) β → Arg]: I. Concentrations of haptoglobin and hemopexin in the serum. *Johns Hopk. med. J.*, **144**, 37–40.

The thalassaemias I: history, heterogeneity, and clinical and haematological features

In this Chapter are described certain hereditary anaemias — the thalassaemias — caused by defects in the synthesis of the globin part of the haemoglobin molecule. These defects lead to the formation of erythrocytes that are low in haemoglobin content and usually very variable in size and shape. The life-span of the most defective corpuscles is considerably reduced and it is for this reason that a discussion of the thalassaemias is included in this book. They are in fact a common and most important, and most interesting, group of disorders; and they are the cause of much chronic ill health in many countries of the world. The relevant literature is correspondingly enormous, and thousands of papers on the clinical, haematological, genetical and molecular-biological aspects of the thalassaemias must have been published since the corresponding Chapter in the 2nd edition of this book (Ch. 5) was written more than 25 years ago.

Synonyms

Erythroblastic anemia (Cooley and Lee, 1932), Mediterranean disease — thalassemia (Whipple and Bradford, 1932, 1936), Cooley's anemia (Kato and Downey, 1933), target-cell anemia (Dameshek, 1940), familial microcytic anemia (Strauss, Daland and Fox, 1941), familial Mediterranean target–oval cell syndromes (Dameshek, 1943), thalassemia major and thalassemia minor (Valentine and Neel, 1944); microcitemia (Silvestroni and Bianco, 1946); Rietti-Greppi-Micheli anaemia (see Marmont and Bianchi, 1948), Mediterranean hemopathic syndrome (Chini and Valeri, 1949), hereditary leptocytosis (Committee for Clarification of the Nomenclature of Cells and Diseases of the Blood and Blood-forming Organs, 1950), hemopathic Mediterranean syndrome (de Muro and Leonardi, 1950).

In some interesting comments on nomenclature, Daland and Strauss, writing in 1948, stated that they felt that none of the titles that had been suggested up to that time were wholly satisfactory and that while thalassaemia major and minor were better than most earlier titles, they preferred Cooley's anaemia and trait, by analogy with sickle-cell anaemia and trait.

EARLY HISTORY

The first description of thalassaemia as a recognizable distinct entity is usually attributed to Dr Thomas B. Cooley and Dr Pearl Lee who reported at a meeting of the American Pediatric Society 'A series of cases of splenomegaly in children, with anemia and peculiar bone changes' (Cooley and Lee, 1925).★

Five children were described, four from the Children's Hospital of Michigan and one 'from Dr Abt's clinic'. All five had presented with the clinical syndrome then known as 'von-Jaksch's disease or pseudoleukemic anemia'. Symptoms attributable to anaemia had been recognized by the 8th month in all five cases. In addition to anaemia the spleen and liver were enlarged

★Thalassaemia must have existed for a long time before this. Zaino (1964), in a review on 'paleontologic thalassemia', suggested that it originated over 50 000 years ago in a now inundated Mediterranean valley south of Italy and Greece.

and the skin and sclerae were discoloured, without bile in the urine. There was also a leucocytosis (not thought to be leukaemic) and normoblastaemia and, in two cases, a reticulocytosis. Osmotic resistance was normal or increased. There appeared to be no evidence of rickets and in only one of the children was congenital syphilis thought to be a contributing factor. The cranial and facial bones of all five children were enlarged, resulting in a peculiar mongoloid appearance. X-ray of the skulls revealed 'peculiar alterations of their structure which the roentgenologist considered pathognomonic of this condition'. Three of the children died; one, given anti-syphilitic treatment improved. The fifth underwent splenectomy without improvement; he had apparently frequent attacks of haemoglobinuria with 'hemoglobin constant in the blood serum'. After splenectomy, very many normoblasts were present in the peripheral blood.

Microscopic study was reported to show 'fibrous hyperplasia of the spleen, pigment deposit in the liver and general leukoblastic hyperplasia of all of the bones, with erythroblastic aplasia'. Cooley and Lee concluded: 'This general aplasia of the red cell-forming tissue seems probably to be the cause of the clinical manifestations, and from the early period at which they were noted, and apparently well advanced, it is suggested that the aplasia is congenital, and the disease to be considered a form of myelophthisic anemia. Case 3 may be considered to show that the body may compensate through secondary hematapoietic areas, for the primary aplasia.'

The racial origin of the children and morphology of the erythrocytes are not mentioned in this brief report, and the histopathological description of the bone marrow hardly fits in with a diagnosis of thalassaemia. Nevertheless, the clinical features — particularly the age of onset, the splenomegaly and hepatomegaly, the acholuric jaundice and the skeletal changes — suggest β-thalassaemia major, and most authors, e.g., Weatherall (1980), have accepted that this was the diagnosis.

Further details of the same patients, and of two additional cases, were given by Cooley, Witwer and Lee (1927). They then suggested that the children were suffering from a form of haemolytic anaemia 'dependent probably on some congenital defect in the hemolyto-poietic system'. They stressed particularly 'the peculiar facies and the changes in the bones, readily demonstrable by the roentgen ray, in connection with a fairly constant blood picture'. The children ranged in age from 11 months to 5 years and their racial origin (where stated) was ? Syrian, English, Italian and Greek. One was a mulatto; two were sibs. Cooley and Lee (1932) published some additional comments under the title 'erythroblastic anaemia': they made the point that the disease was apparently not rare in Mediterranean people, especially in Greeks, and stated that while 'hemolysis is a constant and important feature we are no longer inclined to consider the disease primarily a hemolytic disorder'. They likened the tissues' attempt to make erythrocytes as attempting to make 'bricks without straw'. They added that with only one excep-

tion blood from all their patients had been found to be unusually resistant to lysis by hypotonic saline and that haemolysis might be incomplete even in distilled water.

During the next decade or so quite a large number of similar clinical histories were reported in the American literature, e.g. by Wollstein and Kreidel (1930), Baty, Blackfan and Diamond (1932) and Whipple and Bradford (1932, 1936), and in British (Moncrieff and Whitby, 1934) and European literature (see Chini and Valeri, 1949), and the eponym Cooley's anaemia was widely used for a time in descriptions of the disease.

In 1932, Whipple and Bradford introduced the descriptive terms 'Mediterranean disease' and 'thalassemia', the latter a contraction of the Greek word θαλασσα (the sea) and anaemia. They described three children as suffering from an anaemia which they considered to be the same as that described by Cooley and Lee (1932) as 'erythroblastic', but said they did not like the title. 'Thalassemia' was thought to have some appeal, but 'Mediterranean disease' was considered to be more accurate and comprehensive.

The term 'Mediterranean anemia' (not disease) was in fact at one time extensively employed, but this term, too, has been superseded by 'thalassaemia (thalassemia)' which now seems to be universally used (despite the fact that the Committee for Clarification of the Nomenclature of Cells and Diseases of the Blood and Blood-forming Organs recommended in 1950 the term 'hereditary leptocytosis'!).

A major step forward was the recognition that thalassaemia is a hereditary disease and that Cooley's anaemia is the homozygous (or compound heterozygous) form of a relatively common group of disorders which cause comparatively mild anaemia in heterozygotes. It took, however, more than 10 years from Cooley and Lee's first description in 1925 for this to be realized.

Caminopetros (1938a,b), and in papers published in the Greek literature between 1935 and 1937, working at the Pasteur Institute in Athens, seems to have been the first to realize that both parents and siblings of an infant with erythroblastic anaemia, although apparently healthy in appearance, were carriers of hidden pathological defects ('tares pathologiques cachées'), particularly increased osmotic resistance, and that these defects indicated the existence of a hereditary alteration in haemopoiesis transmitted probably as a Mendelian recessive character. Caminopetros (1938a) gave details in a Table of 14 cases of 'anémie érythroblastique avec facies mongolien parfait (type Cooley)' seen since 1935. He had seen 42 cases between 1927 and 1934. The first patients, a boy and a girl, were seen in a village in Eastern Crete in 1927.

Caminopetros's finding of increased osmotic resistance in the parents and relatives of children with Cooley's anaemia was substantiated almost simultaneously by Panoff (1936) and Angelini (1937). Panoff (1936), who described two cases of Cooley's anaemia in Bulgarian children, wrote: 'only in the father of the first child does the osmotic resistance reach up to the normal: otherwise, as in the children themselves, it is markedly increased'. Angelini, for his part, reported that almost all the available relatives of the six Italian families studied were carriers of the trait.

In America, Atkinson (1939) and Wintrobe and his colleagues (1940) similarly recognized that Cooley's anaemia (as seen in the United States) existed in a less severe inheritable form.

Atkinson studied two young adults aged 20 and 17. Although the blood counts of the parents were considered to be normal, a marked increase in osmotic resistance was demonstrated. Wintrobe and his colleagues reported in detail the findings in 14 patients belonging to three families of Italian parentage. Nearly all the signs that are now recognized to be characteristic of thalassaemia minor were described. In a postscript they mentioned that they had been able to demonstrate similar abnormalities in the blood of both parents of a child with typical Cooley's anaemia.

Strauss, Daland and Fox (1941), under the title 'familial microcytic anemia', described similar findings in a further Italian family. Six out of 21 living members of the family in two generations (and probably four deceased members also) had anaemia of iron-deficiency type (haemoglobin 60–70%) that was completely refractory to treatment. There was marked anisocytosis and poikilocytosis, the MCV was 56–66 fl, osmotic resistance was increased and X-rays of the skull showed a granular appearance.

The observations referred to above were confirmed and elaborated in other families by Smith (1942, 1943), Dameshek (1943) and Daland and Strauss (1948) in America, by Rohr (1943) in Switzerland and by Italian workers (see Chini and Valeri, 1949). In retrospect, patients suffering from the Rietti-Greppi-Micheli anaemia of Italian authors, the 'itteri emolitici con aumento della resistenza globulare' (Greppi, 1935; Rietti, 1937, 1946; Marmont and Bianchi, 1948; Chini and Valeri, 1949; de Muro and Leonardi, 1950) seem to have been thalassaemia heterozygotes.

An important step forward in understanding was the realization that the severe form of the disease could be the homozygous state of a partially dominant autosomal disorder and that the less severe form was the heterozygous condition. This interpretation was supported by many extensive studies carried out between the mid-1940s and the early 1950s (e.g. by Valentine and Neel, 1944; Smith, 1948; Silvestroni, Bianco and Vallisneri, 1949; Astaldi, Tolentino and Sacchetti, 1951; Banton, 1951; Bianco et al., 1952; Ludwin, Limentani and Dameshek, 1952). Silvestroni, Bianco and Vallisneri (1949), for instance, studied 110 sibships: 'microcitemia' was demonstrable in nearly all of the parents of 220 children with Cooley's anaemia; in only four were the signs doubtful or negative. In 1944 Valentine and Neel introduced the terms 'thalassemia minor' for the heterozygous condition ('the milder carrier state') and 'thalassemia major' for the homozygous state ('the full-blown disease'). These terms are still in use.

A further advance was the realization that heterozygosity for thalassaemia could lead to anaemia of a wide range of severity, from a clinically unimportant trait to chronic anaemia of moderate degree. Astaldi, Tolentino and Sacchetti (1951) referred to the mildest form of the disease as 'talassemia minima' and 'intermediate' types of Cooley's anaemia were described by Sturgeon, Itano and Bergren (1955), Erlandson et al. (1958) and Fessas (1959a). Subsequently, the term 'thalassaemia intermedia' has been widely used to describe patients with thalassaemia of moderate clinical severity.

As described on pages 425–429, 'thalassaemia intermedia' has no precise genotype connotation, for patients with thalassaemia of moderate clinical severity may, for instance, be either homozygous or heterozygous for β-thalassaemia or have α-thalassaemia (Hb-H disease) or be compound heterozygotes. Despite its imprecision, the term is useful clinically. An important criterion for its use had been the ability of the patient to lead a reasonably active and useful life and to maintain an adequate (although low) level of haemoglobin without the necessity for regular transfusions (Sturgeon, Itano and Bergren, 1955; Erlandson et al., 1958; Erlandson, Brilliant and Smith, 1964).

By the early 1950s the clinical and genetic basis

of thalassaemia, and the blood picture, had been well described and it was realized that the disorder was a common one — in its heterozygous form — and that it affected in particular certain Mediterranean populations. Virtually nothing was, however, known as to its pathogenesis and no one at that time can have had any inkling of its remarkable genetic diversity or that the disorder had such a world-wide distribution.

As may be imagined, the fascinating story of the early history of thalassaemia has been the subject of many reviews. In the accounts of Lehndorff (1936), Chini and Valeri (1949) and Astaldi, Tolentino and Sacchetti (1951), much of the voluminous early literature is listed. The monograph of Bannerman (1961) is noteworthy also, as are the recent historical accounts by Weatherall in Wintrobe's *Blood, Pure and Eloquent* (1980) and in Weatherall and Clegg's (1981) monumental work, *The Thalassaemia Syndromes*, and by Lehmann (1982). Weatherall's (1965) monograph, too, is a masterly survey; it was written at a time when knowledge of 'The Thalassaemia Syndromes' (a title introduced by Weatherall who realized that the clinical picture of thalassaemia could result from a variety of different inherited defects of globin synthesis) was expanding at a tremendous rate.

Other reviews in which the state of knowledge at the time of writing is ably summarized include those of Hammond *et al.* (1964), Necheles, Allen and Gerald (1969), Weatherall and Clegg (1969), Freedman (1974), Orkin and Nathan (1976), Bank (1978), Weatherall *et al.* (1980) and Kan (1983).

In the remainder of this Chapter, and in Chapters 19 and 20, the clinical manifestations of the various types of thalassaemia will be described along with the corresponding haematological findings. In addition, an attempt will be made to summarize what has been learnt as to its diversity, genetics, geographical distribution, molecular biology and pathogenesis and how this new knowledge has been obtained and by whom. The ways in which the precise diagnosis of the type of thalassaemia may be arrived at, and the possibilities for antenatal diagnosis and for effective treatment, will also be considered.

LATER HISTORY: THE GENETIC BACKGROUND OF THALASSAEMIA — A SUMMARY

Pauling (1955), in his 1954 Harvey Lecture on the relationship between abnormality of haemoglobin molecules and haemolytic anaemia, concluded that thalassemia might be caused by the presence of an abnormal haemoglobin 'with properties so similar to those of normal adult hemoglobin that the differences have escaped detection'. He emphasized that the proportion of Hb S in Hb-S/thalassaemia compound heterozygotes was higher than in simple heterozygotes for Hb S and Hb A and concluded that the hypothetical thalassaemia allele interfered with the manufacture of normal adult haemoglobin while not interfering as seriously with the manufacture of abnormal haemoglobins.

It was Itano (1957), however, who seems to have been the first to suggest that thalassaemia could result from inherited abnormalities of globin production as opposed to the presence of a molecularly abnormal haemoglobin. Ingram and Stretton's paper published in 1959 can, nevertheless, rightly be regarded as the key contribution to the understanding of its nature. They suggested that there were two main types of thalassaemia, α and β, according to whether reduced haemoglobin synthesis was the consequence of an abnormality affecting the α or β chains of haemoglobin, respectively. They drew an analogy with the two groups of structural haemoglobin variants that were then known to exist which affected, respectively, the α- and β-globin chains. They explained the formation of Hb H as the consequence of failure of α-chain synthesis leading to an excess of β chains.

Ingram and Stretton's percipient analysis was particularly based on the accumulating evidence of diversity which was being revealed by the relatively new techniques of quantitative haemoglobin analysis. The discovery by Vecchio (1946) that the haemoglobin of Cooley's-anaemia children was more resistant to alkali denaturation led to the finding that the increase in Hb F was a variable one and that in some cases of thalassaemia minor the proportion might be quite low (Zuelzer,

Robinson and Booker, 1961). Similarly, the finding of Kunkel and Wallenius (1955) that the newly discovered haemoglobin migrating on electrophoresis between Hb C and Hb S (Hb A_2) was present in increased concentration in thalassaemia-minor patients was found not to be always true. There was also the evidence provided by the analysis of the haemoglobin of compound heterozygotes for structural abnormal haemoglobin variants and thalassaemia in which interaction between the two genes might, as in sickle-cell/thalassaemia (Sturgeon, Itano and Valentine, 1953) or might not, as in Hb-C/thalassaemia (Zuelzer and Kaplan, 1954), take place.

The presence, too, of Hb H in the blood of some patients presenting with the clinical picture of thalassaemia (Rigas, Koler and Osgood, 1955) but not in the blood of others was also a strong pointer to diversity, as was the subsequent discovery of a 'new' fast running haemoglobin, Hb Bart's, in the blood of certain anaemic infants (Ager and Lehmann, 1958; Lehmann, 1980–81).

An important further advance was the appreciation that α-thalassaemia appeared to be determined by two distinct abnormal genes, designated α-thalassaemia-1 and α-thalassaemia-2, and that homozygotes for either gene or combined heterozygotes for both genes suffer from thalassaemia of widely different grades of severity, ranging from fatal hydrops fetalis through Hb-H disease to a silent trait, depending upon the combination of abnormal genes present (see p. 447). More recent work has shown that the genes for α globin are duplicated (Lehmann and Carrell, 1968; Lehmann, 1970) and that the different clinical severities of α-thalassaemia reflect the absence or dysfunction of not one or two, but of one, two, three or four genes (see Lehmann and Carrell, 1984) (see also p. 447).

β-thalassaemia also comprises several entities. Evidence for this has stemmed from the discovery that some apparent homozygotes for β-thalassaemia form Hb A, i.e., they synthesize some β chains, while others do not. The former have been designated β^+-thalassaemia, the latter β^0-thalassaemia (see p. 410). Within each group several types have been identified, based on genetic and/or molecular-biological evidence and on Hb-A_2 levels. In addition, there are the δβ (or βδ)-

thalassaemias (at one time referred to as F-thalassaemia), in which the failure to synthesize β chains is accompanied by failure to synthesize δ chains (Zuelzer, Robinson and Booker, 1961; Malamos, Fessas and Stamatoyannopoulos, 1962). In each group the percentage of Hb F present is increased, and where Hb-A production is totally suppressed in homozygotes this may reach almost 100% (Brancati and Baglioni, 1966).

Yet another group of variants leading to thalassaemia syndromes are the Hb Lepores which are the result of δ and β gene fusion leading to the non-α-chain being formed of δ globin at the amino end and β globin at the carboxyl end, and Hb Kenya in which the non-α-chain is a hybrid of γ-chain sequences at the amino end and β-chain sequences at the carboxyl end. And then there are the disorders that have been referred to as hereditary persistence of fetal hemoglobin (HPFH) in which failure to form β and δ chains is compensated by an increased formation of γ chains and hence Hb F.

All the above-mentioned variants, if present in homozygous form or combined with other thalassaemia variants or with structural haemoglobin defects in compound heterozygotes, or with Hb A, lead to a range of clinical syndromes — thalassaemia major, intermedia or minor — which vary widely in their clinical severity according to the nature and extent of the defect in haemoglobin synthesis (Table 18.1). Further details of the syndromes are given in subsequent sections of this Chapter.

α:β globin-chain ratios

In the early 1960s, the elaboration of a novel technique — the assessment of the relative rates at which the α- and β-globin chains of haemoglobin are synthesized within reticulocytes incubated in vitro in the presence of [^{14}C]leucine — provided a new and potent tool in the investigation of the apparent heterogeneity of thalassaemia. In brief, the α:β globin-chain ratio was shown by this technique to be greater than normal in the β-thalassaemias and to be less than normal in the α-thalassaemias.

Early studies by Marks and Burka (1964a,b) and Marks, Burka and Rifkind (1964) led them to conclude

Table 18.1 The β-thalassaemias: the effect of simple and compound heterozygosity and of homozygosity for β-thalassaemia genes on clinical presentation and haemoglobin.

'Genotype'	Clinical presentation	Hb A (%)	Hb A$_2$ (%)	Hb F (%)	Hb Lepore (%)
β^+/β^A	Thal minima or normal	c 95	3.5–7.0	0–6	
β^0/β^A	Thal minor	c 95	3.5–7.0	0–6	
β^+/β^+	Thal intermedia	25–65	1–4	30–70	
β^0/β^0	Thal major	0	1–4	>95	
β^0/β^+	Thal major or intermedia	<20	1–4	>75	
$\delta\beta^0/\beta^A$	Normal	80–85	<2.5	10–18	
$\delta\beta^0/\beta^+$	Thal intermedia	0–50	<2.5	45–95	
$\delta\beta^0/\beta^0$	Thal intermedia	0	0	100	
Lepore/β^A	Normal	80–85	2.0–2.5	1–13	5–18
Lepore/Lepore	Thal intermedia	0	0	70–90	9–30
Lepore/β^0	Thal major or intermedia	0	c 2.5	c 90	5–15

The figures given for percentages of haemoglobin are approximate; their wide range reflects genotypic heterogeneity. The 'genotypes' given are also only approximate: β^0 denotes a thalassaemia gene resulting in complete failure to form β chains; β^+ a thalassaemia gene resulting in partial failure to form β chains. β^A represents the normal haplotype.

that in thalassaemia the capacity of the polyribosomes of erythroid cells to synthesize Hb A was subnormal. Heywood, Karon and Weismann (1964; 1965) carried the research a stage further by demonstrating in four patients with thalassaemia major that when globin being synthesized by reticulocytes was labelled with [^{14}C]amino acids the specific activity of the β chains was consistently lower than that of the α chains. They concluded that their results were consistent with the hypothesis that in thalassaemia there was an increased production of the α-chain peptide relative to that of the β-chain peptide. Technical improvements initiated by Weatherall, Clegg and Naughton (1965) allowed the clear separation of the α, β, γ and δ chains of haemoglobin and the relatively accurate measurement of the total amounts of α and β chains synthesized. These and similar techniques have been widely applied with most fruitful results: a total or partial deficit of β-chain synthesis was soon demonstrated in all forms of β-thalassaemia (Bank and Marks, 1966; Conconi et al., 1968; Pontremoli, Bargellesi and Conconi, 1969; Weatherall et al., 1969; Banks and Marks, 1971; Nathan, 1972) (see also p. 501). Comparable deficiencies of α-chain synthesis have, too, been demonstrated in the α-thalassaemias (Clegg and Weatherall, 1967).

Early in this important and developing work it was found in thalassaemia that the relative rates of synthesis of the α and β chains altered during erythroid-cell maturation. Braverman and Bank (1969), who studied nine thalassaemia-major patients, found that β-chain synthesis was 1.5 times greater in nucleated erythroid precursors than in reticulocytes, and they suggested that this indicated a decay in β-chain synthesizing capacity as the cells developed (see also p. 501). They also found that γ-chain synthesis varied with the cells' maturity. In this case the synthesis in precursor cells was found to be only about half that in reticulocytes, and it was suggested that this might be due to the selective survival of cells with high rates of γ-chain synthesis.

Schwartz (1970) studied two thalassaemia-minor patients and found that the ratio of the synthesis of the α and β chains was normal in marrow nucleated cells; in contrast, the synthesis of β chains was significantly reduced in peripheral-blood reticulocytes. He concluded that β-chain messenger RNA was relatively unstable.

Subsequent work has demonstrated how the clinical severity of β-thalassaemia is closely correlated to the degree to which β-chain synthesis is impaired and to the extent to which the α:β globin-chain synthesis is unbalanced (see p. 501). A great deal of research, too, has been directed to the possible ways in which the synthesis of the globin chains may fail. Here the application of techniques of molecular biology has revealed how remarkably heterogeneous the thalassaemias are at the level of the genes controlling globin synthesis (see also p. 509).

Naturally, all this new and important work has been well documented in numerous reviews. Noteworthy, at the time they were written, were those of Marks and Gerald (1964), Marks (1966), Nathan and Gunn (1966), Silvestroni and Bianco (1966), Weatherall (1969), Bannerman (1972), Nathan (1972), Fessas and Loukopoulos (1974), Schwartz (1974), Benz and Forget (1974, 1975) and the monographs of Weatherall (1965) and Weatherall and Clegg (1972, 1981). Kan's (1983) account is particularly valuable as a summary of recent knowledge of the molecular-biological aspects of thalassaemia.

DISTRIBUTION AND RACIAL INCIDENCE

Thalassaemia was first considered to affect principally people living in the Central and Eastern Mediterranean regions and those who had emigrated (*e.g.* to North America) from these areas. Thus the disorder was considered to be particularly frequently encountered in Italy, Sardinia, Sicily and Greece and elsewhere in the Mediterranean islands and littoral. Later it came to be realized that thalassaemia was also to be found in many countries throughout the world — commonly in some, but less frequently in others — and to affect people of many races (Silver, 1950; March, Schlyen and Schwartz, 1952). Brumpt (1955) called attention to its frequency in the Far East and suggested that the disorder might have originated in China and suggested 'sinémie' as an alternative to 'thalassémie'.

The wide distribution of thalassaemia — a genetically-determined disease — raises some interesting questions. To some extent its distribution could be the consequence of the ancient or more modern migrations of Mediterranean peoples (as from Italy and Greece to the United States). Be this as it may, its marked genetic heterogeneity, and the prevalence of certain types of thalassaemia in particular areas, certainly indicate multiple foci of origin. The mechanism by which the abnormal genes have maintained themselves at a high incidence, despite the disease in homozygotes leading in many cases to early death, and the role of malaria in particular in maintaining this balanced polymorphism, are considered on page 398.

Early reports of the occurrence of thalassaemia in non-Mediterranean populations were listed in the 2nd edition of this book (Dacie, 1960, p. 204). These referred to cases diagnosed (mostly as thalassaemia minor) before the separation of thalassaemia into the α and β categories. In some instances (*e.g.* in certain of the English and Scottish cases) it is difficult to exclude the possibility of remote Mediterranean ancestors.

It is now known that the β- and α-thalassaemias, although found virtually world-wide, differ in their incidence in different regions. β-thalassaemia is particularly frequent in Italy, Sardinia and Sicily and in Greece and the Greek islands and in Cyprus and Malta. It occurs, too, but on the whole less frequently, in North and West Africa and in a broad belt extending eastwards from the Eastern Mediterranean through the Middle East (*e.g.* in Iran, Israel, Saudi Arabia, Syria and Turkey) to Pakistan and India and South-East Asia and China. β-thalassaemia is found, too, in Yugoslavia, particularly in Yugoslavian Macedonia, and in Bulgaria and Russia. It occurs, but is not common, in Southern France and Spain, and isolated cases have been reported from Northern Europe, *e.g.* from the United Kingdom, Germany, Holland, Norway and Finland, and from Switzerland.

In North America, β-thalassaemia occurs mainly in descendants of Italian and Greek immigrants and in blacks originating from West Africa. In Jamaica, the disorder is found chiefly in persons of West-African descent.

As Weatherall and Clegg (1981) pointed out in an extensive review, it is not easy to ascertain gene frequencies from the published data as in some instances the population studied has been small and not all the statistics have been based on data which satisfy the full diagnostic criteria for β-thalassaemia. It is clear, however, that the incidence of thalassaemia varies markedly within individual regions. For instance, in Italy its prevalence varies from well less than 5% to as high as 19% in some villages in the River Po delta while in Southern Sardinia its incidence may reach as high as 30% (Silvestroni and Bianco, 1975). In Greece, too, the percentage varies considerably according to the population group studied (Stamatoyannopoulos and Fessas, 1964).

α-thalassaemia is particularly frequent in South-East Asia, especially perhaps in Thailand. It is common, too, in China. It is also quite frequently met with in West Africa and hence in American blacks; it occurs, too, with varying frequency, in India, the Middle East and in Mediterranean countries. It is occasionally diagnosed in North Europeans.

Selected references to the occurrence of thalassaemia in the areas referred to above are set out below. Additional coverage of the literature is to be found in the reviews of Chernoff (1959), Bannerman (1961) and in Weatherall and Clegg's (1981) book.

SELECTED REFERENCES TO THE DISTRIBUTION AND FREQUENCY OF THALASSAEMIAS IN DIFFERENT POPULATIONS

Arabs

Vella and Hassan (1961): thalassaemia major in a Sudanese Arab family. Pembrey et al. (1975): Hb Bart's in Shiite Saudi Arabians. White et al. (1985): α- and β-thalassaemia common in Southern Peninsular Arabs.

Armenians

Vella (1961): microcythaemia in 27% of Armenians in Khartoum.

Bantu

Stijns and Charles (1956): two families; thalassaemia associated with Hb S

British (English and Scots)

Israels, Suderman and Hoogstraten (1955): thalassaemia minor in three generations of a Scottish family. Israëls and Turner (1955): target-cell anaemia in two British families. Havard, Lehmann and Bodley Scott (1958): thalassaemia minor in an English woman of East Anglian stock. Callender, Mallet and Lehmann (1961): 25 individuals in three families with heterozygous thalassaemia. Buchanan et al. (1963): five cases of thalassaemia major and 11 symptomless carriers in four Scottish families. Roberts (1963): nine members of an English family had thalassaemia trait. Lloyd and Brown (1964): homozygous thalassaemia in an English child. Knox-Macaulay et al. (1973): 116 individuals with various thalassaemia syndromes (83 in 16 families were β-thalassaemia heterozygotes). Cook and Lehmann (1973): 17 cases of thalassaemia minor out of 3968 random blood samples from the Highlands of Scotland.

Bucharan Jews

Schieber (1945): two adults with target-cell anaemia.

Bulgarians

Panoff (1936): two cases of Cooley's anaemia.

Burmese

Perabo (1954): two children; one with thalassaemia major, the other probably with thalassaemia minor.

Canadians

Dauphinee and Langley (1967): four out of six families with thalassaemia minor had no known Mediterranean ancestry. Ing et al. (1968): five cases of Hb-H disease in Oriental-Canadian families.

Ceylonese

de Silva, Jonxis and Wickramasinghe (1959): nine cases of thalassaemia major. Nagaratham and Sukumaran (1967): Hb-H disease as well as β-thalassaemia.

Chinese

Foster (1940): Cooley's syndrome in a child. DeMarsh and Boyce (1950): severe Mediterranean anaemia in a child. Silverberg and Shotton (1951): seven cases of thalassaemia minor. Siddoo et al. (1956): three cases of thalassaemia major and 11 of thalassaemia trait in Chinese Canadians. McFadzean and Todd (1964): 485 families or individual patients with Cooley's anaemia seen in Hong Kong between 1949 and 1963; concluded that the gene is widely distributed throughout China. Lin and Yu (1965): Hb-H disease in two unrelated Chinese families. Lin et al. (1965): Hb-H disease in Taiwan. Choi and Necheles (1983): α-thalassaemia and (to a lesser extent) β-thalassaemia frequent amongst Chinese in Boston. Yang et al. (1985): the incidence of β-thalassaemia and of α-thalassaemia and of positive tests for Hb Bart's in cord blood, based on surveys of many thousands of individuals resident in a wide range of regions.

Cypriots

Fawdry (1944): 20 cases of Cooley's anaemia. Banton (1951): about 20% of 532 children had thalassaemia trait; the incidence in those of Greek and Turkish origin about the same. Plato, Rucknagel and Gershowitz (1964): minimal estimate of thalassaemia trait about 5%. Modell, Benson and Payling Wright (1972): 14% of Cypriots in London have the β-thalassaemia trait. Ashiotis et al. (1973): 15% of Greek and Turkish Cypriots carry β-thalassaemia genes, 10% α-thalassaemia genes.

Dutch

de Vries and van Valkenburg (1953): nine members of

a Dutch family had thalassaemia minor. Schokker, Went and Bok (1966): two Dutch homozygotes about 40 years of age with relatively mild symptoms; their parents and siblings had the blood picture of thalassaemia minor with unusually high Hb-A$_2$ (5.3–7.6) and Hb-F (5.1–14.4) percentages.

Egyptians and Egyptian-Sudanese

Vella and Moussa (1962): thalassaemia minor present in 23% of Egyptian children.

Ethiopians

Vella (1961): microcythaemia in four out of 12 Ethiopians in Khartoum.

Filipinos

Lazar (1956): thalassaemia trait in a Hawaiian family of Filipino extraction.

Germans

Graser (1941): a probable case of Cooley's erythroblastic anaemia in girl. Heilmeyer, Müller and Schubothe (1951): thalassaemia minor in two families. Pribilla (1951): thalassaemia minor in three generations. Middlebrook (1956): thalassaemia minor in three generations. Nowicki et al. (1963): a family from Baden with thalassaemia. Flatz, Hauke and Kleihauer (1964): a case of thalassaemia major. Rönisch and Kleihauer (1967): α-thalassaemia with Hb H and Hb Bart's in a German family.

Greeks

Fessas (1959b): a review — 'thalassaemia is by far the most frequent of the hereditary anaemias in Greece'. Vella and Ibrahim (1961): 29% of 553 Greeks or Greek-Cypriot children had thalassaemia minor. Malamos, Fessas and Stamatoyannopoulos (1962): 7.44% of 1600 healthy Greek males had the thalassaemia trait. Stamatoyannopoulos and Fessas (1964): incidence of thalassaemia varied between 6.1 and 19.3% in five different areas.

Gurkhas

Weatherall and Vella (1960): a thalassaemia-like disease in a young Gurkha girl.

Gypsies

Zilliacus and Ottelin (1963): possible occurrence of thalassaemia trait in six gypsies in Finland. Cabrera and de Pablos (1984): β-thalassaemia minor common in gypsies in the south of Spain.

Indians

Mukherji (1938): Cooley's anaemia in a Hindu child. Napier, Shorten and Das Gupta (1939): a case of Cooley's anaemia. Dhayagude (1944): erythroblastic anaemia of Cooley in a Brahmin boy. Ganguli and Lahiri (1955): 11 cases of Cooley's anaemia in Hindus. Siddoo et al. (1956): thalassaemia in Sikhs in Vancouver. Labie, Rosa and Paviot (1961): 20% of population in Madras region had raised Hb-A$_2$ levels. Chatterjea (1959, 1966): reviews. Chouhan, Sharma and Parekh (1970): α-thalassaemia in India. Walford and Deacon (1976): a mild form of α-thalassaemia in Indians in the United Kingdom. Thein et al. (1984): genetic studies on 64 families with β-thalassaemia living in the United Kingdom. Dash (1985): 3.6% of healthy Punjabi blood donors have β-thalassaemia trait.

Indonesians

Lie-Injo and Jo (1955): three cases of Cooley's anaemia. Lie-Injo et al. (1959): 21 cases of Cooley's anaemia. Lie-Injo (1959b): a review.

Iranians

Nuyken (1954): two cases of thalassaemia major and 73 cases of thalassaemia minor or minima. Pouya (1959): 39 patients with thalassaemia major or minor. Nasab (1979): 141 cases of homozygous β-thalassaemia.

Iraquis

Hindawi and Subhiyah (1962): 14 cases of thalassaemia major. Taj-Eldin et al. (1968): 25 cases of thalassaemia major; one case of probable αβ-thalassaemia.

Italians

Silvestroni and Bianco (1948): frequency of thalassaemia in the Po delta. Silvestroni and Bianco (1959): extensive data on incidence of thalassaemia in different areas in Italy. Silvestroni and Bianco (1975): analysis of results of screening for microcytemia in Italy over a 30-year period; β- to α-thalassaemia ratio in 46 559 students at Rome University approximately 7.4:1.0. Schilirò et al. (1978): haematological and biosynthetic studies of β-thalassaemia in Sicily. Pepe, Lupi and Luzzatto (1980): genetic and biochemical heterogeneity of β-thalassaemia in Naples.

Jamaicans

Ahern et al. (1975): β-thalassaemia intermedia in five adults.

Japanese

Imamura, Ohta and Hanada (1968): α-thalassaemia in a Japanese girl associated with a malignant thymoma and carbonic anhydrase deficiency.

Kurdish Jews

Matoth, Shamir and Freundlich (1955): four severe cases of thalassaemia major and three less severe cases. Ramot et al. (1964): thalassaemia trait common in Kurdish and Indian Jews in Israel. Horowitz et al. (1966): both α- and β-thalassaemia demonstrated in Kurdish Jews in Israel. Cohen et al. (1966): five cases of Hb-H disease; one probable.

Kuwaitis

Ali (1969): Hb-H disease in an adult male.

Liberians

Olesen et al. (1959): two children with thalassaemia major; incidence of thalassaemia minor or minima at least 11%.

Malaysians

Lopez and Lie-Injo (1971): α-thalassaemia in newborns in West Malaysia.

Maltese

Vella (1962): incidence of thalassaemia minor in Malta 4–5%; in Gozo 6–7%. Cauchi (1970): incidence of thalassaemia heterozygotes approximately 3.5%.

Nigerians

Esan (1970): incidence of β-thalassaemia trait low (slightly less than 1%); that of Hb Bart's at birth 4.5%.

Norwegians

Evensen, Jeremic and Hjort (1969): heterozygous β-thalassaemia in three generations of a Scandinavian family.

Oriental Jews

Dreyfuss (1955): thalassaemia minor in three families.

Papua New Guineans

Ryan (1961a,b): four cases of thalassaemia major. Oppenheimer et al. (1984): Hb Bart's detected in 81% of 217 infants born on the north coast of Papua New Guinea.

Pathans

Stern, Kynoch and Lehmann (1968): five out of 129 Pathans had β-thalassaemia minor.

Portuguese

Tamagnini et al. (1983): 10 families with a mild form of β^+-thalassaemia.

Russians

Idelson and Didkowsky (1971): Hb H in two brothers: α-thalassaemia in four relatives.

Sardinians

Carcassi, Ceppellini and Pitzus (1957): frequency of thalassaemia in relation to distribution of malaria. Siniscalco et al. (1961): thalassaemia trait (and favism) and their relationship to malaria. Cao et al. (1978): thalassaemia types and their high incidence in Sardinia. Campanacci, Broccia and Fiumano (1962): Hb-H disease in Sardinia.

Spaniards

Vayá et al. (1983): comparison of haematological and clinical data in F-thalassaemia and A_2-thalassaemia traits.

Sudanese

Hassan and Ziada (1965): a case of thalassaemia major.

Swedes

Hedenberg et al. (1958): Hb-H disease in a Swedish family. Persson et al. (1967): β-thalassaemia minor in two Swedish families. Persson et al. (1969): high prevalence of β-thalassaemia in a third Swedish family.

Swiss

Rohr (1943): anerythroblastic type of Cooley's anaemia in a 60-year-old female and in her son and daughter. Dankwa et al. (1975): 2.6% of 2672 patients with a thalassaemia syndrome diagnosed between 1968 and 1974 were of Swiss origin and were β-thalassaemia heterozygotes.

Syrians

Vella (1961): microcythaemia in 18% of Syrians in Khartoum. Ali (1969): two cases of haemoglobin-H disease. Ibrahim and Barakat (1970): 12 children with β-thalassaemia minor.

Thais

Minnich et al. (1954): 32 patients with Mediterranean anaemia, 17 of whom were splenectomized. Na-Nakorn (1959): a review. Flatz, Pik and Sringam (1965): 11 families with thalassaemia; in 10, Hb E present in addition. Wasi, Na-Nakorn and Suindumrong (1964): Hb-H disease in Thailand; a genetical study. Wasi et al. (1969): α- and β-thalassaemia in Thailand. Poortrakul, Wasi and Na-Nakorn (1973): haematological findings in β-thalassaemia. Wasi et al. (1980): incidence of different types of thalassaemia in Thailand.

Tibetans

Jackson, Lehmann and Sharih (1960): β-thalassaemia in an elderly Sherpa.

Turks

Aksoy et al. (1958): thalassaemia in Turks and Eti-Turks. Aksoy (1959): a review. Dinçol, Aksoy and Erdem (1979): a study of 164 β-thalassaemia heterozygotes.

United States blacks

Schwartz and Mason (1949), Schwartz and Hartz (1955): two families with thalassaemia; comparison with Hb-C disease. Norris, Hanson and Loeffler (1956): Mediterranean anaemia in an adult. Scott, Ferguson and Jenkins (1962): two cases of thalassaemia major. Weatherall (1964a): 54 β-thalassaemia heterozygotes. Pearson (1966): αβ-thalassaemia in a family. McCurdy (1967): thalassaemia in six adult women; one had superimposed auto-immune haemolytic anaemia. Crouch, Maurer and Valdas (1970): probable (mild) homozygous β-thalassaemia in a child. Friedman et al. (1974): α-thalassaemia in infants. Charache et al. (1974): a review. Schwartz

and Atwater (1972): α-thalassaemia in American blacks. Pierce et al. (1977): frequency of thalassaemia in American blacks.

United States Europeans

Neel and Valentine (1945): 4% of people of Southern Italian or Sicilian origin living in Rochester, N.Y., had thalassaemia minor.

Yemenite and Iraqui Jews

Zaizov and Matoth (1972): Hb Bart's present in cord blood of 17% of Yemenite infants and in 11% of Iraqui infants.

Yugoslavians

Efremov et al (1969): two families with β-thalassaemia illustrating different severity of expression in homozygotes.

West Indians

Went and MacIver (1961): five types of thalassaemia identified.

MALARIA AND THALASSAEMIA

Lehmann wrote in 1959 that 'Everything points towards a regulation of the incidence of thalassaemia by a balanced polymorphism similar to that found to determine the incidence of sickling'; he added that it was thalassaemia for which J. B. S. Haldane in 1949 had proposed the relatively greater protection of the heterozygote against malaria. This hypothesis is now generally accepted as being true. Lehmann (1959), however, made the additional point that although there is an association between the severity of malaria (in a geographical location) and the frequency of the thalassaemia gene, the reverse does not apply. That is to say, where thalassaemia is present there is now or has been in the past much malaria; but thalassaemia is not found everywhere where malaria is to be found, 'not even in Italy and Greece, and certainly not in Africa and Asia'. Lehmann also pointed out that abnormal haemoglobins and thalassaemia had not been recorded in Australian aborigines and that Australia was free of malaria until this was introduced by Europeans.

Weatherall and Clegg (1981, p. 312) reviewed the historical and more recent evidence suggestive of a close link between the geographical incidence of thalassaemia and the occurrence of malaria. The literature they cited indicated that this close link is clearly true in, for instance, the Po valley in Italy, and in Sardinia, but less obviously so in Greece, Cyprus, Malta, Sudan, New Guinea and Thailand (see also Choremis et al. 1963; Siniscalco et al., 1966; Carcassi, 1974).

Luzzatto, writing in 1985, stated that in his opinion: 'It seems inconceivable that so many independently arisen mutant genes, each causing severe or total loss of reproductive fitness in the homozygous state, could have increased in frequency in many populations in the absence of a selective agent, and from geographical considerations malaria remains the one and obvious candidate.'

In recent years much research and effort has been directed to the question as to how the presence of malaria could influence the incidence of thalassaemia — in particular, how an infant who is a heterozygote for thalassaemia could have an improved chance of survival in the first year or two of life compared with a normal infant of the same vulnerable age living in the same environment and exposed to a similar risk of contracting and dying from malaria.

The recently acquired ability to culture malaria parasites in vitro has provided a means of testing various hypotheses. One possible factor which might be inimical to the development of the parasites within erythrocytes is the concentration of Hb F. Evidence in favour of this hypothesis has in fact been obtained in short-term culture experiments using Pl. falciparum and the erythrocytes of infants and adults containing increased percentages of Hb F (Pasvol, Weatherall and Wilson, 1977). It is interesting to note that the possible protective role of Hb F had been mentioned by Lehmann as far back as 1953. He had written: 'It may not be a coincidence that the decline in the "natural resistance" of the newborn to malaria takes place when it loses its foetal haemoglobin.'

The presence of high concentrations of Hb F does not seem, however, to be the only factor which helps to protect the thalassaemia erythrocyte from the malarial parasite. Friedman (1979), for instance, obtained evidence of impaired multiplication of Pl. falciparum in thalassaemia-trait erythrocytes (and also in G6PD$^-$ and Hb-F-containing erythrocytes) when the cells were exposed to oxidant damage; and Nurse (1979) stressed the possible protective importance of a low MCH, on the assumption that haemoglobin is an important nutrient for plasmodia and provides the parasites with the ferrous iron they need for their own enzyme systems.

α-thalassaemia. The work cited above has mostly been concerned with the influence of malaria on the occurrence of β-thalassaemia. There is, however, increasing evidence that the frequency of α-thalassaemia has been similarly influenced. Recent epidemiological evidence in favour of this hypothesis includes the studies of Oppenheimer et al. (1984) in relation to Papua New Guinea, Ramsey and Jenkins (1984) in relation to Africa and Bowden et al. (1985) in relation to Melanesia.

Laboratory evidence, too, supports the hypothesis that the presence of endemic malaria has encouraged the persistence of α-thalassaemia. Thus Ifediba and co-workers (1985) studied the growth of Pl. falciparum in erythrocytes of different α genotypes and found that the cells of five black Hb-H disease patients, four of whom were $--/-\alpha$ genotype, supported the growth of the parasites substantially less well than did normal αα/αα cells. Whether growth was impaired in $-\alpha/-\alpha$ cells was uncertain; in $-\alpha/\alpha\alpha$ cells, on the other hand, it was clearly normal. In all the cell samples tested, with the exception of one atypical Hb-H disease case, the Hb-F percentage was less than 1.6.

CLINICAL AND HAEMATOLOGICAL FEATURES OF THE THALASSAEMIAS

The clinical effects of thalassaemia vary greatly according to the degree to which the production of haemoglobin is impaired. At one extreme α-thalassaemia, in its severest form, leads to death *in utero* (the Hb-Bart's fetal hydrops syndrome); at the other extreme, the carrier state for α- and β-thalassaemia (thalassaemia minor or minima) is generally harmless and those affected have few if any symptoms and are likely to be but mildly anaemic or to have no anaemia at all, as judged by haemoglobin level. Between these two extremes are found Cooley's anaemia (β-thalassaemia major), a severe disorder often resulting in death in childhood in the absence of repeated blood transfusions and various grades of thalassaemia intermedia, as well as Hb-H disease, which are accompanied by chronic but generally not life-threatening anaemia.

The essential feature of all types of thalassaemia — failure to synthesize haemoglobin normally — results in the formation of erythrocytes deficient in haemoglobin content and mostly smaller in volume than normal and which vary unusually greatly in size and shape, *i.e.*, there is (in haematological jargon) hypochromasia, microcytosis and excessive anisocytosis and poikilocytosis. As could be anticipated, the worse the defect in haemoglobin synthesis, the more abnormal are the erythrocytes the patient manages to produce.

β-THALASSAEMIA MAJOR (HOMOZYGOUS β-THALASSAEMIA: COOLEY'S ANAEMIA)

The disease is usually diagnosed in the first year of life, anaemia often becoming marked when the infant is a few months old. Pallor is the predominant sign and this is accompanied by swelling of the abdomen due to enlargement of the spleen and liver. There may be slight icterus of the conjunctivae but overt jaundice is unusual. Purpura and lymph-node enlargement do not as a rule occur. Bouts of pyrexia are not infrequent. How the child develops subsequently depends on whether or not

it receives adequate and repeated blood transfusions. If it does not, the signs and symptoms so well recorded in the early reports of Cooley's anaemia develop (see below).

A child (not supported by blood transfusion) fails to thrive and becomes emaciated: body fat is reduced in amount; the limbs become more and more spindly and the abdomen more and more protruberant; as in Hb-SS disease the bones may be tender. Striking skeletal changes occur. As the child grows, widening of the diploe of the cranial and facial bones leads to enlargement and bossing of the skull and often to a mongoloid appearance (Cooley and Lee, 1925: Cooley, Witwer and Lee, 1927; Logothetis *et al.*, 1972; etc.). The teeth in the maxilla become exposed and the bridge of the nose becomes depressed. Maturation of the bones is retarded (Erlandson, Brilliant and Smith, 1964).

According to Logothetis and co-workers (1971), cephalofacial deformities were obvious in 94 out of 138 Greek children with thalassaemia major. They are secondary to enlargement of the bone-marrow cavities as the result of the marked hyperplasia of erythropoietic marrow which dates from early childhood. Three categories of deformity were defined, and could be positively correlated with other stigmata of severity, such as degree of anaemia, age of onset of requirement for blood transfusion and enlargement of the liver and spleen. The deformities were, however, not accompanied by intellectual impairment

Radiological examination of the bones of an inadequately transfused child typically reveals thinning of the cortical compact bone and resorption of trabeculae. The outer table of the skull becomes extremely thin and characteristic perpendicular striae often appear between the inner and outer tables (Cooley, Witwer and Lee, 1927; Baty, Blackfan and Diamond, 1932; Caffey, 1937, 1951, 1957; Baker, 1964; Moseley, 1974; etc.) (Fig. 18.1).

Skeletal fractures occur with unusual frequency. Erlandson, Brilliant and Smith (1964) reported that 10 out of 21 patients with severe Cooley's anaemia had suffered a total of 27 fractures, mostly of the arm or forearm, as the result of falls.

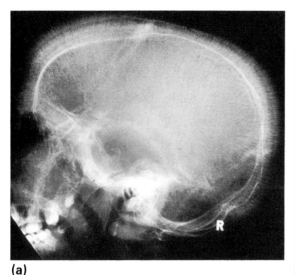

(a)

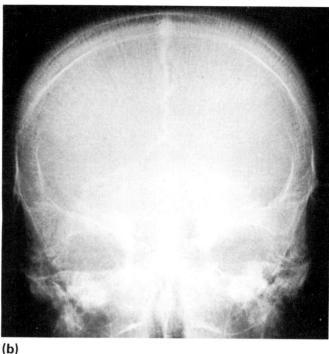

(b)

Fig. 18.1 X-ray photographs of the skull of a child with β-thalassaemia major. (a) Lateral view; (b) antero-posterior view.
  Shows well-marked hair-on-end appearance.
(Reproduced by courtesy of Dr Elizabeth Letsky.)

Irrespective of fractures, skeletal pain is not uncommon and is probably associated with increased erythropoiesis; it can be relieved by blood transfusion (Smith *et al.*, 1955).

Variation in clinical severity

Not all patients who have been diagnosed as suffering from β-thalassaemia major are affected to the same degree. In Italy, for instance, several grades of the disease were at one time recognized. Astaldi, Tolentino and Sacchetti (1951) referred to three degrees of severity: (1) a severe form causing serious anaemia early in infancy and often resulting in death in the first year; (2) a slightly less severe form of the disease usually first becoming manifest in the second half of the first year, the child often surviving until school age; and (3) a milder form usually diagnosed in the second year of life, and compatible with survival until adult life. Bone lesions were particularly conspicuous in patients belonging to the second and third groups.

The early literature dealing with the occurrence of what was considered to be thalassaemia major in patients surviving until adult life was reviewed by March, Schlyen and Schwartz (1952) who added two more (Italian) cases of their own. Currin and Lieberman (1951) and Sansone and Noceto (1955) reported two further cases, also in Italians; and Polosa and Ferreri (1956) described three further patients who survived until 33, 20 and 16 years of age, respectively. Fessas (1959a) gave details of adult patients seen in Greece, apparently homozygous for thalassaemia, whose illness was of 'intermediate' clinical severity

Mildness is also a characteristic feature of the disease as it occurs in American blacks (see below). More recently, too, a mild form has been found to occur in a small area of North Portugal (Tamagnini *et al.*, 1983).

β-thalassaemia in American blacks: a clinically mild form

As mentioned above, β-thalassaemia in American blacks is generally clinically less severe than in heterozygotes or homozygotes of Italian or Greek origin. American blacks thought to be homozygotes have, for instance, lived to adult life without needing to be transfused (Crouch, Maurer and Valdes, 1970; Braverman *et al.*, 1973; Charache *et al.*, 1974). One such adult patient was said to have even undergone 14 pregnancies (Heller *et al.*, 1966). The cause of the mild expression is not wholly clear. Braverman and co-workers (1973) found no significant difference in the degree to which β-chain synthesis was impaired in six American black patients thought to have homozygous β-thalassaemia and seven patients of Mediterranean origin whose illness was much more severe; they suggested that increased γ-chain production might in part be responsible.

Genetic heterogeneity as an explanation for the mild expression of β-thalassaemia

The rapid progress in recent years in the molecular-biological analysis of β-thalassaemia has shown conclusively that some apparent homozygotes are in reality compound heterozygotes for two distinct types of β-thalassaemia, or bear in addition a gene or genes for α-thalassaemia. Thus Kattamis and co-workers (1979) found that certain apparent homozygotes were in fact compound heterozygotes for high Hb-A_2 β-thalassaemia and normal Hb-A_2 β-thalassaemia, the latter being minimally expressed in heterozygotes and commonly referred to as 'silent' thalassaemia. Weatherall and his co-workers (1981b) concluded that about 20% of apparent homozygotes for β-thalassaemia in some Mediterranean and S.E. Asian populations were in addition heterozygotes for a gene for deletion α-thalassaemia (genotype $-\alpha/\alpha\alpha$) or a non-deletion type ($\alpha\alpha^T/\alpha\alpha$), the effect in both cases being less unbalanced chain synthesis and a milder clinical expression.

Weatherall and his co-workers (1985) in a later review emphasized how the localization and nature of the β-thalassaemia mutation within the β-globin gene complex, as well as the patient's α-globin genotype, his ability to form γ globin and his β-globin gene haplotype, all play a part in determining his ultimate phenotype.

Further details of 'silent' β-thalassaemia, δβ-thalassaemia (F-thalassaemia), γβ-thalassaemia, γδβ-thalassaemia and compound heterozygosity for β-thalassaemia and Hb Lepore, or hereditary persistence of fetal haemoglobin (HPFH), and of the effect of the loss of one or more α-globin genes on the clinical severity of β-thalassaemia, are given

in subsequent sections of this Chapter. The discovery, definition and molecular-genetic analysis of all these variants illustrate the vast strides that have been made in the understanding of the complexity of the thalassaemias, particularly in the last two decades.

COMPLICATIONS OF HOMOZYGOSITY FOR β-THALASSAEMIA

A wide range of complications develop in the homozygous β-thalassaemic child, their severity depending essentially on the degree to which β-chain synthesis is impaired and also on how often and how regularly the child is transfused. These complications include (in alphabetical order) cardiac impairment, endocrine dysfunction, gallstone formation, gout, hypersplenism, hypocalcaemia and hypomagnesaemia, impairment of growth and development, iron overload, neuromuscular problems, proneness to infections, ulceration of the leg and vitamin deficiencies. Weatherall and Clegg (1981) reviewed the relevant literature in detail. A brief discussion follows.

Cardiac impairment

As in other chronic anaemias of different pathogenesis, long-standing severe anaemia in an inadequately transfused thalassaemic child is associated with enlargement of the heart and a hyperdynamic circulation. In the second decade, iron overloading of the myocardium becomes, even in the untransfused patient, an important cause of cardiac failure in addition to the anoxia attributable to the anaemia. Cardiac arrhythmias are a common feature in such cases and sudden death may occur (Engle, 1964). Pericarditis, too, has been observed, the incidence being possibly greatest in splenectomized patients (Smith *et al.*, 1955, 1962; Orsini *et al.*, 1970). In the regularly transfused patient iron overloading of the myocardium is a frequent cause of death, and the prevention of this is an important objective of iron chelation therapy (see p. 547).

More recently Ehlers and co-workers (1980) have reported on a longitudinal study of cardiac function in 93 patients, all but three of whom were transfusion-dependent, prior to chelation therapy. Complications included pericarditis and disturbances of conduction. Death, when it occurred, was usually due to cardiac failure. Marni and co-workers (1983) reported on the echocardiographic findings in 32 thalassaemia-major children, aged between 3 and 15 years, who had been treated by long-term blood transfusion. None showed signs of congestive cardiac failure at the time of testing; morphological and functional abnormalities were, however, demonstrated in 56% of them.

Deafness and nasal obstruction

Hazell and Modell (1976) and McIntosh (1976) have described the development of deafness, due apparently to invasion of the middle ear by erythropoietic tissue. Hazell and Modell also recorded nasal obstruction resulting from hypertrophy of the turbinate bones.

Endocrine dysfunction

Impairment of growth is an important accompaniment of thalassaemia major (see p. 404); it is but one consequence of dysfunction which tends to affects most of the endocrine organs. Iron overloading is probably the most important cause and diabetes the most important sequel.

In an early study of 13 patients (six necropsies, seven biopsies) Ellis, Schulman and Smith (1954) found evidence for widespread visceral siderosis plus fibrosis of the liver and pancreas in four cases. In three patients the changes seemed anatomically to be the same as in haemochromatosis; in others, they were less severe. One patient had diabetes. More recent information has been summarized by Weatherall and Clegg (1981, pp. 159–161). Delay of puberty is well documented, but studies of other aspects of pituitary function have given inconsistent results, as have studies of adrenal function. Mild impairment of thyroid or parathyroid function has been detected in some patients. According to Canale and co-workers (1974), pituitary, adrenal, thyroid and gonadal function is, however, normal in most patients, irrespective of whether they have been transfused.

Gallstone formation

As in other chronic haemolytic anaemias, pigment gallstones frequently form (Currin and Lieberman, 1951; Smith and Morgenthau, 1951; Dewey, Grossman and Canale, 1970).

Gout

Secondary gout is a well-documented complication, according to Weatherall and Clegg (1981, p. 167), but it seems to be uncommon. Hyperuricaemia is, on the other hand, commonly present, according to Rosmino, Norelli and Ghidella (1968).

Haemorrhagic symptoms

An abnormal tendency to bleed has been reported in some patients with thalassaemia major. Hilgartner and Smith (1964), for instance, stated that of 66 patients under their care many had experienced epistaxis and in some this had been severe enough to warrent blood transfusion. Bentorello, Pescetto and Bo (1977) instanced a 14-year-old boy who had suffered from severe epistaxis in whom there was some evidence of a consumption coagulopathy. Eldor (1978a) described 15 patients aged between 4 and 21 years, all but two having undergone splenectomy: nine gave a history of easy bruising and 11 had had recurrent epistaxis. In vitro, there was some evidence of impaired platelet aggregation (see p. 408).

Hypersplenism

Progressive enlargement of the spleen is the rule in the inadequately transfused child. Occasionally, massive splenomegaly is associated with marked thrombocytopenia, moderate neutropenia, trapping of the patient's (and transfused) erythrocytes in the spleen pulp and a striking expansion of the total blood volume and plasma volume. In such patients the survival of transfused normal erythrocytes has been shown to be impaired, and to be markedly improved by splenectomy, e.g., by Lichtman et al. (1953), McElfresh, Sharpstein and Akabane (1955) and Smith et al. (1955). Reemstma and Elliott (1956) concluded, as the result of a long-term follow-up study, that splenectomy was more beneficial in this group of patients than in those in whom there was no presumptive evidence of hypersplenism (see also p. 559).

Hypocalcaemia and hypomagnesaemia

Hypocalcaemia and subnormal excretion of calcium in the urine was described by Erlandson *et al.* (1964) in eight out of 11 severely affected patients. The cause of this finding is uncertain. [It is interesting to note that Cooley, Witwer and Lee reported in 1927 a low serum calcium and a negative calcium balance in one patient.] Erlandson and co-workers also reported that serum magnesium might be subnormal, and gave data on lowered magnesium excretion in the urine in eight patients. Later, Hyman and co-workers (1980) described hypomagnesaemia in five of 17 children being treated by transfusion and Desferal. They had complained of muscular pain and spasms and depression and were said to improve on magnesium therapy.

Impairment of growth and development

Growth as a whole is usually retarded, and exceptionally this may lead to dwarfism similar to that resulting from pituitary hypofunction (de Muro and Leonardi, 1950). Erlandson, Brilliant and Smith (1964) made the point that the affected child's height is normal or close to normal early but is likely to be definitely subnormal should the child survive to adolescence. According to Johnston, Hertzog and Malina (1966), the rate of growth is nearly normal in infants up to the age of 4 years. From thereon the growth rate is consistently slower and there is likely to be no pubertal spurt in height or weight.

Extensive studies on 138 Greek patients aged 2–28 years were reported by Logothetis and co-workers (1972). Height and weight were found to be subnormal in most children over 4 years of age, retardation in growth becoming clearly significant in children aged 9 or 10. Subnormal height and weight did not appear to be clearly correlated with anaemia; they were, however, significantly correlated with spleen and liver size.

In children adequately supported by regular blood transfusions some improvement can be expected. Even so, most affected children do not grow as well as do their normal siblings (Weatherall and Clegg, 1981, p. 162).

Iron overload

Generalized iron overloading has been recognized for many years as a frequent and important complication of thalassaemia major. Particularly, of course, is this so in patients who have received many transfusions, as in a child aged 10 who died having received almost 77 litres of blood (Frumin, Waldman and Morris, 1952). However, even in the absence of regular transfusions a moderate or even a marked amount of excess iron may accumulate in the liver, heart, kidneys, pancreas and other organs (Whipple and Bradford, 1936; Astaldi, Tolentino and Sacchetti, 1951; Currin, 1954; etc.). In such cases the iron overloading appears to result from excessive absorption from the intestine (see also Robertson, Maxwell and Elliott, 1963). The harmful effect of iron overloading on cardiac function and the endocrine organs has already been briefly referred to; and its possible role in promoting infections is mentioned on page 405. The effect of iron on the liver is referred to on page 498.

An unusual complication — the sicca syndrome, clinically closely similar to Sjögren's syndrome, was reported by Borgna-Pignatti and co-workers (1984) in a 20-year-old man who had received many blood transfusions. A heavy infiltration of the salivary glands with iron was thought to be the cause.

Recently, Gorodetsky and co-workers (1985) have used X-ray spectrometry, a method based on X-ray fluorescence analysis, to determine in a non-invasive way the concentration of iron (and zinc) in two skin areas, representing predominantly dermal (flexor surface of arm) and epidermal (thenar eminence) tissues, respectively, in 56 patients with thalassaemia major or intermedia. The mean iron levels in both skin areas were increased by more than 200% and 50%, respectively, compared with control values. The method was considered to be potentially useful in monitoring the clearance of iron overload as the result of the use of chelation agents.

For data on serum-iron levels in thalassaemia major, see page 413.

Neuromuscular problems

These are uncommon. However, Logothetis and co-workers (1972) reported that 26 out of 138 patients who were being supported by periodic blood transfusions developed a myopathic syndrome with proximal weakness mainly affecting the legs. Sinniah, Vignaendra and Ahmad (1977) reported the occurrence of transient major motor seizures in two cases, perhaps the consequence of cerebral venous infarction.

Proneness to infections

It is generally believed that children suffering from thalassaemia major are more prone to severe bacterial infections than are normal children. The cause of this is not clear: probably several adverse factors, of which iron overload is one, bring this about (see Weatherall and Clegg, 1981, p. 164). Modell (1976) considered that the incidence of infections was lower in children receiving adequate and regular blood transfusions. Splenectomy, on the other hand, seems without doubt to increase their incidence and to lead in some cases to overwhelming and often fatal septicaemia and/or meningitis. In an early report on this important topic, Smith and co-workers (1962) reported that of 33 children with Cooley's anaemia who had been splenectomized seven had suffered from severe infections and five had died in consequence: in contrast, of 23 non-splenectomized Cooley's-anaemia children, three had had severe infections but none of them had died. Smith and co-workers also stated that, according to the literature, the majority of such infections had occurred within 2 years of splenectomy.

Renal function

This is not usually significantly impaired in β-thalassaemia major. According to Khalifa *et al.* (1985) the blood urea, serum creatinine and urinary β$_2$-microglobulin levels did not differ significantly from normal in a group of 45 Egyptian children and young adolescents being treated by regular blood transfusion. Microscopic haematuria was, however, detected in 67% of the patients and ultrasonography demonstrated abnormal findings in 15.5%, all of whom had haematuria. Renal biopsy in five patients revealed evidence of moderate and diffuse thickening of capillary walls, with segmental and focal cellular proliferation in glomeruli.

Ulceration of the leg

Intractable ulcers of the leg occasionally develop (Estes, Farber and Stickney, 1948; March, Schlyen and Schwartz, 1952; Pascher and Keen, 1957).

Pascher and Keen suggested that ulceration results from a combination of factors, including the effect of stasis, long-continued anaemia and trauma. Their patients (Italians) were aged 14–32 years and it seems likely that they were suffering from thalassaemia intermedia. The same is true of the three Italian patients of Estes, Farber and Stickney (1948) who were aged 19, 23 and 30 years, respectively.

Vitamin deficiencies

Deficiencies of vitamin C (Choremis, Economou-Mavrou and Gregoriou, 1961; Wapnick *et al.*, 1969) and vitamin E (Hyman *et al.*, 1974) have been described, but the clinical significance of these laboratory observations is uncertain. Rachmilewitz, Shifter and Kahane (1979) reported that no benefit appeared to result from the administration of vitamin-E supplements.

Zaino, Yeh and Aloia (1985) assessed vitamin-D metabolism, and serum calcium and parathyroid function, in 16 thalassaemia-major patients of Italian or Greek extraction all of whom were receiving regular transfusion: three had severe hypocalcaemia and most had low serum vitamin D [25 OHD and 1,25-(OH)$_2$D] levels. These changes were thought to be secondary effects of iron overloading on liver function.

Folate deficiency is well known to occur not uncommonly, and benefit has followed the administration of folic acid in some cases (Jandl and Greenberg, 1959; Luhby and Cooperman, 1961; Luhby *et al.*, 1961).

Recently, Kumar and co-workers (1985) reported that while the serum folate levels of 157 patients with homozygous β-thalassaemia living in Northern India tended to be lower than in normal subjects or in the patients' parents, the concentration of folate within the patients' erythrocytes tended to be abnormally high.

Prognosis

All the problems and complications affecting children suffering from thalassaemia major that have been listed in the preceding pages are alleviated to a greater or lesser extent in children receiving regular and adequate transfusions. Growth and development are more normal; the spleen and liver are less enlarged and the children probably suffer, too, from fewer infections. Most will survive well into the second decade, while some, but not many, will live longer. The majority of deaths in the second decade, or later, are caused by iron overload. Before regular transfusion was adopted as the mainstay of therapy, most affected children died within the *first* decade, usually from the consequences of severe anaemia and of infections.

As already repeatedly referred to, an important element in prognosis is the nature of the β-thalassaemia genes present. It is the extent to which β-globin synthesis is impaired that controls the clinical severity of the disease and hence the prognosis.

TREATMENT OF THALASSAEMIA MAJOR

The management of thalassaemia major, including the place of splenectomy, the essential role of blood transfusion and the possibilities of the control of iron overload by chelation therapy are considered in some detail in Chapter 20.

BLOOD PICTURE IN β-THALASSAEMIA MAJOR

Erythrocytes

In the untransfused patient, the erythrocyte count lies as a rule between 1.0 and 3.0 × 10^{12}/1, with the haemoglobin concentration proportionately lower and often less than 5.0 g/dl. The erythrocytes vary greatly in size and shape: the majority are microcytes but a few macrocytes may be present also. The MCV is usually substantially less than normal. According to Daland and Strauss (1948) it varies widely, i.e., between 50 and 100 fl. Irregularly-shaped cell fragments are usually conspicuous. In stained films the majority of the cells stain palely; some appear as mere rings of haemoglobin, a few as target cells (Fig. 18.2). Some of the cell fragments, if contracted, often stain relatively deeply. Punctate basophilia and polycromasia may be conspicuous. Normoblasts are almost invariably present, and are found in the largest numbers in severely affected children, and especially after splenectomy (see below). Some are early forms; others have a pyknotic nucleus and a pale-staining cytoplasm, in which punctate basophilia may be seen.

The reticulocyte count is usually raised and may reach 10% or even more in severely anaemic children. The count tends to increase after splenectomy, in association with the marked normoblastaemia which then develops.

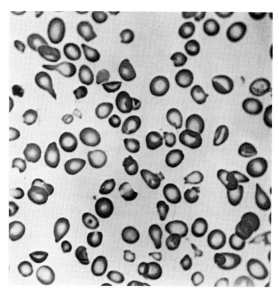

Fig. 18.2 Photomicrograph of a blood film of a patient with thalassaemia major.
The erythrocytes vary greatly in size and shape and many cell fragments are present. Some of the cells are markedly hypochromic. × 700.

Fessas (1963) was the first to describe the presence in peripheral-blood normoblasts, reticulocytes and erythrocytes of thalassaemia-major and thalassaemia-intermedia patients (particularly after splenectomy) of large inclusions which stained with methyl violet, and he postulated that the inclusions consisted of α-globin chains unused because of the failure to synthesize sufficient β chains.

Nathan and Gunn (1966) described the blood picture in Cooley's anaemia in detail; they stressed that what can be seen depends very much upon whether or not the spleen has been removed. They emphasized that before splenectomy tear-drop forms are conspicuous and that the erythrocytes are markedly heterogeneous with respect to haemoglobin content and size, large pale cells and small dense cells being present together with intermediate forms. They reported that, after splenectomy, fewer tear-drop forms, but many more large-diameter hypochromic erythrocytes, are present together with 'small piscine forms which are little more than fragments of stroma' and that anisochromia is markedly increased as is the number of normoblasts. They made the point, however, that the reticulocyte count is elevated after splenectomy to a lesser extent than in other haemolytic anaemias. Nathan and Gunn also reported that many of the large-diameter pale cells contain Heinz bodies and stressed that the inclusions are more irregularly shaped and larger than the Heinz bodies produced in vitro by incubating erythrocytes in the presence of phenylhydrazine; they stressed, too, that many of the erythrocytes could be seen to be 'pocked' with craters when viewed by Nomarski optics (see also p. 83).

Nathan and Gunn found that when the Betke-Kleihauer technique for the demonstration of Hb F was applied to Cooley's-anaemia blood the distribution of Hb F within the erythrocyte population is markedly heterogeneous. They also noted that after splenectomy the largest methyl-violet-staining inclusions are found in the cells containing the least amounts of Hb F.

The erythrocytes in β-thalassaemia have also been extensively studied by electron-microscopic techniques. A brief account of what can be seen is given on page 496.

Leucocytes and platelets

The total leucocyte count is typically increased and may even exceed $25 \times 10^9/l$, and a small percentage of myelocytes is commonly present. The platelet count is usually within the normal range. In the presence of hypersplenism, however, the total leucocyte count and neutrophil count fall significantly, perhaps to less than $5 \times 10^9/l$ and $2 \times 10^9/l$, respectively; and the platelet count falls, too, although usually less in proportion than does the neutrophil count. The counts increase after splenectomy, in association with the marked normoblastaemia which then develops.

Excellent early accounts of the blood picture in the 'erythroblastic anaemia of Cooley' were given by Baty, Blackfan and Diamond (1932) and Bradford and Dye (1936). Both groups remarked, too, on the changes in the blood picture resulting from splenectomy. Baty, Blackfan and Diamond (1932), for instance, reported that very hypochromic macrocytes and many nucleated cells were then present as well as numerous platelets. Bradford and Dye (1936) actually carried out Price-Jones cell diameter distribution curves and recorded increases in mean cell diameter following splenectomy in three cases. In two patients the MCV remained low, and Bradford and Dye concluded that the cells had become thinned following the operation.

Bradford and Dye also reported that the erythrocytes tended to fragment in vitro. In their words: 'Wet preparations [of oxalated blood (1 mg/ml)] revealed a marked degree of fragmentation. Knob-like projections were observed to form and break off the erythrocytes with regularity. One obtained the impression that many of the cells were leaflike and that they were thinner than normal erythrocytes.'

Effect of splenectomy

The blood picture after splenectomy is indeed a remarkable one: normoblastaemia and an apparent extreme flattening of the erythrocytes, as described above, and thrombocytosis, are conspicuous and regular features (Fig. 18.3). In addition, siderotic granules, as well as larger inclusions visible by phase-contrast microscopy and staining (as do Heinz bodies) with methyl violet, will be present in many of the circulating erythroblasts and reticulocytes and in some ripened erythrocytes. The larger inclusions represent unused α-globin chains that would have been removed from the cells by

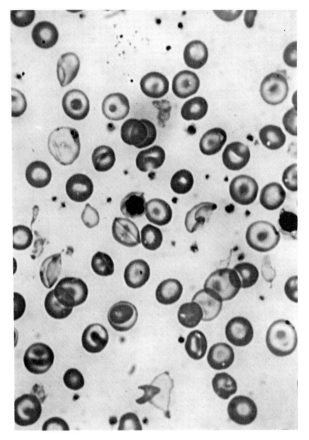

Fig. 18.3 Photomicrograph of a blood film of a patient with β-thalassaemia major after splenectomy.
There is a mixed population of erythrocytes: the patient's cells are strikingly hypochromic and some appear as thin rings; inclusions (Pappenheimer bodies) are present in some of them. Some irregularly-shaped hypochromic fragments can be seen. The darker-staining cells are probably all transfused cells; some appear as target cells. Two pyknotic normoblasts are present as well as numerous platelets. × 900.

the spleen if the organ had been *in situ*. [The same inclusions can sometimes be seen in preparations of peripheral blood taken before splenectomy if carefully looked for, but only in very small numbers.]

Polliack and Rachmilewitz (1973) gave details of the post-splenectomy normoblastaemia and of the frequency of Heinz bodies. In five patients the total nucleated cell count ranged from 40 to 200 × 10^9/l, of which 70–94% of the cells were normoblasts, and 8–12% of the eryth-

rocytes contained Heinz bodies. Before splenectomy in five patients, the total nucleated cell count ranged from 5.4 to 11.2 × 10^9/l of which 0–20% were normoblasts (maximum count 1.26 × 10^9/l), and Heinz bodies were seen in only 2% or less of the cells.

Coagulation-factor activity and platelet aggregation

As already referred to (p. 403), some thalassaemia-major patients do seem to suffer from an excessive tendency to bleed, especially epistaxis. Minor or minimal defects in coagulation-factor activity and platelet response to aggregants have been demonstrated in some of these patients (Hilgartner, Erlandson and Smith, 1963; Hilgartner and Smith, 1964; Caocci et al., 1978; Eldor, 1978b).

Eldor (1978b), who had studied 15 patients, obtained evidence in most of them of diminished aggregation when their platelets were exposed to ADP, collagen, ristocetin or epinephrine. Caocci and co-workers (1978) studied 30 children at least 25 days after their last transfusion. The activity of factors IX, XI and XII was found to be decreased in most of them: that of factors VII, IX and X was slightly reduced in a minority, while that of factor VIII and prothrombin and fibrinogen were found to be normal in the majority. The prothrombin time and partial thromboplastin time were also mostly normal. Caocci *et al.* concluded that liver failure could not explain all the abnormal findings, particularly the markedly reduced activity of factors XI and XII, and they suggested that this might be a consequence of activation of the intrinsic coagulation system following intravascular haemolysis and multiple blood transfusions. High platelet counts (430–960 × 10^9/l) were noted in five splenectomized patients.

NATURE OF HAEMOGLOBIN IN HOMOZYGOUS β-THALASSAEMIA

The main abnormality is the large amount of Hb F present. Hb A_2 is always present in variable but small amounts; Hb A is absent in $β^0$-thalassaemia but present in $β^+$-thalassaemia. A small amount of free α chains may be demonstrable in severe cases (Fessas and Loukopoulos, 1964).

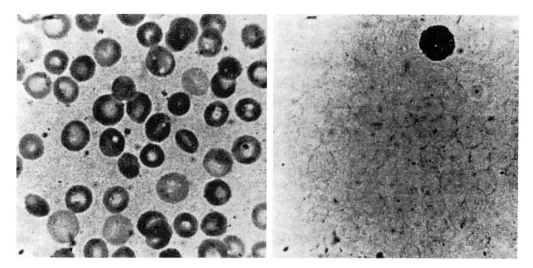

Fig. 18.4 Photomicrograph of a blood film of a newborn infant (left) and from an adult (right) stained by May-Grünwald-Giemsa after acid elution according to the method of Kleihauer, Braun and Betke (1957).
Erythrocytes containing Hb F resist acid elution. The dark staining object in the film of the adult is a lymphocyte.
[Reproduced by permission from Betke and Kleihauer (1958).]

Hb F

The amount of Hb F present is variable: as estimated by alkali denaturation, it usually comprises 50–90% of the total circulating haemoglobin. Acid elution preparations by the method of Kleihauer, Braun and Betke (1957) (Fig. 18.4) or its modifications show that the Hb F is most unevenly distributed amongst the erythrocytes, many cells containing large amounts and staining deeply, other cells containing little or no Hb F. There is every reason to believe that the Hb F present in such large amounts in typical homozygous β-thalassaemia major is chemically the same as that formed normally in fetal life.

The first observations suggesting that the blood in Cooley's anaemia might contain large amounts of Hb F appear to have been made by Vecchio (1946, 1948) and Putignago and Fiore-Donati (1948). They demonstrated in several patients that the rate of denaturation by alkali of their haemoglobin was substantially slowed and resembled that of normal fetal haemoglobin. These observations were soon confirmed and the similarity in reactions between the alkali-resistant haemoglobin of thalassaemia patients and normal Hb F was established. It soon became clear from a variety of experimental approaches that the haemoglobins were in fact identical (Liquori, 1951; Chernoff, 1953; Roche et al., 1953; Huisman, Prins and van der Schaaf, 1956; de Marco and Trasarti, 1957; Sturgeon et al., 1963).

As already mentioned, in thalassaemia major Hb F is usually present in amounts varying between 50 and almost 100% (Rich, 1952; Cutillo and Romagnoli, 1953; Penati, Turco and Lovisetto, 1954; Choremis, Zannos and Dentakis, 1955; etc.). In all probability the percentages of Hb F present are higher than those quoted as estimation by alkali denaturation is known to give falsely low values when Hb F is present at high concentrations and the 1-minute denaturation technique of Singer, Chernoff and Singer (1951) is used without modification (Wood, 1983).

Whether the level of Hb F is ever (or occasionally) less than 50% in untransfused patients who are genuine homozygotes for β-thalassaemia is uncertain. Percentages as low as 20%, or even less, were, for instance, at one time described in patients thought to be homozygotes, e.g., by Choremis, Zannos and Dentakis (1955), Sturgeon, Itano and Bergren, (1955), White and Beaven (1959) and Aksoy and Erdem (1965). Blood transfusions, however, depress the formation of Hb F (Murano, 1955), and Weatherall and Clegg (1981, p. 196) made the point that they have observed children with homozygous β⁰-thalassaemia who had as little as 5% Hb F in their circulation despite 8 weeks having passed since they were last transfused.

There is some evidence that erythrocytes containing a high percentage of Hb F survive longer in the peripheral blood than do cells containing a low percentage. *In vivo*, the turnover of Hb F has been shown to be slower than that of Hb A or Hb A_2 (Gabuzda et al., 1963) and the amount of Hb F to be greater in heavy (old) cells than in light (young) cells separated by centrifugation (Gabuzda *et al.*, 1963; Loukopoulos and Fessas, 1965). However, although it might be expected that the illness of patients whose blood contains the most Hb F would be clearly less severe than that of patients with blood containing lower percentages of Hb F, this does not seem to be borne out in practice (Penati *et al.*, 1955; Josephson *et al.*, 1958).

A relatively recent development has been the demonstration that Hb F exists normally in more than one chemical form: $^{G}\gamma$ has glycine in position 136 in the amino acid chain; $^{A}\gamma$ has alanine in position 136 and $^{A}\gamma^{T}$ has threonine at position 75 while $^{A}\gamma^{I}$ has iso-leucine in this position (see Huisman *et al.*, 1974, 1981).

It has naturally been of interest to see whether in β-thalassaemia the ratio between the types of chain differs from that found normally (see p. 90). According to Huisman *et al.* (1974), who studied Hb F obtained from 84 homozygous β-thalassaemics and 130 heterozygotes, the heterozygous patients could be placed in two groups (regardless of their ethnic background): Group 1 with a $^{G}\gamma$:$^{A}\gamma$ ratio of about 2:3 (as in the traces of Hb F found in normal adult blood); Group 2 with a ratio $^{G}\gamma$:$^{A}\gamma$ of about 3:1 (as in the normal newborn infant). In the homozygotes the ratio was about 3:2, even if both parents belonged to Group 1 or Group 2. The $^{A}\gamma^{T}$ variant was reported by Huisman *et al.* (1981) to be present in the normal newborn infant at a ratio of about 1 in 5 in 150 black Americans of varying thalassaemia genotypes. In Sardinians the percentage of the $^{A}\gamma^{T}$ variant in β⁰-thalassaemia newborn infants was found by Masala *et al.* (1986) to be similar to that in normal newborns with the same $^{A}\gamma^{T}$ phenotype.

$^{G}\gamma$ and $^{A}\gamma$ (and also β-globin) chain synthesis was studied *in vitro* by Saglio *et al.* (1982) in eight patients who were homozygous for β-thalassaemia. In five of them the total γ-chain synthesis was higher in the peripheral blood than in the bone marrow and in seven $^{A}\gamma$-chain synthesis was markedly higher in the bone marrow compared to that in the peripheral blood. These results were interpreted as suggesting that F cells synthesizing the largest amount of $^{G}\gamma$ chains withstood ineffective erythropoiesis better than did $^{A}\gamma$-producing cells.

Hb A₂

In homozygous β-thalassaemia the percentage of Hb A₂ is usually within the normal range; less frequently it is slightly elevated or even slightly reduced. There is some evidence that erythrocytes containing large amounts of Hb F have a relatively low content of Hb A₂ (Weatherall and Clegg, 1981, p. 201).

Crowley and co-workers (1957) had demonstrated an Hb-E-like component by paper electrophoresis in 14 individuals from Cyprus and Turkey suffering from a thalassaemia syndrome: four of these patients had thalassaemia major. Josephson and co-workers (1958) identified Hb A₂ (by starch-block electrophoresis) at a raised concentration (9.4 and 4.3%) in two patients homozygous for thalassaemia.

Fessas (1959a) reported Hb-A₂ values ranging from approximately 1 to 13.3% in 21 Greek patients (his normal range 2.0–3.9%). Silvestroni, Bianco and Graziani (1968) found rather lower values, 0.8–2.8% (mean 2.12%), in 34 out of 38 Italian patients; the remaining four had raised values, as in heterozygotes.

Aksoy and Erdem (1969) reported finding raised Hb-A₂ levels in seven homozygous patients, normal levels in seven patients and subnormal levels in two patients; they emphasized the variability of their findings with respect to Hb A₂ and that the same was true of Hb F (25–94% in their 16 patients).

β⁰ and β⁺-thalassaemia

As already referred to, the extent to which β-chain production is impaired varies in β-thalassaemia from severe impairment resulting in no recognizable production of Hb A in (homozygous) β⁰-thalassaemia to moderate impairment only, allowing the formation of significant amounts of Hb A, in β⁺-thalassaemia. As might be expected, homozygotes for β⁰-thalassaemia tend to have a more serious disease than do homozygotes for β⁺-thalassaemia, many of whom present with the signs and symptoms of thalassaemia intermedia. Compound heterozygotes for β⁰ and β⁺-thalassaemia, too, tend to suffer from an illness of only moderate severity, *e.g.*, the 25-year-old female described by Russo *et al.* (1973). Simple heterozygosity for β⁰-thalassaemia is on average associated with greater abnormality than is simple heterozygosity for β^+-thalassaemia

The relative frequency of the two types of thalassaemia gene is of considerable interest. In Jamaican blacks Millard and co-workers (1977) reported that 29 out of 62 heterozygotes had the β^0 type, 33 the β^+ type. [The two types were identified by the presence or absence of Hb A in close relatives with Hb-S/β-thalassaemia.] Total haemoglobin, MCV and MCH tended to be lower in the β^0 type but the Hb-A$_2$ levels were similar in both types. In some β^+ heterozygotes individual values for MCV, MCH and Hb A$_2$ overlapped with the normal population, and it seemed likely that β^+-thalassaemia heterozygotes were probably under-diagnosed.

Kattamis and co-workers (1978) similarly found both β^+ and β^0 genes to be common in a group of 30 homozygous Greek children studied before transfusion. In 13 (43%), no Hb A could be detected; they were considered to be of the $\beta^0\beta^0$ genotype. In 17, Hb A was present, its distribution being bimodal (range 4–36%). Kattamis et al. suggested that low concentrations of Hb A (4–11%) were associated with the β^0/β^+ (compound) genotype while the higher concentrations (24–76%) were associated with the $\beta^+\beta^+$ genotype. The β^0/β^+ genotype was present in 11 (37%) and the $\beta^+\beta^+$ genotype present in six (20%).

As might be expected, the β^0 and β^+ types are associated with differences in α : non-α globin-synthesis ratios. Schilirò and co-workers (1978), using peripheral-blood reticulocytes, demonstrated a progression of abnormality from normal controls, through β-thalassaemia trait, Rietti-Greppi-Micheli anaemia, β^+-thalassaemia (70% of homozygotes) to (giving the most abnormal ratio) β^0-thalassaemia (30% of homozygotes).

Pepe, Lupi and Luzzatto (1980) reported that of 32 homozygous children five had β^0-thalassaemia, the remainder β^+-thalassaemia. β : α globin-synthesis ratios in the β^+ patients varied from 0.01 to 0.16; the distribution was, however, bimodal, and this was considered to be consistent with there being β^0/β^+ and β^+/β^+ genotypes. The ratios in the children's parents ranged quite widely, too, from 0.24 to 0.73, and this was thought to reflect the presence of multiple alleles, one of which was β^0 and at least one other a β^+.

Agglutinability of thalassaemia-major erythrocytes by anti-i

The first patient who was found to have apparently an increased amount of i antigen on his erythrocytes was a 15-year-old male with thalassaemia major investigated by Dr Ruth Sanger. Subsequently, Giblett and Crookston (1964) reported that they had tested the erythrocytes of 17 further thalassaemia-major patients for agglutinability by anti-i and found that all gave

titration scores only a little less than those that could be obtained with cord-blood erythrocytes, with the exception of a single patient who had received a large transfusion of adult erythrocytes a few days previously.

The interesting phenomenon of increased agglutinability by anti-i is, however, not specific for thalassaemia major, for variably raised anti-i titration scores were later obtained with the erythrocytes of patients suffering from a variety of blood diseases including thalassaemia minor, hypoplastic anaemia, leukaemia and PNH. The cause of the increased agglutinability does not seem to have been determined, but proliferative 'stress' was suggested by Giblett and Crookston as a possible common factor.

ERYTHROCYTE LIFE-SPAN IN β-THALASSAEMIA MAJOR

Survival studies carried out by the Ashby method and later by the use of ^{51}Cr have indicated a considerable shortening of the life-span of patients' erythrocytes. Two-component elimination curves have been reported in some instances and usually excessive accumulation of radioactivity in the spleen in ^{51}Cr studies.

Ashby method

Kaplan, Zuelzer and Hoogana (1950) transfused into normal recipients blood from three children considered to be suffering from severe or moderately severe Mediterranean anaemia. Between 25 and 50% of the transfused erythrocytes disappeared from the recipients' circulation in 20–30 days; later, however, the slope of elimination ran roughly parallel to that expected for normal corpuscles. Frontali and Stegagno (1951) transfused blood from two children with a severe grade of Cooley's anaemia into recipients suffering from mild anaemia not considered to be haemolytic in origin; elimination of the transfused cells was complete in 12 and 19 days, respectively. Frontali (1954) reported that the erythrocyte life-span in normal recipients in the case of five patients with thalassaemia major or minor was between 18–20 and 50–70 days, the longest life-spans being obtained with the blood of two mildly affected children.

Normal erythrocytes transfused into thalassaemia-major patients have usually been found to survive normally, *e.g.*, by Frontali and Stegagno (1951). Considerably shortened survival has, however, been found in some cases, *e.g.* by Lichtman et al. (1953) and Smith et al. (1955) and was attributed to hypersplenism by McElfresh, Sharpstein and Akabane (1955) and Sitarz, Ultmann and Wolff (1963). (See also p. 557, under *Splenectomy*.)

^{51}Cr method

Radioactive chromium has been quite extensively employed.

Sturgeon and Finch (1957) labelled the erythrocytes of three patients and found ^{51}Cr half-times of 10, 9 and 7 days, respectively, corresponding to a calculated rate of destruction of 7–10 times the normal.

Vullo and Tunioli (1958) transfused the ^{51}Cr-labelled erythrocytes of seven children with thalassaemia into a variety of recipients. In the patients themselves the ^{51}Cr half-times were 9–22 days (normal 25–35 days). In four instances it was also possible to transfuse normal recipients (with spleens *in situ*) also; in each case the survival of the patient's erythrocytes was less in the normal subject than in the patient's own circulation. In three further experiments the patient's cells were divided between the patient and a splenectomized but otherwise healthy subject: the rates of elimination were about the same in each pair of recipients.

Erlandson and co-workers (1958) published data on 10 children with homozygous thalassaemia. Six of the children were clinically severely affected (^{51}Cr T_{50} 6.5–16 days); four had thalassaemia intermedia (^{51}Cr T_{50} 11–19.5 days). The shortened survivals could not be correlated either with the Hb-F content of the cells or with the degree of anaemia present and Erlandson *et al.* concluded that increased haemolysis, although it might be markedly increased, did not by itself determine the degree of anaemia present.

Bailey and Prankerd (1958) studied two adult Cypriots and obtained evidence of two populations of erythrocytes, one with a mean life-span of a few days only, the other with a mean life-span of about 30 days (*cf.* Kaplan, Zuelzer and Hoogana, 1950). The short-lived cells appeared to be destroyed in the spleen.

Grinstein and co-workers (1960) used [^{14}C]-2-glycine to label haem, and estimated in two patients with thalassaemia major that the 50% survival time was 36 and 38 days, respectively. [The 50% survival time was calculated by drawing a horizontal line across each radioactivity curve at 50% of the maximum activity and measuring the distance between the points at which this line cuts the ascending and descending limbs of the curve. In two normal subjects the 50% survival time was 118 and 128 days, respectively.]

Malamos and co-workers (1961a) studied three severely affected children, aged 9, 12 and 13 years, respectively: the ^{51}Cr T_{50}s were 13.7, 12.4 and 17.0 days.

Hindawi and Subhiyah (1962) reported on 14 patients with thalassaemia major. The ^{51}Cr T_{50} ranged from 8 to 19 days. Surface counting over the liver and spleen was carried out, and analysis of the data by several methods showed the uptake of radioactivity by the spleen to be abnormally great and that by the liver to be also raised but less markedly so. As just referred to, Bailey and Prankerd (1958), by in-vivo counting with ^{51}Cr, had concluded that the spleen was an important site for the destruction of short-lived cells, although according to Vullo and Tunioli (1958) it is in this respect less active than is a normal spleen.

Hillcoat and Waters (1962) studied five children, two of whom had been splenectomized. Four were considered to have thalassaemia major, one thalassaemia intermedia. The ^{51}Cr T_{50}s were short, 7.5–8.5 days in the pre-splenectomy cases and 8.5 and 11.0 days, respectively, in the post-splenectomy patients. The elimination curves were biphasic, with 30–40% of the ^{51}Cr leaving the circulation in the first 2 days. One patient had a massively enlarged spleen in which excess radioactivity was demonstrated. There was, however, no evidence of an excess accumulation in either spleen or liver in the other two patients with their spleen *in situ*. Excess ^{51}Cr, however, accumulated in the liver in the two post-splenectomy patients.

ERYTHROKINETIC STUDIES IN β-THALASSAEMIA MAJOR

Many studies have been undertaken with the aim of measuring quantitatively the degree to which haemoglobin production is impaired in β-thalassaemia major and intermedia. Crosby and Akeroyd (1952) calculated from published reports of erythrocyte survival that in three cases of Cooley's anaemia haemoglobin production amounted to only 0.18–0.30 g/kg/day, as compared with the normal maximum of 0.60–0.65 g/kg/day. Norris, Hanson and Loeffler (1956) used ^{59}Fe in studying an adult black with moderately severe Mediterranean anaemia and found a rapid plasma clearance but poor incorporation of the iron in erythrocytes. Sturgeon and Finch (1957), in elaborate isotope studies on four children with clinically severe or intermediate Cooley's anaemia, concluded that the delivery of erythrocytes was reduced to 50% of the normal in the mildly anaemic patient and to as little as 15% of the normal in the most severely anaemic patient. Bailey and Prankerd (1958) in somewhat similar studies on two patients concluded that, although erythrocyte production per unit volume of marrow was reduced, total production might be greater than normal because of the expanded marrow volume.

Further studies using radioactive iron were reported by Larizza and co-workers (1958) who investigated eight patients with Cooley's anaemia and three with 'Rietti-Greppi-Micheli' anaemia. Both groups of patients handled intravenously-administered ^{59}Fe in a similar way: the plasma clearance times were rapid and more iron than normal was taken up by the liver. The output of ^{59}Fe-labelled erythrocyes from the marrow was markedly subnormal and unusually slow, the peak output being delayed to the 4th–6th day.

Erlandson and co-workers (1958) also used ^{59}Fe in a study of 10 children, all with Cooley's anaemia. The rate of erythrocyte production was calculated to be from 2.2 to 6.1 times the normal, *i.e.*, it did not reach that attained in patients with most other types of haemolytic anaemia. They stressed that the severity of an individual patient's anaemia depended on his personal balance between erythrocyte formation and haemolysis.

Malamos and co-workers (1961a) carried out simultaneous tracer studies of erythropoiesis and erythrocyte destruction, using ^{59}Fe and ^{51}Cr, in 17 Greek patients with thalassaemia major, four classified as severe (requiring regular transfusion) and 13 as intermediate (not requiring regular transfusion). The plasma iron turnover was calculated to be more than 10 times the normal and the erythrocyte ^{59}Fe uptake at 10 days (the proportion of the injected radioactivity in the circulation 10 days after administration), expressed as a percentage of the amount administered, was markedly subnormal (mean $13.1 \pm 2.5\%$ in the four severely affected patients, $19.1 \pm 2.9\%$ in the 13 intermediate category patients and $82.4 \pm 2.1\%$ in the normal controls).

Included in the paper of Malamos et al, (1961a) are interesting graphs of surface counts showing very rapid initial incorporation of iron in the marrow, failure to achieve the normal expected maximum counting-rate, a slow and irregular fall in counting-rate, indicating retention of iron in the marrow, and a sharp secondary rise in the counting rate over the spleen suggesting an early sequestration there of newly labelled erythrocytes. Further data based on studies on a total of 27 thalassaemia patients were given by Malamos et al (1961b).

Subsequent studies on thalassaemia-major patients using ^{59}Fe include those of Schettini, Meloni and Costa (1967), who also estimated erythrocyte survival using ^{51}Cr, Priolisi, Astaldi and Burgio (1968), Astaldi, Burgio and Priolisi (1969) and Finch et al. (1970). Their conclusions were essentially the same as those of earlier workers: namely, that plasma iron clearance is markedly accelerated and plasma iron turnover markedly raised, that erythrocyte iron turnover is slightly raised and that the amount of radioactivity eventually appearing in the peripheral blood, carried by ^{59}Fe-labelled newly formed erythrocytes, is markedly subnormal, often amounting to well less than 20% of that administered.

The findings listed above are typical of ineffective erythropoiesis, *i.e.*, the death of erythrocyte precursors in the bone marrow (and in extra-medullary foci, if any are present). The conclusion that ineffective erythropoiesis was an important factor in the pathogenesis of the anaemia of thalassaemia major had been reached, too, by Grinstein et al (1960) in an elegant study using a different approach. Three patients with thalassaemia major had been given an oral dose of 100 μci of $[^{14}C]$-2-glycine and the appearance of radioactivity followed in the peripheral blood and in the faecal sterobilin. The findings in three patients were compared with those obtained with two normal subjects and with previously published findings in patients with pernicious anaemia or sickle-cell anaemia: ineffective erythropoiesis was clearly demonstrated in the pernicious-anaemia patient but to nothing like the extent found in the thalassaemia-major patients. In Grinstein and co-workers' thalassaemia patients the appearance of the radioactivity in the circulating blood was delayed; in contrast, radioactivity appeared extremely rapidly in the stercobilin and reached a maximum on the third day when it was over 100 times that of the maximum radioactivity found in the circulating blood haem.

BIOCHEMICAL FINDINGS IN β-THALASSAEMIA MAJOR

Serum bilirubin. This is usually within the range 1–3 mg/dl in thalassaemia major.

Serum iron. This is usually higher than normal even in children who have not received transfusions. In those who are regularly transfused the values are still higher and the serum iron-binding capacity is typically fully saturated.

Cartwright and co-workers (1948) found raised levels in four out of five patients; the fifth patient, in whom the level was normal, had an infection and fever. The findings of Smith et al. (1950) were similar: the mean serum iron concentration in 15 children was grossly elevated: 269.6 ± 62.9 μg/dl and the iron-binding capacity was fully saturated in each case. In a more recent study, Erlandson and co-workers (1964) reported on the serum iron levels in 10 children at the time of initial diagnosis when they were from 5 to 16 months of age: in seven of them the level exceeded 100 μg/dl. In 10 older children, who had received multiple transfusions, the levels ranged between approximately 170 and 230 μg/dl and the iron-binding capacity was fully saturated.

Serum ferritin. Very high values have been reported in thalassaemia major, reflecting the increase in body iron stores as well as the severity of the defect in haemoglobin formation (Piperno et al., 1984; Saraya et al., 1985).

Erythrocyte ferritin. The concentration of erythrocyte ferritin has been reported and to be greatly increased and these increases, too, probably reflect raised body iron stores as well as the degree to which erythropoiesis is impaired (Bauminger et al., 1979; Jacobs et al., 1981; Piperno et al., 1984).

Serum copper. Cartwright and co-workers (1948) measured serum copper levels in three patients and found them elevated in each case. Increased levels have been reported, too, by Prasad et al. (1965).

Serum zinc. Prasad and co-workers (1965) investigated 11 Egyptian patients and found that the serum zinc concentration tended to be subnormal. Doğru, Arcasoy and Gavdar (1979) studied 20 children; plasma, erythrocyte and hair zinc concentrations were all much lower than in a series of 20 control normal children. The excretion of zinc in the urine was increased and it was suggested that this was the cause of the low levels in the blood and tissues. It was suggested, too, that the zinc deficiency might play a part in the children's retardation of growth and sexual development.

Serum proteins

These were studied using paper electrophoresis by Allamanis (1955) in 36 Greek children with Cooley's anaemia: in 11 infants less than 24 months old the patterns were in most cases normal; in older children the albumin concentration was decreased (by an average of 30%); there were minor reductions in the concentrations of α_1, α_2 and β globulins, and flocculation tests often gave abnormal results.

Tovo and co-workers (1981) have quite recently reported the result of a study carried out on 187 β-thalassaemia homozygotes. Compared with age-matched controls, patients with a spleen in situ showed increases in the concentrations of IgG and IgA. Splenectomized patients, compared to those who had not been splenectomized, showed increases in IgG and in IgA (in older patients) and decreases in IgM. The data were considered not to support the hypothesis that chronic liver disease or the transfusion therapy was responsible for the increases in IgG, and it was suggested that excessive exposure to antigens (as the result of an overworked RE system failing to clear antigens effectively) might, on the other hand, be responsible.

Plasma β_2 microglobulin (β_2- MG). Cooper and co-workers (1984) reported that plasma β_2-MG concentrations tended to be abnormally high in 118 transfusion-dependent children with β-thalassaemia major. The raised levels were thought to reflect increased RE cell activity and not to be related to iron overload.

Plasma haemoglobin. This has been estimated by Crosby and Dameshek (1951) and by Das Gupta et al. (1955). According to Crosby and Dameshek it was considerably elevated (12–60 mg/dl) in three out of four patients with severe Mediterranean anaemia (probably thalassaemia major), while in the fourth patient it was normal before splenectomy but rose to 25 mg/dl after splenectomy. Das Gupta and his co-workers reported similar findings: 22 patients with Cooley's anaemia had values between 4.3 and 56.5 mg/dl. Substantially similar figures based on a larger series of patients were reported by Das Gupta et al. (1958).

Haptoglobin and haemopexin. The serum haptoglobin concentration was reported by Priolisi and Giuffrè (1963) to be absent or decreased in 37 patients with thalassaemia major (including 12 who had undergone splenectomy). Cutillo and Meloni (1974) measured by an immunodiffusion technique haptoglobin and haemopexin in 45 children with Cooley's anaemia: haptoglobin was absent in 13 and haemopexin absent in 37. Haemopexin was absent in many cases despite the haptoglobin concentration being as much as half normal.

Erythrocyte enzymes and metabolism

A variety of abnormalities have been described. The activity of most enzymes is increased (Grignani *et al.*, 1962; Belfiore, Meldolesi and Calcara, 1965; Nathan *et al.*, 1969; etc.). Glucose consumption and lactate production and HMP shunt activity are raised, and K^+ flux is increased, particularly in young (light) cells, as separated by centrifugation; the concentration of GSH is normal or slightly raised (Nathan *et al.*, 1969). According to Wiley (1980), Na^+ influx and cation pump activity are markedly increased. Intracellular Na^+ and K^+ concentrations and cell water, in fresh erythrocytes, are generally within the normal range (Wiley, 1980; Choremis, Economou-Mavrou and Tsenghi, 1981). Erythrocyte arginase activity has been reported as markedly increased (Reynolds, Follette and Valentine, 1957) and mean cholinesterase activity significantly reduced (Choremis *et al.*, 1965).

Matioli and Del Piano (1959) reported that more Heinz bodies developed than normal as the result of incubating thalassaemia-major erythrocytes with acetylphenylhydrazine. Grignani and co-workers (1962) found raised methaemoglobin levels (2.8–7.1%) in three thalassaemia-major patients.

Anderson and her co-workers (1979) found that the metabolism of pyridoxine tended to be abnormal in that the rate of conversion of pyridoxine to pyridoxal phosphate was slow or borderline normal in most transfusion-dependent homozygotes, despite the admixture of some abnormal erythrocytes. (The conversion rate was subnormal, too, in 63% of 107 heterozygotes.)

The above abnormalities reflect probably the immaturity of the cell population, damage to the erythrocyte membrane and oxidant stress; they are not specific to thalassaemia major. However, they do probably play a significant role in connection with the shortened life-span of thalassaemia-major erythrocytes (see also p. 502).

Erythrocyte calcium. Shalev and co-workers (1984) measured erythrocyte calcium and Ca^{2+},Mg^{2+}ATPase activity in 18 patients with β-thalassaemia intermedia, nine of whom had been splenectomized. The intracellular Ca^{2+} concentration was found to be substantially increased compared to the normal, particularly in the splenectomized patients. Ca^{2+}, Mg^{2+} ATPase activity was, however, normal in both groups. Shalev *et al.* concluded that the raised Ca^{2+} levels were likely to be secondary to a major defect in the cell membrane, the nature of which was uncertain at the time of their report.

Erythrocyte and serum lipids

Increases in the serum and erythrocyte lipids and phospholipids were described by Erickson and co-workers (1937) and by Schwarz-Tiene, Corda and Careddu (1953), the latter authors reporting, too, low levels of free and combined cholesterol. Choremis, Kyriakides and Papadakis (1961) found that the concentration of all the fractions of serum lipids they studied were below normal.

Giardini, Castro and Maggioni (1974) studied 20 thalassaemia-major children from Sardinia and found increases in the percentages of sphingomyelin and phosphatidylcholine and a reduction in the percentage of phosphatidylethanolamine. They suggested that these deviations from the normal were the result of autoxidation.

In 1976, Rachmilewitz, Lubin and Shohet described the results of a comprehensive study of 17 splenectomized thalassaemia-major patients and eight patients with a spleen *in situ*. The total erythrocyte lipids were nearly twice normal in amount: the percentages of phosphatidylcholine and palmitic acid (a saturated fatty acid) were increased but there were reductions in the percentages of phosphatidylethanolamine and arachidonic acid (a polyunsaturated fatty acid). Serum α-tocopherol (vitamin-E) levels were low. An increase was found in the amount of malonyldialdehyde (MDA) generated when erythrocytes were exposed to H_2O_2, as calculated per g haemoglobin or per cell, but not when calculated per μg membrane P at risk. Rachmilewitz, Lubin and Shohet pointed out that the cells contained more lipid susceptible to oxidation and that the distribution of fatty acids indicated that autoxidation was taking place *in vivo*; they suggested that this was probably being initiated by free radicals which were constantly being formed. The reduction in the cells' content of haemoglobin would, it was postulated, allow potent oxidants to find their way to the cells' membrane; the low content of α-tocopherol would also facilitate this.

Earlier, Stocks, Kemp and Dormandy (1971) had reported finding evidence for a tendency to lipid autoxidation in five patients with auto-immune haemolytic anaemia and in four patients with G6PD deficiency recovering from an acute haemolytic episode as well as in six patients with thalassaemia major. There was, however, no evidence for this in three patients with HS, and it was concluded that increased MDA generation was not invariable in haemolytic states.

Erythrocyte porphyrins

Considerable interest has been taken in the thalassaemia-major erythrocyte's content of porphyrins and in the possibility that protoporphyrin and haem synthesis might be abnormal in thalassaemia. Some abnormalities have in fact been reported, but they seem likely all to be secondary to impaired globin synthesis.

Sturgeon, Chen and Bergren (1958) found in seven thalassaemia-major patients that the concentration of erythrocyte coproporphyrin was greatly increased and that of protoporphyrin was at the upper limit of normal. (The findings in 10 thalassaemia-minor patients were normal.) Sturgeon, Chen and Bergren made the point that similarly high concentrations of the porphyrins may be found in other types of haemolytic anaemia associated with raised reticulocyte counts.

Bannerman, Grinstein and Moore (1959) studied nine thalassaemia-major patients, seven after splenectomy. They used [2-^{14}C]glycine and ^{59}Fe to measure haemoglobin synthesis *in vitro* in peripheral blood containing immature erythrocytes. Synthesis of both haem and globin was lower than normal and there were no consistent differences in the haem:globin ratio. However, the incorporation of [^{14}C]protoporphyrin into haem was brisk and the uptake of ^{59}Fe into haem was greatly increased by the addition of free protoporphyrin. It was concluded that haem synthesis might be impaired in two ways: by a relatively slow rate of protoporphyrin synthesis and by a partial block to the combination of protoporphyrin and iron.

Prato and Mazza (1962) reported on similar studies. Less porphobilinogen than expected was synthesized from α-aminolaevulic acid by thalassaemia-major erythrocytes but the rate of synthesis of porphyrin from porphobilinogen appeared to be greater than in normal or HS erythrocytes. Vavra and Mayer (1964) studied six thalassaemia-major patients and concluded that the enzyme sequence catalyzing porphyrin synthesis was functioning normally. Vavra, Mayer and Moore (1964), in a further study of nine thalassaemia-major patients, reported that the utilization of [^{14}C]glycine to form aminolevulinic acid was defective and a step following the formation of protoporphyrin or haem was defective, too.

Bannerman (1964), in a review, discussed the significance of raised concentrations of erythrocyte porphyrins in thalassaemia. Lyberatos and co-workers (1972) measured the erythrocyte protoporphyrin content in 20 thalassaemia homozygotes and 31 heterozygotes. The levels were consistently raised: 83.3 ± 23.42 in the homozygotes; 70.4 ± 22.9 in the heterozygotes; and 25.6 ± 9.43 μg/dl in normal controls.

Plasma cyclic nucleotides

Peracchi and co-workers (1985) have measured cAMP and cGMP concentrations in the plasma of 20 transfusion-dependent thalassaemia-major and 18 thalassaemia-intermedia patients and compared the levels with those found in 18 post-hepatitis patients and 37 normal subjects. The cAMP concentrations were normal in the thalassaemia patients but the cGMP concentrations were significantly raised, and in the thalassaemia-intermedia patients they were negatively correlated with their haemoglobin level. It was suggested that the raised extracellular cGMP levels reflected the extent of erythroid hyperplasia.

Amino-aciduria in thalassaemia major

According to Choremis, Zannos and Basti (1957) and Choremis *et al* (1959), the excretion of amino acids in the urine in Cooley's anaemia, and in sickle-cell anaemia, is abnormally great.

Hillcoat (1960) reported that β-aminoisobutyric acid (BAIB) was present in large amounts in the urine of three patients with thalassaemia major, but was found in only small quantities in two thalassaemia-major patients who had undergone splenectomy. In one of the patients studied before and after splenectomy the excretion of BAIB fell to one-quarter of the pre-operative level (Hillcoat, 1962). Hillcoat stated that the amino acid is a metabolic derivative of thymine and is excreted whenever there is much breakdown of nucleic acids; he suggested that in the case of thalassaemia major the excretion is due to the excessive destruction of erythrocyte precursors.

Fessas, Koniavitis and Zeis (1969) confirmed Hillcoat's observations in a larger number of patients: 16 thalassaemia-major patients who had not been splenectomized excreted 42–510 mg of BAIB in 24 hours while six previously splenectomized patients excreted from a trace to 88 mg. Transfusion constantly, although temporarily, reduced BAIB excretion. No BAIB was detected in the urine of 50 normal subjects or in 17 thalassaemia-trait patients; traces or moderate amounts were, however, detected in four out of six sickle-cell anaemia patients and small amounts in three out of 12 patients with iron-deficiency anaemia.

Urinary pyrrole pigments

As already referred to (p. 366), dipyrrole (dipyrrol) compounds are often found in large amounts in the urine of patients with unstable haemoglobin haemolytic anaemias. Sometimes their concentration is high enough to blacken the urine. Similar compounds have been identified in the urine in thalassaemia major and other thalassaemias (Kreimer-Birnbaum *et al.*, 1966, 1974; Kreimer-Birnbaum, Bannerman and Pinkerton, 1969). Darkening of the urine due to the presence of dipyrrols seems, however, to be unusual (or seldom noticed) in clinically severe thalassaemia, although this has been recorded. Thus one of Kreimer-Birnbaum, Bannerman and Pinkerton's patients, a 40-year-old man with severe β-thalassaemia intermedia who had undergone splenectomy, passed urine that was 'consistently dark brown in color'. The metabolic origin of the pigments still seems to be somewhat obscure, but that they are derived one way or another from the catabolism of haem molecules seems to be most likely.

β-THALASSAEMIA MINOR AND MINIMA

Most of those who are simple heterozygotes for β+- or β0-thalassaemia have no symptoms attributable to their haemoglobin defect and are clinically well and are usually but mildly anaemic.

Usually the diagnosis of heterozygosity for a thalassaemia gene is arrived at in the course of a family study or occasionally as the result of the investigation of mild anaemia, perhaps discovered in the course of a routine examination.

Details have been reported of the clinical findings in some large series of patients, including those of Gardikas (1968) (Greeks), Pootrakul, Wasi and Na-Nakorn (1973) (Thais), Knox-Macaulay *et al.* (1973) (British) and Mazza *et al.* (1976) (Italians). There were some differences in presentation in the different racial groups but most of the patients had no symptoms or signs attributable to thalassaemia.

CLINICAL PRESENTATION

Splenomegaly. Some heterozygotes have a palpably enlarged spleen and in some series this has been found in quite a high percentage of patients: according to Fessas (1959a) the spleen is palpable in about half the patients, although it rarely extends more than two finger-breadths below the costal margin. In most series, however, *e.g.* in that of Dinçol, Aksoy and Erdem (1979), the percentage has been much lower than this, and Weatherall and Clegg (1981, p. 222) concluded, as the result of a personal experience of more than 200 cases, that if the spleen is palpable an alternative cause than simple heterozygosity for β-thalassaemia should be sought. Weatherall and Clegg also made the point that in their experience the only common clinical presentation of heterozygous β-thalassaemia was refractory, *i.e.* iron-therapy-resistant, anaemia of pregnancy.

Knox-Macaulay and co-workers (1973) had reported that 35 out of the 67 β-thalassaemia heterozygotes (relatives of 16 affected propositi) of apparently British stock had been free from symptoms attributable to anaemia (although most were in fact found to be anaemic); the remaining 32 relatives had been known to be anaemic and had been subjected to various investigations in the past. The only abnormal physical sign common to the whole series was slight pallor. Their spleen were not palpable and there was no clinical or X-ray evidence of bony abnormalities. None gave a history of ulcers affecting the leg.

Pregnancy. In the series of patients of Knox-Macaulay *et al.* (1973) referred to above, a common finding was a worsening of anaemia during pregnancy. Megaloblastic change has been noted, too, particularly in malnourished populations, *e.g.* by Meital, Izak and Rachmilewitz (1961) in oriental Jews and by Ryan (1962) in Papuans.

Bone changes. Some degree of rarefaction, less severe than in thalassaemia major, has been reported in some series of patients. Sfikakis and Stamatoyannopoulos (1963), for instance, found areas of rarefaction, particularly in the skull, in 29 out of 55 healthy Greeks with the thalassaemia trait.

Jaundice. Clinical jaundice is uncommon. However, in a small proportion of patients it is appreciable although other signs of chronic haemolysis, *e.g.* anaemia and splenomegaly, may not be obvious. [Chronic mild jaundice was a feature of the Italian Rietti-Greppi-Micheli syndrome.]

Gallstones. Biliary calculi have not been commonly demonstrated in thalassaemia-minor patients. However, in some patients they have caused symptoms and have led to cholecystectomy. Thus in Spector and Frumin's (1953) early report, operation revealed a gall bladder and bile duct packed with stones up to $\frac{1}{2}$ inch in diameter. Stones are in fact probably formed more frequently than was at one time suspected: for instance, amongst the 262 patients of Gardikas (1968), 22 (8.5%) presented with symptoms that were attributed to gallstones.

Osteoarthropathy. An interesting association — osteoarthropathy — was reported by Gratwick and co-workers (1978). Twenty-five out of 50 patients with thalassaemia minor, aged 5–33 years, experienced periarticular dull aching pain affecting the ankles that was exacerbated by weight bearing. Radiographs showed microfractures in some cases. The cause is obscure.

Thalassaemia minor with unusually severe manifestations

Patients have been described, who seem without doubt to be heterozygotes for β-thalassaemia, who, nevertheless, present with relatively marked clinical manifestations and with other signs indicative of a severely expressed disease.

Stamatoyannopoulos and co-workers (1974a) described a Swiss-French family in which 18 carriers in four generations mostly presented with relatively severe symptoms and signs. A noteworthy and unexpected finding was the presence of inclusions in 30–40% of normoblasts of intermediate size and in 60–70% of small normoblasts, as might be found in genuine homozygotes. It was speculated that the cause of this was the presence of a closely linked gene leading to an unusual degree of α-chain excess or to inhibition of β-chain synthesis.

Friedman and co-workers (1976) described rather similar findings in three families of North-European or Italian origin. An unusual form of heterozygous β-thalassaemia was confirmed by haematological, genetic and peripheral-blood globin-synthesis studies. The diversity of clinical expression within the families was, too, a striking feature: *e.g.*, in certain of the patients chronic haemolysis necessitated splenectomy, gallstones required cholecystectomy, and there was chronic leg ulceration. Laboratory studies showed unbalanced globin synthesis, in contrast to the more balanced synthesis usually found in thalassaemia trait, and the free pool of α chains was markedly increased. Freidman and co-workers considered that their study indicated that undefined acquired and genetic factors play an important role in the expression of β-thalassaemia.

Thalassaemia minima

Almost by definition, individuals labelled as having β-thalassaemia minima will have no signs and symptoms attributable to thalassaemia. Their blood picture is, however, likely to be not strictly normal (see below).

BLOOD PICTURE IN β-THALASSAEMIA MINOR AND MINIMA

Although the majority of heterozygotes for β-thalassaemia are slightly to moderately anaemic, as judged by haemoglobin levels, in some individuals the haemoglobin lies within the normal range. Even so, inspection of stained blood films, as well as measurement of absolute values, almost always, if not always, will reveal definite abnormalities (Fig. 18.5). The characteristic features are: a tendency to a high total erythrocyte count, often exceeding 6.0×10^{12} cells per litre, a markedly subnormal MCV and MCH (but a normal or only slightly subnormal MCHC) and in stained films a moderate to marked degree of hypochromasia, microcytosis and anisopoikilocytosis, as well as slight polychromasia and a variable degree of

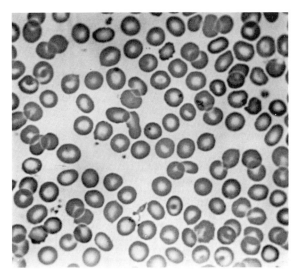

Fig. 18.5 Photomicrograph of a blood film of a patient with β-thalassaemia minor.
The erythrocytes vary moderately in size and shape and tend to be microcytic and hypochromic. Target cells are present in moderate numbers. × 700.

values. Reliable haematological data obtained in this way from several large groups of β-thalassaemia heterozygotes are now available.

Weatherall and Clegg (1981) (their Table 6.1) summarized the data obtained from six different populations, Greek (Malamos, Fessas and Stamatoyannopoulos, 1962), Thai and Chinese (Pootrakul, Wasi and Na-Nakorn, 1973), British (Knox-Macaulay *et al.*, 1973), Italian (Mazza *et al.*, 1976), Turkish (Dinçol *et al.*, 1979) and Sardinian (Galanello *et al.*, 1979). The findings in each series were similar irrespective of race: in adult males the mean haemoglobin ranged from 11.6 ± 1.5 to 13.9 ± 1.2 g/dl and the mean erythrocyte count from 5.2 ± 0.7 to $6.3 \pm 0.4 \times 10^{12}$/l; in adult females the mean haemoglobin ranged from 10.3 ± 1.2 to 11.8 ± 0.9 g/dl and the mean erythrocyte count from 4.7 ± 0.6 to $5.4 \pm 0.4 \times 10^{12}$/l. The minimum mean MCH was 20 ± 3.0 pg and the maximum 23.5 ± 1.0 pg and the minimum mean MCV was 66 ± 4.0 fl and the maximum 76.3 ± 1.0 fl.

punctate basophilia. Except for the fact that normoblasts are usually absent, the changes are similar to those seen in β-thalassaemia major, although less marked. In some films, but not in all, target cells can be seen in quite large numbers and in some films, too, oval and elliptical cells are conspicuous. Beaven and White (1962) in a study of five families of Anglo-Saxon origin made the point that the erythrocyte morphological characters tended to vary markedly between affected individuals belonging to the same family.

The above changes are rather similar to those of an iron-deficiency anaemia of mild to moderate severity. However, in iron-deficiency anaemia the erythrocyte count is usually lower at any level of haemoglobin and the count is seldom in the 'polycythaemic' range. Hence the MCV and MCH tend to be distinctly lower in β-thalassaemia heterozygotes than in iron-deficiency anaemia. On cell morphology alone, however, it is often difficult to separate the two conditions (see p. 530).

The recent development of automated blood-cell counting machines has made it possible to count erythrocytes more accurately than had hitherto been possible and to demonstrate small differences between populations in counts and absolute

Pootrakul, Wasi and Na-Nakorn (1973) reported that of 312 Thai and Chinese asymptomatic carriers of the β-thalassaemia trait 67, 81 and 6%, respectively, had a MCV, MCH or MCHC below the normal range; 54% of 312 carriers had haemoglobin values which fell within the normal range and among those considered to be anaemic 83% had a haemoglobin above 10 g/dl.

Piomelli and Siniscalco (1969) reported on a study of the inhabitants of a Sardinian village in which the thalassaemia trait and G6PD deficiency were present in high frequency. The blood picture of the affected individuals was similar to that reported for other series and the interesting observation was made that the haematological effects of the combination of both traits (*e.g.* on MCV) was equal to the sum of the independent effects of each.

The above recently obtained data have confirmed what had in fact been clearly established in the 1940s and 1950s. Thus, most thalassaemia-minor patients were recognized to have haemoglobin levels above 10 g/dl, with the level in 'minima' cases usually normal. Their erythrocyte counts, too, were known not infrequently to exceed 6.0×10^{12}/l.

Wintrobe and co-workers (1940), who studied 14 male adolescents in three families of Italian descent (whom they considered to be suffering from a less severe form of Cooley's anaemia), had stressed that the degree of anisocytosis and poikilocytosis seemed generally to be out of proportion to the mild anaemia that might be present and that sometimes there might be no anaemia at all, as judged by haemoglobin levels; they also had remarked on the target cells, basophilic stippling, slight polychromasia and the occasional normoblasts that might be present. They recognized that the erythrocyte counts were unexpectedly high in relation to the low PCV and haemoglobin levels. They stressed, too, the increased resistance to hypotonic saline.

Dameshek (1943) had emphasized that high erythrocyte counts, basophilic stippling, elongation of erythrocytes and the presence of target cells, as well as increased resistance to hypotonic saline, were characteristic features of the blood picture of patients with the 'familial Mediterranean target-oval cell syndrome'. Hanlon, Selby and Bayrd (1956) reported similar findings. Thus out of 30 hereditary leptocytosis (thalassaemia minor) patients studied, 22 had erythrocyte counts exceeding $5.0 \times 10^{12}/l$, the highest being $7.5 \times 10^{12}/l$.

It is interesting to note that females seem to be rather more anaemic than males. This had been noted, too, by Valentine and Neel (1948) and these observations are born out by more recent data (Mazza et al. 1976).

The MCV had for many years been recognized to be well below normal, e.g. by Dameshek (1943), Smith (1943), Valentine and Neel (1944, 1948), Daland and Strauss (1948), Heinle and Read (1948) and Gerald and Diamond (1958a). As compared with the substantially reduced MCH, the MCHC was considered to be but slightly lowered (Valentine and Neel, 1948; Gerald and Diamond, 1958a).

The MCD was reported by Mooney (1952) to be usually within the normal range, the presence of macrocytes balancing the effect of the microcytes. Hypochromic macrocytes had earlier been noted by Smith (1942, 1948). The mean cell thickness (MCT) had been recognized to be reduced by Dameshek (1940), Wintrobe et al. (1940) and by Smith (1943) (hence the term 'leptocytosis').

Punctate basophilia had often been commented on, e.g. by Wintrobe et al. (1940), Smith (1942, 1948), Rietti (1950) in cases of Rietti-Greppi-Micheli anaemia, Mooney (1952) and Hanlon, Selby and Bayrd (1956). [Punctate basophilia is not a common feature of simple iron-deficiency anaemia.] Rietti (1950), in referring to the Rietti-Greppi-Micheli anaemia, made the interesting point that punctate basophilia mainly affected elliptical hypochromic cells and was rarely seen in target cells. Mooney (1952) stated that the stippled-cell count varied between 2000 and 19 500/μl in the relatives of Cooley's anaemia patients and concluded that the stippled-cell count and measurement of osmotic resistance together were the best indicators of the trait.

Reticulocytes. The reticulocyte count is often a little raised above the normal but seldom exceeds 3% (Smith, 1943; Valentine and Neel, 1944, 1948; Daland and Strauss, 1948; Hanlon, Selby and Bayrd, 1956; etc.) or $200 \times 10^9/l$ (Mazza et al., 1976). Pootrakul, Wasi and Na-Nakorn (1973) reported a mean value of 1.69% in 193 asymptomatic Thai and Chinese with the β-thalassaemia trait; in 74% the count was < 2%.

Hb A$_2$

As already referred to on page 392, the discovery by Kunkel and Wallenius in 1955 that the then recently described Hb A$_2$ was present in increased amount in patients with thalassaemia minor was an important step in the understanding of the nature of thalassaemia. More data from the Rockefeller Institute were published in 1957. Kunkel and his co-workers then recorded that the mean Hb-A$_2$ percentage in 34 thalassaemia-trait individuals was 5.11 ± 1.36, compared to their normal range of 2.54 ± 0.35. It soon became apparent, however, that raised Hb-A$_2$ percentages, although commonly present, were not a consistent characteristic of β-thalassaemia.

Data on a large series of patients were reported in 1957 by Carcassi, Ceppellini and Siniscalco who compared 157 normal subjects with 78 patients considered to have thalassaemia minima: the mean Hb-A$_2$ concentration in the former was 2.33 ± 0.39% and in the latter (the patients) 5.19 ± 0.68%. In a few of the patients the raised Hb-A$_2$ level was the only abnormality demonstrable and in a few other patients, who presented other manifestations of thalassaemia, the Hb-A$_2$ level was normal. Silvestroni and Bianco (1957), too, published some interesting findings. In two families there were high Hb-A$_2$ levels but no signs of microcythaemia. In one of the families the father had a high Hb-A$_2$ level and the mother microcythaemia: three of their children had high Hb-A$_2$ levels and four microcythaemia; one child, presumably a compound heterozygote, had died.

Marti (1962) reported on 100 individuals with thalassaemia minor observed in Switzerland. Their mean Hb-A$_2$ percentage was 4.9, with a range from 3.3 to 6.5%.

Weatherall (1964a) studied 94 individuals with thalassaemia minor and compared the Hb-A$_2$ levels in populations of different racial origin, i.e., in 54 American blacks, 28 Italians and 12 Greeks. No significant differences were established in the concentration of Hb A$_2$ (and of Hb F) in the different groups. Hb A$_2$

varied between 3.4 and 7.4%, mean 5.16%. Its concentration could not be related to total haemoglobin level, PCV or MCHC, but there was an inverse correlation between MCH and % Hb A_2. The data indicated a content of Hb A_2 per cell of about 1.0 pg, a figure remaining constant from case to case. There appeared to be segregation of Hb-A_2 values from family to family, indicating that genetic factors play a part in determining Hb-A_2 level.

Silverstroni and Bianco (1965) reported details of three families that again emphasized how Hb-A_2 (and Hb-F) levels are controlled by genetic factors. In all three families there were high Hb-A_2 and low Hb-A_2 cases in different sides of the family and in each family there was a patient with Cooley's anaemia who was a compound heterozygote of both types. There appeared, too, to be a reciprocal relationship between Hb A_2 and Hb F.

More recently, cases of thalassaemia with normal Hb-A_2 levels have become to be known as examples of $\delta\beta$-thalassaemia (see p. 430).

Details of Hb-A_2 levels in large series of β-thalassaemia patients in Thailand and Turkey were reported, respectively by Pootrakul, Wasi and Na-Nakorn (1973) and Dinçol, Aksoy and Erdem (1979). In the patients of Thai or Chinese nationality, the Hb-A_2 levels ranged from 3.59 to 7.08%, mean 5.08 ± 0.63%; in those of Turkish nationality 80% had raised Hb-A_2 levels (3.8–6.5%).

Hb F

The percentage of Hb F present in β-thalassaemia heterozygotes is typically small and almost always less than 10%.

White and Beaven (1959) described how they could not detect any Hb F in about 50% of their patients and could find small increases only (1–4%) in the remainder. Fessas's (1959a) figures were similar: usually less than 3% and often a normal content; six out of 50 had 3–7% Hb F.

If stained by the Kleihauer, Braun and Betke technique (1957), or by its modifications, F-containing cells can be demonstrated to persist in the peripheral blood throughout the patient's lifetime. Sansone and Massimo (1959), in an early publication, demonstrated positive staining in thalassaemia major, thalassaemia minima and drepanocytosis. The amount of Hb F present varies markedly from cell to cell (a heterogeneous distribution) (see also p. 431).

Marti (1962) recorded that the Hb-F percentage was increased in only 76% of his 100 cases. Cutillo et al.

(1962), who studied the 32 parents of 16 children with Cooley's anaemia, reported that their Hb-F percentage ranged between 0.7 and 6.8 (and their Hb-A_2 percentage from 1.3 to 7.7).

Weatherall (1964a) reported 2–6% Hb F in a group of 94 blacks, Italians and Greeks, with a continuous distribution but with interfamily segregation also. However, one apparent thalassaemia heterozygote had 17.8% Hb F (with 4.2% Hb A_2). Silvestroni, Bianco and Muratore (1965) found a range for Hb F of 3–14% in heterozygotes belonging to a large Italian family and Silvestroni and Bianco (1965) noted in three families what appeared to be a reciprocal relationship between the levels of Hb A_2 and Hb F.

Pootrakul, Wasi and Na-Nakorn (1973) found in their large series of Thai and Chinese patients a Hb-F concentration ranging from 0% (none demonstrated) to 7.8%, mean 1.54 ± 1.3%; 58% of the values were elevated. In Turks, Dinçol, Aksoy and Erdem (1979) reported that Hb-F values were increased in 15% of 164 thalassaemia heterozygotes: 7.1% of their patients had normal values for both Hb A_2 and Hb F.

Normal Hb-A_2 and Hb-F values had been previously reported in four families by Silvestroni et al. (1978). In three of these families a member had had Cooley's anaemia: one parent had high Hb-A_2 thalassaemia, the other had normal Hb-A_2 and Hb-F levels. The $\alpha : \beta$ chain-synthesis ratio was shown in the normal Hb-A_2 and Hb-F patients to be similar to that found in typical (high Hb-A_2) β-thalassaemia heterozygotes, i.e. to be greater than 1.0.

OSMOTIC FRAGILITY, AUTOHAEMOLYSIS AND MECHANICAL FRAGILITY IN THALASSAEMIA MAJOR AND MINOR

The increased resistance of the erythrocyte in thalassaemia to haemolysis in hypotonic saline has been recognized since the early descriptions of the disease.

In thalassaemia major the resistance of the majority of the erythrocytes is increased but there is, too, often a small percentage of corpuscles that are abnormally fragile. This had been noted as far back as 1932 by Baty, Blackfan and Diamond.

In thalassaemia minor increased osmotic resistance has also been noted for many years to be a characteristic finding. It had, too, been regarded as a diagnostic feature of the Rietti-Greppi-Micheli anaemia of Italian authors (see Rietti, 1946).

Wintrobe and co-workers (1940) and Dameshek (1940) postulated that it was the presence of unusually thin erythrocytes that was responsible for the increased resistance; and it was soon realized that a significant degree of increased resistance, with lysis being incomplete in solutions as hypotonic as 0.20% NaCl, might be present even if anaemia was minimal and the individuals studied free of symptoms (Smith, 1943; Valentine and Neel, 1944; Mooney, 1952; Gatto and Valentino, 1953; Hanlon, Selby and Bayrd, 1956; etc.). Increased osmotic resistance was in fact at one time used quite widely as a criterion for the identification of carriers of thalassaemia, e.g., by Piomelli and Siniscalco (1969), and with the advent of sensitive, rapidly performable and simplified osmotic-fragility tests, e.g., the glycerol lysis-time test of Gottfried and Robertson (1974), renewed interest has been taken in such measurements (e.g., by Rajnoldi et al., 1980)

While there is no question but that increased erythrocyte osmotic resistance is a characteristic feature of β-thalassaemia minor, it seems possible that when the trait is minimally expressed resistance may fall within the normal range. Thus Pootrakul, Wasi and Na-Nakorn (1973) reported normal values using buffered hypotonic saline and a standard technique in 17 out of 188 asymptomatic Thai and Chinese considered to have the β-thalassaemia trait.

The cause of the marked increased resistance to hypotonic saline of thalassaemia erythrocytes is not entirely clear. As mentioned above, both Wintrobe and co-workers (1940) and Dameshek (1940) linked the change with the unusual thinness of the corpuscles.

Haut and co-workers (1962), in studies of the osmotic fragility of incubated normal and abnormal erythrocytes, including leptocytes and iron-deficiency anaemia cells, concluded that the differences they observed were related to the surface area: volume ratio. But whether this is the entire explanation is uncertain. The erythrocytes of four patients with thalassaemia minor were incubated at 37°C for up to 72 hours and the changes in osmotic resistance recorded. The increased resistance that developed was more marked than with the cells of comparably anaemic iron-deficiency anaemia patients. The difference was particularly striking after 12 hours' incubation with the cells then exposed to 0.40% saline.

That the increase in osmotic resistance in thalassaemia minor is generally more marked than in patients with a similar degree of anaemia due to iron deficiency (as measured by haemoglobin levels) was also clearly shown by the data of Buchanan et al. (1963): resistance was outside the normal range in all 15 (Scottish) patients with thalassaemia minor but this was so only in eight of 30 iron-deficient patients.

Autohaemolysis

The scanty evidence available suggests that thalassaemia-major and thalassaemia-minor erythrocytes behave (perhaps not unexpectedly) abnormally on incubation as well as being morphologically abnormal.

Selwyn (1953) observed with the blood of a patient with thalassaemia major: (a) that the rate of autohaemolysis was at the upper limit of the normal (0.8% at 24 hours and 3.3% at 48 hours); (b) that cell volume diminished on incubation for 24 hours instead of increasing as with normal blood; (c) that the loss of potassium from the corpuscles was greater than normal; and (d) that the erythrocyte osmotic fragility was markedly diminished rather than increased at the end of 24 hours' incubation.

Swarup, Ghosh and Chatterjea (1960) studied eight thalassaemia-major patients; lysis at 48 hours (without added glucose) ranged from 1.6 to 12.5%, mean 6.19%. 29 thalassaemia-trait patients were also studied: lysis at 48 hours ranged from 0.4 to 18.7%, mean 3.68%. The normal subjects' lysis at 48 hours ranged from 0.51 to 3.8%, mean 1.53%. Swarup, Ghosh and Chatterjea also investigated seven patients who had iron-deficiency anaemia. Lysis at 48 hours ranged from 0.2 to 5.9%, mean 2.31%.

Scott, Rasbridge and Grimes (1970) studied six patients who had Hb-H disease, two of whom had been splenectomized. The rate of autohaemolysis was variably but slightly increased and not reduced, in fact generally increased, by added glucose.

Knox-Macaulay and co-workers (1972) reported that the rate of autohaemolysis was slightly increased in one patient, and normal in another patient, who were compound heterozygotes for α-thal-1 and β-thalassaemia and that lysis was considerably reduced by adding either glucose or ATP. Lysis was slightly increased, too, in a patient who had Hb-H disease.

Whether thalassaemic erythrocytes behave differently from corpuscles from patients with comparable deficits in haemoglobin as the result of iron deficiency is a question that does not seem to have been clearly answered.

Vanella and co-workers (1980) compared the effect of added polyamines on the autohaemolysis of 25 thalassaemia-major blood samples and 25 normal control blood samples. The polyamines had no effect on the lysis of the normal cells but reduced that of the thalassaemia cells (mean value without additive approximately 7% at 48 hours) by up to almost 50%. It was suggested that this effect was linked to the polyamines acting as antioxidants. (Vanella *et al.* stated that highly activated forms of oxygen are released in abnormally large amounts during the oxidation of haemoglobin in thalassaemia erythrocytes.)

Mechanical fragility

The finding of cell fragments in the peripheral blood in cases of thalassaemia major led at one time to interest in the possibility that the erythrocytes were abnormally mechanically fragile. Attempts to assess this have, however, mostly led to equivocal results.

Tolentino (1951) reported that the mechanical fragility of thalassaemic erythrocytes was normal or even slightly diminished. Chatterjea and co-workers (1956), in contrast, reported slight increases in some Cooley's anaemia patients but generally normal values in patients with the trait. The pathogenesis of erythrocyte fragmentation in thalassaemia is further considered on page 503.

BIOCHEMICAL FINDINGS IN β-THALASSAEMIA MINOR

Plasma haemoglobin and serum haptoglobin and haemopexin. There is little overt evidence of intravascular haemolysis in most cases of thalassaemia minor. Crosby and Dameshek (1951) reported that the plasma haemoglobin level was normal (1–3 mg/dl) in the 23 patients they studied. Das Gupta and co-workers (1955) reported essentially similar findings (0.6–4.3 mg/dl) in 13 patients.

Cutillo and Meloni (1974) reported that the serum haptoglobin and haemopexin concentrations in 25 adults with thalassaemia minor were similar to those of normal controls.

Serum bilirubin. This is usually within the normal range. However, a few heterozygotes with apparently uncomplicated β-thalassaemia have had slightly raised serum bilirubin levels. Thus out of 10 adult Italians studied by Gallo and co-workers (1975) values above 1.0 mg/dl (1.2 and 1.3 mg) were found in three of them.

Faecal urobilinogen. The excretion of urobilinogen is probably always increased, the excess pigment excreted being largely the product of ineffective erythropoiesis. Gallo and co-workers

(1975) found a clear negative correlation between the amount of pigment excreted and the patient's haemoglobin level. In 10 patients studied the excretion was 3–10 times the normal.

Serum cholesterol. As in other anaemias, serum cholesterol and β-lipoprotein levels tend to be unusually low in thalassaemia trait (Fessas, Stamatoyannopoulos and Keys, 1963).

Erythrocyte metabolism and enzymes

In most patients glucose metabolism via the EM pathway and HM shunt has been found to be within the normal range. According to Sass and Spear (1961) erythrocyte glutamic oxaloacetic transaminase activity is increased to about twice the normal, the increase being more marked than in iron-deficiency anaemia.

The DPG concentration in the thalassaemia-minor erythrocyte was reported by Pearson *et al.* (1977) to be higher than normal. A point of interest is whether the increase is higher than would be expected in similarly anaemic, but not thalassaemic, patients. The results of recent studies have been conflicting. Tassiopoulos and co-workers (1982) reported values higher than those expected while Alvarez-Sala *et al.* (1983a,b) reported values within the expected range. Interestingly, Alvarez-Sala *et al.* (1983b) found that the mean DPG concentration in six homozygous patients was significantly less than the theoretical value.

Vives Corrons and co-workers (1984) in a detailed study measured the activity of 18 erythrocyte enzymes and estimated GSH in 50 individuals with the thalassaemia trait as well as in 50 non-thalassaemic patients with a haemolytic anaemia and reticulocytosis and in 70 normal subjects, the latter two groups serving as controls. In addition, the activity of erythrocyte pyrimidine 5' nucleotidase (P5N) was measured in 34 patients who had an iron-deficiency anaemia. The activity of most of the enzymes measured was increased in the β-thalassaemia-trait patients and the findings were in most instances similar to those found in the haemolytic-anaemia controls. However, the activity of 2,3-biphosphoglycerate synthetase and GSH reductase was normal and that of acetylcholinesterase was slightly decreased. A striking finding was that P5N activity was markedly subnormal (less than −2 SD below the mean normal value) in 23 out of the 50 β-thalassaemia-trait patients. Vives Corrons *et al.* suggested that the low P5N activity might be responsible for the erythrocyte punctate basophilia that is so frequently found in thalassaemia trait. In the iron-deficient patients the P5N activity did not differ significantly from normal.

Erythrocyte creatine. Gimferrer and co-workers

(1984) measured erythrocyte creatine in 15 heterozygous β-thalassaemia propositi and in 21 β-thalassaemia relatives, all of whom were otherwise healthy. The mean level was significantly below normal in both groups, and the creatine concentration relative to the reticulocyte count was substantially subnormal, too. Higher values were found in pregnant β-thalassaemia patients but they were not as high as in normal pregnant females. The cause of the low values was not established.

Erythrocyte protoporphyrin. Pootrakul and coworkers (1984) measured erythrocyte protoporphyrin (EP) in a large number of patients suffering from the haemoglobinopathies found in Thailand. Included in the series were 14 patients with thalassaemia minor. The EP concentrations were found to vary rather widely but in a minority of individuals the values were significantly above normal, irrespective of the exact nature of their haemoglobinopathy. In none of the patients, however, were the values raised if the transferrin-iron saturation exceeded 44% of the normal. Pootrakul et al. suggested that the raised values found in some of their patients were causally related to an iron supply that was inadequate for the massive expansion of erythropoiesis. Included in their paper is a useful Table in which are summarized the results of earlier studies.

Serum iron and total iron-binding capacity (TIBC)

The serum iron concentration and TIBC have been reported to be normal in most heterozygotes with β-thalassaemia minor.

Cartwright, Hugeley and Ashenbrucker (1948) stated that the plasma iron was normal in the five thalassaemia-minor patients they investigated. Smith and co-workers (1950), however, reported serum iron concentrations of 126–404 μg/dl in nine adult patients; in four the saturation was 100%.

Crosby and Conrad (1964) studied three adults. The plasma iron concentrations were high, 234, 175 and 175 μg/dl, respectively, and it was calculated that the patients' ability to absorb oral iron was enhanced, 19%, 22% and 17% of single doses being absorbed. Williams and Siemsen (1968) provided further (indirect) evidence for abnormally great iron absorption in thalassaemia minor. Their patient, a French-Italian male aged 30 years, had never been transfused and had not received oral iron therapy. Nevertheless, he had a high serum iron level (192–216 μg/dl), with 83–96% saturation, and his bone marrow and liver were heavily infiltrated with iron.

The more recent data of Knox-Macaulay and co-workers (1973) were based on 53 patients (33 female and 20 male) and 20 of their normal siblings. The serum iron levels, TIBC and percentage saturation did not differ between the male and female patients, in contrast to the lower values for serum iron in the females belonging to the normal control series. The values for the patients were no doubt distorted by iron therapy, for many of them (23 of the females and three of the males) had received repeated courses of iron preparations, so much so that one of the females had a completely saturated TIBC.

Pootrakul, Wasi and Na-Nakorn (1973) reported that the serum iron concentration varied from 6 to 305 μg/dl in 292 Thai and Chinese with the β-thalassaemia trait. The mean value was 108 μg/dl; 11% had values less than 50 μg/dl and 6% values greater than 200 μg/dl. None of the patients had an enlarged spleen or liver or crural ulcers. The very low serum iron concentrations in some of them indicates a considerable incidence of nutritional iron deficiency in the population studied.

Iron deficiency is common, too, in Indian patients with heterozygous β-thalassaemia, particularly in females, according to Saraya et al. (1985) who give data on transferrin saturation and serum-ferritin concentration.

Erythrocyte ferritin has been measured in β-thalassaemia-minor erythrocytes by Jacobs et al. (1981), Peters, Jacobs and Fitzsimmons (1983) and Piperno et al. (1984). Slight to moderate increases have been reported.

Iron overloading and haemochromatosis

The possibility that some thalassaemia-minor patients who are iron-overloaded are heterozygous, too, for a gene for idiopathic haemochromatosis (IH) has been investigated. Bowdler and Huehns (1963) had described a family in which two and possibly three out of five members suffering from thalassaemia minor may have been affected in this way. Some recent evidence in favour of this hypothesis was described by Fargion et al. (1985), who characterized the HLA antigens in 107 carriers of the β-thalassaemia trait. The incidence of the HLA-A3 antigen (which is closely associated with the presence of a gene for IH) was found to be significantly higher in the patients with iron overload compared with those who were not iron-overloaded (an incidence of 50% compared to 18%).

Serum copper

Cartwright, Hugeley and Ashenbrucker (1948) reported that the serum copper level was raised in four out of six thalassaemia-minor patients.

ERYTHROCYTE LIFE-SPAN IN β-THALASSAEMIA MINOR AND MINIMA

A number of studies have shown that the erythrocyte life-span in thalassaemia minor and minima (heterozygous β-thalassaemia) is normal or but slightly shortened.

Ashby method. Kaplan, Zuelzer and Hoogana (1950) transfused the erythrocytes of three women with the thalassaemia trait into normal recipients and found that the transfused cells survived normally. Hamilton and co-workers (1950) reported that the erythrocytes of an individual considered to have thalassaemia minima survived normally in a normal recipient; in contrast, the survival of the corpuscles of a patient with a more severe form of the trait appeared to be slightly impaired (elimination complete in 85 days). Frontali (1954) found the survival of the erythrocytes of five symptomless carriers of the thalassaemia trait to be between 110 and 130 days, *i.e.* to be normal.

^{51}Cr method. McFarland and Pearson (1960), Pearson *et al.* (1960), Malamos *et al.* (1961a), Honetz *et al.* (1968) and Gallo *et al.* (1975) have reported slight reductions in ^{51}Cr T$_{50s}$ in some of the individuals with thalassaemia minor they studied.

Pearson and co-workers (1960) studied nine white adults. Their ^{51}Cr T$_{50s}$ ranged between 15 and 30 days, the mean being 23 days. In five of the nine the T$_{50}$ was considered to be normal (25 days or more). Gallo *et al.* (1975) investigated 10 adult Italians and found the ^{51}Cr T$_{50}$ to range between 21 and 24 days, all slightly subnormal figures. In contrast, Bernini *et al.* (1964), who had studied nine adult Sardinians, had earlier

concluded that their erythrocyte survival was normal.

^{59}Fe method. Cazzola and co-workers (1979) calculated from ferrokinetic data that the mean erythrocyte life-span in eight β-thalassaemia heterozygotes was 25–64 days (normal by the method 109 ± 12 days).

ERYTHROKINETIC STUDIES IN β-THALASSAEMIA MINOR AND MINIMA

Studies in thalassaemia minor have given results similar to those found in thalassaemia major although less abnormal. Thus the plasma iron turnover is increased and iron utilization subnormal.

Pearson and co-workers (1960) studied nine adults with 'classical' thalassaemia trait. The plasma disappearance of ^{59}Fe was abnormally fast in three of them; plasma iron turnover was increased in all of them, averaging 3 times the normal, and iron utilization averaged 58% at 14 days (normally 80–95%). Cazzola *et al.* (1979) investigated eight patients. Erythropoiesis was markedly increased and 10–74% of this was calculated to be ineffective. All the patients were moderately anaemic (haemoglobin 7.1–11.7 g/dl) and the importance of the ineffective haemopoiesis in the causation of their anaemia was emphasized. Haemolysis of mature erythrocytes was thought to be an important factor in the most anaemic patients.

THALASSAEMIA INTERMEDIA

As already indicated (p. 390), the term 'thalassaemia intermedia' has been widely used as a tentative clinical label for thalassaemic patients whose illness is of a severity somewhere between that of thalassaemia major and that of the relatively benign or completely symptomless thalassaemia minor or minima.

An important clinical differentiating point that many physicians have adhered to is the necessity or otherwise for the administration of repeated and regular transfusions. A child that can manage to lead a reasonable life without being transfused has 'thalassaemia intermedia'; one that requires regular transfusions has thalassaemia major (Erlandson, Brilliant and Smith, 1964; etc.).

As discussed, too, the genetic background of thalassaemia intermedia is extremely complicated, a variety of abnormalities affecting haemoglobin

synthesis, in various combinations in compound heterozygotes, resulting in the syndrome (Pearson, Gerald and Diamond, 1959; Pearson, 1964; Aksoy 1970; Braverman *et al.*, 1973; Aksoy, Dinçol and Erdem, 1978; Cividalli *et al.*, 1978; Weatherall *et al.*, 1981b; Aksoy *et al.*, 1982; Fessas *et al.*, 1982; Trent *et al.*, 1982; Musumeci *et al.*, 1983; Wainscoat *et al.*, 1983; Thein, Al-Hakim and Hoffbrand, 1984; Cacace *et al.*, 1985) (Table 18.2).

The clinical effects of the failure of haemoglobin synthesis are, however, much the same irrespective of the exact nature of the genetic cause, *i.e.* they depend more on its severity than its causation.

Clinical presentation

This is very variable. Some patients have become

Table 18.2 Thalassaemia intermedia: some important varieties.

β-*thalassaemias*
  Homozygous β^+/β^+ thalassaemia
  Some cases of β^0/β^+ thalassaemia
  β^0/β^0 or β^0/β^A thalassaemia plus α-thalassaemia
  Some cases of β^0/Hb-Lepore combination
  β^0/Greek HPFH combination

δβ-*thalassaemias*
  Homozygous $\delta\beta^0/\delta\beta^0$ thalassaemia
  $\delta\beta^0/\beta^0$ thalassaemia combination
  $\delta\beta^0$/Hb-Lepore combination

quite markedly anaemic in early childhood; in others, symptoms and signs have been much less obvious so that they have not been investigated until adolescence or later, *e.g.*, the patients of Ahern *et al.* (1975). Nevertheless, the spleen is almost always palpably enlarged, occasionally massively so (Farhangi, Sass and Bank, 1970). Growth and development are usually normal and regular blood transfusions are typically not required. There may or may not be clinical or X-ray evidence of skeletal changes of the type seen in β-thalassaemia major (Fig. 18.6). Fractures seldom occur (Erlandson *et al.*, 1964).

Clinical and haematological evidence of chronic hypersplenism is not uncommon (Rapaport, Reilly and Carpenter, 1957) and gallstones frequently form (Erlandson, Brilliant and Smith, 1964; Aksoy *et al.*, 1970). Acute transient splenic sequestration leading to pancytopenia, similar to that occurring in Hb-SS disease children, is rare, but has been reported (Schilirò *et al.*, 1983a).

According to Weatherall and Clegg (1981, p. 671), hyperbilirubinaemia resulting from ineffective erythropoiesis and increased haemolysis is a common feature of thalassaemia intermedia, many patients being chronically jaundiced. [It seems likely in retrospect that patients who at one time would have been diagnosed as suffering from the Rietti-Greppi-Micheli anaemia of Italian authors would nowadays be labelled as having thalassaemia intermedia.]

Other complications that have been recorded include diabetes secondary to iron overload (Erlandson *et al.*, 1964; Bannerman *et al.*, 1967) and leg ulcers (Estes, Farber and Stickney, 1948;

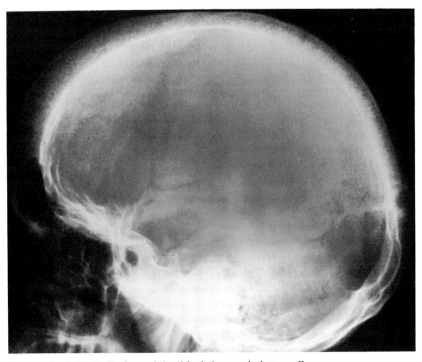

Fig. 18.6 X-ray photograph of the skull of an adult with thalassaemia intermedia.
The vault of the skull is thickened, particularly in the frontal region. (Reproduced by courtesy of Dr Janet Dacie.)

March, Schlyen and Schwartz, 1952; Cooper and Wacker, 1954; Gallo *et al.* 1979; Weatherall and Clegg, 1981, p. 678; Cacace *et al.*, 1987). Hyperuricaemia has been reported (March, Schlyen and Schwartz, 1952) and gout has been recorded but seems to be uncommon (Weatherall and Clegg, 1981, p. 677). A few patients have become pregnant; in some at least this has been associated with a worsening of their anaemia (Walker, Whelton and Beaven, 1969; Gallo *et al.*, 1979). Heart failure and hepatomegaly have been described secondary to iron overload (see p. 499) and it seems quite clear that a clinically important degree of iron overloading can take place even in patients who have not been transfused and have not been treated with iron (Celada, 1982; Frigerio *et al.*, 1984).

Tumour-like masses of bone marrow. These are not uncommon (Knoblich, 1960; Erlandson *et al.*, 1964; Korsten *et al.*, 1970; Ben-Basset *et al.*, 1977) (Fig. 18.7; see also Vol. 1, Fig. 3.44, p. 95); exceptionally, they have led to compression of the spinal cord (Gatto, Terrana and Biondi, 1954; Sorsdahl, Taylor and Noyes, 1964; Papavasiliou, 1965; Bate and Humphries, 1977).

Knoblich's (1960) patient was a 63-year-old Greek man who had been known since the age of 49 to have tumours in the lower lung fields demonstrable by X-ray. Thoracotomy for a ? neurogenic tumour demonstrated a mass the size of two fists and another the size of a golf ball. Sections showed haemopoietic tissue. Subsequent examination revealed the blood picture of thalassaemia intermedia and it later transpired that the patient's sister had had a 700-g spleen excised.

The patient described by Ben-Basset and co-workers (1977) is of unusual interest, too, as he was one of the two patients described in 1945 by Schieber in his report of the first cases of 'target-cell anaemia' recognized in Israel. The patient died aged 69 of cardiac failure associated probably with hepatic cirrhosis. A limited necropsy revealed several masses of bone-marrow tissue (predominantly formed of erythroblasts) varying in size from 7 cm to 2 cm in diameter. Ben-Basset and his co-workers considered that thalassaemia intermedia is the commonest cause of the intrathoracic haemopoietic tumour syndrome.

Papavasiliou and Sandilos (1987) reported that they had treated with small doses of radiation eight patients aged between 14 and 59 years, who were considered to be suffering from thalassaemia major and who had presented with symptoms or signs of spinal-cord compression. The treatment relieved their symptoms and in the three patients followed radiographically the mass of heterotopic marrow regressed completely in two and partially in one.

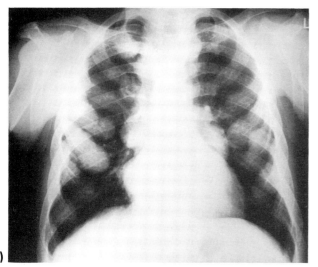

(a)

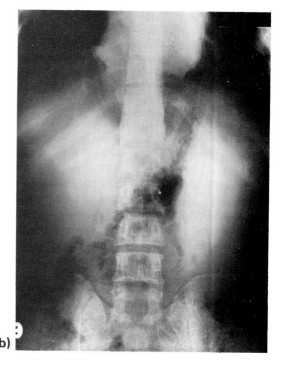

(b)

Fig. 18.7 X-ray photograph of (a) chest and (b) abdomen of a 34-year-old male Turk who had thalassaemia intermedia.
The X-ray of the chest shows paravertebral masses and tumour-like growths from the ribs. The X-ray of the abdomen shows paravertebral masses and massive enlargement of the liver and spleen. (Reproduced by courtesy of Dr Janet Dacie.)

Blood picture

The blood picture in β-thalassaemia intermedia varies from one not distinguishable from that of transfusion-dependent homozygotes for β-thalassaemia to one indistinguishable from that of simple heterozygotes for β-thalassaemia in whom the disorder is well expressed. The haemoglobin, in the absence of transfusion, usually ranges between 5 and 10 g/dl. The erythrocyte count is relatively high; the MCV and MCH are thus markedly lowered.

There is a variable but often very marked microcytosis, hypochromia and anisopoikilocytosis, with a slightly or moderately raised reticulocyte count and a corresponding degree of polychromasia or punctate basophilia (Fig. 18.8). Normoblasts, too, will be almost certainly present in the peripheral blood. Staining with methyl violet may show inclusion bodies in some of them.

The leucocyte and platelet counts are likely to be within the normal range except in patients who have developed hypersplenism.

The changes resulting from splenectomy are

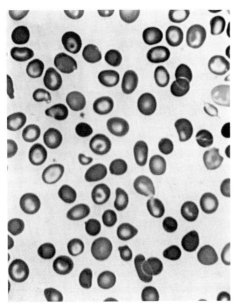

Fig. 18.8 Photomicrograph of a blood film of a patient with β-thalassaemia intermedia.
The erythrocytes vary considerably in size and shape and there is also marked anisochromasia. Cell fragments and target cells are also present. (Film provided by courtesy of Dr Adrian Stephens.)

similar to those seen in β-thalassaemia major, but are likely to be less marked.

Reticulocytes. The counts tend to be, as might be expected, generally between those seen in thalassaemia major and minor. In all variants of thalassaemia the counts are lower at comparable haemoglobin levels than would be expected in haemolytic anaemias in which erythropoiesis is not impaired.

Erythrocyte life-span

As expected, the erythrocyte life-span is shortened to a moderate degree in thalassaemia intermedia. Malamos and co-workers (1961a) recorded ^{51}Cr T_{50s} between 13.5 and 26.4 days (mean 17.4 days) in eight patients. They illustrated the results of surface-counting studies carried out on two adult patients: there was a moderate accumulation of ^{51}Cr in the spleen and rather less in the liver (the ^{51}Cr T_{50s} were 17 and 21 days, respectively). The spleen: liver ratio was normal. More recently, Ahern and co-workers (1975) reported ^{51}Cr T_{50s} of 21–24 days in four patients and Gallo and co-workers (1975) ^{51}Cr T_{50s} of 10–16 days (mean 13.2 days) in five patients. The survival curves in three of the patients of Ahern *et al.* were compatible with two populations of erythrocytes. In two of the patients there was excess uptake of radioactivity in the spleen compared with that in the liver.

Erythrokinetics

The data of Malamos and co-workers (1961a), based on studies carried out on 13 Greek patients considered to have thalassaemia major of intermediate severity, have already been referred to (p. 413). Earlier, Norris, Hanson and Loeffler (1956) had reported a rapid ^{59}Fe clearance, a raised plasma iron concentration and poor incorporation of radioactivity into erythrocytes in the case of an adult American black. Similar observations, *i.e.* rapid plasma clearance and increased plasma iron turnover, but reduced ^{59}Fe utilization (27–41%), were reported by Ahern and co-workers (1975) in four patients. Cavill and co-workers (1978) studied two untransfused patients and calculated that the marrow iron turnover was approximately 6 times the normal. The greater part of the iron, however, was shown to be used for ineffective erythropoiesis. The mean cell life-span of the erythrocytes the patients managed to produce was calculated to be 21 and 36 days, respectively.

More recently, Najean and co-workers (1985) have reported on kinetic studies carried out with ^{59}Fe on 12 patients with β-thalassaemia intermedia, six being adults and six children. The results were compared with those obtained in 17 transfusion-dependent patients with Cooley's anaemia. The intermediate patients were characterized by a higher ^{59}Fe marrow uptake, less ineffective erythropoiesis (i.e. better ^{59}Fe incorporation into erythrocytes) and a greater degree of peripheral haemolysis. Non-α:α chain synthesis was statistically better in the intermediate than in the Cooley's anaemia patients. Najean et al. concluded that kinetic studies provided a useful guide to therapeutic management. Pippard (1985), in discussing their results, doubted whether ferrokinetic studies would be more helpful in arriving at decisions as to therapy than knowledge of the haemoglobin level the patients are able to maintain unaided.

'Inclusion-body β-thalassaemia trait'.

As already emphasized, heterozygosity for β thalassaemia is associated with a wide range of clinical and haematological expression. At one extreme patients present with the syndrome of thalassaemia intermedia, at the other they have no symptoms and their blood picture is distinguishable only with difficulty from the normal — this is so-called silent thalassaemia (see below).

Under the title 'inclusion-body β-thalassaemia trait' Stamatoyannopoulos and co-workers (1974b) described a family of Swiss-French descent in which 18 individuals in three generations were moderately anaemic and had correspondingly abnormal blood pictures. An unexpected feature in line with unusual severity was that about 70% of their late normoblasts contained inclusions of precipitated α chains, a phenomenon normally only found in homozygotes.

'Silent β-thalassaemia'

As already referred to, minimally expressed thalassaemia was at one time referred to by Italian authors as 'microcytemia' (Silvestroni and Bianco, 1946) or thalassaemia minima (Astaldi, Tolentino and Sacchetti, 1951). More recently, it has been recognized that it is not uncommon in minimally expressed cases for the Hb-A$_2$ level not to be raised. Such cases have been labelled 'silent β-thalassaemia' and most have been brought to light in the course of investigating the parents of patients presenting with thalassaemia intermedia, when one parent has been found to have typical high Hb-A$_2$ β-thalassaemia minor and the other an apparently normal blood picture with but minimal microcytosis and a normal Hb-A$_2$ level.

Schwartz (1969) described in detail a family of this sort in which two children (Albanians) had mild thalassaemia major and did not need to be transfused. Their mother had typical high Hb-A$_2$ β-thalassaemia minor, their father had what was thought to be a normal film (possibly slightly hypochomic), MCV 88 fl, MCH 28.0 pg, and normal Hb-A$_2$ and Hb-F levels. That their father really had a β-thalassaemia trait was shown by globin-chain synthesis data carried out on his own erythrocytes and those of four relatives: all were abnormal, β:α 0.60–0.69. (The ratios of the children were 0.32 and 0.24 and that of their mother 0.47).

Aksoy (1970) and Aksoy, Dinçol and Erdem (1978), in a genetic study of thalassaemia intermedia, referred to several families in which the patient under investigation was a compound heterozygote for a gene for high Hb-A$_2$ β-thalassaemia and a (silent) gene for normal Hb-A$_2$ β-thalassaemia.

Kattamis and co-workers (1979) studied nine Greek families and emphasized the heterogeneity of normal Hb-A$_2$ β-thalassaemia. In six families heterozygotes with normal Hb-A$_2$ levels had minimal erythrocyte morphological abnormalities and normal osmotic resistance, yet unbalanced β-globin chain synthesis. Compound heterozygotes (normal A$_2$/high A$_2$) had mild thalassaemia intermedia with 20% Hb F.

In three families heterozygotes for normal Hb-A$_2$ β-thalassaemia had more marked erythrocyte abnormalities and increased osmotic resistance and more unbalanced β-globin chain synthesis. Compound heterozygotes (normal A$_2$/high A$_2$) were more severely affected and were transfusion-dependent. Kattamis and co-workers suggested that the genes for normal Hb-A$_2$ β-thalassaemia comprise about 10% of all thalassaemia genes in Greece.

Sciarratta and co-workers (1985) described the clinical and haematological findings in eight Italian families in which cases of clinically mild thalassaemia major or thalassaemia intermedia had occurred. In each family one parent of the propositus was a silent β-thalassaemia carrier and had a normal blood picture, or only a slightly reduced MCV and MCH, as well as a normal Hb-A$_2$ percentage. One propositus was considered to be homozygous for a silent carrier state.

δβ-THALASSAEMIA

Another variant of thalassaemia which became recognized in the 1960s is δβ-thalassaemia (or βδ-thalassaemia). This, as its title signifies, is characterized by failure to form δ chains as well as β chains. In heterozygotes Hb-A_2 levels are normal and in homozygotes, Hb A_2, as well as Hb A, is absent. Compensating for the failure to form δ chains and β chains is an increased production of γ chains, so much so that in homozygotes the circulating haemoglobin is almost entirely formed of Hb F. Because of this, this type of thalassaemia was at one time referred to as 'F thalassaemia' (Stamatoyannopoulos, Fessas and Papayannopoulou, 1969). Now δβ-thalassaemia is subdivided into [G]γ and [G]γ[A]γ types according to the nature of the Hb F present.

CLINICAL AND HAEMATOLOGICAL PRESENTATION OF δβ-THALASSAEMIA

Heterozygotes. Carriers of β-thalassaemia are usually perfectly normal clinically and their spleen is not normally palpable. Their haemoglobin is within the normal range or slightly below.

Zuelzer, Robinson and Booker (1961) described two Italian families in which in retrospect δβ-thalassaemia was occuring as well as more typical high Hb-A_2 β-thalassaemia. The Hb-A_2 and Hb-F concentrations in heterozygotes in different branches of the families appeared to vary reciprocally, *i.e.*, high Hb-F levels were associated with low Hb-A_2 levels and *vice versa*. There was thus evidence for the presence of two distinct thalassaemia genes, and one individual who presented with thalassaemia major appeared to be the product of the two dissimilar genes.

Other early reports of δβ-thalassaemia include those of Wolff and Ignatov (1963) in Greeks, Silvestroni, Bianco and Brancati (1964) in Italians, Weatherall (1964a) in American blacks, Flatz, Pik and Sringam (1965) in Thais, and Stamatoyannopoulos, Fessas and Papayannopoulou (1969) in Greeks.

The genetic events thought likely to lead to δβ-thalassaemia were reviewed by Stamatoyannopoulos *et al.* (1969) (see also p. 511).

Stamatoyannopoulos, Fessas and Papayannopoulou (1969) recorded the following data based on 68 Greek patients belonging to 31 families: haemoglobin 9.7–15.2 g/dl, mean 12.4 g; erythrocyte count 4.55–6.97 × 10^{12}/1, mean 5.54 × 10^{12}/1; MCH 17.6–26.5 pg, mean 22.4 pg; Hb A_2 0–3.4%, mostly < 2.6%; Hb F 2.2–18.6% (mostly > 10%). All their blood films showed the anisopoikilocytosis, microcytosis and punctate basophilia characteristic of thalassaemia, and osmotic resistance was increased in each case. The Hb F is heterocellularly distributed amongst the erythrocytes (Fig. 18.9).

More recent interesting reports include those of Stamatoyannopoulos *et al.* (1971) in Greeks (heterozygotes formed both [G]γ and [A]γ chains, ratio 2:3), Mann *et al.* (1972) in Chinese (the propositus, a compound heterozygote of δβ-thalassaemia and β-thalassaemia, synthesized [G]γ chains only), Kattamis *et al.* (1973) in Greeks (11 children were compound heterozygotes of δβ-thalassaemia and β-thalassaemia), Efremov *et al.* (1975) in Yugoslavians (two families in which two children were compound heterozygotes for δβ-thalassaemia and β-thalassaemia; both [G]γ and [A]γ chains were formed by heterozygotes, ratio 2:3), Aksoy, Dinçol and Erdem (1978) in Turks (five out of 20 patients were compound heterozygotes of δβ-thalassaemia and β-thalassaemia), Vayá *et al.* (1983) in Spaniards (102 F-thalassaemia heterozygotes were compared with 98 high Hb-A_2 β-thalassaemia heterozygotes), and Wainscoat *et al.* (1984) in Indians (a characterization of an Indian type of δβ-thalassaemia; [G]γ:[A]γ ratio in heterozygotes 7:3).

Homozygotes. Patients who have inherited two genes for δβ-thalassaemia have generally presented with rather mild thalassaemia intermedia. They develop normally, their spleen and liver are but slightly enlarged and they have seldom needed transfusing. Anaemia is mild to moderate, jaundice mild at the most and radiological changes in the bones are minimal.

The first patient to be recognized as homozygous for δβ-thalassaemia was the 31-year-old Southern Italian woman described by Brancati (1965) and Brancati and Baglioni (1966). She had been in good health although anaemic (haemoglobin 62%, erythrocytes 3.9 × 10^{12}/1, MCV 80 fl) and the blood film was typical of that of thalassaemia. Osmotic resistance was markedly increased. The spleen and liver were palpable. Both parents and one brother had a thalassaemia-minor blood picture, with raised Hb-F levels (8.6%, 8.3% and 13.2%) and low Hb-A_2 levels (1.1%, 2.7% and 1.5%). The patient's own haemoglobin appeared to be entirely composed of Hb F; no Hb A_2 could be detected.

Since this description, other homozygotes have been

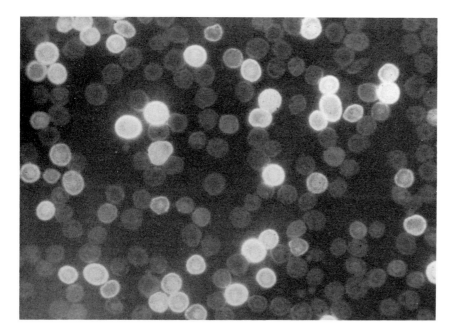

Fig. 18.9 Photomicrograph of F cells demonstrated by an immunofluorescent technique.
The patient was heterozygous for δβ-thalassaemia and only a proportion of the erythrocytes contain significant amounts of Hb F (a heterocellular distribution). (Reproduced by courtesy of Sir David Weatherall.)

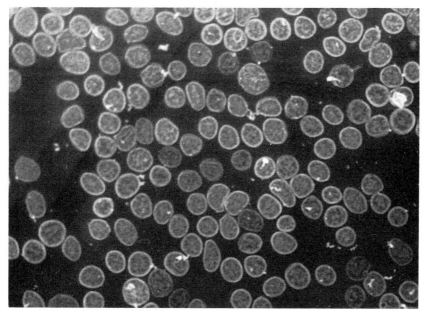

Fig. 18.10 Photomicrograph of F cells demonstrated by an immunofluorescent technique.
The patient was homozygous for δβ-thalassaemia, and all the erythrocytes contain Hb F (a pancellular distribution). (Reproduced by courtesy of Sir David Weatherall.)

reported from different racial groups and the clinical and haematological picture has been well defined (see below). Interesting reports include those of Silvestroni, Bianco and Reitano (1968), Ramot *et al.* (1970), Tsistrakis, Amarantos and Koukouris (1974), Aksoy, Dinçol and Erdem (1978), Amin *et al.* (1979), Gimferrer, Baiget and Rutllant (1979), Dinçol *et al.*, (1981), Aksoy *et al.* (1982), Baiget *et al.* (1983) and George *et al.* (1986).

Weatherall and Clegg (1981; p. 549) summarized the

haematological findings in 11 published cases of homozygous δβ-thalassaemia as follows: haemoglobin 5.9–13.3 g/dl, mean 10.1 g/dl; MCV 66–88 fl, mean 79 fl; MCH 21–28 pg, mean 24.2 pg; reticulocytes 1.5–8.0%, mean 4.7%, *i.e.* findings falling well within those to be expected in patients presenting with rather mild thalassaemia intermedia. The Hb F is distributed amongst the erythrocytes in a pancellular fashion (Fig. 18.10).

As already referred to, an interesting recent development has been the recognition that $\delta\beta$-thalassaemia comprises several entities which differ with respect to the type of Hb F present — whether formed of $^{G}\gamma$ and $^{A}\gamma$ chains or of $^{G}\gamma$ chains only — and the extent of the causal genetic lesion. Amin and co-workers (1979) described a Greek patient who was a homozygote for $^{G}\gamma^{A}\gamma(\delta\beta)$-thalassaemia (who formed both types of γ chains) as well as Arabian and Indian patients who were homozygous for $^{G}\gamma(\delta\beta)$-thalassaemia (who formed only $^{G}\gamma$ chains).

Three more homozygous $^{G}\gamma(\delta\beta)$-thalassaemic patients were described by Matthews et al. (1981) in a Hindu family. Clinically, they were mildly affected and no transfusions had been required. Erythrocyte morphology was, however, markedly abnormal. Brief details of patients with $^{G}\gamma(^{A}\gamma\delta\beta)^{0}$-thalassaemia in five families — Malaysian, Chinese, Bangladeshi, Indian and Kuwaiti — were given by Trent et al. (1984). Analysis of their Hb F revealed only $^{G}\gamma$ chains. Globin-gene mapping revealed four different deletions involving the $^{A}\gamma$, δ and β genes. The clinical and haematological effects were similar despite the different molecular bases for the disorders. A further Malaysian patient with homozygous $^{G}\gamma(^{A}\gamma\delta\beta)^{0}$-thalassaemia was reported by George et al. (1986). The 'new' causal deletion in this case was exceptionally large. Clinically, he suffered from thalassaemia intermedia.

'γ-thalassaemia'

Under the heading *Hypothesis*, Stamatoyannopoulos (1971) suggested that γ-chain thalassaemias should exist, with $^{A}\gamma$-thalassaemia associated with a mild reduction in the amount of Hb F synthesized and $^{G}\gamma$-thalassaemia associated with a moderate redution. Whether in fact impairment of γ-chain synthesis as the sole abnormablity, as envisaged by Stamatoyannopoulos, ever leads to a type of thalassaemia seems doubtful. What is clear is that impaired $^{A}\gamma$-chain synthesis, associated with impaired δ- and β-chain synthesis, is the hallmark of $(^{A}\gamma\delta\beta)^{0}$-thalassaemia. The possibility, too, that impairment of γ-chain production can lead to the syndrome of haemolytic disease of the newborn is suggested by the case reports summarized below.

γ-chain variants are also known to exist that do not apparently have any clinical effects. Thus Huisman and co-workers (1983) described newborn infants from India, China and Japan who if heterozygous formed fewer $^{G}\gamma$ chains than normal and if homozygous no $^{G}\gamma$ chains at all. Two such homozygotes were, nevertheless, clinically normal and were not anaemic despite a decreased percentage of Hb F. Zeng and co-workers (1985) identified the causal lesion as a 5-kb deletion.

'*Haemolytic disease of the newborn' associated with $\gamma\beta$- or $\gamma\delta\beta$-thalassaemia*

Kan, Forget and Nathan (1972) studied a female child

of English-German origin shortly after birth. She had presented with the syndrome of haemolytic disease of the newborn (haemoglobin 10.4 g/dl, MCV 84 fl, MCH 27 pg, bilirubin 13.7 mg/dl, reticulocytes 26%, erythroblasts 400 per 100 leucocytes). The direct antiglobulin test was negative and the G6PD concentration normal. There was 52% Hb F and 1.2% Hb A_2. No Hb Bart's was detected. The infant was transfused and recovered. One year later she was found to have a mild hypochromic microcytic anaemia, which was indistinguishable from that affecting her father and seven other family members. Globin-chain synthesis revealed deficiencies in the synthesis of both β and γ chains in relation to α chains. It was concluded that $\gamma\beta$-thalassaemia was a mild disorder in heterozygotes in postnatal life but could be severe in the neonatal period at a time when the infant was dependent on γ-chain production.

A similar family was described by Oort et al. (1981). Severe neonatal haemolytic anaemia, hyperbilirubinaemia and erythroblastosis affected nine members of a Dutch family. Two infants died soon after birth, five recovered after exchange-transfusion, one improved without transfusion. After 1 year the surviving children were found to have a mild hypochromic microcytic anaemia. The same pattern was found in one parent of affected children. The adults had normal Hb-A_2 and Hb-F levels and $\beta:\alpha$ globin-synthesis ratios of 0.49 and 0.53. Reduced γ-chain synthesis was demonstrated in two of the affected infants at birth and in parallel with the switch to β-chain production a similar reduction in β-chain synthesis was demonstrable. The normal Hb-A_2 levels suggested that δ-chain production was impaired also. Restriction enzyme analysis demonstrated a major deletion at the $\gamma\delta\beta$ gene locus in one chromosome; the β-globin gene appeared, however, to be intact and it was concluded that deletion (of γ and δ genes) far away from the β-globin gene was apparently suppressing its activity.

A further type of $\gamma\delta\beta$-thalassaemia was described by Pirastu and co-workers (1983b). Seven affected members were found in four generations of a Scottish-Irish family; they presented with haemolytic disease of the newborn (with hypochromia and microcytosis) and as adults had a moderately severe hypochromic microcytic anaemia (haemoglobin 11.6–13.2 g/dl, erythrocytes 6.0–6.92 $\times$ 10^{12}/l, MCV 59–65 fl, MCH 19.1–21.1 pg, reticulocytes 1.0–2.2%, Hb A_2 2.9–3.0%, Hb F 0.5–1.3%, α : non-α ratio 1.8–2.3). Investigation of DNA showed that the entire β-globin gene cluster had been deleted.

δ-thalassaemia

A defect in δ-chain synthesis unaccompanied by a defect in β-chain synthesis has been referred to as δ-thalassaemia. Under the title 'Absence of haemoglobin A_2 in an adult', Fessas and Stamatoyannopoulos (1962) described an adult Greek male, aged 60, whom they considered was a compound heterozygote of δβ-thalassaemia and an isolated defect in δ-chain synthesis, δ-thalassaemia. The patient had the blood picture of thalassaemia trait, but Hb A_2 was completely absent. Since then other reports have indicated that the gene for δ-thalassaemia is not uncommon and is quite widely distributed, particularly in Mediterranean populations. It seems mostly to have been reported in families in which other and more important defects were also present (Thompson *et al.*, 1965, 1966; Ohta *et al.*, 1971). By itself δ-thalassaemia is unimportant, for even homozygotes present no clinical or haematological abnormalities (Yasukawa *et al.*, 1980).

A variant of δ-thalassaemia, $δ^+$-thalassaemia, in which δ-globin synthesis is diminished but not absent, was described by Pirastu and co-workers (1983a). 0.7% of a Sardinian population had Hb-A_2 levels less than 3 SD below the normal mean. Compound heterozygosity for $δ^+$-thalassaemia and β-thalassaemia was thought to result in thalassaemia trait with normal Hb-A_2 levels.

Compound heterozygosity for δβ-thalassaemia and β-thalassaemia

As already indicated, δβ-thalassaemia, although less frequently met with than high Hb-A_2 β-thalassaemia, is widespread and affects many races. Many accounts of compound heterozygotes for both traits are to be found in the early reports of δβ-thalassaemia, *e.g.* in those of Zuelzer, Robinson and Booker (1961), Stamatoyannopoulos, Fessas and Papayannopoulou (1969), Stamatoyannopoulos *et al.* (1971), Kattamis *et al.* (1973) and Efremov *et al.* (1975). The syndrome is certainly not a rare one.

Stamatoyannopoulos, Fessas and Papayannopoulou (1969), who reported on 21 individuals from 16 families, stressed how variable the clinical manifestations are. The usual presentation is, however, that of thalassaemia intermedia, and the condition is usually mild compared with homozygous $β^0$-thalassaemia.

Stamatoyannopoulos, Fessas and Papayannopoulou's (1969) youngest patient was 7 months old, the oldest 29 years of age; 12 were more than 10 years old; seven were less than 5 years of age and these could be considered as having thalassaemia major, and some had been transfused (12 of the 21 patients never received a transfusion). Subicterus was a constant finding, even in adults who were not obviously anaemic. The spleen was always enlarged and two patients had undergone splenectomy with benefit. Mongoloid facial abnormalities were obvious in three children only. Stamatoyannopoulos, Fessas and Papayannopoulou (1969) recorded the following haematological data (from 19 patients): haemoglobin 5.3–13.1 g/dl (mean 9.9 g/dl); MCH 20.3–26.7 pg; poikilocytosis, microcytosis, anisocytosis, hypochromasia and normoblastaemia were conspicuous features, particularly in the more anaemic patients. Hb-A_2 concentration varied from very low values to 4.5%, mostly < 2.1%; Hb F 46–96%, mostly > 75%. Hb A was absent in more than one-third of the patients.

The series of patients described by Kattamis and co-workers (1973) comprised 11 Greek children, 1–10 years of age. Again the clinical syndrome was rather variable but generally it was of intermediate severity. The mean haemoglobin level was 9.0 ± 1.9 g/dl, MCH 21.6 ± 3.3 pg, mean MCV 69.3 ± 10.3 fl, mean reticulocyte count 4.0 ± 1.3%, normoblasts 0–14 per 100 leucocytes (120 per 100 leucocytes in one patient after splenectomy), mean bilirubin 1.16 ± 0.76 mg/dl. Osmotic resistance was markedly increased and inclusion bodies were found in the erythrocytes of all but one patient. They were present before splenectomy.

COMPOUND HETEROZYGOSITY BETWEEN β-THALASSAEMIA AND AN ABNORMAL HAEMOGLOBIN; ABNORMAL HAEMOGLOBINS RESULTING IN A THALASSAEMIA-LIKE BLOOD PICTURE

The quite common occurrence of compound heterozygosity for β-thalassaemia and Hb S, Hb C, Hb E and Hb O has already been described in some detail in Chapters 13 and 16. Brief reference is made below (in alphabetical order) to compound heterozygosity for β-thalassaemia and other abnormal haemoglobins. The majority of the abnormal haemoglobins listed, when present in heterozygotes with Hb A, have no obvious effect on the blood picture. Some, however, which result from substitutions in the β-globin chain impair β-chain production sufficiently severely as to cause substantial reductions in the β:α globin-chain ratio and to produce as a result a mild or 'silent' thalassaemia-like effect in simple heterozygotes and thalassaemia intermedia in compound heterozygotes with β-thalassaemia.

Hb B$_2$ ($\alpha_2\delta_2^{16 \text{ Gly} \rightarrow \text{Arg}}$). Hb B$_2$ is an allele of Hb A$_2$. Huisman, Punt and Schaad (1961) described a black American family in which both Hb B$_2$ and β-thalassaemia were present. The total Hb B$_2$ + A$_2$ percentage in compound heterozygotes ranged from 3.5 to 4.5; their blood picture was typical of thalassaemia minor. Comings and Motulsky (1966) described a patient who was a compound heterozygote for Hb B$_2$ and δβ-thalassaemia. Hb A$_2$ was absent, and this led them to conclude that the cis delta gene was completely suppressed.

Hb Beograd ($\alpha_2\beta_2^{121 \text{ Glu} \rightarrow \text{Val}}$). Aksoy et al. (1984) described two Turkish adults who were compound heterozygotes for Hb Beograd and β^0-thalassaemia. They had moderately severe thalassaemia intermedia. Four children of the proposita were simple heterozygotes for Hb Beograd but were not significantly anaemic.

Hb Crete ($\alpha_2\beta_2^{129 \text{ Ala} \rightarrow \text{Pro}}$). Maniatis et al. (1979) described an adult male Greek who was a compound heterozygote for β^0-thalassaemia and Hb Crete, an unstable high O$_2$ affinity haemoglobin. The patient had polycythaemia (erythrocytes $8.9 \times 10^{12}/1$, haemoglobin 19.6 g/dl), MCV 69 fl, reticulocytes 4.9%, bilirubin 1.5 mg/dl, Hb Crete 67%. Hb A was absent; Hb A$_2$ 3.2% and Hb F 30% (heterocellularly distributed).

Hb G Philadelphia ($\alpha_2^{68 \text{ Asn} \rightarrow \text{Lys}}\beta_2$). Grifoni et al (1975) described a 59-year-old Sicilian with β-thalassaemia major who had been living a comparatively normal life. He was, however, also a heterozygote for Hb G Philadelphia and for a γ-chain variant referred to as Hb F Sardinia ($^A\gamma^{75 \text{ Ile} \rightarrow \text{Thr}}$). Stathopoulou, Sulis and Lehmann (1979) identified a mildly affected male Sardinian as being homozygous for β^0-thalassaemia as well as heterozygous for both α-thalassaemia-2 and Hb G Philadelphia.

'Hb I'. Atwater et al. (1960) described a 25-year-old female black whose blood appeared to sickle consistently in 4% sodium metabisulphite (but not in other reducing agents or as the result of deoxygenation). No Hb S was present. However, approximately 70% of her haemoglobin was identified as the fast-moving variant Hb I. The patient was also thought to carry a gene for thalassaemia. The apparent sickling was attributed to the high percentage of the abnormal haemoglobin that was present.

'Hb J'. Sanghvi, Sukumaran and Lehmann (1958) reported finding a variant haemoglobin identified as 'Hb J' in a Gujerati Indian woman, the mother of an infant with thalassaemia major. There was no evidence of interaction between the two abnormalities.

Hb J Baltimore ($\alpha_2\beta_2^{16 \text{ Gly} \rightarrow \text{Asp}}$). Wilkinson et al. (1967b) reported the association of Hb J with β-thalassaemia in an Australian family. The compound heterozygotes were clinically well but had a mild to moderate microcytic anaemia.

Hb J Georgia ($\alpha_2\beta_2^{16 \text{ Gly} \rightarrow \text{Asp}}$). Sydenstrycker et al. (1961) reported the occurrence of a fast-moving variant in an American black family. The Hb J comprised

74–81% of the haemoglobin in the compound heterozygotes; the percentage was lower in simple heterozygotes in the absence of thalassaemia (47–56%).

Hb J Sardegna ($\alpha_2^{50 \text{ His} \rightarrow \text{Asp}}\beta_2$). This haemoglobin is not uncommon in Sardinia and its presence in compound heterozygotes with β-thalassaemia does not influence the blood picture, according to Gallo et al. (1972).

Hb K Woolwich ($\alpha_2\beta_2^{132 \text{ Lys} \rightarrow \text{Gln}}$). This haemoglobin combined in simple heterozygotes with Hb A gives rise to a mild thalassaemia-like blood picture with a raised Hb-A$_2$ percentage. β-chain synthesis is reduced (Lang, Lehmann and King-Lewis, 1974).

Hb Knossos ($\alpha_2\beta_2^{27 \text{ Ala} \rightarrow \text{Ser}}$). This is a particularly interesting example of a variant leading to reduced synthesis of β chains, which, associated with β-thalassaemia trait in compound heterozygotes, leads to thalassaemia intermedia (Arous et al., 1982; Fessas et al., 1982, 1986; Rouabhi et al., 1983). Baklouti and co-workers (1986) have described a patient, a male aged 19, who was homozygous for Hb Knossos; he, too, had a β$^+$-thalassaemia-intermedia syndrome.

Hb Lepore. Pearson, Gerald and Diamond (1959) described three individuals in a family originating from Sicily who had thalassaemia intermedia and were compound heterozygotes for Hb Lepore and β-thalassaemia (see p. 442).

'Hb N'. Silvestroni and Bianco (1961) described twins aged 1½ years who had a moderately severe microcytic anaemia and were compound heterozygotes for β-thalassaemia and Hb N.

'Hb Nicosia'. Fessas et al. (1965) referred to two patients who were compound heterozygotes for β-thalassaemia and Hb Nicosia. There was no evidence of interaction between the two genes.

Hb Norfolk ($\alpha_2^{57 \text{ Gly} \rightarrow \text{Asp}}\beta_2$). Two members of an Italian family living in Australia were found by Wilkinson et al. (1967a) to be compound heterozygotes for Hb Norfolk and β-thalassaemia. There was no evidence of interaction; 35–37% of their haemoglobin was Hb Norfolk.

Hb North Shore ($\alpha_2\beta_2^{134 \text{ Val} \rightarrow \text{Glu}}$). According to Smith et al. (1983) this variant haemoglobin gave rise in the family studied to a mild thalassaemia-minor blood picture with a slightly reduced haemoglobin (11.2–12.3 g/dl), slight microcytosis (MCV 69–80 fl) and a raised Hb-A$_2$ percentage. Hb North Shore is slightly unstable to heat and isopropanol.

Hb P Galveston ($\alpha_2\beta_2^{117 \text{ His} \rightarrow \text{Arg}}$). Di Lorio et al. (1975) described the occurrence of Hb P in a Swiss family who also carried the gene for β-thalassaemia. There was no evidence of interaction between the two genes.

Hb Q ($\alpha_2^{74 \text{ Asp} \rightarrow \text{His}}\beta_2$). Lehmann and Lang (1975) reported the occurrence of Hb Q and β-thalassaemia in a Chinese woman. She was mildly anaemic (Hb 11.2 g/dl) and had a thalassaemic blood picture (MCV 67 fl, MCH 19 pg, Hb A$_2$ 5.3%, Hb F 1.3%) and 22% Hb Q.

Hb Q India ($\alpha_2^{64 \; Asp \to His}\beta_2$). Sukumaran *et al.* (1972b) described the occurrence of Hb Q and β-thalassaemia in three Sindhi families. There was no evidence of interaction between the genes.

Hb San Diego ($\alpha_2\beta_2^{109 \; Val \to Met}$). Loukopoulos *et al.* (1986) have described a 29-year-old male Greek with polycythaemia and a low MCV and MCH. A haemolysate consisted of almost pure Hb San Diego, and the patient was considered to be a compound heterozygote for the variant haemoglobin and β^0-thalassaemia. Hb San Diego has an increased oxygen affinity.

Hb Siriraj ($\alpha_2\beta_2^{7 \; Glu \to Lys}$). An 8-year-old Thai child presented with the clinical and haematological picture of thalassaemia intermedia. On electrophoresis the predominant haemoglobin was Hb Siriraj; there was 4% Hb F and the Hb-A_2 percentage was raised. Other members of the family had β-thalassaemia minor or were heterozygous for Hb Siriraj and Hb A (and had apparently normal blood pictures) (Tuchinda, Beale and Lehmann, 1965).

Hb Tak (the β chain of which is extended by 11 residues). The Thai girl who was the proposita in the family described by Lehmann *et al.* (1975) had a severe thalassaemic blood picture and may have been homozygous for Hb Tak; heterozygous carriers of Hb Tak had a blood picture similar to that of thalassaemia minor.

β-THALASSAEMIA IN ASSOCIATION WITH OTHER DISORDERS

Hereditary elliptocytosis. Several reports of this association are referred to in Volume 1 of this book (p. 247). In most of the patients there appear to have been no indication of any interaction between the two traits. In a few instances, however, the compound heterozygotes appear to have been the most anaemic.

G6PD deficiency. β-thalassaemia and G6PD deficiency occur together in high frequency in the same geographical areas under the influence of endemic malaria (see p. 398). Their occurrence from time to time in the same patient is therefore not unexpected (Vella, 1960). Whether there is a significant degree of interaction between the two genes has been a matter of debate. Piomelli and Siniscalco (1969) concluded that the haematological effects of G6PD deficiency and thalassaemia trait (in Sardinia) represented the summation of two independent effects — G6PD deficiency leading to mild anaemia, and slight macrocytosis, the consequence of chronic mild haemolysis; thalassaemia trait leading to mild anaemia, marked microcytosis and moderate hypochomia. In a similar and more recent large study carried out by Sanna *et al.* (1980), also on Sardinians, in which α- and β-thalassaemia carriers were treated separately, the only abnormality in erythrocyte indices established was a significantly raised MCV in the β-thalassaemia G6PD-deficient group.

Hereditary spherocytosis. Two families were referred to in Volume 1 of this book (p. 163) in which single patients appeared to be heterozygotes for both HS and thalassaemia.

Auto-immune haemolytic anaemia. The occurrence of severe auto-immune haemolytic anaemia super-imposed on homozygosity for β^0-thalassaemia was described by Cividalli *et al.* (1980).

The patient, a female Jewish-Moroccan child, when aged 2 years 4 months, suddenly became severely ill and needed many transfusions. She was subsequently treated fruitlessly with prednisone, cyclophosphamide and methotrexate and by splenectomy. Homozygosity for β^0-thalassaemia was established by family and globin-synthesis studies, and the diagnosis of auto-immune haemolytic anaemia was confirmed by the impaired survival of patient's and transfused normal erythrocytes and by serological studies. Measurement of globin-chain synthesis showed a 50% increase in the $\gamma:\alpha$ ratio during cyclophosphamide therapy.

HEREDITARY PERSISTENCE OF FETAL HAEMOGLOBIN (HPFH)

An interesting group of hereditary disorders in which large amounts of Hb F are formed continuously in post-natal life has been recognized since the late 1950s. Even in the homozygous state they are not accompanied by significant anaemia. There is, however, then some microcytosis and hypochromia, and the relationship between the HPFHs and the β-thalassaemias has proved to be an interesting problem (Weatherall and Clegg, 1981, p. 450).

The story of HPFH starts with the report of Edington and Lehmann (1955a) of two adult West Africans who, despite the fact that they were only forming Hb S and Hb F, were not anaemic and were symptom-free. Also, each of the patients had had a child not bearing Hb S. They could not, therefore, be homozygous for Hb S. Their children, too, were forming abnormally large amounts of Hb F (5–24%) and this led Edington and Lehmann (1955b) later to suggest that the children had inherited a thalassaemia-like gene from their parents. In 1958, Jacob and Raper described four similar patients from Uganda and concluded that they, too, were carrying a gene which led in carriers to the presence of about 20% of Hb F; otherwise, they had a normal blood picture. Jacob and Raper designated the condition 'hereditary persistence of foetal hemoglobin', a title that has been generally accepted. Now the condition is usually referred to simply as HPFH.

HPFH was next detected in Jamaica in three generations of a family of West-African origin in which the gene for Hb S was also present (Went and MacIver, 1958). In compound heterozygotes high levels of Hb F (about 27%) were present along with Hb S; they had little or no disability or anaemia, and Went and MacIver suggested that the high levels of Hb F were protective by inhibiting sickling. Further studies carried out on American blacks established that the gene for HPFH behaves as an allele at the β-globin chain locus and confirmed that heterozygotes usually have 20–30% of Hb F in their peripheral blood but no other haematological abnormalities and no clinical abnormalities (Bradley and Conley, 1960; Herman and Conley, 1960; Bradley, Brawner and Conley, 1961; Kraus, Koch and Burckett, 1961; MacIver, Went and Irvine, 1961; Conley et al., 1963). Homozygotes, on the other hand, present a thalassaemia-like picture with slight to moderate anisocytosis and poikilocytosis, target-cell formation, microcytosis and hypochromia but little or no anaemia. No Hb A or Hb A$_2$ is detectable; all the haemoglobin is Hb F (Wheeler and Krevans, 1961; Baglioni, 1963; Conley et al., 1963; Charache and Conley, 1969).

Charache and Conley (1969) observed a homozygous child from 20 months of age to 8½ years. He had mild polycythaemia and a high haematocrit throughout (40.6–45.6%), and his erythrocytes were shown to have a high oxygen affinity, higher than that of cord blood.

Acquaye, Oldham and Konotey-Ahulu (1977) described a homozygous Ghanaian male aged 32 who was in excellent health and acted as a blood donor. He, too, was mildly polycythaemic. His haemoglobin was 18.2 g/dl, erythrocytes $6.30 \times 10^{12}/1$, reticulocytes 2%, PCV 52%, MCV 79 fl, MCH 28 pg and MCHC 36 g/dl.

An interesting feature of HPFH in blacks is that when erythrocytes are stained by the Kleihauer-Betke acid-elution technique (Kleihauer, Braun and Betke, 1957; Betke and Kleihauer, 1958) the Hb F can be seen to be almost uniformly distributed in the cell population, a homogeneous (pancellular) distribution, in contrast to the findings in thalassaemia (and Hb-SS disease) in which the amount of Hb F differs considerably from cell to cell, a heterogeneous distribution (Bradley and Conley, 1960; Thompson, Mitchener and Huisman, 1961; Shepard, Weatherall and Conley, 1962). A question soon to be asked (and answered) was whether the Hb F in HPFH is the same as the fetal haemoglobin obtained from normal cord blood. Chemical and physical studies established that it is identical (Thompson, Mitchener and Huisman, 1961; Schroeder, Sturgeon and Bergren, 1962).

The next development was the recognition that HPFH is not confined to black populations and that several types of HPFH exist. In 1961 HPFH was reported to occur in Greece by Fessas, Stamatoyannopoulos and Karaklis and to exist there, too, in combination with α- or β-thalassaemia. In 1962 Raper reported that he had found 5.3% Hb F in the blood of a boy aged 9 years suffering from acute thrombocytopenic purpura, 7.5% in the blood of his brother and 4.5% in that of his father. Acid elution showed that the Hb-F-containing cells contained varying amounts of Hb F. There was no evidence of thalassaemia in the family.

A fuller account of the occurrence of HPFH in Greeks, and a comparison with the 'Negro' type was given by Fessas and Stamatoyannopoulos in 1964. In heterozygotes the Hb-F percentage varied from 10 to 19.4%, with a mean of 14.5%, while the mean Hb-A$_2$ percentage was slightly lower than normal. The Hb-F percentages thus appeared to be significantly lower than the previously published Jamaican and American figures. The distribution of Hb F in the erythrocytes of the Greek patients was found to be relatively homogeneous, i.e., although every cell contained Hb F, there was a little variation from cell to cell. The 33 individuals investigated were clinically healthy and their blood picture appeared normal. No homozygotes were available for study. Eight additional patients who were combined heterozygotes for HPFH and β-thalassaemia were also described (see p. 440).

The next advance came from Switzerland. Marti (1963) reported that he had found that 1.1% out of a total of 2845 army personnel had blood in which the Hb-F level was slightly but significantly raised. The values ranged from 0.8 to 3.4% (normal maximum assumed to be 0.75%); otherwise, the individuals forming the Hb F appeared to be haematologically normal. The hereditary nature of the abnormality was established by demonstrating the occurrence of raised levels in two generations in four families. Hb-A$_2$ levels were normal, and Marti concluded that the condition he had discovered was not a form of thalassaemia.

It is now realized that the Swiss-type of HPFH is but one of several benign disorders, present in several racial groups, in which abnormal amounts of Hb F are found in the blood of adults and in which the fetal haemoglobin is distributed in a 'heterocellular' fashion as opposed to being pancellular (Boyer et al., 1975, 1977). The F-containing cells are best demonstrated by an immunofluorescent technique (Fig. 18.11). When combined with the traits for β-thalassaemia or Hb S, the levels of Hb F present are higher than are usually found in either condition alone (Wood, Clegg and Weatherall, 1979).

As already discussed in relation to δβ-thalassaemia, it is now known that normal Hb F exists in genetically distinct forms, which differ in respect of the amino acid occupying the 136th residue of the γ chain. The residue may be either glycine or alanine. Normally, Hb F, as in cord blood, comprises a mixture of $\gamma^{136\,\mathrm{Gly}}$ ($^G\gamma$) and $\gamma^{136\,\mathrm{Ala}}$ ($^A\gamma$) (Schroeder et al., 1968) in the proportion of approximately 3:1 (Huisman et al., 1974). In HPFH the composition of Hb F has been found to vary despite clinical similarity. Huisman and his colleagues (1969) reported on 32 HPFH heterozygotes: in some the Hb F was $^G\gamma$; in others $^A\gamma$; in still others (the most frequent finding) a mixture of the two was present, but in different proportions from that in the normal newborn.

Details of a type of HPFH with $^A\gamma$ chains only were given by Huisman et al. (1970a). The abnormality was present in two generations of a Caucasian family: the affected individuals were not anaemic but 5.0–6.8% of their haemoglobin was Hb F (by alkali denaturation); the distribution of Hb F was heterocellular but the distinction between positive and negative cells was less clear-cut than in artificial mixtures of normal and cord blood.

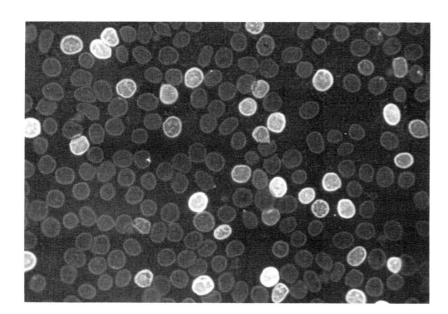

Fig. 18.11 Photomicrograph of F cells demonstrated by an immunofluorescent technique.
The patient was heterozygous for heterocellular HPFH, and only a proportion of the erythrocytes contain significant amounts of Hb F. (Reproduced by courtesy of Sir David Weatherall.)

In the Greek type of HPFH Huisman and co-workers (1970b) found in three families with HPFH evidence for $^A\gamma$ chains only, but in a later study, Clegg and his colleagues (1979) concluded that the Hb F contained about 10% of $^G\gamma$ chains.

Sukumaran and co-workers (1972a) described two Indian and four black American families with HPFH who appeared to be forming $^G\gamma$ chains only. One of the Indians was a homozygote: he was a boy who when aged 7 years had 7.5 g of haemoglobin (100% of it Hb F), 10% reticulocytes, 1.2 mg/dl bilirubin, MCV 69 fl and MCH 21 pg. Thalassaemia had been diagnosed. Weatherall and Clegg (1981, p. 496) referred to this ($^G\gamma$) type as the Georgia type and they labelled the British family described by Weatherall and his colleagues (1975) as having 'British' type of HPFH. In this family 13 members were affected: three had 19.8 ± 0.51% Hb F and were thought to be homozygotes and 10 had 8.9 ± 3.1% Hb F and were thought to be heterozygotes. Their blood picture was normal. The Hb F was mainly of the $^A\gamma$ type but there was about 10% of the $^G\gamma$ type in both homozygotes and heterozygotes; it was heterogeneously distributed. The condition was thought to differ from previously described types of HPFH. The presence of β- and δ-chain synthesis in the homozygotes was consistent with their normal blood picture.

In 1973 a second type of HPFH affecting Indians was described by Schroeder, Huisman and Sukumaran. Six heterozygotes in four families were studied: they formed 25–30% Hb F and the $^G\gamma$:$^A\gamma$ ratio was 70:30. In 1974 a Ghanaian was reported who was homozygous for HPFH and whose Hb F was thought to be formed entirely of $^G\gamma$ chains (Kamuzora et al., 1974). Reinvestigation of this patient has revealed that $^G\gamma$ and $^A\gamma$ chains were both being formed (Kamuzora et al., 1975).

A further type of HPFH (the Atlanta type) was described in two members of a black family by Altay, Huisman and Schroeder (1976–77). The Hb F levels in two heterozygotes were low, 2.3% and 3.8%, and their blood picture was normal. Only $^G\gamma$ chains were formed and the Hb F was heterocellularly distributed (6% of F cells were present). A second family with this type of HPFH was described by Huisman et al. (1985).

The reports summarized above illustrate the complexity and heterogeneity of HPFH (Table 18.3). A further interesting facet is the relationship between HPFH and the small amounts of Hb F that can be commonly demonstrated in the blood of normal adults, if sensitive methods of detection are used. According to Boyer and co-workers (1975), sufficient erythrocytes (F cells) that react with fluorescein-conjugated anti-Hb-F sera are present to account for the small amount (< 0.7%) of Hb F that can be detected in normal

Table 18.3 Hereditary persistence of fetal haemoglobin (HPFH): six types and their expression in heterozygotes and homozygotes.

Type	Clinical presentation	Hb F (%)	Pancellular or heterocellular	γ globin
Black African Heterozygotes	Normal	15–30	Pancellular	$^G\gamma$ plus $^A\gamma$ usually, but $^G\gamma$ type has been described
Homozygotes	Normal, but with minor thalassaemia-like blood changes	100	Pancellular	
Greek Heterozygotes	Normal	10–20	Pancellular but with variation from cell to cell	$^A\gamma$ plus a small proportion of $^G\gamma$
Swiss Heterozygotes	Normal	1–3.5	Heterocellular	
British Heterozygotes	Normal	c 9.0	Heterocellular	$^A\gamma$ plus a small proportion of $^G\gamma$
Homozygotes	Normal	c 20	Heterocellular	
Atalanta Heterozygotes	Normal	2–4.0	Heterocellular	$^G\gamma$
Georgia Heterozygotes	Normal	2.5–6.0	Heterocellular	$^G\gamma$ plus a small proportion of $^A\gamma$

adult blood. Wood and co-workers (1975) reported that the mean F-cell count in adults is $2.7 \pm 1.4\%$ and that there is a good correlation between the percentage of F cells and the amount of Hb F demonstratable by alkali denaturation. In the African (pancellular) variety of HPFH all the erythrocytes fluoresced. Boyer and co-workers (1977) reported the result of an interesting study on two families, one black and one English, with HPFH of heterocellular type which differed in the mean quantity of Hb F per cell and in the $^{G}\gamma{:}^{A}\gamma$ ratio. Approximately 50% of the erythrocytes in heterozygotes contained immunologically demonstrable Hb F and virtually 100% of the cells in homozygotes. Boyer *et al.* pointed out that, although the gene determining Hb-F formation was probably present in all the erythrocyte precursor cells in heterozygotes, it was expressed in only half the cells and that the amount of Hb F in the cells in which it could be demonstrated varied widely. The absence of Hb F in half the cells was regarded as a remarkable example of allelic exclusion, a phenomenon paralleling X-chromosome inactivation.

Zago and co-workers (1979) reported, relevant to the Hb F formed by normal adults, that six out of 750 normal blood donors (0.8%) had Hb-F levels in excess of 1.1%. Evidence was obtained indicating a genetic basis for these occurrences.

RELATIONSHIP BETWEEN HPFH AND β-THALASSAEMIA

A topic of considerable interest and importance is the relationship between the many forms of HPFH and the β-thalassaemias. If it is accepted that globin-chain imbalance is *the* criterion for the diagnosis of thalassaemia, then pancellular $^{G}\gamma^{A}\gamma$ HPFH, as found in black Americans, is a mild form of thalassaemia in which the chain imbalance and the absence of Hb A and Hb A_2 demonstrable in homozygotes is almost completely compensated for by Hb-F formation (Charache, Clegg and Weatherall, 1976).

Wood, Clegg and Weatherall (1979) and Weatherall and Clegg (1981, p. 502) discussed the problem in considerable detail and contrasted the haematological findings in pancellular $^{G}\gamma^{A}\gamma$ HPFH and in the $^{G}\gamma^{A}\gamma$ and $^{G}\gamma$ varieties of δβ-thalassaemia. Wood, Clegg and Weatherall (1979) concluded that $^{G}\gamma^{A}\gamma$ HPFH, $^{G}\gamma^{A}\gamma$ δβ-thalassaemia, $^{G}\gamma$ δβ-thalassaemia and Hb Lepore (as well as possibly Hb Kenya and $^{G}\gamma\beta^{+}$ HPFH) are closely related disorders brought about by deletions within the $^{G}\gamma^{A}\gamma$ δβ globin-gene complex which abolish or reduce the output of normal β-globin chains but which differ in their effect on the affected subject's ability to compensate by increasing γ-chain production. Compensation is least effective in Hb Lepore but becomes more effective in $^{G}\gamma$ δβ-thalassaemia, is still more effective in $^{G}\gamma^{A}\gamma$ δβ-thalassaemia and most effective of all in $^{G}\gamma^{A}\gamma$ HPFH. As increasing amounts of Hb F are formed, erythrocyte morphology becomes less abnormal and globin-chain synthesis more normal, and the distribution of Hb F becomes more obviously pancellular. Wood, Clegg and Weatherall (1979) summarized and contrasted in a Table available data on the absolute amount of Hb F present per cell in $^{G}\gamma^{A}\gamma$ HPFH (3.9–10.0, mean 7.1 ± 1.6 pg) and in $^{G}\gamma^{A}\gamma$ δβ-thalassaemia (0.9–4.5, mean 2.4 ± 0.8 pg). They pointed out that these differences in the amount of Hb F per cell probably explain the fact that Hb F can be demonstrated in all the erythrocytes (a pancellular distribution) when it is present in major amounts as in $^{G}\gamma^{A}\gamma$ HPFH, but can be seen in only some cells when present in relatively small amounts — very small amounts not being detectable by the techniques usually employed.

The heterocellular types of HPFH seem to be disorders which are not related to β-thalassaemia. The responsible molecular defects appear to result in abnormal regulation of Hb-F production without affecting α and β globin-chain balance (see Ch. 19, p. 512).

PANCELLULAR HPFH COMBINED WITH OTHER HAEMOGLOBIN VARIANTS

HPFH/Hb S. The occurrence of compound heterozygosity for HPFH and Hb S has been frequently reported, subsequent to the original reports of Edington and Lehmann in 1955. As already mentioned, affected individuals are as a rule not anaemic and there is no clinical or laboratory evidence of increased haemolysis (Went and MacIver, 1958; MacIver, Went and Irvine, 1961; Thompson and Lehmann, 1962). The Hb-F level has varied between 15 and 35%, percentages that are appreciably higher than in simple heterozygotes for HPFH and Hb A. The Hb F is distributed amongst the erythrocytes more homogeneously than in Hb-S disease. The Hb-A level is normal or slightly low. No Hb A is produced (Herman and Conley, 1960; Conley et al., 1963).

HPFH/Hb C. Compound heterozygosity for HPFH and Hb C has also been reported (McCormick and Humphreys, 1960; Kraus, Koch and Burckett, 1961; MacIver, Went and Irvine, 1961; Thompson and Lehmann, 1962). Some of the affected individuals have been a little anaemic and the reticulocyte count has been slightly raised in a few instances. The erythrocytes possibly vary rather more in size and shape than in the Hb-AC trait. The ^{51}Cr erythrocyte survival was stated by Conley et al. (1963) to be reduced in one instance. The Hb-F level has been reported to vary between 27 and 39%; it is homogeneously distributed. Hb A is absent.

HPFH/Hb E. Three individuals who were compound heterozygotes for HPFH and Hb E were detected by Wasi, Pootrakul and Na-Nakorn (1968) in a Thai family. They were not anaemic but many target cells were present. The MCV ranged from 64 to 77 fl and the MCH from 21 to 26 pg: approximately 40% of Hb E was present, the remainder of the haemoglobin being Hb F; it was homogeneously distributed. (In the Thai families the Hb S and HPFH compound heterozygotes had 21–22% Hb F and a reduced percentage of Hb A$_2$.)

HPFH/β-thalassaemia

This combination has been widely reported. Amongst early descriptions are those of Kraus, Koch and Burckett (1961), Wheeler and Krevans (1961) and Conley et al. (1963) in American blacks, Barkhan and Adinolfi (1962) in an Indian-Portuguese family, Mangenelli, Dalfino and Tannoia (1962) and Hitzig, Marti and Roy (1965) in Italians, Bird et al. (1964) in an Indian family and Fessas and Stamatoyannopoulos (1964) in Greeks.

Most of the American blacks with HPFH/β-thalassaemia have been free of symptoms and as a rule their spleen has not been palpable. Often the patient's haemoglobin has been within the normal range. The blood picture is, however, generally similar to that seen in mild β-thalassaemia minor, the erythrocyte count being high and the MCV and MCH reduced. The reticulocyte count and serum bilirubin may be slightly raised.

Hb F. The percentage of Hb F is characteristically high, usually between 60 and 79%, according to Conley et al. (1963) and Huisman et al. (1971). Higher levels than this, however, have been reported (Fogarty et al. 1974; Rothschild, Bickers and Marcus, 1976). These patients have presumably been HPFH/β^0-thalassaemia compound heterozygotes; Hb A has been present in traces only or has been absent. (Similar findings were reported by Yamak et al. (1973) in the case of a Turkish boy.)

Hb A$_2$. The percentage of Hb A$_2$ in HPFH/β-thalassaemia heterozygotes is normal or elevated as in β-thalassaemia minor. Rothschild, Bickers and Marcus (1976) reported in a review of 28 cases that seven patients had raised levels.

The considerable heterogeneity of both HPFH and β-thalassaemia leads inevitably to many possible genetic combinations, in addition to the pancellular HPFH/β-thalassaemia compound heterozygosity discussed briefly in the preceding paragraphs. Some of the reported combinations are referred to briefly below.

Greek-type HPFH/β-thalassaemia

As already mentioned, HPFH/β-thalassaemia occurs in Greece. Fessas and Stamatoyannopoulos (1964) reported on eight patients derived from four families. Their sclerae were subicteric and their spleen was palpable. They were moderately anaemic: haemoglobin 8.2–11.3 g/dl and MCH 20.4–23.5 pg. Their Hb-F level (26–43%) was lower than in the black American patients; the Hb-A$_2$ percentage was raised (3.8–5.2%).

Clegg and co-workers (1979) gave details of four further Greek compound heterozygotes who were members of four different families. The results were a little different from those of Fessas and Stamatoyannopoulos (1964). The Hb-F levels were higher, 34.5–46%, and the haemoglobin was shown to contain significant amounts of $^{G}\gamma$ chains. The patients were slightly anaemic, their blood picture being similar to that of thalassaemia minor, and they had a low MCV (58–65 fl) and MCH 19.3–21.0 pg). The Hb-A$_2$ percentage ranged from 3.2 to 5.9%. Acid elution preparations showed that Hb F was present in every cell, although in widely differing amounts: some cells were virtually unstained, others (the majority) stained deeply. Clegg and co-workers demonstrated that older cells (as separated by centrifugation) contain more Hb F than do younger cells, an observation implying that the cells that contain the larger amounts of Hb F survive longer in the circulation. The Hb-F $^{G}\gamma{}^{A}\gamma$ ratios did not differ between the two populations.

Swiss-type HPFH/β-thalassaemia

Three families (Italian, Indian and black West-Indian) with the above combination were described by Wood and co-workers (1977). Compound heterozygotes formed 6–15% Hb F, which was heterogeneously distributed. Four individuals with HPFH/β-thalassaemia plus Hb S were clinically very mildly affected. Globin-chain synthesis studies showed less imbalance in HPFH/β-thalassaemia compound heterozygotes than in Hb-A/β-thalassaemia heterozygotes. Older cell populations obtained by centrifugation were shown to contain more Hb F and a higher percentage of Hb-F-containing cells, indicating their preferential survival. Wood and his colleagues suggested that their observations supported the concept that increasing the size of the Hb-F-containing cell population, as achieved by the HPFH gene, is of benefit to the patient.

Capellini, Fiorelli and Bernini (1981) have reported another remarkable combination-interaction between homozygous β^0-thalassaemia and the Swiss-type HPFH. Once again, the presence of the gene for HPFH appeared to be of clinical benefit. The patient, a Sicilian male, aged 52, was only slightly anaemic, despite complete failure to form Hb A. The haemoglobin was 11.6–12.4 g/dl, erythrocytes 5.96–6.12 × 10^{12}/l, MCV 67 fl, MCH 18–21 pg, reticulocyte count 2.4–2.8%, Hb-F 97.2%, Hb A_2 2.8%. There was only slight globin-chain imbalance.

Schilirò and co-workers (1983b) described an even more remarkable Sicilian family in which β-thalassaemia, Hb Lepore Boston-Washington and heterocellular HPFH were present in a variety of combinations. One individual, an adult female, was a Hb-Lepore/HPFH compound heterozygote. She was clinically normal, but had the blood picture of the Hb-Lepore trait and an unusually high level of Hb F and many Hb-F-containing (F) cells. Her haemoglobin was 13 g/dl, MCV 71 fl, MCH 23.6 pg, Hb F 12%, Hb A_2 2%, Hb Lepore 13%; there were 40% F cells, osmotic resistance was increased, and the α:non-α globin-chain ratio was 1.6.

HPFH associated with Hb Kenya

Hb Kenya is a fusion haemoglobin comprising γ-like residues 1–80 and β-like residues 87–146 (Huisman *et al.*, 1972), and individuals carrying Hb Kenya have been found to have raised Hb-F levels, consisting solely of α and $^{G}\gamma$ chains (Smith *et al.*, 1973; Nute *et al.*, 1976). According to Nute *et al.*, Hb F was demonstrable in all the erythrocytes in the Ugandan carriers of the Hb-Kenya trait they had studied.

HPFH combined with a hereditary haemolytic anaemia

Possible hereditary spherocytosis. An interesting Japanese family was described by Shibata *et al.* in 1966. The propositus, a male aged 25, had a congenital haemolytic anaemia, possibly HS, associated with splenomegaly and gallstone formation. He had 17–24.3% Hb F which was heterocellularly distributed. Three other members of the family, including his father, had 2.5–8.4% Hb F; they were free from haemolytic anaemia.

Hereditary elliptocytosis. Ringelhann and co-workers (1970) described the combination of HPFH and HE in a Ghanaian family. The propositus was homozygous for HPFH and had a compensated haemolytic anaemia. Virtually all his haemoglobin was Hb F. Two of his five children had HE, with 25 and 27% Hb F, respectively; three other children had similarly high Hb-F percentages but were free from HE. Ringelhann *et al.* pointed out that 'Our case demonstrates that man can reach the fifth decade in a good physical condition with the haemoglobin of a foetus circulating in his body'!

Swiss type of HPFH associated with auto-immune haemolytic anaemia (AIHA)

Pawlak and Kozlowska (1979) reported that a 32-year-old female with AIHA (direct antiglobulin test positive) had 10–23% Hb F. There were no indications of thalassaemia, and raised, but lower, percentages of Hb F were found in the blood of the patient's mother (2.5%) and daughter (2.2%). The distribution of the Hb F in the patient's erythrocytes was heterocellular.

HAEMOGLOBIN LEPORE

Another variant of β-thalassaemia is caused by the presence of Hb Lepore, in which fusion of the δ- and β-globin chains leads to failure of globin synthesis. The fusion is the consequence of unequal crossing-over between the δ- and β-globin genes.

The 'Lepore trait' was first described by Gerald and Diamond (1958b). In investigating the mother of a male child, who when 7 months of age had been found to be severely anaemic and to have an enlarged spleen, they found that she (and also four of her relatives) were forming an abnormal haemoglobin fraction which on starch-block electrophoresis formed a band running between Hb F and Hb A_2. The abnormal haemoglobin comprised 10–12% of the total haemoglobin and was named Lepore (the family name). The child's father had typical thalassaemia minor, and the child was considered to be doubly heterozygous for the Lepore trait and thalassaemia trait. Both parents were of Italian origin.

It was not long before other patients with thalassaemia syndromes from a wide variety of populations were found to be forming an abnormal haemoglobin component with the characteristics of Hb Lepore. Thus 'Hb Lepore' was described by Pearson, Gerald and Diamond (1959), Silvestroni and Bianco (1963) and Wolff and Ignatov (1963) in further Sicilian and Italian families, by Neeb et al. (1961), Ryan (1961b) and Barnabas and Muller (1962) in Papuans, by Fessas, Stamatoyannopoulos and Karaklis (1962) in Greeks (described as Hb 'Pylos'), by Beaven et al. (1964) in Turkish-Cypriots, by Ranney and Jacobs (1964) in black Americans, by Duma et al. (1968) in Yugoslavian Macedonians and by Rowley, Barnes and Williams (1969) in a Rumanian. More recent references to the occurrence of Hb Lepore in still other racial groups were given by Efremov (1978) and Weatherall and Clegg (1981, p. 414).

As will be discussed below, it is now realized that three different Hb Lepores exist which vary with respect to the site of the δ- and β-chain fusion. This difference is reflected in the suffix appended to the title Lepore. The commonest type is Hb Lepore Boston. This has been identified in a variety of populations, particularly in Italians, Greeks and Yugoslavian Macedonians. However, it has also been reported in families of Scottish and British origin (Cook and Lehmann, 1973; Wilkinson et al., 1975) and in Afro-American

families in Jamaica (Ahern et al., 1972) and Cuba (Martinez and Colombo, 1973). More recently, it has been observed in Iranian (Rahbar, Golban-Moghadam and Saoodi, 1974), Spanish (Gimferrer et al., 1976) and Hungarian (Ringelhann et al., 1979) families.

The other two types of the Lepore are rare: one is Hb Lepore Hollandia (Barnabas and Muller, 1962), which has been identified in several Papuan families; the other is Hb Lepore Baltimore (Ostertag and Smith, 1969), which has been found in a black American family, in a Yugoslavian Macedonian family and in a Spanish family (Villegas et al, 1983). Hb Lepore Washington (Ahern et al., 1972) seems to be identical with Hb Lepore Boston.

In addition to the Hb Lepores, at least four so-called 'anti-Lepore' haemoglobins have been identified. These are the product of βδ-chain fusion (as opposed to δβ-chain fusion in the Lepore haemoglobins). The βδ-chain fusion does not, however, lead to a failure to form β chains.

CLINICAL FEATURES OF Hb-LEPORE SYNDROMES

Heterozygotes. Carriers of the Hb-Lepore trait typically have no symptoms attributable to their abnormal haemoglobin and present no abnormal physical signs.

Homozygotes. A small number of homozygotes have been described (see below). Most of the patients have presented in early childhood as moderately severe cases of thalassaemia major; others have been less severely affected and have needed few, if any, transfusions and can be described as having thalassaemia intermedia. Enlargement of the spleen and liver has been a constant feature and retardation of growth and a mongoloid facies have been reported.

Neeb and co-workers (1961) and Barnabas and Muller (1962) seem to have been the first to report homozygosity (for Hb Lepore Hollandia): two children in a Papuan family presented clinically as cases of thalassaemia major. Fessas, Stamatoyannopoulos and Karaklis (1962) described a Greek patient, homozygous for Hb Lepore Boston, who was also rather severely affected. Quattrin and his co-workers (Quattrin, Ventruto and Dini, 1966; Quattrin et al., 1967; Quattrin and Ventruto, 1974) described several homozygous patients in Italian families resident in Campania where Hb

Lepore is particularly prevalent. More recently, Quattrin, Luzzatto and Quattrin (1980) summarized the clinical and biochemical findings in nine homozygotes (and 214 heterozygotes). They stressed that the majority of the homozygotes are not very severely affected and that splenectomy seems always to be beneficial.

Duma and co-workers (1968) gave details of three homozygous patients found in a study of nine Yugoslavian Macedonian families; all three had been severely anaemic as small children and presented as cases of thalassaemia major. Rahbar, Azizi and Nowzari (1975) described an Iranian male aged 16 with homozygous Hb Lepore Boston. Clinically, he had presented as a rather mild case of thalassaemia major and had undergone splenectomy when 8 years old.

Compound heterozygosity for Hb Lepore and β-thalassaemia

β-thalassaemia. Many examples of compound heterozygosity for Hb Lepore and β-thalassaemia have been described, e.g., by Gerald and Diamond (1958b), Silvestroni and Bianco (1963), Quattrin et al. (1967), Marinucci et al. (1979) and Quattrin, Luzzatto and Quattrin (1980) in Italians, by Fessas, Stamatoyannopoulos and Karaklis (1962) in Greeks, by Beaven et al. (1964) in a Turkish-Cypriot family, by Duma et al. (1968) in Yugoslavian Macedonians, by Zachariadis, Nute and Stamatoyannopoulos (1975) in a Greek-Cypriot family, and by Francina et al. (1985) in an Algerian family. Most of these patients have presented with severe anaemia in early childhood, and the clinical findings have been similar to those of homozygous β-thalassaemia; in a small minority the picture has been that of thalassaemia intermedia.

δβ-thalassaemia. A small number of patients have been compound heterozygotes for Hb Lepore and δβ-thalassaemia.

In the patient described by Efremov et al. (1976) anaemia was moderate (Hb 9.4–11.0 g/dl) and there was no need for regular transfusions. When she was 14, splenectomy was carried out but without apparent benefit. Gallstones formed and she died of cholangitis when aged 24. Quattrin, Luzzatto and Quattrin (1980) referred to another patient, an Italian male, first seen in 1967. He was anaemic but chronically jaundiced and had very marked hepatosplenomegaly. His clinical picture was considered to be similar to that of heterozygous thalassaemia with biliary dyskinesia and mild compensated haemolysis. In both the above patients the haemoglobin pattern was similar to that of homozygous Hb Lepore: Hb F and Hb Lepore were alone present; Hb A and Hb A$_2$ were absent.

Hb Lepore combined with structural haemoglobin variants

Hb S. Ahern and co-workers (1972) reported that a female Jamaican aged 76 was a Hb Lepore/Hb S compound heterozygote. She has never had any symptoms suggestive of vascular occlusion or a haemolytic crisis and had had five successful pregnancies. Her haemoglobin was 10.6 g/dl.

Hb C. Ranney and Jacobs (1964) reported that a 17-year-old female member of an Afro-American family was a compound heterozygote for Hb C and Hb Lepore: 80% of her haemoglobin was Hb C, 6% Hb F and 14% Hb Lepore. Hb A appeared to be absent; Hb A$_2$ was not separated from Hb C. Two members of the Jamaican family described by Ahern et al. (1972) were similarly compound heterozygotes for Hb Lepore and Hb C. They were aged 60 and 59 and had had no symptoms attributable to their haemoglobinopathy. Their haemoglobins were 12.1 and 13.2 g/dl, respectively. A Hb-Lepore/Hb-C combination has more recently been described by Francina et al. (1985) in an Algerian family. Their patient, too, was clinically and haematologically almost normal.

Hb J Oxford. Quattrin and Ventruto (1974) referred to an Italian family in which Hb J Oxford and Hb Lepore had been detected in three generations. One asymptomatic individual was a compound heterozygote.

Hb Peterborough. This haemoglobin, which is unstable, was detected in two generations of an Italian family by King et al. (1972). The propositus was a compound heterozygote of Hb Peterborough and Hb Lepore. He was mildly anaemic (haemoglobin 10 g/dl), had 20% reticulocytes and his spleen was palpable: 67% of his haemoglobin was Hb Peterborough, 26.8% Hb Lepore, 4% Hb A$_2$ and 2.7% Hb F; Hb A was absent.

HAEMATOLOGICAL FINDINGS IN THE Hb-LEPORE SYNDROMES

Heterozygotes

The blood picture is similar to that in heterozy-

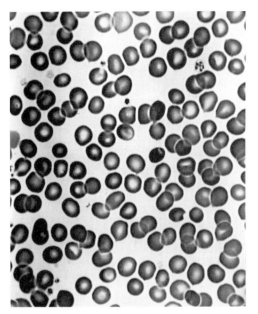

Fig. 18.12 Photomicrograph of a blood film of a patient who was heterozygous for Hb Lepore.
There is slight anisocytosis and microcytosis. × 700. (Film provided by courtesy of Dr Adrian Stephens.)

gous β-thalassaemia, *i.e.*, the haemoglobin is often within the normal range, but some patients are mildly anaemic. The MCH and MCV are subnormal. The erythrocyte morphology is, too, similar in the two conditions (Fig. 18.12).

Marinucci and co-workers (1979), however, have reported some differences. They compared the haematological findings in 59 Italian Hb-Lepore heterozygotes with the findings in 60 Italian β-thalassaemia heterozygotes: the two sets of data overlapped, but the mean erythrocyte count in the β-thalassaemia series was significantly higher and the mean MCV and MCH were significantly lower. The degree of morphological abnormality in the Hb Lepore heterozygotes was thought to be less; and Marinucci *et al.* concluded that globin-chain imbalance was less affected in the Hb Lepore heterozygotes than in β thalassaemia.

Haemoglobin. The amount of Hb Lepore present has generally been close to 10%. The data of Marinucci *et al.* (1979) indicated a range of 5–18% for Hb Lepore, with a mean of 11.9%; Hb F varied between 0.2 and 13.2% (mean 3.1%). According to Weatherall and Clegg (1981, p. 405), Hb A$_2$ ranges between 2.0 and 2.5%, a percentage

which represents an increased output from a single functioning δ-chain locus.

Homozygotes

The blood picture is indistinguishable from that of homozygous β-thalassaemia; and the changes following splenectomy, *e.g.*, the erythroblastaemia and the presence of α-globin chain inclusions, are similar.

Haemoglobin. Hb Lepore and Hb F are alone present; Hb A and Hb A$_2$ cannot be demonstrated. Hb Lepore comprises as a rule about 15% of the total haemoglobin, but the reported percentages have ranged rather widely, *e.g.*, from 8.6% (Duma *et al.*, 1968) to 27.7% and 24.2% in two siblings (Neeb *et al.*, 1961) to 30% (Quattrin *et al.*, 1967).

Hb Lepore/β-thalassaemia compound heterozygotes

The blood picture is similar to that of homozygous β-thalassaemia.

Haemoglobin. Most patients have been transfused and this has complicated haemoglobin analysis. In any case most of the haemoglobin will be Hb F, and this may amount to as much as 90% of the haemoglobin in an untransfused patient. If the β-thalassaemia is of the β^0 variety, Hb A will be absent. The percentage of Hb Lepore present is always low, and is similar to that found in Hb Lepore simple heterozygotes, *i.e.* 5–15%. The Hb-A$_2$ percentage is normal or slightly subnormal.

STRUCTURE OF Hb LEPORE

The nature of Hb Lepore has been determined by finger-printing of tryptic digests of Hb-Lepore globin. Baglioni (1962) showed that the abnormal chain in Hb Lepore Boston was the product of the fusion of part of the β-chain sequence with part of the δ-chain sequence and concluded that this was the result of the non-homologous crossing-over between corresponding points of the β and δ genes. He subsequently demonstrated (Baglioni, 1965) that the length of the abnormal peptide was the same as that of a normal β or δ chain and with

Ventruto (Baglioni and Ventruto, 1968), in a study of Hb Lepore obtained from a homozygous individual, established that the chain comprised a δ-like sequence at the N-terminal end and a β-like sequence at the C-terminal end and that the switch was located between residues 87 and 116.

Labie, Schroeder and Huisman (1966) in a similar analysis of a sample of Hb Lepore Washington (= Boston) obtained from an Italian in Augusta came to the same conclusion as had Baglioni — namely, that the abnormal chain in Hb Lepore was formed of δ-chain residues 1–87 and β chain residues 116–146. The point was made that the exact point of crossing-over could not be determined because residues 88–115 are the same in both chains. The structure and genetics of Hb Lepore were succinctly reviewed by Labie and Rosa (1967).

Hb Lepore Hollandia and Hb Lepore Baltimore differ from each other and from Hb Lepore Boston with respect to the site of fusion. In Hb Lepore Hollandia it is between residues δ22 and β50 (Barnabas and Muller, 1962); in Hb Lepore Baltimore it is between residues δ50 and β86 (Ostertag and Smith, 1969).

Synthesis of Hb Lepore

A considerable number of in-vitro studies have been undertaken with the aim of finding an explanation for the relatively low proportion of Hb Lepore in the peripheral blood of heterozygotes (c 10% of the total haemoglobin) and homozygotes (c 15%). The results have demonstrated that few Hb Lepore chains are in fact synthesized compared with α chains and (in heterozygotes) compared with normal β chains.

In early studies, White and co-workers (1972) found in a Turkish-Cypriot, who was heterozygous for Hb Lepore Boston, that the specific activity of the δβ chains was very low compared to that of the normal β chains and could not be demonstrated in reticulocytes. The result was imbalance of globin synthesis with an excess of α chains. Later, White, Lang and Lehmann (1972) reported a compensatory excess of normal β-chain synthesis by nucleated erythroid cells in two Hb-Lepore Boston heterozygotes.

Forget and co-workers (1978) studied a homozygous patient — an Italian boy who had presented with the clinical syndrome of thalassaemia major. His peripheral-blood cells were found to synthesize only 1.5–3% as many Lepore-globin chains as α chains. Similarly, in an analysis of peripheral-blood globin mRNA only 1–2% of it was identified as δβ Lepore mRNA, the remainder being α-globin mRNA.

Luppis and Ventruto (1979) compared the synthesis of α, δβ and γ chains in two brothers who were Hb-Lepore homozygotes; one brother was severely affected, the other much less severely so. An excess of α-chain production was demonstrated in both cases, but the imbalance was greater in the patient who was more severely affected.

Dobkin and co-workers (1986) cloned the Hb-Lepore gene and analyzed its expression after transference into HeLa cells. They found that the Lepore gene produced less mRNA than a normal β gene but more than that produced by a δ gene, a finding consistent with the apparent relative expression of the genes in erythroid cells in vivo.

ATYPICAL GENETICALLY-DETERMINED DISORDERS ASSOCIATED WITH GLOBIN-CHAIN IMBALANCE

Two interesting disorders with some thalassaemia-like features are referred to briefly below.

'A genetically determined disorder with features of both thalassaemia and congenital dyserythropoietic anaemia'

Weatherall and Clegg (1971) and Wealtherall et al, (1973) described a most unusual Irish family. Six members were affected: they were moderately anaemic and had life-long jaundice, cholelithiasis and splenomegaly. Their erythrocytes varied markedly in size and shape but were mostly well haemoglobinized. In the bone marrow there was erythroblastic hyperplasia and inclusions in normoblasts which stained with methyl violet. Inclusions, too, were present in the peripheral-blood erythrocytes of two of the patients who had undergone splenectomy. Globin-chain synthesis studies revealed a relative excess of α-chain synthesis, the α:β ratio being 2:1. The nature of the basic molecular lesion in the family was not determined but it seemed to lead to a defect in cell division, as well as to an overproduction of α-globin chains. Against a diagnosis of thalassaemia intermedia were the minor degree of globin-chain imbalance, the well-marked inclusion-body formation, the relatively high MCH (25–35 pg) and the erythroblast multinuclearity.

'X-linked syndrome of platelet dysfunction, thrombocytopenia, and imbalanced globin-chain synthesis with hemolysis'

Thompson, Wood and Stamatoyannopoulos (1977) described an unusual family in which four males in three generations had suffered from a bleeding disorder.

As well as thrombocytopenia and markedly prolonged bleeding times, they were found to have elevated reticulocyte counts (4.4–7.5%), a slightly reduced MCH (27.1–28.1 pg) and an $\alpha:\beta$ globin-synthesis ratio of 1.54–1.82:1. Nine additional family members in four generations were studied and found to be normal except for one female who had a reticulocyte count of 3.4% and an $\alpha:\beta$ globin-synthesis ratio of 1.58:1. The males in the family with the bleeding tendency were those with the raised $\alpha:\beta$ globin-synthesis ratios. The exact genetic basis of the disorder could not be determined: a pleiotropic effect of a single mutation or a deletion in the X chromosome affecting closely linked genes influencing platelet survival and function, and globin synthesis, respectively, were considered.

THE α-THALASSAEMIAS

Early history

The concept that Hb-H disease was associated with a failure to form α-globin chains stemmed from the discovery that Hb H is a tetramer of β-globin chains (β_4) (Jones *et al.*, 1959; Ingram and Stretton, 1959) and also from the realization that Hb Bart's is a fetal haemoglobin which lacks α-chains (γ_4) (Hunt and Lehmann, 1959; Ramot *et al.*, 1959; Kekwick and Lehmann, 1960).

As already referred to (p. 392), a 'new' fast-running abnormal haemoglobin, designated Hb Bart's was identified by Ager and Lehmann in 1958. This had been detected in the blood of a 4-week-old anaemic infant, of West-Indian and Chinese parentage (Ager *et al.*, 1960), thought to have thalassaemia, which was under investigation at St Bartholomew's Hospital in London. Subsequently, a small amount (*e.g.* 2–10%) of Hb Bart's was discovered in the cord blood of certain newborn infants belonging to many racial groups: it was found to be particularly common in South-East Asia, especially in Thais (Tuchinda *et al.*, 1959; Todd *et al.*, 1969; Na-Nakorn and Wasi, 1970), but it was also found to be common in Nigerians (Hendrickse *et al.*, 1960) and Shiite Saudi Arabs (Pembrey *et al.*, 1975) and to be present, too, in some American blacks (Minnich *et al.*, 1962; Weatherall, 1963, 1964b). In many instances the Hb Bart's was observed to disappear within the first few months of life (Barrow and Kohler, 1960; Silvestroni and Bianco, 1962); in most cases it had disappeared by 6 months (Weatherall, 1963, 1964b) and was not necessarily replaced by easily detectable amounts of Hb H. Such infants are now known to be heterozygous for α-thalassaemia.

Ager and Lehmann's (1958) discovery and naming of Hb Bart's had probably been antedated by the finding of Fessas and Papaspyrou (1957) of a novel haemoglobin in a Greek newborn infant both of whose parents were thought to have thalassaemia. A similar haemoglobin was subsequently identified by Lie-Injo (1959a), on the basis of its mobility on paper electrophoresis at both alkaline and acid pH, in the blood of 21 out of 633 Chinese newborn infants. There is little doubt, too, but that this haemoglobin was in fact Hb Bart's.

At about the this time a 'new' fetal hydrops syndrome was becoming to be recognized. The special feature of the affected Chinese infant described in Indonesia by Lie-Injo and Jo (1960a, b) was the presence of a large amount of a fast-moving haemoglobin with the characteristics of Hb Bart's.

Subsequent genetical studies, particularly in Thailand (Wasi, Na-Nakorn and Suindumrong, 1964; Poortrakul, Wasi and Na-Nakorn, 1967; Na-Nakorn *et al.*, 1969; Na-Nakorn and Wasi, 1970), led to the concept that there are two genetic types of α-thalassaemia. These were designated, respectively, α-thalassaemia-1 (α-thal-1) (a more serious type) and α-thalassaemia-2 (α-thal-2) (a less serious type). The fetal hydrops syndrome was considered on genetic evidence to be the consequence of homozygosity for α-thal-1 and Hb-H disease to be the result of compound heterozygosity for α-thal-1 and α-thal-2. According to Na-Nakorn *et al.* (1969) and Na-Nakorn and Wasi (1970), heterozygotes for α-thal-1 have 3–14% of Hb Bart's in their blood at birth and continue with a thalassaemia-like blood picture in later life while heterozygotes for α-thal-2 form only a trace (1–2%) of Hb Bart's at birth and have a virtually normal blood picture subsequently. (For further information on the relationship between Hb-Bart's percentages and α-globin genotype, see page 458.)

Geographical distribution

It is now known that α-thalassaemia affects many different racial groups and has a world-wide distribution. As already referred to, it is particularly common in South-East Asia, but it occurs frequently in Mediterranean and Middle-Eastern populations, e.g., in Greeks, Israelis, Italians, Saudi Arabs and Turks, as well as in Chinese, Indians and West Africans and Afro-Americans. It has in fact been reported in almost every racial group. Of particular interest are the recent studies which have shown that the failure of α-chain production leading to the α-thalassaemia syndromes can be brought about by several different mechanisms (see p. 516).

NOMENCLATURE OF THE α-THALASSAEMIAS

The different types of α-thalassaemia were so designated before it was discovered that the α-globin gene is duplicated and that the different severities of α-thalassaemia, from the symptomless and barely detectable carrier state to the fatal fetal hydrops syndrome, result from the absence or failure to function of one, two, three or four genes (Kattamis and Lehmann, 1970a; Koler et al., 1971; Adams and Steinberg, 1977; Ohene-Frempong et al., 1980; Weatherall and Clegg, 1981, p, 536; Lehmann, 1984). It was particularly unfortunate that the term α-thalassaemia-1 referred to a condition now known to be caused by the absence of *two* genes while α-thalassaemia-2 referred to the mildest state of all, caused by the absence of *one* gene. Lehmann and Carrell (1984) have recently suggested a logical revision of the nomenclature. This is incorporated into Table 18.4. (Further details of the genetics of the α-thalassaemias are given in Chapter 19, page 513.)

Table 18.4 Genotypes and nomenclature of the α-thalassaemias and clinical and haematological presentation of the main types.

Genotype	Conventional nomenclature	WHO (1982) nomenclature	Lehmann and Carroll's (1984) nomenclature	Clinical and haematological presentation	Haemoglobins present
αα/αα	Normal	Normal	Normal	Normal	Hb A, Hb A_2 (2–3.5%)
−α/αα	α-thal-2	$α^+$-thalassaemia	1α-thalassaemia	Silent trait. Blood picture: almost normal	Hb A, Hb A_2 Hb Bart's (0–3%, at birth) Hb H trace only
−α/−α (*trans*) −−/αα (*cis*)	α-thal-1	$α^0$-thalassaemia	2α-thalassaemia	Thalassaemia minor (trait). Blood picture: slightly to moderately abnormal	Hb A, Hb A_2 Hb Bart's (2–8%, at birth) Hb H (<2%)
−−/−α	Hb-H disease	$α^0/α^+$-thalassaemia	3α-thalassaemia	Moderately severe haemolytic anaemia. Blood picture: markedly abnormal	Hb A, Hb A_2 (1–2%) Hb Bart's (<5%) Hb H (2–40%)
−−/−−	Hb Bart's fetal hydrops	$α^0/α^0$-thalassaemia	4α-thalassaemia	Death *in utero* or shortly after birth. Blood picture: markedly abnormal	Hb A absent or trace Hb Bart's (70–80%) Hb H (<5%) Hb Portland (10–15%)

The figures for haemoglobin percentages are approximate and have been extracted from the literature quoted in the accompanying text.

THE Hb-BART'S FETAL HYDROPS SYNDROME

Hydrops fetalis accompanied by large amounts of Hb Bart's in the cord blood was first described in Chinese infants in Indonesia by Lie-Injo and Jo (1960a,b), Lie-Injo and Lie (1961) and Lie-Injo et al. (1962) and by Lie-Injo (1962) in Malaya. Subsequently, other cases were reported in Chinese living elsewhere in South-East Asia, e.g., by Banwell and Strickland (1964), Kan, Allen and Lowenstein (1967) and Todd, Lai and Braga (1967). The syndrome was soon recognized in other racial groups, e.g., in a Greek-Cypriot infant (Diamond, Cotgrove and Parker, 1965), in a Filipino infant (Pearson, Shanklin and Brodine, 1965) and in Thai infants (Pootrakul, Wasi and Na-Nakorn, 1967).

While it might be thought that the syndrome would occur wherever α-thalassaemia is to be found, this seems not be so. Thus while α-thalassaemia is common in the black population in the United States, the Hb-Bart's fetal hydrops syndrome seems not to occur or at least to be extremely uncommon (see p. 514). It has, however, been reported in at least one Greek family (Kattamis et al., 1980).

Clinical findings

In an interesting necropsy report on a hydropic Filipino infant delivered in 1955 (retrospectively diagnosed as suffering from α-thalassaemia on the basis of family studies) the major finding of wide-spread extramedullary erythropoiesis was considered by Pearson, Shanklin and Brodine (1965) to be very similar to that seen in haemolytic disease of the newborn due to Rh incompatibility.

Lie-Injo, Lopez and Dutt (1968) reported on 32 infants studied in Thailand. All but two were stillborn and the two that were born alive survived for only a few hours. Most of the fetuses were grossly hydropic and pale and were small for their age if no account was taken of ascites and oedema. The abdomen was typically markedly distended due to the ascites and gross enlargement of the liver. Petechiae or larger haemorrhages were often visible in the skin. The ascitic fluid, 150–800 ml in volume, was yellow in colour. Pericardial effusions were often present. The placenta was always enlarged and oedematous. Death results apparently from tissue anoxia brought about by failure of the transfer of oxygen to the tissues from Hb Bart's and Hb H as the result of the haemoglobins' increased oxygen affinity, compounded by anaemia and heart failure.

Blood picture

No doubt because so many of the affected infants have been stillborn, the blood picture in the Hb-Bart's fetal hydrops syndrome has seldom been described in detail. Anaemia, however is severe and erythrocyte morphology grossly abnormal. Many normoblasts are present in the peripheral blood (Fig. 18.13).

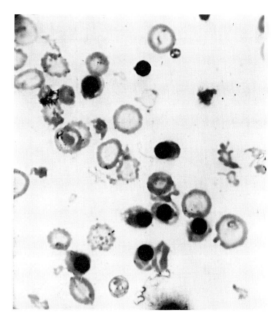

Fig. 18.13 Photomicrograph of a blood film of an infant suffering from Hb Bart's hydrops fetalis.
The erythrocytes vary markedly in size and shape and are hypochromic. Many normoblasts are present. × 700. (Film provided by courtesy of Dr Wanchi Wanachiwanawin.)

According to Thumasathit and co-workers (1968) the mean haemoglobin in a series of 22 hydropic infants from Northern Thailand was 4.9 g/dl, range 3.0–8.5 g/dl and the mean haematocrit 21.3%, range 14.8–36.0%. Blood films from 19 cases were described as showing macrocytosis with moderate hypochromia and polychromasia and moderate to marked anisocytosis and poikilocytosis as well as target-cell formation. Erythroblasts were present in varying stages of development: pronormoblasts averaged 0.3%, basophilic normoblasts 7.8%, polychomatic normoblasts 24.4% and orthochromatic normoblasts 67.3%. Megaloblastic changes were thought to be present in the films from six of the infants. No erythrocyte count data and no values for MCV were given. The total bilirubin in 12 infants ranged from 0.29 to 1.6 mg/dl, mean 0.87 mg/dl. Twenty-seven out of the 31 hydropic infants had almost 100% Hb Bart's; Hb H was not demonstrated but inclusion bodies were noted in a 'few erythrocytes of some infants'.

Gray and co-workers (1972) described the blood picture in a premature Chinese infant studied in Canada who survived for 3 hours after birth. The haemoglobin was 8.7 g/dl, haematocrit 44%, MCHC very low (19.7%), MCV 120 fl, MCH 23.8 pg, reticulocyte count 14%; osmotic fragility a very long span (0.1–0.75 g/dl NaCl). Almost all the haemoglobin was Hb Bart's. No Hb H was demonstrated by electrophoresis and no Hb-H inclusions were seen.

The haemoglobin in the large series of infants from Malaysia, Singapore, Hong Kong and Thàiland reviewed by Wasi, Na-Nakorn and Pootrakul (1974) ranged between 3 and 10 g/dl, the MCV ranged between 100 and 190 fl and up to 60% of reticulocytes were present.

Haemoglobin

As already referred to, a characteristic and diagnostic feature of the Hb-Bart's fetal hydrops syndrome is the presence of large amounts of Hb Bart's. According to Todd *et al.* (1970), Weatherall, Clegg and Wong (1970) and Wasi, Na-Nakorn and Poortrakul (1974), it comprises as a rule about 70–80% of the haemoglobin present. The remainder of the haemoglobin consists of substantial amounts (10–15%) of Hb Portland ($\zeta_2\gamma_2$), an embryonic haemoglobin present in traces in normal cord blood (Capp, Rigas and Jones, 1967), and small amounts of Hb H. Hb A, Hb A_2 and Hb F cannot as a rule be detected. The presence of Hb Portland is probably important as its oxygen-carrying ability helps affected fetuses to survive *in utero* and sometimes even for a few hours after birth (Kamuzora, Jones and Lehmann, 1974).

Lie-Injo (1961) reported an unusual phenomenon, namely, that erythrocytes from Hb-Bart's fetal hydrops infants undergo a type of 'sickling' when blood preparations are allowed to stand between slide and coverglass for 1 hour or more. Deoxygenation did not appear to be the cause, and the sickling was attributed to the presence of Hb Bart's in high concentration. Lie-Injo recalled that erythrocytes containing a high percentage

of Hb I had been reported to undergo a possibly similar type of sickling (see p. 434).

Hb-H DISEASE

The chemical nature of Hb H (β_4) has already been referred to (p. 446). Hb H was the designation give by Rigas, Koler and Osgood (1955) to an abnormal haemoglobin with a higher electrophoretic mobility than Hb A that they had detected in two members of a Chinese family in which thalassaemia appeared to be occurring. The abnormal haemoglobin seemed to be particularly remarkable, for, although found in the two siblings, it could not be detected in either of their parents. Independently, Gouttas and co-workers (1955) described the finding of a fast-moving haemoglobin in four members of a Greek family thought to have thalassaemia, and also in three sporadic cases of thalassaemia. They noted, moreover, a remarkable phenomenon: namely, that when the erythrocytes were suspended in brilliant cresyl-blue solution, as for a reticulocyte count, the haemoglobin appeared to undergo denaturation, for in 35–90% of the cells multiple blue-staining round granules appeared (Fig. 18.14). The inclusions could not be seen in fresh prep-

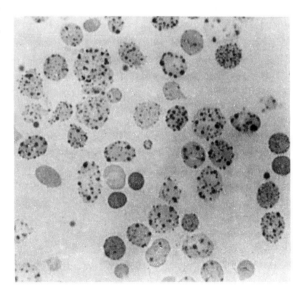

Fig. 18.14 Denaturation of Hb H by brilliant cresyl blue.
The round bodies of varying size consist of precipitated Hb H. [From Dacie and Lewis (1984).]

arations of blood by either conventional optical or phase-contrast microscopy or after staining fixed films with May-Grünwald Giemsa. The presence of brilliant cresyl blue appeared to be essential. The granules started to become visible after 10–15 minutes' exposure to the dye and were most obvious after about 2 hours' incubation.

In 1956, Rigas, Koler and Osgood gave more details of the Chinese family in which they had first found Hb H and reported that they had observed granule formation in reticulocyte preparations similar to that described by Gouttas and his co-workers. There is no doubt but that both groups were studying the same phenomenon, and it is now recognized that 'Hb-H disease' is quite a common disorder, with a particularly high incidence in racial groups living in South-East Asia where it presents as a rule as a milder disease than either homozygous β-thalassaemia or β-thalassaemia/Hb-E disease.

It is interesting to recall that Minnich and her co-workers (1954), in their detailed survey of 32 cases of Mediterranean anaemia in Thailand, had reported that they had noticed inclusion bodies in a large proportion (55.8–83.5%) of the erythrocytes of four of their patients. They were first noticed in platelet-reticulocyte preparations made with a modified Dameshek platelet solution. 'They appeared as blue staining intraerythrocytic coccoid bodies varying in size and number . . . . They were not stained until a lapse of approximately 10 minutes after the preparation was made . . . . In 30 minutes the bodies had fully developed in size and number . . . . Splenectomy had no effect on the numbers present, nor did this operation result in their appearance in other cases.' A photomicrograph shows without doubt that Minnich et al. were observing Hb-H inclusions. They considered that they closely resembled Heinz bodies in their staining properties and realized (and stated) that they had not previously been reported in Mediterranean anaemia. They did not, however, suggest that their presence indicated an abnormal haemoglobin; they came in fact to the erroneous conclusion that the bodies were probably related in some way to the chronic haemolytic anaemia present.

Subsequent studies have shown that Hb-H disease may be found in many racial groups. For example, further early reports included those of Lie-Injo et al. (1957) in two Chinese-Indonesian families, Butikofer et al (1960) in a South Italian family, Dittman et al. (1960) and Campanacci, Broccia and Fiumano (1962) in Sardinians, Ryan,

Campbell and Brain (1961) in a Papuan, Woodrow, Noble and Martindale (1964) in a North Lancashire (English) family, Rönisch and Kleihauer (1967) in a German family and Aksoy and Erdem (1968) in a Eti-Turk family.

Hb-H disease, however, seems sometimes to be rare in populations where α-thalassaemia is common. This is so apparently in Saudi Arabia where Hb Bart's was detected in 52% of 345 Shiite Arab cord-blood samples (Pembrey et al., 1975). In American blacks, too, although α-thalassaemia trait is common, Hb-H disease has seldom been reported (see, however, p. 451).

Genetics

Hb-H disease exists in two genetic forms; most frequently as the result of combined heterozygosity for two types of α-thalassaemia, α-thal-1 and α-thal-2, less frequently (and almost wholly confined to South-East Asia) as the result of combined heterozygosity for α-thalassaemia and a structural haemoglobin α-chain variant Hb Constant Spring (CS) (see p. 456).

The usual pattern is for both parents to show some haematological signs of α-thalassaemia trait, of different severity — one having α-thalassaemia-1 (α-thal-1), the other α-thalassaemia-2 (α-thal-2). Occasionally, one parent will have Hb-H disease, the other an α-thalassaemia trait. Sometimes one parent is phenotypically normal, having presumably silent α-thalassaemia. Rarely, both parents have appeared to be normal or at least indistinguishable from normal (Alessio et al., 1968).

Clinical features

These vary considerably, ranging in severity from that of homozygous β-thalassaemia to a mild illness causing few symptoms and compatible with a long life (Wasi, Na-Nakorn and Pootrakul, 1974). Pallor is the presenting symptom, and affected infants appear normal although they are as a rule slightly anaemic at birth — which is to be expected where there is failure of α-chain formation. The spleen and liver are not then palpably enlarged. By 1 year, however, the disorder is usually fully developed and anaemia is more marked. The spleen is then almost always palpable and the liver is usually enlarged, too. According to Wasi, Na-Nakorn and Pootrakul (1974), who reviewed a large series of Thai children with Hb-H disease, subsequent physical development is usually normal. The most anaemic patients are, however, likely to have a mongoloid facies and in such cases X-rays will show bony changes similar to those of homozygous β-thalassaemia.

As mentioned above, Hb-H disease may be clinically benign. Schwartz and Atwater (1972) described two black American families in which this was so. In the first family the propositus was not diagnosed as suffering from haemolytic anaemia (Hb-H disease) until she was aged 77; her spleen was not palpable and this was true also of the two other members of this family who had Hb-H disease. In this family, and in two other families in one of which the propositus was a combined heterozygote for α-thalassaemia and Hb I, the α:β globin-synthesis ratios determined on peripheral-blood samples were, according to Schwartz and Atwater, less abnormal than those that had been described in Italian or Chinese patients heterozygous for α-thalassaemia or with Hb-H disease. Bellevue, Dosik and Rieder (1979) have more recently described another American black family in which Hb-H disease had occurred. Five members were affected; their illness was similarly mild, the amount of Hb H present and the severity of their anaemia being less than in typical South-East Asia cases. In this family the degree of α:β globin-chain imbalance was, however, approximately the same as in Hb-H disease in other races, and Bellevue, Dosik and Rieder suggested that the milder clinical course was not due to greater α-chain production but rather to the more efficient way in which the excess β-globin chains were being disposed of.

As in other types of thalassaemia, infections lead to an increase in anaemia; this has been recorded, too, following the administration of oxidant drugs (Rigas and Koler, 1961a).

Massive enlargement of the spleen is not uncommon, and many Thai children with Hb-H disease have been splenectomized for hypersplenism (Wasi et al., 1969) (see p. 560). As in β-thalassaemia major, there is an increased tendency to form gallstones, and chronic leg ulceration, too, has been recorded (Daneshmend and Peachey, 1978). According to Weatherall and Clegg (1981, p. 523), overloading with iron is not an important complication of Hb-H disease (see *Iron stores*, p. 453). Pregnancy, on the other hand, may be rather hazardous. It can be uneventful (Ong, White and Sinnathuray, 1977),

but the patients generally become more anaemic and transfusion may be necessary (White and Jones, 1969; Wasi, Na-Nakorn and Pootrakul, 1974).

Possible association of mental retardation with Hb-H disease

An interesting series of reports has been published indicating a possible association of mental disorder with Hb-H disease.

Sjölin, Wallenius and Wranne (1964) described the history of a Swedish boy who suffered from respiratory distress at birth and was found to have an enlarged liver and spleen, petechial haemorrhages and minor congenital abnormalities, namely, low-set and deformed ears, skin folds at the back of neck and undescended testes. His haemoglobin when 1 day old was 20.3 g/dl but there were 15% reticulocytes and many circulating erythroblasts. When 11 days old 19% of Hb Bart's was demonstrated but no Hb H; 5% of the erythrocytes developed inclusions after incubation with brilliant cresyl blue. From 3–9 months, both Hb H and Hb Bart's were present; at 9 months there was 10.1% Hb H but Hb Bart's had by then disappeared. By 1 year 10 months his haemoglobin was 10.8 g/dl and the reticulocyte count had fallen to 2.0%. The MCV was then 79 fl and MCH 23 pg. There was 3.9% of Hb H, 2.3% of Hb A_2 and 2.5% of alkali-resistant haemoglobin (at 1 year 4 months); 49% of the erythrocytes developed inclusions in brilliant cresyl blue. At 1 month of age numerous target cells were noted and at 3 months hypochromia and microcytosis. Osmotic resistance was increased but became normal later.

The boy was mentally retarded and markedly hypotonic, his mental and motor development at 22 months corresponding to that of a normal infant of about 6 months of age. Both parents were of Swedish origin; they were healthy and no haematological abnormalities were demonstrable. However, the mother's reticulocyte count was 4%.

There appeared to be no doubt that the boy was forming Hb H and had produced considerable amounts of Hb Bart's when a small infant. The simultaneous occurrence of malformations (and mental retardation) and the haemoglobinopathy were considered likely to be fortuitous.

Borochovitz and co-workers (1970) described from South Africa a male child of Dutch descent with apparent Hb-H disease and several congenital abnormalities, namely, patent ductus, cryptorchidism and hypospadias, as well as mental retardation. His parents were not anaemic and electrophoresis of their haemoglobin revealed no abnormalities, and no inclusions were demonstrated with brilliant cresyl blue. The father's blood film showed, however, an abnormal degree of anisopoikilocytosis.

Weatherall, Higgs and their co-workers (1981a), under the title 'Hemoglobin H disease and mental retardation. A new syndrome or a remarkable coincidence?', described three families of North-European origin in which one member was a mentally retarded male with Hb-H disease. Patient 2 was the Swedish boy previously described by Sjölin, Wallenius and Wranne in 1964. One parent (the mother) of each patient with Hb-H disease appeared to be a carrier of α-thalassaemia; the other parent was apparently normal. In addition to the Hb-H disease the patients had certain features in common: mild respiratory distress at birth, hypotonia, microcephaly, mental retardation (IQ 76, <50, <50), fits and foot deformities. Weatherall *et al.* suggested that the abnormality resulted from a defect in the α-globin gene cluster in one chromosome 16 and a new mutation in the other chromosome 16 leading to both mental impairment and impairment of α-chain synthesis. [See also Weatherall *et al.* (1982), who also referred to three similar additional but unpublished cases; they also confirmed that typical genetic Hb-H disease is not associated with mental retardation.]

More recently, Bowcock, van Tonder and Jenkins (1984) have described the results of a reinvestigation of the child reported by Borochovitz *et al.* (1970). This indicated that their patient corresponds closely clinically to the three patients described by Weatherall *et al.* (1981a) and corresponds closely, too, to the first patient at the molecular level. The present patient had inherited α-thal-2 (−α) from his mother and from his father a chromosome which had undergone a deletion which included the ζ-(zeta) and α-globin genes. His father was, nevertheless, phenotypically normal.

It is interesting to note that Hjelle, Charache and Phillips (1982) described a Caucasian boy with Hb-H disease who also suffered from multiple congenital abnormalities — spina bifida, myelomeningocoele, congenital cataracts, herniae and femoral-neck abnormalities. He did not, however, suffer from mental retardation, and the conclusion was reached that he did not belong to the same category as the cases described above. Both his parents had α-thalassaemia trait, and although of North-European origin, their α-thalassaemia appeared, by restriction-enzyme analysis, to be of the Asian type.

Blood picture

The degree of anaemia and the blood picture in Hb-H disease conforms closely to that already described (p. 428) as being found in the β-thalassaemia intermedia syndrome: *i.e.*, hypochromia, microcytosis, anisocytosis, poikilocytosis, target cells, cell fragments and punctate basophilia are marked features (Fig. 18.15). A few normoblasts

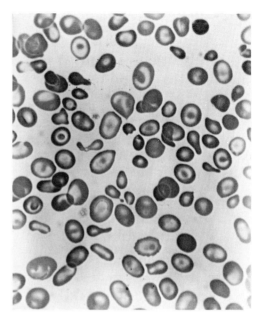

Fig. 18.15 Photomicrograph of a blood film of a patient with Hb-H disease.
There is very marked anisocytosis, poikilocytosis and anisochromasia, as well as target cell formation. × 700. (Film provided by courtesy of Dr Adrian Stephens.)

are likely to be present. The reticulocyte count is slightly to moderately raised in patients in a steady state, but rises considerably in response to episodes of acute haemolysis. The feature which distinguishes the blood picture of Hb-H disease from that of other thalassaemia syndromes is, of course, the development of inclusions of precipitated Hb H in the erythrocytes when they are suspended in brilliant cresyl blue or New methylene blue solutions, as used for reticulocyte counts.

Most patients are moderately anaemic. Thus Wasi and co-workers (1969), who reported on 260 patients seen in Thailand, found that their mean haemoglobin was 7.79 g/dl. Wasi, Na-Nakorn and Pootrakul (1974) emphasized that the haemoglobin level and degree of splenomegaly fluctuate in individual patients, the result, in their view, of environmental influences, *e.g.*, infections and/or drugs, leading to temporary increases in haemolysis. They also stressed that, if the hamoglobin was significantly and persistently lower than 8 g/dl, causes other than Hb-H disease, *e.g.*, iron deficiency, should be sought as an explanation.

The intra-erythrocytic inclusions

As already referred to (p. 450), before Hb H had been recognized as an abnormal fast-moving haemoglobin, intra-erythrocytic inclusions had been recognized in cases of thalassaemia in South-East Asia by Minnich *et al.* (1954). Gouttas and his co-workers (1955), too, had reported similar findings in four members of a Greek family thought to be suffering from thalassaemia, namely, that multiple blue-staining granules appeared in a high proportion of their erythrocytes when the cells were suspended in brilliant cresyl blue solution. Next, Rigas, Koler and Osgood (1956) observed the same phenomenon in the erythrocytes of members of the family in which they had originally detected the fast-moving haemoglobin that they had referred to as Hb H. Further studies of the nature of the inclusions and on the circumstances of their formation were reported by Rigas and Koler (1961a) and Nathan and Gunn (1966).

Rigas and Koler (1961a) studied two patients who underwent splenectomy. In films made after splenectomy, but not before the operation, a small proportion of the erythrocytes in fixed films (2.3 and 4%, respectively) were found to contain inclusions which stained by Wright's stain (as well as vitally by brilliant cresyl blue). Rigas and Koler also reported that multiple Hb-H inclusions were produced immediately by exposure to brilliant cresyl blue, if the cells had been previously exposed to sodium nitrite so as to produce methaemoglobin, *i.e.*, that oxidation increased the instability of Hb H. Rigas and Koler (1961a) and Nathan and Gunn (1966) separated blood from Hb-H patients who had undergone splenectomy into light and heavy fractions by centrifugation. Soluble Hb H was more abundant in the young (light) cell population as compared with the old (heavy) cell population, as shown by the proportion of cells yielding material precipitated by brilliant cresyl blue and also by the amount precipitated. Already precipitated material in the form usually of a single 'Heinz body' was virtually only found in the old cell population.

According to Rachmilewitz and co-workers (1969), the precipitated haemoglobin is in the form of haemichromes; they included, too, in their paper some phase-contrast photomicrographs of erythrocyte ghosts. In a patient with the spleen *in situ* an occasional ghost contained a single inclusion body. However, in ghosts prepared from blood pre-incubated for 12 hours at 37°C the majority, if not all, of the ghosts contained more than one inclusion. All the ghosts prepared from the fresh blood of a splenectomized patient contained many inclusion bodies.

Ultrastructure of Hb-H precipitates. Wickramasinghe and his co-workers (1981) described as golf-ball-like the electron-microscopic appearance of the precipitates that form when Hb-H-containing erythrocytes are suspended in brilliant cresyl blue solution (Fig. 18.16). Spherical or biconvex masses were seen to be attached to and to bulge into the cell membrane, unlike the Heinz bodies present prior to supravital staining (in two splenectomized patients) which were not attached to cell membrane. Wickramasinghe *et al.* suggested that the masses become attached to the cell membrane as the result of disulphide bonds forming between some residual thiol groups in the precipitates and thiol groups of cell membrane proteins.

Bunyaratvej and co-workers (1983) reported some interesting but unexplained electron-microscopic differences in the intracellular distribution of precipitated haemoglobin between the two genotypes of Hb-H disease, α-thal-l/α-thal-2 and α-thal-l/Hb CS: in three cases of the former 62.3% of the inclusions were marginated and 37.7% were 'floating'; in four cases of the latter 31.9% were marginated and 68.1% 'floating'. Under the light microscope the two patterns of precipitation could not be distinguished.

Wickramasinghe and his co-workers (1985) and Gadsdon *et al.* (1986) have more recently reported differences in the electron-microscopic appearances of Hb-H inclusions that form in the presence of brilliant cresyl blue (BCB), methylene blue and New methylene blue, respectively. The inclusions formed in the presence of BCB and New methylene blue were small and were bound to the erythrocyte membrane while those produced by methylene blue were larger and more variable in size and not necessarily membrane-bound (Figs. 18.16 and 18.17).

Iron stores

Pootrakul and co-workers (1981) recorded serum-ferritin concentrations in 71 Thai patients with Hb-H disease. The values ranged widely: 92–3021 ng/ml, mean 527 ng/ml in males and 11–2578 ng/ml, mean 240 ng/ml in females. The means in each sex were close to 5 times the normal. The patients were said not to have been transfused or to have received only minimal amounts of blood. According to Weatherall and Clegg (1981, p. 523), iron loading is, however, not an important feature of Hb-H disease. The data of Galanelllo and co-workers (1983a) who reported that the serum-ferritin levels were normal in 27 out of 30 patients support this conclusion. The raised levels found in three patients were attributed to past iron medication or blood transfusion or to the possession of a gene for haemochromatosis.

The data of Tso, Loh and Todd (1984) obtained from Chinese in Hong Kong do, however, suggest that iron overloading to a moderate degree is common in this

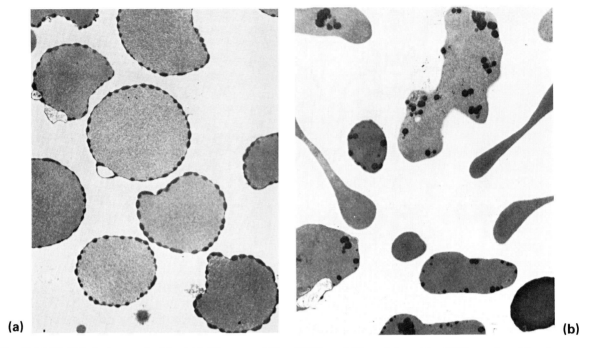

Fig. 18.16 Hb-H inclusions stained by (a) brilliant cresyl blue (BCB), and (b) methylene blue (MB), as viewed by electron microscopy.
The inclusions formed in the presence of BCB are relatively small and uniform in size and are adherent to the erythrocyte membrane. From a patient with Hb-H disease. [Reproduced by permission from Wickramasinghe *et al.* (1985).]

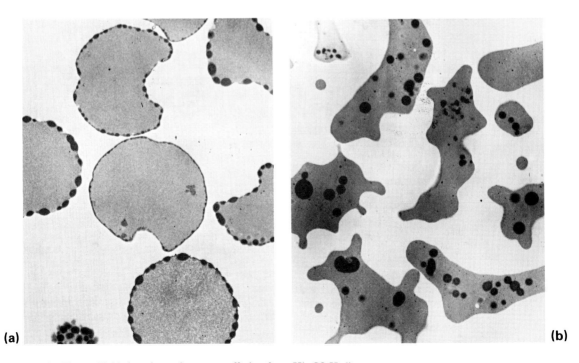

Fig. 18.17 As Figure 18.16, but the patient was suffering from Hb CS-H disease.

population: 14 out of 20 males and 20 out fo 26 females with Hb-H disease had raised serum-ferritin levels compared with controls of the same age-group. None of the patients studied was transfusion-dependent.

ERYTHROCYTE LIFE-SPAN IN Hb-H DISEASE

Studies using ^{51}Cr have established that erythrocyte survival is considerably shortened in Hb-H disease, despite some doubt as to the rate at which the chromium label is eluted from Hb H.

Tso (1972), however, studied eight patients with Hb-H disease in steady state using ^{51}Cr and DF^{32}P as labels simultaneously and found a good correlation between the data obtained by the two methods. Calculating that the rate of chromium elution from the erythrocytes of the Hb-H patients was in fact within the normal range, Tso concluded that ^{51}Cr was a valid label for the estimation of erythrocyte survival in Hb-H disease. Destruction was accelerated and random: the ^{51}Cr T_{50} ranged between 8.1 and 18.1 days and the mean half-life calculated from the DF^{32}P results ranged between 13.8 and 36.3 days.

Earlier, variable but moderately shortened ^{51}Cr T_{50s} had been reported by Rigas, Koler and Osgood (1956), Bingle, Huehns and Prankerd (1958), Rigas and Koler (1961a), Malamos et al. (1962), Gabuzda et al. (1965), Necheles et al. (1966) and others.

The elimination curve obtained with the 32-year-old female studied by Necheles et al. was two-component, with T_{50s} of 4 days and 13 days, respectively.

Erythrokinetics

The turnover of Hb A and Hb H were studied by Gabuzda et al. (1965) using [2-^{14}C]glycine as a label. Hb H was found to have a more rapid fractional turnover rate than Hb A. The study indicated random destruction and the erythrocyte survival time was calculated to be about one-third the normal.

Ferrokinetic studies carried out by Pearson et al. (1962) in one Hb-H disease patient showed that ^{59}Fe was cleared from the plasma at a rate just within the upper limit of normal. However, 62% of the label appeared eventually in the peripheral circulation, indicating that erythropoiesis in the patient they studied was considerably more effective than that found in most patients with β-thalassaemia intermedia. The results

obtained by Malamos et al. (1962) in five patients were similar: the uptake of ^{59}Fe was between 53 and 70%, and their ^{51}Cr T_{50s} were between 12.2 and 19.0 days.

ERYTHROCYTE METABOLISM IN Hb-H DISEASE

Several abnormalities have been demonstrated (Rigas and Koler, 1961b; Gabuzda, 1966; Nathan et al., 1969; Scott, Rasbridge and Grimes, 1970; Knox-Macaulay et al., 1972; Beutler et al., 1977).

As expected with a relatively young cell population, glucose consumption and lactate production are increased. Nathan et al. (1969), who studied five Hb-H disease patients, found that young (light) erythrocytes contained more soluble Hb H and GSH than older (dense) cells and that HMP shunt activity, which was subnormal in young cells, was normal in old cells. K$^+$ flux was increased in old cells.

According to Scott, Rasbridge and Grimes (1970), ATP concentration was low in two out of three patients and GSH low in four out of six patients. Erythrocyte phospholipid was increased in the four patients studied, but was lost, along with ATP, GSH and AChE activity, abnormally rapidly on incubation in vitro. It seems likely that some at least of the observed abnormalities are the consequence of the presence of precipitated Hb H and its interaction with the erythrocyte membrane.

Beutler and his co-workers (1977) found erythrocyte GSH peroxidase activity to be markedly increased in eight Hb-H disease patients and to be less markedly increased in most of the α-thalassaemia carriers studied. This contrasted with only minor increases in individuals with various types of β-thalassaemia. The mechanism and clinical significance, if any, of the increased activity are obscure.

Erythrocyte protoporphyrin

As described on page 424, Pootrakul et al. (1984) measured erythrocyte protoporphyrin (EP) in several different groups of thalassaemic patients: 32 had Hb-H disease. A minority of patients in each group had EP concentrations well above the normal. An inadequate supply of iron in relation to massively expanded erythropoiesis was suggested as the cause.

HAEMOGLOBIN CONSTANT SPRING

Another promoter of α-thalassaemia syndromes is Hb Constant Spring (Hb CS). This interesting haemoglobin was first identified in Jamaica in a Chinese family (Clegg, Weatherall and Milner, 1971; Milner, Clegg and Weatherall, 1971).

The propositus was a young woman aged 19 who had been diagnosed when aged 5 years as having Cooley's anaemia. Splenectomy had been carried out when she was 8 years of age with some improvement. When aged 19, her blood picture was considered to be typical of Hb-H disease after splenectomy. Haemoglobin electrophoresis on starch gel revealed Hb A, Hb H, Hb Bart's and Hb A_2 and an additional fraction migrating slowly between Hb A_2 and the origin. This fraction, Hb Constant Spring (named after a village in Jamaica) was shown subsequently to be an α-chain variant formed of the 141 residues, as in the normal α chain, with, in addition, a further 31 residues attached to the C-terminal end. It was identified in two generations of the family studied: in heterozygotes it did not produce any discernible haematological changes, but combined with an α-thalassaemia gene, as in the propositus, it caused a disorder phenotypically the same as Hb-H disease.

Subsequent studies have shown that Hb CS is not uncommon in Far Eastern populations (Lie-Injo, Lopez and Lopez, 1971; Todd, 1971) and is an important cause of Hb-H disease there when in combination with a gene for α-thalassaemia. Except for apparently a single report of its occurrence in a Greek patient with Hb-H disease (Sofroniadou et al., 1968; Fessas et al., 1972; Clegg and Weatherall, 1974), Hb CS appears not to have been observed in other racial groups.

Todd (1971) found that five out of 43 (11.7%) South-Chinese patients with Hb-H disease had a slow-moving haemoglobin component which he considered to be Hb CS. Lie-Injo, Lopez and Lopez (1971) studied 23 patients with Hb-H disease and their relatives in 17 Chinese or Malaysian families: in 11 of the families a slow-moving component, tentatively referred to as the X component, was present in one parent; some siblings possessed it, too.

Homozygosity for Hb Constant Spring

Lie-Injo (1973) and Lie-Injo and her co-workers (1974) reported that they had investigated eight children belonging to a Malay family whose parents both produced a slow-moving X component (identified as Hb CS) on haemoglobin electrophoresis. Six of the children had the X-component trait: they were healthy and presented no physical abnormalities. Three of them, and their father, had significant erythrocyte microcytosis and anisopoikilocytosis; their mother, grandmother and one of the children had similar slight morphological abnormalities but without microcytosis. Two of them had a blood picture indistinguishable from normal, despite having the X-component trait; one child appeared to be entirely normal. The propositus appeared to be homozygous for Hb CS. He was aged 12 when studied and his liver and spleen were just palpable; he was well nourished but slightly small for his age and was not jaundiced. His haemoglobin was then 11.3 g/dl, erythrocyte count 4.82×10^{12}/l, with 7.6% reticulocytes; MCV 75.7 fl and MCH 22.3 pg. Haemoglobin electrophoresis revealed 5.2% Hb CS (about 10 times the amount in the supposed heterozygotes), 1.8% Hb A_2 and 1.3% Hb F. Hb H and Hb Bart's were not detectable. The remainder of the haemoglobin was Hb A. The presence of so much normal Hb A in association with apparent homozygosity for an α-chain variant haemoglobin was held to provide further evidence for the existence of duplicated α-chain genes.

Since the report summarized above, several additional homozygous cases have been described, e.g., by Pongsamart et al. (1975) and Qin et al. (1985). The findings have been essentially the same as in Lie-Injo's original patient, and there seems little doubt but that homozygosity for Hb CS usually leads to a mild rather than to a severe thalassaemia syndrome.

The homozygous $(\alpha^{CS}\alpha/\alpha^{CS}\alpha)$ patient studied in detail by Derry et al. (1984) was mildly affected. He was a 32-year-old Thai who gave a history of recurrent jaundice as a child but had no symptoms at the time of investigation. His liver and spleen were palpable, 4 and 3 cm, respectively, below the costal margin. His haemoglobin was 11.5 g/dl, erythrocyte count 4.38×10^{12}/l, MCV 87 fl, MCH 26.3 pg and reticulocyte count 11.5%. Deficiency in α-chain synthesis was demonstrated and cessation of synthesis and destruction of excess β chains proceeded unusually rapidly. A ^{51}Cr survival study revealed a double population of erythrocytes: the majority (84.4%) had a calculated mean life-span of 47 days while a significant minority had a much shorter life-span of 5 days. The overall findings were thought to resemble more closely those typical of Hb-

H disease with three α genes inactive rather than those of individuals with two inactive α genes.

Hunt and co-workers (1982) have provided evidence that the presence of the gene for Hb CS results in the production of an unstable ^{CS}mRNA. In two patients with Hb CS-H disease ($--/\alpha^{CS}\alpha^{A}$) the α:β mRNA ratio was higher in RNA extracted from marrow nucleated cells than in that from peripheral-blood reticulocytes. All the α mRNA in the peripheral blood appeared to be derived from the single α^{A} gene present.

Hb-H levels and proportion of erythrocytes containing inclusion bodies in the two types of Hb-H disease

Adirojmanon and Wasi (1980) reported some interesting data, based on a large number of patients, which indicated that the Hb-H percentage and the proportion of erythrocytes developing inclusions when suspended in 1% methylene blue in saline were significantly higher in the α-thal-1/Hb-CS type of Hb-H disease than in the more common α-thal-1/α-thal-2 type. It was suggested that inheritance of the Constant Spring gene in some way activated the synthesis of β chains.

α-THALASSAEMIA TRAIT: CLINICAL AND HAEMATOLOGICAL FINDINGS

As described on page 533, individuals who are obligatory heterozygotes for α-thal-1 or α-thal-2 tend to be slightly anaemic and to have a slightly subnormal MCV and MCH. Microcytosis and slightly increased anisocytosis should be recognizable in blood films (Fig. 18.18). However, the changes are often slight and it is then not easy to be sure that an individual patient's film is in fact abnormal.

Clinically, carriers of α-thalassaemia have no symptoms attributable to the trait. In particular, and in contrast to some heterozygotes for β-thalassaemia, they are not jaundiced and the spleen is not palpable.

Some interesting reports on α-thalassaemia trait in different parts of the world are referred to briefly below (in alphabetical order).

α-thalassaemia trait in Arabia

White and co-workers (1985) recorded haematological findings in 2000 pregnant women living in Abu Dhabi, United Arab Emirates: 18% of them were diagnosed as having the α-thalassaemia trait (compared with 2% diagnosed as having the β-thalassaemic trait). Both groups of patients became more anaemic during pregnancy, the curve of progression of their anaemia paralleling that of normal non-thalassaemic controls. The fall

in haemoglobin appeared mostly to be due to haemodilution. Iron deficiency was as frequent in the α-thalassaemics as in the normal controls; in the β-thalassaemics it was less frequent.

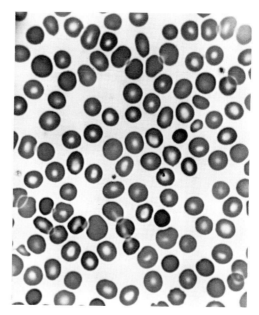

Fig. 18.18 Photomicrograph of a blood film of a patient with α-thalassaemia trait (one α gene deleted).
There is slight anisocytosis and microcytosis. × 700. (Film provided by courtesy of Dr Adrian Stephens.)

α-thalassaemia trait in the Far East

According to Pornpatkul, Wasi and Na-Nakorn (1969), α-thal-1 heterozygotes are likely to be a little more anaemic than α-thal-2 heterozygotes and to have a lower MCV and MCH, a slightly higher erythrocyte count, an abnormal erythrocyte morphology and an increased osmotic resistance. Morphology and osmotic resistance in α-thal-2 heterozygotes were reported to be normal. Hb-F and Hb-A$_2$ percentages were normal in both groups.

α-thalassaemia trait in Greece

Kanavakis and co-workers (1986) looked for evidence of α-thalassaemia in the cord blood of 227 infants and found by gene mapping that 16 (7.05%) were α-thal-2 ($-\alpha/\alpha\alpha$) heterozygotes; Hb Bart's was detected in only two of these. In addition, one infant had the $--/\alpha\alpha$ genotype and one a 20.5-kb deletion; they had Hb-Bart's percentages of 4.8 and 6.6. A further infant with 8% Hb Bart's had α-thal-2 plus a dysfunctional α gene. The overall incidence of α-thalassaemia in Athenian newborns was calculated to be 8.4%.

α-thalassaemia trait in Jamaica

Maude and co-workers (1985) reported from Jamaica on the effect of the number of α-globin genes present on the blood picture of 195 black children, from 6 months to 9 years of age, with a normal Hb-AA genotype. Five of the children were homozygous for α-thal-2 (two genes); 60 were heterozygous for α-thal-2 (three genes) and 130 had the normal complement of four genes. The Hb-F and Hb-A$_2$ percentages did not differ between the groups. Compared to the normal four-gene group, the three-gene α-thal-2 heterozygotes tended to have a significantly lower total haemoglobin, MCHC, MCV and MCH and a higher erythrocyte count. The differences became more obvious with increasing age. There were too few two-gene patients for their data to be compared statistically with the other two groups but the differences between this group and the other two groups seemed likely to be even more marked.

α-thalassaemia trait in North America

The α-thalassaemia trait is found frequently amongst the black population in North America. Friedman and co-workers (1974), who examined the heel blood of 693 full-term black infants, found a moderate or small amount of Hb Bart's in 15% of them: 3% had more than 2% of Hb Bart's; 12% had from 1 to 2%. The former were considered to have the α-thalassaemia trait, and they had, too, microcytosis and iron-resistant hypochromia which persisted over a 5–24-month period.

Those with 1–2% Hb Bart's were thought possibly to have a type of α-thalassaemia. [Recent work has suggested that reliance on the demonstration of small amounts of Hb Bart's grossly underestimates the incidence of α-thalassaemia trait (see p. 535).]

Pierce and co-workers (1977) likewise concluded that α-thalassaemia is a common abnormality in American blacks. They investigated 541 healthy adults: 13.4% were found to have a subnormal MCH (<27.0 pg); 1.4% had heterozygous β-thalassaemia; 2.3% were iron-deficient; 5.7% had α:β globin-synthesis ratios compatible with α-thal-l trait and 2.5%, with synthesis ratios 0.75–0.9, were suspected of having α-thalassaemia.

α-thalassaemia trait in Sicily and Sardinia

Musumeci and co-workers (1979) and Melis and co-workers (1980) have reported haematological and biosynthetic data on α-thalassaemia heterozygotes in Sicily and Sardinia, respectively. In Sicily significant differences were demonstrated between the α-thalassaemia carriers and normal controls with respect to haemoglobin, MCH and MCHC, but not with respect to erythrocyte counts, MCV, and Hb-A$_2$ and Hb-F levels. The mean α:β globin-chain ratio was significantly different, however, although there was some overlap with the normal.

Melis et al. (1980) studied 88 Sardinian adults with thalassaemia-like indices but normal serum iron concentration and normal Hb-A$_2$ and Hb-F levels: 65 developed inclusions when their erythrocytes were incubated in brilliant cresyl blue solution. α:β globin-chain ratios were measured in 23: the results (mean 0.70 ± 0.10) were the same as in obligate α-thalassaemia heterozygotes.

Galanello and co-workers (1983b) described the haematological findings in heterozygotes for non-detection α-thalassaemia in Sardinia. Their MCH and MCV were widely scattered and overlapped the values found in α-thalassaemia patients with deletions of two genes ($--/\alpha\alpha$ or $-\alpha/-\alpha$ genotypes) or those with a single deletion ($-\alpha/\alpha\alpha$). This variability was thought to indicate the possible existence of more than one form of non-deletional α-thalassaemia.

Galanello et al. (1984a) reported on the relationship between the presence of Hb Bart's in the cord blood of newborn infants and their α-thalassaemia genotype. Infants who had two α-globin genes deleted (either of $--/\alpha\alpha$ or $-\alpha/-\alpha$ genotype) had mean Hb Bart's levels of $4.5 \pm 1.6\%$ (range 2.0–7.1%), irrespective of the presence or absence of a gene for β-thalassaemia. A minority of infants (39%) with the $-\alpha/\alpha\alpha$ genotype, with or without a gene for β-thalassaemia, had 0.78–2.5% Hb Bart's; in the majority (61%), however, no Hb Bart's was detectable. Five infants with 1.2–7.4% Hb Bart's had four α genes present and were thought to be heterozygous for a non-deletional α-thalassaemia; three of them were found later to be carriers of β-thalassaemia also.

α-thalassaemia trait in the United Kingdom

Studies by Walford and Deacon (1976) in the United Kingdom on 44 individuals with α-thalassaemia trait suggested that minor differences exist in its expression in different racial groups, as judged by MCV and MCH measurements: the Chinese were more severely affected than the Greeks who were more severely affected than the Indians. Compared with β-thalassaemia heterozygotes, the α-thalassaemia heterozygotes presented with a milder disorder in terms of erythrocyte morphology and indices and in globin-chain synthesis imbalance. The Indians in particular were mildly affected.

More recently, Higgs and co-workers (1985) have provided evidence of the existence of a British type of α-thalassaemia. α-thalassaemia had been diagnosed in 12 people of apparent British lineage and in eight of them a molecular defect was identified which was clearly distinct from the defects found in α-thalassaemics living in Mediterranean or Far-Eastern countries. Three of them had Hb-H disease, the remainder α-thalassaemia trait. Two of the Hb-H patients were compound heterozygotes for the British type of α-thalassaemia and a foreign type. The 12 patients were apparently unrelated, but Higgs *et al.* suggested that those sharing the same molecular defect were probably in fact distantly related. The rarity of the defect could be explained, it was suggested, by the absence in the country of any factor giving α-thalassaemia heterozygotes a selective advantage.

α:β GLOBIN-CHAIN RATIOS IN α-THALASSAEMIA

As expected, α:β globin specific-activity ratios are subnormal in the various types of α-thalassaemia. Kan, Schwartz and Nathan (1968) were able to demonstrate an interesting progression from a very low value in six Hb-H disease patients, 0.41 ± 0.11, to 0.77 ± 0.05 in nine α-thalassaemia trait individuals, to 0.82–0.95 in four silent carriers. (In 11 non-thalassaemic individuals the mean specific-activity ratio was 1.02 ± 0.07.) The

patients were Chinese or Italians and peripheral blood labelled with [^{14}C]leucine was used. Similar data were provided by Schwartz, Kan and Nathan (1969). As previously referred to (p. 451), the α:β chain synthesis ratios in black Americans with Hb-H disease have been found to be less abnormal than the ratios that had previously been obtained in Italian and Chinese Hb-H disease patients (Schwartz and Atwater, 1972).

There is some evidence that globin-chain synthesis is more unbalanced in peripheral-blood reticulocytes than in their nucleated precursors. Zaizov and co-workers (1980) studied eight α-thalassaemic children of Middle-Eastern parentage. Five who were mildly anaemic gave α:non-α globin-chain synthesis ratios of 0.77–0.88. Bone-marrow preparations of the same eight patients gave balanced ratios in six, while in the other two α-chain synthesis, although subnormal, was greater than in peripheral-blood cells.

A next step in the understanding of the mechanism of α-thalassaemia was the demonstration that functional α-globin mRNA activity is decreased (Benz, Swerdlow and Forget, 1973; Grossbard et al. 1973.)

Benz, Swerdlow and Forget (1973) isolated mRNA from the reticulocytes of two patients, of Mediterranean origin, with Hb-H disease and tested the RNA for its capacity to direct the formation of α- and β-globin chains in a RNA-dependent cell-free system prepared from Krebs II mouse ascites tumour cells. A great excess of β chains relative to α chains was demonstrated which was greater than that expected from β:α globin-chain synthesis ratios in intact reticulocytes.

The nature of the lesions responsible for the decreased mRNA formation in Hb-H disease, and in other types of α-thalassaemia, is discussed on page 514.

αβ-THALASSAEMIA

The comparative frequency of the genes for α- and β-thalassaemia in certain populations has led to the birth of individuals who are combined heterozygotes for both abnormalities. A relatively mild

form of thalassaemia is the result, for it seems that the combined heterozygotes do not suffer from a greater degree of difficulty in haemoglobin formation than is associated usually with simple heterozygosity for each separate type of thalassaemia. Cases of this type have been described by Pearson (1966), Wasi *et al.* (1969), Kan and Nathan (1970), Knox-Macaulay *et al.* (1972), Altay *et al.* (1977), Furbetta *et al.* (1979), Kanavakis *et al.* (1982) and Melis *et al.* (1983).

Patients, too, have been observed who are homozygous for β-thalassaemia as well as heterozygous for α-thalassaemia, and in such cases the clinical expression of their disease has been generally mild. Rarer combinations, too, have been reported, *e.g.*, Hb-H/heterozygous β-thalassaemia, homozygous α-thalassaemia (two genes for thalassaemia) plus homozygous β-thalassaemia and heterozygous α-thalassaemia plus the β-thalassaemia/HPFH combination; also triplicated α genes (ααα/αα) plus homozygous β-thalassaemia, and triplicated α genes (ααα/ααα) plus heterozygous β-thalassaemia. In general, the presence of a gene or genes for α-thalassaemia in patients who have β-thalassaemia results in less α:β globin-chain imbalance (*i.e.* fewer free α chains) and a milder than usual clinical state. Reports of the various combinations referred to above are summarized below (in chronological order).

Pearson (1966) gave details of a black American family which possessed the genes for α-thalassaemia, β-thalassaemia and Hb S. Three members of the family were considered to have αβ-thalassaemia, and the point was made that their haematological findings were no more abnormal than in other members of the family who were simple heterozygotes for either trait.

Kan and Nathan (1970) studied two families, one Italian, the other Chinese. The propositus in the first family suffered from what was described as mild Cooley's anaemia; he was believed to possess two genes for β-thalassaemia and one for α-thalassaemia. In the second family two individuals were believed to have a gene for α-thalassaemia, another for a 'silent carrier' (of α-thalassaemia) and a single gene for β-thalassaemia. They had the genotype of Hb-H disease, yet their erythrocytes contained no Hb H and survived normally *in vivo*. This was because, it was suggested, excess β-chain production was being inhibited by the β-thalassaemia gene. Kan and Nathan concluded that the α:β chain imbalance normally present in thalassaemia could be favourably influenced by combinations of α- and β-thalassaemia genes.

Knox-Macaulay and co-workers (1972) investigated a Cypriot family possessing three thalassaemia genes — those for α-thal-1, α-thal-2 and β-thalassaemia. Two siblings were heterozygotes for α-thal-1 and β-thalassaemia; a third had typical Hb-H disease, being

a compound heterozygote for α-thal-1 and α-thal-2. The compound heterozygotes for α-thal-1 and β-thalassaemia were found to have α:β chain-synthesis ratios of 1.05 and 1.03, signifying that chain synthesis was in balance. The compound heterozygote for α-thal-1 and α-thal-2 had the very low ratio of 0.20, as found in the Hb-H disease, and was forming Hb H from the excess of β chains. All three patients had a similar blood picture, with marked hypochromia and much anisocytosis and poikilocytosis, and they were slightly anaemic (haemoglobin 10.2–11.1 g/dl). The ^{51}Cr T_{50} was normal (33 days) in one of the compound heterozygotes for α-thal-1 and β-thalassaemia; it was definitely subnormal (18 days) in the patient with Hb-H disease, whose reticulocyte count (5.2%) was the highest of the three. Knox-Macaulay *et al.* concludad that unbalanced globin-chain synthesis is the primary cause of the short erythrocyte survival in Hb-H disease and that any metabolic abnormalities and changes in membrane permeability are of secondary importance.

Özsoylu, Hiçsönmez and Altay (1973) described a Turkish child who presented with the clinical picture of thalassaemia major. He was considered to have Hb-H disease and to be heterozygous for β-thalassaemia. His father had αβ-thalassaemia, his mother the α-thalassaemia trait.

Altay and co-workers (1977) described a Turkish family in which the genes for β-thalassaemia or δβ-thalassaemia, 'silent' β-thalassaemia and mild and severe α-thalassaemia were considered to be present in different combinations. Three children presented with the clinical syndrome of thalassaemia major. When aged 9, 8 and 2 years old, respectively, they were found to be forming 7–11% of Hb Bart's, but without measurable Hb H. The children were regarded as being compound heterozygotes for α-thal-1 and α-thal-2 as well as for β-thalassaemia and 'silent' β-thalassaemia. The haemoglobin analysis findings were thought to be compatible with the reduction in β-chain synthesis associated with the presence of the β-thalassaemia genes.

Loukopoulos, Loutradi and Fessas (1978) described in detail a Greek-Cypriot child who for the first 5 years of his life was anaemic but had not been transfused and was of normal weight and height and had a normal facies. His haemoglobin fluctuated between 6 and 8 g/dl. The liver was palpable and the spleen extended to the rim of the pelvis. The erythrocytes were extremely hypochromic and markedly resistant to osmotic haemolysis. The MCV was 41–48 fl, the MCH 9.0–9.4 pg[!] and MCHC 22 g/dl. A ^{51}Cr study revealed a T_{50} of 30 days for 80% of the erythrocyte population and a very short life-span (1 day) for the remainder. Up to 40% of the haemoglobin was Hb F and 9.6–12.0% Hb A_2, and there was 0–2% Hb Bart's; the remaining Hb was Hb A. The child's father was thought to possess one gene for β-thalassaemia and one for α-thalassaemia and his mother one gene for β-thalassaemia and two for α-thalassaemia; the child was regarded as being homozygous for both β-thalassaemia and α-thalassaemia. α- and β-chain synthesis, despite being grossly subnormal, appeared to be almost balanced.

Furbetta and co-workers (1979) described the results of the interaction of α- and β-thalassaemia genes in two Sardinian families. The propositus in the first family had at birth 25% Hb Bart's and 75% Hb F and went on to develop the clinical and haematological picture of Cooley's anaemia. He was thought to be a homozygote for β⁰-thalassaemia as well as a compound heterozygote for α-thal-1 and α-thal-2. In the second family two premature twins (who died shortly after birth) were born with haemoglobin patterns similar to that of the propositus in the first family. Their mother was considered to be a compound heterozygote for α-thal-2 and β⁰-thalassaemia and their father a compound heterozygote for α-thal-1 and β⁰-thalassaemia.

Beutler, Turner and Kuhl (1981) investigated a 2-year-old black female child and her family. Her mother was a heterozygote for HPFH and her father a heterozygote for β-thalassaemia. The child appeared to be a compound heterozygote for β-thalassaemia and HPFH. Her haemoglobin was 8.9 g/dl and she had 8.0% reticulocytes, and the spleen was palpable 3.5 cm below the costal margin. She had a brother of apparently the same genotype but he was clinically far less severely affected. Examination of the α-gene status of the family revealed that the brother and his mother were of the α−/αα genotype, and it was suggested that the possession of only three α-gene loci resulted in the accumulation of fewer free α chains and the lesser severity of his illness compared to that of his sister.

Weatherall and co-workers (1981b), in a paper on the molecular basis for mild forms of homozygous β-thalassaemia, described three Cypriots who were heterozygotes for α-thal-2 as well as being homozygotes for β⁺-thalassaemia; they also described two Cypriots who had inherited a gene for a non-deletion type of α-thalassaemia (see p. 516), as well as being homozygous for β⁺-thalassaemia. They concluded that the inheritance of the α-thalassaemia genes had ameliorated the course of the homozygous β⁺-thalassaemia and suggested that such associations were probably not uncommon in some Mediterranean and South-East Asian populations.

Kanavakis and co-workers (1982) determined the α-globin genotype of 55 β-thalassaemic heterozygotes by restriction endonuclease analysis; 42 were Cypriots and 13 Sardinians. Thirty-three had a normal α genotype (αα/αα), 14 had three α genes (α−/αα), four two α genes (α−/α−) and four one gene (α−/−−). The patients with one or two α genes deleted had, progressively, better balanced α:β globin-chain synthesis ratios, higher haemoglobin levels and a higher MCV and MCH. [There was in fact little difference in MCV and MCH between those with four or three α genes.] The four patients with the α−/−− genotype were significantly more anaemic and had very low MCVs and MCHs and a mean α:β globin ratio of 0.5 ± 0.05. The point was made that programmes screening for thalassaemia based on the determination of the MCV could miss cases of α- and β-thalassaemia interaction.

Melis and co-workers (1983), in a further study of Sardinian β-thalassaemia heterozygotes, investigated the α-globin gene states of 10 β⁰-thalassaemics who had normal or virtually normal blood pictures. Eight of them were found by restriction endonuclease gene analysis to possess the −α/−α genotype and two to have the −α/αα genotype.

Melis, Galanello and Cao (1983) have reported further data on the Sardinian child described by Furbetta et al. (1979) as being probably homozygous for β-thalassaemia as well as being a compound heterozygote for α-thal-1 and α-thal-2. This conclusion was confirmed by restriction endonuclease analysis which revealed that three α genes had been deleted. The patient is transfusion-dependent, and Melis, Galanello and Cao pointed out that the failure of the loss of three α genes to ameliorate the effect of homozygosity for β-thalassaemia probably means that the output of β chains is so low that it cannot be compensated for by any decrease in chain imbalance.

In 1983 Furbetta and co-workers reported on a review of the clinical findings in a large series of Sardinian children suffering from homozygous transfusion-dependent β⁰-thalassaemia with particular reference to their α-globin genotype. Six of them had two genes deleted, as determined by restriction enzyme assay: in them the onset of their disease and transfusion dependency occurred significantly later than in the 50 children who possessed the normal complement of four α genes. The clinical history of 35 children in whom only one gene had been deleted did not differ from those with four genes except for a later presentation of their disease. An interesting additional finding was that the Hb-A₂ level was significantly higher (as a percentage or as pg Hb A₂ per cell) in the patients with two α genes deleted than in those with one gene deleted or in those with the normal complement of four genes. Furbetta et al. pointed out that variation in α-globin genotype could explain the previously reported observation that the Hb-A₂ percentage varies widely in homozygous β-thalassaemia.

Effect of triplicated α-globin loci on β-thalassaemia

This combination has been reported in Greek and Sardinian families. The presence of one additional α gene (ααα/αα genotype) appears to have no effect on the clinical or haematological manifestations of β-thalassaemic heterozygotes (Kanavakis et al., 1983; Galanello et al., 1983c). Kanavakis and co-workers recorded, however, that four out of five homozygous β-thalassaemia ααα/αα patients suffered from a mild thalassaemia-intermedia syndrome and suggested that the ααα gene arrangement might be acting as an α-thalassaemia allele. Mild thalassaemia intermedia, too, was the clinical consequence of the concurrence of homo-zygosity for the triplicated α-globin gene (ααα/ααα) and heterozygosity for β-thalassaemia in a Sardinian male aged 28. In this case the α:β globin ratio was markedly unbalanced at 4.56.

Further and more recent reports of αβ-thalas-saemia are cited in Chapter 19 where the results of recent molecular-genetic analyses of the various thalassaemia genotypes are discussed.

α-THALASSAEMIA IN ASSOCIATION WITH OTHER ABNORMAL HAEMOGLOBINS

β-chain variants

The concurrence of a gene or genes for α-thalassaemia and for an abnormal haemoglobin in the same individual is not a rare event. Particularly is this true of α-thalassaemia and Hb S where the presence of both abnor-malities has important consequences. As described in Chapter 13 (p. 137), α-thalassaemia tends to lessen the severity of homozygosity for Hb S and to reduce the proportion of Hb S to Hb A in heterozygotes where it leads to microcytosis and hypochromia [see also Embury (1985) and El-Hazmi (1986) who studied 171 Hb-S heterozygotes in Arabia]. The effect of the interaction between the genes for α-thalassaemia and Hb E has also already been discussed (p. 310). As with Hb S, there is evidence that the percentage of Hb E in the eryth-rocytes of Hb-AE heterozygotes is reduced by the pres-ence of one or more α-thalassaemia genes.

In the case of Hb S and Hb E the reduction in the percentage of the abnormal haemoglobin present in heterozygotes seems to be due to the affinity of the β^S and β^E chains for α chains being less than that of normal β^A chains. This is, however, not necessarily true of all β-chain variants. Natta, Casey and Lehmann (1978), for instance, reported that Hb Camden ($\alpha_2\beta_2^{131 \text{ Gln} \to \text{Glu}}$), which was present in a concentration of 45% in a black American female who was also heterozygous for α-thalassaemia, had the same affinity for α chains as did normal β^A chains.

α-chain variants

Of particular interest are structural variants which appear to be linked to α-thalassaemia gene de-letion and whose presence in heterozygotes is as-sociated with a thalassaemia-like syndrome of varying severity. In some instances the mRNA derived from the abnormal gene is prematurely degraded or the newly synthesized variant chains are unstable. The net result, however caused, is a deficiency of α chains. Variant haemoglobins which have been shown to be (or have been

thought to be) linked to α-gene deletion include the following (in alphabetical order):

Hb Evanston ($\alpha_2^{14 \text{ Try} \to \text{Arg}} \beta_2$) (Honig et al., 1984). This variant was described by Honig et al. in two unrelated black families. The proposita were of geno-type $-\alpha^A/-\alpha^{EV}$ and newly synthesized α^{EV} chains were demonstrated to be unstable. The variant gene appeared to be linked to an α-globin gene deletion.

Hb Hasharon ($\alpha_2^{47 \text{ Asp} \to \text{His}} \beta_2$) (del Senno et al., 1980). This variant is not uncommon in the Ferrara region of Northern Italy. Heterozygotes have approxi-mately 32% Hb Hasharon. The abnormal haemoglobin is probably linked to an α-globin gene deletion.

Hb G Philadelphia ($\alpha_2^{68 \text{ Asn} \to \text{Lys}} \beta_2$) (French and Lehmann, 1971; Surrey et al., 1980b; Martinez, Ferriera and Colombo, 1985). Martinez, Ferriera and Colombo demonstrated linkage of the $\alpha^{G \text{ Philadelphia}}$ locus to α-thalassaemia in three Cuban families of African ancestry. Each family carried the same α-thalassaemic gene deletion.

Hb J Capetown ($\alpha_2^{92 \text{ Arg} \to \text{Gln}} \beta_2$) (Botha et al., 1978). Hb J Capetown was present as 39–43% of the total haemoglobin in the heterozygotes described by Botha et al.; Hb A was absent in a homozygote.

Hb J Tongariki ($\alpha_2^{115 \text{ Ala} \to \text{Asp}} \beta_2$) (Old et al., 1978; Bowden et al., 1982). Bowden et al. studied four families and found that all those who were heterozygous for Hb Tongariki had the α-globin genotype $-\alpha^J/\alpha\alpha$ and a phenotype consistent with that of α^+-thalassaemia trait; c 40% of their haemoglobin was Hb Tongariki.

Hb Nigeria ($\alpha_2^{81 \text{ Ser} \to \text{Cys}} \beta_2$) (Honig et al., 1980). Honig et al. described a Nigerian female who had a thalassaemia-minor blood picture; c 45% of her haemo-globin was Hb Nigeria and c 27% Hb S. Her α-globin genotype was thought to be $-\alpha/-\alpha^{\text{Nigeria}}$.

Hb Q = Mahidol ($\alpha_2^{74 \text{ Asp} \to \text{His}} \beta_2$) (Vella et al., 1958; Dormandy, Lock and Lehmann, 1961; Lie-Injo and van der Hart, 1963; Lie-Injo, Pillay and Thuraisingham, 1966; Lehmann and Lang, 1975; Lie-Injo et al., 1979). The Chinese patient described by Lehmann and Lang (1975) was thought to be a compound heterozygote for α-thalassaemia and β-thalassaemia as well as for Hb Q. Lie-Injo *et al.* (1979) studied a Chinese patient who presented with Hb-H disease: experimental data indicated that the patient's α-globin genotype was $--/-\alpha^Q$ and that the Hb-Q structural gene was located adjacent to a deleted α gene.

Pagnier and co-workers (1982) described a Cambo-dian family in which the proposita was thought to be a compound heterozygote for deletion α-thalassaemia and non-deletional α-thalassaemia as well as being heterozygous for Hb E and Hb Q. She was jaundiced at birth and 3% Hb Bart's was present. An interesting feature was that the α^Q/α^A globin-chain synthesis ratio was consistently 60:40.

α-THALASSAEMIA IN ASSOCIATION WITH OTHER DISORDERS

Not unexpectedly, α-thalassaemia has been reported to occur in association with a variety of other disorders.

G6PD deficiency. Helleman, Punt and Verloop (1964) described a family of mixed European and South-East Asian ancestry in which males had an α-thalassaemia trait and were also hemizygous for G6PD deficiency. There was apparently no interaction between the two abnormalities.

Sulis and co-workers (1968) gave details of five Sardinian families, some members of which were affected with both G6PD deficiency and α-thalassaemia; one patient had Hb-H disease.

Glutathione peroxidase (GPx) deficiency. Vives Corrons, Aguilar and Mateo (1983) in a brief report stated that they had found Hb-H disease and severe GPx deficiency in a mentally retarded child.

Hereditary elliptocytosis (HE). Ahern and Milner (1968) gave a brief description of two brothers of Chinese, black and Caucasian lineage. Both had Hb-H disease and HE. Other members of the family had uncomplicated α-thalassaemia trait or Hb-H disease and still others HE without any evidence of α-thalassaemia. In this family at least the HE gene did not seem to affect the severity of Hb-H disease.

Auto-immune haemolytic anaemia. Kruatrachue and co-workers (1980) reported that they had observed 10 patients with various types of thalassaemia who had developed a warm-antibody-type auto-immune haemolytic anaemia (AIHA). Nine of the patients were females and one was a male, and they were aged between 15 and 50 years. Five had Hb-H disease, four β-thal/Hb E and one Hb-H/Hb E. The direct Coombs test was positive in all, in eight with anti-IgG, in four with anti-IgM and in one with anti-IgA; seven were positive with anti-C sera. Four patients had been transfused 4–17 months before the development of the AIHA; six had never been transfused. All the patients responded to prednisone therapy, with their haemoglobin returning to the pre-AIHA levels. These occurrences are intriguing but their significance is obscure.

REFERENCES

ACQUAYE, C. T. A., OLDHAM, J. H. & KONOTEY-AHULU, F. I. D. (1977). Blood-donor homozygous for hereditary persistence of fetal haemoglobin. *Lancet*, i, 796–797 (Letter).

ADAMS, J. G. III & STEINBERG, M. H. (1977). Alpha-thalassaemia. *Amer. J. Hemat.*, **2**, 317–325.

ADIROJMANON, P. & WASI, P. (1980). Levels of haemoglobin H and preparation of red cells with inclusion bodies in the two types of haemoglobin H disease. *Brit. J. Haemat.*, **46**, 507–509.

AGER, J. A. M., HUNT, J. A., KOHLER, H. G. & LEHMANN, H. (1960). Haemoglobin "Bart's". *Proc. 7th Congr. europ. Soc. Haemat., London, 1959*; Part II, pp. 1112–1116. Karger, Basel.

AGER, J. A. M. & LEHMANN, H. (1958). Observations on some "fast" haemoglobins: K, J, N, and "Bart's". *Brit. med. J.*, i, 929–931.

AHERN, E. J., AHERN, V. N., AARONS, G. H., JONES, R. T. BRIMHALL, B. (1972). Hemoglobin Lepore_Washington in two Jamaican families: interaction with beta chain variants. *Blood*, **40**, 246–256.

AHERN, E., HERBERT, R., McIVER, C., AHERN, V., WARDLE, J. & SEAKINS, M. (1975). Beta-thalassaemia of clinical significance in adult Jamaican negroes. *Brit. J. Haemat.*, **30**, 197–213.

AHERN, E. J. & MILNER, P. F. (1968). Hereditary elliptocytosis in association with HB H disease in two brothers. *Proc. 12th int. Congr. Hemat., New York*, p. 57 (Abstract L-l).

AKSOY, M. (1959). Abnormal haemoglobins in Turkey. *Abnormal Haemoglobins. A Symposium*, pp. 216–235. Blackwell Scientific Publications, Oxford.

AKSOY, M. (1970). Thalassaemia intermedia: a genetic study in 11 patients. *J. med. Genet.* **7**, 47–51.

AKSOY, M., BERMEK, E., ALMIS, G. & KUTLER, A. (1982). β-thalassaemia intermedia homozygous for normal hemoglobin A₂ β-thalassaemia: study of four families. *Acta haemat. (Basel)*, **67**, 57–61.

AKSOY, M., CAMLI, N., DIRVANA, S., ERDEM, S., DINÇOL, K. & AKGÜN, T. (1970). "Porcelain gallbladder" in a case of thalassemia intermedia. *Radiology*, **95**, 265–266.

AKSOY, M., DINÇOL, G. & ERDEM, S. (1978). Different types of beta-thalassaemia intermedia. A genetic study of 20 patients. *Acta haemat. (Basel)*, **59**, 178–189.

AKSOY, M. & ERDEM, S. (1965). The thalassaemia syndromes. V. Cooley' anaemia with low level of fetal haemoglobin. A genetic study in four families. *Acta haemat. (Basel)*, **34**, 291–300.

AKSOY, M. & ERDEM, S. (1968). Haemoglobin H disease. Study of an Eti-Turk family. *Acta genet. (Basel)*, **18**, 12–22.

AKSOY, M. & ERDEM, S. (1969). Some problems of hemoglobin patterns in different thalassemic syndromes showing the heterogeneity of beta-thalassaemia genes. *Ann. N.Y. Acad, Sci.*, **165**, 13–24.

AKSOY, M., IKIN, E. W., MOURANT, A. E. & LEHMANN, H. (1958). Blood groups, haemoglobins, and thalassaemia in Turks in Southern Turkey and Eti-Turks. *Brit. med. J.*, **ii**, 937–939.

AKSOY, M., KUTLAR, A., KUTLAR, F., DINÇOL, G., ERDEM, S., WILSON, J. B. & HUISMAN, T. H. J. (1984). Hb Beograd-β⁰thalassaemia in a Turkish family from Yugoslavia. *Hemoglobin*, **8**, 417–421.

ALESSIO, L., SULIS, E., PABIS, A. & MANNUCCI, M. P. (1968). Unusual pattern of inheritance of haemoglobin-H disease. Family study and report of a case. *Scand. J. Haemat.*, **5**, 454–457.

ALI, S. A. (1969). Haemoglobin H disease in Arabs in Kuwait. *J. clin. Path.*, **22**, 226–228.

ALLAMANIS, J. (1955) Paper electrophoresis of serum proteins in Cooley's anaemia and sickle cell anaemia. *Acta paediat. (Uppsala)*, **44**, 122–127.

ALTAY, C., HUISMAN, T. H. J. & SCHROEDER, W. A. (1976–77). Another form of hereditary persistence of fetal hemoglobin (the Atlanta type)? Hemoglobin, **1**, 125–133.

ALTAY, C., SAY, B., YETGIN, S. & HUISMAN, T. H. J. (1977). α-thalassaemia and β-thalassaemia in a Turkish family. *Amer. J. Hemat.*, **2**, 1–15.

ALVAREZ-SALA, J. L., VILLEGAS, A., ALARCÓN, G. & ESPINÓS, D. (1983a). Intraerythrocytic adaptation to anaemia in thalassaemia. *Nouv. Rev. franç. Hémat.*, **25**, 267–268 (Letter).

ALVAREZ-SALA, J. L., VILLEGAS, A., CALERO, F. & ESPINÓS, D. (1983b). Red-cell 2,3-diphosphoglycerate in thalassaemia. *Haematologica*, **68**, 312–319.

AMIN, A. B., PANDYA, N. L., DIWIN, P. P., DARBOE, P. D., KATTAMIS, C., METAXATOU-MAVROMATI, A., WHITE, J. M., WOOD, W. G., CLEGG, J. B. & WEATHERALL, D. J. (1979). A comparison of the homozygous states for ᴳγ and ᴳγᴬγδβ thalassaemia. *Brit. J. Haemat.*, **43**, 537–548.

ANDERSON, B. B., PERRY, G. M., MODELL, C. B., CHILD, J. A. & MOLLIN, D. L. (1979). Abnormal red-cell metabolism of pyridoxine associated with β-thalassaemia. *Brit. J. Haemat.*, **41**, 497–507.

ANGELINI, V. (1937). Primi risultati di ricerche ematologiche nei familiari di ammalati di anemia di Cooley. *Minerva med. (Torino)*, **28**, 331–332.

AROUS, N., GALACTEROS, F., FESSAS, PH., LOUKOPOULOS, D., BLOUQUIT, Y., KOMIS, G., SELLAYE, M., BOUSSIOU, M. & ROSA, J. (1982). Hemoglobin Knossos, β27 ALA→SER (B9): a new hemoglobinopathy presenting as a silent β-thalassaemia. *Blood*, **60** (Suppl. 1), 51a (Abstract 131).

ASHIOTIS, TH., ZACHARIADIS, Z., SOFRONIADOU, K., STAMATOYANNOPOULOS, G. & LOUKOPOULOS, D. (1973). Thalassaemia in Cyprus. *Brit. med. J.*, **ii**, 38–41.

ASTALDI, G., BURGIO, R. & PRIOLISI, A. (1969). Evaluation of plasma iron turnover in Cooley's anemia. *Ann. N.Y. Acad. Sci.*, **165**, 111–125.

ASTALDI, G., TOLENTINO, P. & SACCHETTI, C. (1951). La Talassemia. *Biblioteca "haematologica"*, Pavia.

ATKINSON, D. W. (1939). Erythroblastic anaemia. Report of two cases in adult siblings. With a review of the theories as to its transmission. *Amer. J. med. Sci.*, **198**, 376–383.

ATWATER, J., SCHWARTZ, I. R., ERSLEV, A. J., MONTGOMERY, T. L. & TOCANTINS, L. M. (1960). Sickling of erythrocytes in a patient with thalassaemia-hemoglobin I disease. *New Engl. J. Med.*, **263**, 1215–1223.

BAGLIONI, C. (1962). The fusion of two peptide chains in hemoglobin Lepore and its interpretation as a genetic deletion. *Proc. natn. Acad. Sci. U.S.A.*, **48**, 1880–1886.

BAGLIONI, C. (1963). A child homozygous for persistence of foetal haemoglobin. *Nature (Lond.)*, **198**, 1177–1179.

BAGLIONI, C. (1965). Abnormal human hemoglobins. X. A study of hemoglobin Lepore_Boston. *Biochim. biophys. Acta*, **97**, 37–46.

BAGLIONI, C. & VENTRUTO, V. (1968). Human abnormal hemoglobins. 11. A chemical study of hemoglobin Lepore from a homozygote individual. *Europ. J. Biochem.*, **5**, 29–32.

BAIGET, M., GIMFERRER, E., FERNANDEZ, I., ROMERO, C., MIRA, Y & PÉREZ, M. L.(1983). Spanish delta-beta-thalassaemia: hematalogical studies and composition of the gamma-chains in ten homozygous patients. *Acta haemat. (Basel)*, **70**, 341–344.

BAILEY, I. S. & PRANKERD, T. A. J. (1958). Studies

in thalassaemia. *Brit. J. Haemat.*, **4**, 150–155.

BAKER, D. H. (1964). Roentgen manifestations of Cooley's anemia. *Ann. N.Y. Acad. Sci.*, **119**, 641–661.

BAKLOUTI, F., DORLÉAC, E., MORLE, L., LASELVE, P., PEYRAMOND, D., AUBRY, M., GODET, J. & DELAUNAY, J. (1986). Homozygous hemoglobin Knossos ($\alpha_2\beta_2$ 27 (B 9) Ala→Ser): a new variety of β^+-thalassemia intermedia associated with δ^0-thalassemia. *Blood*, **67**, 957–961.

BANK, A. (1978). The thalassemia syndromes. *Blood*, **51**, 369–384 (Review).

BANK, A. & MARKS, P. A. (1966). Excess α chain synthesis relative to β chain synthesis in thalassaemia major and minor. *Nature (Lond.)*, **212**, 1198–1200.

BANK, A. & MARKS, P. A. (1971). Hemoglobin synthesis in thalassemia. *Ser. haemat.*, **4**, 97–115.

BANKS, L. O. & SCOTT, R. B. (1953). Thalassemia in negroes; report of case of Cooley's anemia in a Negro child. *Pediatrics*, **11**, 622–627.

BANNERMAN, R. M. (1961). *Thalassemia. A Survey of some Aspects.* 138 pp. Grune and Stratton, New York.

BANNERMAN, R. M. (1964). Abnormalities of heme and pyrrole metabolism in thalassemia. *Ann. N.Y. Acad. Sci.*, **119**, 503–512.

BANNERMAN, R. M. (1972). The thalassemias: recent advances in study and management. In: *Hematologic Reviews* (ed. by J. L. Ambrus), pp. 297–385. Marcel Dekker, New York.

BANNERMAN, R. M., GRINSTEIN, M. & MOORE, C. V. (1959). Haemoglobin synthesis in thalassaemia; in-vitro studies. *Brit. J. Haemat.*, **5**, 102–120.

BANNERMAN, R. M., KENSCH, G., KREIMER-BIRNBAUM, M., VANCE, U.K. & VAUGHAN, S. (1967). Thalassemia intermedia, with iron overload, cardiac failure, diabetes mellitus, hypopituitarism and porphyrinuria. *Amer. J. Med.*, **42**, 476–486.

BANTON, A H. (1951). A genetic study of Mediterranean anaemia in Cyprus. *Amer. J. hum. Genet.*, **3**, 47–64.

BANWELL, G. S. & STRICKLAND, M. (1964). Haemoglobinopathy associated with recurrent stillbirth. *J. Obstet. Gynaec. Brit. Commonwlth*, **71**, 788–790.

BARKHAN, P. & ADINOLFI, M. (1962). Observations on the high foetal haemoglobin gene and its interaction with the thalassaemia gene. *J. clin. Path.*, **15**, 350–356.

BARNABAS, J. & MULLER, C. J. (1962). Haemoglobin-Lepore_Hollandia. *Nature (Lond.)*, **194**, 931–932.

BARROW, D. H. E. & KOHLER, H. G. (1960). Haemoglobin 'Bart's' — a rare abnormality in the newborn. *Arch. Dis. Childh.*, **35**, 360–363.

BATE, C. M. & HUMPHRIES, G. (1977). Alpha-beta thalassaemia. *Lancet*, **i**, 1031–1034.

BATY, J. M., BLACKFAN, K. D. & DIAMOND, L. K. (1932). Blood studies in infants and in children. I.

Erythroblastic anemia; a clinical and pathologic study. *Amer. J. Dis. Child.*, **43**, 667–704.

BAUMINGER, E. R., COHEN, S. G., OFER, S. & RACHMILEWITZ, E. A. (1979). Quantitative studies of ferritin-like iron in erythrocytes of thalassemia, sickle-cell anemia, and hemoglobin Hammersmith with Mössbauer spectroscopy. *Proc. natn. Acad. Sci., U.S.A.*, **76**, 939–943.

BEAVEN, G. H., GRATZER, W. B., STEVENS, B. L., SHOOLER, E. M., ELLIS, M. J., WHITE, J. C. & GILLESPIE, J. E. O'N. (1964). An abnormal haemoglobin (Lepore/Cyprus) resembling haemoglobin-Lepore and its interaction with thalassaemia. *Brit. J. Haemat.*, **10**, 159–169.

BEAVEN, G. H. & WHITE, J. C. (1962). Variability of thalassaemic red cell characters. *Nature (Lond.)*, **193**, 448–449.

BELFIORE, F., MELDOLESI, J. & CALCARA, G. (1965). Erythrocyte enzymes in thalassemia and thalassodrepanocytosis. *Acta haemat. (Basel)*, **34**, 329–337.

BELLEVUE, R., DOSIK, H. & RIEDER, R. F. (1979). Alpha thalassaemia in American Blacks: a study of a family with five cases of haemoglobin H disease. *Brit. J. Haemat.*, **41**, 193–202.

BEN-BASSET, I., HERTZ, M., SELZER, G., RAMOT, B. (1977). Extramedullary hematopoiesis with multiple tumor-simulating mediastinal masses in patient with β-thalassemia intermedia. *Israel J. med. Sci.*, **13**, 1206–1210.

BENTORELLO, C. F., PESCETTO, T. & BO, G. (1977). Manifestazioni emorragiche secondarie a coagulopatia da consumo, in paziente affetto da morbo di Cooley. *Minerva pediat. (Torino)*, **29**, 1423–1426.

BENZ, E. J. JNR, & FORGET, B. G. (1974). The biosynthesis of hemoglobin. *Seminars Hemat.*, **11**, 463–523.

BENZ, E. J. JNR & FORGET B. G. (1975). The molecular genetics of the thalassemia syndrome. In: *Progress in Hematology*, Vol. IX (ed. by E. B. Brown), pp. 107–155. Grune and Stratton, New York.

BENZ, E. J., SWERDLOW, P. S. & FORGET, B. G. (1973). Globin messenger RNA in hemoglobin H disease. *Blood*, **42**, 825–833.

BERNINI, L., LATTE, B., SINISCALCO, M., PIOMELLI, S., SPADA, U., ADINOLFI, M. & MOLLISON, P. L. (1964). Survival of ^{51}Cr-labelled red cells in subjects with thalassaemia-trait or G6PD deficiency or both abnormalities. *Brit. J. Haemat.*, **10**, 171–180.

BERRY, C. L. & MARSHALL, W. C. (1967). Iron distribution in the liver of patients with thalassaemia major. *Lancet*, **i**, 1031–1033.

BETKE, K. & KLEIHAUER, E. (1958). Fetaler und bleibender Blutfarbstoff in Erythrocyten und Erythroblasten von menschlichen Feten und Neugeborenen. *Blut*, **4**, 241–249.

BEUTLER, E., MATSUMOTO, F., POWARS, D. &

WARNER, J. (1977). Increased glutathione peroxidase activity in α-thalassemia. *Blood*, **50**, 647–655.

BEUTLER, E., TURNER, E. & KUHL, W. (1981). The effect of α-thalassemia on the expression of the β-thalassemia/HPFH heterozygote in a black family. *Blood*, **57**, 1132–1134.

BIANCO, I., MONTALENTI, G., SILVESTRONI, E. & SINISCALCO, M. (1952). Further data on genetics of microcythaemia or thalassaemia minor and Cooley's disease or thalassaemia. *Ann. Eugen. (Lond.)*, **16**, 299–315.

BINGLE, J. P., HUEHNS, E. R. & PRANKERD, T. A. J. (1958). Haemoglobin-H disease. *Brit. med. J.*, **ii**, 1389–1390.

BIRD, G. W. G., HASAN, M. I., MALHOTRA, O. P. & LEHMANN, H. (1964). Interaction of β-thalassaemia and hereditary persistence of foetal haemoglobin. *J. med. Genet.*, **1**, 24–26.

BORGNA-PIGNATTI, C., CAMMARERI, V., DE STEFANO, P. & MAGRINI, U. (1984). The sicca syndrome in thalassaemia major. *Brit. med. J.*, **i**, 668–669.

BOROCHOVITZ, D., LEVIN, S. E., KRAWITZ, S., STEVENS, K. & METZ, J. (1970). Haemoglobin-H disease in association with multiple congenital abnormalities. *Clin. Pediat.*, **9**, 432–435.

BOTHA, M. C., STATHOPOULOU, R., LEHMANN, H., REES, J. S. & PLOWMAN, D. (1978). A Hb J Capetown homozygote — association of Hb J Capetown and alpha-thalassaemia. *FEBS Lett.*, **96**, 331–334.

BOWCOCK, A. M., VAN TONDER, S. & JENKINS, T. (1984). The haemoglobin H disease mental retardation syndrome: molecular studies on the South African case. *Brit. J. Haemat.*, **56**, 69–78.

BOWDEN, D. K., HILL, A. V. S., HIGGS, D. R., WEATHERALL, D. J. & CLEGG, J. B. (1985). Relative roles of genetic factors, dietary deficiency, and infection in anaemia in Vanuatu, South-West Pacific. *Lancet*, **ii**, 1025–1028.

BOWDEN, D. K., PRESSLEY, L., HIGGS, D. R., CLEGG, J. B. & WEATHERALL, D. J. (1982). α-globin gene deletions associated with Hb J Tongariki. *Brit. J. Haemat.*, **51**, 243–249.

BOWDLER, A. J. & HUEHNS, E. R. (1963). Thalassaemia minor complicated by excessive iron storage. *Brit. J. Haemat.*, **9**, 13–24.

BOYER, S. H., BELDING, T. K., MARGOLET, L. & NOYES, A. N. (1975). Fetal hemoglobin restriction to a few erythrocytes (F cells) in normal human adults. *Science*, **188**, 361–363.

BOYER, S. H., MARGOLET, L., BOYER, M. L., HUISMAN, T. H. J., SCHROEDER, W. A., WOOD, W. G., WEATHERALL, D. J., CLEGG, J. B. & CARTNER, R. (1977). Inheritance of F cell frequency in heterocellular hereditary persistence of fetal hemoglobin: an example of allelic exclusion. *Amer. J. hum. Genet.*, **29**, 256–269.

BRADFORD, W. L. & DYE, J. (1936). Observations on the morphology of the erythrocytes in Mediterranean disease — thalassemia (erythroblastic anemia of Cooley). *J. Pediat.*, **9**, 312–317.

BRADLEY, T. B. JNR, BRAWNER, J. N. III & CONLEY, C. L. (1961). Further observations on an inherited anomaly characterized by persistence of fetal hemoglobin. *Bull. Johns Hopk. Hosp.*, **108**, 242–257.

BRADLEY, T. B. JNR, & CONLEY, C. L. (1960). Studies of an inherited disorder manifested by persistence of fetal hemoglobin. *Ass. Amer. Phycns*, **73**, 72–79.

BRANCATI, C. (1965). Primo caso di omozigosi per la varietà di microcitemia con quota normale di emoglobina A$_2$ e quota elevata di emoglobina F. *Progr. med. (Napoli)*, **21**, 388–390.

BRANCATI, C. & BAGLIONI, C. (1966). Homozygous βΔthalassaemia (βΔmicrocythaemia). *Nature (Lond.)*, **212**, 262–264.

BRAVERMAN, A. S. & BANK, A. (1969). Changing rates of globin chain synthesis during erythroid cell maturation in thalassemia. *J. mol. Biol.*, **42**, 57–64.

BRAVERMAN, A. S., MCCURDY, P. R., MANOS, O & SHERMAN, A. (1973). Homozygous beta thalassemia in American Blacks: the problem of mild thalassemia. *J. Lab. clin. Med.*, **81**, 857–866.

BRITTENHAM, G., LOZOFF, B., HARRIS, J. W., BAPAT, V., GRAVELY, M. & HUISMAN, T. H. J. (1980). Thalassemia in Southern India. Interaction of genes for β$^+$, β^0 and δ^0/β^0-thalassemia. *Acta haemat. (Basel)*, **63**, 44–48.

BRUMPT, L.-C. (1955). A propos de l'anémie de Cooley: thalassémie ou sinémie. *Bull. Acad. Méd. (Paris)*, **139**, 333–336.

BUCHANAN, K. D., KINLOCH, J. D., HUTCHISON, H. E., PINKERTON, T. H. & CASSIDY, P. (1963). Thalassaemia in Scots. *J. clin. Path.*, **16**, 596–600.

BUNYARATVEJ, A., SAHAPHONG, S., BHAMAROPRAVATI, N. & WASI, P. (1983). Different patterns of intraerythrocytic inclusion body distribution in the two types of haemoglobin H disease. An ultrastructural study. *Acta haemat. (Basel)*, **69**, 314–318.

BUTIKOFER, E., HOIGNE, R., MARTI, H. R. & BETKE, K. (1960). Hämoglobin-H-Thalassämie. Mitteilung eines Falles mit Familienuntersuchung. *Schweiz. med. Wschr.*, **90**, 1214–1217.

CABRERA, A. & DE PABLOS, J. M. (1984). Beta-thalassaemia minor in gypsies from the South of Spain. *Brit. J. Haemat.*, **58**, 377 (Letter).

CACACE, E., FRIGERIO, R., OLLA, N., SOLE, G., MELA, Q., PERPIGNANO, G. & CARCASSI, U. (1985). Genetic heterogeneity of β^0-thalassemia intermedia in Southern Sardinia. *Haematologica*, **70**, 95–100.

CACACE, E., MANCONI, E., BINAGHI, F., PERPIGNANO, G., PITZUS, F. & CARCASSI, U. (1987). Leg ulcers in β-thalassaemia intermedia. In: *Thalassemia Today: the Mediterranen Experience* (ed. by G. Sirchia and A. Zanella), pp. 559–574. Centro Trasfusionale

Ospedale Maggiore Policlinico di Milano Editore.

CAFFEY, J. (1937). The skeletal changes in chronic hemolytic anemias (erythroblastic anemia, sickle cell anemia and chronic hemolytic icterus). *Amer. J. Roentgenol.*, **37**, 293–324.

CAFFEY, J. (1951). Cooley's erythroblastic anemia. Some skeletal findings in adolescents and young adults. *Amer. J. Roentgenol.*, **65**, 547–560.

CAFFEY, J. (1957). Cooley's anemia: a review of roentgenographic findings in the skeleton. Hickey Lecture 1957. *Amer. J. Roentgenol.* **78**, 381–391.

CALLENDER, S. T., MALLET, B. J. & LEHMANN, H. (1961). Thalassaemia in Britain. *Brit. J. Haemat.*, **7**, 1–8.

CAMINOPETROS, J. (1938a). Recherches sur l'anémie érythroblastique infantile, des peuples de la Méditerranée orientale. Premier memoire: étude nosologique. *Ann. Méd.*, **43**, 27–61.

CAMINOPETROS, J. (1938b). Recherches sur l'anémie érythroblastique infantile des peuples de la Méditerranee orientale. Étude anthropologique, étiologique et pathogénique. La transmission héréditaire de la maladie (2e memoire). *Ann. Méd.*, **43**, 104–125.

CAMPANACCI, L., BROCCIA, G., & FIUMANO, R. M. (1962). Lá emoglobinopatia H-talassemia. Studio clinico, ematologico ed eritrocinetico di un caso con anemia a corpi inclusi e tromboflebite migrante. *G. Clin. med.*, **43**, 977–1027.

CANALE, V. C., STEINHERZ, P., NEW, M. & ERLANDSON, M. (1974). Endocrine function in thalassemia major. *Ann. N.Y. Acad. Sci.*, **232**, 333–345.

CAO, A., GALANELLO, R., FURBETTA, M., MURONI, P. P., GARBATO, L., ROSATELLI, C., SCALAS, M. T., ADDIS, M., RUGGERI, R., MACCIONI, L. & MELIS, M. A. (1978). Thalassaemia types and their incidence in Sardinia. *J. med. Genet.*, **15**, 443–447.

CAOCCI, L., ALBERTI, M., BURRAI, P. & CORDA, R. (1978). Screening coagulation tests and clotting factors in homozygous β-thalassaemia. *Acta haemat. (Basel)*, **60**, 358–364.

CAPELLINI, M. D., FIORELLI, G. & BERNINI, L. F. (1981). Interaction between homozygous β⁰ thalassaemia and the Swiss type of hereditary persistence of fetal haemoglobin. *Brit. J. Haemat.*, **48**, 561–572.

CAPP. G. L., RIGAS, D. A. & JONES, R. T. (1967). Hemoglobin Portland 1: a new human hemoglobin unique in structure. *Science*, **157**, 65–66.

CARCASSI, U. E. F. (1974). The interaction between β-thalassaemia, G-6-PD deficiency and favism. *Ann. N.Y. Acad. Sci.*, **232**, 297–305.

CARCASSI, U., CEPPELLINI, R. & PITZUS, F. (1957). Frequenza della talassemia in quattro popolazioni sarde e suoi rapporti con la distribuzione dei gruppi sanguigni e della malaria. *Boll. Ist. sieroter. milan.*, **36**, 206–218.

CARCASSI, U., CEPPELINI, R. & SINISCALCO, M.

(1957). Il tracciato elettroforetico dell'emoglobina per una migliore discriminazione delle talassemie. *Haematologica*, **42**, 1635–1653.

CARTWRIGHT, G. E., HUGULEY, C. M. JNR & ASHENBRUCKER, H. (1948). Studies on free erythrocyte protoporphyrin, plasma iron and plasma copper in normal and anemic subjects. *Blood*, **3**, 501–525.

CAUCHI, M. N. (1970). The incidence of glucose-6-phosphate dehydrogenase deficiency and thalassaemia in Malta. *Brit J. Haemat.*, **18**, 101–106.

CAVILL, I., RICKETTS, C., JACOBS, A. & LETSKY, E. (1978). Erythropoiesis and the effect of transfusion in homozygous β-thalassemia. *New Engl. J. Med.*, **298**, 776–778.

CAZZOLA, M., ALESSANDRINO, P., BAROSI, G., MORANDI, S. & STEFANELLI, M. (1979). Quantitative evaluation of the mechanisms of the anaemia in heterozygous β-thalassaemia. *Scand. J. Haemat.*, **23**, 107–114.

CELADA A. (1982). Iron overload in a non-transfused patient with thalassaemia intermedia. *Scand. J. Haemat.*, **28**, 169–174.

CHARACHE, S., CLEGG, J. B. & WEATHERALL, D. J. (1976). The Negro variety of hereditary persistence of fetal haemoglobin is a mild form of thalassaemia. *Brit. J. Haemat.*, **34**, 527–534.

CHARACHE, S. & CONLEY, C. L. (1969). Hereditary persistence of fetal hemoglobin. *Ann. N.Y. Acad. Sci.*, **165**, 37–41.

CHARACHE, S., CONLEY, C. L., DOEBLIN, T. D. & BARTALOS, M. (1974). Thalassemia in black Americans. *Ann. N.Y. Acad. Sci.*, **232**, 125–134.

CHATTERJEA, J. B. (1959). Haemoglobinopathy in India. In: *Abnormal Haemoglobins. A symposium*, pp. 322–339. Blackwell Scientific Publications, Oxford.

CHATTERJEA, J. B. (1966). Hemoglobinopathies, glucose-6-phosphate dehydrogenase deficiency and allied problems in the Indian sub-continent. *Bull. Wld Hlth Org.*, **35**, 837–856.

CHATTERJEA, J. B., GHOSH, S. K., RAY, R. N. & DAS GUPTA, C. R. (1956). Observations on mechanical fragility of red cells. *Bull. Calcutta Sch. trop. Med.*, **4**, 10–11.

CHERNOFF, A. I. (1953). Immunologic studies of hemoglobins. II. Quantitative precipitin test using anti-fetal hemoglobin sera. *Blood*, **8**, 413–421.

CHERNOFF, A. I. (1959). The distribution of the thalassemia gene: a historical review. *Blood*, **14**, 899–912.

CHINI, V. & VALERI, C. M. (1949). Mediterranean hemopathic syndromes. *Blood*, **4**, 989–1013.

CHOI, E. S. K. & NECHELES, T. F. (1983). Thalassemia among Chinese-Bostonians. Usefulness of the hemoglobin H preparation. *Arch. intern. Med.*, **143**, 1713–1715.

CHOREMIS, C., ECONOMOU-MAVROU, C. &

GREGORIOU, M. (1961). Blood plasma levels and urinary excretion of ascorbic acid before and after a test dose in children with severe thalassemia. *J. Pediat.*, **59**, 361–369.

CHOREMIS, C., ECONOMOU-MAVROU, C. & TSENGHI, C. (1961). Sodium, potassium, water and haemoglobin in the packed red cells of severe thalassaemia. *J. clin. Path.*, **14**, 637–643.

CHOREMIS, C., FESSAS, PH., KATTAMIS, C., STAMATOYANNOPOULOS, G., ZANNOS-MARIOLEA, L., KARAKLIS, A. & BELIOS, G. (1963). Three inherited red-cell abnormalities in a district of Greece. Thalassaemia, sickling, and glucose-6-phosphate-dehydrogenase deficiency. *Lancet*, i, 907–909.

CHOREMIS, C., KIOSSOGLOU, K., MAOUNIS, F. & BASTI, B. (1959). Amino-acid tolerance curves and amino-aciduria in Cooley's and sickle-cell anaemias. *J. clin. Path.*, **12**, 245–253.

CHOREMIS, C., KYRIAKIDES, V. & PAPADAKIS, E. (1961). Studies on the blood lipids and lipoproteins in thalassaemia and sickle cell anaemia. *J. clin. Path.*, **14**, 361–364.

CHOREMIS, C., NICOLOPOULOS, D. METAXOTOU, K. & MOSCHOS, A. (1965). Erythrocyte cholinesterase activity in hemolytic anemia. *Acta paed. scand.*, **54**, 218–224.

CHOREMIS, C., ZANNOS, L. & BASTI, B. (1957). Amino-aciduria in Cooley and sickle cell anaemias. *J. clin. Path.*, **10**, 330–335.

CHOREMIS, C., ZANNOS, L. & DENTAKIS, C. L. (1955). Alkali-resistant haemoglobin in thalassaemia. *Acta paediat.* (*Uppsala*), **44**, 116–121.

CHOUHAN, D. M., SHARMA, R. S. & PAREKH, J. G. (1970). Alpha-thalassaemia in India. *J. Indian med. Ass.*, **54**, 364–367.

CIVIDALLI, G., KEREM, H., EZECKIEL, E. & RACHMILEWITZ, E. A. (1978). β^0-thalassemia intermedia. *Blood*, **52**, 345–349.

CIVIDALLI, G., SANDLER, S. G., YATZIV, S., ENGELHARD, D., RACHMILEWITZ, N. & RACHMILEWITZ, E. A. (1980). β^0-thalassemia complicated by autoimmune hemolytic anemia. Globin synthesis during immunosuppressive therapy *Acta haemat.* (*Basel*), **63**, 37–43.

CLEGG, J. B., METAXATOU-MAVROMATI, A., KATTAMIS, C., SOFRONIADOU, K., WOOD, W. G. & WEATHERALL, D. J. (1979). Occurrence of $^G\gamma$ Hb F in Greek HPFH: analysis of heterozygotes and compound heterozygotes with β thalassaemia. *Brit. J. Haemat.*, **43**, 521–536.

CLEGG, J. B. & WEATHERALL, D. J. (1967). Haemoglobin synthesis in α-thalassaemia (haemoglobin H disease). *Nature* (*Lond.*), **215**, 1241–1243.

CLEGG, J. B. & WEATHERALL, D. J. (1974). Hemoglobin Constant Spring, an unusual α-chain variant involved in the etiology of hemoglobin H disease. *Ann. N.Y. Acad. Sci.*, **232**, 168–178.

CLEGG, J. B., WEATHERALL, D. J. & MILNER, P. F. (1971). Haemoglobin Constant Spring — a chain termination mutant? *Nature* (*Lond.*), **234**, 337–340.

COHEN, T., HOROWITZ, A., ABRAHAMOV, A. & LEVENE, C. (1966). Hemoglobin H disease, alpha- and beta-thalassemia traits in a family of Kurdish Jews. *Israel J. med. Sci.*, **2**, 600–606.

COMINGS, D. & MOTULSKY, A. G. (1966). Absence of cis delta chain synthesis in ($\Delta\beta$) thalassemia (F-thalassemia). *Blood*, **28**, 54–69.

Committee for Clarification of the Nomenclature of Cells and Diseases of the Blood and Blood-forming Organs. Third, fourth and fifth reports. (1950). *Amer. J. clin. Path.*, **20**, 562–579.

CONCONI, F., BARGELLESI, A., PONTREMOLI, S., VIGI, V., VOLPATO, S. & GABURRO, D. (1968). Absence of β-globin synthesis and excess of α-globin synthesis in homozygous β-thalassaemic subjects from the Ferrara region. *Nature* (*Lond.*), **217**, 259–269.

CONLEY, C. L., WEATHERALL, D. J., RICHARDSON, S. N., SHEPARD, M. K. & CHARACHE, S. (1963). Hereditary persistence of fetal hemoglobin: a study of 79 affected persons in 15 Negro families in Baltimore. *Blood*, **21**, 261–281.

COOK, I. A. & LEHMANN, H. (1973). Beta-thalassaemia and some rare haemoglobin variants in the Highlands of Scotland. *Scot. med. J.*, **18**, 14–20.

COOLEY, T. B. & LEE, P. (1925). A series of cases of splenomegaly with anemia and peculiar bone changes. *Trans. Amer. pediat. Soc.*, **37**, 29–30.

COOLEY, T. B. & LEE, P. (1932). Erythroblastic anemia: additional comment. *Amer. J. Dis. Child.*, **43**, 705–708.

COOLEY, T. B., WITWER, E. R., & LEE, P. (1927). Anemia in children, with splenomegaly and peculiar changes in the bones: report of cases. *Amer. J. Dis. Child.*, **34**, 347–363.

COOPER, C. D. & WACKER, W. E. C. (1954). The successful therapy with streptokinase-streptodonase of ankle ulcers associated with Mediterranean anemia. *Blood*, **9**, 241–243.

COOPER, E. H., FORBES, M. A., BOWEN, M., GABUTTI, V. & PIGA, A. (1984). Plasma beta-2-microglobulin and fibronectin levels in beta-thalassaemia. *Acta haemat.* (*Basel*), **71**, 257–262.

CROSBY, W. H. & AKEROYD, J. H. (1952). The limit of hemoglobin synthesis in hereditary hemolytic anemia. *Amer. J. Med.*, **13**, 273–283.

CROSBY, W. H. & CONRAD, M. E. (1964). Iron balance in thalassemia minor. A preliminary report. *Ann. N.Y. Acad. Sci.*, **119**, 616–623.

CROSBY, W. H. & DAMESHEK, W. (1951). The significance of hemoglobinuria and associated hemosiderinuria with particular reference to various types of hemolytic anemia. *J. Lab. clin. Med.*, **38**, 829–841.

CROUCH, E. R. JNR, MAURER, H. M. & VALDES, O. R. (1970). Probable homozygous beta thalassemia in a Negro child. *Amer. J. Dis. Child.*, **120**, 356–359.

CROWLEY, M. F., McSORLEY, J. G. A., AKSOY, M. & LEHMANN, H. (1957). The demonstration of a haemoglobin E-like compound in some cases of thalassaemia. *Vox Sang.*, **2**, 53–59.

CURRIN, J. F. (1954). Occurrence of secondary hemochromatosis in patient with thalassemia major. *Arch. intern. med.*, **93**, 781–786.

CURRIN, J. F. & LIEBERMAN, B. (1951). An unusual case of thalassemia major in an adult. *N.Y. St. J. Med.*, **51**, 1321–1323.

CUTILLO, A. & MELONI, T. (1974). Serum concentrations of haptoglobin and hemopexin in favism and thalassemia. *Acta haemat. (Basel)*, **52**, 65–69.

CUTILLO, S., CANANI, M. B., REA, F., LUPI, L. & DI TORO, R. (1962). Ricerche su un gruppo di portatori della tara talassemica. *Pediatria (Napoli)*, **4**, 641–649.

CUTILLO S. & ROMAGNOLI, A. (1953). Sull'entità dell'emoglobinogenesi di tipo fetale nelle forme thalassemiche. Ossevazioni su 18 casi di morbo di Cooley. *Pediatria (Napoli)*, **61**, 539–563.

DACIE, J. V. (1960). The Haemolytic Anaemias: Congenital and Acquired. Part 1 — The Congenital Anaemias, 2nd edn. 339 pp. Churchill, London.

DACIE, J. V. & LEWIS, S. M. (1984). *Practical Haematology*, sixth edition. 453 pp. Churchill Livingstone, Edinburgh.

DALAND, G. A. & STRAUSS, M. B. (1948). The genetic relation and clinical differentiation of Cooley's anemia and Cooley's trait. *Blood*, **3**, 438–448.

DAMESHEK, W. (1940). "Target cell" anemia. An-erythroblastic type of Cooley's erythroblastic anemia. *Amer. J. med. Sci.*, **200**, 445–454.

DAMESHEK, W. (1943). Familial Mediterranean target–oval cell syndromes. *Amer. J. med. Sci.*, **205**, 643–660.

DANESHMEND, T. K. & PEACHEY, R. D. G. (1978). Leg ulcers in alpha-thalassaemia (haemoglobin H disease). *Brit. J. Dermat.*, **98**, 233–235.

DANKWA, E., KILLER, D., FISCHER, S. & MARTI, H. R. (1975). Die Häufigkeit der Thalassämien in der Schweiz. *Schweiz. med. Wschr.*, **105**, 102–105.

DAS GUPTA, C. R., CHATTERJEA, J. B., RAY, R. N. & GHOSH, S. K. (1955). Plasma haemoglobin in Cooley's anaemia. *Bull. Calcutta Sch. trop. Med.*, **3**, 147.

DAS GUPTA, C. R., CHATTERJEA, J. B., RAY, R. N., GHOSH, S. K. & CHOWDHURY, A. B. (1958). Observations on Cooley's anemia (Thalassemia). *Proc. Sixth Int. Congr. Int. Soc. Hemat., Boston, 1956*, p. 733. Grune and Stratton, New York.

DASH, S. (1985). Beta-thalassaemia trait in the Punjab (North India). *Brit. J. Haemat.*, **61**, 185 (Letter).

DAUPHINEE, D. & LANGLEY, G. R. (1967). Thalassemia in Canadians. *Canad. med. Ass. J.*, **96**, 309–311.

DE MARCO, C. & TRASARTI, F. (1957). Haemoglobin F in Talassemia minor. Amino-acid composition. *Experientia*, **13**, 353–354.

DEMARSH, Q. B. & BOYCE, S. (1950). Severe Mediterranean anemia (Cooley's anemia) in a Chinese child. *Blood*, **5**, 798–803.

DE MURO, P. & LEONARDI, G. (1950). Hemopathic Mediterranean syndrome. *Acta med. scand.*, **138**, 362–373.

DE SILVA, C. C., JONXIS, J. H. P. & WICKRAMASINGHE, R. L. (1959). Haemoglobinopathies in Ceylon. *In: Abnormal Haemoglobins. A Symposium*, pp. 340–356. Blackwell Scientific Publications, Oxford.

DE VIRGILIIS, S., CORNACCHIA, G., SANNA, G., ARGIOLU, F., GALANELLO, R., FIORELLI, G., RAIS, M., COSSU, P., BERTOLINO, F. & CAO, A. (1981). Chronic liver disease in transfusion-dependent thalassemia: liver iron quantitation and distribution. *Acta haemat. (Basel)*, **65**, 32–39.

DE VRIES, S. I. & VAN VALKENBURG, R. A. (1953). Thalassaemia (anaemie van Cooley) bij een Nederlandse familie. *Ned. T. Geneesk.*, **97**, 2789–2797.

DEL SENNO, L., BERNARDI, F., MARCHETTI, G., PERROTTA, C., CONCONI, F., VULLO, C., SALSINI, G., CRISTOFORI, G., CAPPELLOZZA, G., BELLINELLO, F., BEDENDO, B. & MERCURIATI, M. (1980). Organization of α globin genes and RNA translation in subjects carrying hemoglobin Hasharon (α47 Asp → His) from the Ferrara region (Northern Italy). *Europ. J. Biochem.*, **111**, 125–130.

DERRY, S., WOOD, W. G., PIPPARD, M., CLEGG, J. B., WEATHERALL, D. J., WICKRAMASINGHE, S. N., DARLEY, J., FUCHAROEN, S. & WASI, P. (1984). Hematologic and biosynthetic studies in homozygous hemoglobin Constant Spring. *J. clin. Invest.*, **73**, 1673–1682.

DEWEY, K. W., GROSSMAN, H. & CANALE, V. C. (1970). Cholelithiasis in thalassemia major. *Radiology*, **96**, 385–388.

DHAYAGUDE, R. G. (1944). Erythroblastic anemia of Cooley (familial erythroblastic anemia) in an Indian boy. *Amer. J. Dis. Child.*, **67**, 290–293.

DIAMOND, M. P., COTGROVE, I. & PARKER, A. (1965). Case of intrauterine death due to α-thalassaemia. *Brit. med. J.*, ii, 278–279.

DI LORIO, E. E., WINTERHALTER, K. H., WILSON, K., ROSENMUND, A. & MARTI, H. R. (1975). A Swiss family with hemoglobin P Galveston β$^{117\,His \to Arg}$, including two patients with Hb P/β thalassemia. *Blut*, **31**, 61–68.

DINÇOL, G., AKSOY, M. & ERDEM, S. (1979). Beta-thalassaemia with increased hemoglobin A$_2$ in Turkey. A study of 164 thalassaemia heterozygotes. *Hum. Hered.*, **29**, 272–278.

DINÇOL, G., ALTAY, C., AKSOY, M., GURGEY, A., FELICE, A. E. & HUISMAN, T. H. J. (1981). Clinical and hematological evaluation of two δ^{0}β^0-thalassemia homozygotes. *Hemoglobin*, **5**, 153–164.

DITTMAN, W. A., HAUT, A., WINTROBE, M. M. & CARTWRIGHT, C. E. (1960). Hemoglobin-H associated with an uncommon variant of thalassemia trait. *Blood*, **16**, 975–983.

DOBKIN, C., CLYNE J., METZENBERG, A. & BANK, A. (1986). Expression of a cloned Lepore globin gene. *Blood*, **67**, 168–172.

DOĞRU, U., ARCASOY, A., & GAVDAR, A. O. (1979). Zinc levels of plasma, erythrocyte, hair and urine in homozygote beta-thalassemia. *Acta haemat. (Basel)*, **62**, 41–44.

DORMANDY, K. M., LOCK, S. P. & LEHMANN, H. (1961). Haemoglobin Q-alpha-thalassaemia. *Brit. med. J.*, **i**, 1582–1585.

DREYFUSS, F. (1955). La thalassémie mineure (Cooley) dans trois familles juives orientales. *J. Génét. hum.*, **4**, 143–151.

DUMA, H., EFREMOV, G., SADIKARIO, A., TEODOSIJEV, D., MIADENOVSKI, B., VLAŠKI, R. & ANDREEVA, M. (1968). Study of nine families with haemoglobin-Lepore. *Brit. J. Haemat.*, **14**, 161–172.

EDINGTON, G. M. & LEHMANN, H. (1955a). Expression of the sickle-cell gene in Africa. *Brit. med. J.*, **i**, 1308–1311.

EDINGTON, G. M. & LEHMANN, H. (1955b). Expression of the sickle-cell gene in Africa. *Brit. med. J.*, **ii**, 1328 (Letter).

EFREMOV, G. D. (1978). Hemoglobins Lepore and anti-Lepore. *Hemoglobin*, **2**, 197–233.

EFREMOV, G., MLADENOVSKI, B., SADIKARIO, A. & DUMA, H. (1969). Two families with different expression of homozygous β-thalassaemia. *Acta haemat. (Basel)*, **41**, 114–120.

EFREMOV, G. D., NIKOLOV, N., DUNA, H., SCHROEDER, W. A., MILLER, A. & HUISMAN, T. H. J. (1975). δβ-thalassaemia in two Yugoslavian families. *Scand. J. Haemat.*, **14**, 226–232.

EFREMOV, G. D., RUDIVIC, R., NIAZI, G. A., HUNTER, E. JNR, HUISMAN, T. H. J. & SCHROEDER, W. A. (1976). An individual with Hb-Lepore-Baltimore-δβ-thalassaemia in a Yugoslavian family. *Scand. J. Haemat.*, **16**, 81–89.

EHLERS, K., LEVIN, A. R., MARKENSON, A. L., MARCUS, J. R., KLEIN, A. A., HILGARTNER, M. W. & ENGLE, M. A. (1980). Longitudinal study of cardiac function in thalassemia major. *Ann. N.Y. Acad. Sci.*, **334**, 397–404.

EL-HAZMI, M. A. F. (1986). Studies on sickle cell heterozygotes in Saudi Arabia — Interaction with α-thalassaemia. *Acta haemat. (Basel)*, **75**, 100–104.

ELDOR, A. (1978a). Hemorrhagic tendency in β-thalassemia major. *Israel J. med. Sci.*, **14**, 1132–1134.

ELDOR, A. (1978b). Abnormal platelet functions in β thalassaemia. *Scand. J. Haemat.*, **20**, 447–452.

ELLIS, J. T., SCHULMAN, I. & SMITH, C. H. (1954). Generalized siderosis with fibrosis of liver and pancreas in Cooley's (Mediterranean) anemia; with observations on the pathogenesis of the siderosis and fibrosis. *Amer. J. Path.*, **30**, 287–309.

EMBURY, S. H. (1985). The interaction of coexistent α-thalassemia and sickle cell anemia: a model for the clinical and cellular results of diminished polymerization? *Ann. N.Y. Acad. Sci.*, **445**, 37–44.

ENGLE, M. A. (1964). Cardiac involvement in Cooley's anemia. *Ann. N.Y. Acad. Sci.*, **119**, 694–702.

ERICKSON, B. N., WILLIAMS, H. H., HUMMELL, F. C., LEE, P. & MACY, I. G. (1937). The lipid and mineral distribution of the serum and erythrocytes in the hemolytic and hypochromic anemias of childhood. *J. biol. Chem.*, **118**, 569–598.

ERLANDSON, M. E., BRILLIANT, R. & SMITH, C. H. (1964). Comparison of sixty-six patients with thalassemia major and thirteen patients with thalassemia intermedia: including evaluations of growth, development and prognosis. *Ann. N.Y. Acad. Sci.*, **119**, 727–735.

ERLANDSON, M. E., GOLUBOW, J., WEHMAN, J. & SMITH, C. H. (1964). Metabolism of iron, calcium and magnesium in homozygous thalassemia. *Ann. N.Y. Acad. Sci.*, **119**, 769–775.

ERLANDSON, M. E., SCHULMAN, I., STERN, G. & SMITH, C. H. (1958). Studies of congenital hemolytic syndromes. I. Rates of destruction and production of erythrocytes in thalassemia. *Pediatrics*, **22**, 910–922.

ESAN, G. J. F. (1970). The thalassaemia syndromes in Nigeria. *Brit. J. Haemat.*, **19**, 47–56.

ESTES, J. E., FARBER, E. M. & STICKNEY, J. M. (1948). Ulcers of the leg in Mediterranean disease. *Blood*, **3**, 302–306.

EVENSEN, S. A., JEREMIC, M. & HJORT, P. F. (1969). Iron-resistant hypochromic anaemia in a Scandinavian family: heterozygous β-thalassaemia. *Acta med. scand.*, **186**, 331–335.

FARGION, S., PIPERNO, A., PANAIOTOPOULOS, N., TADDEI, M. T. & FIORELLI, G. (1985). Iron overload in subjects with beta-thalassaemia trait: role of idiopathic haemochromatosis gene. *Brit. J. Haemat.*, **61**, 487–490.

FARHANGI, M., SASS, M. D. & BANK, A. (1970). Prolonged survival in homozygous high A$_2$-type beta thalassaemia. *Scand. J. Haemat.*, **7**, 465–470.

FAWDRY, A. L. (1944). Erythroblastic anaemia of childhood (Cooley's anaemia) in Cyprus. *Lancet*, **i**, 171–176.

FESSAS, CH., KARAKLIS, A., LOUKOPOULOS, D., STAMATOYANNOPOULOS, G. & FESSAS, PH. (1965). Haemoglobin Nicosia: an α-chain variant and its combination with β-thalassaemia. *Brit. J. Haemat.*, **11**, 323–330.

FESSAS, PH. (1959a). Thalassaemia and the alterations of the haemoglobin pattern. In: *Abnormal Haemoglobins. A Symposium*, pp. 134–155. Blackwell Scientific Publications, Oxford.

FESSAS, PH. (1959b). The hereditary anaemias in Greece. In: *Abnormal Haemoglobins. A Symposium*, pp. 260–289. Blackwell Scientific Publications, Oxford.

FESSAS, PH. (1963). Inclusions of hemoglobin in erythroblasts and erythrocytes of thalassemia. *Blood*, **21**, 21–32.

FESSAS, PH, KONIAVITIS, A. & ZEIS, P. M. (1969). Urinary beta-aminoisobutyric acid excretion in thalassaemia. *J. clin. Path.*, **22**, 154–157.

FESSAS, PH., LIE-INJO, L. E., NA-NAKORN, S. F, TODD, D., CLEGG, J. B. & WEATHERALL, D. J. (1972). Identification of slow-moving haemoglobins in haemoglobin H disease from different racial groups. *Lancet*, i, 1308–1310.

FESSAS. PH. & LOUKOPOULOS, D. (1964). Alpha-chain of human hemoglobin, occurrence in vivo. *Science*, **143**, 590–591.

FESSAS, PH. & LOUKOPOULOS, D. (1974). The β thalassaemias. *Clinics Haemat.* 3, 411–435.

FESSAS, PH., LOUKOPOULOS, D., KOKKINOU, S., PAPASOTIRIOU, Y. & KARAKLIS, A. (1986). Hemoglobin Knossos: a clinical, laboratory, and epidemiological study. *Amer. J. Hemat.*, **21**, 119–133.

FESSAS, PH., LOUKOPOULOS, D., LOUTRADI-ANAGNOSTOU, A. & KOMIS, G. (1982). 'Silent' β-thalassaemia caused by a 'silent' β-chain mutant: the pathogenesis of a syndrome of thalassaemia intermedia. *Brit. J. Haemat.*, **51**, 577–583.

FESSAS, PH. & PAPASPYROU, A. (1957). New 'fast' hemoglobin associated with thalassemia. *Science*, **126**, 1119.

FESSAS, PH. & STAMATOYANNOPOULOS, G. (1962). Absence of haemoglobin A_2 in an adult. *Nature (Lond.)*, **195**, 1215–1216.

FESSAS, PH, & STAMATOYANNOPOULOS, G. (1964). Hereditary persistence of fetal hemoglobin in Greece. A study and a comparison. *Blood*, **24**, 223–240.

FESSAS, P., STAMATOYANNOPOULOS, G. & KARAKLIS, A. (1961). Hereditary persistence of foetal haemoglobin and its combination with alpha and beta-thalassaemia. *8th Congr. Europ. Soc. Haemat.*, *Vienna.* Proceedings (1962), p. 302. Karger, Basel.

FESSAS, P., STAMATOYANNOPOULOS, G. & KARAKLIS, A. (1962). Hemoglobin 'Pylos': study of a hemoglobinopathy resembling thalassemia in the heterozygous, homozygous and double heterozygous state. *Blood*, **19**, 1–22.

FESSAS, PH, STAMATOYANNOPOULOS, G. & KEYS, A. (1963). Serum-cholesterol and thalassaemia trait. *Lancet*, i, 1182–1183.

FINCH, C. A., DEUBELBEISS, K., COOK, J. D., ESCHBACH, J. W., HARKER, L. A., FUNK, D. D., MARSAGLIA, G., HILLMAN, R. S., SLICHTER, S., ADAMSON, J. W., GANZONI, A. & GIBLETT, E. R. (1970). Ferrokinetics in man. *Medicine (Baltimore)*, **49**, 17–53.

FLATZ, G., HAUKE, H. & KLEIHAUER, E. (1964). Thalassaemia major in Deutschland. *Klin. Wschr.*, **42**, 850–852.

FLATZ, G., PIK, C. & SRINGAM, S. (1965). Haemoglobinopathies in Thailand. I. A study of patients with the thalassaemia syndrome and their families. *Brit. J. Haemat.*, **11**, 216–226.

FOGARTY, A. M. JNR, VEDVICK, T. S. & ITANO, H. A. (1974). Absence of haemoglobin A in an individual simultaneously heterozygous in the genes for hereditary persistence of foetal haemoglobin and β-thalassaemia. *Brit. J. Haemat.*, **26**, 527–533.

FORGET, M. G., CAVALLESCO, C., BENZ, E. J. JNR, MCCLURE, P. D., HILLMAN, D. G., KRIEGER, H., CLARKE, B. & HOUSMAN, D. (1978). Studies of globin chain synthesis and globin mRNA content in a patient homozygous for hemoglobin Lepore. *Hemoglobin*, **2**, 117–128.

FORNARA, P. & GENESI, M. (1955). Rilieri anatomo-patologici ed istologici nelle talassemie (major e minor). *Minerva med. (Torino)*, **46**, 1891–1916.

FOSTER, L. P. (1940). Cooley's syndrome (erythoblastic anemia) in a Chinese child. *Amer. J. Dis. Child.*, **59**, 828–834.

FRANCINA, A., DORLEAC, E., AUBRY, M., BAKLOUTI, F., ELWAN, S., RHODA, L., PHILLIPE, N. & DELAUNAY, J. (1985). Hb Lepore-Hb C and Hb Lepore-$β^0$-thalassaemia compound heterozygotes in an Algerian family. *Hemoglobin*, **9**, 505–508.

FREEDMAN, M. L. (1974). Thalassemia: an abnormality in globin chain synthesis. *Amer. J. med. Sci.*, **267**, 256–265.

FRENCH, E. A. & LEHMANN, H. (1971). Is haemoglobin Gα Philadelphia linked to α-thalassaemia? *Acta haemat. (Basel)*, **46**, 149–156.

FRIEDMAN, M. J. (1979). Oxidant damage mediates variant red cell resistance to malaria. *Nature (Lond.)*, 280, 245–247.

FRIEDMAN, S., ATWATER J., GILL, F. M. & SCHWARTZ, E. (1974). α-thalassemia in Negro infants. *Pediat. Res.*, **8**, 955–959.

FRIEDMAN, SH., ÖZSOYLU, S., LUDDY, R. & SCHWARTZ, E. (1976). Heterozygous beta thalassaemia of unusual severity. *Brit. J. Haemat.*, **32**, 65–77.

FRIGERIO, R., MELA, Q., PASSIU, G., CACACE, E., LA NASA, G., PERPIGNANO, G. & CARCASSI, U. E. F. (1984). Iron overload and lysosomal stability in $β^0$-thalassaemia intermedia and trait: correlation between serum ferritin and serum N-acetyl-β-D-glucosaminidase levels. *Scand. J. Haemat.*, 33, 252–255.

FRONTALI, G. (1954). Die Lebensdauer der roten Blutkörperchen bei der Mittelmeer Anämie. *Med. Klinik.*, **49**, 509–511.

FRONTALI, G. & STEGAGNO, G. A. (1951). Durée de vie du globule rouge dans l'anémie Méditerraneénne. *Helvet. paediat. Acta*, **6**, 271–280.

FRUMIN, A. M., WALDMAN, S. & MORRIS, P. (1952). Exogenous hemochromatosis in Mediterranean anemia. *Pediatrics*, **9**, 290–294.

FURBETTA, M., GALANELLO, R., XIMENES, A., ANGIUS, A., MELIS, M. A., SERRA, P. & CAO, A. (1979). Interaction of alpha and beta thalassaemia genes in two Sardinian families. *Brit. J. Haemat.*, **41**, 203–210.

FURBETTA, M., TUVERI, T., ROSATELLI, C., ANGIUS, A., FALCHI, A. M., COSSU, P., MELONI, A., GIAGU, N. & CAO, A. (1983). Molecular mechanisms accounting for milder types of thalassemia major. *J. Pediat.*, **103**, 35–39.

GABUZDA, T. G. (1966). Hemoglobin H and the red cell. *Blood*, **27**, 568–579.

GABUZDA, T. G., NATHAN, D. G. & GARDNER, F. H. (1964). Thalassemia trait: genetic combinations of increased fetal and A2 hemoglobins. *New Engl. J. Med.*, **270**, 1212–1217.

GABUZDA, T. G., NATHAN, D. G., GARDNER, F. H., COUNCIL, A. & LIMAURO, A. (1963). The turnover of hemoglobins A, F, and A2 in the peripheral blood of three patients with thalassemia. *J. clin. Invest.*, **42**, 1678–1688.

GABUZDA, T. G., NATHAN, D. G., GARDNER, F H., COUNCIL, A. & LIMAURO, A. (1965). The metabolism of the individual C^{14}-labeled hemoglobins in patient with H-thalassemia, with observations on radiochromate binding to the hemoglobins during red cell survival. *J. clin. Invest.*, **44**, 315–325.

GADSDON, D., HUGHES, M., DEAN, A. & WICKRAMASINGHE, S. N. (1986). Morphology of redox-dye-treated HbH-containing red cells: confusion caused by wrongly-identified dyes. *Clin. lab. Haemat.*, **8.**, 365–366.

GALENELLO, R., MACCIONI, L., RUGGERI, R., PERSEU, D. & CAO, A. (1984a). Alpha thalassaemia in Sardinian newborns. *Brit. J. Haemat.*, **58**, 361–368.

GALANELLO, R., MELIS, M. A., PAGLIETTI, E., CORNACCHIA, G., DE VIRGILIIS, S. & CAO, A. (1983a). Serum ferritin levels in hemoglobin H disease. *Acta haemat. (Basel)*, **69**, 56–58.

GALANELLO, R., MELIS, M. A., RUGGERI, R., ADDIS, M., SCALAS, M. T., MACCIONI, L. FURBETTA, M., ANGIUS, A., TUVERI, T. & CAO, A. (1979). β^0 thalassaemia trait in Sardinia. *Hemoglobin*, **3**, 33–46.

GALANELLO, R., PAGLIETTI, E., GIAGU, L., MELIS, M. A., SCALES, M. T. & CAO, A. (1983b). Phenotypic manifestations of heterozygous non-deletion α-thalassaemia (αα/(αα)th) in Sardinians. *Brit. J. Haemat.*, **55**, 711–713 (Letter).

GALANELLO, R., PAGLIETTI, E., MELIS, M. A., GIAGU, L. & CAO, A. (1984b). Hemoglobin inclusions in heterozygous alpha-thalassaemia according to their alpha-globin genotype. *Acta haemat. (Basel)*, **72**, 34–36.

GALANELLO, R., RUGGERI, R., PAGLIETTI, E., ADDIS, M., MELIS, M. A. & CAO, A. (1983c). A family with segregating triplicated alpha globin loci and beta thalassaemia. *Blood*, **62**, 1035–1040.

GALLO, E., MASSARO, P., MINIERO, R., DAVID, D. & TARELLA, C. (1979). The importance of the genetic picture and globin synthesis in determining the clinical and haematological features of thalassaemia intermedia. *Brit. J. Haemat.*, **41**, 211–221.

GALLO, E., PICH, P., RICCO, G., SAGLIO, G., CAMASCHELLA, C. & MAZZA, U. (1975). The relationship between anemia, fecal stercobilinogen, erythrocyte survival, and globin synthesis in heterozygotes for β-thalassaemia. *Blood*, **46**, 693–698.

GALLO, E., PUGLIATTI, L., RICCO, G., PICH, P. G., PINNA, G. & MAZZA, U. (1972). A case of haemoglobin J Sardegna/beta-thalassaemia double heterozygosis. *Acta haemat. (Basel)*, **47**, 311–320.

GANGULI, H. & LAHIRI, S. C. (1955). Observations on Cooley's anaemia. *J. Indian med. Ass.*, 24, 453–457

GARDIKAS, C. (1968). Modes of presentation of thalassaemia minor. *Acta haemat. (Basel)*, **40**, 34–36.

GATTO, I., TERRANA, V. & BIONDI, L. (1954). Compressione sul midollo spinale da proliferazione di midollo osseo nello spazio epidurale in soggetto affetto da malattia di Cooley splenectomizzato. *Haematologica*, **38**, 61–76.

GATTO, I. & VALENTINO, L. (1953). Thalassemia (microcarterocitosis) minima. *Pediatria (Napoli)*, **61**, 313–335.

GEORGE, E., FARIDAH, K., TRENT, R. J., PADENILAM, B. J., HUANG, H.-j & HUISMAN, T. H. J. (1986). Homozygosity for a new type of $^G\gamma(^A\gamma\delta\beta)^0$-thalassaemia in a Malaysian male. *Hemoglobin*, **10**, 353–363.

GERALD, P. G. & DIAMOND, L. K. (1958a). The diagnosis of thalassemia trait by starch block electrophoresis of the hemoglobin. *Blood*, **13**, 61–69.

GERALD, P. G. & DIAMOND, L. K. (1958b). A new hereditary hemoglobinopathy (the Lepore trait) and its interaction with thalassemia trait. *Blood*, **13**, 835–844.

GIARDINI, O., CASTRO, M. & MAGGIONI, G. (1974). Increased susceptibility of red-blood-cell lipids to autoxidation in thalassaemia major. *Lancet*, **i**, 33 (Letter).

GIBLETT, E. R. & CROOKSTON, M. C. (1964). Agglutinability of red cells by anti-i in patients with thalassaemia major and other haematological disorders. *Nature (Lond.)*, **201**, 1138–1139.

GIMFERRER, E., BAIGET, M., BARCELÓ, M. J., MARIGÓ, ROJAS, E. & DEL RIO, E. (1984). Erythrocyte creatine concentration and its relationship with reticulocyte counts. I. Studies in normal subjects and in heterozygous β-thalassemia. *Biol. clin. Hemat.*, **6**, 15–25.

GIMFERRER, E., BAIGET, M., DARBRE, P. A. & LEHMANN, H. (1976). Haemoglobin Lepore Boston in a Spanish family. *Acta haemat. (Basel)*, **56**, 234–240.

GIMFERRER, E., BAIGET, M. & RUTLLANT, M. L. (1979). Homozygous delta-beta-thalassaemia in a Spanish woman. *Acta haemat. (Basel)*, **61**, 226–229.

GORODETSKY, R., GOLDFARB, A., DAGAN, I. & RACHMILEWITZ, E. A. (1985). Noninvasive analysis of skin iron and zinc levels in β-thalassemia major and intermedia. *J. Lab. clin. Med.*, **105**, 44–51.

GOTTFRIED, E. L. & ROBERTSON, N. A. (1974). Glycerol lysis time as a screening test for erythrocyte disorders. *J. Lab. clin. Med.*, **83**, 323–333.

GOUTTAS, A., FESSAS, PH., TSEVRENIS, H. J. & XEFTERI, E. (1955). Description d'une nouvelle varieté d'anémie hémolytique. *Sang*, **26**, 911–919.

GRASER, E. (1941). Erythroblastenanämie Typ Cooley bei einem deutschen Kinde. *Z. Kinderheilk.*, **62**, 698–713.

GRATWICK, G. M., BULLOUGH, P. G., BOHNE, W. H. O., MARKENSON, A. L. & PETERSON, C. M. (1978). Thalassemic osteoarthropathy. *Ann. intern. Med.*, **88**, 494–501.

GRAY, G. R., TOWELL, M. E., WRIGHT, V. J. & HARDWICK, D. F. (1972). Thalassemic hydrops fetalis in two Chinese-Canadian families. *Canad. med. Ass. J.*, **107**, 1186–1190.

GREPPI, E. (1935). Sugli itteri emolitici con aumento della resistenza globulare, e sui microciti massimoresistenti come figura ematologica sui generis. *Minerva med. (Torino)*, **26**(**I**), 409–415.

GRIFONI, V., KAMUZORA, H., LEHMANN, H. & CHARLESWORTH, D. (1975). A new Hb variant: Hb F Sardinia $\gamma^{75\ (E\ 19)\ Isoleucine\ \rightarrow\ Threonine}$ found in a family with Hb G Philadelphia, β-chain deficiency and a Lepore-like haemoglobin indistinguishable from Hb A_2. *Acta haemat. (Basel)*, **53**, 347–355.

GRIGNANI, F., LOEHR, G. W., BRUNETTI, P. & WALLER, H. D. (1962). Le métabolisme énergétique de l'érythrocyte thalassémique. *Acta haemat. (Basel)*, **28**, 293–305.

GRINSTEIN, M., BANNERMAN, R. M., VAVRA, J. D. & MOORE, C. V. (1960). Hemoglobin metabolism in thalassemia. *In vivo* studies. *Amer. J. Med.*, **29**, 18–32.

GROSSBARD, E., TERADA, M., DOW, L. W. & BANK, A. (1973). Decreased α globin messenger RNA activity associated with polyribosomes in α thalassaemia. *Nature new Biol.*, **241**, 209–211.

HALDANE, J. B. S. (1949). Disease and evolution. *Ricerca scient.*, **19** (Suppl. 1), 3–13.

HAMILTON, H. E., SHEETS, R. F., DeGOWIN, E. L. & DAHLIN, R. E. (1950). Studies with inagglutinable erythrocyte counts. II. Analysis of mechanisms of Cooley's anemia. *J. clin. Invest.*, **29**, 693–722.

HAMMOND, D., STURGEON, P., BERGREN, W. & CAVILES, A. JNR (1964). Definition of Cooley's trait or thalassemia minor: classical, clinical and routine laboratory hematology. *Ann. N.Y. Acad. Sci.*, **119**, 372–389.

HANLON, D. G., SELBY, J. B. & BAYRD, E. D.

(1956). Hereditary leptocytosis (thalassemia minor). *J. Amer. med. Ass.*, **161**, 1132–1135.

HASSAN, M. M. & ZIADA, M. A. R. (1965). Thalassaemia major in the Sudan. *Brit. med. J.*, **i**, 295.

HAUT, A., TUDHOPE, G. R., CARTWRIGHT, G. E. & WINTROBE, M. M. (1962). Studies on the osmotic fragility of incubated normal and abnormal erythrocytes. *J. clin. Invest.*, **41**, 1766–1775.

HAVARD, C. W. H., LEHMANN, H. & BODLEY SCOTT, R. (1958). Thalassaemia minor in an Englishwoman. *Brit. med. J.*, **i**, 304–305.

HAZELL, J. W. P. & MODELL, C. B. (1976). Complications in thalassaemia major. *J. Laryng. Otol.*, **90**, 877–881.

HEDENBURG, F., MÜLLER-EBERHARD, U., SJÖLIN, S. & WRANNE, L. (1958). Haemoglobin H and inclusion-body anaemia in a Swedish family. *Acta paediat. (Uppsala)*, **47**, 652–665.

HEILMEYER, L., MÜLLER, W. & SCHUBOTHE, H. (1951). Uber eisenrefraktäre, Kobaltsensible anämien und zur Frage des Vorkommem der Thalassaemia minor in Deutschland. *Klin. Wschr.*, **29**, 333–335.

HEINLE, R. W. & READ, M. R. (1948). Study of thalassemia minor in three generations of an Italian family. *Blood*, **3**, 449–456.

HELLEMAN, P. W., PUNT, K. & VERLOOP, M. C. (1964). Occurrence of haemoglobin H and haemoglobin Bart's in alpha-thalassaemia: a family with two possible homozygous cases and with G-6-PD-deficiency. *Nature (Lond.)* **201**, 1039–1040.

HELLER, P., YAKULIS, V. J., ROSENZWEIG, A. I., ABILDGAARD, C. F. & RUCKNAGEL, D. L. (1966). Mild homozygous beta-thalassemia: further evidence for the heterogeneity of beta thalassemia genes. *Ann. intern. Med.*, **64**, 52–61.

HENDRICKSE, R. G., BOYO, A. E., FITZGERALD, P. A. & RANSOME KUTI, S. (1960). Studies on the hemoglobins of newborn Nigerians. *Brit. med. J.* **i**, 611–614.

HERMAN, E. C. JNR & CONLEY, C. L. (1960). Hereditary persistence of fetal hemoglobin. A family study. *Amer. J. Med.*, **29**, 9–17.

HEYWOOD, D., KARON, M. & WEISSMAN, S. (1965). Asymmetrical incorporation of amino acids in the alpha and beta chains of hemoglobins synthesized by thalassemic reticulocytes. *J. Lab. clin. Med.*, **66**, 476–482.

HEYWOOD, J. D., KARON, M. & WEISSMAN, S. (1964). Amino acids: incorporation into α- and β-chains of hemoglobin by normal and thalassemic reticulocytes. *Science*, **146**, 530–531.

HIGGS, D. R., AYYUB, H., CLEGG, J. B., HILL, A. V. S., NICHOLLS, R. D., TEAL, H., WAINSCOAT, J. S. & WEATHERALL, D. J. (1985). α thalassaemia in British people. *Brit. med. J.*, **i**, 1303–1306.

HILGARTNER, M. W., ERLANDSON, M. E. & SMITH, C. H. (1963). The coagulation mechanism in patients with thalassemia major. *J. Pediat.*, **63**, 36–45.

HILGARTNER, M. W. & SMITH, C. H. (1964). Coagulation studies as a measure of liver function in Cooley's anemia. *Ann. N. Y. Acad. Sci.*, **119**, 631–640.

HILLCOAT, B. L. (1960). Occurrence of β-amino-isobutyric acid in the urine of patients with thalassemia major. *Aust. J. exp. Biol. med. Sci.*, **38**, 441–446.

HILLCOAT, B. L. (1962). Altered urinary excretion of beta-amino-isobutyric acid after splenectomy. *Lancet*, **i**, 74–75.

HILLCOAT, B. L. & WATERS, A. G. (1962). The survival of ^{51}Cr labelled autotransfused red cells in patients with thalassaemia. *Aust. Ann. Med.*, **11**, 55–58.

HINDAWI, A. Y. & SUBHIYAH, B. W. (1962). Study by radiochromium of red-cell survival and the role of the spleen in red-cell elimination in thalassaemia. *Brit. J. Haemat.*, **8**, 266–273.

HITZIG, W. H., MARTI, H. R. & ROY, I. (1965). Kombination von Thalassaemia minor und hereditärer HbF-Persistenz. *Schweiz. med. Wschr.*, **95**, 1459–1461.

HJELLE, B., CHARACHE, S. & PHILLIPS, J. A. III (1982). Hemoglobin H disease and multiple congenital anomalies in a child of Northern European origin. *Amer. J. Hemat.*, **13**, 319–322.

HONETZ, N., MOSER, K., NEUMANN, E. & SEIPEL, H. (1968). Untersuchungen über Erythrokinetik und Erythrozytenstoffwechsel bei Thalassaemia minor. *Acta haemat.(Basel)*, **39**, 333–344.

HONIG, G. R. & 18 CO-AUTHORS (1984). Hemoglobin Evanston (α 14 Trp → Arg). An unstable α-chain variant expressed as α-thalassemia. *J. clin. Invest.*, **73**, 1740–1749.

HONIG, G. R., SHAMSUDDIN, M., MASON, R. G., VIDA, L. N., TREMAINE, L. M., TARR, G. E. & SHAHIDI, N. T. (1980). Hemoglobin Nigeria (α-81 Ser→Cys): a new variant associated with α-thalassemia. *Blood*, **55**, 131–137.

HOROWITZ, A., COHEN, T., GOLDSCHMIDT, E. & LEVENE, C. (1966). Thalassemia types amongst Kurdish Jews in Israel. *Brit. J. Haemat.*, **12**, 555–568.

HUISMAN, T. H. J., CHEN, S. S., NAKATSUJI, T. & KUTLAR, F. (1985). A second family with the Atlanta type of HPFH. *Hemoglobin*, **9**, 393–398.

HUISMAN, T. H. J., GRAVELY, M. E., WEBBER, B., OKONJO, K., HENSON, J. & REESE, A. L. (1981). The gamma chain heterogeneity of fetal hemoglobin in black β-thalassemia and HPFH. *Blood*, **58**, 62–70.

HUISMAN, T. H. J., PRINS, H. K. & VAN DER SCHAAF, P. C. (1956). Is alkali-resistant haemoglobin in Cooley's anaemia different from foetal haemoglobin? *Experientia*, **12**, 107–108.

HUISMAN, T. H. J., PUNT, K. & SCHAAD, J. D. G.

(1961). Thalassemia minor associated with hemoglobin-B$_2$ heterozygosity. A family report. *Blood*, **17**, 747–757.

HUISMAN, T. H. J., REESE, A. L., GARDINER, M. B., WILSON, J. B., LAM, H., REYNOLDS, A., NAGLE, S., TROWELL, P., YI-TAO, Z., SHU-ZHENG, H., SUKUMARAN, P. K., MIWA, S., EFREMOV, G. D., PETKOV, G., SCIARRATTA, G. V. & SANSONE, G. (1983). The occurrence of different levels of $^{G}\gamma$ chain and of the $^{A}\gamma^{T}$ variant of fetal hemoglobin in newborn babies from several countries. *Amer. J. Hemat.*, **14**, 133–148.

HUISMAN, T. H. J., SCHROEDER, W. A., ADAMS, H. R., SHELTON, J. R., SHELTON, J. B. & APELL, G. (1970a). A possible subclass of the hereditary persistence of fetal hemoglobin. *Blood*, **36**, 1–9.

HUISMAN, T. H. J., SCHROEDER, W. A., CHARACHE, S., BETHLENFALVAY, N. C., BOUVER, N., SHELTON, J. R., SHELTON, J. B. & APELL, G. (1971). Hereditary persistence of fetal hemoglobin. Heterogeneity of fetal hemoglobin in homozygotes and in conjunction with β-thalassemia. *New Engl. J Med.*, **285**, 711–716.

HUISMAN, T. H. J., SCHROEDER, W. A., DOZY, A. M., SHELTON, J. R., SHELTON, J. B., BOYD, E.M. & APPEL, G. (1969). Evidence for multiple structural genes for the chain of human fetal hemoglobin in hereditary persistence of fetal hemoglobin. *Ann. N.Y. Acad. Sci.*, **165**, 320–331.

HUISMAN, T. H. J., SCHROEDER, W. A., EFREMOV, G. D., DUMA, H., MLADENOVSKI, B., HYMAN, C. B., RACHMILEWITZ, E. A., BOUVER, N., MILLER, A., BRODIE, A., SHELTON, J. R., SHELTON, J. B. & APPELL, G. (1974). The present status of the heterogeneity of fetal hemoglobin: an attempt to unify some observations in thalassemia and related conditions. *Ann. N.Y. Acad. Sci.*, **232**, 107–124.

HUISMAN, T. H. J., SCHROEDER, W. A., STAMATOYANNOPOULOS, G., BOUVER, N., SHELTON, J. R., SHELTON, J. B. & APELL, G. (1970b). Nature of fetal hemoglobin in the Greek type of hereditary persistence of fetal hemoglobin with and without concurrent β-thalassemia. *J. clin. Invest.*, **49**, 1035–1040.

HUISMAN, T. H. J., WRIGHTSTONE, R. N., WILSON, J. B., SCHROEDER, W. A. & KENDALL, A. G. (1972). Hemoglobin Kenya, the product of fusion of γ and β polypeptide chains. *Arch. Biochem. Biophys.*, **153**, 850–853.

HUNT, D. M., HIGGS, D. R., WINICHAGOON, P., CLEGG, J. B. & WEATHERALL, D. J. (1982). Haemoglobin Constant Spring has an unstable α chain messenger RNA. *Brit. J. Haemat.*, **51**, 405–413.

HUNT, J. A. & LEHMANN, H. (1959). Abnormal human haemoglobins. Haemoglobin 'Bart's': a foetal haemoglobin without α-chains. *Nature (Lond.)*, **184**, 872–873.

HYMAN, C. B., LANDING, B., ALFIN-SLATER, R., KOZAK, L., WEITZMAN, J. & ORTEGA, J. A. (1974). dl-α-tocopherol, iron and lipofuscin in thalassemia. *Ann. N. Y. Acad. Sci.*, **232**, 211–220.

HYMAN, C. B., ORTEGA, J. A., COSTIN, G. & TAKAHASHI, M. (1980). The clinical significance of magnesium depletion in thalassemia. *Ann. N.Y. Acad. Sci.*, **344**, 436–443.

IBRAHIM, S. A. & BARAKAT, S. M. (1970). Thalassaemia and high F-gene in Aleppo. *Acta haemat. (Basel)*, **44**, 287–291.

IDELSON, L. I. & DIDKOVSKY, N. A.(1971). Haemoglobin H disease in a Russian family. *Haematologia*, 5, 241–248.

IFEDIBA, T. C., STERN, A., IBRAHIM, A. & RIEDER, R. F. (1985). *Plasmodium falciparum* in vitro: diminished growth in hemoglobin H disease erythrocytes. *Blood*, **65**, 452–455.

IMAMURA, T., OHTA, Y. & HANADA, M. (1968). The occurrence of hemoglobins Bart's and F associated with carbonic anhydrase deficiency in a patient with alpha-thalassemia and malignant thymoma. *Blood*, **32**, 71–82.

ING, R. Y. K., CROOKSTON, J. H., DWORATZEK, J. A. & BURNIE, K. (1968). Alpha thalassemia: five cases of hemoglobin H disease in three Oriental-Canadian families. *Canad. med. Ass. J.*, **99**, 49–56.

INGRAM, V. M. & STRETTON, A. O. W. (1959). Genetic basis of the thalassaemia diseases. *Nature (Lond.)*, **184**, 1903–1909.

ISRAELS, L. G., SUDERMAN, H. J. & HOOGSTRATEN, J. (1955). Thalassaemia in a Scottish family. *Lancet*, ii, 1318–1320.

ISRAËLS, M. C. G. & TURNER, R. L. (1955). A British target-cell anaemia. *Lancet*, ii, 1363–1365.

ITANO, H. A. (1957). The human hemoglobins: their properties and genetic control. *Advanc. Protein Chem.*, **12**, 215–268.

JACKSON, F. S., LEHMANN, H. & SHARIH, A. (1960). Thalassaemia in a Tibetan discovered during a haemoglobin survey among the Sherpas. *Nature (Lond.)*, **188**, 1121–1122.

JACOB, G. F. & RAPER, A. B. (1958). Hereditary persistence of foetal haemoglobin production, and its interaction with the sickle-cell trait. *Brit. J. Haemat.*, **4**, 138–149.

JACOBS, A., PETERS, S. W., BAUMINGER, E. R., EIKELBOOM, J., OFER, S. & RACHMILEWITZ, E. A. (1981). Ferritin concentration in normal and abnormal erythrocytes measured by immunoradiometric assay with antibodies to heart and spleen ferritin and Mössbauer spectroscopy. *Brit. J. Haemat.*, **49**, 201–207.

JANDL, J. H. & GREENBERG, M. S. (1959). Bone-marrow failure due to relative nutritional deficiency in Cooley's hemolytic anemia. Painful "erythropoietic crises" in response to folic acid. *New Engl. J. Med.* **260**, 461–468.

JOHNSTON, F. E., HERTZOG, K. P. & MALINA, R. M.

(1966). Longitudinal growth in thalassemia major: relationship to hemoglobin level. *Amer. J. Dis. Child.*, **112**, 396–401.

JONES, R. T., SCHROEDER, W. A., BALOG, J. E. & VINOGRAD, J. R. (1959). Gross structure of hemoglobin H. *J. Amer. chem. Soc.*, **81**, 3161.

JOSEPHSON, A. M., MASRI, M. S., SINGER, L., DWORKIN, D. & SINGER, K. (1958). Starch block electrophoretic studies of human hemoglobin solutions. II. Results in cord blood, thalassemia and other hematologic disorders: comparison with Tiselius electrophoresis. *Blood*, **13**, 543–551.

KAMUZORA, H., JONES, R. T. & LEHMANN, H. (1974). The ζ-chain, an α-like chain of human embryonic haemoglobin. *FEBS Lett.*, **46**, 195–199.

KAMUZORA, H., RINGELHANN, B., KONOTEY-AHULU, F. I. D., LEHMANN, H. & LORKIN, P. A. (1974), The γ-chain in a Ghanaian adult, homozygous for hereditary persistence of fetal haemoglobin. *Acta haemat.*, (Basel), **51**, 179–184.

KAMUZORA, H., RINGELHANN, B., KONOTEY-AHULU, F. I. D., LEHMANN, H. & LORKIN, P. A. (1975). Further investigations of the γ-chain in a Ghanaian adult, homozygous for hereditary persistence of fetal haemoglobin. Isolation of γ CB-3 peptides and $^{G}\gamma:^{A}\gamma$ ratio determination in human Hb F. *Acta haemat. (Basel)*, **53**, 315–320.

KAN, Y. W. (1983). The thalassemias. In: *The Metabolic Basis of Inherited Disease*, 5th edn (ed. by J. B. Stanbury, J. B. Wyngaarden, D. S. Fredrickson, J. L. Goldstein and M. S. Brown), pp. 1711–1725. McGraw-Hill Book Company, New York.

KAN, Y. W., ALLEN, A. & LOWENSTEIN, L. (1967). Hydrops fetalis with alpha thalassemia. *New Engl. J. Med.*, **276**, 18–23.

KAN, Y. W., FORGET, B. G. & NATHAN, D. G. (1972). Gamma-beta thalassemia: a cause of hemolytic disease of the newborn. *New Engl. J. Med.*, **286**, 129–134.

KAN, Y. W. & NATHAN, D. G. (1970). Mild thalassemia: the result of interactions of alpha and beta thalassemia genes. *J. clin. Invest.*, **49**, 635–642.

KAN, Y. W., SCHWARTZ, E. & NATHAN, D. G. (1968). Globin chain synthesis in the alpha thalassemia syndromes. *J. clin. Invest.*, **47**, 2515–2522.

KANAVAKIS, E., METAXOTOU-MAVROMATI, A., KATTAMIS, C., WAINSCOAT, J. S. & WOOD, W. G. (1983). The triplicated α gene locus and β thalassaemia. *Brit. J. Haemat.*, **54**, 201–207.

KANAVAKIS, E., TZOTZOS, S., LIAPAKI, A., METAXOTOU-MAVROMATI, A. & KATTAMIS, C. (1986). Frequency of α-thalassemia in Greece. *Amer. J. Hemat.*, **22**, 225–236.

KANAVAKIS, E., WAINSCOAT, J. S., WOOD, W. G., WEATHERALL, D. J., CAO, A., FURBETTA, M., GALANELLO, R., GEORGIOU, D. & SOPHOCLEOUS, T. (1982). The interaction of α thalassaemia with heterozygous β thalassaemia. *Brit. J. Haemat.*, **52**, 465–473.

KAPLAN, E., ZUELZER, W. W. & HOOGANA, L. (1950). Erythrocyte survival studies in childhood. II. Studies in Mediterranean anaemia. *J. Lab. clin. Med.*, **36**, 517–523.

KATO, K. & DOWNEY, H. (1933). The hematology of erythroblastic anemia (type Cooley). *Folia haemat. (Lpz.)*, **50**, 55–67.

KATTAMIS, C., KARAMBULA, K., METAXOTOU-MAVROMATI, A., LADIS, V. & CONSTANTOPOULOS, A. (1978). Prevalance of β⁰ and β⁺ thalassemia genes in Greek children with homozygous β-thalassemia. *Hemoglobin*, **2**, 29–46.

KATTAMIS, C. & LEHMANN, H. (1970a). The genetical interpretation of haemoglobin H disease. *Hum. Hered.*, **20**, 156–164.

KATTAMIS, C. & LEHMANN, H. (1970b). Duplication of alpha-thalassaemia gene in three Greek families with haemoglobin H disease. *Lancet*, **ii**, 635–637.

KATTAMIS, C., METAXOTOU- MAVROMATI, A., KARAMBOULA, K., NASIKA, E. & LEHMANN, H. (1973). The clinical and haematological findings in children inheriting two types of thalassaemia: high-A₂ type β-thalassaemia, and high-F type or δβ-thalassaemia. *Brit. J. Haemat.*, **25**, 375–384.

KATTAMIS, C., METAXOTOU-MAVROMATI, A., TSIARTA, E., METAXATOU, C., WASI, P., WOOD, W. G., PRESSLEY, L., HIGGS, D. R., CLEGG, J. B. & WEATHERALL, D. J. (1980). Haemoglobin Bart's hydrops syndrome in Greece. *Brit. med. J.*, **ii**, 268–270.

KATTAMIS, C., METAXOTOU-MAVROMATI, A., WOOD, W. G., NASH, J. R. & WEATHERALL, D. J. (1979). The heterogeneity of normal Hb A₂-β thalassaemia in Greece. *Brit. J. Haemat.*, **42**, 109–123.

KEKWICK, R. A. & LEHMANN, H. (1960). Sedimentation characteristic of the γ-chain haemoglobin (haemoglobin 'Bart's'). *Nature (Lond.)*, **187**, 158.

KHALIFA, A. S., SHEIR, S., EL MAGD, L. A., EL TAYEB, H., EL LAMIE, O., KHALIFA, A. & MOKHTAR, G. (1985). The kidney in beta-thalassaemia major. *Acta haemat. (Basel)*, **74**, 60.

KING, M. A. R., WILTSHIRE, B. G., LEHMANN, H. & MORIMOTO, H. (1972). An unstable haemoglobin with reduced oxygen affinity: haemoglobin Peterborough, β111 (G13) valine → phenylalanine, its interaction with normal haemoglobin and with haemoglobin Lepore. *Brit. J. Haemat.*, **22**, 125–134.

KLEIHAUER, E., BRAUN, H. & BETKE, K. (1957). Demonstration von fetalen Hämoglobin in den Erythrocyten eines Blutausstrichs. *Klin. Wschr.*, **35**, 637–638.

KNOBLICH, R. (1960). Extramedullary hematopoiesis presenting as intrathoracic tumours. Record of a case in a patient with thalassemia minor. *Cancer*, **13**, 462–468.

KNOX-MACAULAY, H. H. M., WEATHERALL, D. J., CLEGG, J. B., BRADLEY, J. & BROWN, M. J. (1972). The clinical and biosynthetic characterization of αβ-thalassaemia. *Brit. J. Haemat.*, **22**, 497–512.

KNOX-MACAULAY, H. H. M., WEATHERALL, D. J., CLEGG, J. B. & PEMBREY, M. E. (1973). Thalassaemia in the British. *Brit. med. J.*, **iii**, 150–155.

KOLER, R. D., JONES, R. T., WASI, P. & POOTRAKUL, S. (1971), Genetics of haemoglobin H and α-thalassemia. *Ann. hum. Genet.*, **34**, 371–377.

KORSTEN, J., GROSSMAN, H., WINCHESTER, P. H. & CANALE, V. C. (1970). Extramedullary hematopoiesis in patients with thalassemia anemia. *Radiology*, **95**, 257–263.

KRAUS, A. P., KOCH, B. & BURCKETT, L. (1961). Two families showing interaction of haemoglobin C or thalassaemia with high foetal haemoglobin in adults. *Brit. med. J.*, **i**, 1434–1436.

KREIMER-BIRNBAUM, M., BANNERMAN, P. M. & PINKERTON, P. H. (1969). Recent studies on pyrrole metabolism in thalassemia. *Ann. N.Y. Acad. Sci.*, **165**, 185–193.

KREIMER-BIRNBAUM, M., PINKERTON, P. H., BANNERMAN, R. M. & HUTCHISON, H. E. (1966). Dipyrrolic urinary pigments in congenital Heinz-body anaemia due to Hb Köln and in thalassaemia. *Brit. med. J.*, **ii**, 396.

KREIMER-BIRNBAUM, M., RUSNAK, P. A. & BANNERMAN, R. M. (1974). Urinary pyrrole pigments in thalassemia and unstable hemoglobin diseases. *Ann. N.Y. Acad. Sci.*, **232**, 283–292.

KRUATRACHUE, M., SIRISINHA, S., PACHAREE, P., CHANDARAYINGYONG, D. & WASI, P. (1980). An association between thalassaemia and autoimmune haemolytic anaemia (AIHA). *Scand. J. Haemat.*, **25**, 259–263.

KUMAR, R., SARAYA, A. K., CHOUDHYR, V. P., SUNDARAM, K. R., KAILASH, S. & SEHGAL, A. K. (1985). Vitamin B₁₂, folate and iron studies in homozygous beta thalassemia. *Amer. J. clin. Path.*, **84**, 668–671.

KUNKEL, H. G., CEPPELLINI, R., MÜLLER-EBERHARD, U. & WOLF, J. (1957). Observations on the minor basic hemoglobin component in the blood of normal individuals and patients with thalassemia. *J. clin. Invest.*, **36**, 1615–1625.

KUNKEL, H. G. & WALLENIUS, G. (1955). New hemoglobin in normal adult blood. *Science*, **122**, 288.

LABIE, D., PAGNIER, J., MALLARME, J. & BOIVIN, P. (1971). Un cas d'hémoglobine Lepore chez un malade d'origine française. *Ann. Biol. clin.*, **29**, 343–345.

LABIE, D. & ROSA, J. (1967). Structure et génétique des hémoglobines Lepore. *Nouv. Rev. franç. Hémat.*, **7**, 683–696.

LABIE, D., ROSA, J. & PAVIOT, J.-J. (1961). Sur l'existence de différentes anomalies de l'hémoglobine dans une population du sud de l'Inde. *Nouv. Rev. franç. Hémat.*, **1**, 562–568.

LABIE, D., SCHROEDER, W. A. & HUISMAN, T. H. J. (1966). The amino acid sequence of the δ-β chains of hemoglobin Lepore$_{\text{Augusta}}$ = Lepore$_{\text{Washington}}$. *Biochim. biophys. Acta*, **127**, 428–437.

LANG, A., LEHMANN, H. & KING-LEWIS, P. A. (1974). Hb K Woolwich: the cause of a thalassaemia. *Nature (Lond.)*, **249**, 467–469.

LARIZZA, P., VENTURA, S., MATIOLI, G., SULIS, E. & ARESU, G. (1958). Contributo alla conoscenza dell'anemia talassemica (Ricerche condotte con l'ausilio del Fe^{59}). *Haematologica*, **43**, 517–621.

LAZAR, H. P. (1956). Thalassemia in a Hawaiian family of Filipino extraction. *Blood*, **11**, 1019–1023.

LEHMANN, H. (1953). Sickle-cell anaemia. *Brit. med. J.*, **ii**, 1217 (Letter).

LEHMANN, H. (1959). The maintenance of the haemoglobinopathies at high frequency: a consideration of the relation between sickling and malaria and of allied problems. In: *Abnormal Haemoglobins. A Symposium* (ed. by J. H. P. Jonxis and J. F. Delafresnaye), pp. 307–321. Blackwell Scientific Publications, Oxford.

LEHMANN, H. (1970). Different types of alpha-thalassaemia and significance of haemoglobin Bart's in neonates. *Lancet*, **ii**, 78–80.

LEHMANN, H. (1980–81). Hemoglobins we have known. *Texas Rep. Biol. Med.*, **40**, 471–477.

LEHMANN, H. (1982). The history of thalassemia. In: *Birth Defects: Original Article Series*, **18**, 1–11. March of Dimes Birth Defects Foundation.

LEHMANN, H. (1984). The gradual understanding of thalassemia. In: *The Red Cell: Sixth Ann Arbor Conference*, pp. 121–136. Alan R. Liss, New York.

LEHMANN, H. & CARRELL, R. W. (1968). Differences between α- and β-chain mutants of human haemoglobin and between α- and β-thalassaemia. Possible duplication of the α-chain gene. *Brit. med. J.*, **iv**, 748–750.

LEHMANN, H. & CARRELL, R. W. (1984). Nomenclature of the α-thalassaemias. *Lancet*, **i**, 552–553.

LEHMANN, H., CASEY, R., LANG, A., STATHOPOULOU, R., IMAI, K., TUCHINDA, S., VINAI, P. & GLATZ, G. (1975). Haemoglobin Tak: a β-chain elongation. *Brit. J. Haemat.*, **31** (Suppl.), 119–131.

LEHMANN, H. & LANG, A. (1975). Haemoglobin Q and thalassaemia. *J. Sci. Soc. Thailand*, **1**, 41–48.

LEHNDORFF, H. (1936). Die Erythroblastenanämie. *Ergebn. inn. Med. Kinderheilk.*, **50**, 568–619.

LICHTMAN, H. C., WATSON, R. J., FELDMAN, F., GINSBERG, V. & ROBINSON, J. (1953). Studies in thalassemia. Part I. An extracorpuscular defect in thalassemia major. Part II. The effects of splenectomy in thalassemia major with an associated acquired hemolytic anemia. *J. clin. Invest.*, **32**, 1229–1235.

LIE-INJO, L. E. (1959a). Haemoglobin of new-born infants in Indonesia. *Nature (Lond.)*, **183**, 1125–1126.

LIE-INJO, L. E. (1959b). Pathological haemoglobins in Indonesia. In: *Abnormal Haemoglobins. A Symposium*, pp. 368–384. Blackwell Scientific Publications, Oxford.

LIE-INJO, L. E. (1961). Haemoglobin 'Bart's' and the sickling phenomenon. *Nature (Lond.)*, **191**, 1314.

LIE-INJO, L. E. (1962). Alpha-chain thalassemia and hydrops fetalis in Malaya: report of five cases. *Blood*, **20**, 581–590.

LIE-INJO, L. E. (1973). Haemoglobin Bart's and slow-moving haemoglobin X components in newborns. The homozygous state for the slow-moving X components in a Malay boy. *Acta haemat. (Basel)*, **49**, 25–35.

LIE-INJO, L., DOZY, A. M., KAN, Y. W., LOPES, M. & TODD, D. (1979). The α-globin gene adjacent to the gene for HbQ-α74 Asp → His is deleted, but not that adjacent to the gene for HbG-α30 Glu→Gln; three-fourths of the α-globin genes are deleted in HbQ-α-thalassaemia. *Blood*, **54**, 1407–1416.

LIE-INJO, L. E., GANESAN, J., CLEGG, J. B. & WEATHERALL, D. J. (1974). Homozygous state for Hb Constant Spring (slow-moving Hb X component). *Blood*, **43**, 251–259.

LIE-INJO, L. E. & JO, B. H. (1960a). A fast-moving haemoglobin in hydrops foetalis. *Nature (Lond.)*, **185**, 698.

LIE-INJO, L. E. & JO, B. H. (1960b). Hydrops foetalis with a fast-moving haemoglobin. *Brit. med. J.*, **ii**, 1649–1650.

LIE-INJO, L. E. & JO, K. T. (1955). Cooley's anaemia in children in Indonesia. *Docum. Med. geogr. trop. (Amst.)*, **7**, 30–42.

LIE-INJO, L. E., KHO, L. K., LIEM, D. L. & OEI, O. B. (1959). Further cases of Cooley's anaemia in Indonesia. *Acta haemat. (Basel)*, **21**, 102–108.

LIE-INJO, L. E. & LIE, H. G. (1961). Abnormal haemoglobin production as a probable cause of erythroblastosis and hydrops foetalis in uniovular twins. *Acta haemat. (Basel)*, **25**, 192–199.

LIE-INJO, L. E., LIE, H. G., AGER, J. A. M. & LEHMANN, H. (1962). α-thalassaemia as a cause of hydrops foetalis. *Brit. J. Haemat.*, **8**, 1–4.

LIE-INJO, L. E., LOPEZ, C. G. & DUTT, A. K. (1968). Pathological findings in hydrops foetalis due to alpha-thalassaemia: a review of 32 cases. *Trans. roy. Soc. trop. Med. Hyg.*, **62**, 874–879.

LIE-INJO, L. E., LOPEZ, C. G. & LOPEZ, M. (1971). Inheritance of haemoglobin H disease. A new aspect. *Acta haemat. (Basel)*, **46**, 106–120.

LIE-INJO, L. E., PILLAY, R. P. & THURAISINGHAM, V. (1966). Further cases of Hb Q-H disease (Hb Q-α thalassaemia). *Blood*, **28**, 830–839.

LIE-INJO, L. E., POEY, S. H., KHO, L. K. & ENDENBERG, P. M. (1957). Chronic hypochromic microcytic anaemia associated with haemoglobin H. *Acta haemat. (Basel)*, **18**, 156–167.

LIE-INJO, L. E. & VAN DER HART, P. L. (1963). Splenectomy in two cases of haemoglobin Q-H-disease (Hb Q-α-thalassaemia). *Acta haemat. (Basel)*, **29**, 358–367.

LIN, H.-C. & YU, C.-F. (1965). Haemoglobin H associated with hemoglobin Bart's in two unrelated Chinese families. *Chin. med. J.*, **84**, 100–106.

LIN, K.-S., LEE, T.-C., LU, T.-C., HUANG, J. T.-H. & BLACKWELL, R. Q. (1965). Haemoglobin H disease among Chinese residents of Taiwan. *Acta haemat. (Basel)*, **33**, 178–185.

LIQUORI, A. M. (1951). Presence of foetal haemoglobin in Cooley's anaemia. *Nature (Lond.)*, **167**, 950–951.

LLOYD, J. K. & BROWN, G. A. (1964). Homozygous thalassaemia in an English child. *Arch. Dis. Childh.*, **39**, 625–629.

LOGOTHETIS, J., ECONOMIDOU, J., CONSTANTOULAKIS, M., AUGOUSTAKI, O., LOEWENSON, R. B. & BILEK, M. (1971). Cephalofacial deformities in thalassaemia major (Cooley's anemia). A correlative study among 138 cases. *Amer. J. Dis. Child.*, **121**, 300–306.

LOGOTHETIS, J., LOEWENSON, R. B., AUGOUSTAKI, O., ECONOMIDOU, J. & CONSTANTOULAKIS, M. (1972). Body growth in Cooley's anemia (homozygous beta-thalassaemia) with a correlative study as to other aspects of the illness in 138 cases. *Pediatrics*, **50**, 92–99.

LOPEZ, C. G. & LIE-INJO, L. E. (1971). Alpha-thalassaemia in newborns in West Malaysia. *Hum. Hered.*, **21**, 185–191.

LOUKOPOULOS, D. & FESSAS, PH. (1965). The distribution of hemoglobin types in thalassemic erythrocytes. *J. clin. Invest.*, **44**, 231–240.

LOUKOPOULOS, D., LOUTRADI, A. & FESSAS, PH. (1978). A unique thalassaemic syndrome: homozygous α-thalassaemia + homozygous β-thalassaemia. *Brit. J. Haemat.*, **39**, 377–389.

LOUKOPOULOS, D., POYART, C., DELANOE-GARIN, J., MATSIS, C., AROUS, N., KISTER, J., LOUTRADI-ANAGNOSTOU, A., BLOUQUIT, Y., FESSAS, PH., THILLET, J., ROSA, J. & GALACTEROS, F. (1986). Hemoglobin San Diego β⁰ thalassaemia in a Greek adult. *Hemoglobin*, **10**, 143–159.

LUDWIN, I., LIMENTANI, D. & DAMESHEK, W. (1952). Linkage tests of Mediterranean anemia with blood groups, blood types, Rh factors and eye color. *Amer. J. hum. Genet.*, **4**, 182–193.

LUHBY, A. L. & COOPERMAN, J. M. (1961). Folic-acid deficiency in thalassaemia major. *Lancet*, ii, 490–491 (Letter).

LUHBY, A. L., COOPERMAN, J. M., FELDMAN, R., CERAOLO, J., HERRARO, J. & MARLEY, J. F. (1961). Folic-acid deficiency as a limiting factor in the anemias of thalassaemia major. *Blood*, **18**, 786–787 (Abstract).

LUPPIS, B. & VENTRUTO, V. (1979). Synthesis of alpha, delta-beta and gamma chains by reticulocytes from two brothers homozygous for haemoglobin Lepore. *Acta haemat. (Basel)*, **61**, 216–221.

LUZZATTO, L. (1985). Malaria and the red cell. In: *Recent Advances in Haematology* (ed. by A. V. Hoffbrand). pp. 109–126. Churchill Livingstone, Edinburgh.

LYBERATOS, C., CHALEVELAKIS, G., PLATIS, A., STATHAKIS, N., PANANI, A. & GARDIKAS, C. (1972). Erythrocyte content of free protoporphyrin in thalassaemia syndromes. *Acta haemat. (Basel)*, **47**, 164–167.

MCCORMICK, W. F. & HUMPHREYS, E. W. (1960). High fetal-hemoglobin C disease: a new syndrome. *Blood*, **16**, 1736–1744.

MCCURDY, P. R. (1967). Thalassemia in negroes. *Arch. intern. Med.*, **119**, 86–91.

MCELFRESH, A. E., SHARPSTEIN, J. R. & AKABANE, T. (1955). Secondary hypersplenism occurring in a seven-month-old infant with thalassemia major. *J. Pediat.*, **47**, 347–350.

MCFADZEAN, A. J. S. & TODD, D. (1964). The distribution of Cooley's anaemia in China. *Trans. roy. Soc. trop. Med. Hyg.*, **58**, 490–499.

MCFARLAND, W. & PEARSON, H. A. (1960). Thalassemia in 'non-Mediterranean' families. *Ann. intern. Med.*, **53**, 510–522.

MCINTOSH, N. (1976). Beneficial effects of transfusing a patient with nontransfusion-dependent thalassaemia major. *Arch. Dis. Childh.*, **51**, 471–472.

MACIVER, J. E., WENT, L. N. & IRVINE, R. A. (1961). Hereditary persistence of foetal haemoglobin: a family study suggesting allelism of the F gene to the S and C haemoglobin genes. *Brit. J. Haemat.*, **7**, 373–381.

MALAMOS, B., BELCHER, E. H., GYFTAKI, E. & BINOPOULOS, D. (1961a). Simultaneous radioactive tracer studies of erythropoiesis and red-cell destruction in thalassaemia. *Brit. J. Haemat.*, **7**, 411–429.

MALAMOS, B., BELCHER, E. H., GYFTAKI, E. & BINOPOULOS, D. (1961b). Simultaneous studies with Fe⁵⁹ and Cr⁵¹ in congenital haemolytic anaemias. *Nucl. Med. (Stuttgart)*, **2**, 1–20.

MALAMOS, B., FESSAS, PH. & STAMATOYANNOPOULOS, G. (1962). Types of thalassaemia-trait carriers as revealed by a study of their incidence in Greece. *Brit. J. Haemat.*, **8**, 5–14.

MALAMOS, B., GYFTAKI, E., BINOPOULOS, D. & KESSE, M. (1962). Studies of haemoglobin synthesis and red cell survival in haemoglobinopathy H. *Acta haemat. (Basel)*, **28**, 124–134.

MANGANELLI, F., DALFINO, G. & TANNOIA, N. (1962). Su di un caso associazione tra talassemia e "persistenza ereditaria di emoglobina fetale". *Haematologica*, **47**, 353–366.

MANIATIS, A., BOUSIOS, T., NAGEL, R. L., BALAZS, T., UEDA, Y., BOOKCHIN, R. M. & MANIATIS, G. M. (1979). Hemoglobin Crete (β129 Ala →Pro): a new high-affinity variant interacting with β⁰ and

$\delta\beta^0$-thalassemia. *Blood*, **54**, 54–63.

MANN, J. R., MacNEISH, A. S., BANNISTER, D., CLEGG, J. B., WOOD, W. G. & WEATHERALL, D. J. (1972). $\delta\beta$-thalassaemia in a Chinese family. *Brit. J. Haemat.*, **23**, 393–402.

MARCH, H. W., SCHLYEN, S. M. & SCHWARTZ, S. E. (1952). Mediterranean hemopathic syndromes (Cooley's anaemia) in adult. Study of a family with unusual complications. *Amer. J. Med.*, **13**, 46–57.

MARINOZZI, V. (1958). Aspetti insoliti dell'iperplasia midollare nelle anemie emolitiche. *Haematologica*, **43**, 737–759.

MARINUCCI, M., MAVILIO, F., MASSA, A., GABBIANELLI, M., FONTANAROSA, P. P., SAMOGGIA, P. & TENTORI, L. (1979). Haemoglobin Lepore trait: haematological and structural studies on the Italian population. *Brit. J. Haemat.*, **42**, 557–565.

MARKS, P. A. (1966). Thalassemia syndromes: biochemical, genetic and clinical aspects. *New. Engl. J. Med.*, **275**, 1363–1369.

MARKS, P. A. & BURKA, E. R. (1964a). Hemoglobins A and F: formation in thalassemia and other hemolytic anemias. *Science*, **144**, 552–553.

MARKS, P. A. & BURKA, E. R. (1964b). Hemoglobin synthesis in human reticulocytes: a defect in globin formation in thalassemia major. *Ann. N.Y. Acad. Sci.*, **119**, 513–522.

MARKS, P. A., BURKA, E. R. & RIFKIND, R. A. (1964). Control of protein synthesis in reticulocytes and the formation of hemoglobins A and F in thalassemia syndromes and other hemolytic anemias. *Medicine (Baltimore)*, **43**, 769–778.

MARKS, P. A. & GERALD, P. (1964). The thalassemia syndromes. Biochemical, genetic and clinical considerations. *Amer. J. Med.*, **36**, 919–935 (Combined staff clinic).

MARMONT, A. & BIANCHI, V. (1948). Mediterranean anemia. Clinical and haematological findings, and pathogenetic studies in the milder form of the disease (with report of cases). *Acta haemat. (Basel)*, **1**, 4–28.

MARNI, E., BORGNA-PIGNATTI, C., DE STEFANO, P., DELL'ACQUA, S., NOÉ, G. P., BARZIZZA, F., GRANDI, A. & VENCO, A. (1983). Evaluation of cardiac status in thalassemia major: a study of 32 patients. *Haematologica*, **68**, 517–522.

MARTI, H. R. (1962). Hämoglobinuntersuchungen bei 100 in der Schweiz gefundenen Fallen von Thalassaemia minor. *Schweiz. med. Wschr.*, **92**, 403–405.

MARTI, H. R. (1963). *Normale und anomale menschliche Hämoglobine*, pp. 85–89. Springer, Berlin.

MARTINEZ, G. & COLOMBO, B. (1973). Hemoglobina Lepore Washington (Boston) y su interaccion con la β thalasemia en un niño cubano. *Rev. Invest. clín. (Revista di investigacíon clinica)*, **25**, 359–366.

MARTINEZ, G., FERREIRA, R. & COLOMBO, B. (1985). Linkage of the α^G Philadelphia locus to α-thalassemia in the Cuban population. *Acta haemat. (Basel)*, **74**, 186–188.

MASALA, B., MANCA, L., FORMATO, M. & MATERA, A. (1986). The level of Hb F-Sardinia ($\alpha_2 {}^A\gamma_2 {}^{75\ \text{Ile}}_{\text{Thr}}$) in the fetal hemoglobin of Sardinian β-thalassemic homozygotes determined by isoelectric focusing. *Amer. J. Hemat.*, **21**, 367–376.

MATIOLI, G. & DEL PIANO, E. (1959). Emazie talassemiche e corpi di Heinz. *Haematologica*, **64**, 739–748.

MATOTH, Y., SHAMIR, Z. & FREUNDLICH, E. (1955). Thalassemia in Jews from Kurdistan. *Blood*, **10**, 176–189.

MATTHEWS, J. H., ROWLANDES, D., WOOD, J. K. & WOOD, W. G. (1981). Homozygous ${}^G\gamma\delta\beta$ thalassemia. *Clin. lab. Haemat.*, **3**, 121–127.

MAUDE, G. H., HIGGS, D. R., BECKFORD, M., GRANDISON, Y., MASON, K., TAYLOR, B., SERJEANT, B. E. & SERJEANT, G. R. (1985). Alpha thalassaemia and the haematology of normal Jamaican children. *Clin. lab. Haemat.*, **7**, 289–295.

MAZZA, U., SAGLIO, G., CALIGARIS CAPPIO, F., CAMASCHELLA, C., NERETTO, G. & GALLO, E. (1976). Clinical and haematological data in 254 cases of beta-thalassaemia trait in Italy. *Brit. J. Haemat.*, **33**, 91–99.

MEITAL, V., IZAK, G. & RACHMILEWITZ, M. (1961). L'effet de la grossesse sur la thalassémie. *Nouv. Rev. franç. Hémat.*, **1**, 389–409.

MELIS, M. A., GALANELLO, R. & CAO, A. (1983). Alpha globin gene analysis in a Sardinian family with interacting alpha and beta thalassaemia genes. *Brit. J. Haemat.*, **53**, 667–671.

MELIS, M. A., PIRASTU, M., GALANELLO, R., FURBETTA, M., TUVERI, T. & CAO, A. (1983). Phenotypic effect of heterozygous α and β^0-thalassemia interaction. *Blood*, **62**, 226–229.

MELIS, M. A., ROSATELLI, C., FALCHI, A. M., ANGIUS, A., FURBETTA, M., GALANELLO, R. & CAO, A. (1980). Hematological characteristics of Sardinian α-thalassaemia carriers detected in a population study. *Acta haemat. (Basel)*, **63**, 32–36.

MIDDLEBROOK, J. E. (1956). Thalassemia in a family of pure German extraction. *New Engl. J. Med.*, **255**, 815–817.

MILLARD, D. P., MASON, K., SERJEANT, B. E. & SERJEANT, G. R. (1977). Comparison of the haematological features of the β^0 and β^+ thalassaemia traits in Jamaican Negroes. *Brit. J. Haemat.*, **36**, 161–170.

MILNER, P. F., CLEGG, J. B. & WEATHERALL, D. J. (1971). Haemoglobin H disease due to a unique haemoglobin variant with an elongated α-chain. *Lancet*, **i**, 729–732.

MINNICH, V., CORDONNIER, J. K., WILLIAMS, W. J. & MOORE, C. V. (1962). Alpha, beta and gamma hemoglobin polypeptide chains during the neonatal period with description of the fetal form of hemoglobin D$_{\text{a St. Louis}}$ *Blood*, **19**, 137–167.

MINNICH, V., NA-NAKORN, S., CHONGCHAREONSUK, S. & KOCHASENI, S.-E. (1954). Mediterranean anemia. A study of thirty-two cases in Thailand. *Blood*, **9**, 1–23.

MODELL, B. (1976). Management of thalassaemia major. *Brit. med. Bull.*, **32**, 270–276.

MODELL, C. B., BENSON, A. & PAYLING WRIGHT, C. R. (1972). Incidence of β-thalassaemia trait among Cypriots in London. *Brit. med. J.*, **iii**, 737–738.

MONCRIEFF, A. & WHITBY, L. E. H. (1934). Cooley's anaemia. *Lancet*, **ii**, 648–649.

MOONEY, F. S. (1952). The diagnosis of carriers of Cooley's anaemia. *J. clin. Path.*, **5**, 154–160.

MOSELEY, J. E. (1974). Skeletal changes in the anemias. *Seminars Roentgen.*, **9**, 169–184.

MUKHERJI, M. (1938). Cooley's anaemia (erythroblastic or Mediterranean anaemia). *Ind. J. Pediat.*, **5**, 1–7.

MURANO, G. (1955). Qualche rilievo sull'impiego della trasfusione di sangue nella anemia di Cooley. *Pediatria (Napoli)*, **63**, 529–559.

MUSUMECI, S., SCHILIRO, G., PIZZARELLI, G., D'AGATA, A., FISHER, A. & RUSSO, G. (1979). Alpha thalassaemia in Sicily: haematological and biosynthetic studies. *Brit. J. Haemat.*, **43**, 413–422.

MUSUMECI, S., SCHILIRO, G., ROMEO, M. A., DI GREGORIO, F., PIZZARELLI, G., TESTA, R. & RUSSO, G. (1983). Heterogeneity of β-thalassemia intermedia. *Haematologica*, **68**, 503–516.

NAGARATHAM, N. & SUKUMARAN, P. K. (1967). Thalassaemia in Ceylon. *Acta haemat. (Basel)*, **38**, 209–218.

NAJAEN, Y., DESCHRYVER, F., HENNI, T. & GIROT, R. (1985). Red cell kinetics in thalassaemia intermedia: its use for a prospective prognosis. *Brit. J. Haemat.*, **59**, 533–539.

NA-NAKORN, S. (1959). Haemoglobinopathies in Thailand. In: *Abnormal Haemoglobins. A Symposium*, pp. 357–367. Blackwell Scientific Publications, Oxford.

NA-NAKORN, S. & WASI, P. (1970). Alpha-thalassemia in Northern Thailand. *Amer. J. hum. Genet.*, **22**, 645–651.

NA-NAKORN, S., WASI, P., PORNPATKUL, M. & POOTRAKUL, S.-N. (1969). Further evidence for a genetic basis of haemoglobin H disease from newborn offspring of patients. *Nature (Lond.)*, **223**, 59–60.

NAPIER, L. E., SHORTEN, J. A. & DAS GUPTA, C. R. (1939). Cooley's erythroblastic anaemia. *Indian med. Gaz.*, **74**, 660–664.

NASAB, A. H. (1979). Clinical and laboratory findings in the initial diagnosis of homozygous beta thalassaemia in Fars Province, Iran. *Brit. J. Haemat.*, **43**, 57–61.

NATHAN, D. G. (1972). Thalassemia. *New Engl. J. Med.*, **286**, 586–594.

NATHAN, D. G. & GUNN, R. B. (1966). Thalassemia: the consequence of unbalanced hemoglobin synthesis. *Amer. J. Med.*, **41**, 815–830.

NATHAN, D. G., STOSSEL, T. B., GUNN, R. B., ZARKOWSKY, H. S. & LAFORET, M. T. (1969). Influence of hemoglobin precipitation on erythrocyte metabolism in alpha and beta thalassemia. *J. clin. Invest.*, **48**, 33–41.

NATTA, C., CASEY, R. & LEHMANN, H. (1978). Double heterozygosity for hemoglobin Camden (β^{131} Gln → Glu) and alpha thalassemia. *Hemoglobin*, **2**, 463–468.

NECHELES, T. F., ALLEN, D. M. & GERALD, P. S. (1969). The many forms of thalassemia: definition and classification of the thalassemia syndromes. *Ann. N.Y. Acad. Sci.*, **165**, 5–12.

NECHELES, T. F., CATES, M., SHEEHAN, R. G. & MEYER, H. J. (1966). Hemoglobin H disease. A family study. *Blood*, **38**, 501–512.

NEEB, D. H., BEIBOER, J. L., JONXIS, J. H. P., SIJPESTEIJN, J. A. K. & MULLER, C. J. (1961). Thalassemie met Lepore hemoglobine bij twee Papoea-kinderen in Nederlands Nieuw-Guinea. *Ned. T. Geneesk.*, **105**, 8–14.

NEEL, J. V. & VALENTINE, W. N. (1945). The frequency of thalassemia. *Amer. J. med. Sci.*, **209**, 568–572.

NORRIS, J. E., HANSON, H. H. & LOEFFLER, R. K. (1956). Mediterranean anemia in an adult negro. *Arch. intern. Med.*, **98**, 356–364.

NOWICKI, L., HOLZMANN, A., MARTIN, H. & WÖRNER, W. (1963). Thalassämie in Deutschland (mit Bericht über eine weitere Sippe). *Klin. Wschr.*, **41**, 841–848.

NURSE, G. T. (1979). Iron, the thalassaemias, and malaria. *Lancet*, **ii**, 938–940.

NUTE, P. E., WOOD, W. G., STAMATOYANNOPOULOS, G., OLWENY, C. & FAILKOW, P. J. (1976). The Kenya form of hereditary persistence of fetal haemoglobin: structural studies and evidence for homogeneous distribution of haemoglobin F using fluorescent anti-haemoglobin F antibodies. *Brit. J. Haemat.*, **32**, 55–63.

NUYKEN, G, (1954). Thalassämie in Iran. *Med. klin. Berl.*, **49**, 1955–1956.

OHENE-FREMPONG, K., RAPPAPORT, E., ATWATER, J., SCHWARTZ, E. & SURREY, S. (1980). Alpha-gene deletions in black newborn infants with Hb Bart's. *Blood*, **56**, 931–933.

OHTA, Y., YAMAOKA, K., SUMIDA, I., FUJITA, S., FUJIMURA, T. & YANASE, T. (1971). Homozygous delta-thalassemia first discovered in a Japanese family with hereditary persistence of fetal hemoglobin. *Blood*, **37**, 706–715.

OLD, J. M., CLEGG, J. B., WEATHERALL, D. J. & BOOTH, P. B. (1978). Haemoglobin J Tongariki is associated with α thalassaemia. *Nature (Lond)*, **273**, 319–320.

OLESEN, E. B., LIVINGSTONE, F. B., COHEN, F., ZUELZER, W. W., ROBINSON, A. R. & NEEL, J. V.

(1959). Thalassaemia in Liberia. *Brit. med J.* i, 1385–1387.

ONG, H. C., WHITE, J. C. & SINNATHURAY, T. A. (1977). Haemoglobin H disease and pregnancy in a Malaysian woman. *Acta haemat. (Basel)*, 58, 229–233.

OORT, M., HEERSPINK, W., ROOS, D., FLAVELL, R. A. & BERNINI, L. F. (1981). Haemolytic disease of the newborn and chronic anaemia induced by $\gamma\delta\beta$ thalassaemia in a Dutch family. *Brit. J. Haemat.*, 48, 251–262.

OPPENHEIMER, S. J., HIGGS, D. R., WEATHERALL, D. J., BARKER, J. & SPARK, R. A. (1984). α thalassaemia in Papua New Guinea. *Lancet*, i, 424–426.

ORKIN, S. H. & NATHAN, D. G. (1976). Current concepts in genetics: the thalassemias. *New Engl. J. Med.*, 295, 710–714.

ORSINI, A., LOUCHET, E., RAYBAND, C., BRUSQUET, Y. & PERRIMOND, H. (1970). Les pericardites de la maladie de Cooley. *Pédiatrie*, 25, 831–842.

OSTERTAG, W. & SMITH, E. W. (1969). Hemoglobin Lepore$_{Baltimore}$, a third type of $\delta\beta$ crossover $(\delta^{50}, \beta^{86})$. *Europ. J. Biochem.*, 10, 371–376.

ÖZSOYLU, S., HIÇSÖNMEZ, G. & ALTAY, C. (1973). Hemoglobin H-β-thalassemia. *Acta haemat. (Basel)*, 50, 184–190.

PAGNIER, J., ELION, J., LAPOUMÉROULIE, C., VIGNERON, C. & LABIE, D. (1982). Homozygous deletional α^{+} thalassaemia associated with unequal expression of the two remaining α_1 genes ($\alpha_1{}^A$ and $\alpha_1{}^Q$). *Brit. J. Haemat.*, 52, 115–125.

PANOFF, A. (1936). Beitrag zur Cooley-Anämie (mit Beschreibung von 2 Fällen). *Mschr. Kinderkeilk.*, 73, 184–194.

PAPAVASILIOU, C. G. (1965). Tumor-simulating intrathoracic extramedullary hemopoiesis. Clinical and roetgenologic considerations. *Amer. J. Roentgenol.*, 93, 695–702.

PAPAVASILIOU, C. & SANDILOS, P. (1987). Effect of radiotherapy on symptoms due to heterotopic marrow in β-thalassaemia. *Lancet*, i, 13–14.

PASCHER, F., & KEEN, R. (1957). Ulcers of the leg in Cooley's anemia. *New Engl. J. Med.*, 256, 1220–1222.

PASVOL, G., WEATHERALL, D. J. & WILSON, R. J. M. (1977). Effects of foetal haemoglobin on susceptibility of red cells to *Plasmodium falciparum*. *Nature (Lond.)*, 270, 171–173.

PAULING, L. (1955). Abnormality of haemoglobin molecules in hereditary hemolytic anemias. *The Harvey Lectures (1953–1954)*, pp. 216–241. Academic Press, New York.

PAWLAK, A. L. & KOZLOWSKA, F. (1979). Swiss type of hereditary persistence of foetal haemoglobin in a case of acquired haemolytic anaemia. *Acta haemat. (Basel)*, 43, 184–191.

PEARSON, H. A. (1964). Thalassemia intermedia: genetic and biochemical considerations. *Ann. N.Y.*

Acad. Sci., 119, 390–401.

PEARSON, H. A. (1966). Alpha-beta thalassemia in a Negro family. *New Engl. J. Med.*, 275, 176–181.

PEARSON, H. A., GERALD, P. S. & DIAMOND, L. K. (1959). Thalassemia intermedia due to interaction of Lepore trait with thalassemia trait. Report of three cases. *J. Dis. Child.*, 97, 464–472.

PEARSON, H. A., MCFARLAND, W., KING, E. R., BECKNER, W. & PETROFF, C. (1960). Erythrokinetic studies in the thalassemia trait. *J. Lab. clin. Med.*, 56, 866–873.

PEARSON, H. A., MCFARLAND, W., VERTREES, K. M. & BECKNER, W. (1962). Erythrokinetics in thalassemia. II. Studies in Lepore trait and hemoglobin H disease. *J. Lab. clin. Med.*, 59, 147–157.

PEARSON, H. A., MOTOYAMA, E., GENEL, M., KRAMER, M. & ZIGAS, C. J. (1977). Intraerythrocytic adaptation (2, 3-DPG, P_{50}) in thalassemia minor. *Blood*, 49, 463–465.

PEARSON, H. A., SHANKLIN, D. R. & BRODINE, C. R. (1965). Alpha-thalassemia as cause of nonimmunological hydrops. *Amer. J. Dis. Child.*, 109, 168–172.

PEMBREY, M. E., WEATHERALL, D. J., CLEGG, J. B., BUNCH, C. & PERRINE, R. P. (1975). Haemoglobin Bart's in Saudi Arabia. *Brit. J. Haemat.*, 29, 221–234.

PENATI, F., AMBROZINO, C., LIBERATORI, J., LOVISETTO, P. & TURCO, G. L. (1955). Studi sulla emoglobina in condizioni normali e patologiche (talassemie). Nota X, ricerche mediante elettroforesi. *Haematologica*, 39, 597–634.

PENATI, F., TURCO, G. L. & LOVISETTO, P. (1954). Studi sulli emoglobina in condizioni normali et patologiche (talassemie). Nota III. Ricerche mediante denaturazione alcalina frazionata. *Haematologica*, 38, 1411–1431.

PEPE, G., LUPI, L. & LUZZATTO, L. (1980). Genetic and biochemical heterogeneity of β-thalassaemia in Naples. *Brit. J. Haemat.*, 45, 417–429.

PERABO, F. (1954). Über das Vorkommen von Cooley-Anämie in Burma. *Helvet. paediat. Acta*, 9, 339–350.

PERACCHI, M., TOSCHI, V., LOMBARDI, L., BAMONTI-CATENA, F., MAIOLO, A. T., BAREGGI, B., MASSARO, P. & POLLI, E. E. (1985). Plasma cyclic nucleotide levels in patients with homozygous beta-thalassaemia. *Scand. J. Haemat.*, 34, 348–352.

PERSSON, S., SAMUELSON, G., SJÖLIN, S. & WALLENIUS, G. (1967). β-thalassaemia minor in two Swedish families. *Scand. J. Haemat.*, 4, 361–370.

PERSSON, S., SAMUELSON, G., SJÖLIN, S. & WALLENIUS, G. (1969). Beta-thalassaemia minor with an unusually high prevalence among siblings. *Acta haemat. (Basel)*, 41, 234–238.

PETERS, S. W., JACOBS, A. & FITZSIMMONS, E. (1983). Erythrocyte ferritin in normal subjects and patients with abnormal iron metabolism. *Brit. J. Haemat.*, **53**, 211–216.

PIERCE, H. I., KURACHI, S., SOFRONIADOU, K. & STAMATOYANNOPOULOS, G. (1977). Frequencies of thalassemia in American blacks. *Blood*, **49**, 981–986.

PIOMELLI, S. & SINISCALCO, M. (1969). The haematological effects of glucose-6-phosphate dehydrogenase deficiency and thalassaemia trait: interaction between the two genes at the phenotype level. *Brit. J. Haemat.*, **16**, 537–549.

PIPERNO, A., TADDEI, M. T., SAMPIETRO, M., FARGIOU, S., AROSIO, P. & FIORELLI, G. (1984). Erythrocyte ferritin in thalassemia syndromes. *Acta haemat. (Basel)*, **71**, 251–256.

PIPPARD, M. J. (1985). Red cell kinetics in thalassaemia intermedia. *Brit. J. Haemat.*, **60**, 765–766 (Letter).

PIRASTU, M., GALANELLO, R., MELIS, M. A., BRANCATI, C., TAGARELLI, A., CAO, A. & KAN, Y. W. (1983a). δ^+-thalassaemia in Sardinia. *Blood*, **62**, 341–345.

PIRASTU, M., KAN, Y. W., LIN, C. C., BAINE, R. M. & HOLBROOK, C. T. (1983b). Hemolytic disease of the newborn caused by a new deletion of the entire β-globin cluster. *J. clin. Invest.*, **72**, 602–609.

PLATO, C. C., RUCKNAGEL, D. L. & GERSHOWITZ, H. (1964). Studies on the distribution of glucose-6-phosphate dehydrogenase deficiency, thalassemia, and other genetic tracts in the coastal and mountain districts of Cyprus. *Amer. J. hum. Genet.*, **16**, 267–283.

POLLIACK, A. & RACHMILEWITZ, E. A. (1973). Ultrastructural studies in β-thalassaemia major. *Brit. J. Haemat.*, **24**, 319–326.

POLOSA, P. & FERRERI, L. (1956). Il morbo di Cooley nell'adulto. *Haematologica*, **41**, 81–115; 303–333.

PONGSAMART, S., POOTRAKUL, S., WASI, P. & NA-NAKORN, S. (1975). Hemoglobin Constant Spring: hemoglobin synthesis in heterozygous and homozygous states. *Biochem. biophys. Res. Commun.* **64**, 681–686.

PONTREMOLI, S., BARGELLESI, A. & CONCONI, F. (1969). Globin chain synthesis in the Ferrara thalassemia population. *Ann. N.Y. Acad. Sci.*, **165**, 253–269.

POOTRAKUL, P., VONGSMASA, V., LA-ONGPANICH, P. & WASI, P. (1981). Serum ferritin levels in thalassemias and the effect of splenectomy. *Acta haemat. (Basel)*, **66**, 244–250.

POOTRAKUL, P., WASI, P. & NA-NAKORN, S. (1967). Haemoglobin Bart's hydrops foetalis in Thailand. *Ann. hum. Genet.*, **30**, 293–311.

POOTRAKUL, P., WASI, P. & NA-NAKORN, S. (1973). Haematological data in 312 cases of β-thalassaemia trait in Thailand. *Brit. J. Haemat.*, **24**, 703–712.

POOTRAKUL, P., WATTANASAREE, J., ANUWATANAKULCHAI, M. & WASI, P. (1984). Increased red blood cell protoporphyrin in

thalassemia: a result of relative iron deficiency. *Amer. J. clin. Path.*, **82**, 289–293.

PORNPATKUL, M., WASI, P. & NA-NAKORN, S. (1969). Hematologic parameters in obligatory alpha-thalassemia. *J. med. Ass. Thailand*, **52**, 801 [quoted by Weatherall and Clegg (1981)].

POUYA, Y. (1959). Thalassaemia in Iran. In: *Abnormal Haemoglobins. A Symposium*, pp. 236–241. Blackwell Scientific Publications, Oxford.

PRASAD. S. A., DIWANY, M., GABR, M., SANDSTEAD, H. H., MOKHTAR, N. & EL HEFNY, A. (1965). Biochemical studies in thalassemia. *Ann. intern. Med.*, **62**, 87–96.

PRATO, V. & MAZZA, U. (1962). Some aspects of porphyrin metabolism in thalassaemia. *Panminerva med. (Torino)*, **4**, 344–350.

PRIBILLA, W. (1951). Thalassaemia minor. *Dtsch. Arch. klin. Med.*, **198**, 223–235.

PRIOLISI, A., ASTALDI, G. & BURGIO, R. (1968). Sobre la eritro y ferrocinetica en la talasemia major. *Sangre*, **13**, 167–186.

PRIOLISI, A. & GIUFFRÈ, L. (1963). Studio immunoelettroforetico del siero nella thalassemia major, anche in rapporto alla splenectomia. *Haematologica*, **48**, 269–304.

PUTIGNAGO, T. & FIORE-DONATI, L. (1948). La resistenza emoglobinica nel M. di Cooley (del bambino e del l'adulto) e forme affini. *Boll. Soc. Ital. biol. sper.*, **24**, 277–280.

QIN, W.-B., JU, T.-L., YUE, X.-L., YAN, X.-L., QIN, L.-Y., ZHAO, J.-B. & CHEN, C.-B. (1985). Hemoglobin Constant Spring in China. *Hemoglobin*, **9**, 69–71.

QUATTRIN, N., BIANCHI, P., CIMINO, R., DE ROSA, L., DINI, E. & VENTRUTO, V. (1967). Study on nine families with haemoglobin Lepore in Campania. Hb Lepore trait, heterozygosity for Hb Lepore and β-thalassaemia, homozygosity for Hb Lepore. *Acta haemat. (Basel)*, **37**, 266–275.

QUATTRIN, N., LUZZATTO, L. & QUATTRIN, S. JNR (1980). New clinical and biochemical findings from 235 patients with hemoglobin Lepore. *Ann. N.Y. Acad. Sci.*, **334**, 364–374.

QUATTRIN, N. & VENTRUTO, V. (1974). Hemoglobin Lepore: its significance for thalassemia and clinical manifestations. *Ann. N.Y. Acad. Sci.* **232**, 65–75.

QUATTRIN, N., VENTRUTO, V. & DINI, E. (1966). Prima osservacione Italiana di malattia da omozugosi di Hb Lepore. *Haematologica*, **51**, 189–196.

RACHMILEWITZ, E. A., LUBIN, B. H. & SHOHET, S. B. (1976). Lipid membrane peroxidation in β-thalassemia major. *Blood*, **47**, 495–505.

RACHMILEWITZ, E. A., PEISACH, J., BRADLEY, T. B. JNR & BLUMBERG, W. E. (1969). Role of haemichromes in the formation of inclusion bodies in haemoglobin H disease. *Nature (Lond.)*, **222**, 248–250.

RACHMILEWITZ, E. A., SHIFTER, A. & KAHANE, I.

(1979). Vitamin E deficiency in β thalassemia major: changes in hematological parameters following a therapeutic trial with α-tocopherol. *Amer. J. clin. Nutr.*, **32**, 1850–1858.

RAHBAR, S., AZIZI, M. & NOWZARI, G. (1975). A case of homozygous haemoglobin Lepore_Boston in Iran. *Acta haemat. (Basel)*, **53**, 60–64.

RAHBAR, S., GOLBAN-MOGHADAM, N. & SAOODI, H. (1974). Hemoglobin Lepore_Boston in two Iranian families. *Blood*, **43**, 79–83.

RAJNOLDI, A. C., FERRARI, M., PIETRI, S. & TRAVI, M. (1980). Glycerol lysis time for screening for β-thalassaemia trait. *Lancet*, **ii**, 638 (Letter).

RAMOT, B., ABRAHAMOV, A., FRAYER, Z. & GAFNI, D. (1964). The incidence and type of thalassaemia-trait carriers in Israel. *Brit. J. Haemat.*, **10**, 155–158.

RAMOT, B., BEN-BASSAT, I., GAFNI, D. & ZAANOON, R. (1970). A family with three βδ-thalassemia homozygotes. *Blood*, **35**, 158–165.

RAMOT, B., SHEBA, CH., FISHER, S., AGER, J. A. M. & LEHMANN, H. (1959). Haemoglobin H disease with persistent haemoglobin "Bart's" in an oriental jewess and her daughter. A dual alpha-chain deficiency of human haemoglobin. *Brit. med. J.*, **ii**, 1228–1230.

RAMSEY, M. & JENKINS, T. (1984). α-thalassaemia in Africa: the oldest malaria protective trait? *Lancet*, **ii**, 410 (Letter).

RANNEY, H. M. & JACOBS, A. S. (1964). Simultaneous occurrence of haemoglobins C and Lepore in an Afro-American. *Nature (Lond.)*, **204**, 163–166.

RAPAPORT, S. I., REILLY, E. B. & CARPENTER, G. (1957). Clinically "intermediate" thalassemia due to hypersplenism complicating thalassemia minor: a case report illustrating relief of anemia by splenectomy. *Ann. intern. Med.*, **46**, 1199–1207.

RAPER, A. B. (1962). Persistence of haemoglobin F. *Brit. med. J.*, **ii**, 1758–1759.

REEMTSMA, K. & ELLIOTT, R. H. E. JNR (1956). Splenectomy in Mediterranean anemia; an evaluation of long-term results. *Ann. Surg.*, **144**, 999–1007.

REYNOLDS, J., FOLLETTE, J. H. & VALENTINE, W. N. (1957). The arginase activity of erythrocytes and leukocytes with particular reference to pernicious anemia and thalassemia major. *J. Lab. clin. Med.*, **50**, 78–92.

RICH, A. (1952). Studies on the hemoglobin of Cooley's anemia and Cooley's trait. *Proc. natn. Acad. Sci. (Wash.)*, **38**, 187–196.

RIETTI, F. (1937). Les ictères hémolytiques avec augmentation de la resistance globulaire. *Ann. Méd.*, **41**, 405–416.

RIETTI, F. (1946). Haemolytic anaemias with increased osmotic resistance of the erythrocytes. *Acta med. Scand.*, **125**, 451–464.

RIETTI, F. (1950). Punctate basophilia in the erythrocyte with special reference to Rietti-Greppi-Micheli's anemia. *Acta med. Scand.*, **138**, 293–300.

RIGAS, D. A. & KOLER, R. D. (1961a). Decreased erythrocyte survival in hemoglobin H disease as a result of the abnormal properties of hemoglobin H: the benefit of splenectomy. *Blood*, **18**, 1–17.

RIGAS, D. A. & KOLER, R. D. (1961b). Erythrocyte enzymes and reduced glutathione (GSH) in hemoglobin H disease: relation to cell age and denaturation of hemoglobin H. *J. Lab. clin. Med.*, **58**, 417–424.

RIGAS, D. A., KOLER, R. D. & OSGOOD, E. E. (1955). New hemoglobin possessing a higher electrophoretic mobility than normal adult hemoglobin. *Science*, **121**, 372.

RIGAS, D. A., KOLER, R. D. & OSGOOD, E. E. (1956). Hemoglobin H. Clinical laboratory and genetic studies of a family with a previously undescribed hemoglobin. *J. Lab. clin. Med.*, **47**, 51–64.

RINGELHANN, B., EFREMOV, G. D., CSAK, E. & REVICZKY, A. (1979). Hemoglobin Lepore Washington and hemochromatosis in a Hungarian patient. *Hemoglobin*, **3**, 193–204.

RINGELHANN, B., KONOTEY-AHULU, F. I. D., LEHMANN, H. & LORKIN, P. A. (1970). A Ghanaian adult, homozygous for hereditary persistence of foetal haemoglobin and heterozygous for elliptocytosis. *Acta haemat. (Basel)*, **43**, 100–110.

ROBERTS, P. D. (1963). The thalassaemia trait in an English family. *J. clin. Path.*, **16**, 593–595.

ROBERTSON, E. F., MAXWELL, G. M. & ELLIOTT, R. B. (1963). Studies in thalassaemia major. *Med. J. Aust.*, **2**, 705–707.

ROBINSON, S., VANIER, T., DESFORGES, J. F. & SCHMID, R. (1962). Jaundice in thalassemia minor: a consequence of "ineffective erythropoiesis". *New Engl. J. Med.*, **267**, 523–529

ROCHE, J., DERRIEN, Y., DIACONO, G. & ROQUES, M. (1953). Sur les hémoglobines humaines au cours des thalassémies mineure (maladie de Rietti-Greppi-Micheli). *C. R. Soc. Biol. (Paris)*, **147**, 771–774.

ROHR, K. (1943). Familiäre hämolytische hypochrome Anämie (Anämie vom Cooleytypus beim Erwachsenen). *Helv. med. Acta*, **10**, 31–38.

RÖNISCH, P. & KLEIHAUER, E. (1967). Alpha-Thalassämie mit Hb H und Hb Bart's in einer deutschen Familie. *Klin. Wschr.*, **45**, 1193–1200.

ROSMINO, G. C., NORELLI, M. T. & GHIDELLA, G. (1968). L'uricemia in eta pediatrica. Nota III. — Nei soggetti affetti da morbo di Cooley. *Minerva pediat. (Torino)*, **20**, 308–312.

ROTHSCHILD, H., BICKERS, J. & MARCUS, R. (1976). Regulation of the β-and δ-hemoglobin genes. A family with hereditary persistence of fetal hemoglobin and β-thalassemia. *Acta haemat. (Basel)*, **56**, 285–291.

ROUABHI, F., CHARDIN, P., BOISSEL, J. P., BEGHOUL, F., LABIE, D. & BENABADJI, M. (1983). Silent β-thalassemia associated with Hb Knossos β27 (B9)

Ala → Ser in Algeria. *Hemoglobin*, 7, 555–561.

ROWLEY, P. T., BARNES, F. & WILLIAMS, E. (1969). A Lepore hemoglobin in a Rumanian family. *Hum. Hered.*, 19, 48–56.

RUSSO, G., MOLLICA, F., PAVONE, L., MUSUMECI, S. & BAGLIONI, C. (1973). Genetic implication of the interaction of two types of beta-thalassemia genes in a patient with thalassemia major. *Blood*, 42, 763–769.

RUVIDIC, R., EFREMOV, D., JURIČIĆ, D., ROLOVIĆ, Z., RUŽDIĆ, I. & PENDIC, S. (1975). Haemoglobin Beograd ($\alpha_2\beta_2$121 Glu → Val) interacting with β-thalassaemia. *Acta haemat. (Basel)*, 54, 180–187.

RYAN, B. (1961a). Thalassemia in Melanesia. *Nature (Lond.)*, 192, 75–76.

RYAN, B. P. K. (1961b). Thalassaemia major in New Guinea. *Med. J. Aust.*, 2, 753–757.

RYAN, B. P. K. (1962). Thalassaemia and anaemia of pregnancy in Papua. *Med. J. Aust.*, 1, 514–517.

RYAN, B. P., CAMPBELL, A. L. & BRAIN, P. (1961). Haemoglobin H disease in a Papuan. *Med. J. Aust.*, 2, 901–902.

SAGLIO, G., CAMASCHELLA, C., GUERRASIO, A., REGE, CAMBRIN, G., CAPALDI, A., PICH, P. G., TRENTO, M. & MAZZA, U. (1982). $^{G}\gamma$ and $^{A}\gamma$ globin chain synthesis in bone marrow and peripheral blood of β-thalassaemia homozygotes. *Brit. J. Haemat.*, 52, 225–231.

SANGHVI, L. D. & SUKUMARAN, P. K. & LEHMANN, H. (1958). Haemoglobin J trait in two Indian women, associated with thalassaemia in one. *Brit. med. J.*, ii, 828–830.

SANNA, G., FRAU, F., MELIS, M. A., GALANELLO, R., DE VIRGILIIS, A. & CAO, A. (1980). Interaction between glucose-6-phosphate dehydrogenase deficiency and thalassaemia genes at phenotype level. *Brit. J. Haemat.*, 44, 555–561.

SANSONE, G. & MASSIMO, L. (1959). Riconoscimento dei globuli rossi a diverso tipo emoglobinico su strisci di sangue fissati. Importanza del metodo nello studio delle talassemie. Nota preliminare. *Minerva pediat. (Torino)*, 11, 245–247.

SANSONE, G. & NOCETO, L. (1955). Considerazioni sulla malattia di Cooley nell'adulto. *Minerva pediat. (Torino)*, 7, 1154–1158.

SANSONE, G., ROSSO, C., ZUNIN, C. & SALOMONE, P. (1955). Studio clinico ed anatomo-patologico di due bambini con anemia di Cooley deceduti per reazione trasfusionale. *Minerva pediat. (Torino)*, 7, 1005–1031.

SARAYA, A. K., KUMAR, R., CHOUDHRY, V. P., KAILASH, S. & SEHGAL, A. K. (1985). A study of serum ferritin in beta thalassemia, iron deficiency and overload. *Amer. J. clin. Path.*, 84, 103–107.

SASS, M. D. & SPEAR. P. W. (1961). Red cell transaminase levels in anemia. II. Thalassemia minor. *J. Lab. clin. Med.*, 58, 580–585.

SCHETTINI, F., MELONI, T. & COSTA, S. (1967). Erythrokinetic studies in thalassemia with simultaneous radioactive tracers (Fe^{59} and Cr^{51}). *Acta haemat. (Basel)*, 37, 65–87.

SCHIEBER, C. (1945). Target-cell anaemia. Two cases in Bucharan Jews. *Lancet*, ii, 851–852.

SCHILIRÒ, G., LI VOLTI, S., MUSUMECI, S. & ROMEO, M. A. (1983a). Acute splenic sequestration in a child with β^{+}-thalassaemia intermedia. *Haematologica*, 68, 110–113.

SCHILIRÒ, G., MUSUMECI, S., PIZZARELLI, G., DI GREGORIO, L., FISCHER, A. & RUSSO, G. (1978). β-thalassaemia in Sicily. Hematological and biosynthetic studies. *Acta haemat. (Basel)*, 60, 193–200.

SCHILIRÒ, G., MUSUMECI, S., ROMEO, M. A., DI GREGORIO, F., RUSSO, A. TESTA, R. & RUSSO, G. (1983b). Unusual combination of genetic defects in Sicilian family: β-thalassaemia, haemoglobin Lepore Boston-Washington and heterocellular hereditary persistence of fetal haemoglobin. *Brit. J. Haemat.*, 55, 473–477.

SCHOKKER, R. C., WENT, L. N. & BOK, J. (1966). A new genetic variant of β-thalassaemia. *Nature (Lond.)*, 209, 44–46.

SCHROEDER, W. A., HUISMAN, T. H. J., SHELTON, J. T., SHELTON. J. B., KLEIHAUER, E. F., DOZY, A. M. & ROBBERSON, B. (1968). Evidence for multiple structural genes for the γ chain of human fetal hemoglobin. *Proc. natn. Acad. Sci. (U.S.A.)*, 60, 537–544.

SCHROEDER, W. A., HUISMAN, T. H. J. & SUKUMARAN, P. K. (1973). A second type of hereditary persistence of foetal haemoglobin in India. *Brit. J. Haemat.*, 25, 131–135.

SHROEDER, W. A., STURGEON, P. & BERGREN, W. R. (1962). Chemical investigation of haemoglobin F from an individual with persistent foetal haemoglobin. *Nature (Lond.)*, 193, 1161–1162.

SCHWARTZ, E. (1969). The silent carrier of beta thalassemia. *New Engl. J. Med.*, 281, 1327–1333.

SCHWARTZ, E. (1970), Heterozygous beta thalassemia: balanced globin synthesis in bone marrow cells. *Science*, 167, 1513–1514.

SCHWARTZ, E. (1974). Abnormal globin synthesis in thalassemic red cells. *Seminars Hemat.*, 11, 549–567.

SCHWARTZ, E. & ATWATER, J. (1972). Alpha-thalassemia in the American Negro. *J. clin. Invest.*, 51, 412–418.

SCHWARTZ, E., KAN, Y. W. & NATHAN, D. G. (1969). Unbalanced globin chain synthesis in alpha-thalassemia heterozygotes. *Ann. N.Y. Acad. Sci.*, 165, 288–294.

SCHWARTZ, S. O. & HARTZ, W. H. (1955). Mediterranean anemia in the Negro. A re-evaluation of four patients and their families. *Blood*, 10, 1256–1266.

SCHWARTZ, S. O. & MASON, J. (1949). Mediterranean anemia in the negro. A report of four cases and their families. *Blood*, 4, 706–721.

SCHWARZ-TIENE, E., CORDA, G. & CAREDDU, P. (1953). Modificazioni del metabolismo dei lipidi e delle porfirine nell'anemia mediterranea. *Minerva pediat. (Torino)*, **5**, 829–836.

SCIARRATTA, G. V., PARODI, M. I., AGOSTI VALLERINO, S. F. & SANSONE, G. (1985). The silent carrier of β-thalassemia. *Ann. N.Y. Acad. Sci.*, **445**, 111–118.

SCOTT, G. L., RASBRIDGE, M. R. & GRIMES, A. J. (1970). *In vitro* studies of red cell metabolism in haemoglobin H disease. *Brit. J. Haemat.*, **18**, 13–28.

SCOTT, R. B., FERGUSON, A. D. & JENKINS, M. E. (1962). Thalassemia major (Mediterranean or Cooley's anemia). Report of two cases in negro children. *Amer. J. Dis. Child.*, **104**, 74–81.

SELWYN, J. G. (1953). Unpublished observations.

SFIKAKIS, P. & STAMATOYANNOPOULOS, G. (1963). Bone changes in thalassaemia trait. An X-ray appraisal of 55 cases. *Acta haemat. (Basel)*, **29**, 193–201.

SHALEV, O., MOGILNER, S., SHINAR, E., RACHMILEWITZ, E. A. & SCHRIER, S. L. (1984). Impaired erythrocyte calcium homeostasis in β-thalassemia. *Blood*, **64**, 564–566.

SHEPARD, M. K., WEATHERALL, D. J. & CONLEY, C. L. (1962). Semi-quantitative estimation of the distribution of fetal hemoglobin in red cell populations. *Bull. Johns Hopk. Hosp.*, **110**, 293–310.

SHIBATA, S., MIYAJI, T., MATSUDA, N. & OHBA, Y. (1966). A family of high fetal hemoglobin with incidental occurrence of an unclassified hemolytic anemia. *Proc. Jap. Acad.*, **42**, 847–852.

SIDDOO, J. K., COADY, C. J., MORGAN-DEAN, L. & PERRY, W. H. (1956). Mediterranean anaemia in Chinese Canadians. *Canad. med. Ass. J.*, **74**, 124–130.

SIDDOO, J. K., SIDDOO, S. K., CHASE, W. H., MORGAN-DEAN, L. & PERRY, W. H. (1956). Thalassemia in Sikhs. *Blood*, **11**, 197–210.

SILVER, H. K. (1950). Mediterranean anemia in children of non-Mediterranean ancestry. *Amer. J. Dis. Child.*, **80**, 767–778.

SILVERBERG, J. H. & SHOTTON, D. (1951). Mediterranean anemia (hereditary leptocytosis) in a Chinese family. *New Engl. J. Med.*, **245**, 688–690.

SILVESTRONI, E. & BIANCO, I. (1946). Una particolare anomalia ematologica: la "microcitemia" *Minerva med. (Torino)*, **37**, 206–211.

SILVESTRONI, E. & BIANCO, 1. (1948). Sulla frequenza della microcitemia nel Ferrarese ed in alcune altre regioni d'Italia. *Policlinico (Sez. prat.)*, **55**, 417–420.

SILVESTRONI, E. & BIANCO, I. (1957). Sulla resistenza nella popolazione italiana di soggetti non microcitemici portatori di un'elevata quota di emoglobina adulta lenta (Hb A₂) e sui loro rapporti con i malati di anemia microcitica. *Policlinico (Sez. prat.)*, **64**, 1868–1872.

SILVESTRONI, E. & BIANCO, I. (1959). The distribution of microcythaemias (or thalassaemias) in Italy. Some aspects of the haematological and haemoglobinic picture in these haemopathies. In: *Abnormal Haemoglobins. A Symposium*, pp. 243–259. Blackwell Scientific Publications, Oxford.

SILVESTRONI, E. & BIANCO, I. (1961). Association of haemoglobin N and microcythaemia in a Sardinian family. *Nature (Lond.)*, **191**, 1208–1209.

SILVESTRONI, E. & BIANCO, I. (1962). Haemoglobin Bart's in Italy. *Nature (Lond.)*, **195**, 394.

SILVESTRONI, E. & BIANCO, I. (1963). Primo caso di malattia da Hb Lepore-microcitemia osservato in Italia. *Policlinico (Sez. prat.)*, **70**, 1513–1517.

SILVESTRONI, E. & BIANCO, I. (1965). Microcitemia con abbondante Hb F ed Hb A₂ normale in the famiglie pugliesi. *Polinclinico (Sez. prat.)*, **72**, 1381–1388.

SILVESTRONI, E. & BIANCO, I. (1966). Pluralità delle microcitemie (O thalassaemia). *Policlinico (Sez. prat.)*, **73**, 41–71.

SILVESTRONI, E. & BIANCO, I. (1975). Screening for microcytemia in Italy: analysis of data collected in the last 30 years. *Amer. J. hum. Genet.*, **27**, 198–212.

SILVESTRONI, E., BIANCO, I. & BRANCATI, C. (1964). Presenza di microcitemia con quota normale di emoglobina A₂ e quota elevata di emoglobina F in una famiglia calabrese (terza varietà di microcitemia). *Policlinico (Sez. prat.)*, **71**, 1543–1545.

SILVESTRONI, E., BIANCO, I. & GRAZIANI, B. (1968). The haemoglobin picture in Cooley's disease. *Brit. J. Haemat.*, **14**, 303–308.

SILVESTRONI, E., BIANCO, I. GRAZIANI, B. & CARBONI, C. (1978). Heterozygous β-thalassaemia with normal haemoglobin pattern. Haematologic, haemoglobin and biosynthesis study of 4 families. *Acta haemat. (Basel)*, **59**, 332–340.

SILVESTRONI, E., BIANCO, I. & MURATORE, F. (1965). Su un nuovo tipo di microcitemia con alta Hb A₂ ed alta Hb F. Descrizione di una famiglia. *Progr. med. (Roma)*, **21**, 491–495.

SILVESTRONI, E., BIANCO, I. & REITANO, G. (1968). Three cases of homozygous βδ-thalassaemia (or microcythaemia) with high haemoglobin F in a Sicilian family. *Acta haemat. (Basel)*, **40**, 220–229.

SILVESTRONI, E., BIANCO, I. & VALLISNERI, E. (1949). Nuovo contributo allo studio della questione genetica del morbo di Cooley. *Minerva paediat. (Torino)*, **1**, 136–141.

SINGER, K., CHERNOFF, A. I. & SINGER, L. (1951). Studies on abnormal hemoglobins. I. Their demonstration in sickle-cell anemia and other hematologic disorders by means of alkali denaturation. *Blood*, **6**, 413–435.

SINISCALCO, M., BERNINI, L., FILIPPI, G., LATTE, B., MEERA KAHN, P., PIOMELLI, S. & RATTAZZI, M. (1966). Population genetics of haemoglobin variants, thalassaemia and glucose-6-phosphate dehydrogenase deficiency, with particular reference to the malaria hypothesis. *Bull. Wld Hlth Org.*, **34**, 379–393.

SINISCALCO, M., BERNINI, L., LATTE, B. & MOTULSKY, A. G. (1961). Favism and thalassaemia in Sardinia and their relationship to malaria. *Nature (Lond.)*, **190**, 1179–1180.

SINNIAH, D., VIGNAENDRA, V. & AHMAD, K. (1977). Neurological complications of β-thalassaemia major. *Arch. Dis. Childh.*, **52**, 977–979.

SITARZ, A. L., ULTMANN, J. E. & WOLFF, J. A. (1963). Erythrocyte life-span and sites of destruction in thalassaemia major. Relation to clinical and laboratory findings. *Acta haemat. (Basel)*, **30**, 204–214.

SJÖLIN, S., WALLENIUS, G. & WRANNE, L. (1964). Haemoglobin Bart's and H in a Swedish boy. *Acta haemat. (Basel)*, **32**, 239–249.

SMITH, C. H. (1942). Mediterranean (Cooley's) anemia in a youth of nineteen years observed since early childhood. *J. Pediat.*, **20**, 370–382.

SMITH, C. H. (1943). Familial blood studies in cases of Mediterranean (Cooley's) anemia. Diagnosis of the trait, or mild form of the disease. *Amer. J. Dis. Child.*, **65**, 681–701.

SMITH, C. H. (1948). Detection of mild types of Mediterranean (Cooley's) anemia. *Amer. J. Dis. Child.*, **75**, 505–527.

SMITH, C. H., ERLANDSON, M. E., STERN, G. & HILGARTNER, M. W. (1962). Postsplenectomy infection in Cooley's anemia: an appraisal of the problem in this and other blood disorders, with a consideration of prophylaxis. *New Engl. J. Med.*, **266**, 737–743.

SMITH, C. H. & MORGENTHAU, J. E. (1951). Cholelithiasis in severe Mediterranean (Cooley's) anemia. *Blood*, **6**, 1147–1151.

SMITH, C. H., SCHULMAN, I., ANDO, R. E. & STERN, G. (1955). Studies in Mediterranean (Cooley's) anemia. I. Clinical and hematologic aspects of splenectomy, with special reference to fetal hemoglobin synthesis. *Blood*, **10**, 582–599.

SMITH, C. H., SISSON, T. R. C., FLOYD, W. H. JNR & SIEGAL, S. (1950). Serum iron and iron-binding capacity of the serum in children with severe Mediterranean (Cooley's) anemia. *Pediatrics*, **5**, 799–807.

SMITH, C. M. II, HEDLUND, B., CICH, J. A., TUKEY, D. P., OLSON, M., STEINBERG, M. H. & ADAMS, J. G. III (1983). Hemoglobin North Shore: a variant hemoglobin associated with the phenotype of β-thalassemia. *Blood*, **61**, 378–383.

SMITH, D. H., CLEGG, J. B., WEATHERALL, D. J. & GILLIS, H. M. (1973). Hereditary persistence of foetal haemoglobin associated with γβ fusion variant, haemoglobin Kenya. *Nature new Biol.*, **246**, 184–186.

SOFRONIADOU, K., KALTSOYA, A., LOUKOPOULOS, D.

& FESSAS, PH. (1968). Hemoglobin "Athens": an alpha-chain variant with unusual properties. *XII Congr. int. Soc. Hemat., New York*. Plenary Session papers, p.56 (Abstract K-13).

SORSDAHL, O. S., TAYLOR, P. E. & NOYES, W. D. (1964). Extramedullary hematopoiesis, mediastinal masses and spinal cord compression. *J. Amer. med. Ass.*, **189**, 343–347.

SPECTER, J. & FRUMIN, A. M. (1953). Cholelithiasis in hereditary leptocytosis (Mediterranean trait). *Gastroenterology*, **23**, 493–494 .

STAMATOYANNOPOULOS, G. (1971). Gamma-thalassaemia. *Lancet*. **ii**, 192–193.

STAMATOYANNOPOULOS, G. & FESSAS, PH. (1964). Thalassaemia, glucose-6-phosphate dehydrogenase deficiency, sickling, and malaria endemicity in Greece: a study of five areas. *Brit. med. J.*, **i**, 875–879.

STAMATOYANNOPOULOS, G., FESSAS, PH. & PAPAYANNOPOULOU, TH. (1969). F-thalassemia. A study of thirty-one families with simple heterozygotes and combinations of F-thalassemia with A$_2$-thalassemia. *Amer. J. Med.*, **47**, 194–208.

STAMATOYANNOPOULOS, G., PAPAYANNOPOULOU, T., FESSAS, P. & MOTULSKY, A. G. (1969). The beta-delta thalassemias. *Ann. N.Y. Acad. Sci.*, **165**, 25–36.

STAMATOYANNOPOULOS, G., PAPAYANNOPOULOU, T., WOODSON, W., HEYWOOD, D. & KURACHI, S. (1974a). A new form of β-thalassemia trait. *Ann. N.Y. Acad. Sci.*, **232**, 159–167.

STAMATOYANNOPOULOS, G., SCHROEDER, W. A., HUISMAN, T. H. J., SHELTON, J. R., SHELTON, J. B., APELL, G. & BOUVER, N. (1971). Nature of foetal haemoglobin in F-thalassaemia. *Brit. J. Haemat.*, **21**, 633–642.

STAMATOYANNOPOULOS, G., WOOD, W. G., PAPAYANNOPOULOU, T. & NUTE, P. E. (1975). A new form of hereditary persistence of fetal hemoglobin in blacks and its association with sickle cell trait. *Blood*, **46**, 683–692.

STAMATOYANNOPOULOS, G., WOODSON, R., PAPAYANNOPOULOU, TH., HEYWOOD, D. & KURACHI, S. (1974b). Inclusion-body β-thalassemia trait. *New Engl. J. Med.*, **290**, 939–943.

STATHOPOULOU, R., SULIS, E. & LEHMANN, H. (1979). Interaction between β-thalassaemia and Hb G Philadelphia associated with α-thalassaemia. *Acta haemat. (Basel)*, **62**, 106–111.

STERN, M. A., KYNOCH, P. A. M. & LEHMANN, H. (1968). β-thalassaemia, glucose-6-phosphate-dehydrogenase deficiency, and haemoglobin D-Punjab in Pathans. *Lancet*, **ii**, 1284–1285.

STIJNS, J. & CHARLES, P. (1956). La tare thalassémique chez les Bantous d'Afrique centrale. *Ann. Soc. belge. Med. trop.*, **36**, 763–780.

STOCKS, J., KEMP, M. & DORMANDY, T. L. (1971). Increased susceptibility of red-blood-cell lipids to autoxidation in haemolytic states. *Lancet*, **i**, 266–269.

STRAUSS, M. S., DALAND, G. A. & FOX, H. J. (1941). Familial microcytic anemia. Observations on 6 cases of a blood disorder in an Italian family. *Amer. J. Med. Sci.*, **201**, 30–34.

STURGEON, P., CHEN, L. P. L. & BERGREN, W. R. (1958). Free erythrocyte porphyrins in thalassemia: preliminary observations. *Proc. sixth int. Congr. Hemat., Boston*, p. 730. Grune and Stratton, New York.

STURGEON, P. & FINCH, C. A. (1957). Erythrokinetics in Cooley's anemia. *Blood*, **12**, 64–73.

STURGEON, P., ITANO, H. A. & BERGREN, W. R. (1955). Genetic and biochemical studies of 'intermediate' types of Cooley's anaemia. *Brit. J. Haemat.*, **1**, 264–276.

STURGEON, P., ITANO, H. A. & VALENTINE, W. N. (1953). Chronic hemolytic anemia associated with thalassemia and sickling traits. *Blood*, **7**, 350–357.

STURGEON, P., SCHROEDER, W. A., JONES, R. T. & BERGREN, W. R. (1963). The relation of alkali-resistant haemoglobin in thalassaemia and abnormal haemoglobin syndromes to foetal haemoglobin. *Brit. J. Haemat.*, **9**, 438–445.

SUKUMARAN, P. K., HUISMAN, T. H. J., SCHROEDER, W. A., McCURDY, P. R., FREEHAFER, J. T., BOUVER, N., SHELTON, J. R., SHELTON, J. B. & APELL, G. (1972a). A homozygote for the Hb$_{G\gamma}$ type of foetal haemoglobin in India: a study of two Indian and four Negro families. *Brit. J. Haemat.*, **23**, 403–417.

SUKUMARAN, P. K., MERCHANT, S. M., DESAI, M. P., WILTSHIRE, B. G. & LEHMANN, H. (1972b). Haemoglobin Q India (β64 (E13) aspartic acid → histidine) associated with β-thalassaemia observed in three Sindhi families. *J. med. Genet.*, **9**, 436–442.

SULIS, E., FIORELLI, G., ALESSIO, L. & PABIS, A. (1968). G-6-PD Mangel mit Hämoglobinopathie und alpha-Thalassämie. *Acta haemat. (Basel)*, **39**, 167–173.

SURREY, S., OHENE-FREMPONG, K., RAPPAPORT, E., ATWATER, J. & SCHWARTZ, E. (1980a). α thalassaemia and the expression of hemoglobin G-Philadelphia. *Ann. N.Y. Acad. Sci.*, **334**, 62–72.

SURREY, S. K., OHENE-FREMPONG, K., RAPPAPORT, E., ATWATER, J. & SCHWARTZ, E. (1980b). Lingkage of α$^{G-Philadelphia}$ to α-thalassaemia. *Proc. natn. Acad. Sci. U.S.A.*, **77**, 4885–4889.

SWARUP, S., GHOSH, S. K. & CHATTERJEA, J. B. (1960). Observations on autohaemolysis in thalassaemia syndrome. *Proc. nat. Inst. Sci. India*, **26**, B (Suppl. 1), 158–164.

SYDENSTRYCKER, V. P., HORTON, B., PAYNE, R. A. & HUISMAN, T. H. J. (1961). Studies on a fast hemoglobin variant found in a negro family in association with thalassemia. *Clin. chim. Acta*, **6**, 677–685.

TAJ-ELDIN, S., AL-RABII, H., JAWAD, J. & FAKHRI, G. (1968). Thalassemia in Iraq. *Ann. trop. Med. Parasit.*, **62**, 147–153.

TAMAGNINI, G. P., LOPES, M. C., CASTANHEIRA, M. E., WAINSCOAT, J. S. & WOOD, W. G. (1983). β$^+$ thalassaemia — Portuguese type: clinical, haematological and molecular studies of a newly defined form of β thalassaemia. *Brit. J. Haemat.*, **54**, 189–200.

TASSIOPOULOS, TH., KALTSOYA-TASSIOPOULOS, A., ALCHANATI, N., ROMBOS, J., POURNARAS, N. & FESSAS, PH. (1982). Anémie, 2,3-DPG et oxygénation tissulaire chez les heterozygotes de β-thalassémie. *Nouv. Rev. franç. Hémat.*, **24**, 359–362.

THEIN, S. L., AL-HAKIM, I. & HOFFBRAND, A. V. (1984). Thalassaemia intermedia: a new molecular basis. *Brit. J. Haemat.*, **56**, 333–337.

THEIN, S. L., OLD, J. M., WAINSCOAT, J. S., PETROU, M., MODELL, B. & WEATHERALL, D. J. (1984). Population and genetic studies suggest a single origin for the Indian deletion β° thalassaemia. *Brit. J. Haemat.*, **57**, 271–278.

THOMPSON, A. R., WOOD, W. G. & STAMATOYANNOPOULOS, G. (1977). X-linked syndrome of platelet dysfunction, thrombocytopenia, and imbalanced globin chain synthesis with hemolysis. *Blood*, **50**, 303–316.

THOMPSON, G. R., & LEHMANN, H. (1962). Combinations of high levels of haemoglobin F with haemoglobins A, S, and C in Ghana. *Brit. med. J.*, **i**, 1521–1523.

THOMPSON, R. B., HEWITT, B. JNR, ARD, E., ODOM, J. & BELL, W. N. (1966). A new thalassemic syndrome: homozygous hemoglobin S disease delta thalassemia. *Acta haemat. (Basel)*, **36**, 412–417.

THOMPSON, R. B., MITCHENER, J. W. & HUISMAN, T. H. J. (1961). Studies on the fetal hemoglobin in the persistent high Hb-F anomaly. *Blood*, **18**, 267–283.

THOMPSON, R. B., WARRINGTON, R., ODOM, J. & BELL, W. N. (1965). Interaction between genes for delta thalassaemia and hereditary persistence of foetal hemoglobin. *Acta genet. (Basel)*, **15**, 190–200.

THUMASATHIT, B., NONDASUTA, A., SILPISORNKOSOL, S., LOUSUEBSAKUL, B., UNCHALIPONGSE, P. & MANGKORNKANOK, M. (1968). Hydrops fetalis associated with Bart's hemoglobin in Northern Thailand. *J. Pediat.*, **73**, 132–138.

TODD, D. (1971). Slow-moving haemoglobin bands in haemoglobin-H disease. *Lancet*, **ii**, 439 (Letter).

TODD, D., LAI, M. C. S., BEAVEN, G. H. & HUEHNS, E. R. (1970). The abnormal haemoglobins in homozygous α-thalassaemia. *Brit. J. Haemat.*, **19**, 27–31.

TODD, D., LAI, M. & BRAGA, C. A. (1967). Thalassaemia and hydrops foetalis — family studies. *Brit. med. J.*, **ii**, 347–349.

TODD, D., LAI, M. C. S., BRAGA, C. A. & SOO, H. N. (1969). Alpha-thalassaemia in Chinese: cord blood studies. *Brit. J. Haemat.*, **16**, 551–556.

TOLENTINO, P. (1951). Mechanical fragility of thalassaemic erythrocytes. *Nature (Lond.)*, **167**, 905.

TOVO, P. A., MINIERO, R., BARBERA, C., SACCHETTI, L. & SAITTA, M. (1981). Serum immunoglobulins in homozygous β-thalassaemia. *Acta haemat. (Basel)*, **65**, 21–25.

TRENT, R. J., JONES, R. W., CLEGG, J. B., WEATHERALL, D. J., DAVIDSON, R. & WOOD, W. G. (1984). (Aγδβ)° thalassaemia: similarity of phenotype in four different molecular defects, including one newly described. *Brit. J. Haemat.*, **57**, 279–289.

TRENT, R. J., WAINSCOAT, J. S., HUEHNS, E. R., CLEGG, J. B. & WEATHERALL, D. J. (1982). The molecular basis for β° thalassaemia intermedia in an Iranian individual. *Brit. J. Haemat.*, **52**, 511–516.

TSISTRAKIS, G. A., AMARANTOS, S. P. & KOUKOURIS, L. L. (1974). Homozygous βδ-thalassaemia. Description of a case and review of the literature. *Acta haemat. (Basel)*, **51**, 185–191.

TSO, S. C. (1972). Red cell survival studies in haemoglobin H disease using [51Cr]chromate and [32P]diisopropyl phosphofluoridate. *Brit. J. Haemat.*, **23**, 621–629.

TSO, S. C., LOH, T. T. & TODD, D. (1984). Iron overload in patients with haemoglobin H disease. *Scand. J. Haemat.*, **32**, 391–394.

TUCHINDA, S., BEALE, D. & LEHMANN, H. (1965). A new haemoglobin in a Thai family. A case of haemglobin Siriraj-β thalassaemia. *Brit. med. J.*, **i**, 1583–1585.

TUCHINDA, S., VAREENIL, C., BHANCHIT, P. & MINNICH, V. (1959). Fast hemoglobin component found in umbilical-cord blood of Thai babies. *Pediatrics*, **24**, 43–49.

VALENTINE, W. N. & NEEL, J. V. (1944). Hematologic and genetic study of the transmission of thalassemia (Cooley's anemia; Mediterranean anemia). *Arch. intern. Med.*, **74**, 185–196.

VALENTINE, W. N. & NEEL, J. V. (1948). A statistical study of the hematologic variables in subjects with thalassemia minor. *Amer. J. med. Sci.*, **215**, 456–460.

VAN DER PLOEG, L. H. T., KONINGS, A., OORT, M., ROOS, D., BERNINI, L. & FLAVELL, R. A. (1980). γ-β-thalassaemia studies showing that deletion of the γ- and δ-genes influences β-globin gene expression in man. *Nature (Lond.)*, **283**, 637–642.

VANELLA, A., RIZZA, V., LI VOLTI, R., PINTURO, R., MUSUMECI, S. & MOLLICA, F. (1980). Effect of polyamines on autohemolysis: studies on normal and thalassemic children. *Acta haemat. (Basel)*, **63**, 226–229.

VAVRA, J. D. & MAYER, V. K. (1964). In vitro porphyrin synthesis by human blood: porphyrin synthesis by thalassemic erythrocytes. *J. Lab. clin. Med.*, **63**, 754–771.

VAVRA, J. D., MAYER, V. K. & MOORE, C. V. (1964). In vitro heme synthesis by human blood: abnormal heme synthesis in thalassemia major. *J. Lab. clin. Med.*, **63**, 736–753.

VAYÁ, A., CARRATALÁ, A., MARTINEZ, C. & AZNAR, J. (1983). Haematological and clinical data in 200 cases of thalassaemia trait in Eastern Spain. *Nouv. Rev. franç. Hémat.*, **25**, 369–373.

VECCHIO, F. (1946). Sulla resistenza della emoglobina alla denaturazione alcalina in alcune sindromi emopatiche. *Pediatria (Napoli)*, **54**, 545–554.

VECCHIO, F. (1948). Sulla resistenza dell'emoglobina alla denaturazione alcalina negli ammalati di anemia di Cooley e nei loro familiari. *Progr. med. (Napoli)*, **4**, 201–206.

VELLA, F. (1960). Erythrocyte glucose-6-phosphate dehydrogenase deficiency and thalassaemia. *Experientia (Basel)*, **16**, 284–285.

VELLA, F. (1961). La microcitemia costituzionale fra Siriani, Armeni, Indiani, Italiani e Etiopici a Khartoum. *Policlinico (Sez. prat.)*, **68**, 625–627.

VELLA, F. (1962). The frequency of thalassaemia minor in the Maltese islands. *Acta haemat. (Basel)*, **27**, 278–288.

VELLA, F. & HASSAN, M. M. (1961). Thalassaemia major in a Sudanese Arab family. *J. trop. Med. Hyg.*, **64**, 199–201.

VELLA, F. & IBRAHIM, S. A. (1961). The frequency of thalassaemia minor in a Greek community. *J. trop. Med. Hyg.*, **64**, 202–206.

VELLA, F. & MOUSSA, W. G. (1962). Thalassaemia minor in school children of Egyptian and Egyptian-Sudanese parentage. *Trans. roy. Soc. trop. Med. Hyg.*, **56**, 70–73.

VELLA, F., WELLS, R. H. G., AGER, J. A. M. & LEHMANN, H. (1958). A haemoglobinopathy involving haemoglobin H and a new (Q) haemoglobin. *Brit. med. J.*, **i**, 752–755.

VILLEGAS, A., ESPINOS, D., ALVAREZ-SALA, J. L., CALERO, F., VALVERDE, F., ROBB, L. & LEHMANN, H. (1983). Haemoglobin Lepore_Baltimore in a Spanish family. *Acta haemat. (Basel)*, **69**, 192–194.

VIVES CORRONS, J. LL., AGUILAR, J. LL. & MATEO, M. (1983). Haemoglobin H (Hb H) disease and severe glutathione peroxidase deficiency: an undescribed association in a mentally retarded child. *Brit. J. Haemat.*, **54**, 160–161 (Letter).

VIVES CORRONS, J. L., PUJADES, M. A., AQUILAR I BASCOMPTE, J. L., JOU, J. M., ROZMAN, C. & ESTER, A. (1984). Pyrimidine 5'nucleotidase and several other red cell enzyme activities in β-thalassaemia trait. *Brit. J. Haemat.*, **56**, 483–494.

VULLO, C. & TUNIOLI, A. M. (1958). Survival studies of thalassemic erythrocytes transfused into donors, into subjects with thalassemia minor and into normal and splenectomized subjects. *Blood*, **13**, 803–810.

WAINSCOAT, J. S., KANAVAKIS, E., WOOD, W. G., LETSKY, E. A., HUEHNS, E. R., MARSH, G. W., HIGGS, D. R., CLEGG, J. B. & WEATHERALL, D. J.

(1983). Thalassaemia intermedia in Cyprus: the interaction of α and β thalassaemia. *Brit. J. Haemat.*, **53**, 411–416.

WAINSCOAT, J. S., OLD, J. M., WOOD, W. G., TRENT, R. J. & WEATHERALL, D. J. (1984). Characterization of an Indian (δβ)° thalassaemia. *Brit. J. Haemat.*, **58**, 353–360.

WALFORD, D. M. & DEACON, R. (1976). Alpha-thalassaemia trait in various racial groups in the United Kingdom: characterization of a variant of alpha-thalassaemia in Indians. *Brit. J. Haemat.*, **34**, 193–206.

WALKER, E. H., WHELTON, M. J. & BEAVEN, G. H. (1969). Successful pregnancy in a patient with thalassaemia major. *J. Obstet. Gynaec. Brit. Commonwlth*, **76**, 549–553.

WAPNICK, A. A., LYNCH, S. R., CHARLTON, R. W., SEFTEL, H. C. & BOTHWELL, T. H. (1969). The effect of ascorbic acid deficiency on desferrioxamine-induced urinary iron excretion. *Brit. J. Haemat.*, **17**, 563–568.

WASI, P., NA-NAKORN, S. & POOTRAKUL, S.-N. (1974). The α thalassaemias. *Clinics Haemat.*, **3**, 383–410.

WASI, P., NA-NAKORN, S., POOTRAKUL, S., SOOKANEK, M., DISTHASONGCHAN, P., PORNPATKUL, M. & PANICH, V. (1969). Alpha- and beta-thalassaemia in Thailand. *Ann. N.Y. Acad. Sci.*, **165**, 60–82.

WASI, P., NA-NAKORN, S. & SUINDUMRONG, A. (1964). Haemoglobin H disease in Thailand: a genetical study. *Nature (Lond.)*, **204**, 907–908.

WASI, P., POOTRAKUL, S. & NA-NAKORN, S. (1968). Hereditary persistence of foetal haemoglobin in a Thai family: the first instance in the mongol race and in association with haemoglobin E. *Brit. J. Haemat.*, **14**, 501–506.

WASI, P., POOTRAKUL, S., POOTRAKUL, P., PRAVATMUANG, P., WINICHAGOON, P. & FUCHAROEN, S. (1980). Thalassemia in Thailand. *Ann. N.Y. Acad. Sci.*, **334**, 352–363.

WEATHERALL, D. J. (1963). Abnormal haemoglobins in the neonatal period and their relationship to thalassaemia. *Brit. J. Haemat.*, **9**, 265–277.

WEATHERALL, D. J. (1964a). Biochemical phenotypes of thalassemia in the American negro population. *Ann. N.Y. Acad. Sci.*, **119**, 450–462.

WEATHERALL, D. J. (1964b). Relationship of hemoglobin Bart's and H to alpha thalassemia. *Ann. N.Y. Acad. Sci.*, **119**, 463–473.

WEATHERALL, D. J. (1965). *The Thalassaemia Syndromes*. 272 pp. Blackwell Scientific Publications, Oxford.

WEATHERALL, D. J. (1969). The genetics of the thalassaemias. *Brit. med. Bull.*, **25**, 24–29.

WEATHERALL, D. J. (1980). Towards an understanding of the molecular biology of some common inherited anemias: the story of thalassemia. In: *Blood, Pure and Eloquent: a Story of Discovery, of People, and of Ideas* (ed. by M. M. Wintrobe), pp. 373–414. McGraw-Hill, New York.

WEATHERALL, D. J., CARTNER, R., CLEGG, J. B., WOOD, W. G., MACRAE, I. A. & MACKENZIE, A. (1975). A form of hereditary persistence of fetal haemoglobin characterized by uneven cellular distribution of haemoglobin F and the production of haemoglobins A and A₂ in homozygotes. *Brit. J. Haemat.*, **29**, 205–220.

WEATHERALL, D. J. & CLEGG, J. B. (1969). Disordered globin synthesis in thalassemia. *Ann. N.Y. Acad. Sci.*, **165**, 242–252.

WEATHERALL, D. J. & CLEGG, J. B. (1971). Haemoglobin synthesis in thalassaemia: two new molecular mechanisms for the production of the clinical picture of thalassaemia. *Hämat. Bluttransfusion*, **10**, 237–239.

WEATHERALL, D. J. & CLEGG, J. B. (1972). *The Thalassaemia Syndromes*, 2nd edn. 374 pp. Blackwell Scientific Publications, Oxford.

WEATHERALL, D. J. & CLEGG, J. B. (1981). *The Thalassaemia Sydnromes*, 3rd edn. 875 pp. Blackwell Scientific Publications, Oxford.

WEATHERALL, D. J., CLEGG, J. B., KNOX-MACAULAY, H. H. M., BUNCH, C., HOPKINS, C. R. & TEMPERLEY, I. J. (1973). A genetically determined disorder with features both of thalassaemia and congenital dyserythropoietic anaemia. *Brit. J. Haemat.*, **24**, 681–702.

WEATHERALL, D. J. CLEGG, J. B., NA-NAKORN, S. & WASI, P. (1969). The pattern of disordered haemoglobin synthesis in homozygous and heterozygous β-thalassaemia. *Brit. J. Haemat.*, **16**, 251–267.

WEATHERALL, D. J., CLEGG, J. B. & NAUGHTON, M. A. (1965). Globin synthesis in thalassaemia: an *in vitro* study. *Nature (Lond.)*, **208**, 1061–1065.

WEATHERALL, D. J., CLEGG, J. B. & WONG, H. B. (1970). The haemoglobin constitution of infants with the haemoglobin Bart's hydrops foetalis syndrome. *Brit. J. Haemat.*, **18**, 357–367.

WEATHERALL, D. J., CLEGG, J. B., WOOD, W. G., OLD, J. M., HIGGS, D. R., PRESSLEY, L. & DARBRE, P. D. (1980). The clinical and molecular heterogeneity of the thalassemia syndromes. *Ann N.Y. Acad. Sci.* **334**, 83–100.

WEATHERALL, D. J., HIGGS, D. R., BUNCH, C., OLD, J. M., HUNT, D. M., PRESSLEY, L., CLEGG, J. B., BETHLENFALVAY, N., SJOLIN, S., KOLER, R. D., MAGENIS, E., FRANCIS, J. L. & BEBBINGTON, D. (1981a). Hemoglobin H disease and mental retardation. A new syndrome or a remarkable coincidence? *New Engl. J. Med.*, **305**, 607–612.

WEATHERALL, D. J., HIGGS, D. R., CLEGG, J. B. & WOOD, W. G. (1982). The significance of haemoglobin H in patients with mental retardation or myeloproliferative disease. *Brit. J. Haemat.*, **52**, 351–355 (Annotation).

WEATHERALL, D. J., PRESSLEY, L., WOOD, W. G.,

HIGGS, D. R. & CLEGG, J. B. (1981b). Molecular basis for mild forms of homozygous beta-thalassaemia. *Lancet*, i, 527–529.

WEATHERALL, D. J. & VELLA, F. (1960). Thalassaemia in a Gurkha family. *Brit. med. J.*, i, 1711–1713.

WEATHERALL, D. J., WAINSCOAT, J. S., THEIN, S. L., OLD, J. M., WOOD, W. G., HIGGS, D. R. & CLEGG, J. B. (1985). Genetic and molecular analysis of mild forms of homozygous β-thalassaemia. *Ann. N.Y. Acad. Sci.*, 445, 68–80.

WENT, L. N. & MACIVER, J. E. (1958). An unusual type of hemoglobinopathy resembling sickle cell-thalassaemia in a Jamaican family. *Blood*, 13, 559–568.

WENT, L. N. & MACIVER, J. E. (1961). Thalassemia in the West Indies. *Blood*, 17, 166–181.

WHEELER, J. T. & KREVANS, J. R. (1961). The homozygous state of persistent fetal hemoglobin and the interaction of persistent fetal hemoglobin with thalassemia. *Bull. Johns Hopk. Hosp.*, 109, 217–233.

WHIPPLE, G. H. & BRADFORD, W. L. (1932). Racial or familial anemia of children associated with fundamental disturbances of bone and pigment metabolism (Cooley-von Jaksch). *Amer. J. Dis. Child.*, 44, 336–365.

WHIPPLE, G. H. & BRADFORD, W. L. (1936). Mediterranean disease — thalassemia (erythroblastic anemia of Cooley): associated pigment abnormalities simulating hemochromatosis. *J. Pediat.*, 9, 279–311.

WHITE, J. C. & BEAVEN, G. H. (1959). Foetal haemoglobin. *Brit. med. Bull.*, 15, 33–39.

WHITE, J. M., BYRNE, M., RICHARDS, R., BUCHANON, T., SHEIK-YOUSOUF, I., WHITE, Y. S. & FROST, B. (1985). Thalassaemia genes in Peninsular Arabs. *Brit. J. Haemat.*, 60, 269–278.

WHITE, J. M. & JONES, R. W. (1969). Management of pregnancy in a woman with Hb H disease. *Brit. med. J.*, iv, 473–474.

WHITE, J. M., LANG, A. & LEHMANN, H. (1972). Compensation of β chain synthesis by the single β chain gene in Hb Lepore trait. *Nature new Biol.*, 240, 271–273.

WHITE, J. M., LANG, A., LORKIN, P. A., LEHMANN, H. & REEVE, J. (1972). Synthesis of haemoglobin Lepore. *Nature new Biol.*, 235, 208–210.

WHITE, J. M., RICHARDS, R., BYRNE, M., BUCHANAN, T., WHITE, Y. S. & JELENSKI, G. (1985). Thalassaemia trait and pregnancy. *J. clin. Path.*, 38, 810–817.

WHO WORKING GROUP (1982). Hereditary anaemias: genetic basis, clinical features, diagnosis, and treatment. *Bull. Wld Hlth Org.*, 60, 643–660.

WICKRAMASINGHE, S. N., HUGHES, M., FUCHAROEN, S. & WASI, P. (1985). The morphology of redox-dye-treated HbH-containing red cells: differences between cells treated with brilliant cresyl blue, methylene blue and new methylene blue. *Clin. lab. Haemat.*, 7, 353–358.

WICKRAMASINGHE, S. N., HUGHES, M., HIGGS, D. R. & WEATHERALL, D. J. (1981). Ultrastructure of red cells containing haemoglobin H inclusions induced by redox dyes. *Clin. lab. Haemat.*, 3, 51–60.

WILEY, J. S. (1980). Increased erythrocyte cation permeability in thalassemia and conditions of marrow stress. *J. clin. Invest.*, 67, 917–922.

WILKINSON, T., GOUGH, P., OWEN, M. C., CARRELL, R. W. & KRONENBERG, H. (1975). The isolation and identification of haemoglobin Lepore Boston (Washington) in an Australian family. *Med. J. Aust.*, 2, 706–709.

WILKINSON, T., KRONENBERG, H., BEALE, D. & LEHMANN, H. (1967a). The second observation of haemoglobin Norfolk occurring in an Italian family together with beta-thalassaemia. *Med. J. Aust.*, 1, 910–913.

WILKINSON, T., KRONENBERG, H., ISAACS, W. A. & LEHMANN, H. (1967b). Haemoglobin J Baltimore interacting with beta-thalassaemia in an Australian family. *Med. J. Aust.*, 1, 907–910.

WILLIAMS, C. E. & SIEMSEN, A. W. (1968). Hemosiderosis in association with thalassemia minor. *Arch. intern. Med.*, 121, 356–360.

WINTROBE, M. M., MATTHEWS, E., POLLACK, R. & DOBYNS, B. M. (1940). A familial hemopoietic disorder in Italian adolescents and adults, resembling Mediterranean anemia (thalassemia). *J. Amer. med. Ass.*, 114, 1530–1538.

WOLFF, J. A. & IGNATOV, V. G. (1963). Heterogeneity of thalassemia major. *Amer. J. Dis. Child.*, 105, 234–242.

WOLLSTEIN, M. & KREIDEL, K. V. (1930). Familial hemolytic anemia of childhood — von Jaksch. *Amer. J. Dis. Child.*, 39, 115–130.

WOOD, W. G. (1983). Hemoglobin analysis. In: *The Thalassemias* (ed. by D. J. Weatherall), pp. 31–53. Churchill Livingstone, Edinburgh.

WOOD, W. G., CLEGG, J. B. & WEATHERALL, D. J. (1979). Hereditary persistence of fetal haemoglobin (HPFH) and δβ thalassaemia. *Brit. J. Haemat.*, 43, 509–520 (Annotation).

WOOD, W. G., STAMATOYANNOPOULOS, G., LIM, G. & NUTE, P. E. (1975). F-cells in the adult: normal values and levels in individuals with hereditary and acquired elevations of Hb F. *Blood*, 46, 671–681.

WOOD, W. G., WEATHERALL, D. J., CLEGG, J. B., HAMBLIN, T. J., EDWARDS, J. H. & BARLOW, A. M. (1977). Heterocellular hereditary persistence of fetal haemoglobin (heterocellular HPFH) and its interaction with β thalassaemia. *Brit. J. Haemat.*, 36, 461–473.

WOODROW, J. C., NOBLE, R. L. & MARTINDALE, J. H. (1964). Haemoglobin H disease in an English family. *Brit. med. J.*, i, 36–38.

YAMAK, B., OZSOYLU, S., ALTAY, Ç., HIÇSÖNMEZ, G. & SAY, B. (1973). Hereditary persistence of fetal hemoglobin and β-thalassemia in a Turkish child. *Acta haemat. (Basel)*, **50**, 124–128.

YANG, T.-Y., YANG, X.-Y., CH'EN, W.-C., QI, S.-L., JIN, Y.-J., GAN, W.-J. & QU, Q. (1985). Thalassemia in China. *Ann. N.Y. Acad. Sci.*, **445**, 92–105.

YASUKAWA, M., SAITO, S., FUJITA, S., OHTA, Y., IKEDA, K., MATSUMOTO, I. & KOBAYASHI, Y. (1980). Five families with homozygous δ-thalassaemia in Japan. *Brit. J. Haemat.*, **46**, 199–206.

ZACHARIADIS, Z., NUTE, P. E. & STAMATOYANNOPOULOS, G. (1975). Haemoglobin Lepore in Cyprus. *J. med. Genet.*, **12**, 275–279.

ZAGO, M. A., WOOD, W. G., CLEGG, J. B., WEATHERALL, D. J., O'SULLIVAN, M. & GUNSON, H. (1979). Genetic control of F-cells in human adults. *Blood*, **53**, 977–986.

ZAINO, E. C. (1964). Paleontologic thalassemia. *Ann. N.Y. Acad. Sci.*, **119**, 402–412.

ZAINO, E. C., YEH, J. K. & ALOIA, J. (1985). Defective vitamin D metabolism in thalassemia major. *Ann. N.Y. Acad. Sci.*, **445**, 127–134.

ZAIZOV, R. & MATOTH, Y. (1972). α-thalassemia in Yemenite and Iraqi Jews. *Israel J. med. Sci.*, **8**, 11–17.

ZAIZOV, R., STEINHERZ, M., WOLLACH, B. & KIRSCHMANN, C. (1980). Balanced bone marrow globin studies in mideastern α-thalassaemia. *Acta haemat. (Basel)*, **64**, 136–140.

ZENG, Y.-C., HUANG, S.-Z., NAKATSUJI, T. & HUISMAN, T. H. J. (1985). $-^{G}\gamma^{A}\gamma$-thalassaemia and γ-chain variants in Chinese newborn babies. *Amer. J. Hemat.*, **18**, 235–242.

ZILLIACUS, H. & OTTELIN, A.-M. (1963). A thalassaemic trait in gipsies? *Acta med. Scand.*, **174**, 261–263.

ZUELZER, W. W. & KAPLAN, E. (1954). Thalassemia–hemoglobin C disease. A new syndrome presumably due to the combination of the genes for thalassemia and hemoglobin C. *Blood*, **9**, 1047–1054.

ZUELZER, W. W., ROBINSON, A. R. & BOOKER, C. R. (1961). Reciprocal relationship of hemoglobins A_2 and F in beta chain thalassemia, a key to the genetic control of hemoglobin F. *Blood*, **17**, 393–408.

The thalassaemias II: pathology, pathogenesis and molecular genetics

MORBID ANATOMY AND HISTOPATHOLOGY

The cytological and histological changes that are found in thalassaemia are primarily those associated with long-standing anaemia and with the bone-marrow hyperplasia secondary to the anaemia. In addition, the reticulo-endothelial cell system and organs undergo hyperplasia in response to the increased turnover of erythrocytes and to the overloading with iron which results from increased absorption and, more importantly, from misguided iron therapy (occasionally) and from blood transfusion. The accumulation of iron, if sufficiently great, leads to organ damage and fibrosis closely similar to that of idiopathic haemochromatosis.

Much of the literature on the morbid anatomical and histopathological findings in thalassaemia deals with post-mortem findings in thalassaemia major (Whipple and Bradford, 1936; Sansone *et al.*, 1955, Witzleben and Wyatt, 1961; etc.), where the findings are grossly abnormal. Block (1969), however, has given a valuable account of the histopathological findings in thalassaemia minor (17 patients) and thalassaemia intermedia (two patients). Bone marrow was aspirated or cores were obtained in 17 patients and liver biopsies were carried out in 13 patients.

BONE MARROW

The extent to which the bone marrow undergoes hyperplasia varies directly with the severity of the defect in haemoglobin formation irrespective of its exact cause. In thalassaemia major the hyperplasia of the marrow is so great that the marrow cavity becomes greatly expanded, producing in the growing child the deformities of the facial bones and skull, and the characteristic accompanying X-ray changes, that have already been described (p. 400). Red hyperplastic marrow will be found, too, throughout the developing long bones. The development in certain patients of paravertebral extramedullary masses of marrow has, too, been referred to (p. 427). Films or sections of the marrow show very active (although ineffective) erythropoiesis and an erythroid: myeloid ratio that often exceeds unity. In thalassaemia intermedia and in thalassaemia minor and minima the hyperplasia is naturally less intense than in thalassaemia major.

Erythropoiesis is typically normoblastic and the normoblasts tend to be smaller than normal (micronormoblasts). This is mostly due to diminution in the amount of cytoplasm and is most marked in the most ripened cells. Detailed measurements were given by Astaldi, Tolentino and Sacchetti (1951b). In thalassaemia major the percentage of basophilic normoblasts is often unusually high: in thalassaemia minor polychromatic and pyknotic normoblasts predominate.

Megaloblastic change. This has almost always been the result of folate deficiency. Folate deficiency is in fact not uncommon in thalassaemia major in certain populations, but the morphological changes affecting the erythroblasts that are usually found in folate deficiency may not be obvious (Chanarin, Dacie and Mollin, 1959). 'Giant' metamyelocytes should, however, always be present.

Crosby and Sacks (1949) reported under the title 'The coincidence of Mediterranean anemia and pernicious anemia in a young Sicilian' a patient with mild thalassaemia trait whose haemoglobin rose to 16.5 g/dl after treatment with liver. The diagnosis in this case is, however, uncertain.

Goldberg and Schwartz (1954) described a black American female with Mediterranean anaemia who developed megaloblastic anaemia in each of three pregnancies. In retrospect, this patient seems likely to have suffered from folate deficiency.

Chanarin, Dacie and Mollin's (1959) patient was proved to have folate deficiency and responded well to the administration of folic acid. He was an Arab, aged 22, who had been known to have thalassaemia since the age of 5 years. He had been unusually anaemic for the last 2 years and during this time had been transfused with 10 litres of blood. Before folic-acid therapy, his

haemoglobin was 4.4 g/dl and the spleen extended to the umbilicus: after therapy (40 mg of folic acid daily) the haemoglobin rose to 8.0 g/dl and the reticulocyte count reached 25%. His history and blood findings suggest that he had thalassaemia intermedia. The cause of the folate deficiency was not exactly determined. The increased erythropoiesis consequent on life-long thalassaemia plus possibly a more recent failure of folate absorption appeared possible (Figs. 19.1 and 19.2).

Jandl and Greenberg's (1959) patient was of very great interest. She was 36 years old and was considered to have Cooley's anaemia. On three occasions she had experienced subacute episodes of bone-marrow failure that had responded to treatment with folic acid. On each occasion, however, she had experienced severe bone pains locally in her spine, pelvis, ribs and occiput following the administration of folic acid. These started about 12 hours after taking the drug and lasted for the next 24 hours or so. Jandl and Greenberg, who referred to the pains as painful 'erythropoietic crises', suggested that they were brought about by expansion of the intramedullary cell mass as the result of the erythroid cells dividing in response to the folic acid.

Robinson and Watson (1963), too, have described a patient who responded to folic-acid therapy in a similar

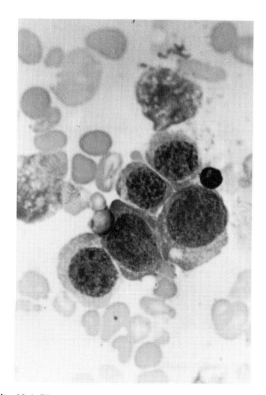

Fig. 19.1 Photomicrograph of bone-marrow cells from a patient with thalassaemia intermedia.
Erythropoiesis is megaloblastic. × 1100. [From Chanarin, Dacie and Mollin (1959).]

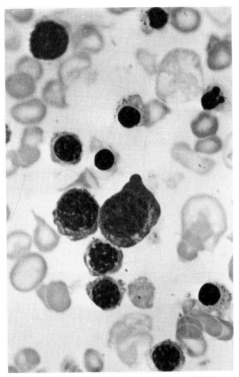

Fig. 19.2 Photomicrograph of bone-marrow cells from a patient with thalassaemia intermedia.
The same patient as in Figure 19.1, after folic-acid therapy. Erythropoiesis is now normoblastic. × 1100. [From Chanarin, Dacie and Mollin (1959).]

fashion. He was a $13\frac{1}{2}$-year-old male Italian who had received many transfusions and had been splenectomized when $7\frac{1}{2}$ years old. He later developed heart failure and signs of haemochromatosis and bone-marrow aspiration showed megaloblastic changes. Folic-acid therapy led to the development of bone pains, first in his spine and pelvis, which later became generalized. His peripheral-blood nucleated cell count, 29 700/μl before therapy, responded dramatically: it rose to 100 000/μl on the 6th day after therapy and later to 350 000–600 000/μl, 70–95% of the cells being normoblasts. The exceptionally great nucleated cell response seems likely to be a reflection of the hyperplasia of the bone marrow and the absence of the spleen. His transfusion requirement decreased after the folic-acid therapy.

Further information concerning folate deficiency in thalassaemia patients was provided by Luhby and Cooperman (1961) and Luhby *et al.* (1961) who concluded that it was an important and common complication of thalassaemia major that could lead to sudden crises of anaemia. More recently, Vatanavicharn and co-workers (1979)

demonstrated reduced serum and erythrocyte folate levels in large series of Hb-H and β-thal/ Hb-E patients in Thailand.

Aplastic crises. According to Fessas (1959), aplastic crises with prolonged arrest of erythroblast maturation are common during intercurrent infections.

Abnormalities in erythroblasts

Inclusions. In thalassaemia major, in bone-marrow films stained with Romanowsky dyes, the haemoglobin in some of the developing normoblasts may be seen to be formed in a patchy fashion in the cells' cytoplasm, which often, too, contains fine or coarse basophilic granules (Fig. 19.3). In striking contrast to the findings in haemoglobin deficiency based upon a lack of iron, siderotic granules are present in marrow normoblasts. Typically, they are more numerous than in health and, although larger than normal, are not arranged in a 'ring' pattern. Abundant iron will be found, too, in marrow phagocytes, particularly if many transfusions have been given.

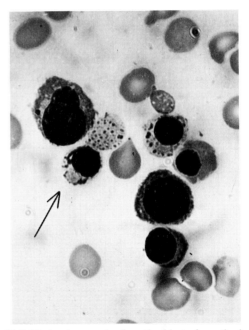

Fig. 19.3 Photomicrograph of erythroblasts from the bone marrow of a child with severe thalassaemia major.
Punctate basophilia is conspicuous in the cells' cytoplasm. The rounded mass marked with the arrow represents haemoglobin or precipitated α chains. × 1100.

Fessas (1963) reported that unusual large, usually single, inclusions, having the staining propeties of Heinz bodies, *i.e.*, staining supravitally with methyl violet, were present within the cytoplasm of a proportion of the normoblasts in the marrow of patients with thalassaemia major or intermedia. After splenectomy, similar inclusions were to be found in many of the reticulocytes and in some of the erythrocytes in the peripheral blood (Fig. 19.4). Fessas suggested that the inclusions most probably 'represent aggregates of the excess of α-chains of the hemoglobin molecule which have remained uncombined due to the deficiency in the β-chains and which have not been taken up by γ- or δ-chains'.

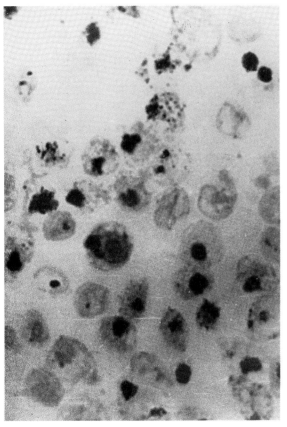

Fig. 19.4 Photomicrograph of a film made from the top layer of blood from a splenectomized patient with thalassaemia intermedia, stained vitally with methyl violet.
Most of the cells contain inclusions and in the centre there is an inclusion-carrying normoblast; two bare inclusions are to be seen in the top right of the field. [Reproduced by permission from Fessas (1963).]

Fessas (1963) had studied the blood of 24 patients: 12 had been splenectomized and 12 had their spleen *in situ*. 10–60% of the normoblasts contained inclusions and they were demonstrable, too, in the more mature erythroblasts in the bone marrow. With the spleen *in situ*, a very small proportion of the erythrocytes or reticulocytes were, too, found to contain an inclusion: after splenectomy, inclusions were found in as many as 9–28% of the reticulocytes and in 3–16% of mature erythrocytes. The striking increase in the number of peripheral-blood erythrocytes containing inclusions in the patients who had undergone splenectomy led Fessas to suggest that before splenectomy many of the inclusions were being removed from erythrocytes during their passage through the spleen, as has been thought to happen also in the case of siderotic granules (Vol. 1, p. 88).

Fessas, Loukopoulos and Kaltsoya (1966) showed by peptide mapping that the inclusions that they had isolated from peripheral-blood erythrocytes were formed to a great extent, if not exclusively, of precipitated α chains. Yataganas and Fessas (1969) reported that the precipitated material was more likely to be found in mature erythroblasts than in younger forms and that inclusions could be found, too, in erythroblasts from patients with β-thalassaemia intermedia; a smaller proportion of cells was, however, affected, and the inclusions were generally smaller in size than those seen in β-thalassaemia major. Yataganas, Gahrton and Thorell (1974) showed that the material could be found in the nuclei of erythroblasts as well as in their cytoplasm. Rachmilewitz and Thorell (1972) reported that the inclusions contained haemichromes. Earlier, Rachmilewitz (1969) had suggested that it was the instability of haemichromes that accounted for the presence of intra-erythrocytic inclusions in the various forms of thalassaemia.

Glycogen in erythroblasts. It has been known for many years that material staining positively with PAS (periodic-acid-Schiff reagent) can be demonstrated in the cytoplasm of erythroblasts in thalassaemia (as well as in erythroleukaemia and other conditions). The results of staining with PAS was first described by Astaldi *et al.* (1954): positive reactions were obtained in 20 cases of thalassaemia major and negative reactions in 10 cases of thalassaemia minima. The material was usually demonstrable as pink-staining granules, less often as a diffuse staining, and was considered to be a glucomucoprotein or mucopolysaccharide.

Fessas and Papayannopoulou (1965) concluded that the positively-staining material was glycogen and they found a rough correlation between the apparent severity of β-thalassaemia and the degree of PAS positivity. The reaction was negative in the normoblasts of adults with the β-thalassaemia trait, and they suggested that the accumulated glycogen functioned as a store of energy not utilized because of the severe reduction in haemoglobin synthesis. Yataganas and co-workers (1973) came to a similar conclusion, postulating that the accumulation of glycogen represented a store of unutilized energy in erythroblasts blocked in the G_1 phase of the cell cycle. Dörmer and Betke (1978) suggested that the accumulation of PAS-positive material in cells in the G_1 phase corresponds to the degree to which their growth is retarded. In relation to the cause of the accumulation, Eylar and Matioli (1965) had found that the rate of incorporation of glucosamine into the glycoprotein of reticulocyte stroma was greatly increased in thalassaemia major.

Ultrastructural studies of erythroblasts and erythrocytes

In early studies Hoffman and co-workers (1956) described the results of an electron-microscopic study of the membranes of thalassaemia-major and thalassaemia-minor erythrocytes. In thalassaemia minor the appearances could not be distinguished from the normal: in thalassaemia major, however, the surface texture appeared to be distinct and unusual high-density particles could be seen. Bessis and his co-workers (Bessis and Breton-Gorius, 1957; Bessis, Alagille and Breton-Gorius, 1958; Bessis and de Boisfleury, 1970), Marinone et al. (1958) and Polliack and Rachmilewitz (1973) reported further abnormalities, e.g., unusual accumulations in thalassaemic erythrocytes and erythroblasts of dense iron-containing granules ('micelles ferrugineuses'), either dispersed or in mitochondria, as well as the presence of vacuoles, amorphous material and denser spherules.

Bessis and de Boisfleury (1970) described and illustrated the appearance of poikilocytes in wet suspension and in dried films under the interference and scanning electron microscopes as well as the artifacts produced by dehydration.

Polliack and Rachmilewitz (1973) studied 11 patients, six of whom had had their spleens removed. A 'wide spectrum' of intracellular changes was observed, particularly in the splenectomized patients. The erythrocytes were found to be grossly distorted and deformed with indentations and infolding of the plasma membrane and vacuole formation. A great deal of iron was present, either as free particles or as aggregates of ferritin or haemosiderin within membrane-bound particles or mitochondria. The ultrastructural changes were regarded as the consequence of multiple defects involving the synthesis of globin, haem, glycoprotein and cell membrane.

Polliack and co-workers (1974) reported on an electron-microscopic study of normoblasts in the peripheral blood of 20 patients who had been splenectomized for thalassaemia major. A variety of abnormalities were demonstrated, including widening of nuclear pores, partial absence and areas of reduplication of the nuclear membrane, and intranuclear inclusions referred to as Heinz bodies. The nuclear abnormalities appeared to be most prominent when inclusions were abundant in the cells' cytoplasm and when they were close to, or in contact with, nuclear material.

α-globin precipitates. The ultrastructure of the precipitated α-globin chains has, too, been carefully studied. These appear as multiple electron-dense amorphous foci which tend to coalesce. As can be seen, too, under the light microscope, they occur most frequently in the more mature erythroblasts (Polliack and Rachmilewitz, 1973; Wickramasinghe and Bush, 1975), but unlike Heinz bodies artifically generated by the use of phenylhydrazine they are not attached to the cell membrane (Polliack, Yataganas and Rachmilewitz, 1974). Inclusions of α-globin chains have also been shown to be present within nuclei (Polliack, Yataganas and Rachmilewitz, 1974; Wickramasinghe, 1976).

Wickramasinghe and Hughes (1984) described how the electron-microscopic appearance of β-chain inclusions in the erythroblasts in Hb-H disease differ from the α-chain inclusions seen in β-thalassaemia. Precipitated β chains present a stellate appearance with bifurcating branches of electron-dense material radiating outwards from a central point while precipitated α chains appear as rounded masses of amorphous electron-dense material which tend to fuse into larger masses (Figs. 19.5 and 19.6). Wickramasinghe et al. (1984) compared the incidence of erythroblasts and marrow reticulocytes bearing inclusions demonstrable by electron microscopy in four different varieties of α thalassaemia: they occurred in 0.6–1.3% of the cells in two patients with α-thal-1 trait (presumed genotype $--/\alpha\alpha$), in 2.1–13.7% of the cells in five patients with Hb-H disease (presumed genotype $--/-\alpha$) and in 6.2% of the cells in a patient with Hb Q-H disease (presumed genotype $--/-\alpha^Q$); very few such cells were present in a single patient with α-thal-2 trait (presumed genotype $-\alpha/\alpha\alpha$).

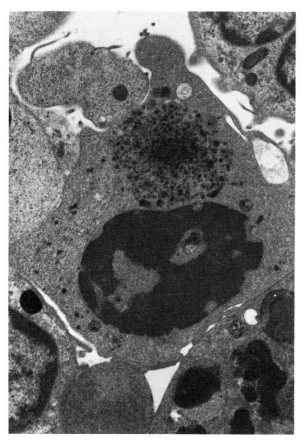

Fig. 19.5 Electronmicrograph of a late erythroblast from a patient with homozygous β-thalassaemia.
   The cytoplasm contains precipitated α chains. × 10 900. [Reproduced by permission from Wickramasinghe and Hughes (1984).]

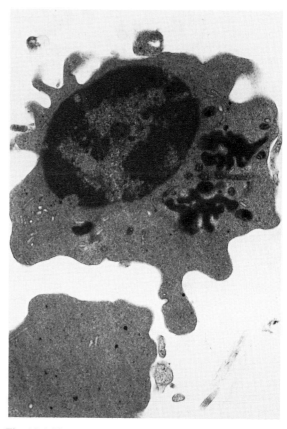

Fig. 19.6 Electronmicrograph of a late erythroblast from a patient with Hb-H disease.
   The cytoplasm contains a stellate inclusion probably composed of precipitated β chains. × 6700. [Reproduced by permission from Wickramasinghe and Hughes (1984).]

Phagocytic cells in bone marrow

Electron-microscopic studies of marrow phagocytic cells have revealed within their cytoplasm remnants of immature and mature erythrocytes and in addition sometimes whole erythroblasts and extruded nuclei (Wickramasinghe and Bush, 1975). Some of these cells, under the light microscope, resemble Gaucher cells according to Zaino *et al.* (1971). Wickramasinghe and Hughes (1978), however, considered that the cells differ in their ultrastructure.

It is interesting to recall that foamy cells were described in the bone marrow of fatal cases of Cooley's disease many years previously, *e.g.*, by Whipple and Bradford (1936) and Sansone *et al.* (1955). They were recorded, too, by Mukherjee and Sen Gupta (1963) as being present in the bone marrow of some Indian patients.

Block (1969) pointed out that phagocytic cells (described as reticular cells, *not* as Gaucher cells), containing excessive amounts of cellular breakdown products, can be seen in sections or smears of the marrow in thalassaemia minor, and that in some cells remnants of nuclei or cytoplasm are clearly recognizable.

SPLEEN

In thalassaemia major the spleen is substantially enlarged in relation to the patient's age (see Mukherjee, Sen Gupta and Chatterjea, 1959; Mukherjee and Sen Gupta, 1963; Okon, Levij and Rachmilewitz, 1976). Sections show congestion with blood, slight to marked extramedullary haemopoiesis (mainly consisting of normoblasts), a thickened reticular framework, an increased iron content and Gamna-Gandi bodies (Okon, Levij and Rachmilewitz, 1976). The amount of iron present depends upon the number of times, if any, the patient has been transfused. In the absence of transfusions only small amounts are usually present.

In thalassaemia minor the changes are far less marked; in thalassaemia intermedia they lie, as might be expected, some way between those of the major and minor disorders.

Phagocytic cells. Foamy cells were described by Whipple and Bradford (1936) in the spleen in fatal cases of Cooley's erythroblastic anaemia (as well as in the bone marrow and lymph nodes). Small collections of 'foam' cells were, too, reported by Mukherjee, Sen Gupta and Chatterjea (1959) and Sen Gupta et al. (1960) as being present in 27 out of 30 spleens removed from patients with homozygous thalassaemia (six cases) or Hb-E/thalassaemia. The cytoplasm of the foam cells, which were considered to be histiocytes, stained deep red with PAS and the material thus stained was thought to be an acidic mucopolysaccharide, derived possibly from the lysis of abnormal erythroid cells. More recently, cells, referred to as being 'Gaucher-like', with intracytoplasmic tubular structures visible on electron microscopy, have been reported in the spleens of thalassaemia-major patients by Zaino et al. (1971), Zaino and Rossi (1974), Resegotti et al. (1975) and Zaino (1980).

LIVER

The liver is enlarged in fatal cases of thalassaemia major. The main pathological changes (excluding those associated perhaps with terminal cardiac failure) are the deposition of iron, which may be massive, and fibrosis, which in some patients may be marked also. In young children especially, and particularly after splenectomy, there may be massive extramedullary haemopoiesis.

Early accounts of the histopathology of the liver in thalassaemia major include those of Whipple and Bradford (1936), Astaldi, Tolentino and Sacchetti (1951b), Howell and Wyatt (1953), Ellis, Schulman and Smith (1954) and Sansone et al. (1955).

Mukherjee, Sen Gupta and Chatterjea (1960) studied 18 livers (in 16 patients biopsy specimens had been obtained at the time of splenectomy) and reported finding histiocytic cells containing granules of muco-polysaccharide in the portal tracts in five cases. Besides haemosiderin, lipofuscin or haemofuscin was found in Kupffer cells as well as in liver cells in 16 cases.

Howell and Wyatt (1953) and Ellis, Schulman and Smith (1954) had discussed the relationship between their finding of fibrosis of the liver (and other organs) and those of idiopathic haemochromatosis and transfusional siderosis. Ellis, Schulman and Smith (1954) concluded that there appeared to be no correlation between the fibrosis and siderosis and the severity and chronicity of the anaemia. However, in some cases the amount of iron present exceeded that which could be accounted for by transfusion and it seemed to them probable that the amount absorbed from the gastro-intestinal tract might have been unusually large.

Accumulation of iron. Witzleben and Wyatt (1961) reported on the findings at necropsy in four Italians who had survived for between $8\frac{1}{2}$ and 13 years. In each patient the liver was massively loaded with iron, the organ's iron content being recorded as 2.77–8.14 g per 100-g dry weight. In addition, the livers were variably cirrhotic. Witzleben and Wyatt suggested that cirrhosis develops late following the attainment of a critical level of iron in the liver cells. They considered that the iron was predominately derived from increased absorption from the gut; they pointed out that iron in the liver increases markedly after splenectomy and suggested that the operation may accelerate the onset of cirrhosis. [The same possible link between splenectomy and cirrhosis was referred to by Okon, Levij and Rachmilewitz (1976).]

Accounts of secondary haemochromatosis associated with repeated transfusions include those of Fink (1964) and Chaptal et al. (1967). Fink, whose data were based on 49 spleens removed for hypersplenism or spacial encroachment and 11 necropsies, compared the distribution of iron with that in idiopathic haemochromatosis. [Fink's patients had received 20–25 blood transfusions.] The distribution was comparable except that more iron was proportionately present in the spleen in thalassaemia (where blood destruction was taking place).

Berry and Marshall (1967) studied liver biopsy specimens from 17 patients and distinguished two types of iron distribution: *parenchymal*, in which the parenchymal cells were heavily loaded with iron and in which there was iron, too, in distended macrophages in portal areas and in Kupffer cells; and *non-parenchymal*, in which the Kupffer cells and macrophages were heavily loaded and there was iron, too, lying free in portal tracts, with relatively little involvement of parenchymal cells. The parenchymal pattern was found in 10 patients who had been splenectomized and the non-parenchymal pattern in seven patients whose spleen had not been removed. The factors responsible for these two contrasting patterns were not established. The site of storage could not be correlated with age, sex, diet or severity of disease as judged by transfusion requirements.

Iancu and Neustein (1977) described the sequence of events, as revealed by electron microscopy, when liver cells are subjected to progressive iron loading. Their findings were based on liver biopsies carried out on 10 patients with homozygous β-thalassaemia who were being treated by a hypertransfusion regime. The number of iron-laden lysosomes was found to increase with time and Iancu and Neustein considered that segregation of iron in this way helped to prevent the concentration of ferritin in the cell sap from rising above a plateau level, so preserving the functional capacity of most of the liver parenchyma cells until the most advanced stages of iron overload.

De Virgiliis and co-workers (1981) have more recently stressed the importance of another hazard in thalassaemia patients who need to be repeatedly transfused: this is chronic infective liver disease. Of 81 transfusion-dependent patients, 31 were considered to have chronic active hepatitis and 23 chronic persistent hepatitis. Hepatitis B virus and hepatitis non-A, non-B virus were implicated as infective agents.

Excess absorption of iron from the gastro-intestinal tract

The effect of β-thalassaemia on the intestinal absorption of iron was studied in depth by Heinrich *et al.* (1973), who found that absoprtion of inorganic iron ($^{59}Fe^{2+}$) was increased by 70–100% in four homozygous β-thalassaemia children when measured 64–300 days after blood transfusion and that absorption of labelled food iron was increased 2–4 times. In each case the absorption was normal if tested soon after the children were transfused. Eight heterozygous β-thalassaemia children were found to absorb inorganic iron normally unless they had depleted iron stores, in which case the absorption was increased. Heinrich and his co-workers concluded that haemosiderosis was inevitable in homozygous β-thalassaemia patients either as the result of blood transfusions or, if they managed to survive without transfusions, as the result of the increased absorption of iron from

food consequent on the presence of markedly ineffective erythropoiesis. The latter mechanism would result, according to Heinrich *et al.*, in an accumulation of about 19 g of iron by the time the child was 18 years old. They added that the mechanism by which the intestinal absorption of iron is increased in the presence of markedly ineffective erythropoiesis was unknown. Pippard and co-workers (1979) similarly obtained objective evidence of increased iron absorption in non-transfusion-dependent thalassaemia patients. They had studied 15 patients with thalassaemia intermedia and found that the absorption of a 5-mg test dose of iron labelled with ^{59}Fe was strikingly increased, from 17 to 89% of the dose being absorbed. [The normal mean absorption by iron-replete controls was $14.8 \pm 9.5\%$.] It was calculated that patients surviving to the 3rd and 4th decades would by then be likely to have an iron load similar to that of transfusion-dependent thalassaemia-major patients.

PATHOLOGICAL CHANGES IN OTHER ORGANS

The main pathological change that has been reported is widespread deposition of iron, with the pancreas, endocrine glands and kidneys being amongst the organs most affected (Whipple and Bradford, 1936; Sansone *et al.*, 1955; Covey *et al.*, 1960; Witzleben and Wyatt, 1961; etc.). Covey and co-workers (1960) gave details of the necropsy findings in a patient who survived for 35 years. He had been diagnosed as suffering from thalassaemia major and had been splenectomized when 9 years old. Unusual features included obliterative pulmonary endoarteritis and widespread demineralization of bones (but without involvement of the skull).

PATHOGENESIS

Three interrelated factors are responsible for the anaemia of the thalassaemias: failure of haemoglobin formation, the primary factor, ineffective

erythropoiesis and an increased rate of destruction of the erythrocytes after they have left the bone marrow. The ineffective erythropoiesis is itself a consequence of a partial or complete failure of synthesis of one or other of the globin chains of haemoglobin; the increased rate of erythocyte destruction appears mainly to be the indirect result of unbalanced globin-chain formation.

In the discussion that follows ineffective erythropoiesis is dealt with first, as quantitative studies on erythropoiesis preceded those on haemoglobin formation. Most of the studies that are quoted refer to patients with thalassaemia major or intermedia. The pathogenesis of the Hb-Bart's fetal hydrops syndrome and Hb-H disease is dealt with briefly in separate short sections.

INEFFECTIVE ERYTHROPOIESIS

Early reports emphasized delay in the maturation of erythroblasts (Astaldi, Tolentino and Sacchetti, 1951a; Hamilton and Fowler, 1951; Astaldi and Tolentino, 1952), failure to acquire a minimal complement of haemoglobin until the late normoblast stage (Hamilton and Fowler, 1951) and possible difficulty in the enucleation of erythroblasts (Astaldi and Tolentino, 1952). Hamilton and Fowler, who studied three families in which cases of Cooley's anaemia had occurred, also stressed the importance of periodic depression of erythropoiesis rather than haemolysis as the cause of severe episodes of anaemia and recorded reticulocyte counts in two patient as low as 0.00 and 0.1%

More recent studies of erythropoiesis in thalassaemia have employed radioisotope labelling techniques. The results of an interesting metabolic study carried out on a patient with β-thalassaemia intermedia following the administration of $[^{14}C\text{-}2]$-glycine were reported by Kreimer-Birnbaum and Bannerman (1968). A notable feature was a marked and abnormal increase in the early-labelled fraction of faecal bile pigment, the labelling being maximal at 5 days, in advance of the haem peak in the peripheral blood. The urine contained a brown (dipyrrole) pigment and this labelled, too; in this case the maximal labelling was in the first sample passed. These data were interpreted as being the consequence of the early breakdown of redundant haem, perhaps the haem of excess α chains. At all times Hb F was more

highly labelled in the peripheral blood than was Hb A.

Other workers have used labelling techniques to study the proliferation and maturation of bone-marrow cells. Wickramasinghe and his co-workers (1970) studied nine Cypriot children, eight of whom had thalassaemia major and one thalassaemia intermedia, using Feulgen micro-spectrophotometry and ^{3}H-thymidine autoradiography. Early polychromatic erythroblasts were found to accumulate in the G_1 phase (with diploid DNA content), DNA synthesis was markedly decreased and cells were failing to enter mitosis. Death of the arrested cells was thought possibly to account for the ineffectiveness of erythropoiesis. The data of Queisser et al. (1971), using similar techniques, were similar. They had studied six patients suffering from thalassaemia of differing severity. An abnormal distribution of DNA and ^{3}H incorporation was demonstrated, which was most marked in thalassaemia major and not discernible in thalassaemia minima. Amongst the polychromatic erythroblasts, there was an abnormal accumulation of cells in the G_1 phase, a decreased proportion of cells in the S (synthetic) phase and a decreased $S:G_2$ (unlabelled tetraploid cells) ratio. Their data were thought to indicate a direct relationship between ineffective erythropoiesis and the degree of anaemia.

Dörmer and Betke (1978) studied the kinetics of erythropoiesis in four homozygous β-thalassaemia patients and two heterozygotes. In both states the erythroblasts were found to proceed through the compartments at a reduced rate. In the homozygotes only 15–30% of the erythroblasts appeared to escape desctruction; in the heterozygotes it seemed that cell death was confined to cells in the non-proliferating stages.

FAILURE TO FORM Hb A

As already referred to (p. 392), the early studies of Marks and his co- workers (Burka and Marks, 1963; Marks and Burka, 1964; etc.) had led them to conclude that in thalassaemia the capacity of the ribosomes of reticulocytes to synthesize Hb A was subnormal. In contrast, the ability to synthesize Hb F appeared to be unimpaired. These observations were confirmed by Necheles, Steiner and Baldini (1965) who had studied the rate of incorporation of [2-^{14}C]glycine into erythroid precursors obtained from the bone marrow of seven patients suffering from various forms of thalassaemia. The synthesis of Hb A was found to be markedly reduced in thalassaemia major and reduced to a lesser extent in thalassaemia minor. Subsequently, the elaboration of techniques that enable the rate of formation of the different globin chains of haemoglobin to be separately assessed was a major step forward in thalassaemia research, for it soon became clear that globin-chain imbalance is a most important factor in the pathogenesis of thalassaemia.

Some of the early work demonstrating globin-chain synthesis imbalance in β-thalassaemia has been referred to in Chapter 18 (p. 392). Further noteworthy reports of similar and confirmatory studies carried out on patients suffering from a variety of types of thalassaemia include those of Modell et al. (1969), Clegg and Weatherall (1972), Kan, Nathan and Lodish (1972), Natta et al. (1976), Kinney et al. (1978), Cividalli, Kerem and Rachmilewitz (1980), Musumeci et al. (1981), Ritchey et al. (1981) and Sampietro et al. (1983).

The problem discussed in the following sections is how the imbalance affects erythropoiesis and the viability of the erythrocytes that are produced. The β-thalassaemias and α-thalassaemias are dealt with separately.

Excess of α-globin chains in β-thalassaemia

Failure to form adequate numbers of β chains leads to a relative excess of α chains. The γ chains that are produced fail to bind all the excess α chains and the latter accumulate and eventually precipitate and form relatively rigid insoluble inclusions. This is because free α chains are unable to combine with themselves and form soluble tetramers, as can β chains and γ chains (see p. 5).

Precipitation of excess α chains takes place at an early stage of erythroblast development and it appears that their presence leads to the death within the bone marrow of many erythroblasts, particularly at the late polychromatic stage (Yataganas and Fessas, 1969; Wickramasinghe, Letsky and Moffatt, 1973; Wickra-

masinghe, 1976; Wickramasinghe and Hughes, 1982, 1984).

Wickramasinghe and Bush (1975) considered that arrest of polychromatic erythroblasts at the G_1 phase of the cell cycle could be brought about not only by the presence of α-chain precipitates but also by free α chains. It seems likely that the erythroblasts that do survive are those that manage to form relatively large amounts of Hb F, thus reducing the number of free α chains present. Exactly how free α chains are damaging is an interesting question. Wickramasinghe and Hughes (1982) found in electron micrographs prepared from erythroblasts from cases of homozygous β-thalassaemia and Hb-E/β-thalassaemia that some of the excess α chains was precipitated around microtubules and centrioles; they suggested that this would hinder the separation of centrioles in early prophase, hinder spindle formation and thus prevent the progress of mitosis.

Proteolysis of excess α-chains. A mechanism which is potentially protective is the ability of human bone-marrow erythroblasts to bring about proteolysis of free α chains (Bank and O'Donnell, 1969; Yataganas, Fessas and Gahrton, 1972). This probably explains why in β-thalassaemia heterozygotes, where the α:β globin-chain synthesis ratio in reticulocytes is clearly unbalanced (ratio 2:1 approximately), the ratio in bone-marrow erythroblasts may appear to be balanced (Chalevelakis, Clegg and Weatherell, 1975; Wood and Stamatoyannopoulos, 1975; Hanash and Rucknagel, 1978; Vissers, Winterbourn and Carrell, 1983; Benz et al., 1984).

The excess α chains that persist and are precipitated are thought to be responsible, at least in part, for the thalassaemia erythrocyte's shortened life-span. According to Rachmilewitz et al. (1969), Rachmilewitz and Thorell (1972) and Rachmilewitz (1974), the free (excess) α chains become oxidized to haemichromes and then precipitate forming inclusions with the appearance and staining characteristics of Heinz bodies. The 'Heinz bodies' produced in this way do not, however, attach themselves to the cell membrane as do the inclusions in other Heinz-body haemolytic anaemias (Polliack and Rachmilewitz, 1973). Nevertheless, the inclusions appear to be removed from the erythrocytes harbouring them during the cells' passage from the pulp of the spleen into the splenic sinuses, and it seems highly likely that the erythrocytes are damaged and become distorted during the process. As far back as 1968, Slater, Muir and Weed wrote 'many of the small, fragmented and distorted cells in non-splenectomized thalassemia major blood may arise from fragmentation pitting of intracellular precipitates secondary to splenic passage'.

Indirect support for the hypothesis that the presence of an excess of α chains has a deleterious affect on erythrocyte survival was provided by Vigi et al. (1969). They transfused ^{51}Cr-labelled blood from patients with thalassaemia major or minor, and from healthy donors, into healthy group-compatible recipients and were able to demonstrate a clear negative correlation between erythrocyte survival and excess α-chain formation.

Aside from the damage to the erythrocyte resulting from the removal of α-chain precipitates during the cell's passage through the spleen, the α-chain precipitates probably affect the integrity of the cell's membrane in other ways. These are discussed below.

POSSIBLE MECHANISMS OF INCREASED HAEMOLYSIS

Abnormal permeability of erythrocytes to cations

Several studies carried out on thalassaemia erythrocytes have demonstrated increased permeability to potassium in vitro (Nathan and Gunn, 1966; Nathan et al., 1969; Cividalli, Locker and Russell, 1971; Gunn, Silvers and Rosse, 1972; Knox-Macaulay et al., 1972; Chapman, Allison and Grimes, 1973; Vettore et al., 1974).

Cividalli, Locker and Russell (1971) studied 11 Kurdish Jews with thalassaemia major and 14 with thalassaemia minor. The intracellular content of K^+ and Na^+ in freshly withdrawn erythrocytes was virtually normal. On incubation for 24 hours, however, the thalassaemia-major cells gained substantial amounts of Na^+ and lost even more K^+; the changes in the thalassaemia-minor cells were, on the other hand, much less abnormal. Cividalli, Locker and Russell concluded that inability to maintain a normal composition of cations and water might play a part in the pathogenesis of haemolysis in thalassaemia major.

Gunn, Silvers and Rosse (1972) incubated the erythrocytes of 10 thalassaemia-minor patients for 24 hours. Abnormal amounts of K^+ were lost without compensatory increase in Na^+. This was attributed to a selective increased permeability to K^+ following depletion of sources of energy, and the membrane of thalassaemia-minor erythrocytes was considered to be functionally different from that of normal cells.

Vettore and co-workers (1974) studied 20 β-thalassaemia heterozygotes. Loss of K^+ was found to be much greater than in normal erythrocytes after 24 hours' incubation, and K^+ loss, decrease in MCV and increase in osmotic resistance appeared to be directly related to clinical severity. The addition of glucose largely prevented the abnormal responses to incubation.

Other membrane abnormalities. Rachmilewitz and Kahane (1980) and Rachmilewitz et al. (1985) have listed in reviews a number of other observations indicative of membrane abnormality or damage: for instance, ultrastructural abnormalities (Hoffman et al., 1956); an increase in membrane phospholipids, a decrease in the percentage of phosphatidylethanolamine, a decrease in the level of the polyunsaturated arachidonic acid and an increase in the level of saturated palmitic acid (Rachmilewitz, Lubin and Shohet, 1976); abnormally high levels of malonyldialdehyde (MDA) following oxidant stress (H_2O_2) (Stocks et al., 1972; Rachmilewitz, Lubin and Shohet, 1976); a reduced number of titratable SH groups (Kahane and Rachmilewitz, 1976); more prominent than usual cross-linking of several membrane proteins following oxidant stress used to generate MDA (Kahane, Shifter and Rachmilewitz, 1978); a reduced number (Kahane and Rachmilewitz, 1976) and uneven distribution of sialic acid residues (Kahane et al., 1978); and an increased susceptibility to phagocytosis by mouse macrophages (Knyszynski et al., 1979) and human macrophages (Rachmilewitz, Treves and Treves, 1980). In addition, several studies have indicated low serum vitamin-E levels in thalassaemia (Rachmilewitz, Lubin and Shohet, 1976; Rachmilewitz, Shifter and Kahane, 1979). Then it seems likely that superoxide, a potent oxygen radical, is generated during the conversion of free α chains to haemichromes and their precipitation (Brunori et al., 1975), while the presence of excess intracellular iron may by itself be harmful by encouraging the formation of free oxygen radicals (Rachmilewitz and Kahane, 1980). Also, the reduced haemoglobin content in thalassaemic erythrocytes may facilitate the action of free oxygen radicals on membrane components (Vettore and Tedesco, 1975).

It is interesting to note that Gerli and co-workers (1980), who compared the superoxide dismutase (SOD), catalase and glutathione peroxidase (GPx) activities in the erythrocytes from 11 thalassaemia-major and 24 thalassaemia-minor patients with those from 40 normal adults, reported raised values in the thalassaemia-minor patients, but not in the thalassaemia-major patients. The latter had, however, received multiple transfusions.

Recently, Joshi and co-workers (1983) have reported that isolated α subunits of normal haemoglobin are unusually sensitive to oxidative damage and cross-linkage with spectrin; they suggested that in β-thalassaemia this cross-linkage would contribute significantly to the premature senescence of the erythrocytes.

Another mechanism possibly leading to shortening of the life-span of thalassaemia erythrocyte is the presence on the cells' membrane of abnormal amounts of IgG. Galili and co-workers (1983) identified the IgG as anti-galactosyl: by means of a sensitive antiglobulin test making use of the FC receptors on cells of the myeloid K562 line, 73 out of 80 patients with thalassaemia major or intermedia gave positive results.

Some at least of the abnormalities listed above clearly result from the presence of free or precipitated α chains. But it is unlikely that they can all be explained in this way or that the erythrocytes' shortened life-span depends entirely upon the presence of the excess chains. It is known for instance that the severely hypochromic erythrocytes of post-haemorrhagic iron-deficiency anaemia patients have, too, a shortened life-span (Layrisse, Linares and Roche, 1965), and it also seems that the abnormal erythrocyte cation movements referred to above as being demonstrable when thalassaemia erythrocytes are incubated at 37°C in vitro also occur with the erythrocytes of hypochromic anaemias of quite different origin, i.e., in iron-deficiency anaemia and sideroblastic anaemia (Chapman, Allison and Grimes, 1973; Knox-Macaulay and Weatherall, 1974).

The cause of the increased haemolysis in the severe forms of thalassaemia is clearly complicated and multifactorial. A question often asked is whether, or to what extent, the morphological abnormalities that are so obvious in thalassaemia blood films — the marked variation in size and shape of the erythrocytes and the presence of cell fragments — by themselves lead to increased haemolysis. The shape changes and the fragmen-

tation are clearly the consequences of imperfect erythrocyte formation as well as the result of interaction between the erythrocytes and the spleen (see p. 506). It is certainly difficult to believe that cells of markedly abnormal shape and cell fragments can have a normal life-span, but abnormalities of shape or size per se seem to be less important than the membrane and metabolic changes that underlie the shape abnormalities and fragmentation.

Fragmentation

The obvious occurrence of erythrocyte fragmentation, as seen in fresh thalassaemia blood in suspension or in films of freshly withdrawn blood, has led many investigators in the past to study the occurrence of fragmentation under various in-vitro conditions.

As far back as 1936, Whipple and Bradford recognized that Mediterranean-anaemia erythrocytes appeared to undergo fragmentation in vitro unusually readily. Marmont and Bianchi (1948) found in three cases of Rietti-Greppi-Micheli anaemia that fragmentation was particularly marked if the cells were suspended in brilliant cresyl blue solution; 'dumb-bell' erythrocytes with two spheres of haemoglobin united by a colourless membrane appeared to be a stage in the fragmentation process. According to Marmont and Bianchi, only in Mediterranean anaemia is the fragmentation so striking, but it is interesting to note that they added that in iron-deficiency anaemia, if severe, the fragmentation may be almost as great.

Astaldi and Tolentino (1952) stressed the importance of fragmentation in the pathogenesis of the haemolysis in thalassaemia. They concluded that the bizarre forms of erythrocytes and small microcytes to be seen in peripheral-blood films were not caused by increased mechanical fragility but were the result of unspecified intrinsic causes. In vitro, resistance to mechanical trauma was reported by them to be increased.

Zintl (1954) reported similar observations to those of Marmont and Bianchi (1948), i.e., that bell-like and umbrella-like erythrocytes developed in supravitally-stained wet preparations in a case of thalassaemia minor, type Rietti-Greppi-Mecheli.

Perosa and Dell'Aquila (1955) claimed that a rise in body temperature increases haemolysis in patients with Mediterranean anaemia. In vitro, they reported that citrated thalassaemia blood kept at 42°C underwent an abnormal degree of fragmentation and haemolysis after 5–6 hours' incubation.

In vivo, the occurrence of significant and abnormal fragmentation of circulating erythrocytes is supported by the finding of raised plasma haemoglobin levels in thalassaemia major, although not in thalassaemia minor (see p. 414).

Deformability

The rheological properties of the erythrocytes from 12 heterozygous and nine homozygous β-thalassaemia patients was studied by Tillmann and Schröter (1979). They used 5-μm 'Nucleopore' polycarbonate sieves to measure flow-rates and estimated the viscosity of suspensions of whole erythrocytes and of erythrocyte ghosts. Erythrocyte deformability was decreased in all the patients studied: in the heterozygotes this was attributed to the microcytosis; in the homozygotes to shape alterations, to diminished fluidity of haemoglobin associated with the presence of excess α chains and in splenectomized patients to the presence of inclusions.

ABSENCE OF ANAEMIA IN HPFH: THE EXPLANATION

In contrast to β-thalassaemia, globin-chain synthesis is balanced in HPFH. Natta and co-workers (1974) studied eight HPFH simple heterozygotes, and a Hb-S/HPFH compound heterozygote, who were members of two black families. The α : β+γ synthesis ratio was approximately 1.0 in the simple heterozygotes but definitely abnormal (1.7) in the Hb-S/HPFH individual. Natta *et al.* attributed the absence of anaemia in uncomplicated HPFH to globin-chain synthesis being balanced. The absence of significant changes in erythrocyte morphology is, too, a reflection of the lack of chain imbalance.

MECHANISM OF ANAEMIA IN β-THALASSAEMIA: A SUMMARY

The major shortening of erythrocyte life-span which is a feature of β-thalassaemia major and of some cases of thalassaemia intermedia is the consequence of ineffective erythropoiesis, itself secondary to failure of β-globin chain formation.

This leads to the production of hypochromic erythrocytes of varying size and shape, with defective cell membranes, impaired deformability and a tendency to spontaneous fragmentation. The spleen, too, plays a part: it removes from the circulation the most defective cells as well as intracellular inclusions, *e.g.*, precipitated α chains, from cells that survive passage through the spleen (see also p. 506).

PATHOGENESIS OF THE α-THALASSAEMIAS

Hb-Bart's hydrops fetalis

A total failure of α-chain synthesis prevents the fetus from forming any Hb F. γ chains are, however, produced and combine together to form Hb Bart's ($\gamma_2\gamma_2$). In addition, small amounts of Hb H ($\beta_2\beta_2$) may be formed, and some γ chains combine with persisting embryonic zeta chains to form Hb Portland ($\gamma_2\zeta_2$) — according to Weatherall, Clegg and Wong (1970), Hb Portland comprises 10–15% of the haemoglobin in Hb-Bart's hydrops fetuses. Hb Bart's has a high O_2 affinity and there is no Bohr effect; Hb Portland, on the other hand, although it has a higher O_2 affinity than Hb A, has a smaller n value and the alkaline Bohr effect is nearly halved (Tuchinda, Nagai and Lehmann, 1975). It can, therefore, supply oxygen to the tissues, and its presence may explain why infants, unable to produce α chains, can survive at all, even for a few hours after birth.

As already referred to, infants suffering from the Hb-Bart's hydrops syndrome are severely anaemic and the reticulocyte count is raised. There is also marked hypochromia and anisocytosis and poikilocytosis. The anaemia is presumably due to a failure of haemoglobin production leading to ineffective erythropoiesis as well as to increased haemolysis, but the exact mechanisms are obscure. Hb Bart's is a relatively stable haemoglobin and does not denature readily and form easily visible inclusions as does Hb H. Death *in utero* results probably from anoxia secondary to the chronic anaemia and the failure of Hb Bart's to act as an effective oxygen transporter; the oedema seems likely to be mainly due to cardiac failure (itself a consequence of anoxia).

Hb-H disease

This is a less severe disorder than is β-thalassaemia major and the peripheral-blood erythrocyte abnormalities are usually less marked. Erythropoiesis is more effective than in β-thalassaemia major but the formed erythrocytes are nevertheless destroyed at a considerably accelerated rate (see p. 455). Hb H is a soluble haemoglobin but it is unstable. Its denaturation and precipitation within erythroblasts (Fessas and Yataghanas, 1968; Wickramasinghe et al., 1980) does not seem, however, to be associated with any substantial impairment of erythroblast proliferation as is the case when α chains are precipitated in erythroblasts in the β-thalassaemias (Wickramasinghe et al., 1981b). According to Wickramasinghe et al. (1980) the ultrastructure of the inclusions in Hb-H disease is quite different from that in β-thalassaemia (see Figs. 19.5 and 19.6, p. 497).

It is interesting to note that there is evidence that a proportion of the newly formed excess β chains are probably destroyed by proteolysis in much the same way as excess α chains are destroyed in β-thalassaemia. In an adult female black American with Hb-G Philadelphia/Hb-H disease the α:β globin-synthesis ratio was shown by Sancar, Cedeno and Rieder (1981) to increase significantly as incubation continued: the ratio was 0.89 at 30 minutes; at zero time it was calculated to be 0.35. It was suggested that degradation of the excess β chains was responsible for the low levels of circulating Hb H (5–8%) and for the mildness of the patient's illness (see also Wickramasinghe et al., 1984).

As already referred to (p. 453), Rigas and Koler (1961) studied two patients with Hb-H disease who were splenectomized. They stressed that the instability of Hb H was enhanced by environmental factors, particularly chemicals and drugs; and they found that erythrocyte survival improved following splenectomy. Rigas and Koler, noting that conversion of Hb H to methaemoglobin accelerated its denaturation, suggested that the gradual formation of methaemoglobin as the cells aged was an important factor in the denaturation and precipitation of Hb H in vivo. They also found that denaturation was promoted by anoxia. They concluded that the spleen, if present, would filter off the precipitated material, and that in its absence the precipitates would persist in the older erythrocytes in the form of Heinz bodies easily visible under the light microscope.

As in the unstable haemoglobin haemolytic anaemias, the precipitated material appears to coalesce (in the absence of the spleen) and tends to form single large inclusions.

Gabuzda and co-workers (1965) centrifuged blood samples from two Hb-H disease patients who had not been splenectomized. At least twice as much Hb H was found in the top fraction compared with the bottom (older-cell) fraction. Nathan and Gunn (1966) also made some interesting observations. Centrifugation of the blood of splenectomized Hb-H patients revealed two populations. The top 10% of cells (the youngest) contained few Heinz bodies but much soluble Hb H which could be precipitated with brilliant cresyl blue: the bottom 10% of cells contained much less total haemoglobin and precipitable Hb H and in many of the cells there was a single large round Heinz body. K$^+$ flux was greater in cells from the bottom layer than in cells from the top layer and it was suggested that this was due to membrane damage resulting from the Heinz-body formation.

Wennberg and Weiss (1968) reported on a light- and electron-microscopic study of the spleen of a 29-year-old patient with Hb-H disease. They found evidence of two patterns of splenic action: the removal of intracellular precipitates from the erythrocytes as they squeezed their way through the slits between adjacent sinus-lining cells and, less commonly, the splitting of erythrocytes into two or more fragments during their passage from splenic cord to sinus. The latter mechanism, Wennberg and Weiss suggested, could explain how a hypochromic macrocyte could be split into 'two small, dense cells leaving behind a small fragment to be phagocytosed by splenic macrophages'. Wennberg and Weiss postulated that the presence of the abnormal haemoglobin would make the erythrocytes abnormally rigid and suggested that (if this was so) the cells would not regain their original shape once the deforming force exerted on them during their passage through the sinus wall was removed. The presence of much iron in the sinus-lining cells and numerous macrophages in the splenic cords was interpreted as further evidence of the spleen's haemolytic activity.

How exactly the precipitation of Hb H within erythrocytes leads to their premature senescence is an interesting problem. In the absence of the spleen, membrane damage caused by factors similar to those that have been demonstrated in β-thalassaemia probably play a significant part. With the spleen in situ, the same factors plus cumulative damage sustained by the cells in passing through the organ presumably operate. The favourable results of removing the spleen in Hb-H disease illustrate its importance in curtailing erythrocyte life-span.

ROLE OF THE SPLEEN IN THALASSAEMIA: A SUMMARY

The spleen plays a significant role in the pathogenesis of thalassaemia, and its enlargement is an important clinical feature in thalassaemia major and intermedia and in Hb-H disease. Histopathological studies and in-vivo counting after labelling erythrocytes with ^{51}Cr provide evidence that the spleen removes severely defective erythrocytes from the circulation; in addition, it removes inclusions (precipitated α-globin chains, Hb H, siderotic granules) from erythrocytes which manage to escape from the spleen pulp. The histopathological findings (p. 497) and the accumulation of ^{51}Cr after erythrocyte labelling (p. 412) are in accord with the slight to moderate improvement which may follow splenectomy, particularly where the spleen in greatly enlarged. Removal of the spleen profoundly affects the blood picture in all types of thalassaemia (p. 407), although it does not alter the essential basis of the disorders — namely, failure of globin-chain synthesis.

MOLECULAR GENETICS OF THE THALASSAEMIAS

Ever since it was considered that the basis of thalassaemia appeared to be a complete or partial failure to form one or other of the globin chains of haemoglobin, the cause and mechanism of this failure have been the subjects of much research and speculation.

In 1957, Itano wrote that he could not exclude the possibility that the product of the thalassaemia allele 'is an abnormal form [of haemoglobin] having the same electrophorettic mobility as haemoglobin A', this suggestion being based on the knowledge that the mutant haemoglobins that had been studied up to that time were all synthesized in amounts smaller than was normal adult haemoglobin. Itano's concept had to be discarded when it became clear that the amino-acid composition of globin chains obtained from thalassaemic blood was normal in all respects. With this in mind Ingram and Stretton (1959), in the same paper in which they proposed that there were two types of thalassaemia according to whether the synthesis of the α or β peptide chain was affected, suggested that lowered production of a peptide chain could be due to the incomplete switching on of a genetic element which controls the turning on (or off) of the structural genes for the α and β chains. This was their 'tap' hypothesis.

Ingram (1964) introduced a new idea, namely, that 'the basic defect in thalassaemia is the production of a defective messenger RNA molecule for either the α peptide chain in the case of a α-thalassaemia or for the β peptide chain'. He went on to suggest that the messenger RNA molecule might combine with ribosomes in the usual way but because it was defective it might block the synthetic activity of the ribosomes so that very few or even no peptide chains were produced.

Weatherall (1968) discussed the mechanisms that might result in peptide-chain synthesis being defective, according to knowledge then available. They were: total or partial reduction in the rate of production of messenger RNA (mRNA); the rate of production of mRNA might be normal but it might be qualitatively altered so that globin-chain assembly on the mRNA-ribosomal template was retarded, or chain initiation or termination might be defective.

By 1981, Steinberg and Adams were able to list a far larger number of mechanisms that had actually been shown to produce the haematological findings of thalassaemia. They were: gene deletions; impaired processing of nuclear RNA; nonsense mutations; fusion genes; elongated globin chains resulting from termination codon mutants, and, rarely, very unstable globins such as that of Hb Indianapolis. They suggested, too, that gene transcription defects secondary to mutation in 5' promotor sequences would eventually be discovered. Since 1981 progress has been even more rapid, as recent reviews illustrate.

In a review dedicated to the mutation and polymorphism of the human β-globin gene and its surrounding DNA, Orkin and Kazazian (1984) listed no less than 30 specific mutations known (up to the time of writing) to lead to β^0- or β^+-thalassaemia. The sequence changes, ethnic group of the affected individuals and references were tabulated. Orkin and Kazazian pointed out, too, that because of the extensive genetic heterogeneity most patients considered on clinical grounds to have thalassaemia major are in reality genetic compounds rather than homozygotes (except for those individuals living in isolated geographical areas). Their tabulation referred to what they termed 'simple thalassaemia', *i.e.*, to cases in which β-globin synthesis alone is affected. [The term complex β-thalassaemia was used for cases in which the formation of β-like globins is affected also — as in the various types of δβ-thalassaemia and the HPFH syndromes.] In relation to the mutations causing simple (*sic*) β-thalassaemia, they discussed and gave references to mutations resulting in impairment of transcription, premature chain termination leading to the production of non-functional mRNAs, and errors in mRNA splicing resulting from sequence changes at splice junctions or within introns or from enhancement of a cryptic splice site.

Nienhuis, Anagnou and Ley's (1984) review entitled 'Advances in thalassemia research' also included a comprehensive survey of the molecular mechanisms of thalassaemia: the remarkable complexity of the structure of the globin genes, and of mRNA transcription, processing and translation, and the multitude of mutations known to affect almost every stage in the process and to lead to thalassaemia, are well documented.

The progress that has been made since the mid-1960s towards the complete understanding of the causes and mechanisms of the thalassaemias has indeed been startling, in parallel with the remarkable strides that have been made in the knowledge of gene structure and molecular genetics. The newly emerging techniques of molecular biology have been applied with great effect. The result has been that thalassaemia has been demonstrated to be heterogeneous to a degree that was undreamed of in the 1960s and earlier. In the account that follows an attempt will be made to refer to the highlights of a remarkable and complicated story

that has not yet been completed. The literature on the molecular-genetic aspects of thalassaemia is now extensive, and it is impossible in a book of this size and scope to refer to more than a proportion of the papers that have been published. Brief reference will, however, first be made to the molecular-biological techniques that have enabled the new work to be carried out and to the arrangement of the human globin genes in health, before summarizing what has been found out about the thalassaemias.

The following are readily available reviews the present author has found particularly valuable as records of the state of knowledge at the time they were written: Weatherall (1968, 1979), Marks and Bank (1971), Nienhuis and Anderson (1974), Nienhuis and Benz (1977), Bank *et al.* (1980), Benz *et al.* (1980), Jackson and Williamson (1980), Orkin (1980), Bank (1981, 1985), Steinberg and Adams (1981), Benz and Forget (1982), Weatherall and Clegg (1982), Kan (1983), Orkin, Antonarakis and Kazazian (1983), Nienhuis, Anagnou and Ley (1984), Orkin and Kazazian (1984), Weatherall and Wainscoat (1985) and Bunn and Forget (1986).

Analysis of the globin genes

The first step in the analysis is to obtain DNA. Leucocytes from 10–20 ml of blood should provide sufficient DNA for the analysis. The next step is to extract the DNA from the blood's buffy coat and to submit the extract to the action of a restriction endonuclease (of bacterial origin) which will cut up the DNA into small fragments, different enzymes cleaving the DNA nucleotide sequence at specific places known as restriction sites. The product of this enzyme digestion can then be separated by electrophoresis in agarose gel, the migration rates of the fragments being inversely proportional to their molecular size. Next, the fragments are transferred from the agarose gel to a sheet of nitrocellulose by the blotting technique originally described by Southern (1975). The fragments can then be submitted to possible hybridization with ^{32}P-labelled complementary DNA (cDNA) probes, prepared in the case of probes for α- or β-globin genes from messenger RNA obtained from reticulocytes, using enzymes referred to as reverse transcriptase that can synthesize DNA on an RNA template. [Such enzymes were first described by Baltimore (1970) and Temin and Mizutani (1970).] In this way it is possible to locate the α- or β-globin genes amongst the isolated and separated fragments of DNA, the bound labelled cDNA being demonstrated by autoradiography after placing an emulsion sensitive to the β particles of ^{32}P adjacent to the nitrocellulose filter. [Old and Higgs (1983) give a detailed account of how exactly these complicated and exacting manoeuvres can be carried out.]

It is possible, too, to clone globin genes. In order to achieve this, fragments of DNA containing the genes are introduced into the DNA of certain bacteria by the use of plasmids or bacteriophages. Replication of the bacteria in a successful experiment generates large amounts of the introduced gene or genes. The above techniques, of which the above account is the merest sketch, and the use of a range of restriction enzymes capable of cleaving DNA at different sites, have enabled a complete map of the organization of the human globin genes to be constructed. Weatherall (1979) and Jackson and Williamson (1980) give excellent summaries of the technical procedures through and by which most of the new knowledge has been gained.

Arrangement of the globin genes

In man, the globin genes are situated in clusters on two different chromosomes: the δ, β, γ and epsilon (ε) genes are located in chromosome 11 and the two α genes and the zeta (ζ) genes are in chromosome 16 (Deisseroth et al., 1977, 1978; Proudfoot et al., 1980). Kan (1983) gave a valuable summary account of, and references to, the evidence which has enabled the precise order and location of the genes on the chromosomes, and the distance between them, measured in thousands of base pairs (kb), to be determined.

In each chromosome 16 there are normally two α-globin gene loci separated by approximately 3700 base pairs (3.7 kb): one is named α1, the other upstream or leftward (in the 5′ direction) α2. Further upstream are two pseudo (non-functional) α genes, ψα1 and ψα2, and further upstream still are a pseudo zeta (ψ ζ) gene and a zeta (ζ) gene. Downstream or rightward (in the 3′ direction) is a theta (θ)1 gene (Fig. 19.7).

In each chromosome 11 the δ-globin locus lies approximately 7 kb upstream or leftward (in the 5′ direction) from the β-globin gene locus. Further upstream (approximately 15 kb) is the ^{A}γ-gene locus with a pseudo β gene (ψβ) in between. Approximately 5 kb upstream from the ^{A}γ gene is the ^{G}γ gene; the epsilon (ε) gene is further upstream still (Fig. 19.7).

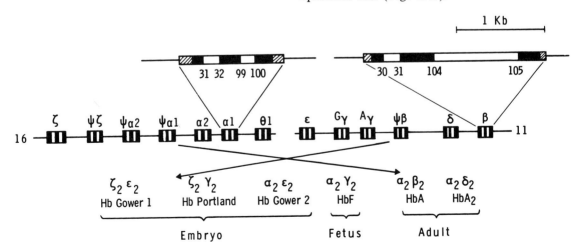

Fig. 19.7 Arrangement of the human globin genes on chromosome 16 (left) and chromosome 11 (right).
　The figure includes an enlargement of the α$_1$ and β genes, the black areas being exons and the white areas introns; the hatched areas are non-coding regions; the figures refer to codon numbers. The scale (1 kb) refers to the enlarged genes. The figure illustrates, too, the constitution of the haemoglobins found normally in the human embryo, fetus and adult. (Reproduced by courtesy of Sir David Weatherall.)

It is interesting to recall Neel's (1961) prescient analysis of the likely arrangement of the globin genes based on the genetic information then available to him. He concluded that the loci determining the specificity of the α and β chains were not closely linked and that 'the simplest interpretation would place the β, γ and δ structural or "template" genes on the same chromosome'.

MOLECULAR GENETICS OF THE β-THALASSAEMIAS

The most commonly met with lesion is a nucleotide mutation which affects in one way or the other the amount of mRNA available for β-globin synthesis. Deletions at the β-gene locus do, however, occur.

Early work suggested that defective regulation of β-chain mRNA production rather than defective translation was responsible for a reduced rate of β-chain synthesis (Clegg et al., 1968; Cividalli, Nathan and Lodish, 1974). Forget and co-workers (1974) and Benz, Swerdlow and Forget (1975) studied two unrelated β^0-thalassaemia homozygotes and reported that functional β-globin-specific mRNA was absent; they suggested that the DNA sequences coding for the mRNA were deleted. Ottolenghi and co-workers (1975) analysed the globin genes in a patient with $\beta^0/\delta\beta^0$-thalassaemia: mRNA specific for β globin was not detected but the β-globin genes did not appear to be deleted; partial deletion could, however, not be excluded.

Orkin and co-workers (1979b) reported on an analysis of the β-globin gene complex in 17 individuals with β^+- or β^0-thalassaemia and were able to demonstrate in three Indian patients with β^0-thalassaemia a consistent deletion of 0.6 kb of DNA, i.e. the β-globin gene was partially deleted. In the remaining patients, mostly of Mediterranean origin, the β-gene complex appeared to be intact.

Flavell and co-workers (1979) independently reported similar findings. Twenty-one patients with β^0- or β^+-thalassaemia were studied and in almost all cases no deletions in the vicinity of the

β- or δ-globin genes were detected. However, in a single Asian patient with homozygous β-thalassaemia they were able to demonstrate a deletion of approximately 600 bp which involved most or all of the 3' end of the β-globin gene.

Chang and Kan (1979) and Chang et al. (1980) identified a nonsense mutation in a Chinese patient with β^0-thalassaemia. The mutation (resulting in the production of a termination codon) caused premature termination of the β chain.

The report of the Fourth Cooley's Anemia Symposium held at the New York Acadamy of Sciences on 21st–23rd May 1979 contained several papers and reviews devoted to β-globin gene analysis in β-thalassaemia phenotypes. Bank and co-workers (1980), reporting that β genes were present in β^+- and β^0-thalassaemia, looked forward to globin-gene cloning providing material which would enable specific DNA defects to be defined. Tuan et al. (1980) stated that they had failed to find any evidence of gene deletion in three cases of homozygous β^0-thalassaemia. Mears et al. (1980) similarly reported that they had detected no differences from the normal gene map in several patients homozygous for β^+- or β^0-thalassaemia.

Conconi and co-workers (1980) reported on their investigation of β^0-thalassaemia as it occurs in the Ferrara district of Italy; they concluded that the translation of the mRNA is defective, and suggested that it decays faster than normal. In 1980, too, it was reported that in seven patients with β-thalassaemia (of diverse ethnic origin) the cause of the β-globin deficiency was a failure in the processing of nuclear mRNA precursor to mature cytoplasmic mRNA (Kantor, Turner and Nienhuis, 1980; Maquat et al., 1980).

In 1981, further interesting information illustrating the heterogeneity of β-thalassaemia was reported. Westaway and Williamson (1981) and Spritz et al. (1981) detected in Turkish-Cypriot and Greek-Cypriot patients, respectively, an intervening sequence (intron) nucleotide base change in cloned β^+-thalassaemia genes. Trecartin and co-workers (1981) reported that β^0-thalassaemia is caused in the great majority of Sardinians by a nonsense mutation: at the position corresponding to amino acid 39 the glutamine codon (CAG) is converted to an amber termination codon (UAG). They had earlier reported a nonsense mutation in the β-globin mRNA at the position corresponding with amino acid 17 in a Chinese patient with β⁰-thalassaemia (Chang and Kan, 1979) and they predicted that other β⁰-thalassaemias with mutations at various points along the β-globin gene would comprise a discrete subgroup of β⁰-thalassaemias.

Moschonas *et al.* (1981) and Orkin and Goff (1981) found in Italian patients with β⁰-thalassaemia the same single nucleotide substitution in the codon for amino acid 39 as had Trecartin *et al.* (1981). Orkin and Goff also discovered in a Turkish patient a dinucleotide deletion in the codon for amino acid 8; this frameshift mutation, too, produced a termination codon. They concluded that mutations such as they had described that lead to premature termination of β-globin synthesis were probably common causes of β-thalassaemia.

Baird and co-workers (1981), too, obtained evidence for an IVS splice junction mutation in an Italian patient and in two Iranian patients with homozygous β⁰-thalassaemia, and Maquat *et al.* (1981) found the mRNA to be very unstable in a variety of β⁰-thalassaemia occurring in Kurdish Jews.

Further evidence indicating that the mutation at codon 39 is a common cause of β⁰-thalassaemia was reported by Pergolizzi *et al.* (1981), Humphries *et al.* (1984) and Takeshita *et al.* (1984). Both the latter groups demonstrated that cloned β⁰-39 thalassaemia genes transfected into tissue-cultured cells generated far less β-mRNA than did normal genes. Takeshita and co-workers summarized the molecular-genetic causes of β-thalassaemia known to them at the time they wrote their paper as including partial gene deletions, impaired function of the transcription promotor region, errors in processing (splicing) of β-mRNA precursors and the creation of premature translation termination codons that abolish translation of β-mRNA into β globin.

The remarkable heterogeneity of the molecular lesions responsible for β-thalassaemia was further underlined by the report of Kazazian *et al.* (1984) who, investigating 44 Asian Indians, found evidence for seven different mutations — one

nonsense, three frameshift, one affecting an acceptor splice site and two affecting a donor splice site. None of these mutations had, it was thought, been identified in Mediterranean populations. About one-third of the patients investigated had the Indian-type (619 bp) deletion.

β-thalassaemias associated with gene deletions

As previously stated, in a minority of individuals with β-thalassaemia part or all of the β-globin gene in chromosome 11 appears to be deleted. Partial deletion (0.6 kb) towards the 3′ end was demonstrated by Orkin *et al.* (1979b, 1980) in three patients of Indian origin. Similar observations in thalassaemic Indians were described independently by Flavell *et al.* (1979). An 'Indian' deletion type of thalassaemia was thus designated. According to Spritz and Orkin (1982) duplication followed by deletion accounts for the loss of part of the β⁰-thalassaemia gene.

Deletion types of β-thalassaemia have also been identified in other racial groups. Gilman, Huisman and Abels (1984) obtained evidence for the complete loss (a 10-kb deletion) of the β-globin gene (but not of the δ-globin gene) in a 57-year-old Dutchman. He had relatively few symptoms. 98% of his haemoglobin was Hb F, 2% Hb A_2, and no Hb A was detectable. Padanilam, Felice and Huisman (1984) described the partial (1.35 kb) deletion of the β-globin gene in an American black patient with Hb-S/β⁰-thalassaemia and also in his uncle who was a β⁰-thalassaemia heterozygote. The site of the deletion was shown to be different from that in Indian-type deletion β⁰-thalassaemia.

An interesting recent development has been the assay of cloned genes in heterologous cell cultures (Treisman, Orkin and Maniatis, 1983), a technique that provides the possibility of comparing gene effectiveness *in vitro* with clinical expression *in vivo*. Treisman, Orkin and Maniatis, however, concluded that such comparisons might not be meaningful. It is interesting to note, nevertheless, that the IVS-1 position-6 mutant gene was associated with only mild RNA processing abnormalities — *in vivo*, this is the gene that has been identified in Portuguese and Cypriots who suffer from a relatively benign form of thalassaemia (Tamagnini *et al.*, 1983; Wainscoat *et al.*, 1983). Another mutant gene that was found to impair function only moderately in the cultured cell assay was that associated with a mild type of thalassaemia occurring in American blacks (Antonarakis *et al.*, 1984). These findings reinforce the concept that mild clinical expression is in many instances associated with the presence of particular mutant genes.

[Another cause is the presence, too, of α-thalassaemia genes; see p. 459.]

The rapid growth of knowledge concerning the basic genetic lesions responsible for β-thalassaemia has been recently vividly illustrated by the publication in the journal *Hemoglobin* under the title 'The Thalassemia Repository' (Lanclos and Kutlar, 1986) of an up-to-date listing of all the mutations that have been described as being responsible for β^0- and β^+-thalassaemia. Thirty-six are in fact listed under the following headings — deletions (three types), nonsense and/or frameshift mutations (11 types), promotor defects (five types) and splicing defects (17 types). The nucleotide substitution responsible for each type is given along with the haplotype (if known), as well as the ethnic origin of the patient, his or her phenotype (whether β^0 or β^+) and the corresponding reference in the literature. In addition, the mechanism is given by which the mutation is thought to affect β-globin synthesis. The mutations have been recorded in 14 different populations: seven different mutations have been so far identified in Asian-Indian and American black populations, respectively, six in Mediterranean populations, four in Chinese, and a lesser number in the remaining groups.

Reports of further 'new' mutations, not included in Lanclos and Kutlar's list, include those of Boehm et al. (1986) (β^0-thalassaemia in a Saudi-Arabian family), Padanilam and Huisman (1986) (β^0-thalassaemia in a black American family) and Takihara et al. (1986) (β^+-thalassaemia in a Japanese patient).

MOLECULAR GENETICS OF $\delta\beta$-THALASSAEMIA AND HPFH

Major deletions present

It is now known that extensive deletions within the δ- and β-gene cluster are responsible for most types of $\delta\beta$-thalassaemia and HPFH. Typically, in the $^{G}\gamma^{A}\gamma\delta\beta$ variety the deletion starts downstream to the β-globin gene, includes the whole of the β-globin gene and extends to, and involves, part only of the δ-globin gene (Fig. 19.7) (Bernards, Kooter and Flavell 1979; Fritsch,

Lawn and Maniatis, 1979; Ottolenghi et al., 1979; Bank et al., 1980). In other variants the deletion involves the whole of the β-globin gene and extends to about 3.8 kb 5' to the δ-globin gene (Jagadeeswaran et al., 1982; Ottolenghi and Giglioni, 1982).

$^{G}\gamma^{A}\gamma$ **HPFH.** More extensive deletions lead to $^{G}\gamma^{A}\gamma$ HPFH: they involve the β-globin gene and the whole of the δ-globin gene and extend further upstream towards the pseudo $\beta1$ gene (Bethlenfalvay et al., 1975; Mears et al., 1978; Bernards and Flavell, 1980; Tuan et al., 1980) (Fig. 19.7).

Tuan and her co-workers (1980) concluded that at least two types of extensive DNA deletions, differing in their 5' and 3' end-points lead to the common $^{G}\gamma^{A}\gamma$ variety of HPFH that occurs in blacks: in HPFH-1 a relatively small amount of inter γ-δ-gene DNA is deleted; in HPFH-2 the amount deleted is approximately 5 kb greater. The additional deletion does not, however, appear to affect the HPFH phenotype.

Further specific types of deletion have been identified in other populations. Saglio and co-workers (1986), who described a 'new' deletion in three different Southern-Italian families, gave the probable dimensions of the deletions in three other types of $^{G}\gamma^{A}\gamma$ HPFH and compared the findings with the deletions present in several types of $(\delta\beta)^0$-thalassaemia.

$(^{A}\gamma\delta\beta)^0$-**thalassaemia.** This is the condition originally referred to as $^{G}\gamma(\delta\beta)$-thalassaemia. The responsible deletions are even more extensive. Loss of the β- and δ-globin genes is accompanied by deletion of part or all of the $^{A}\gamma$-globin gene (Fritsh, Lawn and Maniatis, 1979; Orkin, Alter and Altay, 1979; Jones et al., 1981a). In another variant (identified in Indian families) deletions are accompanied by an inversion involving the $^{A}\gamma$-, δ- and β- globin genes (Jones et al., 1981b; Nakatsuji et al., 1984).

Trent and co-workers (1984), who described the clinical and haematological findings in five families with $(^{A}\gamma\delta\beta)^0$-thalassaemia, of Malaysian, Chinese, Bangladeshi, Indian and Kuwaiti origin, were able to demonstrate four different deletions, including one not hitherto reported. Despite the molecular differences the clinical and haematological phenotypes were similar.

Henthorn and co-workers (1985) reported on a study carried out on $(^{A}\gamma\delta\beta)^0$-thalassaemia individuals who were members of 10 black families. A large 34-kb deletion was identified which appeared to be different from those previously described in similar cases. Part of the $^{A}\gamma$ gene and all of the $\psi\beta$, δ and β genes were deleted.

γβ-thalassaemia. Still more extensive are the deletions which have been described in this rare condition (Kan, Forget and Nathan, 1972; Van der Ploeg et al., 1980; Orkin, Goff and Nathan, 1981; Fearon et al., 1983). In the Mexican-American family studied by Fearon and his co-workers, the deletion extends for more than 105 kb, resulting in the loss of the entire β-globin gene cluster.

Curtin and co-workers (1985) described a most unusual family, four members of which presented with a microcytic hypochromic anaemia. Atypical γδβ-thalassaemia was diagnosed; the Hb-A$_2$ percentage was normal. Gene mapping revealed an extensive deletion which extended upstream for at least 100 kb from the 3rd exon of the $^{G}\gamma$ gene. The $^{A}\gamma$-,$\psi\beta$-, δ- and β-globin genes in *cis* were intact. Despite this the patients presented a thalassaemia-minor-like phenotype, and Curtin et al. concluded that this suggested 'that chromatin structure and conformation are important for globin gene expression'. None of the affected members of the family gave a history of haemolytic disease requiring transfusion in the neonatal period, as had been the case in previously reported cases.

Major deletions absent

Types of HPFH have been described in which the γδβ gene cluster appears to be largely intact. Balsley and co-workers (1982), for instance, found no evidence of a major deletion in a black American family diagnosed as having $^{G}\gamma\beta^{+}$-HPFH; and British (Jones et al., 1982; Wood et al., 1982) and Greek (Bernards and Flavell, 1980; Papayannopoulou et al., 1982) $^{A}\gamma$ variants have been reported in which most of the γ chains formed are of the $^{A}\gamma$ variety and in which there appear to be no major deletions. These conditions appear to be the result of mutations leading to a regulatory abnormality affecting the repression of γ-chain synthesis which normally takes place in post-natal life, and in an interesting study of West-Indian and American blacks with $^{G}\gamma\beta^{+}$-HPFH, Collins et al.

(1984a,b) were able to demonstrate a point mutation, guanosine for cytosine, 202 bp 5' to the $^{G}\gamma$ gene.

A further interesting type of HPFH, described by Jensen et al. (1984) as occurring in a mother and her daughter, was found to be associated with chromosomal translocations involving chromosomes 6, 9, 11 and 20. One of the breakpoints was in band p 12 in the short arm of chromosome 11 where the γδβ-globin gene cluster is situated. The percentage of Hb F in the peripheral blood was moderately raised, but neither subject was anaemic and their MCV and MCH were normal. There was no evidence of any gene deletion.

In the case of the Greek ($^{A}\gamma\beta^{+}$) type of HPFH, recent studies suggest that this is brought about by a sequence change in the first 200 nucleotides 5' of the $^{A}\gamma$ gene (Waber et al., 1986).

γ-thalassaemia

In this condition, as described by Sukumaran and co-workers (1983), an Indian infant was born with Hb F formed of $^{A}\gamma^{T}$ chains but no $^{G}\gamma$ chains. Analysis of the DNA of the infant's father suggested the presence of a hybrid $^{G}\gamma^{A}\gamma$ gene resulting from homologous but unequal crossing-over between the $^{G}\gamma$ and $^{A}\gamma$ genes.

β-GLOBIN DNA POLYMORPHISMS

A perhaps not unexpected development has been the demonstration of DNA polymorphisms in the β-globin gene cluster, i.e., significant differences have been shown to exist in gene structure in healthy individuals when their DNA is submitted to restriction enzyme analysis (Kan and Dozy, 1978; Lawn et al., 1978, 1980; Orkin, Antonarakis and Kazazian, 1983; Orkin and Kazazian, 1984).

Orkin and Kazazian (1984) illustrated in a figure the location of 17 polymorphic sites located from 5' to the ε gene to 3' to the β gene, and they pointed out that since most of the polymorphisms are present in all racial groups they can be considered as ancient markers of β-globin gene clusters. Orkin and co-workers (1982) had suggested that as the disease-producing mutations are primarily restricted to particular ethnic groups, such mutations must have occurred relatively recently. Whether specific mutations are associated with particular DNA polymorphisms (haplotypes) is an interesting question, and Orkin and co-workers (1982) have provided some evidence in favour of this. For instance, 47% of 91 individuals of Mediterranean origin with β-thalassaemia were found to have haplotype-1 chromosomes. They demonstrated also, however, that the same thalassaemia-causing mutation could be found within different haplotypes in the same population, probably it was suggested as the result of crossing over; and they isolated from the 91 individuals eight different mutant thalassaemia genes within nine different β-globin gene haplotypes. Seven of the eight mutant genes were found in Italians from various places in Italy; six were present in Greeks.

Additional reports on the relationship between DNA haplotypes and β-thalassaemia include those of Kazazian et al. (1984) on people of Mediterranean origin, Giampaolo et al. (1984) on Southern Italians, Cheng et al. (1984) on Chinese (living in Hong Kong or New York), Aksoy et al. (1985) on Turkish Cypriots, Turks, Macedonians and Bulgarians, and Harano et al. (1985) on black Americans. These reports emphasized the heterogeneity of β-thalassaemia, even in limited geographical areas, and the close association between haplotype and specific mutations.

Kazazian and co-workers (1984) concluded that a different mutation had arisen within each haplotype and they recorded the incidence of 10 haplotypes in β^A and β^{thal} chromosomes: on average, 86% of the thalassaemia mutations within a particular haplotype were found to be identical. Their data were based on the chromosomes of 156 individuals. Of the thalassaemia-major patients investigated by Aksoy et al. (1985), the majority of those living in North Cyprus were homozygous for haplotype 1; those from other racial groups were mostly compound heterozygotes for two different haplotypes.

MOLECULAR GENETICS OF THE α-THALASSAEMIAS

The genetic abnormalities responsible for the α-thalassaemias are many and varied. Both gene deletion and non-deletion types exist, the former being the commoner. The extent of the deletions, in the region of the α genes, can be correlated with the degree to which α-globin production is impaired: deletion of a single gene leads to α-thalassaemia-2 (α-thal-2); a deletion involving both genes (on the same chromosone or a single gene on both chromosomes) results in α-thalassaemia-1 (α-thal-1) (Table 18.4, p. 447). The deletions are the consequences of misalignment of the strands of DNA during meiosis and unequal (non-homologous) interchromosomal crossing-over. This process leads (when one α gene is lost) to the occurrence of chromosomes bearing three α genes (see p. 517).

The non-deletion varieties of α-thalassaemia are the consequence of mutations within, or in the vicinity of, the α genes; the mutations affect α-globin production although the genes themselves are intact. The clinical syndromes that result from the mutations depend upon the degree to which α-globin production is interfered with.

Recent reviews of the molecular pathology of the α-thalassaemias and the responsible molecular rearrangements within the α-globin gene cluster include those of Kan (1985) and Higgs et al. (1985).

As in the β-thalassaemias, some of the molecular abnormalities that lead to the α-thalassaemias have a much higher incidence in (or are only found in) certain ethnic groups. As in the β-thalassaemias, too, many of the individuals who at first sight appear to be homozygous for a particular genetic abnormality can be shown on further investigation to be compound heterozygotes for two different abnormalities. It is hardly to be wondered at that the clinical phenotype of such individuals is highly variable.

GENE DELETIONS AS THE CAUSE OF α-THALASSAEMIA

In 1974 two papers appeared in the same issue of the journal *Nature* in which it was suggested that gene deletion was responsible for the severe form of α-thalassaemia that led to hydrops fetalis: Ottolenghi and co-workers (1974) concluded that 'a substantial, in all probability complete, deletion of the genes for α globin is the molecular mechanism which produces α-thal-1 disorder and hence, in its homozygous state, the Hb Bart's hydrops syndrome', and Taylor and co-workers (1974), who had studied two Chinese infants with hydrops fetalis, found that their DNA contained less than 2% of the α-chain sequences detectable in normal DNA; they concluded that part or all of the α-chain gene was deleted and that both loci must be affected.

In 1975 Kan and his co-workers reported that in a Chinese patient with Hb-H disease only one-quarter the number of α genes was present, as determined by the rate of annealment of cDNA with mRNA derived from the patient's reticulocytes; they concluded that their data supported the hypothesis that the four syndromes of α-thalassaemia — the silent carrier state (α-thal-2), heterozygous α-thalassaemia (α-thal-1), Hb-H disease, and hydrops fetalis — are the result of involvement of one, two, three or four α genes. Kan and his co-workers (1979) went on to study Hb-H disease in individuals of Mediterranean origin. Of 12 patients (from Cyprus and Sardinia), eight had a deletion defect with a single α-globin gene remaining, three had a non-deletion-type defect and one a 'dysfunctional' gene. They concluded that a deletion is the common cause of Hb-H disease in the area: the percentage of cDNA annealed was subnormal, the values being similar to those obtained with Asian patients. The three patients with the non-deletion lesion (and two α-globin genes present) gave a normal 23.0-kb fragment on restriction enzyme mapping with the *Eco* R1 enzyme, as did Asian patients with non-deletion Hb-H disease; the nine patients with low hybridization values gave a 19.0-kb fragment.

Dozy and co-workers (1979) reported on the α-globin gene organization in blacks with particular regard to the rarity of severe forms of α-thalassaemia. The α-globin genotype was measured in 211 American blacks: 149 were αα/αα, 58 −α/αα, four −α/−α. Not a single individual had the genotype −−/αα, commonly found in Asians (and in the homozygous form (−−/−−) responsible for hydrops fetalis). It was pointed out that

these findings explained why hydrops fetalis is unlikely to occur in blacks and why Hb-H disease (−−/−α) is so rare. Dozy and co-workers pointed out, too, that Hb-H disease would not be uncommon in the West Indies where there is a mixture of people of Asian and African origin. Higgs and co-workers (1979), reporting independently on two black West-Indian families with α-thalassaemia, came to the same conclusions. Two phenotypes were defined which resembled the (severe) α-thal-1 and (mild) α-thal-2 forms of α-thalassaemia seen in orientals. Genetic analysis indicated that the individuals who had α-thal-1 were homozygous for the α-thal-2 determinant and that α-thal-2 heterozygotes had the genotype −α/αα. Phillips and co-workers (1979) illustrated the pedigrees of two black American families with α-thalassaemia and gave details of the MCV and α:β globin-synthesis ratios of affected individuals. Three had Hb-H disease: this was clinically mild and the percentages of Hb H (4%, 1% and 10%) in the peripheral blood were low. Genetic analysis indicated that three α genes had been deleted and it was concluded that the single α gene could have originated by crossing-over of mispaired α genes leading to a deletion of about 4.2 kb.

Further details of the organization of α-globin genes in oriental α-thalassaemia were given by Embury *et al.* (1979). They found that in Chinese with Hb-H disease the 5′α-globin locus is deleted and that a single 3′α-globin locus is present on a 19.0-kb restriction enzyme-derived fragment; in α-thal-2 two α-globin genes are present on a 23.0-kb fragment and one on a 19-kb fragment, while in α-thal-1 (and in the non-deletion type of Hb-H disease) two α-globin genes are at two loci on one chromosome and none is present on the other chromosome. In a review, Embury, Dozy and Kan (1980) summarized the knowledge then available as to the molecular mechanisms of α-thalassaemia and contrasted the findings in two racial groups — the Chinese and American blacks. In both groups the common mechanism is a deletion, but the deletions differ. In Chinese the −−/ haplotype is the usual cause of α-thalassaemia trait, the two remaining genes being in *cis* (−−/αα): in blacks the common haplotype is −α/; it occurs in approximately one in four individuals and homozygosity results in an α-thalassaemia in which the remaining genes are in *trans* $(-\alpha/-\alpha)$.

Sancar, Cedeno and Rieder (1980) stressed how variable was the arrangement of the α-globin genes in α-thalassaemia and illustrated this with details of a short series of seven American blacks, two of whom had Hb-H disease. Six different genotypes were proposed! The series included patients with the triple ααα gene, Hb-G Philadelphia, Hb S, non-deletion thalassaemia (ααth) as well as the $-\alpha/$ and $--/$ haplotypes.

Altay, Gurgey and Tuncbilek (1980) investigated five Turkish families in which cases of Hb-H disease had occurred by means of restriction endonuclease DNA mapping. Four different α-gene haplotypes were demonstrated, and Altay, Gurgey and Tuncbilek concluded that the variation in the clinical and haematological findings in the Hb-H patients reflected the way in which the haplotypes were combined. According to Phillips and co-workers (1980), most patients with Hb-H disease have, however, the same genetic lesion: all 12 patients investigated — five black Americans, two Chinese and five Filipinos — gave identical restriction endonuclease fragment patterns indicative of the $--/-\alpha$ genotype, the result, it was considered, of unequal crossing-over. This is, however, not the mechanism in certain Saudi Arabians, in whom Pressley and co-workers (1980b) have reported that the $--/$ haplotype seems not to be present. The two common haplotypes identified by them in 11 families from the Qatif oasis in Eastern Saudi Arabia were a deletion one $(-\alpha)$ and a non-deletion one (αα^T). Interaction between these haplotypes and the αα haplotype produces a variety of phenotypes, the most severe of which is Hb-H disease caused by homozygosity for the non-deletion haplotype αα^T. The absence of the $--/$ haplotype precludes the occurrence of the Hb-Bart's hydrops fetalis syndrome. The syndrome does, however, occur in Greece. Kattamis and co-workers (1980) described such an occurrence (and gave three references to earlier reports of hydrops fetalis in Mediterranean populations). The particular interest of their report is that they demonstrated that the deletion responsible resulted in the loss of a ζ embryonic gene, too. The deletion was thus more extensive than the common deletion found in South-East Asia and had presumably arisen independently. An identical molecular defect was reported by Sophocleous et al. (1981) in a Greek-Cypriot infant with hydrops fetalis. An even larger deletion which included both ζ genes was identified by Orkin and Michelson (1980). This, it was suggested, would cause in homozygotes early fetal loss rather than the hydrops syndrome.

Further evidence of heterogeneity was furnished by Embury and co-workers (1980), who identified two different deletions, designated 'leftward' and 'rightward', respectively, which resulted in the loss of one α gene and led to α-thal-2. The rightward deletion genotype was found in all nine blacks and in all eight Mediterranean subjects investigated and in four out of 13 Chinese; the leftward deletion was found in four Chinese (the remaining five having a non-deletion lesion).

A still more extensive, hitherto undescribed, deletion was described by Pressley et al. (1980a), in a Greek family with α-thalassaemia of the α-thal-1 type. The deletion involved the α-2 globin gene and extended to, and removed part of, the 5′ end of the α-1 globin gene. The affected chromosome produced no α chains.

The remarkable genetic and molecular diversity of α-thalassaemia was well illustrated by Higgs and co-workers (1981) in a paper primarily concerned with non-deletion Hb-H disease; 13 α-thalassaemia haplotypes were known to them at the time of writing and these were calculated to be capable in theory of producing 105 different genotypes! Four haplotypes were considered to lead to the α⁰ phenotype (α-thal-1) and nine to the α⁺ phenotype (α-thal-2), amongst which were three non-deletion haplotypes and four haplotypes in which one α gene was a chain termination mutant gene.

A further variant capable of causing Hb-H disease was reported by Orkin, Goff and Hechtman (1981). This was a pentanucleotide deletion within the 5′ splice junction of the first intervening sequence. The result was failure to form stable mRNA.

Pirastu and co-workers (1982) reported on the frequency of α-thalassaemia haplotypes in two Mediterranean populations. The $-\alpha/$ haplotype causing α-thal-2 was relatively common: its frequency was 0.18 in Sardinians and 0.07 in Greek Cypriots — all the deletions were of the rightward type. The deletion $--/$ haplotype was not detected in any of the 119 randomly selected Greek Cypriots and Sardinian blood donors tested.

Sancar and co-workers (1983) gave details of the α-gene haplotypes in α-thalassaemia occurring in Ashkenazi Polish Jews, and Mathew et al. (1983) and Rousseau et al. (1985) reported on the α-thalassaemia genotypes in Cape coloured South Africans. Lie-Injo and her co-workers (1985) have reported similar studies employing α- and ζ-globin gene probes on Malaysian patients with α-thalassaemia, including patients with Hb-H disease and Hb-Bart's fetal hydrops cases. Most had deletions of the α1 and α2 globin genes which did not extend to the ψζ1 and ζ2 genes. Two newborns had non-deletion α-thal-1.

Felice and co-workers (1984) described and compared the clinical, haematological and molecular-genetic findings in two unusual and complicated cases of Hb-H disease. One of the patients was a 5-year-old black girl who was described as having an $\alpha^0\alpha^0/\alpha^0\alpha$; β/β^S genotype; the other, a 4-year-old Laotion boy, was thought to have an $\alpha^0\alpha^0/\alpha\alpha^{CS}$;$\beta/\beta^E$ genotype. Both were moderately anaemic and had markedly lowered MCVs and MCHs. The $\alpha^0\alpha^0(--/)$ haplotype of the black girl was shown to be the result of a major deletion involving the ζ gene and extending to and including the α_1 gene. According to Felice et al., this deletion, of rare occurrence in blacks, is the fifth variant resulting, in heterozygotes, in α-thal-1 (or, more accurately, $\zeta\alpha$-thal-1). The girl's Hb-H disease, of moderate severity, was the consequence of her inheriting the α-thal-2 trait ($\alpha^0\alpha$) (and Hb S) from her mother. The deletion giving rise to α-thal-1 ($\alpha^0\alpha^0$) in the Laotian boy was inherited, along with Hb E, from his mother. This deletion, although extensive, leaves the ζ gene intact. The boy inherited Hb Constant Spring from his father.

Recent technical advances have permitted more precise analysis of the extent of the deletions; the data, too, have underlined the remarkable heterogeneity of α-thalassameia. This is illustrated in the four publications quoted below.

Aksoy et al. (1985) described two Turkish patients with Hb-H disease due to a combination of a 3.7-kb deletion with a 25-kb deletion.

Nicholls et al. (1985) described four Cypriots with Hb-H disease and two infants with fetal hydrops. All had an uncommon $\alpha^0\alpha^0$ thalassaemia determinant designated α thal$^{2.6}$ that gives rise to a 20.5-kb deletion.

Wong et al. (1985) reported the results of haematological, biosynthetic and DNA studies on two black Canadian families with α-thalassaemia. Both propositi were compound heterozygotes for two α-thal-2 genotypes ($-\alpha^{3.7}$ and $-\alpha^{4.2}$).

Steinberg et al. (1986) described a black boy with the Hb-AS trait who had in addition a deletion affecting both α genes in one chromosome as well as the $\psi\alpha$ and $\varphi\zeta$ genes.

NON-DELETION α-THALASSAEMIA

The existence of non-deletion types of α-thalassaemia has been referred to in the previous section.

Kan and co-workers (1977) obtained evidence for such a lesion in members of a Chinese family, nine of whom were phenotypically α-thal-1 and two of whom had Hb-H disease. One parent gave a normal result on molecular hybridization with cDNA, despite presenting an α-thal-1 phenotype, and it was postulated that the combination of a deletion defect ($--$) and a non-deletion defect ($\alpha\alpha^T$) had led to Hb-H disease.

Orkin and co-workers (1979a), who had studied Hb-H disease patients belonging to a variety of racial groups, obtained evidence that in non-Asian patients (Italian, Turkish and Israeli) Hb-H disease might be associated with one, two or three α-gene loci in contrast to the one-gene (deletion) pattern demonstrable in Asians. They concluded that defective, not deleted, α genes led to α-thalassaemia in certain non-Asian individuals.

As already mentioned, a non-deletion haplotype ($\alpha\alpha^T$) is of common occurrence in the Qatif oasis in Eastern Saudi Arabia (Pressley et al., 1980b), and this was one of the three non-deletion haplotypes referred to by Higgs et al. (1981) — the other two types were designated $\alpha\alpha^{T(LM)}$ and $\alpha\alpha^{T(HM)}$, the superscripts LM and HM referring to the production of low levels and high levels, respectively, of non-functioning mRNA.

Details of the molecular lesions responsible for non-deletion α-thalassaemia have been given by del Senno et al. (1981) in Italians living in the Po river delta, by Goosens et al. (1982) in a Chinese patient, by Felber, Orkin and Hamer (1982) in an Italian patient and by Higgs et al. (1983) in Saudi-Arabian patients [see also Weatherall and Wainscoat (1985)].

The novel mechanism described by Goosens et al. (1982) was a nucleotide mutation in the α-2 globin gene which resulted in proline being substituted for leucine ($\alpha^{125\ Leu \to Pro}$) in a position critical for the $\alpha1$-$\beta1$ contact. The formation of $\alpha1$-$\beta1$ dimers is impeded and this leads to an α-thalassaemia-like phenotype. The variant was named Quong Sze.

Three recent reports confirming that the possession of a gene for a non-deletion α-thalassaemia, in combination with a gene giving rise to a deletion, is likely to lead to a clinical syndrome of unusual severity, are summarized below.

Di Marzo et al. (1986) reported that two Sicilian children had a severe form of Hb-H disease requiring transfusion. Their genotype included the non-deletion α-thalassaemia determinant $\alpha\alpha^{thal}$. The severity of the children's illness was attributed to the very low output of α globin associated with the α^{thal} determinant.

Trent *et al.* (1986) described two children who had a severe grade of Hb-H disease. Both had inherited non-deletion types of α-thalassaemia from one parent and a deletion haplotype (− −) from the other parent. One child died in the neonatal period; the other was trans-fusion-dependent.

Chan *et al.* (1985) reported that a Chinese infant with hydrops fetalis had one parent with a non-deletion α-thalassaemia trait and that the other parent had a complete deletion of the ζα gene cluster (genotype ζζαα/− − − −).

TRIPLICATED α GENES

As already mentioned, one result of chromosome misalignment and non-homologous crossing-over is the occurrence of three α-globin genes on one chromosome — the counterpart of the deletion of an α gene on the other chromosome. Normally, the presence of five α genes is not associated with any haematological abnormality.

Higgs and co-workers (1980) identified five α genes in three members of a Welsh family and raised the question as to whether some cases of 'silent' β-thalassaemia are caused by the presence of the ααα/αα (or ααα/ααα) genotype resulting in chain imbalance as the result of an increased output of α mRNA. In the case of the family they had studied, Higgs *et al.* suggested that the excess α-chain synthesis was being compensated for by proteolysis.

Goosens and co-workers (1980) identified 12 individuals who were similarly heterozygous for triplicated α genes (ααα/αα). Five were members of two black families and were found in screening 280 unrelated blacks, five were found in screening 50 unrelated Greeks; none was found in screening 125 Sardinians. In addition, one Sicilian and one Caucasian American were found to have a triplicated gene. The presence of the three α genes did not seem to lead to any haematological abnormality and no inclusions developed in blood exposed to brilliant cresyl blue or methyl violet. Not unexpectedly perhaps, more than one type of triplicated gene has subsequently been described, corresponding to deletions of different extent (Lie-Injo, Herrera and Kan, 1981; Trent *et al.*, 1981).

Some interesting effects of the presence of the ααα/αα genotype on individuals who are also heterozygous or homozygous for β-thalassaemia have, however, been described. Kanavakis and co-workers (1983) referred to five families in which both abnormalities were present. The presence of the ααα/αα genotype did not seem to affect those who were heterozygous for β-thalassaemia either clinically or haematologically, but the illness of four out of five of those who were homozygotes was unusually mild and conformed to the criteria of thalassaemia intermedia. It was suggested that the triplicated gene could act as an α-thalassaemia allele.

Sampietro *et al.* (1983), on the other hand, described a 32-year-old Italian woman with thalassaemia intermedia who had the ααα/αα genotype and was apparently heterozygous for β-thalassaemia. Three rather similar cases were described by Henni *et al.* (1985). Five sibs in an Algerian family had heterozygous β-thalassaemia: three who had a relatively severe illness with features of thalassaemia intermedia had inherited the ααα gene from their father; two sibs with typical mild heterozygous β-thalassaemia had normal α-globin genes.

REFERENCES

AKSOY, M., KUTLAR, A., EFREMOV, G. D., NIKOLOV, N., PETKOV, G., REESE, A. L., HARANO, T., CHEN, S. S. & HUISMAN, T. H. J. (1985). Haplotypes and levels of fetal hemoglobin and ᴳγ to ᴬγ ratios in Mediterranean patients with thalassaemia minor and major. *Amer. J. Hemat.*, **20**, 7–16.

AKSOY, M., KUTLAR, A., KUTLAR, F., HARENO, T., CHEN, S. S. & HUISMAN, T. H. J. (1985). Hemoglobin H disease in two Turkish females and one Iranian newborn. *Hemoglobin*, **9**, 373–384.

ALTAY, G., GURGEY, A. & TUNCBILEK, E. (1980). Hematological evaluation of patients with various combinations of α-thalassemia. *Amer. J. Hemat.*, **9**, 261–267.

ANTONARAKIS, S. E., ORKIN, S. K., CHENG, T.-C., SCOTT, A. F., SEXTON, J. P. & TRUSKO, S., CHARACHE, S. & KAZAZIAN, H. H. JNR (1984). β-thalassemia in American blacks: novel mutations in the TATA box and an acceptor splice site. *Proc. natn. Acad. Sci. U.S.A.*, **81**, 1154–1158.

ASTALDI, G., RONDANELLI, E. G., BERNARDELLI, E. & STROSSELLI, E. (1954). An abnormal substance present in the erythroblasts of thalassaemia major. Cytochemical investigations. *Acta haemat. (Basel)*, **12**, 145–153.

ASTALDI, G. & TOLENTINO, P. (1952). Studies on the pathogenesis of thalassaemia. *J. clin. Path.*, **5**, 140–144.

ASTALDI, G., TOLENTINO, P. & SACCHETTI, C. (1951a). Untersuchungen über die Biologie des Erythroblasten in der Thalassaemia major. *Helv. paediat. Acta*, **6**, 50–61.

ASTALDI, G., TOLENTINO, P. & SACCHETTI, C. (1951b). La Talassemia. *Biblioteca "haematologica"*, Pavia.

BAIRD, M., DRISCOLL, C., SCHREINER, H., SCIARRATTA, G. V., SANSONE, G., NIAZI, G., RAMIREZ, F. & BANK, A. (1981). A nucleotide change at a splice junction in a human β-globin gene is associated with $β^0$-thalassemia. *Proc. natn. Acad. Sci. U.S.A.*, **78**, 4218–4221.

BALSLEY, J. F., RAPPAPORT, E., SCHWARTZ, E. & SURREY, S. (1982). The γ-δ-β-globin gene region in $^Gγ$-β$^+$-hereditary persistence of fetal hemoglobin. *Blood*, **59**, 828–831.

BALTIMORE, D. (1970). RNA-dependent DNA polymerase in virions of RNA tumour viruses. *Nature (Lond.)*, **226**, 1209–1211.

BANK, A. (1981). Globin gene structure in disorders of hemoglobin. In: *Progress in Hematology*, Vol. XII (ed. by E. B. Brown), pp. 25–42. Grune and Stratton, New York.

BANK, A. (1985). Genetic defects in the thalassemias. *Curr. Top. Haemat.*, **5**, 1–23.

BANK, A., MEARS, J. G., RAMIREZ, F., BURNS, A. L., FELDENZER, J. & SPENCE, S. (1980). Detection of gene defects in the thalassemias and related disorders. *Ann. N.Y. Acad. Sci.*, **344**, 1–11.

BANK, A. & O'DONNELL, J. V. (1969). Intracellular loss of free α chains in β thalassaemia. *Nature (Lond.)*, **222**, 295–296.

BENZ, E. J. JNR, & FORGET, B. G. (1982). The thalassemia syndromes: models for the molecular analysis of a human disease. *Ann. Rev. Med.*, **33**, 363–373.

BENZ, E. J., GLASS, J., TSISTRAKIS, G. A., HILLMAN, D. G., CAVALLESCO, C., COUPAL, E., FORGET, B. G., TURNER, P. A., KANTOR, J. A. & NIENHUIS, A. W. (1980). Heterogeneity of messenger RNA defects in the thalassemia syndromes. *Ann. N.Y. Acad. Sci.*, **344**, 101–112.

BENZ, E. J. JNR, PRITCHARD, J., HILLMAN, D., GLASS, J. & FORGET, B. G. (1984). β globin messenger RNA content of bone marrow erythroblasts and heterozygous β-thalassemia. *Amer. J. Hemat.*, **16**, 33–45.

BENZ, E. J. JNR, SWERDLOW, P. S. & FORGET, B. G. (1975). Absence of functional messenger RNA activity for beta globin chain synthesis in $β^0$-thalassaemia. *Blood*, **45**, 1–10.

BERNARDS, R. & FLAVELL, R. A. (1980). Physical mapping of the globin gene deletion in hereditary persistence of foetal haemoglobin (HPFH). *Nucl. Acids Res.*, **8**, 1521–1534.

BERNARDS, R., KOOTER, J. M. & FLAVELL, R. A. (1979). Physical mapping of the globin gene deletion in $(δβ)^0$-thalassaemia. *Gene*, **6**, 265–280.

BERRY, C. L. & MARSHALL, W. C. (1967). Iron distribution in the liver of patients with thalassaemia major. *Lancet*, **i**, 1031–1033.

BESSIS, M., ALAGILLE, D. & BRETON-GORIUS, J. (1958). Particularités des érythroblastes et des érythrocytes dans la maladie de Cooley. Étude au microscope electronique. *Rev. Hémat.*, **13**, 538–551.

BESSIS, M. & BRETON-GORIUS, J. (1957). Étude au microscope electronique des granulations ferrugineuses des érythrocytes normaux et pathologiques. Anémias hémolytiques. Hémoglobinopathies. Saturnisme. *Rev. Hémat.*, **12**, 43–63.

BESSIS, M. & DE BOISFLEURY, A. (1970). Étude sur les poikilocytes au microscope à balayage, en particulier dans la thalassémie. *Nouv. Rev. franç. Hémat.*, **10**, 515–534.

BETHLENFALVAY, N. C., MOTULSKY, A. G., RINGELHANN, B., LEHMANN, H., HUMBERT, J. R., & KONOTEY-AHULU, F. I. D. (1975). Hereditary persistence of fetal hemoglobin, β thalassemia, and the hemoglobin δ-β locus: further family data and genetic interpretations. *Amer. J. hum. Genet.*, **27**, 140–154.

BLOCK, M. (1969). Histopathologic studies in beta-thalassemia minor and intermedia. *Ann. N.Y. Acad. Sci.*, **165**, 126–147.

BOEHM, C. D., DOWLING, C. E., WABER, P. G., GIARDINA, P. J. V. & KAZAZIAN, H. H. JNR (1986). Use of oligonucleotide hybridization in the characterization of a $β^0$-thalassemia gene ($β^{37\ TGG→TGA}$) in a Saudi Arabian family. *Blood*, **67**, 1185–1188.

BRUNORI, M., FALCIONI, G., FIORETTI, E., GIARDINA, B. & ROTILIO, J. (1975). Formation of superoxide in the autoxidation of the isolated α and β chains of human hemoglobin and its involvement in hemichrome precipitation. *Eur. J. Biochem.*, **53**, 99–104.

BUNN, H. F. & FORGET, B. G. (1986). *Hemoglobin: Molecular, Genetic and Clinical Aspects*, pp. 223–321. W. B. Saunders, Philadelphia.

BURKA, E. R. & MARKS, P. A. (1963). Ribosomes active in protein synthesis in human reticulocytes: a defect in thalassaemia major. *Nature (Lond.)*, **199**, 706–707.

CHALEVELAKIS, G., CLEGG, J. B. & WEATHERALL, D. J. (1975). Imbalanced globin chain synthesis in heterozygous β-thalassemic bone marrow. *Proc. natn. Acad. Sci. U.S.A.*, **72**, 3853–3857.

CHAN, V., CHAN, T. K., LIANG, S. T., GHOSH, A., KAN, Y. W. & TODD, D. (1985). Hydrops fetalis due to an unusual form of Hb H disease. *Blood*, **66**, 224–228.

CHANARIN, I., DACIE. J. V. & MOLLIN, D. L. (1959). Folic-acid deficiency in haemolytic anaemia. *Brit. J. Haemat.*, **5**, 245–256.

CHANG, J. C. & KAN, Y. W. (1979). β^0 thalassemia, a nonsense mutation in man. *Proc. natn. Acad. Sci. U.S.A.*, **76**, 2886–2889.

CHANG, J. C., KAN. Y. W., TRECARTIN, R. F. & TEMPLE, G. F. (1980). Nonsense mutation as a cause of β^0 thalassemia. *Ann. N.Y. Acad. Sci.*, **344**, 113–119.

CHANG, T-C., ORKIN, S. H., ANTANORAKIS, S. E., POTTER, M. J., SEXTON, J. P., MARKHAM, A. F., GIARDINA, P. J. V., LI, A. & KAZAZIAN, H. H. JNR (1984). β-thalassemia in Chinese: use of *in vivo* RNA analysis and oligonucleotide hybridization in systematic characterization of molecular defects. *Proc. natn. Acad. Sci.*, **81**, 2821–2825.

CHAPMAN, S. J., ALLISON, J. V. & GRIMES, A. J. (1973). Abnormal cation movements in human hypochromic red cells incubated in vitro. *Scand. J. Haemat.*, **10**, 225–231.

CHAPTAL, J., JEAN, R. PAYÈS, A., LLORET, R. & ROUSTAN, J. (1967). Hémochromatose secondaire de la maladie de Cooley, étude clinique, biologique et anatomique. *Pédiatrie*, **19**, 677–693.

CIVIDALLI, G., KEREM, H. & RACHMILEWITZ, E. A. (1980). Globin synthesis in severe and intermediate homozygous β thalassemia in Israel. *Ann. N.Y. Acad. Sci.*, **344**, 132–140.

CIVIDALLI, G., LOCKER, H. & RUSSELL, A. (1971). Increased permeability of erythrocyte membrane in thalassemia. *Blood*, **37**, 716–724.

CIVIDALLI, G., NATHAN, D. C. & LODISH, H. F. (1974). Translation control of hemoglobin synthesis in thalassemic bone marrow. *J. clin. Invest.*, **53**, 955–963.

CLEGG, J. B. & WEATHERALL, D. J. (1972). Haemoglobin synthesis during erythroid maturation in β-thalassemia. *Nature new Biol.*, **240**, 190–192.

CLEGG, J. B., WEATHERALL, D. J., NA-NAKORN, S. & WASI, P. (1968). Haemoglobin synthesis in β-thalassemia. *Nature (Lond.)*, **220**, 664–668.

COLLINS, F. S., BOEHM, C. D., WABER, P. G., STOECKERT, J, JNR, WEISSMAN, S. M., FORGET, B. G. & KAZAZIAN, H. H. JNR (1984a). Concordance of a point mutation 5′ to the $^G\gamma$ globin gene with $^G\gamma\beta^+$ hereditary persistence of fetal hemoglobin. *Blood*, **64**, 1292–1296.

COLLINS, F. S., STOECKERT, C. J., SERJEANT, G. R., FORGET, B. G. & WEISSMAN, S. M. (1984b). $^G\gamma\beta^+$ hereditary persistence of fetal hemoglobin: cosmid cloning and identification of a specific mutation 5′ to the $^G\gamma$ gene. *Proc. natn. Acad. Sci. U. S. A.*, **81**, 4894–4894.

CONCONI, F., BERNARDI, F., BUZZONI, D., CASONI, I., DEL, SENNO, L., MARCHETTI, G. & PERROTTA, C. M. (1980). β-globin messenger RNA in Ferrara

β^0 thalassemia. *Ann. N.Y. Acad. Sci.*, **344**, 120–131.

COVEY, M. C., MERIGAN, T. C., PETRAKIS, N. L. & LUCIA, S. P. (1960). Thalassemia major. Thirty-five year survival, with obliterative pulmonary endarteritis and atypical bone changes. *Amer. J. Med.*, **28**, 482–486.

CROSBY, W. H. & SACKS, H. J. (1949). The coincidence of Mediterranean anemia and pernicious anemia in a young Sicilian. *Blood*, **4**, 1267–1270.

CURTIN, P., PIRASTU, M., KAN, Y. W., GOBERT-JONES, J. A., STEPHENS, A. D. & LEHMANN, H. (1985). A distant gene deletion affects β-globin gene function in an atypical γδβ-thalassemia. *J. clin. Invest.*, **76**, 1554–1558.

DE VIRGILIIS, A., CORNACCHIA, G., SANNA, G., ARGIOLU, F., GALANELLO, R., FIORELLI, G., RAIS, M., COSSU, P., BERTOLINO, F. & CAO, A. (1981). Chronic liver disease in transfusion dependent thalassemia: liver iron quantitation and distribution. *Acta haemat. (Basel)*, **65**, 32–39.

DEISSEROTH, A., NIENHUIS, A., LAWRENCE, J., GILES, R., TURNER, P. & RUDDLE, F. H. (1978). Chromosomal localization of human β globin gene on human chromosome 11 in somatic cell hybrids. *Proc. natn. Acad. Sci. U.S.A.*, **75**, 1456–1460.

DEISSEROTH, A., NIENHUIS, A., TURNER, P., VELEZ, R., ANDERSON, W. F., RUDDLE, F., LAWRENCE, J. CREAGAN, R. & KUCHERLAPATI, R. (1977). Localization of the human α-globin structural gene to chromosome 16 in somatic cell hybrids by molecular hybridization assay. *Cell*, **12**, 205–218.

DEL SENNO, L., BERNARDI, F., BUZZONI, D., MARCHETTI, G., PERROTA, C. & CONCONI, F. (1981). Molecular characteristics of a non-deletion α-thalassemia of the Po river delta. *Europ. J. Biochem.*, **116**, 127–130.

DI MARZO, R., LO GIOCO, P., GIAMBONA, A., ACUTO, S., SAMMARCO, P., ODDO, G. & MAGGIO, A. (1986). Clinical severity of non-deletion form of HbH disease $(- -^{Med}/\alpha\alpha^{thal})$. *Scand. J. Haemat.*, **36**, 39–43.

DÖRMER, P. & BETKE, K. (1978). Erythroblast kinetics in homozygous and heterozygous beta-thalassemia. *Brit. J. Haemat.*, **38**, 5–14.

DOZY, A. M., KAN, Y. W., EMBURY, S. H., MENTZER, W. C., WANG, W. C., LUBIN, B., DAVIS, J. R. JNR & KOENIG, H. M. (1979). α-globin gene organization in blacks precludes the severe form of α-thalassemia. *Nature (Lond.)*, **280**, 605–607.

ELLIS, J. T., SCHULMAN, I. & SMITH, C. H. (1954). Generalized siderosis with fibrosis of liver and pancreas in Cooley's (Mediterranean) anemia: with observations on the pathogenesis of the siderosis and fibrosis. *Amer. J. Path.*, **30**, 287–309.

EMBURY, S. H., DOZY, A. M. & KAN, Y. W. (1980). Molecular mechanisms in α thalassemia: racial differences in α-globin gene organization. *Ann.*

N.Y. Acad. Sci., **344**, 31–40.

EMBURY, S. H., LEBO, R. V., DOZY, A. M. & KAN, Y. W. (1979). Organization of the α-globin genes in the Chinese α-thalassemia syndromes. *J. clin. Invest.*, **63**, 1307–1310.

EMBURY, S. H., MILLER, J. A., DOZY, A. M., KAN, Y. W., CHAN, V. & TODD, D. (1980). Two different molecular organizations account for the single α-globin gene of the α-thalassemia-2 genotype. *J. clin. Invest.*, **66**, 1319–1325.

ESTES, J. E., FARBER, E. M. & STICKNEY, J. M. (1948). Ulcers of the leg in Mediterranean disease. *Blood*, **3**, 302–306.

EYLAR, E. H. & MATIOLI, G. T. (1965). Glycoprotein biosynthesis in human reticulocytes: a lesion in thalassemia. *Science*, **147**, 869–870.

FEARON, E. R., KAZAZIAN, H. H. JNR, WABER, P. G., LEE, J. I., ANTONARAKIS, S. E., ORKIN, S. H., VANIN, E. F., HENTHORN, P. S., GROSVELD, F. G., SCOTT, A. F. & BUCHANON, G. R. (1983). The entire β-globin gene cluster is deleted in a form of γδβ-thalassaemia. *Blood*, **61**, 1269–1273.

FELBER, B. K., ORKIN, S. H. & HAMER, D. H. (1982). Abnormal RNA splicing causes one form of α thalassemia. *Cell*, **29**, 895–902.

FELICE, A. E., CLEEK, M. P., McKIE, K., McKIE, V. & HUISMAN, T. H. J. (1984). The rare α-thalassemia-1 of blacks is a ζβ-thalassemia-1 associated with deletion of all α- and ζ-globin genes. *Blood*, **63**, 1253–1257.

FESSAS, PH. (1959). Thalassaemia and the alterations of the haemoglobin pattern. *Abnormal Haemoglobins. A Symposium*, p. 136. Blackwell Scientific Publications, Oxford.

FESSAS, PH. (1963). Inclusions of hemoglobin in erythroblasts and erythrocytes of thalassemia. *Blood*, **21**, 21–32.

FESSAS, PH., LOUKOPOULOS, D. & KALTSOYA, A. (1966). Peptide analysis of the inclusions of erythroid cells in β-thalassemia. *Biochim. biophys. Acta*, **124**, 430–432.

FESSAS, PH. & PAPAYANNOPOULOU, T. (1965). Cytochemical observations on β-thalassaemia. I. The PAS positive substance of erythroblasts. *Acta haemat. (Basel)*, **34**, 1–19.

FESSAS, PH. & YATAGHANAS, X. (1968). Intraerythroblastic instability of hemoglobin β_4 (Hgb H). *Blood*, **31**, 323–331.

FINK, H. (1964). Transfusion hemochromatosis in Cooley's anemia. *Ann. N.Y. Acad. Sci.*, **119**, 680–685.

FLAVELL, R. A., BERNARDS, R., KOOTER, J. B., DE, BOER, E., LITTLE, P. F. R., ANNISON, G. & WILLIAMSON, R. (1979). The structure of the human β-globin gene in β-thalassaemia. *Nucl. Acids Res.*, **6**, 2749–2760.

FORGET, B. G., BENZ, E. J. JNR, SKOULTCHI, A., BAGLIONI, C. & HOUSMAN, D. (1974). Absence of messenger RNA for beta globin chain in β^0-

thalassaemia. *Nature (Lond.)*, **247**, 379–381.

FRITSCH, E. F., LAWN, R. M. & MANIATIS, T. (1979). Characterization of deletions which affect the expression of fetal globin genes in man. *Nature (Lond.)*, **279**, 598–603.

GABUZDA, T. G., NATHAN, D. G., GARDNER, F. H., COUNCIL, A. & LIMAURO, A. (1965). The metabolism of the individual C^{14}-labelled hemoglobins in patients with H-thalassemia, with observations on radiochromate binding to the hemoglobins during red cell survival. *J. clin. Invest.*, **44**, 315–325.

GALILI, U., KORKESH, A., KAHANE, I. & RACHMILEWITZ, E. A. (1983). Demonstration of a natural anti-galactosyl IgG antibody on thalassemic red blood cells. *Blood*, **61**, 1258–1264.

GERLI, G. C., BERETTA, L., BIANCHI, M., PELLEGATTA, A. & AGOSTONI, A. (1980). Erythrocyte superoxide dismutase, catalase and glutathione peroxidase activities in β-thalassaemia (major and minor). *Scand. J. Haemat.*, **25**, 87–92.

GIAMPAOLO, A., MAVILIO, F., MASSA, A., GABBIANELLI, M., GUERRIERO, R., SPOSI, N. M., CARÉ, A., CIANCIULLI, P., TENTORI, L. & MARINUCCI, M. (1984). Molecular heterogeneity of beta thalassaemia in the Italian population. *Brit. J. Haemat.*, **56**, 79–85.

GILMAN, J. G., HUISMAN, T. H. J. & ABELS, J. (1984). Dutch β^0-thalassaemia: a 10 kilobase DNA deletion associated with significant γ-chain production. *Brit. J. Haemat.*, **56**, 339–348.

GOLDBERG, M. A. & SCHWARTZ, S. O. (1954). Mediterranean anemia in a negro complicated by pernicious anemia of pregnancy. *Blood*, **9**, 648–654.

GOOSENS, M., DOZY, A. M., EMBURY, S. H., ZACHARIADES, Z., HADJIMINAS, M. G., STAMATOYANNOPOULOS, G. & KAN, Y. W. (1980). Triplicated α-globin loci in humans. *Proc. natn. Acad. Sci. U.S.A.*, **77**, 518–521.

GOOSENS, M., LEE, K. Y., LIEBHABER, S. A. & KAN, Y. W. (1982). Globin structural mutant $\alpha^{125 \text{ Leu} \rightarrow \text{Pro}}$ is a novel cause of α-thalassaemia. *Nature (Lond.)*, **296**, 864–865.

GUNN, R. B., SILVERS, D. N. & ROSSE, W. F. (1972). Potassium permeability in β-thalassemia minor red blood cells. *J. clin. Invest.*, **51**, 1043–1050.

HAMILTON, H. E. & FOWLER, W. M. (1951). Familial leptocytosis (Cooley's anemia and Cooley's trait). Observations on three families with a related study of bone marrow activity. *Arch. intern. Med.*, **87**, 825–834.

HANASH, S. M. & RUCKNAGEL, D. L. (1978). Proteolytic activity in erythrocyte precursors. *Proc. natn. Acad. Sci. U.S.A.*, **75**, 3427–3431.

HARANO, T., REESE, A. L. RYAN, R., ABRAHAM, B. L. & HUISMAN, T. H. J. (1985). Five haplotypes in Black β-thalassaemia heterozygotes: three associated with high and two with low $^G\gamma$ values in fetal haemoglobin. *Brit. J. Haemat.*, **59**, 333–342.

HEINRICH, H. C., GABBE, E. E., OPPITZ, K. H., WHANG, D. H., BENDER-GÖTZE, CH., SCHÄFER, K. H., SCHRÖTER, W. & PFAU, A. A. (1973). Absorption of inorganic and food iron in children with heterozygous and homozygous β-thalassaemia. *Z. Kinderheilk.*, **115**, 1–22.

HENNI, T., BELHANI, M., MORLE, F., BACHIR, D., TABONE, P., COLONNA, P. & GODET, J. (1985). Alpha globin gene triplication in severe heterozygous beta thalassemia. *Acta haemat. (Basel)*, **74**, 236–239.

HENTHORN, P. S., SMITHIES, O., NAKATSUJI, T., FELICE, A. E., GARDINER, M. B., REESE, A. L. & HUISMAN, T. H. J. (1985). ($^A\gamma\delta\beta^0$)-thalassaemia in blacks is due to a deletion of 34 kbp of DNA. *Brit. J. Haemat.*, **59**, 343–356.

HIGGS, D. R., GOODBOURN, S. E. Y., LAMB, J., CLEGG, J. B., WEATHERALL, D. J. & PROUDFOOT, N. J. (1983). α-thalassaemia caused by a polyadenylation signal mutation. *Nature (Lond.)*, **306**, 398–400.

HIGGS, D. R., HILL, A. V. S., NICHOLLS, R., GOODBOURN, S. E. Y., AYYUB, H., TEAL, H., CLEGG, J. B. & WEATHERALL, D. J. (1985). Molecular rearrangements of the human α-globin gene cluster. *Ann. N.Y. Acad. Sci.*, **445**, 45–56.

HIGGS, D. R., OLD, J. M. PRESSLEY, L., CLEGG, J. B. & WEATHERALL, D. J. (1980). A novel α-globin gene arrangement in man. *Nature (Lond.)*, **284**, 632–635.

HIGGS, D. R., PRESSLEY, L., ALDRIDGE, B., CLEGG, J. B., WEATHERALL, D. J., CAO, A., HADJIMINAS, M. G., KATTAMIS, C., METAXATOU-MAVROMATI, A., RACHMILEWITZ, E. A. & SOPHOCLEOUS, T. (1981). Genetic and molecular diversity in nondeletion Hb H disease. *Proc. natn. Acad. Sci. U.S.A.*, **78**, 5833–5837.

HIGGS, D. R., PRESSLEY, L., OLD, J. M., HUNT, D. M., CLEGG, J. B., WEATHERALL, D. J. & SERJEANT, G. R. (1979). Negro α-thalassaemia is caused by the deletion of a single α-gene. *Lancet*, **ii**, 272–276.

HOFFMAN, J. F., WOLMAN, I. J., HILLIER, J. & PARPART, A. K. (1956). Ultrastructure of erythrocyte membranes in thalassemia major and minor. *Blood*, **11**, 946–956.

HOWELL, J. & WYATT, J. P. (1953). Development of pigmentary cirrhosis in Cooley's anemia. *Arch. Path.*, **55**, 423–431.

HUMPHRIES, R. K., LEY, T. J., ANAGNOU, N. P., BAUR, A. W. & NIENHUIS, A. W. (1984). $β^0$-39 thalassemia gene: a premature termination codon causes β-mRNA deficiency without affecting cytoplasmic β-mRNA stability. *Blood*, **64**, 23–32.

IANCU, T. C. & NEUSTEIN, H. B. (1977). Ferritin in human liver cells of homozygous β-thalassaemia: ultrastructural observations. *Brit. J. Haemat.*, **37**, 527–535.

INGRAM, V. M. (1964). A molecular model for thalassemia. *Ann. N.Y. Acad. Sci.*, **119**, 485–495.

INGRAM, V. M. & STRETTON, A. O. W. (1959). Genetic basis of the thalassaemia diseases. *Nature (Lond.)*, **184**, 1903–1909.

ITANO, H. A. (1957). The human hemoglobins: their properties and genetic control. *Advanc. Protein Chem.*, **12**, 215–268.

JACKSON, I. J. & WILLIAMSON, R. (1980). Mapping of human globin genes. *Brit. J. Haemat.*, **46**, 341–349 (Annotation).

JAGADEESWARAN, P., TUAN, D., FORGET, B. G. & WEISSMAN, S. M. (1982). A gene deletion ending at the midpoint of a repetitive DNA sequence in one form of hereditary persistence of fetal haemoglobin. *Nature (Lond.)*, **296**, 469–470.

JANDL, J. H. & GREENBERG, M. S. (1959). Bone-marrow failure due to relative nutritional deficiency in Cooley's hemolytic anemia. Painful "erythropoietic crises" in response to folic acid. *New Engl. J. Med.*, **260**, 461–468.

JENSEN, M., WIRTZ, A., WALTHER, J.-U., SCHEMKEN, E. M., LARYEA, M. D. & DRIESEL, A. J. (1984). Hereditary persistence of fetal haemoglobin (HPFH) in conjunction with a chromosomal translocation involving the haemoglobin β locus. *Brit. J. Haemat.*, **56**, 87–94.

JONES, R. W., OLD, J. M., TRENT, R. J., CLEGG, J. B. & WEATHERALL, D. J. (1981a). Restriction mapping of a new deletion responsible for $^G\gamma(\delta\beta)^0$ thalassaemia. *Nucl. Acids Res.*, **9**, 6813–6825.

JONES, R. W., OLD, J. M., TRENT, R. J., CLEGG, J. B. & WEATHERALL, D. J. (1981b). Major rearrangement in the human β-globin gene cluster. *Nature (Lond.)*, **291**, 39–44.

JONES, R. W., OLD, J. M., WOOD, W. G., CLEGG, J. B. & WEATHERALL, D. J. (1982). Restriction endonuclease maps of the β-like globin gene cluster in the British and Greek forms of HPFH, and for one example of $^G\gamma\beta^+$ HPFH. *Brit. J. Haemat.*, **50**, 415–422.

JOSHI, W., LEB, L., PIOTROWSKI, J., FORTIER, N. & SNYDER, L. M. (1983). Increased sensitivity of isolated alpha subunits of normal human hemoglobin to oxidative damage and crosslinkage with spectrin. *J. Lab. clin. Med.*, **102**, 46–52.

KAHANE, I., POLLIACK, A., RACHMILEWITZ, E. A., BAYER, E. A. & SKUTELSKY, E. (1978). Distribution of sialic acids on the red blood cell membrane in β thalassaemia. *Nature (Lond.)*, **271**, 674–675.

KAHANE, I. & RACHMILEWITZ, E. A. (1976). Alterations in red blood cell membrane and the effect of vitamin E on osmotic fragility in β-thalassemia major. *Israel J. med. Sci.*, **12**, 11–15.

KAHANE, I., SHIFTER, A. & RACHMILEWITZ, E. A. (1978). Cross-linking of red blood cell membrane proteins induced by oxidant stress in β thalassemia. *FEBS Lett.*, **85**, 267–270.

KAN, Y. W. (1983). The thalassemias. In: *The Metabolic Basis of Inherited Disease*, 5th edn (ed. by J. B. Stanbury, J. B. Wyngaarden, D. S. Fredrickson, J. C. Goldstein and M. S. Brown), pp. 1711–1725. Mcgraw-Hill Book Co., New York.

KAN, Y. W., (1985). Molecular pathology of α-thalassaemia. *Ann. N.Y. Acad. Sci.*, 445, 28–35.

KAN. Y. W. & DOZY, A. M. (1978). Polymorphism of DNA sequence adjacent to human β-globin structural gene: relationship to sickle mutation. *Proc. natn. Acad. Sci. U.S.A.*, 75, 5631–5635.

KAN, Y. W., DOZY, A. M., STAMATOYANNOPOULOS, G., HADJIMINAS, M. G., ZACHARIADES, Z., FURBETTA, M. & CAO, A. (1979). Molecular basis of hemoglobin-H disease in the Mediterranean population. *Blood*, 54, 1434–1438.

KAN, Y. W., DOZY, A. M., TRECARTIN, R. & TODD, D. (1977). Identification of a nondeletion defect in α-thalassaemia. *New Engl. J. Med.*, 297, 1081–1084.

KAN, Y. W., DOZY, A. M., VARMUS, H. E., TAYLOR, J. M., HOLLAND, J. P., LIE-INJO, L. E., GANESAN, J. & TODD, D. (1975). Deletion of α-globin genes in haemoglobin-H disease demonstrates multiple α-globin structural loci. *Nature (Lond.)*, 255, 255–256.

KAN, Y. W., FORGET, B. G. & NATHAN, D. G. (1972). Gamma-beta thalassaemia: a cause of hemolytic disease of newborns. *New Engl. J. Med.*, 286, 129–134.

KAN, Y. W., NATHAN, D. G. & LODISH, H. F. (1972). Equal synthesis of α- and β-globin chains in erythroid precursors in heterozygous β-thalassaemia. *J. clin. Invest.*, 51, 1906–1909.

KANAVAKIS, E., METAXOTOU-MAVROMATI, A., KATTAMIS, C., WAINSCOAT, J. S. & WOOD, W. G. (1983). The triplicated α gene locus and β thalassaemia. *Brit. J. Haemat.*, 54, 201–207.

KANTOR, J. A., TURNER, P. H. & NIENHUIS, A. W. (1980). Beta thalassemia: mutations which affect processing of the β-globin mRNA precursor. *Cell*, 21, 149–157.

KATTAMIS, C., METAXOTOU-MAVROMATI, A., TSIARTA, E., METAXATOU, C., WASI, P., WOOD, W. G., PRESSLEY, L., HIGGS, D. R., CLEGG, J. B. & WEATHERALL, D. J. (1980). Haemoglobin Bart's hydrops syndrome in Greece. *Brit. med. J.*, ii, 268–270.

KAZAZIAN, H. H. JNR, ORKIN, S. H., ANTONARAKIS, S. E., SEXTON, J. P., BOEHM, C. D., GOFF, S. C. & WABER, P. G. (1984). Molecular characterization of seven β-thalassaemia mutations in Asian Indians. *EMBO J.*, 3, 593–596.

KAZAZIAN, H. H. JNR, ORKIN, S. H., MARKHAM, A. F., CHAPMAN, C. R., YOUSSOUFIAN, H. A. & WABER, P. G. (1984). Quantitation of the close association between DNA haplotypes and specific β-thalassaemia mutations in Mediterraneans. *Nature (Lond.)*, 310, 152–154.

KINNEY, T. R., FRIEDMAN, S. H., CIFUENTES, E., KIM, H. C. & SCHWARTZ, E. (1978). Variations in globin synthesis in delta-beta-thalassaemia. *Brit. J. Haemat.*, 38, 15–22.

KNOX-MACAULAY, H. H. M. & WEATHERALL, D. J. (1974). Studies of red-cell membrane function in heterozygous β thalassaemia and other hypochromic anaemias. *Brit. J. Haemat.*, 28, 277–297.

KNOX-MACAULAY, H. H. M., WEATHERALL, D. J., CLEGG, J. B., BRADLEY, J. & BROWN, M. J. (1972). The clinical and biosynthetic characterization of αβ-thalassaemia. *Brit. J. Haemat.*, 22, 497–512.

KNYSZYNSKI, A., DANON, D., KAHANE, I. & RACHMILEWITZ, E. A. (1979). Phagocytosis of nucleated and mature β thalassaemic red blood cells by mouse macrophages *in vitro*. *Brit. J. Haemat.*, 43, 251–255.

KREIMER-BIRNBAUM, M. & BANNERMAN, R. M. (1968). Interrelationship of pyrrole and globin metabolism in β-thalassaemia. *Brit. J. Haemat.*, 15, 7–22.

LANCLOS, K. D. & KUTLAR, A. (1986). The thalassaemia repository. *Hemoglobin*, 10, 533–558.

LAWN, R. M., EFSTRATIADIS, A., O'CONNELL, C. & MANIATIS, T. (1980). The nucleotide sequence of the human β-globin gene. *Cell*, 21, 647–651.

LAWN, R. M., FRITSCH, E. F., PARKER, R. C., BLAKE, G. & MANIATIS, T. (1978). The isolation and characterization of linked δ-and β-globin genes from a cloned library of human DNA. *Cell*, 15, 1157–1174.

LAYRISSE, M., LINARES, J. & ROCHE, M. (1965). Excess hemolysis in subjects with severe iron deficiency anemia associated and non-associated with hookworm infection. *Blood*, 25, 73–91.

LIE-INJO, L. E., HERRERA, A. R. & KAN, Y. W. (1981). Two types of triplicated α-globin gene loci in humans. *Nucl. Acids Res.*, 9, 3707–3717.

LIE-INJO, L. E., HERRERA, A. R., LEBO, R. V., HASSAN, K. & LOPEZ, C. G. (1985). Gene mapping of Malaysian α thalassemias with α and ζ globin gene probes. *Amer. J. Hemat.*, 18, 289–296.

LUHBY, A. L. & COOPERMAN, J. M. (1961). Folic-acid deficiency in thalassaemia major. *Lancet*, ii, 490–491 (Letter).

LUHBY, A. L., COOPERMAN, J. M., FELDMAN, R., CERAOLO, J., HERRARO, J. & MARLEY, J. F. (1961). Folic-acid deficiency as a limiting factor in the anemias of thalassemia major. *Blood*, 18, 786–787 (Abstract).

MAQUAT, L. E., KINNIBURGH, A. J., BEACH, L. R., HONIG, G. R., LAZERSON, J., ERSHLER, W. B. & ROSS, J. (1980). Processing of the human β-globin mRNA precursor to mRNA is defective in three patients with β⁺-thalassaemia. *Proc. natn. Acad. Sci, U.S.A.*, 77, 4287–4291.

MAQUAT, L. E., KINNIBURGH, A. J., RACHMILEWITZ, E. A. & ROSS, J. (1981). Unstable β-globin mRNA in mRNA-deficient β⁰ thalassemia. *Cell*, 27, 543–553.

MARINONE, G., BERNASCONI, C., GAUTIER, A. &

MARCOVICI, I. (1958). Studi di citologia elettronica nella talassemia. I. Ultrastruttura degli eritociti del sangue circolante. *Haematologica*, **43**, 1123–1144.

MARKS, P. A. & BANK, A. (1971). Molecular pathology of thalassemia syndromes. *Fed. Proc.*, **30**, 977–982.

MARKS, P. A. & BURKA, E. R. (1964). Hemoglobins A and F: formation in thalassemia and other hemolytic anemias. *Science*, **144**, 552–553.

MARMONT, A. & BIANCHI, V. (1948). Mediterranean anemia. Clinical and haematological findings, and pathogenetic studies in the milder form of the disease (with report of cases). *Acta haemat. (Basel)*, **1**, 4–28.

MATHEW, C. G. P., ROUSSEAU, J., REES, J. S. & HARLEY, E. H. (1983). The molecular basis of alpha thalassaemia in a South African population. *Brit. J. Haemat.*, **55**, 105–111.

MEARS, J. G., RAMIREZ, F., FELDENZER, J., BURNS, A. L. & BANK. A. (1980). Changes in gene organization in the thalassaemias. *Ann. N.Y. Acad. Sci*, **334**, 41–47.

MEARS,. J. G., RAMIREZ, F., LEIBOWITZ, D., NAKAMURA, F., BLOOM, A., KONOTEY-AHULU, F. I. D. & BANK, A. (1978). Changes in restricted human cellular DNA fragments containing globin gene sequences in thalassemias and related disorders. *Proc. natn. Acad. Sci. U.S.A.*, **75**, 1222–1226.

MODELL, C. B., LATTER, A., STEADMAN, J. H. & HUEHNS, E. R. (1969). Haemoglobin synthesis in β-thalassaemia. *Brit. J. Haemat.*, **17**, 485–501.

MOSCHONAS, N., DE BOER, E., GROSVELD, F. G., DAHL, H. H. M., WRIGHT, S., SHEWMAKER, C. K. & FLAVELL, R. A. (1981). Structure and expression of a cloned β⁰ thalassaemia gene. *Nucl. Acids Res.*, **9**, 4391–4401.

MUKHERJEE, A. M. & SEN GUPTA, P. C. (1963). Pathology of haemoglobinopathy. *J. Ass. Phycns India*, **11**, 911–916.

MUKHERJEE, A. M., SEN GUPTA, P. C. & CHATTERJEA, J. B. (1959). The spleen in thalassaemia. *J. Ind. med. Ass.*, **33**, 451–459.

MUKHERJEE, A. M., SEN GUPTA, P. C. & CHATTERJEA, J. B. (1960). Histopathology of the liver in thalassaemia syndrome. *J. Ind. med. Ass.*, **35**, 291–296.

MUSUMECI, S., SCHILIRÒ, G., ROMEO, A., PIZZARELLI, G., FISCHER, A. & RUSSO, G. (1981). Haemoglobin synthesis in bone marrow of patients with β⁰ and β⁺-thalassaemia. *Acta haemat. (Basel)*, **65**, 170–176.

NAKATSUJI, T., GILMAN, J. G., SUKUMARAN, P. K. & HUISMAN, T. H. J. (1984). Restriction endonuclease gene mapping studies of an Indian (ᴬγ δβ)⁰-thalassaemia, previously identified as ᴳγ-HPFH. *Brit. J. Haemat.*, **57**, 663–670.

NATHAN, D. G. & GUNN, R. B. (1966). Thalassemia: the consequences of unbalanced hemoglobin synthesis. *Amer. J. Med.*, **41**, 815–830.

NATHAN, D. G., STOSSEL, T. B., GUNN, R. B., ZARKOWSKY, H. S. & LAFORET, M. T. (1969). Influence of hemoglobin precipitation on erythrocyte metabolism in alpha and beta thalassemia. *J. clin. Invest.*, **48**, 33–41.

NATTA, C. L., NIAZI, G. A., FORD, S. & BANK, A. (1974). Balanced globin chain synthesis in hereditary persistence of fetal hemoglobin. *J. clin. Invest.*, **54**, 433–438.

NATTA, C. L., RAMIREZ, F., WOLFF, J. A. & BANK, A. (1976). Decreased α globin mRNA in nucleated red cell precursors in α thalassaemia. *Blood*, **47**, 899–907.

NECHELES, T. F., STEINER, M. & BALDINI, M. (1965). The in vitro synthesis of hemoglobin by human bone marrow in thalassemia. *Blood*, **25**, 897–906.

NEEL, J. V. (1961). The hemoglobin genes: a remarkable example of the clustering of related genetic functions on a single mammalian chromosome. *Blood*, **18**, 769–777.

NICHOLLS, R. D., HIGGS, D. R., CLEGG, J. B. & WEATHERALL, D. J. (1985). α⁰-thalassaemia due to recombination between the α1-globin gene and an *Alu* 1 repeat. *Blood*, **65**, 1434–1438.

NIENHUIS, A. W., ANAGNOU, N. P. & LEY, T. J. (1984). Advances in thalassemia research. *Blood*, **63**, 738–758 (Review).

NIENHUIS, A. W. & ANDERSON, W. F. (1974). The molecular defect in thalassaemia. *Clinics Haemat.*, **3**, 447–466.

NIENHUIS, A. W. & BENZ, E. J. JNR (1977). Regulation of hemoglobin synthesis during the development of the red cell. *New Engl. J. Med.*, **297**, 1318–1328.

OKON, E., LEVIJ, I. S. & RACHMILEWITZ, E. A. (1976). Splenectomy, iron overload and liver cirrhosis in β-thalassemia major. *Acta haemat. (Basel)*, **56**, 142–150.

OLD, J. M. & HIGGS, D. R. (1983). Gene analysis. In: *The Thalassemias (Methods in Hematology*, Vol. 6), pp. 74–102. Churchill Livingstone, Edinburgh, London, Melbourne and New York.

ORKIN, S. H. (1980). Specific abnormalities of globin gene organization in thalassemia syndromes. *Ann. N.Y. Acad. Sci.*, **334**, 48–61.

ORKIN, S. H., ALTER, B. P. & ALTAY, C. (1979). Deletion of the ᴬγ globin gene in ᴳγ-δβ-thalassaemia. *J. clin. Invest.*, **64**, 866–869.

ORKIN, S. H., ANTONARAKIS, S. E. & KAZAZIAN, H. H. JNR (1983). Polymorphism and molecular pathology of the human beta-globin gene. In: *Progress in Hematology*, Vol. XIII (ed. by E. B. Brown), pp. 49–73. Grune and Stratton, New York.

ORKIN, S. H. & GOFF, S. C. (1981). Nonsense and frameshift mutations in β⁰-thalassaemia detected in cloned β-globin genes. *J. biol. Chem.*, **256**, 9782–9784.

ORKIN, S. H., GOFF, S. C. & HECHTMAN, R. L. (1981). Mutation in an intervening sequence splice junction in man. *Proc. natn. Acad. Sci. U.S.A.*, **78**, 5041–5045.

ORKIN, S. H., GOFF, S. C. & NATHAN, D. G. (1981). Heterogeniety of DNA deletion in γδβ-thalassaemia. *J. clin. Invest.*, **67**, 878–884.

ORKIN, S. H. & KAZAZIAN, H. H. JNR (1984). The mutation and polymorphism of the human β-globin gene and its surrounding DNA. *Ann. Rev. Genet.*, **18**, 131–171.

ORKIN, S. H., KAZAZIAN. H. H. JNR, ANTONARAKIS, S. E., GOFF, S. C., BOEHM, C. D., SEXTON, J. P., WABER, P. G. & GIARDINA, P. J. V. (1982). Linkage of β-thalassaemia mutations and β-globin gene polymorphisms with DNA polymorphisms in human β-globin gene cluster. *Nature (Lond.)*, **296**, 627–631.

ORKIN, S. H., KOLODNER, R., MICHELSON, A. & HUSSON, R. (1980). Cloning and direct examination of a structurally abnormal human β⁰-thalassaemia globin gene. *Proc. natn. Acad. Sci. U.S.A.*, **77**, 3558–3562.

ORKIN, S. H. & MICHELSON, A. (1980). Partial deletion of the α-globin structural gene in human α-thalassaemia. *Nature (Lond.)*, **286**, 538–540.

ORKIN, S. H., OLD, J., LAZARUS, H., ALTAY, C., GURGEY, A., WEATHERALL, D. J. & NATHAN, D. G. (1979a). The molecular basis of α-thalassaemias: frequent occurrence of dysfunctional α loci among non-Asians with Hb H disease. *Cell*, **17**, 33–42.

ORKIN, S. H., OLD, J. M., WEATHERALL, D. J. & NATHAN, D. G. (1979b). Partial deletion of β-globin gene DNA in certain patients with β⁰-thalassaemia. *Proc. natn. Acad. Sci. U.S.A.*, **76**, 2400–2404.

OTTOLENGHI, S. & GIGLIONI, B. (1982). The deletion in a type of δ⁰-β⁰-thalassaemia begins in an inverted Alu I repeat. *Nature (Lond.)*, **300**, 770–771.

OTTOLENGHI, S., GIGLIONI, B., COMI, P., GIANNI, A. M., POLLI, E., ACQUAYE, C. T. A., OLDHAM, J. H. & MASERA, G. (1979). Globin gene deletion in HPFH δ⁰β⁰ thalassaemia and Hb Lepore disease. *Nature (Lond.)*, **278**, 654–657.

OTTOLENGHI, S., LANYON, W. G., PAUL, J., WILLIAMSON, R., WEATHERALL, D. J., CLEGG, J. B. & PRITCHARD, J. (1974). The severe form of α thalassaemia is caused by a haemoglobin gene deletion. *Nature (Lond.)*, **251**, 389–392.

OTTOLENGHI, S., LANYON, W. G., WILLIAMSON, R., WEATHERALL, D. J., CLEGG, J. B. & PITCHER, C. S. (1975). Human globin gene analysis for a patient with β⁰/δβ⁰ thalassaemia. *Proc. natn. Acad. Sci. U.S.A.*, **72**, 2294–2299.

PADANILAM, B. J., FELICE, A. E. & HUISMAN, T. H. J. (1984). Partial deletion of the 5′β-globin gene region causes β⁰-thalassaemia in members of an American black family. *Blood*, **64**, 941–944.

PADANILAM, B. J. & HUISMAN, T. H. J. (1986). The β⁰-thalassaemia in an American black family is due to a single nucleotide substitution in the acceptor splice junction of the second intervening sequence. *Amer. J. Hemat.*, **22**, 259–263.

PAPAYANNOPOULOU, TH., LAWN, R. M., STAMATOYANNOPOULOS, G. & MANIATIS, T. (1982). Greek (ᴬγ) variant of hereditary persistence of fetal haemoglobin: globin gene organization and studies of expression of fetal haemoglobins in clonal erythroid cultures. *Brit. J. Haemat.*, **50**, 387–399.

PERGOLIZZI, R., SPRITZ, R. A., SPENCE, S., GOOSENS, M., KAN, Y. W. & BANK, A. (1981). Two cloned β thalassaemia genes are associated with amber mutations at codon 39. *Nucl. Acids Res.*, **9**, 7065–7072.

PEROSA, L. & DELL'AQUILA, M. D. (1955). Fever and heat as causes of fragmentation of red cells in patients with Mediterranean anemia. *Acta haemat. (Basel)*, **14**, 209–214.

PHILLIPS, J. A. III, SCOTT, A. F., SMITH, K. D., YOUNG, K. E., LIGHTBODY, K. L., JIJI, R. M. & KAZAZIAN, H. H. JNR (1979). A molecular basis for hemoglobin-H disease in American blacks. *Blood*, **54**, 1439–1445.

PHILLIPS, J. A. III, VIK, T. A., SCOTT, A. F., YOUNG, K. E., KAZAZIAN, H. H. JNR, SMITH, K. D., FAIRBANKS, V. F. & KOENIG, H. M. (1980). Unequal crossing-over: a common basis of single α-globin genes in Asians and American blacks with hemoglobin H disease. *Blood*, **55**, 1066–1069.

PIPPARD, M. J., CALLENDER, S. T., WARNER, G. T. & WEATHERALL, D. J. (1979). Iron absorption and loading in β-thalssaemia intermedia. *Lancet*, **ii**, 819–821.

PIRASTU, M., LEE, K. Y., DOZY, A. M., KAN, Y. W., STAMATOYANNOPOULOS, G., HADJIMINAS, M. G., ZACHARIADES, Z., ANGIUS, A., FURBETTA, M., ROSATELLI, C. & CAO, A. (1982). Alpha-thalassaemia in two Mediterranean populations. *Blood*, **60**, 509–512.

POLLIACK, A. & RACHMILEWITZ, E. A. (1973). Ultrastructural studies in β-thalassaemia major. *Brit. J. Haemat.*, **24**, 319–326.

POLLIACK, A., YATAGANAS, X. & RACHMILLEWITZ, E. A. (1974). Ultrastructure of the inclusion bodies and nuclear abnormalities in β-thalassemic erythroblasts. *Ann. N.Y. Acad. Sci.*, **232**, 261–282.

POLLIACK, A., YATAGANAS, X., THORELL, B. & RACHMILEWITZ, E. A. (1974). An electron microscopic study of the nuclear abnormalities in erythroblasts in beta-thalassaemia major. *Brit. J. Haemat.*, **26**, 201–204.

PRESSLEY, L., HIGGS, D. R., ALDRIDGE, B., METAXATOU-MAVROMATI, A., CLEGG, J. B. & WEATHERALL, D. J. (1980a). Characterization of a new α thalassaemia 1 defect due to a partial deletion of the α globin gene complex. *Nucl. Acids Res.*, **8**, 4889–4898.

PRESSLEY, L., HIGGS, D. R., CLEGG, J. B., PERRINE, R. P., PEMBREY, M. E. & WEATHERALL, D. J. (1980b). A new genetic basis for hemoglobin-H disease. *New Engl. J. Med.*, **303**, 1383–1388.

PRESSLEY, L., HIGGS, D. R., CLEGG, J. B. & WEATHERALL, D. J. (1980). Gene deletions in α thalassemia prove that the 5'ζ locus in functional. *Proc. natn. Acad. Sci. U.S.A.*, **77**, 3586–3589.

PROUDFOOT, N. J., SHANDER, M. H. M., MANLEY, J. L., GEFTER, M. L. & MANIATIS, T. (1980). Structure and in vitro transcription of human globin genes. *Science*, **209**, 1329–1336.

QUEISSER, W., BETZLER, M., HEIMPEL, H. & KLEIHAUER, E. (1971). Erythropoietic cell proliferation in different clinical states of β-thalassaemia. *Acta haemat. (Basel)*, **45**, 303–311.

RACHMILEWITZ, E. A. (1969). Formation of hemichromes from oxidized hemoglobin subunits. *Ann. N.Y. Acad. Sci.*, **165**, 171–184.

RACHMILEWITZ, E. A. (1974). Denaturation of the normal and abnormal hemoglobin molecule. *Seminars Hemat.*, **11**, 441–462.

RACHMILEWITZ, E. A. & KAHANE, I. (1980). The red blood cell membrane in thalassaemia. *Brit. J. Haemat.*, **46**, 1–6 (Annotation).

RACHMILEWITZ, E. A., LUBIN, B. H. & SHOHET, S. B. (1976). Lipid membrane peroxidation in β-thalassemia major. *Blood*, **47**, 495–505.

RACHMILEWITZ, E. A., PEISACH, J., BRADLEY, T. B. JNR, & BLUMBERG, W. E. (1969). Role of haemichromes in the formation of inclusion bodies in haemoglobin H disease. *Nature (Lond.)*, **222**, 248–250.

RACHMILEWITZ, E. A., SHIFTER, A. & KAHANE, I. (1979). Vitamin E deficiency in β thalassemia major: changes in hematological parameters following a therapeutic trial with α-tocopherol. *Amer. J. clin. Nutr.*, **32**, 1850–1858.

RACHMILEWITZ, E. A., SHINAR, E., SHALEV, O., GALILI, U. & SCHRIER, S. L. (1985). Erythrocyte membrane alterations in β-thalassaemia. *Clinics Haemat.*, **14**, 163–182.

RACHMILEWITZ, E. A. & THORELL, B. (1972). Hemichromes in single inclusion bodies in red cells of beta thalassemia. *Blood*, **39**, 794–800.

RACHMILEWITZ, E. A., TREVES, A. & TREVES, A. J. (1980). Susceptibility of thalassemic red blood cells to phagocytosis by human macrophages *in vitro*. *Ann. N.Y. Acad. Sci.*, **334**, 314–322.

RESEGOTTI, L., DALFORNO, S., ROSSI, M. & INFELISE, V. (1975). Cellule simil-Gaucher nella milza di un individuo adulto con morbo di Cooley. *Minerva med. (Torino)*, **66**, 1156–1160.

RIGAS, D. A. & KOLER, R. D. (1961). Increased erythrocyte survival in hemoglobin H disease as a result of the abnormal properties of hemoglobin H: the benefit of splenectomy. *Blood*, **18**, 1–17.

RITCHEY, A. K., HOFFMAN, R., COUPAL, E., FLOYD, V., PEARSON, H. A. & FORGET, B. G. (1981). Imbalanced globin chain synthesis in cultured erythroid progenitor cells from thalassemic bone marrow and peripheral blood. *Blood*, **57**, 788–793.

ROBINSON, M. G. & WATSON, R. J. (1963). Megaloblastic anemia complicating thalassemia major. *Amer. J. Dis. Child.*, **105**, 275–280.

ROUSSEAU, J., MATHEW, C. G. P., REES, J. S. DU TOIT, E., BOTHA, M. C. & HARLEY, E. H. (1985). Incidence of Hb Bart's and α-thalassaemia genotypes in a South African population. *Acta haemat. (Basel)*, **73**, 159–162.

SAGLIO, G., CAMASCHELLA, C., SERRA, A., BERTERO, T., CAMBRIN, G. R., GUERRASIO, A., MAZZA, U., IZZO, P., TERTAGNI, F., GIGLIONI, B., COMI, P. & OTTOLENGHI, S. (1986). Italian type of deletional hereditary persistence of fetal hemoglobin. *Blood*, **68**, 646–651.

SAMPIETRO, M., CAPPELLINI, M. D., TADDEI, M. T. & FIORELLI, G. (1983). Heterogeneity of beta/alpha ratio in Italian beta-thalassaemia heterozygotes. *Haematologica*, **68**, 703–711.

SAMPIETRO, M., CAZZOLA, M., CAPPELLINI, M. D. & FIORELLI, G. (1983). The triplicated alpha-gene locus and heterozygous beta thalassaemia: a case of thalassaemia intermedia. *Brit. J. Haemat.*, **55**, 709–717 (Letter).

SANCAR, G. B., CEDENO, M. M. & RIEDER, R. F. (1980). The varied arrangement of the α globin genes in α thalassemia and Hb H disease in American blacks. *Johns Hopk. med. J.*, **146**, 264–269.

SANCAR, G. B., CEDENO, M. M. & RIEDER, R. F. (1981). Rapid destruction of newly synthesized excess β-chains in HbH disease. *Blood*, **57**, 967–971.

SANCAR, G. B., RAUSHER, D. B., BAINE, R. M., PLATICA, O., CEDENO, M. M., NAWABI, I. & RIEDER, R. F. (1983). Alpha-thalassemia in Ashkenazi jews. *Ann. intern. Med.*, **98**, 933–936.

SANSONE, G., ROSSO, C., ZUNIN, C. & SALOMONE, P. (1955). Studio clinico ed anatomo-patologico di due bambini con anemia di Cooley deceduti per reazione trasfusionale. *Minerva pediat. (Torino)*, **7**, 1005–1031.

SEN GUPTA, P. C., CHATTERJEA, J. B., MUKHERJEE, A. M. & CHATTERJI, A. (1960). Observations on the foam cell in thalassemia. *Blood*, **16**, 1039–1044.

SLATER, L. M., MUIR, W. A. & WEED, R. I. (1968). Influence of splenectomy on insoluble hemoglobin inclusion bodies in β thalassemic erythrocytes. *Blood*, **31**, 766–777.

SOPHOCLEOUS, T., HIGGS, D. R., ALDRIDGE, B., TRENT, R. J., PRESSLEY, L., CLEGG, J. B. & WEATHERALL, D. J. (1981). The molecular basis for the haemoglobin Bart's hydrops fetalis syndrome in Cyprus. *Brit. J. Haemat.*, **47**, 153–156.

SOUTHERN, E. M. (1975). Detention of specific sequences among DNA fragments separated by gel electrophoresis. *J. mol. Biol.*, **98**, 503–517.

SPRITZ, R. A., JAGADEESWARAN, P., CHOUDARY, P. V., BIRO, P. A., ELDER, J. T., deRIEL, J. K., MANLEY, J., GEFTER, M. L., FORGET, B. G. & WEISSMAN, S. M. (1981). Base substitution in an intervening sequence of a β^+-thalassemic human globin gene. *Proc. natn. Acad. Sci. U.S.A.*, **78**, 2455–2459.

SPRITZ, R. A. & ORKIN, S. H. (1982). Duplication followed by deletion accounts for the structure of an Indian deletion β^0-thalassemia gene. *Nucl. Acids Res.*, **10**, 8025–8029.

STEINBERG, M. H. & ADAMS, J. G. III (1981). Thalassemia: recent insights into molecular mechanisms. *Amer. J. Hemat.*, **12**, 81–92.

STEINBERG, M. H., COLEMAN, M. B., ADAMS, J. G. III, HARTMANN, R. C., SABA, H. & ANAGNOU, N. P. (1986). A new gene deletion in the α-like globin gene cluster as the molecular basis for the rare α-thalassemia-1($--/\alpha\alpha$) in blacks: HbH disease in sickle cell trait. *Blood*, **67**, 569–473.

STOCKS, J., OFFERMAN, E. L., MODELL, C. B. & DORMANDY, T. L. (1972). The susceptibility to autooxidation of human red cell lipids in health and disease. *Brit. J. Haemat.*, **23**, 713–724.

SUKUMARAN, P. K., MAKATSUJI, T., GARDINER, M. B., REESE, A. L., GILMAN, J. G. & HUISMAN, T. H. J. (1983). Gamma thalassemia resulting from the deletion of a γ-globin gene. *Nucl. Acids Res.*, **11**, 4635–4643.

TAKESHITA, K., FORGET, B. G., SCARPA, A. & BENZ, E. J. JNR (1984). Intranuclear defect in β-globin mRNA accumulation due to a premature translation termination codon. *Blood*, **64**, 13–22.

TAKIHARA, Y., NAKAMURA, T., YAMADA, H., TAKAGI, Y. & FUKUMAKI, Y. (1986). A novel mutation in the TATA box in a Japanese patient with β^+-thalassemia. *Blood*, **67**, 547–550.

TAMAGNINI, G. P., LOPES, M. C., CASTANHEIRA, M. E., WAINSCOAT, J. S. & WOOD, W. G. (1983). β^+ thalassemia — Portuguese type: clinical, haematological and molecular studies of a newly defined form of β thalassaemia. *Brit. J. Haemat.*, **54**, 189–200.

TAYLOR, J. M., DOZY, A., KAN, Y. W., VARMUS, H. E., LIE-INJO, L. E., GANESAN, J. & TODD, D. (1974). Genetic lesion in homozygous α thalassaemia (hydrops fetalis). *Nature (Lond.)*, **251**, 392–393.

TEMIN, H. M. & MIZUTANI, S. (1970). RNA-dependent DNA polymerase in virions of Rous sarcoma virus. *Nature (Lond.)*, **226**, 1211–1213.

TILLMAN, W. & SCHRÖTER, W. (1979). Rheological properties of erythrocytes in heterozygous and homozygous β thalassaemia. *Brit. J. Haemat.*, **43**, 401–411.

TRECARTIN, R. F., LIEBHABER, S. A., CHANG, J. C., LEE, K. Y., KAN, Y. W., FURBETTA, M., ANGIUS, A. & CAO, A. (1981). β^0 thalassemia in Sardinia is caused by a nonsense mutation. *J. clin. Invest.*, **68**, 1012–1017.

TREISMAN, R., ORKIN, S. H. & MANIATIS, T. (1983). Specific transcription and RNA splicing defects in five cloned β-thalassaemic genes. *Nature (Lond.)*, **302**, 591–596.

TRENT, R. J., HIGGS, D. R., CLEGG, J. B. & WEATHERALL, D. J. (1981). A new triplicated α-globin gene arrangement in man. *Brit. J. Haemat.*, **49**, 149–152.

TRENT, R. J., JONES, R. W., CLEGG, J. B., WEATHERALL, D. J., DAVIDSON, R. & WOOD, W. G. (1984). $(^A\gamma\ \delta\beta)^0$ thalassaemia: similarity of phenotype in four different molecular defects, including one newly described. *Brit. J. Haemat.*, **57**, 279–289.

TRENT, R. J., WILKINSON, T., YAKAS, J., CARTER, J., LAMMI, A. & KRONENBERG, H. (1986). Molecular defects in 2 examples of severe Hb H disease. *Scand. J. Haemat.*, **36**, 272–279.

TUAN, E., BIRO, P. A., deRIEL, J. K. & FORGET, B. G. (1980). Analysis of β-globin genes in β^0-thalassemia. *Ann N.Y. Acad. Sci.*, **334**, 12–30.

TUAN, D., MURNANE, M. J., deRIEL, J. K. & FORGET, B. G. (1980). Heterogeneity in the molecular basis of hereditary persistence of fetal haemoglobin. *Nature (Lond.)*, **285**, 335–337.

TUCHINDA, S., NAGAI, K. & LEHMANN, H. (1975). Oxygen dissociation curve of haemoglobin Portland. *FEBS Lett.*, **49**, 390–391.

VAN DER PLOEG, L. H. T., KONINGS, A., OORT, M., ROOS, D., BERNINI, L. & FLAVELL, R. A. (1980). $\gamma\beta$-thalassaemia studies showing that deletion of the γ- and δ-genes influences β-globin gene expression in man. *Nature (Lond.)*, **283**, 637–642.

VATANAVICHARN, S., AVUNATANKULCHAI, M., NA-NAKORN, S. & WASI, P. (1979). Serum and erythrocyte folate levels is thalassaemia patients in Thailand. *Scand. J. Haemat.*, **22**, 241–245.

VETTORE, L., FALEZZA, C., CETTO, G. L. & DE MATTEIS, M. C. (1974). Cation content and membrane deformability of heterozygous β-thalassaemic red blood cells. *Brit. J. Haemat.*, **27**, 429–437.

VETTORE, L. & TEDESCO, CH. J. G. (1975). Membrane lipid peroxidation in hypochromic red blood cells. *Haematologica*, **60**, 250.

VIGI, V., VOLPATO, S., GABURRO, D., CONCONI, F., BARGELLESI, A. & PONTREMOLI, S. (1969). The correlation between red-cell survival and excess of α-globin synthesis in β-thalassaemia. *Brit. J. Haemat.*, **16**, 25–30.

VISSERS, M. C. M., WINTERBOURN, C. C. & CARRELL, R. W. (1983). Rapid proteolysis of unstable globins in human bone marrow. *Brit. J. Haemat.*, **53**, 417–422.

WABER, P. G., BENDER, M. A., GELINAS, R. E., KATTAMIS, C., KARAKLIS, A., SOFRONIADOU, K.,

STAMATOYANNOPOULOS, G., COLLINS, F. S., FORGET, B. G. & KAZAZIAN, H. H. JNR (1986). Concordance of a point mutation 5' to the $^A\gamma$-globin gene with $^A\gamma$ β^+ hereditary persistence of fetal hemoglobin in Greeks. *Blood*, **67**, 551–554.

WAINSCOAT, J. S., OLD, J. M., WEATHERALL, D. J. & ORKIN, S. H. (1983). The molecular basis for the clinical diversity of β thalassaemia in Cypriots. *Lancet*, **i**, 1235–1237.

WEATHERALL, D. J. (1968). The biochemical lesion in thalassaemia. *Brit. J. Haemat.*, **15**, 1–5 (Annotation).

WEATHERALL, D. J. (1979). Mapping haemoglobin genes. *Brit. med. J.*, **ii**, 352–354 (Review).

WEATHERALL, D. J. (1983). The diagnostic features of the different forms of thalassemia. In: *The Thalassemias (Methods in Hematology)*, Vol. 6, pp. 1–26. Churchill Livingstone, Edinburgh.

WEATHERALL, D. J. & CLEGG, J. B. (1982). Thalassemia revisited. *Cell*, **29**, 7–9.

WEATHERALL, D. J., CLEGG, J. B. & WONG, H. B. (1970). The haemoglobin constitution of infants with the haemoglobin Bart's hydrops foetalis syndrome. *Brit J. Haemat.*, **18**, 357–367.

WEATHERALL, D. J. & WAINSCOAT, J. S. (1985). The molecular pathology of thalassaemia. In: *Recent Advances in Haematology* (ed. by A. V. Hoffbrand), pp. 63–88. Churchill Livingstone, Edinburgh.

WENNBERG, E. & WEISS, L. (1968). Splenic erythroclasia: an electron microscopic study of hemoglobin H disease. *Blood*, **31**, 788–790.

WESTAWAY, D. & WILLIAMSON, R. (1981). An intron nucleotide sequence variant in a cloned β⁺-thalassaemia globin gene. *Nucl. Acids Res.*, **9**, 1777–1788.

WHIPPLE, G. H. & BRADFORD, W. L. (1936). Mediterranean disease — thalassemia (erythroblastic anemia of Cooley). *J. Pediat.*, **9**, 279–311.

WHO WORKING GROUP (1982). Hereditary anaemias: genetic basis, clinical features, diagnosis, and treatment. *Bull. WHO*, **60**, 643–660.

WICKRAMASINGHE, S. N. (1976). The morphology and kinetics of erythropoiesis in homozygous β-thalassaemia. In: *Congenital Disorders of Erythropoiesis*, pp. 221–243. Ciba Foundation Symposium 37 (new series). Elsevier/Excerpta Medica/North Holland, Amsterdam.

WICKRAMASINGHE, S. N. & BUSH, V. (1975). Observations on the ultrastructure of erythropoietic cells and reticulum cells in the bone marrow of patients with homozygous β-thalassaemia. *Brit. J. Haemat.*, **30**, 395–399.

WICKRAMASINGHE, S. N. & HUGHES, M. (1978). Some features of bone marrow macrophages in patients with homozygous β-thalassaemia. *Brit. J. Haemat.*, **38**, 23–28.

WICKRAMASINGHE, S. N. & HUGHES, M. (1982). Precipitation of α-chains on the centrioles of erythroblasts in β-thalassaemia. *Brit. J. Haemat.*, **52**, 681–682 (Letter).

WICKRAMASINGHE, S. N. & HUGHES, M. (1984). Globin chain precipitation, deranged iron metabolism and dyserythropoiesis in some thalassaemia syndromes. *Haematologia*, **17**, 35–55.

WICKRAMASINGHE, S. N., HUGHES, M., FUCHAROEN, S. & WASI, P. (1984). The fate of excess β-globin chains within erythropoietic cells in α-thalassaemia 2 trait, α-thalassaemia 1 trait, haemoglobin H disease and haemoglobin Q-H disease: an electron microscope study. *Brit. J. Haemat.*, **56**, 473–482.

WICKRAMASINGHE, S. N., HUGHES, M., HIGGS, D. R. & WEATHERALL, D. J. (1981a). Ultrastructure of red cells containing haemoglobin H inclusions induced by redox dyes. *Clin. lab. Haemat.*, **3**, 51–60.

WICKRAMASINGHE, S. N., HUGHES, M., HOLLÁN, S. R., HORÁNYI, M. & SZELÉNYI, J. (1980). Electron microscope and high resolution autoradiographic studies of the erythroblasts in haemoglobin H disease. *Brit. J. Haemat.*, **45**, 401–404.

WICKRAMASINGHE, S. N., HUGHES, M., WASI, P. & FUCHAROEN, S. (1981b). Morphology and kinetics of erythropoiesis in haemoglobin H disease. *Brit. J. Haemat.*, **49**, 185–188.

WICKRAMASINGHE, S. N., LETSKY, E. & MOFFATT, B. (1973). Effect of α-chain precipitates on bone marrow function in homozygous β-thalassaemia. *Brit. J. Haemat.*, **25**, 123–129.

WICKRAMASINGHE, S. N., McELWAIN, T. J., COOPER, E. H. & HARDISTY, R. M. (1970). Proliferation of erythroblasts in beta-thalassaemia. *Brit. J. Haemat.*, **19**, 719–727.

WITZLEBEN, C. L. & WYATT, J. P. (1961). The effect of long survival on the pathology of thalassaemia major. *J. Path. Bact.*, **82**, 1–12.

WONG, S. C., CHANG, L. S., OLIVIERI, N. F., POON, A. O., ALI, M. A. M. & GROVES, D. J. (1985). Compound heterozygosity for two genotypes of α-thalassaemia-2: hematological, biosynthetic and DNA studies. *Hemoglobin*, **9**, 111–126.

WOOD, W. G., MacRAE, I. A., DARBRE, P. D., CLEGG, J. B. & WEATHERALL, D. J. (1982). The British type of non-deletion HPFH: characterization of developmental changes *in vivo* and erythroid growth *in vitro*. *Brit. J. Haemat.*, **50**, 401–414.

WOOD, W. G. & STAMATOYANNOPOULOS, G. (1975). Globin synthesis in fractionated normoblasts of β-thalassemia heterozygotes. *J. clin. Invest.*, **55**, 567–578.

YATAGANAS, X. & FESSAS, PH. (1969). The pattern of hemoglobin precipitation in thalassemia and its significance. *Ann. N.Y. Acad. Sci.*, **165**, 270–287.

YATAGANAS, X., FESSAS, P. & GAHRTON, G. (1972). Quantitation of α-chain excess in erythrocytes in β-thalassaemia by microinterferometry. *Brit. J. Haemat.*, **22**, 117–123.

YATAGANAS, X., GAHRTON, G., FESSAS, PH., KESSE-ELIAS, M. & THORELL, B. (1973). Proliferative activity and glycogen accumulation of erythroblasts in β-thalassaemia. *Brit. J. Haemat.*, **24**, 651–659.

YATAGANAS, X., GAHRTON, G. & THORELL, B. (1974). Intranuclear hemoglobin in erythroblasts of β-thalassemia. *Blood*, **43**, 243–250.

ZAINO, E. C. (1980). Pathophysiology of thalassemia. *Ann. N.Y. Acad. Sci.*, **334**, 284–304.

ZAINO, E. C. & ROSSI, M. B. (1974). Ultrastructure of the erythrocytes in β-thalassemia. *Ann. N.Y. Acad. Sci.*, **232**, 238–260.

ZAINO, E. C., ROSSI, M. B., PHAM, T. D. & AZAR, H. A. (1971). Gaucher's cells in thalassemia. *Blood*, **38**, 457–462.

ZINTL, F. (1954). Ein weiterer Fall familiärer Thalassaemia minor Typus Rietti-Greppi-Micheli. *Z. Kinderheilk.*, **74**, 251–274.

The thalassaemias III: differential diagnosis, antenatal diagnosis and treatment

The clinical manifestations of thalassaemia are many and varied, as outlined in Chapter 18. Important pointers to the diagnosis of thalassaemia major or intermedia are, however, a long history of anaemia, extending back perhaps to infancy, a palpable spleen and the occurrence of anaemia in relatives. The patient's racial origin, too, may be a pointer to the diagnosis.

The blood picture is in many ways characteristic. The erythrocytes in stained dried films are hypochromic; they tend to be microcytic but vary markedly in size and shape; some cells are clearly fragments; target cells may be present, too, and cells showing punctate basophilia. Osmotic resistance is increased. The MCV and MCH are usually substantially less than normal; the MCHC is, on the other hand, often within the normal range or at the most slightly subnormal. The changes are most marked in homozygotes or compound heterozygotes. In simple heterozygotes, however, the blood picture is in many ways similar to that in haemoglobin deficiency due to causes other than thalassaemia, and the distinction between heterozygous thalassaemia and iron-deficiency anaemia (and the rare hereditary sideroblastic anaemia) is of practical importance.

The serum iron concentration is characteristically above normal in thalassaemia (and below normal in iron-deficiency anaemia) and the total iron-binding capacity (TIBC) is normal in thalassaemia (but raised in iron-deficiency anaemia). The percentage saturation of the TIBC is raised in thalassaemia. The percentages of Hb F and Hb A_2 are often increased in thalassaemia and raised levels are pointers to the type of thalassaemia, *e.g.*, to β-thalassaemia. The presence of Hb Bart's in cord blood and of Hb H subsequently indicates α-thalassaemia.

The findings outlined above suggest that the diagnosis of thalassaemia can be easily made. This is true in many cases, but relatively 'silent' carriers of both α- and β-thalassaemia exist and the diagnosis in such cases can be difficult, and may depend on the results of a globin-chain synthesis study; and in many cases the exact genotype of the patient can only be determined by a detailed family study and globin-gene analysis.

DISTINCTION BETWEEN THALASSAEMIA TRAIT (HETEROZYGOUS β- or α-THALASSAEMIA) AND IRON-DEFICIENCY ANAEMIA

As mentioned above, it is important not to misdiagnose thalassaemia trait as iron-deficiency anaemia and to condemn the patient possibly to long-term oral iron therapy. It is true that a misdiagnosis is unlikely if the examination includes the estimation of serum iron and Hb F and Hb A_2. But if the diagnosis is based on the blood picture alone, mistakes can occur. The distinction between iron-deficiency anaemia and the reliability of screening tests for thalassaemia has been the subject of considerable study (see below).

Erythrocyte morphology

It is difficult to make a confident diagnosis of heterozygous β- or α-thalassaemia on morphological changes alone, although it seems generally to have been believed, *e.g.*, by Rowley (1976), that in β-thalassaemia trait there is more cell-to-cell variation than in iron-deficiency anaemia at comparable haemoglobin levels.

The presence of basophilic stippling is, too, a strong pointer to the presence of β-thalassaemia [see Joishy, Shafer and Rowley (1986)].

Coulter-counter data

The introduction of automated cell counting methods awakened interest in the possibility of using volumetric data in screening for thalassaemia and in distinguishing thalassaemia from iron-deficiency anaemia.

Erythrocyte volume distribution curves

Torlontano, Tata and Camagna (1972) and Cazzavillan *et al.* (1973) studied volumetric distribution data provided by a Coulter counter and reported that thalassaemia-minor erythrocytes gave a peak which they considered to be separable from the peaks produced by normal or iron-deficiency cells. England and Down (1974) made a similar observation. In a paper concerned primarily with the variations of erythrocyte volume in health they illustrated a curve from a patient with Hb-H disease and another from a patient with heterozygous β-thalassaemia. The volume range was less than normal in the latter patient. England and Down concluded that a 'volume ratio' is the best index of anisocytosis and that it is generally higher in iron-deficiency anaemia than in heterozygous β-thalassaemia. Bessman and Feinstein (1979) extended this work. They calculated the coefficient of variation (CV) of erythrocyte volume from Coulter-counter-derived volume frequency distribution curves, which they referred to as erythrograms and concluded that 'erythrography' provided an excellent means of rapidly distinguishing between iron-deficiency anaemia and thalassaemia minor. In 53 patients with iron deficiency the CV was always greater than 14%, while in 22 out of 25 patients with heterozygous β-thalassaemia it was less than 14% and in the three remaining patients it was between 14.0 and 14.9%; in seven patients with heterozygous α-thalassaemia it was less than 14%. The MCV in the patients in all three groups was less than 70 fl.

Johnson, Tegos and Beutler (1983) compared several methods of using erythrocyte measurements in the differential diagnosis of iron-deficiency anaemia and heterozygous thalassaemia and concluded that analysis of erythrocyte volume measurements provided the best means of discriminating between the two conditions. Using as a criterion (EVR_{50}) the width in fl between the ascending and descending limbs of the distribution curve at half the maximum height of the curve, all of 36 iron-deficient patients (with an EVR_{50} >27 fl) and 57 β-thalassaemics (with an EVR_{50} <26 fl) were correctly identified.

MCV, MCH, erythrocyte count and haemoglobin

The possibility, too, that measurement of the MCV alone (without regard to the distribution of volumes around the mean value) could be used as a criterion for the diagnosis of thalassaemia has been carefully considered, *e.g.*, by McPhedran *et al.* (1973), Pearson, O'Brien and McIntosh (1973) and Pearson *et al.* (1974). Their extensive data indicated that microcytosis (MCV < 79 fl) can be used as an important pointer towards the diagnosis of thalassaemia if iron deficiency is excluded by measurement of serum iron.

McPhedran and co-workers (1973) analysed 1000 patients whose MCV was less than 75 fl. The chances of the diagnosis being β-thalassaemia trait (with Hb-A_2 percentage = or > 3.5) increased as the MCV became less; 47% of those with an MCV of 61–65 fl had the trait, 30% of those with an MCV of 66–70 fl and 16% of those with an MCV of 71–75 fl.

Whether it is possible to exclude iron-deficiency anaemia by using Coulter-counter-derived values alone was investigated by England and Fraser (1973). They used a discriminant function which they had derived from the MCV, erythrocyte count and haemoglobin level and obtained an almost complete separation between 25 patients with iron-deficiency anaemia and 28 patients with β-thalassaemia trait. England, Bain and Fraser (1973) later reported that the discriminant function would correctly indicate thalassaemia even if iron deficiency was present also. They conceded, however, that haemodilution, as in pregnancy or following haemorrhage, could give misleading results and that in thalassaemia complicated by iron deficiency the function would indicate iron deficiency if this was severe. The experience of other workers has suggested that the function is less reliable than it first appeared to be (Hamblin, 1973; Schriever, 1973; Srivastava, 1973).

Hamlin (1973) referred to patients with polycythaemia and iron deficiency who gave results in the β-thalassaemia range.

Schriever (1973), too, found that the formula gave misleading results in pregnant women with thalassaemia and claimed that it is possible to differentiate thalassaemia trait from iron-deficiency anaemia from knowledge of the erythrocyte indices and by examination of stained films. The point was made that in thalassaemia trait the MCV is almost always in the 54–71 fl range and the MCHC is normal; and the presence of punctate basophilia was accepted to be strong evidence, too, in favour of thalassaemia minor.

Srivastava (1973) considered that England and Fraser's formula, although giving correct results in straightforward cases of thalassaemia minor, was unreliable in thalassaemia associated with advanced pregnancy or iron deficiency or when complicated by protein deficiency or rheumatoid arthritis, or by renal insufficiency or tuberculosis, or in hypochromic polycythaemia. He suggested a simpler formula — the MCH in pg divided by the erythrocyte count in millions per μ1, and stated that in nine out of 10 cases the product was less than 3.8 in thalassaemia minor and more than 3.8 in iron-deficiency anaemia. Mentzer (1973) reported that a simple MCV:erythrocyte count ratio was as accurate as England and Fraser's discriminant function. He applied the formula in 53 patients with mild iron-deficiency anaemia and in 50 patients with either α- or β-thalassaemia traits: 87 out of the 103 patients were correctly identified by the MCV:erythrocyte count ratio compared with 86 by England and Fraser's formula. He, too, cautioned that complicating disease or pregnancy might lead to erroneous classification.

Gimferrer and co-workers (1975), however, reported that England and Fraser's function had given more reliable results in their hands than had Mentzer's ratio. They had tested 48 patients with β-thalassaemia trait and 195 iron-deficient patients and found that the results with 14.5% of the thalassaemia patients fell within the zone of uncertainty using England and Fraser's function compared to 39.5% using Mentzer's ratio.

The early results of the use of formulae based on the erythrocyte count and indices that have been outlined above are interesting, if slightly discordant. It is hardly to be expected, however, that in disorders as variable in expression as heterozygous thalassaemia the morphological characteristics of the erythrocytes will always be decisively different from those of iron-deficiency anaemia. The success of the formulae stems, of course, from the rather remarkable and not easily explained tendency for the erythrocyte count in the thalassaemias to be higher in relation to the haemoglobin level, and for the MCV to be lower, than in iron deficiency. Some more recent studies are referred to briefly below.

Klee and co-workers (1976) compared the results given by England and Fraser's function and the ratios of Srivastava and of Mentzer in 122 patients who were iron-deficient and in 66 with β-thalassaemia minor: they concluded that none of the formulae gave sufficiently accurate results for a final diagnosis. Measurement of the MCHC was confirmed as being of little value, being only consistently low in severe iron deficiency. Using England and Fraser's formula, 20% of patients with thalassaemia minor and 4% with iron deficiency were misdiagnosed. The ratio of MCV or MCH to erythrocyte count did not seem to improve the accuracy of diagnosis — in fact, the erythrocyte count alone was thought to identify patients with uncomplicated thalassaemia minor almost as well!

The use of a further formula based on erythrocyte indices was described by Shine and Lal (1977). The product of $(MCV)^2 \times MCH \div 100$ was tested out on 138 blood samples from patients with β-thalassaemia minor: using 1530 as the determining limit, only 4.4% gave false-positive results (i.e., scores less than this). Cappellini, Sampietro and Fiorelli (1977) applied this formula in 245 cases of thalassaemia minor, and in 116 patients with miscellaneous anaemias in which the MCV was less than 80 fl and in 150 normal subjects. They found that the formula did not discriminate well between the patients with thalassaemia trait or other microcytic anaemias and that there was a small overlap with the results in healthy subjects. Shine and Lal's formula, however, appeared to perform better than did those of England and Fraser and of Mentzer tested on the same series of patients.

The control of hereditary anaemias (including thalassaemia) was the subject of a meeting of a WHO Working Group held in Geneva in November 1981 (Boyo et al., 1983). It is interesting to note that none of the formulae utilizing the MCV that have been discussed above were mentioned. Instead, the Group recommended as screening tests the measurement of MCV or MCH or osmotic resistance and indicated that individuals with an MCH of less than 24 pg should be investigated further. MCH measurements, cellulose acetate electrophoresis and Hb-A_2 estimation were considered to be the ideal test combination, as with these tests only the relatively unimportant silent β-thalassaemia trait (with normal Hb A_2) would be missed while abnormal haemoglobins such as Hb S, Hb C and Hb E would be picked up.

Borgna-Pignatti and co-workers (1983) recorded Coulter-counter erythrocyte indices in 137 adult and 132 children with heterozygous β-thalassaemia. The mean MCV in the adults was 67.6 ± 4.36 fl (range 56–79 fl) and in the children 62.8 ± 4.05 fl (range 55–71 fl). Only 0.7% of the adults had a MCV greater than 79 fl while 98% of the children had a MCV less than 72 fl. The MCV in the β-thalassaemic children did not

increase with age, whereas the mean MCV of 172 control normal children increased steadily from 77.5 fl at the age of 2 years to 83.0 at the age of 13. Borgna-Pigatti concluded that the MCV is a valuable indicator of thalassaemia and that the indices of Shine and Lal, England and Fraser and of Mentzer, do not help to discriminate between β-thalassaemia and other disorders associated with microcytosis.

Stephens (1985), in discussing simple ways in which β-thalassaemia may be diagnosed, stressed the value of the MCV and MCH and of a one-tube osmotic fragility test, and of measurement of Hb-F and Hb-A_2 percentage; he emphasized that the various formulae that could be used were useful as guides but should never be used to make a definitive diagnosis.

Aghai and co-workers (1986) investigated 119 children with microcytic anaemia who were apparently not responding to iron therapy: 75 were diagnosed as having heterozygous β-thalassaemia; 40 were in fact iron-deficient. In all the 75 β-thalassaemia children, one parent had a MCV less than 79 fl; 11 of the children had a normal Hb-A_2 percentage until they were treated with iron. Aghai et al. concluded that measurement of the parents' MCV was a valuable means of discriminating between β-thalassaemia and iron deficiency in children and was more reliable than the measurement of Hb A_2.

Osmotic resistance

As referred to in Chapter 18 (p. 421), increased erythrocyte osmotic resistance has been looked upon for many years as a characteristic feature of thalassaemia. But how reliable is the measurement of osmotic resistance as a screening test and how does the increased resistance in thalassaemia compare with that found in iron deficiency?

For screening purposes a multi-tube hypotonic saline test is clearly inappropriate. Silvestroni and Bianco (1975) reviewed the results of screening for thalassaemia trait (microcytemia) in Italy over a 30-year period and concluded that a one-tube test gave an abnormal result in 93% of blood samples from individuals diagnosed as having thalassaemia trait by other criteria. An additional 5% gave an abnormal result despite having apparently normal erythrocyte morphology. Malamos, Fessas and Stamatoyannopoulos (1962) studied 109 Greeks considered to be carriers of a thalassaemia trait: 101 had increased osmotic resistance as judged by less than 75% lysis in 0.4% NaCl. These results clearly supported the concept that increased osmotic resistance is an almost invariable accompaniment of thalassaemia trait. They did not, however, answer the question as to whether the test helps in the distinction between thalassaemia trait and iron deficiency.

More recently, Kattamis, Efremov and Pootrakul (1981) reported on a study of β-thalassaemia heterozygotes in Greece, Yugoslavia and Thailand. They used a 0.36% Tyrode's solution and found that 98% of 431 heterozygotes for β-thalassaemia gave results judged to be abnormal. There were, however, some false-positive results (9.1%) in individuals thought to be normal, and the test was positive, too, in 80% of iron-deficient subjects and in 68% of Hb-E trait carriers. Kattamis, Efremov and Pootrakul concluded, nevertheless, that the test was valuable as a screening test in a laboratory with limited resources. Kattamis and co-workers (1981), in a further report, described the usefulness of the one-tube test in the Island of Lesbos. 428 individuals were submitted to a haematological study: 72 were found to be β-thalassaemia heterozygotes (71 had increased osmotic resistance); 11 had α-thalassaemia (9 had increased osmotic resistance); 25 were suspected of having α-thal-2 trait (20 had increased osmotic resistance); 5 had iron-deficiency anaemia (all had increased osmotic resistance), and 308 were classified as normal (29 had increased osmotic resistance). Kattamis et al. concluded that their screening test had proved to be practical, inexpensive and reasonably effective, and that it provided a means of detecting thalassaemia heterozygotes in areas where comprehensive laboratory facilities and experienced personnel were unavailable.

A recently introduced variant of the hypotonic saline method of measuring osmotic resistance is the glycerol lysis time test (see Vol. 1, p. 101). As used by Posteraro and Gottfried (1978), normal erythrocytes give glycerol lysis times (GLT$_{50}$) of 26–73 seconds. Of 100 consecutive patients with times greater than 73 seconds, 72 had a haemoglobinopathy and of these 65 had a thalassaemia trait; nine individuals had an iron-deficiency anaemia. More recently, Zanella and co-workers (1983) reported on an even larger series of patients: 513 had β-thalassaemia trait, 25 α-thalassaemia trait, 170 were iron-deficient and 217 had a blood disorder classified as miscellaneous. It was concluded that although the test was highly sensitive in detecting β- or α-thalassaemia trait, it could not be used to distinguish between β-thalassaemia and iron-deficiency anaemia because of a large overlap of results; the traditional 0.35% NaCl test, which gave fewer false positives, appeared to be superior as a screening test.

It seems clear from the reports cited above that measurement of one-tube osmotic resistance can provide a useful screening test for heterozygous β- and α-thalassaemia. It cannot, however, be used to distinguish between the two major groups of thalassaemia or between thalassaemia and other types of haemoglobinopathy, and it cannot be used to distinguish between a haemoglobinopathy and iron deficiency. The results overlap too much, although it seems likely that the changes in iron deficiency are usually intermediate between those of thalassaemia and the normal, as had been indicated by Reimann and Arkun in 1955.

Measurement of free erythrocyte protoporphyrin (FEP)

The FEP concentration tends to be above normal in iron deficiency but normal in thalassaemia trait. Stockman and co-workers (1975) measured FEP in 70 normal subjects and in 52 patients with iron deficiency and in 29 with β-thalassaemia trait: 90% of the iron-deficient patients had increased FEP levels while in 97% of the β-thalassaemia patients the result was normal.

DIAGNOSIS OF α-THALASSAEMIA TRAIT

As already referred to (p. 457), the effect of α-thalassaemia on erythrocyte morphology may be minimal in α-thal-2 (α$^+$-thalassaemia) trait, and blood films even from individuals identified on genetic grounds as obligatory heterozygotes may be difficult to separate from normal. The same applies to blood indices. The MCV and MCH are, however, subnormal in the majority of carriers of α-thalassaemia and the practical question arises as to how to establish or exclude the diagnosis of α-thalassaemia in individuals who have a subnormal MCV and MCH but normal Hb-F and Hb-A levels and a normal serum-iron concentration. Then there is the question of how much time should be spent on searching for erythrocytes containing Hb-H inclusions.

There is by now a considerable amount of literature on the above-mentioned problems, and the general conclusion seems to be that in some cases diagnosis can only be arrived at by measurement of the α:β globin-chain synthesis ratio — clearly an impracticable procedure in screening studies. In individual cases genetic information can be of great help, but sometimes the diagnosis of α-thalassaemia can only be presumed not proved. Looking for Hb-H inclusions in heterozygotes is time-consuming, and it is unreliable in that failure to find any inclusions does not exclude α-thalassaemia. However, even one characteristic cell is sufficient for a diagnosis to be made, that is if acquired Hb-H disease (a rarity) can be excluded. According to Wasi, Pravatmuang and Winichagoon (1979), in Thailand very occasional erythrocytes containing Hb-H inclusions (1 cell in 50 000–100 000 perhaps) can always be found in α^0-thalassaemia (α-thal-1) heterozygotes, but none can be found in α^+-thalassaemia (α-thal-2) heterozygotes. According to Wasi (1983), inclusions are always to be found in the Saudi-Arabian variant of α-thalassaemia which phenotypically is intermediate between α^0-thalassaemia and α^+-thalassaemia.

Walford and Deacon (1976) and Walford (1977) reviewed the criteria for the diagnosis of heterozygous α-thalassaemia and described findings in individuals belonging to several racial groups living in Great Britain. The mean $\alpha:\beta$ globin-chain synthesis ratio in 35 patients of Indian, Greek or Chinese origin was 0.79 $\pm$ 0.07 (normal mean 1.06 $\pm$ 0.08). The Hb-H screening test was usually negative in Indian and black individuals but positive in all the Chinese tested and in three-quarters of the Greeks. The erythrocyte indices were significantly less abnormal in the Indians than in the Chinese, with the Greeks giving values in between. Walford and Deacon also compared the erythrocyte indices in Indian, Greek and Chinese patients with either α- or β-thalassaemia. In each sex in each racial group the MCV and MCH were less abnormal in those with α-thalassaemia than in those with β-thalassaemia.

Hegde and his co-workers (1977) studied 66 people of Mediterranean or Asian origin who had microcytic and hypochromic erythrocytes and in whom iron deficiency and β-thalassaemia had been excluded. The Coulter-counter-derived indices were similar to those of obligatory α-thalassaemia heterozygotes, and it was concluded that the group studied had in fact α-thalassaemia. Globin-chain synthesis was carried out in nine individuals: the $\alpha:\beta$ ratio was 0.6–0.8 in seven and 0.84 in two. Hb-H inclusions were found in 16 out of 46 individuals, but in some instances only after 'prolonged search'. The inclusions were found only in those with markedly abnormal blood pictures. Hegde *et al.* applied England and Fraser's discriminant function to their data and found this of value in separating iron-deficiency anaemia from cases considered to be α-thal-1, but it failed to discriminate between α-thal-2 and iron-deficiency.

Melis and co-workers (1980) reported on 88 Sardinian adults who had a thalassaemia-like blood picture and indices, normal Hb-A_2 and Hb-F levels and a normal serum iron concentration. Globin-chain synthesis gave a mean $\alpha:\beta$ ratio of 0.7 $\pm$ 0.10, the same as in obligate α-thalassaemia carriers. Hb-H inclusions were found in 65 out of the 88 patients (74%) but only as the result of up to 1 hour's search.

Diagnosis of α-thalassaemia trait by immunological means

Wasi, Pravatmuang and Winichagoon (1979) described the results of testing for Hb Bart's by exposing haemoglobin derived from patients suspected of having the α-thalassaemia trait to a Hb-Bart's antibody. The antiserum was derived from rabbits immunized against Hb Bart's obtained from hydropic fetuses. Tests were carried out in capillary tubes: precipitation was obvious in 82% of 87 obligatory α-thalassaemia heterozygotes, *i.e.*, in parents of infants with hydrops or in parents or offspring of patients with Hb-H disease. Positive results were obtained in 86% of α-thal-1 trait carriers and in 79% of α-thal-2 carriers, and positive results, too, were obtained in 21% of the general population in Bangkok, *i.e.*, at a percentage corresponding to the believed prevalence of α-thalassaemia trait. The antibody did not cross-react with Hb F. The results were also positive in 16 out of 17 adults who were heterozygotes for Hb Constant Spring, who thus appeared to have small amounts of Hb Bart's in their blood.

Effect of iron deficiency on $\alpha:\beta$ globin-chain synthesis ratios

Not only may iron deficiency accompany α-thalassaemia and complicate diagnosis from haematological findings but is also influences the $\alpha:\beta$ globin-chain synthesis ratio. Both conditions lower the ratio. El-Hazmi and Lehmann (1978) reviewed the relevant literature and described their findings in 12 patients who had α-thalassaemia or were iron-deficient or had both conditions. Four patients had $\alpha:\beta$ globin-synthesis ratios in the α-thal-1 range. On the addition of haemin to the test system, the ratio rose to within the α-thal-2 range — α-thal-2 was presumed to be the diagnosis. The other eight patients gave ratios within the α-thal-2 range. On the addition of haemin the ratio rose to within the normal range, and these patients were considered to be suffering from iron-deficiency anaemia alone.

DIAGNOSIS OF THALASSAEMIA IN THE NEWBORN

β-thalassaemia. It is not possible to diagnose homozygous or heterozygous β-thalassaemia from the examination of cord blood carried out in a routine way. It is certainly wiser to wait until the infant is at least 2–3 months old when, in the case of homozygosity, the diagnosis is usually by then becoming obvious. It has, nevertheless, proved possible to diagnose both the heterozygous and homozygous states by carrying out β-globin-chain synthesis studies using the reticulocytes in cord blood. Thus Kan and Nathan (1968) demonstrated half-normal β-globin-chain synthesis in a heterozygous infant and Gaburro, Volpato and Vigi (1970) complete failure of synthesis in two infants subsequently shown to be homozygous.

Heterozygotes for β-thalassaemia can, according to Weatherall (1983), usually be distinguished from normal infants by the time the infant is 3–6 months old. The Hb-A_2 percentage is raised to above the normal adult level within 3–6 months. The Hb-F level tends to be higher than normal throughout the first year. The MCH and MCV fall within the first 3 months to levels below those of normal infants. In summary, in typical high Hb-A_2 β-thalassaemia the diagnosis is usually clear by the time the infant is about 6 months of age.

α-thalassaemia. In contrast to β-thalassaemia, the diagnosis of α-thalassaemia can be established, or at least suspected, in most affected infants by examining cord blood.

As already described, homozygosity for α-thal-1 ($α^0$-thalassaemia) leads to the fetal hydrops syndrome. Compound heterozygosity for α-thal-1 and α-thal-2, or another combination (see p. 450), leads to Hb-H disease; the infant is born anaemic, has relatively hypochromic and microcytic erythrocytes and has Hb Bart's and 15–25% of Hb H in its blood. There is usually no difficulty in diagnosis and one or both parents should show clear signs of heterozygous α-thalassaemia.

Heterozygosity for α-thalassaemia is less easily diagnosed at birth although the presence of Hb Bart's is an important pointer to the diagnosis. The blood picture may provide important clues, too. The presence of hypochromic and microcytic erythrocytes and 2–8% Hb Bart's suggests heterozygosity for $α^0$-thalassaemia (α-thal-1) or homozygosity for $α^+$-thalassaemia (α-thal-2) (Weatherall, 1983). The blood picture in $α^+$-thalassaemia (α-thal-2) heterozygotes is less easy to distinguish from normal and, although small amounts of Hb Bart's may be present, Hb Bart's cannot always be

clearly demonstrated. According to Schmair et al. (1973), a lowered MCV (= or < 94 fl) and MCH (= or < 29.5 pg) are, too, useful pointers to α-thalassaemia trait.

The recent availability of sophisticated methods of gene analysis has made it possible to study the sensitivity of tests for Hb Bart's and the relationship between the amount of Hb Bart's present and the infant's genotype, i.e., whether one or more α genes are missing.

Ohene-Frempong and co-workers (1980) used restriction endonuclease analysis to compare the number of active α genes and the amount of Hb Bart's in cord blood in a series of black American infants. Four had more than 2% Hb Bart's in their blood; they were shown to have two α genes present, one in each chromosome. Of the remaining 19, all of whom had less than 2% Hb Bart's, eight had three α genes and 11 four α genes — all the latter had 1% or less Hb Bart's. Ohene-Frempong et al. concluded that infants with three α genes (αα/−α) may or may not have elevated Hb-Bart's levels while those with more than 2% Hb Bart's are likely to have two α genes only (−α/−α). The results of a more extensive study on black West-Indian infants were reported by Higgs and co-workers (1980). Approximately 7% of 2191 infants had Hb Bart's in their cord blood. Infants with 3–8% Hb Bart's were found by restriction-enzyme mapping of their DNA to be homozygous (−α/−α) for the α-thal-2 determinant. Those with 0.1–2% Hb Bart's were shown to be heterozygotes, i.e., to have the −α/αα genotype. Higgs et al. concluded, however, that not all black infants with α-thalassaemia have detectable levels of Hb Bart's in their cord blood, and in a later publication on the same population (Higgs et al., 1982) it was emphasized that the use as a diagnostic criterion of Hb Bart's visible on cellulose acetate strips in the 0.1–2% range grossly underestimates the incidence of the −α/αα genotype. Whereas the frequency of this genotype, based on the quantitative estimation of small amounts of Hb Bart's, was 3.1%, the frequency of the genotype determined by DNA analysis was as high as 29.5%, a figure close to the predicted −α/ haplotype frequency.

The results of an extensive study carried out on an Asian population were reported by Lie-Injo et al. in 1982. Hb Bart's was demonstrated in 58 out of 843 Malaysian newborn infants. DNA was prepared from 17 samples of blood containing a trace of Hb Bart's (< 3%): 16 samples were found to have one α gene deleted (α-thal-2) and one sample had two α genes deleted (α-thal-1). Most of the single gene deletions were of the rightward type. Two 'new' deletions were identified; these were thought to be the result of polymorphism in an area outside the α-globin gene. Of 16 blood samples containing a moderate amount of Hb

Bart's (3.5–8.5%), 14 were found to have two α-globin genes deleted and one to have a single gene deleted. In three samples containing Hb Bart's, but in which the α-globin genes appeared to be intact, Hb Constant spring was present.

HAEMOGLOBIN ANALYSIS AS AID TO DIAGNOSIS

As has been repeatedly mentioned, it has been realized for many years that the different thalassaemia syndromes are associated with characteristic changes in Hb-A_2 and Hb-F percentages and that these changes are most helpful in diagnosis. In Tables 18.1 (p. 393) and 18.4 (p. 447) are summarized what may be expected to be found in the more important syndromes. Table 18.4 also includes the percentages of Hb H, Hb Bart's (and Hb Portland) that may be found in the fetal hydrops syndrome and in Hb-H disease.

ANTENATAL DIAGNOSIS OF THALASSAEMIA

An important recent development in the history of thalassaemia has been the development of methods for the diagnosis of the disorder in an affected fetus, at a stage of its development early enough for therapeutic abortion to be considered. Several technical advances have made this possible: in particular, improvements in fetal blood sampling resulting in the possibility of obtaining fetal blood with little or no contamination by maternal blood and the application of molecular-genetic techniques to the analysis of fetal DNA obtained from amniotic fluid cells or chorionic villi (fetal trophoblast).

Obtaining fetal blood (containing reticulocytes) has made possible the measurement of the relative rates of β to γ chain production using [^{3}H]leucine and the separation of the labelled globin chains by carboxymethylcellulose (CMC) chromatography or similar techniques. Normally, there is a small but definite amount of β-chain production, *i.e.*, formation of Hb A, in the second trimester of pregnancy when fetal blood sampling is usually carried out. In homozygous β-thalassaemia few if any β-globin chains are synthesized and the β:γ ratio is substantially lower than normal; in heterozygous thalassaemia the ratio is subnormal but higher than in homozygotes or compound heterozygotes. Despite the technical difficulties inherent in the analysis and in the interpretation of the results, the method has been quite widely applied and there have been few errors in diagnosis. The success of the method, however, depends upon skilled fetal-blood sampling, and although fetal loss attributable to the procedure is low in experienced hands it is not negligible. Amniocentesis is a safer procedure. According to the National Registry for Amniocentesis Study Group (NICHD, 1976), midtrimester amniocentesis is a highly accurate and safe procedure that does not significantly increase the risk of fetal loss or injury. But it may not be possible to obtain sufficient DNA from uncultured amniotic cells; and culturing cells, although a successful technique, takes several weeks, so that a result may not be possible until the 18th–20th week of pregnancy.

Fetal blood sampling

Hollenberg, Kaback and Kazazian (1971) seem to be the first to have demonstrated that reticulocytes obtained from 8–9-week-old human fetuses form Hb A at about 10% of the rate at which Hb F is formed. They concluded that in consequence of this it should be possible to diagnose β-thalassaemia syndromes before birth by demonstrating the absence of β^A-chain formation and sickle-cell disease from the presence of β^S chains. It was not until 1974, however, that the results were published of the first successful attempts to obtain fetal blood samples from living fetuses with the object eventually of applying the method to the diagnosis of thalassaemia or sickle-cell disease

Kan and his co-workers (1974b) carried out transabdominal puncture of the anterior-situated placenta using a 20-gauge spinal needle in 19 patients due to have elective interruption of pregnancy at 18–22 weeks. 0.1–0.2 ml of blood was withdrawn. This proved to be a mixture of fetal and maternal blood, but sufficient fetal cells were obtained in 11 out of the 19 cases for a β-globin chain synthesis study to be practicable.

Hobbins and Mahoney (1974) aspirated fetal blood from a vessel on the chorionic plate of posterior or fundal-situated placentas in eight women undergoing therapeutic abortion at the 15–20th week of pregnancy. The placenta was located ultrasonically and the vessel punctured with the help of an endoscope inserted transabdominally. The fetal blood was in each instance diluted in amniotic fluid and in four cases the majority of erythrocytes present were of maternal origin. These or similar blood-sampling methods have been widely used and new and improved techniques reported, *e.g.* by Daffos, Capella-Pavlovsky and Forestier (1983).

An important disadvantage of all blood-sampling techniques is that they cannot be applied to very young fetuses and so have generally not been attempted before the 16th week of pregnancy. Fetal blood sampling is, too, not free from risk. Thus Fairweather, Ward and Modell (1980) and Ward *et al.* (1981) in large series of patients recorded a fetal loss rate of 9 and 10%, respectively. A further disadvantage is contamination of the fetal blood sample with maternal blood, and several ingenious manoeuvres have been employed to reduce the proportion of maternal erythrocytes present. For example, Kan and his co-workers (1974a) used an anti-i serum which would agglutinate fetal cells in preference to adult cells, while Boyer, Noyes and Boyer (1976) and Alter and her co-workers (1979) utilized the sensitivity of adult erythrocytes to haemolysis by ammonium chloride and ammonium bicarbonate as the result of the adult cells' relatively high content of carbonic anhydrase (the Ørskov procedure) (see also Alter (1983)).

The development of improved fibreoptic fetoscopes has made it possible to aspirate blood from a fetal blood vessel under direct vision, and in skilled hands it has proved possible to obtain fetal blood in this way without any contamination by amniotic fluid or maternal blood. (Rodeck and Campbell, 1978; Rodeck and Nicolaides, 1983). This technique has rendered 'blind' placental aspiration obsolete.

Fetal erythrocytes have a MCV that is considerably larger than that of normal adult cells and this is even more true if the maternal cells, possibly contaminating the sample, are from a patient with heterozygous thalassaemia. A useful and very rapid method of demonstrating contaminating maternal erythrocytes is to use a Coulter Channelyzer. Alter (1983) illustrated a series of strikingly different cell size distribution curves artificially produced by adding increasing proportions of fetal cells to maternal thalassaemia-trait cells of MCV approximately 70 fl. Uncontaminated samples of fetal blood give a single-peak almost symmetrical curve with a MCV in the region of 140 fl. Another but less rapid but also accurate method of determining contamination with maternal erythrocytes is to expose films of the aspirated blood to the acid elution procedure (see p. 409).

Chorionic villus sampling

The recently introduced technique of chorionic villus sampling provides as a rule sufficient DNA for testing (20–50 μg), and it has the great advantage that the sampling can be carried out in very young fetuses, *i.e.*, at the 9–12th week of pregnancy (Niazi, Coleman and Loeffler, 1981; Williamson *et al.*, 1981). It is, too, usually possible to obtain fetal tissue free from maternal contamination (Elles *et al.*, 1983). The technique has been widely used (Rodeck and Morsman, 1983) and the risk to the mother is minimal.

Fetal loss, however, is a possibility. According to Mibashan and his co-workers (1985), recent data collated from an EEC conference gave a loss rate from all causes of 4.1% based on 4054 samplings; the loss rate from the sampling itself was thought, however, to be less than 3% in experienced hands. Unfortunately, despite a good chance of an adequate sample, diagnosis by DNA analysis is not always possible — success depends upon the nature of the molecular lesion responsible for the thalassaemia.

Details of the development and application of antenatal testing for thalassaemia are outlined below. Important reviews include those of Kan (1977), Kan, Trecartin and Dozy (1980), Alter (1981, 1983, 1984, 1985), Modell and Berdoukas (1984), Orkin (1984), Loukopoulos (1985), Nicolaides, Rodeck and Mibashan (1985) and Weatherall (1985).

Globin-chain synthesis

Most workers have separated the globin chains,

after labelling with [^{3}H]leucine by means of CMC chromatography, but this is not the only way in which good separation of the chains can be achieved (see Dubart *et al.*, 1980; Blouquit *et al.*, 1982; Cossu *et al.*, 1982; Ferrari *et al.*, 1984).

Details of the CMC column technique, and of some other methods including electrophoretic techniques and iso-electric focusing were given by Alter (1983). What is aimed at is a reliable figure for the β:γ globin-chain synthesis ratio. In normal fetuses of 18–20 weeks' maturity the β:γ ratio is approximately 0.11; in β-thalassaemia heterozygotes it is approximately 0.06 and in homozygotes less than 0.025.

The above-mentioned techniques have been widely used and Alter (1984), writing for the *WHO International Registry for Prenatal Monitoring of Hereditory Anemias*, listed 24 centres in 12 countries where the prenatal diagnosis of blood diseases was being carried out. Many papers in which the results of chain-synthesis studies used in the diagnosis of heterozygous or homozygous thalassaemia are described have now been published. A selection of the more important reports are referred to briefly below.

Chang and co-workers (1974) demonstrated the feasibility of the technique in nine patients having a therapeutic abortion and established a range of β:γ globin-chain synthesis ratios. Alter and co-workers (1976) reviewed their experience of 15 cases, 11 tested for thalassaemia, four for sickle-cell disease. In eight, blood was obtained by placental aspiration, in seven by fetoscopy. The predicted diagnosis was correct in 10 of the cases.

Kan and co-workers (1977) reported on 22 fetuses at risk for β-thalassaemia and two for sickle-cell anaemia. The placenta was localized by ultrasound and sufficient fetal blood for analysis was obtained in 22 of the cases by placental aspiration. The β:γ globin-chain ratio indicated homozygous β-thalassaemia in four cases and sickle-cell anaemia in two. Three fetuses were lost.

Fairweather and co-workers (1978) investigated 22 fetuses at risk for homozygous β-thalassaemia. A presumptive diagnosis of homozygosity was made in four instances and the pregnancies were terminated; two fetuses were lost and one result was inconclusive. In the remaining cases normal or heterozygous fetuses were delivered. The mothers had been transfused 7–10 days before the fetal blood was obtained in order to suppress erythropoiesis and reduce the reticulocyte count.

Matsakis and co-workers (1980) reported on 200 cases. The patients were Greek, Cypriot or Italian and fetal blood was obtained at 18–22 weeks: 29% of the pregnancies were terminated for thalassaemia major and 9.5% of the non-homozygous fetuses were lost. In eight cases Hb S or Hb E was diagnosed. 96% of the remaining fetuses were followed up and there appeared to be only three misdiagnoses.

Aleporou-Marinou and co-workers (1980) described their experience in 140 cases, 135 fetuses being at risk of thalassaemia and five of Hb-S/thalassaemia: 14 fetuses were lost, mainly at an early stage in the study. There was, however, apparently only one misdiagnosis: thalassaemia major was missed probably because the placental sample was heavily contaminated with maternal erythrocytes.

Alter and Orkin (1980) reviewed the results they had obtained on 58 fetal blood samples studied in Boston: 50 were derived from fetuses at risk of thalassaemia; 27 samples were obtained by placental aspiration, 23 by fetoscopy; seven out of the 58 fetuses were lost. Homozygosity was established in five fetuses which were aborted and of the fetuses that were delivered at term none was a homozygote.

Cao and co-workers (1980) reported on their experience in Sardinia. Fetal blood was obtained from 130 cases by placental aspiration; 10 fetuses were lost. With 34 of the samples no β-chain radioactivity was demonstrated; homozygosity was diagnosed and abortion carried out. Of 91 infants born, none was a homozygote.

Further data from Sardinia were cited by Cao *et al.* (1985) who described the results of having tested 1000 women at risk. In 976, globin-chain synthesis was carried out on fetal blood; in 24, amniocyte DNA was analysed. There were only two misdiagnoses, and the fetal mortality consequent on placental aspiration was 6.1%. Similar impressive data were reported by Loukopoulos *et al.* (1985) from Athens: 1493 women had been investigated, in the great majority of cases by means of globin-chain analysis on fetal blood samples. There were 16 errors of diagnosis in all, representing 1.1% of the whole series and 57 out of the 1493 fetuses (3.8%) were lost.

DNA analysis

As already mentioned, molecular-genetic techniques of DNA analysis are now being quite widely used in the antenatal diagnosis of thalassaemia. Reviews include those of Orkin, Antonarakis and Kazazian (1983), Alter (1984), Orkin (1984), Kazazian, Boehm and Dowling (1985) and Old *et al.* (1986). Details of technical procedures were given by Old and Higgs (1983). The choice of technique depends upon the type of molecular lesion likely to be present. Three approaches are outlined below.

1. DNA probes can be used directly to identify major deletions of genes or gene rearrangements in the fetal DNA.

Orkin and co-workers (1978) applied endonuclease mapping to DNA derived from a hydrops-fetalis fetus and observed a total absence of α-thalassaemia genes. They also demonstrated deletion of particular β and β-like sequences in DNA derived from patients thought to be homozygous for HPFH of the black variety and δβ-thalassaemia, respectively. They applied their method of analysis, too, to DNA derived from amniotic-fluid fibroblasts obtained from a 19-week-old fetus at risk from β-thalassaemia. The results of hybridization were found to be compatible with β-thalassaemia trait, which was the established diagnosis.

Koenig and co-workers (1978) carried out amniocentesis on a 13-week-old fetus at risk from Hb-H disease. They obtained DNA from fibroblasts after 6 weeks' incubation. Hybridization with cDNA established the diagnosis of Hb-H disease by comparing the results obtained with those with DNA obtained from a hydropic fetus, α-thal-1 carriers and Hb-H disease patients and normal controls.

Chan and co-workers (1984) reported on their experience of diagnosing α-thalassaemia antenatally by direct DNA analysis of uncultured amniotic cells. Eight pregnant Chinese women were studied who gave a history of having had a hydropic infant. Amniocentesis was performed between 16 and 23 weeks. The presence or absence of the α gene was determined by restriction-endonuclease mapping and hybridization with cloned α- and β-globin probes: it was found to be absent in three of the fetuses and present in five. Abortion was carried out in the three cases in which the α gene could not be demonstrated: the blood of the fetuses contained 81.5–86.6% Hb Bart's.

Zeng and Huang (1985) reported on a large-scale survey of haemoglobinopathies carried out by the Chinese Haemoglobinopathy Study Group. Cord blood samples from 11 821 infants had been screened by electrophoresis and α-thalassaemia detected in 2.76%. Zeng and Huang studied 60 cases of Hb-H disease. Using a restriction-enzyme mapping technique, they demonstrated the existence of both rightward and leftward deletions and a non-deletion type as well as Hb Constant Spring. DNA derived from amniotic-fluid cells or from chorionic villi was obtained from seven women at risk of hydrops fetalis and in three of them no α genes could be demonstrated.

Rubin and Kan (1985) described a technical advance in testing for α-globin genes. They used a very sensitive 'slot-blot' technique which is simpler and more feasible for use in South-East Asia than Southern-blot analysis. It has the advantage, too, that the relatively long life isotope ^{35}S can be used instead of ^{32}P as a label for the probes.

As new restriction enzymes become available, the possibility of using specific enzymes to diagnose particular variants of β-thalassaemia increases. One such enzyme is that referred to as *Mae* 1. Thein and co-workers (1985a) described how its use allows the $\beta^0 39$ mutation responsible for the great majority of β-

thalassaemia cases in Sardinia to be detected directly; they emphasized that the enzyme should be very useful in antenatal diagnosis.

2. Restriction-fragment polymorphisms, of which many are present in normal DNA, can be used to determine the chromosome that carries the mutant gene for thalassaemia if the polymorphism is closely adjacent to a globin gene so that they are not likely to be separated by crossing-over in meiotic division. The analysis necessitates investigating the parents of the fetus under study and if possible, too, a sibling of the fetus. The aim is to determine whether a particular restriction-fragment polymorphism can be identified on the chromosome in the (heterozygous) parents that carries the gene for thalassaemia. Then, if the fetus is found to be homozygous for the particular polymorphism, homozygous thalassaemia can be diagnosed with confidence.

Little and co-workers (1980) discussed the possibility of undertaking the antenatal diagnosis of thalassaemia and other monogenic disorders by the molecular analysis of linked DNA polymorphisms. They studied an Asian-Indian family comprising a mother and father and a child who was homozygous for β-thalassaemia. Amniocentesis and fetal sampling carried out in a subsequent pregnancy established clearly by direct gene linkage as well as by the β:γ globin-chain synthesis ratio that the fetus was a heterozygote.

Kazazian and co-workers (1980) investigated 12 families with thalassaemia (two had Hb S as well). They were of Greek (5), Italian (4), Italian-Greek (1), black (1) and West Punjabi (1) origin. DNA was obtained from both parents and one previous offspring in each family and analysed for four polymorphic restriction-endonuclease sites. Their experience suggested to Kazazian *et al.* that it should be possible to diagnose β-thalassaemia prenatally by linkage analysis of polymorphic restriction-endonuclease sites in approximately 75% of pregnancies at risk.

Old and co-workers (1982) described the results of using the above technique in three cases. DNA was extracted from fetal trophoblast obtained from three fetuses 9–11 weeks of age. Two were at risk from homozygous β-thalassaemia and one was at risk from sickle-cell anaemia. One fetus was diagnosed as having homozygous β-thalassaemia via a linked polymorphism, one was diagnosed as being heterozygous for a deletion type β-thalassaemia by restriction-enzyme analysis and one was diagnosed as being heterozygous for Hb S via a linked polymorphism.

Boehm and co-workers (1983) attempted the prenatal diagnosis of β-thalassaemia by analysis of restriction-site polymorphism of amniocyte DNA in 95 pregnancies: in 32 the fetus was at risk for β-thalassaemia, in 57 for Hb-S disease and in six for another haemoglobinopathy. Prenatal diagnosis was correct in all 78 pregnancies in which the delivered fetus was available for study, as well as in a further six cases investigated by fetoscopy and globin-chain analysis. In 70% of the cases sufficient DNA was obtained from uncultured amniocytes (derived from 20 ml of amniotic fluid) and the analysis was completed within 3 weeks: in the remaining 30% it was necessary to culture the amniocytes so as to obtain sufficient DNA for exposure to more than one endonuclease.

The major disadvantage of using restriction-fragment polymorphisms in antenatal diagnosis, leaving aside the large amount of detailed and expert laboratory testing necessary, is that the frequency of useful polymorphisms varies in different racial groups. According to Old and co-workers (1984), who tested for seven polymorphic restriction-endonuclease sites, the method can be used in not more than about 35% of Cypriot and 76% of Asian families with β-thalassaemia. The occurrence of restriction-fragment polymorphisms within and in the region of the δ- and β-globin genes is not random and a variety of haplotypes exist (Antonarakis et al., 1982; Orkin et al., 1982). Recently it has been discovered that a few haplotypes are strongly associated with particular thalassaemia mutations. In such cases it is possible to establish the presumptive diagnosis of thalassaemia without the necessity of establishing linkage between the thalassaemia gene and a restriction-site polymorphism in the family of the fetus to be studied. An example of a mutation-linked polymorphism is the *Bam* H1 polymorphism and the common β⁰-thalassaemia variant found in Sardinia (Kan et al., 1980); another is the *Ava* II polymorphism in the ψβ gene of the β-globin cluster which occurs in Mediterranean populations (Wainscoat et al., 1984).

3. Short synthetic probes of DNA (oligonucleotides or oligomers) can be constructed which will hybridize with homologous sequences but not with sequences that differ with respect to even a single base change. They were first used successfully in the diagnosis of the sickle-cell mutation (see p. 271). Analogous probes specific for several β-thalassaemia mutations have, however,

been made and these provide an additional direct if technically difficult method of diagnosis (Orkin, Markham and Kazazian, 1983).

Pirastu and co-workers (1983) described how they had used two oligonucleotide probes, one homologous to the βᴬ gene and the other to the β-thalassaemia gene at the β³⁹ location. Four Sardinian fetuses were tested, DNA being prepared from amniotic fluid withdrawn at the 18th or 16th week. In one case both probes hybridized with the DNA indicating heterozygosity; in three cases only the βᴬ probe hybridized indicating normality. The results agreed with those obtained by fetal-blood analysis.

Rosatelli and co-workers (1985) reported from Sardinia how they had used two oligonucleotide probes in screening for the β⁰39 (nonsense) mutation. One probe was homologous for normal gene sequences at the codon corresponding to amino acid β39 (the βᴬ probe), the other was complementary to the β⁰39 mutant at the same position (the βᵗʰ probe). In 94 couples both parents were heterozygotes. Analysis using DNA from uncultivated amniocytes was successful in 19 out of 61 pregnancies (31%) and in 34 out of 38 pregnancies using DNA prepared from cultivated cells. Rosatelli et al. concluded that synthetic oligonucleotides can be used successfully in monitoring pregnancies in populations in which one or a small number of β-thalassaemia lesions exists.

Thein and co-workers (1985b) described the use of two pairs of synthetic DNA probes in the diagnosis of β-thalassaemia in families from Milan and from Cypriot families living in London. One pair of probes was directed at position 110 of the 1st intervening sequence, the other at codon 39. One probe from each pair was directed at normal sequences, the other at thalassaemia sequences. Using these probes it proved possible to diagnose thalassaemia in 12 out of 16 North-Italian families and in 13 out of 20 Cypriot families. Analysis of the data suggested that antenatal diagnosis would have been possible, using the probes, in 75% of the Italian families and in 65% of the Cypriot families.

The impressive work outlined above has demonstrated the feasibility and relative safety, and the accuracy, with which the antenatal diagnosis of thalassaemia can be undertaken at the present time. Chorionic villus sampling has the great advantage that it can be undertaken at an earlier stage of pregnancy than fetal blood sampling or amniocentesis and the procedure is relatively safe with respect to both mother and fetus. This method of sampling, coupled with DNA analysis by one means or the other, seems likely to be more and more widely undertaken. In experienced hands the procedure has, too, the potential of being remarkably accurate. Old and co-workers (1986), for instance, reported that 200 chorionic villus samplings, followed by DNA analysis, had led to the correct diagnosis in 196 of the samplings (133 of which had been undertaken for possible thalassaemia).

Antenatal diagnosis of thalassaemia by immuno-fluorescence of fetal erythrocytes

It is possible to separate thalassaemia erythrocytes containing Hb F from maternal erythrocytes not containing Hb F by means of their different reactions when exposed to anti-γ-chain and anti-β-chain antisera, respectively.

Thorpe and Huehns (1983) reported the results of a study of 100 fetuses at risk of thalassaemia from which blood samples had been obtained for the measurement of the β:γ globin-chain synthesis ratio. They used an anti-γ-chain serum prepared in guinea-pigs and labelled it with rhodamine isothiocyanate so as to give a red fluorescence and an anti-β-chain serum prepared in rabbits labelled with fluorescein isothiocyanate so as to give a green fluorescence. The antibodies were then applied to air-dried fixed blood films of fetal blood. It was established that blood, in films of which β-chain fluorescence was not observed, gave β:γ ratios of 0–0.026 — in the homozygous range; while blood, in films of which β-chain fluorescence could be clearly seen, gave ratios of 0.07–0.12 — in the heterozygous range. Thorpe and Huehns concluded that, in screening for thalassaemia, if β chains were detectable immunochemically the fetus would be normal or a heterozygote.

An advantage of the method is that it is possible to obtain a result in 6 hours; disadvantages are difficulty in preparing the specific antisera and the possibility of misdiagnosing as homozygotes heterozygotes with low β-chain synthesis and with cells which in consquence fail to give an appreciable reaction with the anti-β-chain serum. The method is, however, a quick and comparatively simple way of establishing heterozygosity or normality. The presence of maternal cells reacting with the anti-β-chain serum does not necessarily invalidate the technique, as positively-reacting maternal cells should not fluoresce with the anti-γ-chain serum while fetal cells reacting with the anti-β-chain serum will also react with the anti-γ-chain serum. Maggio and Castellano (1984), however, made the point that maternal cells would react with the anti-γ-chain serum if the mother was a carrier, too, of Swiss-type HPFH.

Antenatal diagnosis of β-thalassaemia by detection of Hb A by iso-electric focusing

It is possible so to increase the sensitivity of the detection of small percentages of Hb A in fetal blood as to make it possible to diagnose homozygous β-thalassaemia (or exclude it) by means of the estimation of Hb A without the necessity of carrying out globin-chain synthesis. Manca and co-workers (1986) described a method based on iso-electric focusing in immobilized pH gradients by which as little as 0.5% Hb A can be detected in a mixture of haemoglobins. In practice, 0% Hb A would mean homozygous β⁰-thalassaemia and more than 3% Hb A heterozygous thalassaemia or normality. The method, however, has the disadvantages of requiring uncontaminated fetal blood and a delay in sampling until about the 18th week of pregnancy.

MANAGEMENT OF THALASSAEMIA

Although thalassaemia major is a most serious and potentially lethal disorder, the outlook for patients has been improving steadily, particularly since the early 1960s when it was realized that if affected children were regularly transfused and their haemoglobin maintained at a sufficiently high level, their symptoms would largely disappear, their rate of growth would be restored and they would become virtually indistinguishable from normal, at least until they reached 12–13 years of age when symptoms of iron overload were likely to develop.

Research with the aim of improving the prognosis of thalassaemia has been carried out in many centres throughout the world, and major efforts have been directed at improving transfusion regimes, developing means of controlling iron overload, assessing the value of splenectomy and controlling infections.

As already discussed (pp. 536–540), the development of methods of antenatal diagnosis has, too, been a most important step forward, and a major reduction in the number of homozygotes born can be anticipated where this facility is available. A further important recent development is the possibility of treating established thalassaemia major by bone-marrow transplantation. This is at present still a formidable procedure, but successes have been reported and with the further improvements in transplantation techniques and in their safety and effectiveness, which may reasonably be expected in the near future, transplantation holds out real promise (see p. 563).

The literature on the management of thalassaemia is now extensive and many excellent reviews are available: they include those of Pearson and O'Brien (1975), Modell (1976, 1977), Propper (1980), Weatherall and Clegg (1981), Ley, Griffiths and Nienhuis (1982), Modell and Berdoukas (1984) and Piomelli et al. (1985). The discussions held at the Fifth Cooley's Anemia Symposium held in New York in 1984 and published in the *Annals of the New York Academy of Sciences* [edited by Badman, Levine and Anderson (1985)] provide, too, a valuable record of the participants' experience and views at the time the Symposium was held. An excellent recent brief guide to management is that based on a meeting held in Milan on 27th November 1985 by members of the Mediterranean Committee for Thalassemia with the involvement of the WHO Working Party on Community Control of Hereditary Anemias (Cao et al., 1987).

BLOOD TRANSFUSION, INCLUDING HYPERTRANSFUSION

In an interesting review, Propper (1980) described how clinicians in the 1940s and 1950s were reluctant to transfuse severely anaemic children suffering from Cooley's anaemia, and there is no doubt that fear of iron overload played a part in determining this attitude. According to Propper, 'children who were no longer able to function as a result of their peripheral hemoglobin levels falling as low as 3 to 4 g% were transfused begrudgingly, and then only to 6 to 7 g% hemoglobin'. Not everyone, however, subscribed to this view. Thus the author (Dacie, 1954, p. 123) wrote 'The use of repeated transfusion will in time lead to marked haemosiderosis, but this in the author's opinion should not be used as an argument against

the use of periodic transfusion in cases where, without transfusion, the degree of anaemia leads to serious symptoms.' The question of what haemoglobin level to aim at in transfusing was not, however, settled in the 1950s, and it was not until 1964 that Wolman's impressive data illustrating the value of maintaining a relatively high level of haemoglobin were published.

Wolman's (1964) data comprised the records of 35 children up to the age of 12 years who had been diagnosed as having Cooley's anaemia and who had been repeatedly transfused. The group of 10 children with the highest pre-transfusion haemoglobin level (8.0–9.9 g/dl) seemed to be in better health and physical condition than 13 children in the intermediate haemoglobin group and 12 in the lowest group, despite receiving more blood. The children in the high haemoglobin group were the tallest; they had the smallest livers and spleens, had the least obvious frontal bone thickening and changes in the long bones, had not sustained any fractures, had less dental caries, periodontal disease, maxillary overgrowth or other orthodontic abnormalities and had less cardiac enlargement. Wolman suggested that, although maintaining the haemoglobin at a high level meant the transfusion of more blood, such patients might accumulate less iron in the long run as the result of the higher haemoglobin level preventing undue iron absorption from the intestine.

Wolman's data were based on children suffering from Cooley's anaemia who had been studied at the Children's Hospital in Philadelphia. At the same meeting of the New York Acadamy of Sciences at which his paper was delivered, Schorr and Radel (1964), of New York, described how they had submitted two infants newly diagnosed as having Cooley's anaemia to a similar high transfusion regime so as to maintain their haemoglobin between 10.0 and 14.5 g/dl. Growth and development of these children were reported to be excellent over a 3-year period: their facies was normal and the X-ray appearance of skull and long bones was likewise normal: their spleens were but moderately enlarged and their livers only slightly enlarged.

Since the reports of Wolman and of Schorr and Radel, similar transfusion regimes have been widely adopted; they are still in use, and there is no doubt that the children do excellently for a time. However, by the time they become adolescent signs of iron overload start to appear and iron overloading eventually almost inevitably leads to death, as a rule in the second half of the second decade. As will be outlined later (p. 547), an important advance has been the development and introduction of iron-chelating chemicals. Their use has undoubtedly prolonged life, but, at the time of writing, a really effective agent that can be taken orally is still required. Some of the more recent literature dealing with intensive transfusion therapy is reviewed briefly below.

Beard, Necheles and Allen (1967, 1969) described how six children had benefited from a transfusion regime aimed at keeping their haemoglobin above 9.5 g/dl at all times. They improved strikingly clinically, the best results being seen in the younger children; and their liver and spleen markedly diminished in size. It was noted that the improvements were attained at the cost of an extra 2–4 g of iron transfused per year.

Wolman and Ortolani (1969) gave further details of the series of children first treated by various transfusion regimes at Philadelphia. Since the programme had been started 15 years previously, 17 children had been entered into the high haemoglobin schedule. Six died aged between 9 and 21 years, and five between 13 and 21 years of disorders related to iron overload, namely, heart failure, diabetes and liver dysfunction.

Piomelli and co-workers (1969) reported from New York on four infants 4–12 months of age with severe Cooley's anaemia. After their haemoglobin had been raised to 14 g they were transfused every 4 weeks. Over a 20–45-month period their growth was within the 20–50th percentile and none of them developed bone changes or the typical facies. There were no signs of cardiac failure and their liver and spleen were small. Desferrioxamine was given at the time of admission and in two patients, too, at home 5–6 times a week by intramuscular injection.

Kattamis and co-workers (1970) contrasted the growth of 74 children with homozygous β-thalassaemia, aged between 1 and 11 years, who were being treated by different transfusion regimes. The 38 children whose haemoglobin was maintained at 8 g/dl or above grew normally, in contrast to the 14 children whose haemoglobin had fallen to between 6–8 g/dl before transfusion and the 22 children whose haemoglobin had been allowed to drop below 6 g/dl; their growth was retarded, and this was particularly so in most anaemic children.

O'Brien, Pearson and Spencer (1972) described a 2½-year-old child with thalassaemia major and illustrated by means of [^{99}Tc]sulphur colloid scans the major shrinkage in size of both liver and spleen that followed

maintaining the child's haemoglobin above 10 g/dl.

Necheles and his co-workers (1974) gave details of five β-thalassaemia patients studied in Boston over a 6–8-year period, their ages at the end of the study being 9–20 years. The aim was to maintain their haemoglobin above 10 g/dl. There was a striking improvement in general health and activity, which was particularly marked in the younger patients. Several of the older patients showed some evidence of haemochromatosis or endocrine dysfunction.

Piomelli and co-workers (1974) gave further details of the four very young patients reported in 1969 and of three additional patients. They summarized their experience by stating that the hypertransfusion regime appered to be feasible and well tolerated by the patients and that, if started in early life, it prevents bone malformation and cardiomegaly.

Pearson and O'Brien (1975) reviewed recent published experience and concluded that hypertransfusion had clearly been proved to be clinically superior to older practices; they added, however, that at the time of writing large series of patients managed in this way from early life had not been followed for long enough for firm conclusions as to prognosis to be reached.

Modell (1976, 1977) in two important reviews described, too, her personal experience. In her 1976 paper she illustrated how the publication of Wolman's (1964) recommendations had resulted in a dramatic change in British practice, with the result that from the mid-1960s onwards most patients in the United Kingdom were transfused so as to maintain a haemoglobin level between 9 and 14 g/dl. She stated that children so treated from birth were likely to be indistinguishable from normal until they were 12 years old when they would start to show symptoms of iron overload. She stressed that it was important to look out for signs of hypersplenism which, by causing an increased transfusion requirement, would accelerate the onset of iron overload. Modell's (1977) paper was based on an experience of 196 individuals between 1 year and 23 years of age of whom 116 were fully documented. The majority had homozygous β$^+$-thalassaemia. Indications for transfusion were basically an inability to maintain a haemoglobin level of 7 g/dl; but failure to gain weight, anorexia and sleeplessness were important indicators, too. She stressed that care should be taken to differentiate between patients who clinically have thalassaemia intermedia and those who have thalassaemia major and that to start transfusing a child in the former category would be a serious error. If it was decided that transfusion was necessary, then a high-transfusion maintenance scheme (mean haemoglobin 11.5 g/dl) should be started, accompanied by long-term iron-chelation therapy. She concluded that it was realistic to promise good health for 13 years and to give a minimum prognosis of 20 years. She stressed again the importance of recognizing hypersplenism, and of carrying out splenectomy in selected cases (see p. 556), and of the risks of intercurrent illness resulting in acute iron toxicity in patients who are heavily overloaded with iron.

Weiner and his co-workers (1978) at the New York University Medical Center reviewed the clinical progress of the eight children under their care who had been supported on a high-transfusion regime for the longest period of time (3–12 years). They had all managed to live normal, active lives without evidence of hypersplenism or cardiac dysfunction. Echocardiography revealed, however, increased thickness of the left ventricular wall. All the children had received deferoxamine intramuscularly.

Transfusion with blood enriched with young erythrocytes

Propper (1980), in his review of the overall management of thalassaemia, considered, too, the value of using blood for transfusion that had been enriched in its reticulocyte content. In theory, if blood consisting entirely of 1-day-old cells of lifespan almost uniformly 120 days was removed from the recipient by exchange-transfusion 119 days after being transfused (just before the abrupt demise of all the transfused cells) and replaced by a further cohort of 1-day-old cells, the patient could benefit by regular transfusion without any iron accumulating. In practice, such an ideal arrangement would be impossible to organize. Propper stated, however, that, using an Aminco 'celltrifuge', he and his colleagues had been able to prepare from normal donors units of blood of mean age as low as 12 days which they referred to as 'neocytes' (Propper, Button and Nathan, 1980). Using the same machine, it would be possible to remove a proportion of the recipient's older heavier cells ('gerocytes') before replacing them with neocytes. In this way, with an exchange carried out every 7 weeks, it was calculated that the patient would gain not more than an average of 3.5 mg of iron per day, a quantity which was thought could be easily dealt with by an iron chelator given orally.

Further details of the use of young cells in the treatment of patients with thalassaemia major were given by Propper, Button and Nathan (1980). The cells had a ^{51}Cr T_{50} of 43.8 days and the interval between transfusions (necessary to maintain haematocrits above 35%) in the two patients treated with the 'neocytes' lengthened from 30 $\pm$ 4.5 days to 43 $\pm$ 4.5 days. Propper, Button and

Nathan also provided interesting data on whole blood volumes in 20 splenectomized patients with thalassaemia major and on the effect on the blood volume of 'supertransfusion' aimed at maintaining the patients' haematocrits always higher than 35%. On a normal transfusion regime the haematocrits varied from 22 to 44% and the mean total blood volume in ml/kg was 33.8 $\pm$ 3.3% greater than that predicted, due to a major increase in plasma volume: on the supertransfusion regime the total blood volume of 12 patients diminished by a mean of 21 $\pm$ 2%. Plasma iron turnover was also measured: on the supertransfusion regime this became normal or even subnormal, indicative of a substantial reduction in erythropoiesis. Propper, Button and Nathan were also able to show in six patients followed for 6 months on a normal transfusion regime, followed by 12 months on the supertransfusion regime, that they were able, after a period of 1–4 months, to maintain their raised haematocrits without needing larger or more frequent transfusions. This was thought to be due to the fall in plasma volume and total blood volume associated with the supertransfusion regime.

Propper, Button and Nathan concluded that the supertransfusion regime, and the use of neocytes, too, would markedly alter the prognosis of patients with thalassaemia major. Decreasing the rate of iron accumulation in this way, yet achieving a high haemoglobin level, would allow iron balance to be achieved on less aggressive and expensive chelation regimes.

Gabutti and co-workers (1980) reported on the relationship between the blood volume, mean haemoglobin level maintained and the requirement for blood of 166 patients with homozygous β-thalassaemia. They, too, found that patients maintained at haemoglobin levels varying between 10 and 14 g/dl required approximately the same amount of blood, and they attributed this, as had Propper, Button and Nathan (1980), to the total blood volume being less at the higher haemoglobin levels, thus allowing a higher haemoglobin to be reached for the same amount of blood transfused.

Masera and co-workers (1982) discussed the practicability of using blood enriched with young erythrocytes for the transfusions of children with β-thalassaemia major and concluded that technical and organizational problems would render it unlikely that the method could be widely used.

They advocated a supertransfusion regime, aimed in their clinic at achieving a mean pre-transfusion level as high as 12.3 g/dl, and found that, after an initial 5 months, no more blood was required for its maintenance than had been required by their standard regime which aimed at a pre-transfusion haemoglobin level of 10.2 g/dl.

More recent accounts of the use of blood enriched with young erythrocytes include those of Wolfe, Sallan and Nathan (1985), who gave a detailed account of the management by transfusion and splenectomy of a patient over a 23-year period, and Cohen, Mizanin and Schwartz (1985), who compared the annual blood requirement of six splenectomized thalassaemia patients treated by a conventional frozen-thawed erythrocyte regime with their requirement when they received instead a concentrate of young erythrocytes prepared from fresh whole blood. The demand for blood was diminished by 8–24% on the latter regime. A drawback was the need to use 2 units of fresh blood to prepare 1 unit of young-cell concentrate.

Marcus and co-workers (1985) reported that in their hands the benefit from administering blood enriched in young erythrocytes was slight. In a controlled trial they gave blood enriched in reticulocytes (by an average of 2.4 times) to 23 transfusion-dependent thalassaemia-major patients; they found, however, that this resulted in only a minor decrease in blood consumption, and they concluded that the regime was hardly worthwhile. Other centres have concentrated on devising simple methods of enriching blood with neocytes [e.g., Hogan, Blanchette and Rock (1986)]. Frozen erythrocytes, too, have their advocates. Avanzi and co-workers (1983) reported in a series of thalassaemia-major patients a marked reduction in non-haemolytic reactions following the transfusion of frozen cells (only two reactions in 1934 transfusions) as well as a significant reduction in leucocyte and platelet immunization, compared with patients who had received leucocyte-poor blood prepared in other ways.

Reduction in size of the spleen following blood transfusion

As already mentioned, one of the favourable consequences of regularly transfusing a child with thalas-

saemia major is reduction in the size of the spleen. In order to determine the cause of this, Karpathios and co-workers (1982) studied 18 thalassaemic children aged between 3.5 and 13 years who were being regularly transfused. Fourteen of them were examined daily. In nine of them the spleen started to decrease in size 1–3 days after a transfusion and continued to do so up to the 10th post-transfusion day; it then increased in size again to a maximum just before the next transfusion. In one child the spleen enlarged following the transfusion and then decreased in size over the next 4 days; in four children the spleen did not appear to change in size. Decrease in spleen size was accompanied by increase in haematocrit and platelet count, and vice versa. The uptake by the spleen and liver of [$^{99\,m}$Tc]sulphur colloid was measured in 10 children before and 7–10 days after transfusion. The surface area of the spleen was significantly smaller and the uptake of colloid significantly greater after transfusion than before transfusion. Karpathios and his co-workers concluded that the spleen shrinks after transfusion as the result of diminished trapping of erythrocytes (and platelets) and that the improved colloid uptake reflects a better intrasplenic circulation.

Survival of transfused normal erythrocytes

Many laboratory studies have been carried out on the effectiveness and consequences of blood transfusion in thalassaemia. Early work was centred on the survival of the transfused erythrocytes. As expected, this was shown to be normal in uncomplicated cases (Hamilton, Sheets and DeGowin, 1950; Frontali and Stegagno, 1951). Considerable shortening was, however, reported by Lichtman *et al.* (1953) in children with thalassaemia major who had been repeatedly transfused: the half-life of the transfused normal erythrocytes, determined by the Ashby method, was between 5 and 9 days in six children and 35 days in a seventh child. An extracorpuscular defect was postulated but no abnormal antibodies could be demonstrated.

Impaired survival of transfused normal blood is unfortunately not rare: it has been usually attributed to 'hypersplenism', and is an important indication for splenectomy (see p. 559).

Inhibition of erythropoiesis

An important consequence of blood transfusion is partial inhibition of erythropoiesis as the result of the anoxic stimulus being reduced. Smith and co-workers (1955b), who studied five patients with

Cooley's anaemia and one with microdrepanocytic disease, used Hb F as a marker of erythropoiesis. They found that the total circulating Hb F was reduced to about one-half of its former value following transfusions; the patient's erythrocyte volume was, too, shown to diminish and to reach a minimum value 1–2 weeks after a transfusion. This was followed by a gradual rise as the transfused blood was eliminated.

Rewald (1964), of Argentina, had described how a boy aged $2\frac{1}{2}$ years with severe Mediterranean anaemia was maintained almost without reticulocytes as the result of being transfused at regular 2-week intervals. His spleen diminished in size and by 3 months from the start of treatment his previously enlarged frontal and parietal skull bosses had regressed. His return for a further transfusion was delayed, and 16 days after his last transfusion he experienced severe pains in his bones, particularly in those of the skull and pelvis. Two days later his haemoglobin was found to be 11.6 g/dl and the reticulocyte count was still low (0.3%). However, the bone marrow was intensely hypercellular, with erythropoiesis predominating. He was transfused; the haemoglobin rose to 15 g/dl and 2 days later his bone pains — caused presumably by the intense erythroblastic hyperplasia — disappeared.

More recently, Cavill and co-workers (1978) described the results of a ferrokinetic study of 14 patients with homozygous β-thalassaemia, including two with thalassaemia intermedia who had not been transfused. As expected, erythrocyte production was inversely correlated with the haemoglobin concentration, but the suppressive effect of regular transfusions was found to be greater than expected and erythropoietic activity was less than normal at normal haemoglobin concentrations. It was concluded that maintaining a haemoglobin at a level greater than 12 g/dl is sufficient to reduce erythropoiesis to a subnormal level.

Development of allo-antibodies

One important consequence of transfusing any patient repeatedly is an increasing likelihood as time passes for the recipient to develop allo-antibodies directed against erythrocytes, leucocytes, platelets or plasma proteins. Fortunately, children with thalassaemia do not seem to be particularly prone to develop anti-erythrocyte antibodies. Thus, according to Schorr and Radel, writing in 1964, only 5% of 150 children with Cooley's anaemia who were receiving transfusions had developed atypical erythrocyte antibodies at the time they were studied. Moreover, almost half of

these antibodies were of anti-D specificity and had resulted from errors in Rh-typing Rh-negative children.

Antibodies other than those directed against erythrocyte antigens appear, however, to be developed more frequently. Blumberg and co-workers (1964) tested for precipitins against serum lipoprotein antigens and found them to be more frequent in thalassaemia patients (29% of 47 patients) than in non-thalassaemia patients (3.9% of 102 patients) who had received comparable numbers of transfusions. The results of a more comprehensive investigation were reported by Economidou et al. (1971). The sera investigated were derived from 147 patients who had each received from 10 to 287 transfusions over a 2–18-year period. Antibodies reactive with leucocyte and platelet antigens and with protein and lipoprotein (GM, Inv and Ag) antigens were commonly identified, 29–71% of the sera reacting positively. Anti-erythrocyte antibodies were, however, detected in only four of the sera (2.7%), and it was suggested that the rarity of the antibodies was a reflection of immune tolerance perhaps induced by repeated blood transfusions often started during the first year of life.

It seems likely that antibodies (of all types) can lead to transfusion reactions. According to Economidou et al. (1971), who reported that reactions are more likely to occur in patients who have multiple antibodies in their sera, the use of washed erythrocytes abolishes or reduces significantly the incidence and severity of the reactions. [Frozen cells are also associated with few reactions (see p. 545).]

Metabolism of transfused erythocytes

Erythrocyte 2,3-DPG concentration is generally increased in anaemic patients and the O_2-dissociation curve is shifted to the right, resulting in improved delivery of oxygen to the tissues (see Vol. 1, p. 18). However, in patients with thalassaemia (and it seems also in patients with other types of anaemia who are chronically transfused) the 2,3-DPG concentration and the p_{50} O_2 are inappropriately low in relation to the erythrocyte mass (de Furia, Miller and Canale, 1974; Correra, et al., 1984). The cause of this apparent failure of function of transfused blood seems to be obscure; it is, however, an important matter, as the relatively high O_2 affinity may result in tissue hypoxia, tissue damage and ultimately fibrosis as well as requiring an increase in cardiac output.

Transmission of viral infections

Patients receiving repeated blood transfusions are at risk of the transmission of virus infections, irrespective of the nature of their illness. Some data on the prevalence of the Australia antigen and antibody (of hepatitis-B virus) are available. Economidou and her co-workers (1970) detected hepatitis-associated antigen in five out of 181 patients (2.7%) and the antibody in 71 patients (39.2%). The frequency at which the antibody could be detected increased with the number of transfusions received, rising from 21.7% in those who had received 10–25 transfusions to 50% in those receiving 101 to more than 200 transfusions. Antibody was demonstrated in 45% of 60 patients who had been splenectomized.

Kattamis and co-workers (1974) reported similar findings based on study of 196 children of 10 months to 14 years of age. Australia antigen was detected in 7% and antibody in 32%. The prevalence of the antibody was directly related to the age of the patients and the number of units of blood received.

The increasing prevalence throughout the world of the human immune viruses (HIV) raises the spectre of the possibility of transmitting AIDS to transfusion-dependent thalassaemic children. Hopefully, the vigilant application of sensitive screening tests will reduce this risk to a remote possibility. Unfortunately, some thalassaemic children who were receiving transfusions before the introduction of the routine screening of blood donors have become infected. Mozzi and co-workers (1987) have, for instance, reported that four out of 40 such children were found to give positive ELISA and Western blot tests for anti-HIV antibodies.

Role of splenectomy. It is uncertain whether the removal of the spleen increases the risk of the transmission of a virus infection by blood transfusion. It is possible that it does, and it is possible, too, that the severity of any infection is increased (see vol. 1, p. 119). There seems to be little doubt, however, that splenectomy does increase the risk of contracting malaria from blood transfusion as well as increasing the severity of the infection (see Vol. 1, p. 119). Several case reports of its occurrence in splenectomized thalassaemia-major patients are available (Edrissian, 1974; Joishy and Lopez, 1980).

USE OF CHELATING AGENTS IN CONTROLLING IRON OVERLOAD

An inevitable, important and potentially lethal complication of administering repeated blood transfusions to a child with β-thalassaemia major is a gradual overloading of the body with iron. Unchecked, transfusional siderosis produces a syndrome closely similar to that of idiopathic haemochromatosis, and this leads remorselessly to death usually towards the end of the second decade, the immediate cause being as a rule cardiac failure. Fortunately, there are ways in which iron can be removed from the body, and since the early 1960s practical regimes employing iron-chelating drugs have been employed for this purpose. The chemical that has been most widely and successfully used has been desferrioxamine (DF), also referred to as deferoxamine. Unfortunately, the drug is relatively ineffective when given by mouth.

Many careful studies have been carried out in which the amount of iron excreted has been correlated with DF dosage and route of administration and related, too, to the accumulation of iron derived from the transfused blood. DF was at first added to transfused blood or administered by daily intramuscular injection or by intravenous infusion; later it has been given even more successfully by continuous subcutaneous infusion via a portable pump. If given in sufficient dosage and with persistence, DF has been shown to be capable of preventing serious iron overload and even of reversing to some extent existing overload. The financial cost, unfortunately, is high — DF is expensive — and the regime is exacting. Nevertheless, most patients have tolerated it well, and there is no doubt that a high-haemoglobin transfusion regime coupled with the regular subcutaneous administration of DF have together greatly improved the outlook for sufferers from thalassaemia major.

The literature on the use of chelating agents in the treatment of iron overload, in disorders such as thalassaemia major where venesection is inappropriate, is now considerable. Selected papers are referred to below. Reviews include those of Waxman and Brown (1969), Pearson and O'Brien (1975), Modell (1976, 1977, 1979), Weatherall,

Pippard and Callender (1977, 1983), Jacobs (1979), Propper (1980), Ley, Griffiths and Nienhuis (1982), Pippard and Callender (1983) and Modell and Berdoukas (1984).

Early attempts at treating iron overload

Waxman and Brown (1969) listed in their important review the chelating agents that had been used in early attempts to bring about the excretion of iron. Included under the heading 'Iron chelating agents of historical interest' were dimercaprol (BAL) (Ohlsson, Kullendorff and Ljungberg, 1953), edetate (Versene, Versenol) (Seven et al., 1954) and several other synthetic chelating agents with relatively high affinities for iron. None, however, appeared to be particularly effective and they appear not to have been widely used. Two compounds had, however, been shown to be of major value, diethylenetriaminepentaacetic acid (DTPA) and desferrioxamine (DF).

Trisodium calcium diethylenetriaminepentaacetate (DTPA)

DTPA was introduced as an agent for the treatment of iron overload by Fahey and co-workers (1961). The compound, which binds iron with a greater affinity than does EDTA, forms a colourless iron chelate; it binds, too, several other metals. In man, DTPA has usually been administered by intravenous injection. Intramuscular injection leads to severe pain at the site even if procaine is injected at the same time. The drug is poorly absorbed if given by mouth and has led to vomiting and diarrhoea. Its intravenous use is, too, unfortunately accompanied by undesirable side-effects, and for this reason, although an effective drug, it has been superseded by desferrioxamine, which is at least as effective as an iron chelator as is DTPA and is far less toxic.

Fahey and his co-workers' (1961) account of their use of DTPA was based on their experience with four patients suffering from idiopathic haemochromatosis and an adult female who had thalassaemia major and who had undergone splenectomy; she had received more than 100 blood transfusions and presented with the clinical picture of haemochromatosis. DTPA (2.5–3.0 g), given intravenously on four occasions, led to the ex-

cretion of 30.4, 47.3, 55.5 and 66.8 mg of iron. Fahey et al. suggested that DTPA could be used as a means of dealing with iron storage disease in patients who were not suitable for phlebotomy.

Recently, Pippard and co-workers (1986) reported that they had administered DTPA experimentally to two iron-loaded thalassaemia patients by continuous subcutaneous infusion. In one patient a daily infusion of the calcium salt of DTPA was well tolerated and was found to be as effective as desferrioxamine (DF) in causing iron excretion. Unfortunately, the drug also caused depletion of zinc which could not be controlled by zinc therapy. Zinc DTPA proved to be an ineffective iron chelator. DF and calcium DTPA were shown to have additive effects, perhaps by removing iron from different sites, and Pippard et al. suggested that calcium DTPA (which is a relatively cheap chemical) might prove to be useful as a supplement for the much more expensive desferrioxamine.

Desferrioxamine (deferoxamine), Desferal

A group of iron-containing metabolites, with growth-promoting properties for a number of micro-organisms, which were referred to as 'ferrioxamines', were isolated from the actinomyces Streptomyces pilosus by Bickel and co-workers (1960). The iron-free compound desferrioxamine, a trihydroxyamic acid derivative, has a high affinity for iron. According to Waxman and Brown (1969), 100 mg of deferoxamine hydrochloride can in theory bind 9.3 mg of iron and 100 mg of deferoxamine methane sulfonate (Desferal) 8.5 mg of iron.

Desferrioxamine (DF) removes useful quantities of iron from iron-overloaded subjects without depleting the body seriously of trace metals of biological importance. The drug removes iron apparently from parenchymal cells, e.g., hepatocytes, and from phagocytic cells; it does not seem to remove iron from transferrin or from haemoglobin. Iron bound to DF, ferrioxamine, is red in colour; it is excreted mainly by the kidney but a significant and usually unappreciated amount is excreted in the faeces, via the bile and probably via other intestinal secretions, too. DF is poorly absorbed when given by mouth; it binds inorganic iron, although not haemoglobin or muscle iron, when given in this way. As will be discussed below, DF is effective in man when given by intramuscular (bolus) injection or intravenously or by slow subcutaneous infusion. It causes few reactions, although cataracts have been recorded in dogs, cats and rats given high doses of DF over long periods (Brückner *et al.*, 1967) and also in three human patients (Waxman and Brown, 1969). Waxman and Brown, too, listed as possibly attributable to therapy with DF, dysuria, tachycardia, abdominal pain, a lowering of the blood sugar, diarrhoea, fever and thrombocytopenia. The general experience has been, however, that its use has been accompanied by remarkably few side-effects.

The first clinical reports on the use of DF and DTPA in thalassaemia date from 1962. At a round table conference, summarized in the *Schweizerische medizinische Wochenschrift* of 20th October 1962, Wöhler illustrated in a chart the response of a patient with thalassaemia who had been given DF at a dose of 1200 mg daily, first by intravenous infusion and later by intramuscular injection: 20–40 mg of iron per 24 hours were excreted in the urine.

A relatively large series of patients studied in London were reported on by Sephton Smith (1962). He had used DTPA or DF in 17 children with thalassaemia major and in one child with a pure red-cell aplasia. The drugs were given in 100–2000-mg doses (5–104-mg/kg body weight) intramuscularly or intravenously. The results with both drugs were considered together, as sufficient data had not been compiled to allow the drugs to be compared. Children with more than 80% saturation of the plasma iron-binding capacity excreted (with one exception) 11–40 mg Fe per g DTPA or DF, while those with less than 60% saturation of the plasma iron-binding capacity excreted usually less than 8 mg/g; those with 60–80% saturation of plasma iron-binding capacity excreted intermediate amounts of iron. Thus, as was perhaps to be expected, children with the highest iron overload — who had received the largest number of transfusions — excreted most iron. Sephton Smith concluded that the chelators that he had used only cause the mobilization and excretion of stored iron when it is present in great excess and do not influence the normal iron metabolic pathways and, in particular, do not remove iron from plasma transferrin or from erythrocytes or their precursors.

Heilmeyer and Wöhler (1963) and Wöhler (1963), in papers primarily concerned with the treatment of haemochromatosis with DF, referred to the good results they had obtained in two thalassaemic patients. Up to the time of writing 14 g of iron had been removed from one of them and liver biopsy after therapy revealed a 'striking decrease' in haemosiderin. This was the same patient as had been described briefly by Wöhler (1962).

Muller-Eberhard and her co-workers (1963) described how they had used DTPA in the treatment of seven patients, aged between 3 and 25 years, with thalassaemia major, who were considered to have secondary haemochromatosis. All had had their spleens removed. The drug was given intramuscularly in doses of 20–25 mg/kg. Up to 40 mg of iron were excreted in the urine in 24 hours (a $\times$ 16 increase) and the excretion of copper and magnesium was increased, too. The plasma Mg^{2+} concentration was found to be low in all the patients and the levels fell transiently following the administration of the DTPA. This, it was suggested, might be a hazard. Muller-Eberhard *et al.* concluded that DTPA was effective in removing iron; they reported, however, that the injections were painful, even when procaine was administered at the same time.

Sephton Smith (1964) gave further details of his personal experience in using DF and DTPA in 21 children aged 3 months to 15 years. He recommended as a practical regime that large doses (up to 6 g) of DTPA should be given intravenously at the time of transfusions and intramuscular injections of DF should be given daily between transfusions. He reported, too, that three patients had been given DF by daily subcutaneous injection of 0.5 g of DF methansulfonate. This resulted in the excretion of 5–15 mg of iron per day in the urine over a 3-month period.

Additional reports describing the successful use of intramuscular DF in transfusion-dependent patients with thalassaemia include those of Kirimlidis *et al.* (1966), McDonald (1966), Diwany *et al.* (1968), Waxman and Brown (1969), Constantoulakis *et al.* (1974) (who used DTPA as well), Modell and Beck (1974), Seshadri, Colebatch and Fisher (1974) and Seshadri *et al.* (1974).

Diwany and co-workers (1968) reported that the daily injection of 1 g of DF appeared to be followed by a rise in reticulocyte count in five out of the six children studied. Their haemoglobin levels were very low, 3.5–7.0 g/dl. An improvement in haemoglobin synthesis was postulated.

Seshadri, Colebatch and Fisher (1974) treated 26 children with thalassaemia major. The DF-induced urinary excretion of iron was positively correlated with the volume of blood that had been transfused, and with the plasma iron level and the size of the spleen. Splenectomized patients excreted less iron than did those with their spleen *in situ*. Seshadri and co-workers (1974) described long-term benefit in three patients who had been treated for 5–8 years and in a further seven patients treated for 10–22 months. Their symptoms improved and there was objective evidence of improvement in liver and cardiac function, as shown by a fall in SGOT and return of the ECG towards normal.

Letsky (1976) reviewed the long-term results of a trial of Desferal and DTPA given to 10 homozygous β-thalassaemia children who had been regularly transfused at the Hospital for Sick Children, Great Ormond Street, in London over a 10-year period. The progress of these children was compared with that of 10 similar children, closely matched for age, sex and transfusion requirement and splenectomy status, who had not been given the chelator drugs. The Desferal (0.5 g) was given by intramuscular injection on 6 days each week; the DTPA (2 g) was given with each unit of blood. The study showed that the chelation therapy had reduced the accumulation of iron in the liver and the rise in serum-ferritin levels and had retarded the progress of hepatic fibrosis. But the incidence and severity of endocrine and cardiac complications appeared to be much the same in both groups of patients; some of the patients were, however, heavily loaded with iron before the chelation therapy was started.

Continuous subcutaneous infusion of desferrioxamine

An important practical advance in the use of DF in the treatment of iron overload in transfusion-dependent patients with thalassaemia has been its administration by continuous subcutaneous infusion, using a portable pump designed to give a slow but continuous flow. With experience the technique has been refined and at the time of writing DF is widely administered by a light-weight syringe driver [e.g. that designed by Wright and Callan (1979)], usually during the night-time while the child is (hopefully) asleep. The amount of iron that can be removed in this way is not far short of that achieved by bolus intramuscular injection and if persisted in and combined with DF given intravenously at the same time as a blood transfusion it is possible for the child to remain in iron balance. If the rate of delivery of the DF is properly adjusted, the procedure is virtually painless. An important disadvantage of the technique is, however, the expense of the pump.

Reports on the value of administering DF by slow continuous subcutaneous infusion emanated from Boston in 1976 (Propper, Shurin and Nathan, 1976a,b; Propper et al., 1976).

The first two patients treated in this way excreted 21–60 mg of iron when given a daily dose of 0.75 g of DF, a 2–4-fold increase over the excretion achieved when the drug was given by bolus intramuscular injection (Propper, Shurin and Nathan, 1976a).

Propper and co-workers (1976) reported on a comparison between DF administered intravenously or subcutaneously. DF given slowly subcutaneously resulted in an iron excretion of 81% of that achieved

when similar doses were given intravenously. Eight patients had been on the subcutaneous regime for 3–10 months without any untoward side-effects. In three there was some evidence of cardiac improvement; one had improved dramatically clinically.

Hussain and co-workers (1976) compared the responses of 11 patients with thalassaemia major to bolus intramuscular injections of 0.75 g of DF or continuous subcutaneous infusion of the same dose given over a 24-hour period. The subcutaneous regime was shown to be clearly superior, 62–136% more iron being excreted than when the same dose was given intramuscularly. Hussain and co-workers (1977) compared in 13 patients the iron excretion achieved by 12 and 24 hours of continuous subcutaneous infusion of the same dose of DF: when 750 mg was given there was little difference; with 1500 mg, the 24 hours' infusion produced a significant increase. Higher doses, e.g. 2000 mg, produced even greater excretion. Hussain et al. concluded that in most patients with transfusional-iron overload a 12-hour subcutaneous infusion of 2–4 g of DF daily, combined with ascorbic acid saturation (see p. 552), would be the most satisfactory way to remove excess iron.

Propper and co-workers (1977) reported further details of their own experience. They had compared the results of subcutaneous infusion of DF with those obtained when the same dose of the drug was administered intravenously in 24 iron-overloaded patients (17 of whom had thalassaemia) whose iron output was known when DF was administered intramuscularly. The mean excretion of iron per month was more than 3 times greater when the drug was given intravenously than when it was given intramuscularly. Constant subcutaneous infusion was approximately 90% as effective as intravenous administration on a dose-for-dose basis. The cumulative output of iron in the urine exceeded the input of transfused iron in all the patients on the subcutaneous infusion regime and Propper et al. concluded that the method was both practical and effective.

The early descriptions of the value of administering DF by the subcutaneous route cited above have been followed by reports from other centres specializing in the treatment of transfusion-dependent children with thalassaemia major (Cohen and Schwartz, 1978, 1980; Graziano et al., 1978; Pippard, Callender and Weatherall, 1978; Pippard et. al., 1978; Weiner et al., 1978; Hoffbrand et al., 1979; Silvestroni et al., 1982; Pippard and Callender, 1983; Cohen, Mizanin and Schwartz, 1985; Giardina et al., 1985; Hyman et al., 1985). All who have administered DF subcutaneously have been impressed with its effectiveness.

Graziano and co-workers (1978) found that subcutaneous infusion was almost (79%) effective as the intravenous route. Most of their patients had the pump working for 8 hours whilst they were asleep: 20–40 mg/kg of DF was found generally to be the maximum that could be tolerated without local irritation at the needle site. The subcutaneous route was, however, 'overwhelmingly' preferred by the patients.

Pippard and co-workers (1978) compared 12-hour subcutaneous infusion with intramuscular bolus injection in 16 patients with homozygous β-thalassaemia aged 10 months to 23 years. At all ages subcutaneous infusion resulted in greater iron loss than did intramuscular injection and eight of nine children who were under 6 years of age, with a total iron load calculated to be less than 10 g, achieved iron balance when given 0.50–1.0 g of DF daily. Pippard et al. recommended that chelation therapy should be started in early life.

Silvestroni and co-workers (1978) also reported favourably. Twenty transfusion-dependent children with homozygous β-thalassaemia were studied of whom seven (mainly older) children had been splenectomized. Their haemoglobin was maintained above 9 g/dl and DF was administered 3–4 times a week subcutaneously in 0.5–1.0 g (in a few patients 2.0 g) doses. Their iron balance was monitored over a 2–9-month period. This remained positive in five of the (mainly young) children who had not undergone splenectomy but became negative in the remainder; and Silvestroni et al. concluded that splenectomy plus DF given subcutaneously, if suitably combined, should be able to prevent iron loading.

Hoffbrand and his co-workers (1979) described the effect of the long-term administration of DF by the subcutaneous route in 31 patients with transfusion-dependent β-thalassaemia major. The serum-ferritin concentration fell in all the patients after 5–12 months of treatment; in some the level became almost normal. Liver function improved, too; and serum aspartate transaminase levels fell in all 17 patients tested.

Silvestroni and co-workers (1982) administered DF by subcutaneous infusion for 10 hours, four to five nights a week, at a dose of 1 g to children who were under 6 years of age and 1.5–2.0 g to older patients. In nine patients with their spleen in situ, the mean 24-hour urine iron excretion was 15.4 ± 1.7 mg, 10.2 mg in urine, 5.2 mg in faeces; in five splenectomized patients the mean excretion was 25.9 ± 4.3 mg, 18.9 mg in urine, 7.0 mg in faeces. Negative iron balance with respect to transfused iron was achieved in seven out of 18 patients with their spleen in situ (all but one 6 years or more in age) and in 14 out of 16 splenectomized patients (all over 9 years of age).

Cohen and Schwartz (1980) described the results of an intensive study of two 1-year-old boys with homozygous β-thalassaemia who had received intensive DF therapy by the intravenous, intramuscular and continuous subcutaneous routes. Serum-ferritin levels and SGOT and SGPT were substantially reduced and it was calculated that the children's iron load had been reduced from 35 g and 34 g, respectively (calculated from the amount of blood transfused), to 19.5 g in each case. Cohen, Martin and Schwartz (1981) referred to four children with thalassaemia major who had received intensive DF therapy for 36–53 months. The amount of iron excreted in the urine fell progressively with time, by more than 80% in three children and by 45% in the fourth. Serum ferritin fell to normal or near normal values. It was suggested that the decreasing excretion of iron was the result of the reduction in the originally very high iron stores.

Modell and her co-workers (1982) considered the effect that DF therapy had had on survival. They obtained the records up to the end of 1980 of 92 children, all with homozygous β-thalassaemia, who had been born in the United Kingdom in or before 1963. Fewer of those who had received at least 4 g of DF weekly during the previous few years had died, compared to those who had received smaller doses of DF or none at all. Of 19 children treated at the Hospital for Sick Children, Great Ormond Street, in London, six of the 10 who had not received DF therapy had died, compared with one only of the nine children who had been treated.

Pippard, Callender and Finch (1982) reported studies on 25 iron-overloaded patients of whom seven had thalassaemia major and three thalassaemia intermedia. The patients were all receiving 1–2 g of DF in a 12-hour infusion daily and usually, too, a daily dose of 200 mg of ascorbic acid. The main aim of the investigation was to determine how the state of erythropoiesis affected iron excretion. Pippard, Callender and Finch's data indicated that the urinary iron content varied directly with the level of erythropoiesis while faecal iron varied inversely; also that ascorbic acid greatly enhanced urinary iron excretion but had a less constant effect on faecal iron. The data, too, underlined the importance of not omitting from one's calculation biliary iron in monitoring the effect of DF and also that large doses of the chelator removed established iron overload more rapidly than had been previously realized.

Capra and co-workers (1983) described how chelation therapy was preventing the onset of diabetes in transfusion-dependent thalassaemia-major patients. They had instituted chelation therapy in their clinic in Ferrara in 1973. Eighteen of 197 patients receiving regular transfusions had developed diabetes: four had received chelation irregularly; 14 had not accepted the recommended therapy. Only one patient with an impaired glucose tolerance test had been complying regularly with the chelation regime.

Pippard and Callender (1983) recommended that long-term chelation should be carried out in the following way. Treatment with DF should be started when the children are between 2 and 4 years old. In those less than 6 years of age 1 g of

DF should be given daily by slow subcutaneous infusion, at a concentration not greater than 0.5 g in 2 ml. Those over 6 years of age should receive 2 g in 12 hours and heavily iron-overloaded children up to 4 g. Vitamin C should be given, too, but not in doses exceeding 100–200 mg daily (see below).

Cohen, Mizanin and Schwartz (1985) reviewed the responses of 25 transfusion-dependent thalassaemia-major patients to DF administered subcutaneously over a 1–8-year period. They stressed the critical importance of keeping to the treatment programme, which if complied with made it possible, they stated, to reduce to normal or near-normal levels the iron stores of children who had accumulated as much as 50 g of excess iron. Their data illustrate the value of serum-ferritin measurements in assessing progress. Six of Cohen, Mizanin and Schwartz's patients also received 9–16 g of DF given intravenously over a 24-hour period following their 3-weekly blood transfusion.

As has been mentioned, DF is relatively impotent when taken by mouth. It is, however, not completely ineffective. Callender and Weatherall (1980) reported on the excretion of iron following taking 1 g or 3 g of DF in solution 3 times a day by mouth with that brought about by comparable doses given by a 12-hour subcutaneous infusion. All 14 patients tested showed some response to oral DF. This varied from widely from less than 1 mg to 18.5 mg. In each case, however, the excretion following taking the drug by mouth was only a fraction of that brought about by the subcutaneous infusion. Callender and Weatherall suggested, however, that giving DF by mouth might be a useful and acceptable adjunct to treatment when the patient's compliance to the infusion regime was poor.

Ascorbic acid enhancement of desferrioxamine-induced excretion of iron

It is generally agreed that if ascorbic acid (vitamin C) is given to children receiving DF therapy the amount of iron excreted in the urine is substantially increased. There is, however, evidence that large doses of ascorbic acid are potentially toxic and may lead, for instance, to failure of the iron-laden heart (Henry, 1979; Nienhuis et al., 1980).

Pippard and Callender (1983), while advocating the administration of ascorbic acid, recommended that the daily dose should not exceed 100–200 mg. Nienhuis (1981) reviewed the evidence that large doses of ascorbic acid are toxic and suggested that this might result from the mobilization of the iron from the spleen and liver and by the vitamin enhancing the effect that iron has in bringing about the peroxidation of lipids.

Wapnick and co-workers (1969) appear to be the first to have demonstrated that the administration of ascorbic acid increases the excretion in the urine of iron in iron-loaded patients to whom DF has been given. In a previous study (Wapnick et al., 1968), it had been shown that ascorbic-acid deficiency, as determined by measurement of leucocyte ascorbic acid, is commonly found in individuals suffering from overloading with iron. Amongst the patients studied by Wapnick et al. (1969) were eight who had thalassaemia major and five with other transfusion-dependent anaemias. DF was given at a daily dose rate of 10 mg/kg intramuscularly and ascorbic acid, 500 mg 3 times a day, was given by mouth for a 7-day trial period. The mean excretion of iron increased by 88% after 7 days of ascorbic-acid therapy. (The leucocyte ascorbic acid concentration increased by 164%.) No change was noted in the iron excretion in the urine or in the ascorbic-acid concentration in the leucocytes of the normal white or Bantu subjects who served as controls.

O'Brien (1974) reported that he had administered 500 mg of ascorbic acid daily for 7 days to 12 transfusion-dependent patients with thalassaemia major who were being treated with intramuscular DF. The iron excreted in the urine increased by 25–200% during the period the ascorbic acid was being given. In one adult patient the daily iron excretion increased from 18–23 mg to 30–45 mg when he took 100 mg of ascorbic acid daily; the increased excretion was maintained for at least 1 year.

Subsequent reports have confirmed these early findings although the improvement in iron excretion following taking ascorbic acid has varied rather widely from patient to patient (Hussain et al, 1977; Propper et al., 1977; Pippard, Callender and Weatherall, 1978; Piomelli et al., 1980; Pippard, Callender and Finch, 1982).

Serum-ferritin levels and liver histology following therapy with desferrioxamine

Careful studies on the effect of long-term DF therapy on serum-ferritin levels and liver histology have been carried out. The serum-ferritin levels fall if the therapy is persisted in and liver haemosiderosis and damage are arrested, if not improved.

Letsky and her co-workers (1974) measured serum ferritin and liver iron in two groups of 20 transfusion-dependent children with thalassaemia: one group received regular iron-chelation therapy, the other group did not. The serum-ferritin levels and liver-iron content were lower in the treated as compared with the untreated group. The results of both estimations, however, remained high, in the untreated idiopathic haemochromatosis range. The serum-ferritin levels and liver-iron concentrations ran closely parallel, and Letsky *et al.* suggested that estimation of serum ferritin is a valuable and practical alternative to the measurement of liver iron in biopsy specimens.

Barry and co-workers (1974) reported the results of a similar study in which liver-iron concentration (% dry weight of liver), liver histology and clinical progress were compared in two groups of nine thalassaemia-major patients who had been maintained on a high-transfusion regime. One group had been treated for 5.2–6.3 years with DF or DTPA; the other group did not receive the chelators. The liver samples were obtained by biopsy and 49 specimens were available. In those from the patients receiving the chelators the liver-iron concentration did not increase with time and hepatic fibrosis remained essentially unchanged: in those not receiving the chelators there was a significant increase in liver iron and a progressive increase, too, in fibrosis. At the end of the trial there was no overlap between the two groups. Puberty was delayed in four out of five of the controls but in only one of the four children who had been treated with the chelators. More details of liver histology and its relation to liver-iron content were described by Risden, Barry and Flynn (1975). Liver damage ranged from a very slight increase in fibrosis to severe fibrosis and cirrhosis. The severity of the change was positively correlated with the patient's age and the liver-iron concentration. Treatment with the chelators reduced the amount of iron present and resulted in a predictable retardation in the progression of the fibrosis. The stainable iron was, in general, uniformly distributed between parenchymal and phagocytic reticulo-endolthelial (RE) cells from an early stage of loading with iron. Iron loading in parenchymal cells was heavier in splenectomized patients than in those with a spleen *in situ*. Fibrosis was found to develop slowly and appeared to take at least 16 years to become severe.

Further evidence that it is possible to reverse iron loading in the liver as the result of intensive DF therapy was provided by Cohen, Martin and Schwartz (1984). They carried out liver biopsies in four transfusion-dependent children with thalassaemia major and examined the tissue histologically. In three patients in whom biopsies were available after 53–77 months of therapy the iron content, as judged by Prussian-blue staining, was virtually normal. The liver's content of iron was also estimated *in vivo* by magnetic susceptibility: it was found to be normal after therapy in three of the patients and but mildly elevated in the fourth patient.

In the 1960s and 1970s, too, in addition to reports illustrating the value of DF in treating patients suffering from iron overload, the results of a number of studies on its mechanism of action were published. These centred particularly on the source of the iron mobilized and the routes of the excretion of the chelated iron.

Source of iron mobilized by desferrioxamine

As the result of a careful study, Hallberg and Hedenberg (1965) concluded that DF did not take significant amounts of iron from transferrin. They established that DF did not affect plasma iron turnover and that ^{59}Fe bound to transferrin was not excreted following the administration of DF and that DF had no effect on the incorporation into erythroblasts of ^{59}Fe bound to transferrin.

Brown, Hwang and Allgood (1967) described the results of an elaborate study. ^{59}Fe incorporated into dextran was found not to be mobilized from storage depots and the same was found to be true of haemoglobin iron recently deposited in phagocytic cells (using heat-damaged erythrocytes as a source of this iron). Increasing the amount of iron in storage depots or decreasing this by phlebotomy had little effect on DF-induced excretion of iron in the urine. Brown, Hwang and Allgood nevertheless concluded that iron in iron stores was the ultimate source of the iron excreted following the administration of DF; they also pointed out, however, that the amount excreted in patients overloaded with iron seemed to be poorly correlated with the degree of iron overloading.

Karabus and Fielding (1967) administered DF to 44 patients suffering from a variety of blood disorders including one patient who had thalassaemia major. They used a 'differential ferrioxamine test' designed to estimate chelatable body iron and concluded that, in addition to storage iron (ferritin–haemosiderin) that is chelated with difficulty, there is a compartment of readily chelatable iron derived from the breakdown of haem within RE cells.

Harker, Funk and Finch (1968), who studied a large number of patients overloaded with iron (mainly suffering from haemochromatosis), concluded that although there was some correlation between the total iron stores and iron excreted following the administration of DF, this relationship applied more specifically to iron in the liver parenchymal cells rather than to iron stored in phagocytic cells.

Lipschitz and co-workers (1971) concluded that in rats neither ferritin nor haemosiderin is an important direct donor of iron to DF. They confirmed that iron bound to transferrin in the plasma is not bound by the chelate and suggested that some compound on the pathway between the iron stores and plasma is probably the major immediate source.

Hershko, Cook and Finch (1973) used a variety of ^{59}Fe-labelled probes to study the mode of action of DF in the rat. The studies confirmed generally what had been found out in man, namely, that administration of DF produces a marked increase in the excretion of labelled parenchyma-cell iron, whereas the excretion of iron derived from probes taken up by RE cells is no greater than can be accounted for by iron recirculating to parenchyma cells after release from transferrin.

Pollack and co-workers (1976) demonstrated in in-vitro experiments that DF does not deplete transferrin of iron, even when in stoichiometric excess.

Evidence in favour of there being an easily chelatable iron pool, distinct from the total iron storage pool, was reported by Hershko and Rachmilewitz (1978) who studied 16 patients with homozygous β-thalassaemia. Following the intravenous injection of DF, chelated iron accumulated in the plasma and reached peak levels approximately 2 hours after the injection. The rise in the plasma concentration of chelated iron was attributed to iron being released from the tissues at a rate exceeding the renal clearance of chelated iron. The high-specific activity of the chelated urinary iron in patients to whom ^{59}Fe had been administered suggested to Hershko and Rachmilewitz that this iron is derived from the catabolism of non-viable erythrocytes within RE cells, particularly in the spleen and bone marrow, i.e. that recently catabolized haemoglobin, contrary to most earlier reports, is the main source of easily chelatable iron. Hershko and Rachmilewitz pointed out that previous studies had indicated the presence in rats, too, of an easily chelatable iron pool in RE cells (Lipschitz et al., 1971; Hershko, 1978).

A source of chelatable iron additional to that present in parenchyma cells and RE cells is, according to Hershko et al. (1978), 'non-specific' iron in the plasma of individuals whose transferrin has become completely saturated with iron. In patients with thalassaemia major receiving regular transfusions this (dialysable) iron was present in concentrations of 2.7–7.1 μmol/l. This iron, which could be bound to transferrin or chelated, was thought to be potentially toxic and a cause of tissue damage.

Summers and co-workers (1979) reported on the metabolism of ^{59}Fe-labelled desferrioxamine and ferrioxamine in normal subjects and in iron-loaded patients. They concluded that the amount of iron chelated in vivo is related to the increase in size of an intermediate chelatable iron pool rather than to the total extent of the iron load.

Faecal excretion of iron

It was not at first realized that significant amounts of chelated iron were excreted in the faeces after therapy with DF. Gevirtz and co-workers (1965) seem to have been the first to report this. They administered DF to two patients with red-cell aplasia who had been transfused with ^{59}Fe-labelled erythrocytes. The iron excreted in the faeces of one of the patients averaged approximately 13 mg/day per g DF compared with approximately 20 mg/day per g DF in the urine. The results in the second patient were similar. Brown, Hwang and Allgood (1967) accepted that a considerable amount of iron was excreted in the faeces after the administration of DF and concluded that excretion in the bile did not account for all of this. Harker, Funk and Finch (1968) compared the output in urine and faeces in four patients with haemochromatosis; the mean faecal excretion was 42.0 ± 3.7% of that in the urine. In one patient they were able to demonstrate by duodenal aspiration that bile was in fact the major source of the chelated iron.

Cumming and co-workers (1969), too, were able to show in four patients with haemochromatosis being treated with DF that faecal iron comprised 30–50%, mean 40%, of the total iron excreted. There seems no reason to suppose that patients with thalassaemia who are heavily loaded with iron behave differently with respect to routes of excretion of iron from patients with idiopathic haemochromatosis following the administration of DF. This must mean, therefore, that measuring iron excretion in urine alone, as is usually done, substantially underestimates the amount of iron lost and hence the effectiveness of the chelating agent used. Support for this contention was provided by Beard, Necheles and Allen (1969) and Silvestroni et al. (1982).

Beard, Necheles and Allen (1969) reported on five patients: in two the parenteral administration of DTPA or DF resulted in an increase in faecal iron; in one of them, whose day-by-day excretion is recorded, the amount of iron in the faeces sometimes exceeded that in the urine. No increase in faecal iron was noted in the other three patients who were not so heavily iron-loaded.

Silvestroni and co-workers' (1982) data were based on a study of 14 children with thalassaemia major who were being treated by the subcutaneous infusion of DF. The mean 24-hour excretion of iron in the urine in nine children who had not been splenectomized was 10.2 mg and in the faeces 5.2 mg: in the five who had been splenectomized the figures were 18.9 mg and 7.0 mg, respectively.

Earlier work on DF-treated rats (Hershko, 1978) had shown that iron is excreted by two pathways. Intracellular iron in hepatocytes appeared to be excreted exclusively via the bile into the faeces while iron in RE cells was excreted, after saturation of plasma transferrin, via the kidneys. The amount of iron excreted in the faeces exceeded that in the urine. In this respect, at least, Hershko's results differ from those obtained in man in whom the biliary excretion of DF-chelated iron appears usually to be considerably less than half that in the urine (Harker, Funk and Finch, 1968).

Effect on cardiac function of iron chelation

As already referred to, cardiac failure is the usual cause of death in the heavily iron-overloaded patient. In thalassaemia major this usually occurs towards the end of the second decade.

A number of studies based on quite large numbers of patients have been carried out in order to evaluate to what extent, if any, the usual deterioration in cardiac function can be arrested by vigorous and persistent iron-chelation therapy. The answer seems to be that iron loading of the heart can be arrested and even probably to some extent reversed and that cardiac function can be substantially improved in consequence. Not every patient, however, responds well.

Nienhuis and his co-workers (1980) reviewed the cardiac well-being of 42 regularly transfused patients with thalassaemia major who were receiving chelation therapy. Echocardiography, 24-hour monitoring of cardiac rhythm and radionuclide cineangiography were being used to assess the patients' progress. The follow-up period was too short to determine the value of the iron chelation, but it was clearly established that high doses of ascorbic acid (e.g., 500 mg a day) might be positively harmful.

Propper, Clarke and Nathan (1982) reviewed the effect of 'supertransfusion' and nightly subcutaneous DF on the development of cardiac disease in 45 patients treated within the previous 7 years. Their haemoglobin was maintained above 12 g/dl and DF was given subcutaneously for 8–12 hours each night. Cardiac function was assessed and urine iron excretion and serum-ferritin levels were estimated. None of the patients accumulated iron during the period they were being treated, as assessed by the amount of iron excreted in the urine, and the serum-ferritin levels declined in all but two of them. The results with respect to cardiac disease were, however, on the whole rather disappointing, at least in children who were over 5 years of age when treatment was started. None of five patients who started treatment before the age of 6 years developed cardiac disease. Of 20 patients aged 6–11 years when treatment was started,

two had existing cardiac disease and one of these died; three developed cardiac disease whilst on treatment and one died. Ten patients were aged 12–16 years when treatment was started: two had existing cardiac disease and one died; three other patients developed cardiac disease of whom one died. Ten patients were over 17 years of age when treatment was started: five had existing cardiac disease of whom two died, and one more developed cardiac disease.

The report of Marcus and co-workers (1984) was a little more encouraging. Five thalassaemia-major patients with existing signs of impaired cardiac function were treated with high doses of DF (up to 200 mg/kg per day). Two died, but in three there was subjective and objective evidence that their cardiac function had improved.

A later report from Boston and Toronto (Wolfe et al., 1985) is even more encouraging. It was based on 36 transfusion-dependent patients with thalassaemia major, all over 10 years of age, who were being treated with subcutaneous DF. Of 19 who did not comply with the treatment, 12 acquired cardiac disease and seven died. In stark contrast, of 17 patients who did manage to comply with the treatment only one developed cardiac disease (and died). The serum-ferritin and aspartate aminotransferase levels of the 16 survivors fell, indicating a reduction in iron stores and improvement, too, in liver function.

The reports of Giardina et al. (1985) and Hyman et al. (1985) given to the Fifth Cooley's Anemia Symposium, were based on 36 and 25 children and young adults, respectively, being treated on hypertransfusion regimes and receiving daily DF subcutaneously or daily DF subcutaneously supplemented by DF given intravenously at the time of blood transfusions. Both groups emphasized the importance from the point of view of preserving cardiac function of starting therapy at as early an age as practicable. Giardina et al. demonstrated a significant reduction in the incidence of cardiac arrythmias in patients started on DF therapy before they were 13 years of age; the effect in older (and more heavily iron-overloaded) adolescents was, however, much less obvious. Most of their patients who had had arrythmias before treatment was started died of congestive heart failure despite vigorous iron chelation. Hyman et al. raised the question of the value of having a spleen in situ in relation to iron overloading of the heart; they suggested that the spleen performed a valuable function in processing and storing iron and in this respect was more efficient and protective than the liver.

Possible therapeutic use of desferrioxamine entrapped in erythrocytes

Desferrioxamine can be entrapped in resealed erythrocyte ghosts without much difficulty. Green, Miller and Crosby (1981) administered DF-loaded rat erythrocyte ghosts intravenously to rats whose RE iron stores had been labelled with ^{59}Fe. Four to 5 times as much iron was excreted as when DF alone was injected intravenously. DF-loaded human erythrocyte ghosts have also been prepared and were administered by Green, Lamon and Curran (1980) to 10 patients suffering from various types of iron overload. The resultant excretion of iron in the urine was then compared with that following the subcutaneous injection of the same dose of DF. More iron was excreted following the administration of the ghosts in each instance, the increase varying from 7 to 379%.

New iron-chelating drugs

As already mentioned (p. 548), of all the drugs that have been tested for their ability to remove iron from iron-loaded patients, none has approached DF and DTPA in efficiency. What is of course required is an effective and safe drug that can be administered by mouth. Unfortunately, at the time of writing no such drug appears to be available.

Amongst the newer drugs that have been tested in animals or in man are the following: rhodotorulic acid (derived from the yeast *Photorula pilimanae*) (Grady *et al.*, 1974); 2,3-dihydroxybenzoic acid [2,3-DHB (Graziano *et al.*, 1975; Peterson *et al.*, 1976)]; cholyhydroxamic acid (CHA) and ethylenediamine-*N*, *N'*-bis (*o*-hydroxyphenylglycine) (EHPG), a polyanionic amine used in agriculture as an iron chelate (Cerami *et al.*, 1980).

Graziano and co-workers (1975) administered 2,3-DHB orally to five iron-overloaded β-thalassaemia patients at a dose rate of 25 mg/kg daily for 8 days. This resulted in the rather small average increase in urine iron excretion of 5 mg/day. Three patients given 25 mg/kg 4 times daily excreted 4.5–13.0 mg daily. No adverse effects were noted. Some younger patients, aged between 9 and 14 years, were also treated, but they did not seem to respond so well; they were, however, not so heavily loaded with iron.

Peterson and co-workers (1976) gave 2,3-DHB by mouth to five transfusion-dependent thalassaemia-major patients at a dose of 25 mg/kg per day for 8 days. An average of 4.5 mg per day of iron was excreted; this increased to 6.5 mg per day when the same dose of drug was taken 4 times a day. It was well tolerated if taken with food.

SPLENECTOMY

Splenectomy has been carried out for many years as a possible means of treating thalassaemia, indeed long before the nature of the disorder was recognized [*e.g.*, Case 1 of Stillmann (1917)]. Although the operation has, of course, no effect on the fundamental cause of thalassaemia it can be helpful, particularly when the spleen is greatly enlarged and is causing physical discomfort or has led to hypersplenism with the result that the survival of transfused normal blood is impaired and the neutrophil and platelet counts are probably subnormal. Another indication for removing the spleen is when the patient's own erythrocytes are being destroyed at a substantially increased rate, as for instance in Hb-H disease.

Now that children with β-thalassaemia major are so often being treated by regular blood transfusions intended to maintain the haemoglobin at a high level, it is particularly important to be on the lookout for an increase in the amount of blood required to maintain the desired level. In such patients a ^{51}Cr study is likely to substantiate the clinical diagnosis of hypersplenism. In any case, if the need for blood is clearly increasing and the spleen is enlarged and easily palpable, splenectomy should be seriously considered. Splenectomy should, however, not be lightly undertaken for, leaving aside the immediate risks of the operation which are low but not negligible, the later risk of increased susceptibility to serious bacterial infections and to malaria must not be forgotten (see p. 561). For these, if for no other reasons, most physicians are reluctant to recommend splenectomy in very young children, *i.e.* they prefer to postpone the operation until the child is at least 5–6 years old. An additional possible risk is the increased rate of loading of the liver with iron once the spleen has been removed.

Early literature on splenectomy in β-thalassaemia major

Cooley (1928) in a paper entitled 'Likenesses and contrasts in the hemolytic anemias in childhood' referred to the possible value of splenectomy in erythroblastic anaemia. He concluded that there was likely to be little benefit. In his own words: 'splenectomy is followed by a remarkable increase of erythroblasts in the blood, lasting over years; but so far as available reports are concerned, there seems to be little definite improvement in the patient. Hemolysis and jaundice, if present, may be temporarily lessened, but they return and the disease process continues as before. The benefit to the patient lies mostly in the removal of the heavy drag of the spleen.'

Penberthy and Cooley (1935), too, had no illusions about the value of splenectomy for what they also termed 'erythroblastic anemia'. However, they considered that the operation was worth undertaking. They wrote: 'The organ becomes so large, however, that it seems worthwhile to remove it . . . there is no particular change in the anemia after the operation. We have felt so far as our cases are concerned that the patients were more comfortable and lived somewhat longer after splenectomy than we would have expected without the operation. We have operated on five patients. We believe that it is worth doing.'

Other favourable reports were published in the 1940s and 1950s. Govan (1946), for instance, described how the transfusion requirements of two identical twins submitted to splenectomy were reduced after the operation and how their clinical improvement lasted for at least 2 years in one twin and for 9 months in the other. Govan gave references to earlier reports, some describing benefit, others not. Chini and Valeri (1949) in their review gave a number of references, too, to early attempts at splenectomy, mainly in the Italian literature. Referring to severe 'classic' Cooley's anaemia as having a rapidly fatal course, they did not commit themselves for or against the operation but stated simply that 'therapeutic attempts have been made with splenectomy'.

Shapiro, Schneck and Etess (1952) described the effect of the removal of a 'huge' spleen from two Chinese siblings. The first child, aged $3\frac{1}{2}$ years, who was described as deriving some benefit, developed *E. coli* septicaemia 6 weeks after the operation; the younger sibling, aged $2\frac{1}{2}$ years, did better, however, and episodes of cardiac failure which had occurred before splenectomy did not recur.

Lichtman and co-workers (1953) observed in children suffering from thalassaemia major who had received repeated transfusions that it was quite common for the transfusions to be required at increasingly frequent intervals if the patients' haemoglobin levels were to be maintained. They studied by means of the Ashby method the fate of the blood transfused to seven children and found a shortened survival in each case; in six of them the half-life of the transfused cells was reduced to between 5 and 9 days and in the seventh child it was 35 days. This suggested a superadded extracorpuscular mechanism of cell destruction. However, no abnormal antibodies, the presence of which might have explained the findings, could be identified. Splenectomy was carried out in five of the patients; in four of them the volumes of blood required to be transfused after splenectomy were reduced to 19, 21, 28 and 36%, respectively, of the volumes necessary before splenectomy. The fifth patient was not improved. It was concluded that a good case could be made out for removal of the spleen when transfusion studies indicated an abnormal rate of erythrocyte destruction. This seemed likely to occur most commonly in patients in whom the spleen was greatly enlarged.

The detailed observations and conclusions of Lichtman *et al.* referred to above have been largely confirmed by subsequent reports. Splenectomy has been most successful in children who have had particularly large spleens and in whom there was evidence of markedly subnormal survival of transfused normal erythrocytes or other evidence of hypersplenism such as neutropenia or thrombocytopenia.

Reports published in the 1950s describing the effects of splenectomy include those of Gatto and Lo Jacono (1953), Glenn *et al.* (1954), Clement and Taffel (1955), Smith *et al.* (1955a), Reemtsma and Elliott (1956), Fusco, Bouroncle and Doan (1958) and Mainzer and O'Connor (1958).

Glenn and co-workers (1954) and Smith and co-workers (1955a) (who reported the same series of nine patients) described how all of them had improved haemoglobin levels after splenectomy and needed less blood post-operatively than before. The longest follow-up was 51 months. One patient died of encephalitis 14 months after the operation and four patients developed pericarditis of obscure origin from which, however, they recovered.

Clement and Taffel (1955) described four children

each of whom had a large spleen and required massive transfusions. All benefited from splenectomy and their transfusion requirement (to maintain the same haemoglobin level) fell to 25–50% of what it had been before the operation.

Reemtsma and Elliott (1956) reported on the follow-up of a relatively large series of 25 patients who were followed from 6 to 25 years or until death. Thirteen of them underwent splenectomy. The best results were obtained in the older patients or in those in whom there were signs of 'hypersplenism'. The results in children less than 4 years of age were generally disappointing. All the patients who were receiving transfusions had diminished requirements after operation, but the duration of the favourable response was variable and there seemed to be a tendency to relapse. Six of the splenectomized patients died within the next 10 years, but there were no immediate post-operative deaths or serious complications.

Fusco, Bouroncle and Doan (1958) described how five patients with Cooley's anaemia were all apparently improved by splenectomy, the blood transfusion requirement being reduced in each case.

Mainzer and O'Connor (1958) reported the results of splenectomy in 15 patients ranging in age from 18 months to 16 years. There was no immediate post-operative mortality and in five of 11 patients who were followed up for a relatively long period (4–8 years) the requirement of blood for transfusion appeared to be definitely decreased, i.e. to be less than 50% of the pre-operative figures. Mainzer and O'Connor mentioned that one patient developed pneumococcal meningitis post-operatively and two others pathological fractures.

More recent publications on the indications for, and the results of splenectomy in, β-thalassaemia major include those of Smith *et al.* (1960), Wolff, Sitarz and Von Hofe (1960), Bouroncle and Doan (1964), Wahidijat, Markum and Adang (1972), Engelhard, Cividalli and Rachmilewitz (1975), Pearson and O'Brien (1975) and Modell (1976, 1977).

Smith and his co-workers (1960) reviewed the progress of 58 children with Cooley's anaemia, half of whom had been splenectomized. The survival of transfused normal blood appeared to be permanently improved by the operation (see p. 562). However, splenectomy did not seem to help the children to grow or to mature sexually or, most importantly, to prevent death from cardiac failure in the 2nd decade. Smith *et al.* stressed the 'need for an effective method by which the heart can be made to unload its iron deposits'; they stressed, too, the children's increased susceptibility to infections after splenectomy and mentioned that 11 attacks of acute pericarditis had been experienced by eight patients, seven of whom had had their spleen removed.

Wolff, Sitarz and Von Hofe (1960) reported on the effect of splenectomy in 18 children with thalassaemia who had been followed post-operatively for 5 months to 28 years. One patient died during induction of anaesthesia, but all the others benefited initially and required less blood to maintain a higher level of haemoglobin. Seven of the 17, however, ultimately died, all but two of chronic cardiac failure. Pericarditis developed in three of them.

Bouroncle and Doan (1964) discussed the indications for splenectomy in Cooley's anaemia and referred to five patients who had developed signs of hypersplenism and had had their spleens removed in consequence. Erythrocyte survival became normal as judged by their transfusion requirements and the platelet count increased substantially. Follow-up for 7–29 years confirmed that the patients had derived long-term benefit; none of them had been troubled with a serious infection post-operatively. Bouroncle and Doan concluded that splenectomy was worthwhile if there was secondary hypersplenism or if the enlarged spleen was mechanically interfering with normal functions.

Wahidijat, Markum and Adang (1972) reviewed the results of splenectomy carried out in Djakarta on 33 transfusion-dependent children who had thalassaemia major: the operation was undertaken in 19 children because they had shown signs of hypersplenism and haemosiderosis and in 14 slightly younger children because of an increasing blood transfusion requirement only. The latter (younger) children did much better post-operatively than the older hypersplenic and haemosiderotic children: one only of the former group died during a follow-up of 24–188 months compared with 12 of the latter group during a follow-up of 0–70 months. The conclusion was reached that it was unwise to wait for major signs of hypersplenism and that splenectomy should be undertaken earlier rather than later (but not before the child was 2 years of age). Infections seem to have been the major cause of death in this series.

Engelhard, Cividalli and Rachmilewitz (1975) reported on the results of splenectomy carried out in Israel on 30 patients with homozygous β-thalassaemia. Six patients were judged to have thalassaemia intermedia; 24 were transfusion-dependent. The latter could be divided into two groups: those who needed monthly transfusions from the time of diagnosis and those who needed few transfusions before the age of 1–2 years but whose transfusion requirement subsequently increased associated with signs of hypersplenism. Splenectomy in the former group resulted in improvement in general well-being but only a temporary reduction, lasting for 1–2 years, in their requirement for blood transfusion. In the latter group the results were better, particularly in those patients who had developed hypersplenism relatively late in childhood. They usually derived long-term benefit. No significant post-operative infections were recorded in either group, and Engelhard, Cividalli and Rachmilewitz concluded that the risk of post-operative infections should not be considered a contra-indication to splenectomy in children over 2 years of age.

Pearson and O'Brien (1975) in their review of the role of splenectomy in the management of thalassaemia major concluded that 'most patients with thalassaemia major ultimately require surgical removal of the spleen' and that, although in some patients the operation becomes necessary because of the size of the spleen, the most common indication is a progressive shortening of the survival of transfused blood. The operation should, in their opinion, however, be deferred as long as possible, at least until the child is 5–6 years of age. ^{51}Cr studies were considered to be of uncertain value in predicting response to splenectomy.

Recent views on splenectomy in thalassaemia major

Modell (1976, 1977) discussed splenectomy in two important reviews. She stressed, in particular, how important it is to be aware of hypersplenism as a cause of an increasing blood requirement in β-thalassaemia major. In her view the extent of hypersplenism is more sensitively measured by relating the observed volume of blood required by the patient to that of a splenectomized individual on the same transfusion regime than by estimating erythrocyte survival using ^{51}Cr. According to Modell, severe hypersplenism, leading to as much as double the expected blood requirement, is common in β^{+}-thalassaemia major; and added that low-transfusion regimes may precipitate hypersplenism while high-transfusion regimes started from the time of diagnosis may help to prevent its development. According to Modell, too, blood-group incompatibility has not been a common problem in the the United Kingdom. She pointed out that the incidence of serious infections after splenectomy has varied in different parts of the world and recommended that prophylactic penicillin (and anti-malarial drugs, too, where malaria is endemic) should be given indefinitely post-operatively. She stated that severe infections occur less frequently in children on high-transfusion regimes than in those given less blood.

Modell referred to two groups of patients with hypersplenism: a group with very large spleens and a gross (e.g. double) increase in blood requirement for which splenectomy is mandatory, and another group with a smaller increase in blood requirement. Splenectomy was recommended for this group, too, if the blood requirement is greater by 50% or more than that indicated by a standard curve [illustrated by Modell (1976)] relating haemoglobin levels achieved to the annual blood requirement in ml/kg. After splenectomy, she suggested that the physician should wait to see whether the patient can maintain his or her haemoglobin level before embarking on a regular transfusion regime.

Weatherall and Clegg (1981, p. 692), after weighing up carefully the results of splenectomy as recorded in the literature they reviewed, concluded that it was still difficult to determine its true benefit. They pointed out that if a child had been maintained on a high-transfusion regime from an early age the operation may never be necessary; on the other hand, in children on lower-transfusion regimes in whom an apparent increased transfusion requirement can be substantiated on the basis of their mean annual haemoglobin level, splenectomy is indicated and is likely to be followed by a sustained reduction in their need for blood. According to Weatherall and Clegg, post-operative enlargement of the liver, which in the past commonly developed after splenectomy, is not an important problem in children who are maintained on a high-transfusion regime.

Splenectomy in β-thalassaemia intermedia

Patients with thalassaemia intermedia not infrequently develop large spleens in the course of time. Such patients usually benefit from splenectomy and subsequently maintain their haemoglobin well above their pre-operative level. Case reports illustrating the results of splenectomy include those of Virdis (1951), Greppi and di Guglielmo (1955), Rapaport, Reilly and Carpenter (1957), Thompson, Odom and Bell (1965) and Engelhard, Cividalli and Rachmilewitz (1975).

Rapaport, Reilly and Carpenter's (1957) patient, a 34-year-old Sicilian, who was considered to have thalassaemia minor, had a haemoglobin of 6.8 g/dl before splenectomy and a platelet count of 20×10^9/l. After splenectomy the haemoglobin was maintained at 14.5–15.2 g/dl and the erythrocyte count rose to 6.0×10^{12}/l.

One of Thompson, Odom and Bell's (1965) patients

was a man aged 68 who was submitted to laporatomy for suspected gallstones. No gallstones were found but the gall bladder was distended with sludged bile. However, a 550-g spleen was removed. Subsequently he had repeated attacks of thrombophlebitis in his legs and later developed a serious lung infection. He died 11 months after splenectomy. Necropsy revealed bilateral pneumonia with abscess formation and multiple small pulmonary emboli. His platelet count was $700 \times 10^9/1$ at 7 months after splenectomy.

Engelhard, Cividalli and Rachmilewitz's (1975) six patients were considered to be homozygotes for β-thalassaemia. They were aged between $4\frac{1}{2}$ and 19 years and had received 0–4 transfusions per year. Splenectomy was carried out in four of them for severe abdominal discomfort, in one because of repeated haemolytic episodes and in one for a splenic abscess complicating septicaemia. After splenectomy they required fewer transfusions and their haemoglobin increased by 2–3 g/dl.

Splenectomy for Hb-H disease

Patients with Hb-H disease have often been submitted to splenectomy. In most of them the haemoglobin seems to have risen after the operation and the patients' general well-being has been improved.

Early reports describing the effect of the operation include those of Gouttas *et al.* (1955), Minnich *et al.* (1958), Lie-Injo, Tjoa and Kho (1961), Woodrow, Noble and Martindale (1964) and Rosner, Pfenninger and Marti (1965) in Greek, Chinese, English and Italian patients, respectively.

Wasi and co-workers (Wasi *et al.*, 1969; Wasi, Na-Nakorn and Pootrakul, 1974) have given detailed descriptions of the effect of splenectomy in Hb-H disease based on a study of a large number of Thai patients. Wasi *et al.* (1969) referred to 50 patients and stated that their haemoglobin had risen by 2–3 g/dl following splenectomy. Wasi, Na-Nakorn and Pootrakul (1974) gave further details. They stated that the results in Hb-H disease 'are definitely better than in the β-thalassaemia disorders' and that in most cases the haemoglobin was elevated after splenectomy to 9–10 g/dl, the rise being more dramatic in patients with hypersplenism and in those who were severely anaemic before the operation. They cautioned that splenectomy should not be performed in patients who could maintain without transfusion a haemoglobin as high as 8 g/dl, for such patients were felt to be able usually to manage well without splenectomy and because a haemoglobin at that level was unlikely to be raised much by removal of the

spleen. Their patients with Hb-H disease do not seem to have suffered from an excessive incidence of serious post-splenectomy infections as compared with those with β-thalassaemia/Hb-E disease. Wasi, Na-Nakorn and Pootrakul attributed this relative freedom to the iron overload in Hb-H disease being less than in other forms of thalassaemia. They stated that patients with Hb-H disease splenectomized as long as 10 or more years previously do not show signs of liver damage (from iron overload) and have normal serum-albumin levels. Their patients do not seem to have received prophylactic penicillin after splenectomy as a routine; they recommended, however, that this should be given to some patients.

Yang and co-workers (1985) in a review of the incidence of β- and α-thalassaemia in China referred to 29 Hb-H disease patients who had been submitted to splenectomy. The mean rise in haemoglobin after the operation was recorded as 3.5 g/dl (range 0.5–7.0 g) and the mean increase in $^{51}CrT_{50}$ 4.79 days (range 3.03–7.33).

The changes that splenectomy bring about to the blood picture of Hb-H disease patients have already been described (p. 453). In summary, the erythrocytes become thinner and more macrocytic, anisocytosis and poikilocytosis become less marked and large inclusions can be seen in some of the erythrocytes without the necessity for incubation with methylene blue or brilliant cresyl blue.

Persistent thrombocytosis after splenectomy

Rises in platelet count after splenectomy, as recorded by Thompson, Odom and Bell (1965) appear to be a common consequence of the absence of the spleen in any patient in whom anaemia and active erythropoiesis persist after splenectomy (Hirsh and Dacie, 1966) (see also Vol. 1, p. 120). This seems to be true irrespective of whether the erythropoiesis is effective or ineffective. In such cases anaemia appears to stimulate thrombocytopoiesis as well as erythropoiesis; this, however, becomes obvious only when the spleen has been removed (Fig. 20.1). Hirsh and Dacie (1966) recorded mean platelet counts of $683 \times 10^9/1$ in three patients with thalassaemia major 3 or more months after splenectomy [see also Fig. 3.63 (Vol. 1)]; they also referred to a patient with Hb-H disease who developed recurrent thrombophlebitis and pulmonary embolism 1 year after splenectomy and to a patient with thalassaemia major

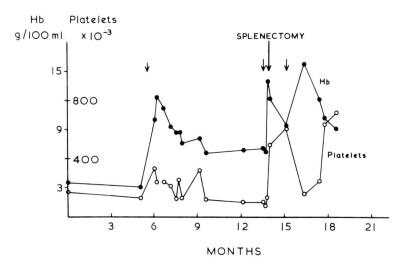

Fig. 20.1 Hemoglobin levels and platelet counts before and after splenectomy in a patient with thalassaemia major.
 ● haemoglobin; ○ platelet count per μl. Note the contrasting effect of blood transfusions (↓) on the platelet count before and after splenectomy. [From Hirsh and Dacie (1966).]

who developed thrombophlebitis and persistent leg oedema 5 years after splenectomy.

Tso, Chan and Todd (1982) reported the occurrence of thrombophlebitis in two out of nine Chinese patients with Hb-H disease who had undergone splenectomy. One was a 24-year-old female who experienced thrombophlebitis in her legs in two successive pregnancies — she had had her spleen removed for traumatic rupture 2 years before her first pregnancy. The other patient, a 35-year-old male, died of pulmonary embolism 19 months after splenectomy. He had developed thrombophlebitis in his left leg 9 months earlier; his platelet count was persistently high (700–1247 × 10⁹/l). (Two more of the Hb-H disease patients had platelet counts of 700 and 920 × 10⁹/l, respectively, 6 and 5 years after splenectomy; they had, however, apparently not experienced thrombo-embolic episodes.) Tso, Chan and Todd stated that of 16 further patients, who had other types of thalassaemia (β-thalassaemia major and trait and Hb-E/β-thalassaemia etc.), 13 had persistent thrombocytosis after splenectomy. None had, however, developed thrombo-embolic complications; seven had platelet counts in excess of 500 × 10⁹/l, the maximum count being 1050 × 10⁹/l in a patient splenectomized 23 years previously. Tso, Chan and Todd concluded that in Hb-H disease thrombocytosis, intravascular haemolysis and depression of RE-cell function contribute in some patients to a hypercoagulable state.

It seems clear that many patients with thalassaemia develop persistent thrombocytosis after splenectomy, particularly if anaemia persists or is allowed to persist. But it is not clear how important a factor thrombocytosis is in the development of thrombophlebitis and thrombo-embolism. Most patients with persistent thrombocytosis do not develop these potentially dangerous complications and their possible occurrence should not be used as an argument against splenectomy in thalassaemia when the operation is otherwise strongly indicated. In 'borderline' cases, however, the possible complications of splenectomy — operative mortality, post-operative infections and thrombo-embolism — must not be forgotten about in coming to a decision as to whether the operation should be recommended.

Serious infections after splenectomy

The effect that absence of the spleen has in increasing the incidence of serious infections has been reviewed in some detail earlier in this book (Vol. 1, pp. 116–119). Attention was first drawn to this potentially lethal complication of splenectomy in the 1950s, with thalassaemia major being mentioned as one of the disorders in which fulminating septicaemia or meningitis might be anticipated. Carl H. Smith and his co-workers of New York have paid particular attention to the problem. Smith and co-workers (1957) described a series of 19 children who had been submitted to splenectomy and who had developed severe infections subsequently. Ten of them had been diagnosed as suffering from Cooley's anaemia and four had died as a result of their infection. Later, Smith et al. (1962) reported that seven out of 33 children with Cooley's anaemia who had undergone splenectomy had suffered from severe infections subsequently and that five had died. (In contrast, three out of 23 children with their spleen in situ developed a severe infection but none of them had died.) The commonest offending organism was Str. pneumoniae, the next most frequent being E. coli and H. influenzae. Most of the serious infections developed in the first 2 years following splenectomy. Similar but slightly expanded data based on 58 patients with Cooley's anaemia seen between 1944 and 1963 were given by Smith et al. (1964). Smith and his colleagues recommended in these papers that antibiotics should be given prophylactically after splenectomy for the first 2 years, if not for longer. At the present time most physicians recommend that an oral penicillin preparation should be taken daily indefinitely and that splenectomy should be postponed if possible until the child is 5–6 years old.

As already remarked on, the incidence of serious infections following splenectomy seems to vary between the different centres specializing in the management of thalassaemia. This seems probably to be connected with the standard of living and hygiene in the environment in which the individual patients live. It seems likely too, that the incidence and severity of infections are related to some extent to the type of thalassaemia the patient suffers from. Thus, as already referred to, in Thailand serious infections have been less frequent in patients with Hb-H disease submitted to splenectomy than in those who have β-thalassaemia/Hb-E disease (Wasi, Na-Nakorn and Pootrakul, 1974).

Effect of splenectomy on immunoglobulin levels in serum

Wasi, Wasi and Thongcharoen (1971) measured the serum immunoglobulin concentration in 128 Thai patients with various types of thalassaemia, mostly Hb-E/β-thalassaemia or Hb-H disease: 42 of the patients had undergone splenectomy. Before splenectomy, the mean IgG, IgA and IgM levels were all greater than normal: after splenectomy the IgA levels rose and IgM levels fell. It was suggested that the spleen is an important source of IgM production and that the deficit in IgM might play a part in the occurrence of postsplenectomy infections.

Effect of splenectomy on erythrocyte survival

β-thalassaemia. Reference has already been made to the improved survival of transfused erythrocytes following splenectomy (p. 558). Some additional studies are summarized below.

Smith and co-workers (1960) referred to 58 patients with severe Cooley's anaemia of which 29 had been splenectomized. Before splenectomy in nine patients, the ^{51}Cr T_{50} of normal donor erythrocytes ranged from 10 to 29 days; in seven the survival was subnormal (10–22 days). In six patients who were studied from 3 months to 20 years after splenectomy, the ^{51}Cr T_{50} of normal donor erythrocytes was 25–43 days, the erythrocyte lifespan being apparently prolonged in five of the patients. It was possible to study the survival of the erythrocytes of 10 patients in their own circulation. The ^{51}Cr T_{50s} ranged between 6.5 and 19.5 days. Two of these patients had been splenectomized: their ^{51}Cr T_{50s} were 7 and 14 days, respectively. Smith et al. concluded that splenectomy removes an extracorpuscular haemolytic mechanism which is responsible for the shortened life-span of donor erythrocytes and that the improvement in survival is long lasting. On the other hand, the survival of the patient's own erythrocytes is not significantly affected by the operation.

The data reported by Wolff, Ultmann and Sitarz (1964) were similar to those of Smith et al. (1960) described above. Before splenectomy, the ^{51}Cr T_{50s} of donor erythrocytes transfused to nine thalassaemia-major recipients were 11–29 days. In two patients before splenectomy the ^{51}Cr T_{50s} of their own erythrocytes were 19 and 21 days and in six patients after splenectomy 5–20 days.

Shahid and Sahli (1971) studied 15 patients with thalassaemia. Ten were considered to have thalassaemia major. The survival of autologous erythrocytes was invariably shortened, and there was evidence, too, of splenic sequestration: that of donor erythrocytes was normal, or decreased in patients who had been transfused repeatedly. In three patients studied in detail before and after splenectomy the survival of the patients' own cells was virtually unaltered by splenectomy while that of donor cells became normal.

Blendis and co-workers (1974) described the results of an interesting study carried out on two patients with thalassaemia major and four with thalassaemia intermedia (one studied only after splenectomy). The ^{51}Cr T_{50} of the erythrocytes of five patients was 8–16 days before splenectomy and 14–20 days after splenectomy, the operation resulting in some improvement in each patient. Their spleens weighed between 510 and 975 g and the spleen pool of erythrocytes was calculated to represent between 8.6 and 39% of the total erythrocyte mass. The total blood volume before splenectomy was 86.3–108.6 ml/kg; after splenectomy it was 90.9–108.6 ml/kg. The erythrocyte mass was 8.5–26 ml/kg before splenectomy and 21.2–26.5 ml/kg after splenectomy, there being an increase in three out of the four patients in which it was possible to make the comparison. The plasma volume was 60.1–80.1 ml/kg before splenectomy and 67–92 ml/kg after splenectomy, still grossly expanded. It was suggested that the persistence of the high plasma volume was associated with the continuing large expansion in bone-marrow volume.

Effect of splenectomy on transfusion requirements

Patients with thalassaemia major who are transfusion-dependent generally require less blood after the operation than before. Not unexpectedly as the result of this, it is easier to achieve a negative iron balance in a transfusion-dependent patient on a chelation regime when his spleen has been removed than when it is in situ, that is if he has responded favourably to the operation. Graziano et al. (1981) described their findings in 79 thalassaemia-major patients who were being transfused so as to maintain their haemoglobin level greater than 10 g/dl. The mean blood requirement of 46 whose spleen had not been removed was 258 ml/kg/year, while that of 33 splenectomized patients was 203 ml/kg/year. In this series it was found that the splenectomized patients generally achieved a negative iron balance as the result of chelation with a daily dose of 20 mg/kg deferoxamine, whereas those with a spleen in situ were unable to do this. Graziano et al. concluded that in order to prevent haemosiderosis splenectomy should be carried out when a patient's transfusion requirement exceeds 250 ml of blood per kg/year. In their experience this was usually when the patient was aged between 6 and 8 years.

Effect of splenectomy on iron overload in the liver

It has been suggested that splenectomy may be followed by an increase in the rate at which iron is deposited in the liver and thus increases the risk of cirrhosis (Witzleben and Wyatt, 1961; Risden, Barry and Flynn, 1975; Okon, Levij and Rachmilewitz, 1976). This possibility is an added reason why patients who have undergone splenectomy should continue to receive effective chelation therapy, even if they require less blood following the operation.

BONE-MARROW TRANSPLANTATION FOR β-THALASSAEMIA MAJOR

The relative success in recent years of bone-marrow transplantation as a means of treating patients with aplastic anaemia or a haematological malignancy has naturally raised the question as to whether transplantation should be attempted in patients who have severe β-thalassaemia major. The outlook for the two categories of patients of course differs markedly. The haematological malignancies are disorders with a high potential mortality and commonly result in death within a few years of diagnosis and in the case of aplastic anaemia within a year of onset. β-thalassaemia major is at least as likely to cause death eventually, but not usually until the patient is well into the 2nd decade of life, and with the improvements in transfusion and iron-chelation therapy that have taken place within the last few years a patient's expectation of life seems likely to be substantially improved. There is thus not the same urgency to treat the patient by marrow transplantation — a potentially radical and curative, yet hazardous procedure — as there is with patients who have aplastic anaemia or a haematological malignancy. Most physicians responsible for the management of patients with thalassaemia would probably agree or have agreed with the short paragraph that Weatherall and Clegg wrote on transplantation in 1981.

This what they wrote: 'We believe that the time is not yet ripe for marrow transplantation in the treatment of thalassaemia. However, once the problem of graft-versus-host reaction is overcome the whole question will have to be seriously reconsidered.' Since they wrote that comment (presumably in 1979 or 1980) much has happened in the transplantation field; GVH disease, if not eradicated, has to some extent become controllable; much has been learnt as to how to eradicate the patient's bone marrow and to achieve the degree of immunosuppression required for the graft to be accepted, and much has been learnt, too, as to how to avoid and control post-transplant infections and to avoid radiation damage in cases in which irradiation has been used to prepare the patient for the graft. The consequence of the progress briefly outlined above has been that bone marrow has by now been transplanted in patients with β-thalassaemia major, with in some cases at least, complete success, *i.e.*, the thalassaemic marrow has been replaced apparently in its entirety by normal (or thalassaemia-minor) marrow. A heavy price has, however, been paid and the mortality attributable to the attempts at transplantation has been high. But with more experience this has been declining.

The first documented transplantation was reported from Seattle by Thomas and his co-workers in 1982. This was successful. Their patient was a 16-month-old Italian boy who was homozygous for β-thalassaemia. He was transplanted with bone marrow withdrawn from a normal HLA-identical elder sister and was prepared for the transplant by being given a single dose of 5 mg/kg of dimethyl busulphan intravenously followed by 50 mg/kg of cyclophosphamide on 4 successive days. 1.7×10^9 nucleated marrow cells per kg body weight were given without complication. After the transplant, immunosuppression was maintained with methotrexate. GVH disease was transient and fever was controlled with antibiotics. On the 47th post-transplant day the haematocrit was 32%, the leucocyte count 3×10^9/l and platelet count 247×10^9/l. The child's spleen and liver became impalpable by the 60th day and 6 months after the transplant his haemoglobin was 14.4 g/dl and Hb F appeared to be absent. The α/non-α globin-chain ratio determined on peripheral-blood reticulocytes between the 20th and 81st post-transplantation day was normal (0.92–1.2).

Thomas and his co-workers (1985) described how they had transplanted five transfusion-dependent homozygous β-thalassaemia children, aged between 6 and 24 months, between December 1981 and July 1983. They were prepared for the transplant by dimethyl busulphan and cyclophosphamide and received HLA-identical sibling marrow. Three of the children survived the procedure (including the boy described in 1982) and

appeared at the time of the report to be cured; two died of complications following the transplant (infection and interstitial pneumonia, respectively).

Lucarelli and co-workers (1984) described how they transplanted 13 children with homozygous β-thalassaemia with bone marrow from HLA-matched sibling donors, employing as preparative treatment busulphan, cyclophosphamide and irradiation in several doses and combinations. Six of the patients, aged 7–15 years, had undergone splenectomy and were advanced cases; seven were between 1 and 6 years of age and had not been splenectomized. Six of the patients died, five of transplant-related problems, one of cardiac failure. Seven children survived, but in five of them the graft failed to take: the two in which it did take were alive 363 and 491 days, respectively, after their transplant without evidence of thalassaemia. Lucarelli *et al.* emphasized that their experience demonstrated the difficulty of eradicating thalassaemic marrow without employing a highly toxic preparatory regime.

Lucarelli and co-workers' (1985a,b) results were more encouraging. Thirty consecutive homozygous β-thalassaemia patients under 8 years of age were transplanted between January 1983 and December 1984 and their progress was evaluated on 1st March 1985. They were prepared for the transplant with busulphan and cyclophosphamide only, and post-transplantation immunosupression was maintained with methotrexate. Three of the first six patients died of transplant-related complications; three survived without evidence of thalassaemia for between 701 and 762 days, respectively. The 24 subsequent patients received slightly less busulphan but the same dose of cyclophosphamide: one child died without evidence of engraftment; 23 children survived, 19 without evidence of thalassaemia, four with thalassaemia reappearing 32–46 days after the transplant. Approximately one-quarter of the children had transient acute GVH disease. Actuarial survival was calculated to be 86%, with disease-free survival 73%. Lucarelli *et al.* concluded that transplantation could be regarded as a realistic therapeutic option; they pointed out that the four children in whom thalassaemia recurred did not seem to be harmed by the attempt at transplantation, all haemopoietic cell lines recovering rapidly and completely.

Shaw, Poynton and Barrett (1985), writing in response to Lucarelli and co-workers' (1985a) report, stated that they had transplanted seven children with thalassaemia major in London, using busulphan and cyclophosphamide as preparatory treatment. All seven achieved stable grafts but four of the children developed CMV infection and three of them died. They warned against transplanting young children who would be particularly sensitive to CMV.

Lucarelli and co-workers' (1987) report was based on the experience of 40 patients with advanced homozygous β-thalassaemia aged between

8 and 15 years. They received HLA-identical allogeneic bone marrow after being treated with busulphan and cyclophosphamide. Thirty of the patients survived the transplant procedure and 28 were alive and free from disease 260–939 days after their transplant; two patients were alive with signs of persistent thalassaemia 372 and 1133 days after transplantation. Ten patients died, three shortly after the transplantation, of cardiac failure, interstitial pneumonia or septicaemia, and five later of acute or chronic GVH disease. Two patients rejected the transplant and died of marrow aplasia. The actuarial probability of grade 2 or higher acute GVH disease in the 32 patients in which the graft was initially successful was 35%. These results are clearly encouraging, and underline the point that bone-marrow transplantation has the potential to provide a really effective treatment for serious cases of thalassaemia. Whether this potential will be realizable in the near future depends upon the finding of effective means of controlling the problems consequent on immunological incompatibility.

OTHER POSSIBLE MEANS OF TREATING THALASSAEMIA

Vitamin C (ascorbic acid)

The effect of ascorbic acid in increasing the output of iron in the urine of iron-loaded patients being treated with desferrioxamine has already been referred to (see p. 552). There is, however, no evidence that administration of the vitamin affects the synthesis of haemoglobin in thalassaemia in any way or the life-span of the erythrocytes.

Vitamin E (α-tocopherol)

There is some evidence that vitamin E may become deficient in β-thalassaemia major, at least in certain populations (Zannos-Mariolea et al., 1974; Vatanavicharn, Yenchitsomas and Siddhikol, 1985). This, it has been suggested, may be due to excessive catabolism of the vitamin mediated by free oxygen radicals (Ley, Griffiths and Nienhuis, 1982).

Rachmilewitz, Shifter and Kahane (1979) gave 750–1000 i.u. of the vitamin to eight transfusion-dependent Kurdish-Jewish patients for an average of 16 months: the serum and erythrocyte levels of the vitamin increased approximately 4 times and in three out of the seven patients erythrocyte survival was increased, although their requirement for transfusion appeared to be unaltered.

Giardini, Cantani and Donfrancesco (1981) gave vitamin E in 300-mg doses daily to 10 children orally and to 20 children parenterally. Erythrocyte malonyldialdehyde (MDA) and vitamin-E concentrations were measured before and after the vitamin was given. No changes were recorded in the children taking the vitamin orally but in those receiving it by injection the concentration of erythrocyte MDA fell and that of vitamin E in the serum and in erythrocytes rose. In the parenterally treated group the intervals between transfusion were reported to be increased.

Ley, Griffiths and Nienhuis, in their 1982 review, recommended that, while further study was required, vitamin E should be administered to thalassaemia patients who were iron-loaded in order to correct possible deficiency of the vitamin and because of its potential to act as a scavenger of free radicals.

5-azacytidine as a possible stimulator of Hb-F formation

As already referred to (p. 268), 5-azacytidine has been administered to patients with Hb-SS disease in an attempt to raise the concentration of circulating Hb F and in this way to alleviate their symptoms. Ley and co-workers (1982) and Nienhuis and co-workers (1985) described how they had tried the drug in three severely affected homozygous β-thalassaemia patients. Each patient responded by a 4–7-fold increase in γ-globin synthesis, which was sufficient in one patient at least to balance the α:non-α globin-synthesis ratio. The reticulocyte count of the first patient treated rose from 5000 to 22 000/μl and total haemoglobin from 8.0 to 10.8 g/dl. Cech and co-workers (1982), too, recorded an interesting response to chemotherapy in a patient who was a compound heterozygote for β-thalassaemia and the Swiss type of heterocellular HPFH. The patient had developed Hodgkin's disease, and following MOPP therapy the percentage of circulating Hb F rose from 4.7 to just over 30 and that of Hb A_2 fell from 4.5 to approximately 2.0.

Nienhuis and co-workers (1985) also tried the effect of hydroxyurea on two of their homozygous β-thalassaemia patients, one of whom had responded to 5-azacytidine. Their haemoglobin level and reticulocyte count were not, however, affected by the hydroxyurea in the doses given and γ-globin synthesis, too, did not appear to be significantly altered.

Whether the use of a cytotoxic immunosuppressive and potentially mutagenic drug in a patient with thalassaemia is justified can be argued (Clegg, Weatherall and Bodmer, 1983; Ley *et al.*, 1983; Heller and DeSimone, 1984). A major difficulty is that experimental treatments can hardly be ethically justified unless the patient is in the last stage of his or her disease. This is, unfortunately, the time when the chances of a favourable outcome, perhaps mainly because of overloading of the myocardium with iron, are very slight indeed.

THALASSAEMIA — FUTURE PROSPECTS

The story of thalassaemia is a remarkable one: it is a story of a disorder, hardly recognized 50 or so years ago, that is now known to be one of the commonest genetically-determined diseases and distributed throughout the world, and remarkable for its clinical severity in homozygotes and compound heterozygotes and remarkable, too, for its molecular heterogeneity. It has proved to be a 'happy hunting ground' for physicians (paediatricians in particular) and haematologists, geneticists and epidemiologists and haemoglobin chemists, and in the last decade particularly, molecular geneticists. Diagnosis can now be precise — the exact lesion in the globin genes responsible for the patient's illness can often be identified. It can be diagnosed, too, in the unborn child, early enough in pregnancy for termination to be offered. For children born with β-thalassaemia major effective palliative treatment can now be provided, but this is expensive and exacting. It is possible, if blood transfusions are given at about 4-weekly intervals and the child's haemoglobin is maintained at a relatively high level (which is not too difficult to do), to convert a severely anaemic and grossly handicapped child into a child who grows normally and leads an almost normal life, only limited by his or her requirement for regular blood transfusions and perhaps daily subcutaneous infusions of an iron chelator such as desferrioxamine. Most children tolerate this rather traumatic regime remarkably well. There is, however, a real need for an iron chelator that can be given by mouth and which is both safe and effective and well tolerated.

Is there any prospect that more radical, even curative, treatments will become available within the next few years? Is bone-marrow transplantation for the severely affected child likely to become a procedure that can be widely applied and will it ever be possible to affect gene expression so as to improve globin-chain synthesis substantially or even to carry out gene transplantation? Within the next decade answers to these questions should be forthcoming. Marx (1980), Anderson (1984) and Williams and Orkin (1986) have summarized in valuable recent reviews current knowledge in relation to the possibilities of the genetic treatment of inherited disorders; they include realistic appraisals of the prospects for, and the ethical problems associated with, gene therapy applied to the human species.

As already referred to, bone-marrow transplantation has been carried out successfully, and judging by the increasing success of transplantation for the haematological malignancies, it should, too, became a safer and surer procedure for children with thalassaemia. As the only radical and potentially fully curative treatment as yet available it seems likely to be more frequently attempted.

In the meanwhile, many of those responsible for the management of children with thalassaemia are thankful for the possibility of diagnosing the major form of the disease *in utero* in an early stage of pregnancy. This is a feeling shared by some at least of the mothers of affected fetuses. According to Modell and her co-workers (1984), the thalassaemia-major birth-rate has fallen in recent years by 60% amongst Cypriots and by 20% amongst East-African Asians (in the United Kingdom); Modell *et al.* stressed, however, the need for better facilities for population screening and more adequate counselling of couples at risk.

REFERENCES

AGHAI, E., SHABBAD, E., QUITT, M. & FROOM, P. (1986). Discrimination between iron deficiency and heterozygous beta-thalassemia in children. *Amer. J. clin. Path.*, **85**, 710–712.

ALEPOROU-MARINOU, V., SAKARELOU-PAPAPETROU, N., ANTSAKLIS, A., FESSAS, PH. & LOUKOPOULOS, D. (1980). Prenatal diagnosis of thalassemia major in Greece: evaluation of the first large series of attempts. *Ann. N.Y. Acad. Sci.*, **344**, 181–188.

ALTER, B. P. (1981). Prenatal diagnosis of haemoglobinopathies: a status report. *Lancet*, **ii**, 1152–1155.

ALTER, B. P. (1983). Antenatal diagnosis using fetal blood. In: *The Thalassemias (Methods in Hematology*, Vol. 6) (ed. by D. J. Weatherall), pp. 114–133. Churchill Livingstone, Edinburgh.

ALTER, B. P. (for the WHO International Registry for Prenatal Monitoring of Hereditary Anemias) (1984). Advances in the prenatal diagnosis of hematologic diseases. *Blood*, **64**, 329–340 (Review).

ALTER, B. P. (for the WHO International Registry for Prenatal Monitoring of Hereditary Anemias) (1985). Antenatal diagnosis of thalassemia: a review. *Ann. N.Y. Acad. Sci.*, **445**, 393–407.

ALTER, B. P., METZGER, J. B. YOCK, P. G., ROTHCHILD, S. B. & DOVER, G. J. (1979). Selective hemolysis of adult red blood cells: an aid to prenatal diagnosis of hemoglobinopathies. *Blood*, **53**, 279–287.

ALTER, B. P., MODELL, C. B., FAIRWAEATHER, D., HOBBINS, J. C., MAHONEY, M. J., FRIGOLETTO, F. D., SHERMAN, A. S. & NATHAN, D. G. (1976). Prenatal diagnosis of hemoglobinopathies. A review of 15 cases. *New Engl. J. Med.*, **295**, 1437–1443.

ALTER, B. P. & ORKIN, S. H. (1980). Prenatal diagnosis of hemoglobinopathies. *Ann. N.Y. Acad. Sci.*, **344**, 151–164.

ANDERSON, W. F. (1984). Prospects for human gene therapy. *Science*, **226**, 401–409.

ANTONARAKIS, S. E., BOEHM. C. D., GIARDINA, P. J. V. & KAZAZIAN, H. H. JNR (1982). Nonrandom association of polymorphic restriction sites in the β-globin gene cluster. *Proc. natn. Acad. Sci. U.S.A.*, **79**, 137–141.

AVANZI, G., BACIGALUPO, A., STRADA, P., MELEVENDI, C., TRAVERSO, T., ADAMI, R., SOLDA, A. M. & REALI, G. (1983). Frozen red blood cell transfusion in patients with Cooley's disease. *Haematologica*, **68**, 646–655.

BARRY, M., FLYNN, D. M., LETSKY, E. A. & RISDON, R. A. (1974). Long-term chelation therapy in thalassaemia major: effect on liver iron concentration, liver histology, and clinical progress. *Brit. med. J.*, **ii**, 16–20.

BEARD, M. E. J., NECHELES, T. F. & ALLEN, D. M. (1967). Intensive transfusion therapy in thalassemia major. *Pediatrics*, **40**, 911–915.

BEARD, M. E. J., NECHELES, T. F. & ALLEN, D. M. (1969). Clinical experience with intensive transfusion therapy in Cooley's anemia. *Ann. N.Y. Acad. Sci.*, **165**, 415–422.

BESSMAN, J. D. & FEINSTEIN, D. I. (1979). Quantitative anisocytosis as a discriminant between iron deficiency and thalassemia minor. *Blood*, **53**, 288–293.

BICKEL, H., GÄUMANN, E., KELLER-SCHIERLEIN, W., PRELOG, V., VISCHER, E., WETTSTEIN, A. & ZÄHNER, G. (1960). Über eisenhaltige Wachstumsfaktoren, die Sideramine, und ihre Antagonisten, die. eisenhaltigen Antibiotika Sideromycine. *Experientia*, **16**, 128–133.

BLENDIS, L. M., MODELL, C. B., BOWDLER, A. J. & WILLIAMS, R. (1974). Some effects of splenectomy in thalassaemia major. *Brit. J. Haemat.*, **28**, 77–87.

BLOUQUIT, Y., BEUZARD, Y., VARNAVIDES, L., CHABRET, C., DUMEZ, Y., JOHN, P. N., RODECK, C. & WHITE, J. M. (1982). Antenatal diagnosis of haemoglobinopathies by Biorex chromatography of haemoglobin. *Brit. J. Haemat.*, **50**, 7–15.

BLUMBERG, B. S., ALTER, H. J., RIDDELL, N. M. & ERLANDSON, M. (1964). Multiple antigenic specificities of serum lipoproteins detected with sera of transfused patients. *Vox Sang.*, **9**, 128–145.

BOEHM, C. D., ANTONARAKIS, S. E., PHILLIP, J. A. III, STRETTON, G. & KAZAZIAN, H. H. (1983). *New Engl. J. Med.*, **308**, 1054–1058.

BORGNA-PIGNATTI, C., ZONTA, L., BONGO, I. & DE STEFANO, P. (1983). Red blood cell indices in adults and children with heterozygous beta-thalassemia. *Haematologica*, **68**, 149–156.

BOURONCLE, B. A. & DOAN, C. A. (1964). Cooley's anemia: indications for splenectomy. *Ann. N.Y. Acad. Sci.*, **119**, 709–721.

BOYER, S. H., NOYES, A. N. & BOYER, M. L. (1976). Enrichment of erythrocytes of fetal origin from adult–fetal blood mixtures via selective hemolysis of adult blood cells: an aid to antenatal diagnosis of hemoglobinopathies. *Blood*, **47**, 883–897.

BOYO, A. *et al.* (WHO Working Group, 14 members) (1983). Community control of hereditary anaemias. *Bull. WHO*, **61**, 63–80.

BROWN, E. B., HWANG, Y.-F. & ALLGOOD, J. W. (1967). Studies of the site of action of deferoxamine. *J. Lab. clin. Med.*, **69**, 382–404.

BRÜCKNER, R., HESS, R., KEBERLE, H., PERICIN, C. & TRIPOD, I. (1967). Tierexperimentelle pathologische Linsenveränderungen nach langdauernder Verabreichung hoher Dosen von Desferal. *Helv. Physiol. Pharmacol. Acta*, **25**, 62–77.

CALLENDER, S. T. & WEATHERALL, D. J. (1980). Iron chelation with oral desferrioxamine. *Lancet*, **ii**, 689 (Letter).

CAO, A., COSSU, P., FALCHI, A. M., MONNI, G.,

PIRASTU, M., ROSATELLI, C., SCALES, M. T. & TUVERI, T. (1985). Antenatal diagnosis of thalassemia major in Sardinia. *Ann. N.Y. Acad. Sci.*, **445**, 380–392.

CAO, A., FURBETTA, A., ANGIUS, A., XIMENES, A., ANGIONI, G. & CAMINITI, F. (1980). Prenatal diagnosis of β thalassemia: experience with 133 cases and the effect of fetal blood sampling on child development. *Ann. N.Y. Acad. Sci.*, **344**, 165–180.

CAO, A., MASERA, G., SIRCHIA, G., GABUTTI, V., MODELL, B. & VULLO, A. (members of the Mediterranean Committee for Thalassemia) (1987). A short guide to the management of thalassemia. In: *Thalassemia Today: the Mediterranean Experience* (ed. by G. Sirchia and A. Zanella), pp. 635–670. Centro Trasfusionale Ospedale Maggiore Policlinico di Milano Editore.

CAPPELLINI, M. D., SAMPIETRO, M. & FIORELLI, G. (1977). Screening for thalassaemia. *Lancet*, i, 1100 (Letter).

CAPRA, L., ATTI, G., DE SANCTIS, V. & CANDINI, G. (1983). Glucose tolerance and chelation therapy in patients with thalassaemia major. *Haematologica*, **68**, 63–68.

CAVILL, I., RICKETTS, C., JACOBS, A. & LETSKY, E. (1978). Erythropoiesis and the effect of transfusion in homozygous beta-thalassemia. *New Engl. J. Med.*, **298**, 776–778.

CAZZAVILLAN, M., BARBUI, T., FRANCHI, F., CHIESI, T. & DINI, E. (1973). Comparison of Price-Jones curves obtained with an electronic corpuscle counter in normal subjects and in patients with thalassaemia and iron deficiency. *Haematologia*, **7**, 333–337.

CECH, P., TESTA, U., DUBART, A., SCHNEIDER, PH., BACHMANN, F., GUERRASIO, A., BEUZARD, Y., SCHMID, P. M., CLÉMENT, F. & ROSA, J. (1982). Lasting Hb F reactivation and Hb A₂ reduction induced by the treatment of Hodgkin's Disease in a woman heterozygous for beta-thalassemia and the Swiss type of heterocellular hereditary persistence of Hb F. *Acta haemat. (Basel)*, **67**, 275–284.

CERAMI, A., GRADY, R. W., PETERSON, C. M. & BHARGAVA, K. K. (1980). The status of the new iron chelators. *Ann. N.Y. Acad. Sci.*, **344**, 425–435.

CHAN, V., GHOSH, A., CHAN, T. K., WONG, V. & TODD, D. (1984). Prenatal diagnosis of homozygous α thalassaemia by direct DNA analysis of uncultured amniotic fluid cells. *Brit. med. J.*, i, 1327–1329.

CHANG, H., HOBBINS, J. C., CIVIDALLI, G., FRIGOLETTO, F. D., MAHONEY, M. J., KAN, Y. W. & NATHAN, D. G. (1974). In utero diagnosis of hemoglobinopathies: hemoglobin synthesis in fetal red cells. *New Engl. J. Med.*, **290**, 1067–1068.

CHINI, V. & VALERI, C. M. (1949). Mediterranean hemopathic syndromes. *Blood*, **4**, 989–1013.

CLEGG, J. B., WEATHERALL, D. J. & BODMER, W. F. (1983). 5-azacytidine for beta-thalassaemia. *Lancet*, i, 536 (Letter).

CLEMENT, D. H. & TAFFEL, M. (1955). Splenectomy in Mediterranean anemia. *Pediatrics*, **16**, 353–362.

COHEN, A., MARTIN, M. & SCHWARTZ, E. (1981). Response to long-term deferoxamine therapy in thalassemia. *J. Pediat.*, **99**, 689–694.

COHEN, A., MARTIN, M. & SCHWARTZ, E. (1984). Depletion of excessive liver iron stores with desferrioxamine. *Brit. J. Haemat.*, **58**, 369–373.

COHEN, A., MIZANIN, J. & SCHWARTZ, E. (1985). Treatment of iron overload in Cooley's anemia. *Ann. N.Y. Acad. Sci.*, **445**, 274–281.

COHEN, A. & SCHWARTZ, E. (1978). Iron chelation therapy with deferoxamine in Cooley anemia. *Pediatrics*, **92**, 643–647.

COHEN, A. & SCHWARTZ, E. (1980). Decreasing iron stores during intensive chelation therapy. *Ann. N.Y. Acad. Sci.*, **344**, 405–417.

CONSTANTOULAKIS, M., ECONOMIDOU, J., KAVAGIORGA, M., KATSANTONI, A. & GYFTAKI, E. (1974), Combined long-term treatment of hemosiderosis with desferrioxamine and DTPA in homozygous β-thalassemia. *Ann. N.Y. Acad. Sci.*, **232**, 193–200.

COOLEY, T. B. (1928). Likenesses and contrasts in the hemolytic anemias of childhood. *Amer. J. Dis. Child.*, **36**, 1257–1262.

CORRERA, A., GRAZIANO, J. H., SEAMAN, C. & PIOMELLI, S. (1984). Inappropriately low red cell 2,3-diphosphoglycerate and p50 in transfused β-thalassemia. *Blood*, **63**, 803–806.

COSSU, G., MANCA, M., PIRASTRU, M. G., BULLITTA, R., BOSISIO, B. A., GIANAZZA, E. & RIGHETTI, P. G. (1982). Neonatal screening of β-thalassemias by thin layer isoelectric focusing. *Amer. J. Hemat.*, **13**, 149–157.

CUMMING, R. L. C., MILLAR, J. A., SMITH, J. A. & GOLDBERG, A. (1969). Clinical and laboratory studies on the action of desferrioxamine. *Brit. J. Haemat.*, **17**, 257–263.

DACIE, J. V. (1954). *The Haemolytic Anaemias*. 525 pp. Churchill, London.

DAFFOS, S., CAPPELLA-PAVLOVSKY, M. & FORESTIER, F. (1983). A new procedure for fetal blood sampling in utero: preliminary results of fifty-three cases. *Amer. J. Obstet. Gynec.*, **146**, 985–986.

DE FURIA, F. G., MILLER, D. R. & CANALE, V. C. (1974). Red blood cell metabolism and function in transfused β-thalassemia. *Ann. N.Y. Acad. Sci.*, **232**, 323–332.

DIWANY, M., GABR, M., EL HEFNI, A. & MOKHTAR, N. (1968). Desferrioxamine in thalassaemia. *Arch. Dis. Childh.*, **43**, 340–343.

DUBART, A., GOOSENS, M., MONTPLAISER, N., TESTA, U., BASSET, P. & ROSA, J. (1980). Prenatal diagnosis of hemoglobinopathies: comparison of the results obtained by isoelectric focusing of hemoglobins and by chromatography of radioactive globin chains. *Blood*, **56**, 1092–1099.

ECONOMIDOU, J., CONSTANTOULAKIS, M., AUGOUSTAKI, O. & ADINOLFI, M. (1971). Frequency of antibodies to various antigenic determinants in polytransfused patients with homozygous thalassaemia in Greece. *Vox Sang.*, **20**, 252–258.

ECONOMIDOU, J., CONSTANTOULAKIS, M., AUGUSTAKI, O., TAYLOR, P. E., ZUCKERMAN, A. J., BAINES, P. M. & BRYCESON, M. A. (1970). The incidence of hepatitis-associated antigen and antibody in patients with thalassaemia in Greece. *Vox Sang.*, **19**, 401–403.

EDRISSIAN, GH. H. (1974). Blood transfusion induced malaria in Iran. *Trans. roy. Soc. trop. Med. Hyg.*, **68**, 491–493.

EL-HAZMI, M. A. F. & LEHMANN, H. (1978). Interaction between iron deficiency and α-thalassaemia: the *in vitro* effect of haemin on α-chain synthesis. *Acta haemat. (Basel)*, **60**, 1–9.

ELLES, R. G., WILLIAMSON, R., NIAZI, M., COLMAN, D. V. & HORWELL, D. (1983). Absence of maternal contamination of chorionic villi used for fetal-gene analysis. *New Engl. J. Med.*, **308**, 1433–1435.

ENGELHARD, D., CIVIDALLI, G. & RACHMILEWITZ, E. A. (1975). Splenectomy in homozygous beta thalassaemia. a retrospective study of 30 patients. *Brit. J. Haemat.*, **31**, 391–403.

ENGLAND, J. M., BAIN, B. J. & FRASER, P. M. (1973). Differentiation of iron deficiency from thalassaemia trait. *Lancet*, i, 1514 (Letter).

ENGLAND, J. M. & DOWN, M. C. (1974). Red-cell-volume distribution curves and the measurement of anisocytosis. *Lancet*, i, 701–703.

ENGLAND, J. M. & FRASER, P. M. (1973). Differentiation of iron deficiency from thalassaemia trait by routine blood-count. *Lancet*, i, 449–452.

FAHEY, J. L., RATH, C. E., PRINCIOTTO, J. V., BRICK, I. B. & RUBIN, M. (1961). Evaluation of trisodium calcium diethylenetriaminepenta-acetate in iron storage disease. *J. Lab. clin. Med.*, **57**, 436–449.

FAIRWEATHER, D. V. I., MODELL, B., BERDOUKAS, V., ALTER, B. P., NATHAN, D. G., LOUKOPOULOS, D., WOOD, W., CLEGG, J. B. & WEATHERALL, D. J. (1978). *Brit. med. J.*, i, 350–353.

FAIRWEATHER, D. V. I., WARD, R. H. T. & MODELL, B. (1980). Obstetric aspects of mid-trimester fetal blood sampling by needling or fetoscopy. *Brit. J. Obstet. Gynaec.*, **87**, 87–99.

FERRARI, M., CREMA, A., CANTÙ-RAJNOLDI, A., PIETRI, S., TRAVI, M., BRAMBATI, B. & OTTOLENGHI, S. (1984). Antenatal diagnosis of haemoglobinopathies by improved method of isoelectric focusing of haemoglobins. *Brit. J. Haemat.*, **57**, 265–270.

FRONTALI, G. & STEGAGNO, G. A. (1951). Durée de vie du globule rouge dans l'anémie Méditerranéenne. *Helv. paediat. Acta*, **6**, 271–280.

FUSCO, F. A., BOURONCLE, B. A. & DOAN, C. A. (1958). Considerazioni su c nque casi di morbo di Cooley e uno di malattia talasso-drepanocitica sottoposti a splenectomia. *Minerva med. (Torino)*, **49**, 185–201.

GABURRO, D., VOLPATO, S. & VIGI, V. (1970). Diagnosis of beta thalassaemia in the newborn by means of haemoglobin synthesis. *Acta paediat. scand.*, **59**, 523–528.

GABUTTI, V., PIGA, A., FORTINA, P., MINIERO, R. & NICOLA, P. (1980). Correlation between transfusion requirement, blood volume and haemoglobin level in homozygous β-thalassaemia. *Acta haemat. (Basel)*, **64**, 103–108.

GATTO, I. & LO JACONO, F. (1953). Ulteriori ricerche sugli effetti a distanza della splenectomia nella malattia di Cooley. *Pediatria (Napoli)*, **61**, 27–39.

GEVIRTZ, N. R., TENDLER, D., LURINSKY, G. & WASSERMAN, L. R. (1965). Clinical studies of storage iron with desferrioxamine. *New Engl. J. Med.*, **273**, 95–97.

GIARDINA, P. J. V., EHLERS, K. H., ENGLE, M. A., GRADY, R. W. & HILGARTNER, M. W. (1985). The effect of subcutaneous deferoxamine on the cardiac profile of thalassemia major: a five-year study. *Ann. N.Y. Acad. Sci.*, **445**, 282–292.

GIARDINI, O., CANTANI, A. & DONFRANCESCO, A. (1981). Vitamin E therapy in homozygous β-thalassemia. *New Engl. J. Med.*, **305**, 644 (Letter).

GIMFERRER, E., MARIGO, G., RUTLLANT, M. L. & VIÑAS, J. (1975). Differentiation of iron deficiency from thalassaemia trait. *Lancet*, i, 114 (Letter).

GLENN, F., CORNELL, G. N., SMITH, C. H. & SCHULMAN, I. (1954). Splenectomy in children with idiopathic thrombocytopenic purpura, hereditary spherocytosis, and Mediterranean anemia. *Surg. Gynec. Obstet.*, **99**, 689–702.

GOUTTAS, A., FESSAS, PH., TSEVRENIS, H. & XEFTERI, E. (1955). Description d'une nouvelle varieté d'anémie hémolytique congénitale (Etude hématologique, électrophorétique et génétique). *Sang*, **26**, 911–919.

GOVAN, C. D. (1946). Erythroblastic anemia of Cooley. Observations on the effect of splenectomy performed on identical twins. *J. Pediat.*, **29**, 504–511.

GRADY, R. W., GRAZIANO, J. H., AKERS, H. & CERAMI, A. (1974). The identification of rhodotorulic acid as a potentially useful iron-chelating drug. *Blood*, **44**, 911 (Abstract).

GRAZIANO, J. H., MARKENSON, A., MILLER, D. R., CHANG, H., BESTAK, M., MEYERS, P., PISCIOTTO, P. & RIFKIND, A. (1978). Chelation therapy in β-thalassemia major. I. Intravenous and subcutaneous deferoxamine. *J. Pediat.*, **92**, 648–652.

GRAZIANO, J. H., PETERSON, C. M., GRADY, R. W., JONES, R. L., DE CIUTIS, A., CANALE, V. C., MILLER, D. R. & CERAMI, A. (1975). Clinical evaluation of 2,3-dihydroxybenzoic acid as an oral iron-chelating drug in β-thalassemia major. *Ped. Res.*, **9**, 322 (Abstract 391).

GRAZIANO, J. H., PIOMELLI, S., HILGARTNER, M., GIARDINA, P., KARPATKIN, M., ANDREW, M., LOLACONO, N. & SEAMAN, C. (1981). Chelation therapy in β-thalassemia major. III. The role of splenectomy in achieving iron balance. *J. Pediat.*, **99**, 695–699.

GREEN, R., LAMON, J. & CURRAN, D. (1980). Clinical trial of desferrioxamine entrapped in red cell ghosts. *Lancet*, **ii**, 327–330.

GREEN, R., MILLER, J. & CROSBY, W. (1981). Enhancement of iron chelation by desferrioxamine entrapped in red blood cell ghosts. *Blood.* **57**, 866–872.

GREPPI, E. & DI GUGLIELMO, R. (1955). Résultats de la splénectomie dans deux cas de thalassaemia minor. *Sang*, **26**, 242–244.

HALLBERG, L. & HEDENBERG, L. (1965). The effect of desferrioxamine on iron metabolism in man. *Scand. J. Haemat.*, **2**, 67–79.

HAMBLIN, T. J. (1973). Differentiation of iron deficiency from thalassaemia trait. *Lancet*, **ii**, 455 (Letter).

HAMILTON, H. E., SHEETS, R. F. & DeGOWIN, E. L. (1950). Studies with inagglutinable counts. II. Analysis of mechanism of Cooley's anemia. *J. clin. Invest.*, **29**, 714–722.

HARKER, L. A., FUNK, D. A. & FINCH, C. A. (1968). Evaluation of storage iron by chelates. *Amer. J. Med.*, **45**, 105–115.

HEGDE, U. M., WHITE, J. M., HART, G. H. & MARSH, G. W. (1977). Diagnosis of α-thalassaemia trait from Coulter Counter 'S' indices. *J. clin. Path.*, **30**, 884–889.

HEILMEYER, L. & WÖHLER, F. (1963). The treatment of haemochromatosis with desferrioxamine. *Germ. med. Monthly.*, **8**, 133–136.

HELLER, P. & DeSIMONE, J. (1984). 5-Acacytidine and fetal hemoglobin. *Amer. J. Hemat.*, **17**, 439–447.

HENRY, W. (1979). Echocardiographic evaluation of the heart in thalassemia major. In: Nienhuis, A. W. (Moderator). Thalassemia major: molecular and clinical aspects (NIH Conference). *Ann. intern. Med.*, **91**, 892–894.

HERSHKO, C. (1978). Determinants of fecal and urinary iron excretion in desferrioxamine-treated rats. *Blood*, **51**, 415–423.

HERSHKO, C., COOK, J. D. & FINCH, C. A. (1973). Storage iron kinetics. III. Study of desferrioxamine action by selective radioiron labels of RE and parenchymal cells. *J. Lab. clin. Med.*, **81**, 876–886.

HERSHKO, C., GRAHAM, G., BATES, G. W. & RACHMILEWITZ, E. A. (1978). Non-specific serum iron in thalassaemia: an abnormal serum iron fraction of potential toxicity. *Brit. J. Haemat.*, **40**, 255–263.

HERSHKO, C. & RACHMILEWITZ, E. A. (1978). Iron chelation in thalassemia: mechanism of desferrioxamine action. *Israel J. med. Sci.*, **14**, 1111–1115.

HIGGS, D. R., LAMB, J., ALDRIDGE, B. E., CLEGG, J. B., WEATHERALL, D. J., SERJEANT, B. E. &
SERJEANT, G. R. (1982). Inadequacy of Hb Bart's as an indicator of α thalassaemia. *Brit. J. Haemat.*, **51**, 177–178.

HIGGS, D. R., PRESSLEY, L., CLEGG, J. B., WEATHERALL, D. J., HIGGS, S., CAREY, P. & SERJEANT, G. R. (1980). Detection of alpha thalassaemia in negro infants. *Brit. J. Haemat.*, **46**, 39–46.

HIRSH, J. & DACIE, J. V. (1966). Persistent post-splenectomy thrombocytosis and thrombo-embolism: a consequence of continuing anaemia. *Brit. J. Haemat.*, **12**, 44–53.

HOBBINS, J. C. & MAHONEY, M. J. (1974). In utero diagnosis of hemoglobinopathies. Technic for obtaining fetal blood. *New Engl. J. Med.*, **290**, 1065–1067.

HOFFBRAND, A. V., GORMAN, A., LAULICHT, M., GARIDI, M., ECONOMIDOU, J., GEORGIPOULOU, P., HUSSAIN, M. A. M. & FLYNN, D. M. (1979). Improvement in iron status and liver function in patients with transfusional iron overload with long-term subcutaneous desferrioxamine. *Lancet*, **i**, 947–949.

HOGAN, V. A., BLANCHETTE, V. S. & ROCK, G. (1986). A simple method for preparing neocyte-enriched leukocyte-poor blood for transfusion-dependent patients. *Transfusion*, **26**, 253–257.

HOLLENBERG, M. D., KABACK, M. M. & KAZAZIAN, H. H. JNR, (1971). Adult hemoglobin synthesis by reticulocytes from the human fetus at midtrimester. *Science*, **174**, 698–702.

HUSSAIN, M. A. M., FLYNN, D. M., GREEN, N. & HOFFBRAND, A. V. (1977). Effect of dose, time and ascorbate on iron excretion after subcutaneous desferrioxamine. *Lancet*, **i**, 977–979.

HUSSAIN, M. A. M., FLYNN, D. M., GREEN, N., HUSSEIN, S. & HOFFBRAND, A. V. (1976). Subcutaneous infusion and intramuscular injection of desferrioxamine in patients with iron overload. *Lancet*, **ii**, 1278–1280.

HYMAN, C. B., AGNESS, C. L., RODRIGUEZ-FUNES, R. & ZEDNIKOVA, M. (1985). Combined subcutaneous and high-dose intravenous deferoxamine therapy of thalassemia. *Ann. N.Y. Acad. Sci.*, **445**, 293–303.

JACOBS, A. (1979). Iron chelation therapy for iron loaded patients. *Brit. J. Haemat.*, **43**, 1–5 (Annotation).

JOHNSON, C. S., TEGOS, C. & BEUTLER, E. (1983). Thalassemia minor: routine erythrocyte measurements and differentiation from iron deficiency. *Amer. J. clin. Path.*, **80**, 31–36.

JOISHY, S. K. & LOPEZ, C. G. (1980). Transfusion-induced malaria in a splenectomized β-thalassemia major patient and review of blood donor screening methods. *Amer. J. Hemat.*, **8**, 221–229.

JOISHY, S. K., SHAFER, J. A. & ROWLEY, P. T. (1986). The contribution of red cell morphology to the diagnosis of beta-thalassemia trait. *Blood Cells*, **11**, 367–371.

KAN, Y. K. (1977). Prenatal diagnosis of hemoglobin disorders. In: *Progress in Hematology*, Vol. X (ed. by E. B. Brown), pp. 91–104. Grune and Stratton, New York.

KAN, Y. W., GOLBUS, M. S., TRECARTIN, R. F., FILLY, R. A., VALENTI, C., FURBETTA, M. & CAO, A. (1977). Prenatal diagnosis of β-thalassaemia and sickle-cell anaemia. Experience with 24 cases. *Lancet*, i, 269–271.

KAN, Y. W., LEE, K. Y., FURBETTA, M., ANGIUS, A. & CAO, A. (1980). Polymorphism of DNA sequence in the β-globin gene region: application to prenatal diagnosis of β⁰ thalassaemia in Sardinia. *New Engl. J. Med.*, 302, 185–188.

KAN, Y. W. & NATHAN, D. G. (1968). Beta thalassemia trait: detection at birth. *Science*, 161, 589–590.

KAN, Y. K., NATHAN, D. G., CIVIDALLI, G. & FRIGOLETTO, F. (1974a). Intrauterine diagnosis of thalassemia. *Ann. N.Y. Acad. Sci.*, 232, 145–151.

KAN, Y. W., TRECARTIN, R. F. & DOZY, A. M. (1980). Prenatal diagnosis of hemoglobinopathies. *Ann. N.Y. Acad. Sci.*, 334, 141–150.

KAN, Y. W., VALENTI, C., GUIDOTTI, R., CARNAZZA, V. & RIEDER, R. F. (1974b). Fetal blood sampling in utero. *Lancet*, i, 79–80.

KARABUS, C. D. & FIELDING, J. (1967). Desferrioxamine chelatable iron in haemolytic, megaloblastic and sideroblastic anaemias. *Brit. J. Haemat.*, 13, 924–933.

KARPATHIOS, TH., ANTYPAS, A., DIMITRIOU, P., NICOLAIDOU, P., FRETZAYAS, A., THOMAIDIS, TH. & MATSANIOTIS, N. (1982). Spleen size changes in children with homozygous β-thalassaemia in relation to blood transfusion. *Scand. J. Haemat.*, 28, 220–226.

KATTAMIS, C., EFREMOV, G. & POOTRAKUL, S. (1981). Effectiveness of one tube osmotic fragility screening in detecting β-thalassaemia trait. *J. med. Genet.*, 18, 266–270.

KATTAMIS, C., MALLIAS, A., METAXOTOU-MAVROMATI, A. & MATSANIOTIS, N. (1981). Screening for beta-thalassaemias. *Lancet*, ii, 930 (Letter).

KATTAMIS, C., SYRIOPOULOU, V., DAVRI-KARAMOUZI, Y., DEMETRIOU, D. & MATSANIOTIS, N. (1974). Prevalence of Au-Ag and Au-Ab in transfused children with thalassaemia in Greece. *Arch. Dis. Childh.*, 49, 450–453.

KATTAMIS, C., TOULIATIS, N., HAIDAS, S. & MATSANIOTIS, N. (1970). Growth of children with thalassaemia: effect of different transfusion regimes. *Arch. Dis. Childh.*, 45, 502–505.

KAZAZIAN, H. H. JNR, BOEHM, C. D. & DOWLING, C. E. (1985). Prenatal diagnosis of hemoglobinopathies by DNA analysis. *Ann. N.Y. Acad. Sci.*, 445, 337–348.

KAZAZIAN, H. H. JNR, PHILLIPS, J. A. III, BOEHM, C. D., VIK, T. A., MAHONEY, M. J. & RITCHES, A. K. (1980). Prenatal diagnosis of β-thalassaemias by amniocentesis: linkage analysis using multiple polymorphic restriction endonuclease sites. *Blood*, 56, 926–930.

KIRIMLIDIS, ST., PHILIPPIDIS, PH., DROSSOS, CH., & ECONOMIDIS, J. (1966). The treatment of hemosiderosis in thalassaemia major with desferrioximine-B. *Helv. paediat. Acta*, 21, 343–350.

KLEE, G. G., FAIRBANKS, V. F., PIERRE, R. V. & O'SULLIVAN, M. B. (1976). Routine erythrocyte measurements in diagnosis of iron-deficiency anemia and thalassemia minor. *Amer. J. clin. Path.*, 66, 870–877.

KOENIG, H. M., VEDVICK, T. S., DOZY, A. M., GOLBUS, M. S. & KAN, Y. W. (1978). Prenatal diagnosis of hemoglobin H disease. *J. Pediat.*, 92, 278–281.

LETSKY, E. A. (1976). A controlled trial of long-term chelation therapy in homozygous β-thalassaemia. *Birth Defects*, 12, 31–41.

LETSKY, E. A., MILLER, E., WORWOOD, M. & FLYNN, D. M. (1974). Serum ferritin in children with thalassaemia regularly transfused. *J. clin. Path.*, 27, 652–655.

LEY, T. J., ANAGNOU, N. P., YOUNG, N. S., NIENHUIS, A. W., DESIMONE, J. & HELLER, P. (1983). 5-Azacytidine for beta-thalassaemia? *Lancet*. i, 467 (Letter).

LEY, T. J., DESIMONE, J., ANAGNOU, N. P., KELLER, G. H., HUMPHRIES, R. K., TURNER, P. T., YOUNG, N. S., HELLER, P. & NIENHUIS, A. W. (1982). 5-azacytidine selectively increases γ-globin synthesis in a patient with β⁺-thalassaemia. *New Engl. J. Med.*, 307, 1469–1475.

LEY, T. J., GRIFFITHS, P. & NIENHUIS, A. W. (1982). Transfusion haemosiderosis and chelation therapy. *Clinics Haemat.*, 11, 437–464.

LICHTMAN, H. C., WATSON, R. J., FELDMAN, F., GINSBERG, V. & ROBINSON, J. (1953). Studies in thalassemia. Part I. An extracorpuscular defect in thalassemia major. Part II. The effects of splenectomy in thalassemia major with an associated acquired hemolytic anemia. *J. clin. Invest.*, 32, 1229–1235.

LIE-INJO, L. E., SOLAI, A., HERRERA, A. R., NICOLAISEN, L., KAN, Y. W., WAN, W. P. & HASAN, K. (1982). Hb Bart's level in cord blood and deletions of α-globin genes. *Blood*, 59, 370–376.

LIE-INJO, L. E., TJOA, G. T. & KHO, L. K. (1961). Splenectomy in a case of chronic haemolytic anaemia associated with haemoglobin H. *J. trop. Med. Hyg.*, 64, 136–139.

LIPSCHITZ, D. A., DUGARD, J., SIMON, M. O., BOTHWELL, T. H. & CHARLTON, R. W. (1971). The site of action of desferrioxamine. *Brit. J. Haemat.*, 20, 395–404.

LITTLE, P. F. R., ANNISON, G., DARLING, S., WILLIAMSON, R., CAMBA, L. & MODELL, B. (1980). Model for antenatal diagnosis of β-thalassaemia and other monogenic disorders by molecular analysis of linked DNA polymorphisms. *Nature (Lond.)*, **285**, 144–147.

LOUKOPOULOS, D. (1985). Prenatal diagnosis of thalassemia and of the hemoglobinopathies; a review. *Hemoglobin*, **9**, 435–459.

LOUKOPOULOS, D., KARABABA, P., ANTSAKLIS, A., PANOURGIAS, J., BOUSSIOU, M., KARAYANNOPOULOS, K., POLITIS, J., ROMBOU, D., KALTSOYA-TASSIOPOULOU, A. & FESSAS, PH. (1985). Prenatal diagnosis of thalassemia and Hb S syndromes in Greece: an evaluation of 1500 cases. *Ann. N.Y. Acad. Sci.*, **445**, 357–375.

LUCARELLI, G., GALIMBERTI, M., POLCHI, P., GAIRDINI, C., POLITI, P., BARONCIANI, D., ANGELUCCI, E., MANENTI, F., DELFINI, C., AURELI, G. & MURETTO, P. (1987). Marrow transplantation in patients with advanced thalassemia. *New Engl. J. Med.*, **316**, 1050–1055.

LUCARELLI, G., POLCHI, P., GALIMBERTI, M., IZZI, T., DELFINI, C., MANNA, M., AGOSTINELLI, F., BARONCIANI, D., GIOGI, C., ANGELUCCI, E., GIARDINI, C., POLITI, P. & MANENTI, F. (1985a). Marrow transplantation for thalassaemia following busulphan and cyclophosphamide. *Lancet*, **i**, 1355–1357.

LUCARELLI, G., POLCHI, P., IZZI, T., MANNA, M., AGOSTINELLI, F., DELFINI, C., PORCELLINI, A., GALIMBERTI, M., MORETTI, L., MANNA, A., SPARAVENTI, G., BARONCIANI, D., PROIETTI, A. & BUCKNER, C. D. (1984). Allogeneic marrow transplantation for thalassemia. *Expl Hemat.*, **12**, 676–681.

LUCARELLI, G., POLCHI, P., IZZI, T., MANNA, M., DELFINI, C., GALIMBERTI, M., PORCELLINI, A., MORETTI, L., MANNA, A. & SPARAVENTI, G. (1985b). Marrow transplantation for thalassaemia after treatment with busulfan and cyclophosphamide. *Ann. N.Y. Acad. Sci.*, **445**, 428–431.

MCDONALD, R. (1966). Deferoxamine and diethylenetriaminepentaacetic acid (DTPA) in thalassemia. *J. Pediat.*, **69**, 563–571.

MCPHEDRAN, P., WEINSTEIN, J., BARNES, M. G. & GELOSO, G. (1973). Mass screening for the detention of β-thalassemia trait. *Ann. intern. Med.*, **78**, 823 (Abstract).

MAGGIO, A. & CASTELLANO, S. (1984). Antenatal diagnosis of β thalassemia. *Brit. J. Haemat.*, **58**, 202–203 (Letter).

MAINZER, R. A. & O'CONNOR, W. J. (1958). Evaluation of splenectomy in the treatment of Cooley's anemia. *Ann. Surg.*, **148**, 44–50.

MALAMOS, B., FESSAS, PH. & STAMATOYANNOPOULOS, G. (1962). Types of thalassaemia-trait carriers as revealed by a study of their incidence in Greece. *Brit. J. Haemat.*, **8**, 5–14.

MANCA, M., COSSU, G., ANGIONI, G., GIGLIOTTI, B., BOSISIO, A. B., GIANAZZA, E. & RIGHETTI, P. G. (1986). Antenatal diagnosis of β-thalassemia by isoelectric focusing in immobolized pH gradients. *Amer. J. Hemat.*, **22**, 285–293.

MARCUS, R. E., DAVIES, S. C., BANTOCK, H. M., UNDERWOOD, S. R., WALTON, S. & HUEHNS, E. R. (1984). Desferrioxamine to improve cardiac function in iron-overloaded patients with thalassaemia major. *Lancet*, **i**, 392–393 (Letter).

MARCUS, R. E., WONKE, B., BANTOCK, H. M., THOMAS, M. J. G., PARRY, E. S., TAITE, H. & HUEHNS, E. R. (1985). A prospective trial of young red cells in 48 patients with transfusion-dependent thalassaemia. *Brit. J. Haemat.*, **60**, 153–159.

MARX, J. L. (1980). Gene transfer moves ahead. *Science*, **210**, 1334–1336 (Research News).

MASERA, G., TERZOLI, A., AVANZINI, A., FONTANELLI, G., MAURI, R. A., PIACENTINI, G. & FERRARI, M. (1982). Evaluation of the supertransfusion regimen in homozygous beta-thalassaemia children. *Brit. J. Haemat.*, **52**, 111–113.

MATSAKIS, M., BERDOUKAS, V. A., ANGASTINIOTIS, M., MOUZOURAS, M., IOANNOU, P., FERRARI, M., MODELL, B., FAIRWEATHER, D. V. I., WARD, R. H. T., LOUKOPOULOS, D. & SAKARELLOU, N. (1980). Haematological aspects of antenatal diagnosis for thalassaemia in Britain. *Brit. J. Haemat.*, **46**, 185–197.

MELIS, M. A., ROSATELLI, C., FALCHI, A. M., ANGIUS, A., FURBETTA, M., GALANELLO, R. & CAO, A. (1980). Hematological characteristics of Sardinian α-thalassaemia carriers detected in a population study. *Acta haemat. (Basel)*, **63**, 32–36.

MENTZER, W. C. JNR (1973). Differentiation of iron deficiency from thalassaemia trait. *Lancet*, **i**, 882 (Letter).

MIBASHAN, R. S., RODECK, C. H., NICOLAIDES, K. H., WARREN, R., OLD, J. M. & WEATHERALL, D. J. (1985). Antenatal diagnosis of inherited blood disorders. *8th Congr. Europ. Afric. Div. int. Soc. Haemat.*, *Sept. 1985, Warsaw* (Plenary lecture).

MINNICH, V., NA-NAKORN, S., TUCHINDA, S., PRAVIT, W. & MOORE, C. V. (1958). Inclusion body anemia in Thailand (hemoglobin H-thalassemia disease). *Proc. 6th Congr. int. Soc. Hemat.*, *Boston* (Aug. 27 — Sept 1, 1956), pp. 743–747. Grune and Stratton, New York.

MODELL, B. (1976). Management of thalassaemia major. *Brit. med. Bull.*, **32**, 270–276.

MODELL, B. (1977). Total management of thalassaemia major. *Arch. Dis. Childh.*, **52**, 489–500.

MODELL, B. (1979). Advances in the use of iron-chelating agents for the treatment of iron overload. In: *Progress in Hematology*, Vol. XI (ed. by E. B. Brown), pp. 267–312. Grune and Stratton, New York.

MODELL, C. B. & BECK, J. (1974). Long-term desferrioxamine therapy in thalassemia. *Ann. N.Y. Acad., Sci.*, **232**, 201–210.

MODELL, B. & BERDOUKAS, V. (1984). *The Clinical Approach to Thalassaemia.* 453 pp. Grune and Stratton, London.

MODELL, B., LETSKY, E. A., FLYNN, D. M., PETO, R. & WEATHERALL, D. J. (1982). Survival and desferrioxamine in thalassaemia major. *Brit. med. J.*, i, 1081–1084.

MODELL, B., PETROU, M., WARD, R. H. T., FAIRWEATHER, D. V. I., RODECK, C., VARNAVIDES, L. A. & WHITE, J. M. (1984). Effect of fetal diagnostic testing on birth-rate of thalassaemia major in Britain. *Lancet*, ii, 1383–1387.

MOZZI, F., VIANELLO, L., ZANELLA, A., ZANETTI, A. & SIRCHIA, G. (1987). Anti-HIV antibodies screening in blood donors and multitransfused patients. In: *Thalassemia Today: the Mediterranen Experience* (ed. by G. Sirchia and A. Zanella), pp. 575–579. Centro Trasfusionale Ospedale Maggiore Policlinico di Milano Editore.

MULLER-EBERHARD, U., ERLANDSON, M. E., GINN, H. E. & SMITH, C. H. (1963). Effect of trisodium calcium diethylenetriaminepentaacetate on bivalent cations in thalassemia major. *Blood*, 23, 209–217.

NECHELES, T. F., CHUNG, S., SABBAH, R. & WHITTEN, D. (1974). Intensive transfusion therapy in thalassemia major: an eight-year follow-up. *Ann. N.Y. Acad. Sci.*, 232, 179–185.

NIAZI, M., COLEMAN, D. V. & LOEFFLER, F. R. (1981). Trophoblast sampling in early pregnancy. Culture of rapidly dividing cells from immature placental villi. *Brit. J. Obstet., Gynaec.*, 88, 1081–1085.

The NICHD National Registry for Amniocentesis Study Group (1976). Midtrimester amniocentesis for prenatal diagnosis: safety and accuracy. *J. Amer. med. Ass.*, 236, 1471–1476.

NICOLAIDES, K. H., RODECK, C. H. & MIBASHAN, R. S. (1985). Obstetric management and diagnosis of haematological disease in the fetus. *Clinics Haemat.*, 14, 775–805.

NIENHUIS, A. W. (1981). Vitamin C and iron. *New Engl. J. Med.*, 304, 170–171.

NIENHUIS, A. W., GRIFFITH P., STRAWCZYNSKI, H., HENRY, W., BORER, J., LEON, M. & ANDERSON, W. F. (1980). Evaluation of cardiac function in patients with thalassemia major. *Ann. N.Y. Acad. Sci.*, 334, 384–395.

NIENHUIS, A. W., LEY, T. J., HUMPHRIES, R. K., YOUNG, N. S. & DOVER, G. (1985). Pharmacological manipulation of fetal hemoglobin synthesis in patients with severe β-thalassemia. *Ann. N.Y. Acad. Sci.*, 445, 198–211.

O'BRIEN, R. T. (1974). Ascorbic acid enhancement of desferrioxamine-induced urinary iron excretion in thalassemia major. *Ann. N.Y. Acad. Sci.*, 232, 211–225.

O'BRIEN, R. T., PEARSON, H. A. & SPENCER, R. P. (1972). Transfusion-induced decrease in spleen size in thalassemia major: documentation by radioisotopic scan. *J. Pediat.*, 81, 105–107.

OHENE-FREMPONG, K., RAPPAPORT, E., ATWATER, J., SCHWARTZ, E. & SURREY, S. (1980). Alpha-gene deletions in black newborn infants with Hb Bart's. *Blood*, 56, 931–933.

OHLSSON, W. T. L., KULLENDORFF, G. T. & LJUNGBERG, L. K. (1953). Transfusion hemosiderosis. Report of a case treated with BAL. *Acta med. scand.*, 145, 410–418.

OKON, E., LEVIJ, I. S. & RACHMILEWITZ, E. A. (1976). Splenectomy, iron overload and liver cirrhosis in β-thalassemia major. *Acta haemat. (Basel)*, 56, 142–150.

OLD, J. M., FITCHES, A., HEATH, C., THEIN, S. L., WEATHERALL, D. J., WARREN, R., McKENZIE, C., RODECK, C. H., MODELL, B., PETROU, M. & WARD, R. H. T. (1986). First-trimester fetal diagnosis for haemoglobinopathies: report on 200 cases. *Lancet*, ii, 763–767.

OLD, J. M. & HIGGS, D. R. (1983). Gene analysis. In: *The Thalassemias (Methods in Hematology)*, Vol. 6 (ed. by D. J. Weatherall), pp. 74–102. Churchill Livingstone, Edinburgh.

OLD, J. M., PETROU, M., MODELL, B. & WEATHERALL, D. J. (1984). Feasibility of antenatal diagnosis of thalassaemia by DNA polymorphisms in Asian Indian and Cypriot populations. *Brit. J. Haemat.*, 57, 255–263.

OLD, J. M., WARD, R. H. T., PETROU, M., KARAGÖZLÜ, F., MODELL, B. & WEATHERALL, D. J. (1982). First-trimester fetal diagnosis for haemoglobinopathies: three cases. *Lancet*, ii, 1413–1416.

ORKIN, S. H. (1984). Prenatal diagnosis of hemoglobin disorders by DNA analysis. *Blood*, 63, 249–253 (Brief review).

ORKIN, S. H., ALTER, B. P., ALTAY, C., MAHONEY, M. J., LAZARUS, H., HOBBINS, J. C. & NATHAN, D. G. (1978). Application of endonuclease mapping to the analysis and prenatal diagnosis of thalassemias caused by globin-gene deletion. *New Engl. J. Med.*, 299, 166–172.

ORKIN, S. H., ANTONARAKIS, S. E. & KAZAZIAN, H. H. JNR (1983). Polymorphism and molecular pathology of the human beta-globin gene. In: *Progress in Hematology*, Vol. XIII (ed. by E. B. Brown), pp. 49–73. Grune and Stratton, New York.

ORKIN, S. H., KAZAZIAN, H. H. JNR, ANTONARAKIS, S. E., GOFF, S. C., BOEHM, C. D., SEXTON, J. P., WABER, P. G. & GIARDINA, P. J. V. (1982). Linkage of β-thalassaemia mutations and β-globin gene polymorphisms with DNA polymorphisms in human β-globin gene cluster. *Nature (Lond.)*, 296, 627–631.

ORKIN, S. H., MARKHAM, A. F. & KAZAZIAN, H. H. JNR (1983). Direct detection of the common Mediterranean β-thalassemia gene with synthetic

DNA probes: an alternative approach for prenatal diagnosis. *J. clin. Invest.*, **71**, 775–779.

PEARSON, H. A., MCPHEDRAN, P., O'BRIEN, R. T., ASPNES, G. T., MCINTOSH, S. & GUILIOTIS, D. K. (1974). Comprehensive testing for thalassemia trait. *Ann. N.Y. Acad., Sci.*, **232**, 135–144.

PEARSON, H. A. & O'BRIEN, R. T. (1975). The management of thalassemia major. *Seminars Hemat.*, **12**, 255–265.

PEARSON, H. A., O'BREIN, R. T. & MCINTOSH, S. (1973). Screening for thalassemia trait by electronic measurement of mean corpuscular volume. *New Engl. J. Med.*, **288**, 351–353.

PENBERTHY, G. C. & COOLEY, T. B. (1935). Results of splenectomy in childhood. *Ann. Surg.*, **102**, 645–655.

PETERSON, C. M., GRAZIANO, J. H., GRADY, R. W., JONES, R. L., VLASSARA, H. V., CANALE, V. C., MILLAR, D. R. & CERAMI, A. (1976). Chelation studies with 2,3-dihydroxybenzoic acid in patients with β-thalassaemia major. *Brit. J. Haemat.*, **33**, 477–485.

PIOMELLI, S., DANOFF, S. T., BEDER, M. H., LIPERA, M. J. & TRAVIS, S. F. (1969). Prevention of bone malformations and cardiomegaly in Cooley's anemia by early hypertransfusion regimen. *Ann. N.Y. Acad. Sci.*, **165**, 427–436.

PIOMELLI, S., GRAZIANO, J., KARPATKIN, M., DUDELL, G. G., HART, D., HILGARTNER, M., KHANNA, K., VALDES-CRUZ, L. M. & VORA, S. (1980). Chelation therapy, transfusion requirement, and iron balance in young thalassemic patients. *Ann. N.Y. Acad. Sci.*, **334**, 409–417.

PIOMELLI, S., HART, D., GRAZIANO, J., GRANT, G., KARPATKIN, M. & MCCARTHY, K. (1985). Current strategies in the management of Cooley's anemia. *Ann. N.Y. Acad. Sci.*, **445**, 256–267.

PIOMELLI, S., KARPATKEIN, M. H., ARZANIAN, M., ZAMANI, M., BECKER, M. H., GENEISER, N., DANOFF, S. J. & KUHNS, W. J. (1974). Hypertransfusion regimen in patients with Cooley's anemia. *Ann. N.Y. Acad. Sci.*, **232**, 186–192.

PIPPARD, M. J. & CALLENDER, S. T. (1983). The management of iron chelation therapy. *Brit. J. Haemat.*, **54**, 503–507 (Clinical annotation).

PIPPARD, M. J., CALLENDER, S. T. & FINCH, C. A. (1982). Ferrioxamine excretion in iron-loaded man. *Blood*, **60**, 288–294.

PIPPARD, M. J., CALLENDER, S. T. & WEATHERALL, D. J. (1978). Intensive iron-chelation therapy with desferrioxamine in iron-loading anaemias. *Clin. Sci. mol. Med.*, **54**, 99–106.

PIPPARD, M. J., JACKSON, M. J., HOFFMAN, K., PETROU, M. & MODELL, C. B. (1986). Iron chelation using subcutaneous infusions of diethylene triamine penta-acetic acid (DTPA). *Scand. J. Haemat.*, **36**, 466–472.

PIPPARD, M. J., LETSKY, E. A., CALLENDER, S. T. & WEATHERALL, D. J. (1978). Prevention of iron

loading in transfusion-dependent thalassaemia. *Lancet*, i, 1178–1181.

PIRASTU, M., KAN, Y. W., CAO, A., CONNER, B. J., TEPLITZ, R. L. & WALLACE, R. B. (1983). Prenatal diagnosis of β-thalassaemia: detection of a single nucleotide mutation in DNA. *New Engl. J. Med.*, **309**, 284–287.

POLLACK, S., AISEN, P., LASKY, F. D. & VANDERHOFF, G. (1976). Chelate mediated transfer of iron from transferrin to desferrioxamine. *Brit. J. Haemat.*, **34**, 231–235.

POSTERARO, A. JNR & GOTTFRIED, E. L. (1978). The diagnostic significance of a prolonged erythrocytic glycerol lysis time (GLT_{50}). *Amer. J. clin. Path.*, **70**, 637–641.

PROPPER, R. D. (1980). Current concepts in the overall management of thalassemia. *Ann. N.Y. Acad. Sci.*, **334**, 375–383.

PROPPER, R. D., BUTTON, L. N. & NATHAN, D. G. (1980). New approaches to the transfusion management of thalassemia. *Blood*, **55**, 55–60.

PROPPER, R. D., CLARKE, D. & NATHAN, D. G. (1982). Cooley's anemia: the effect of supertransfusion and nightly subcutaneous Desferal (DF) on the development of cardiac disease (CD). *Blood*, **60** (Suppl. 1), 57a (Abstract 156).

PROPPER, R. D., COOPER, B., RUFO, R. R., NIENHUIS, A. W., ANDERSON, W. F., BUNN, H. F., ROSENTHAL, A. & NATHAN, D. G. (1977). Continuous subcutaneous administration of deferoxamine in patients with iron overload. *New Engl. J. Med.*, **297**, 418–423.

PROPPER, R. D., NATHAN, D. G., COOPER, B., RUFO, R. R., NIENHUIS, A. W. & ANDERSON, W. F. (1976). Continuous subcutaneous (SC) infusion of desferrioxamine (DF) in patients with iron(Fe) overload. *Blood*, **48**, 964 (Abstract).

PROPPER, R., SHURIN, S. & NATHAN, D. (1976a). Constant subcutaneous (SC) infusion of desferrioxamine (DF) in transfused beta thalassemia patients (Thals). *Pediat. Res.*, **10**, 380 (Abstract 475).

PROPPER, R. D., SHURIN, S. B. & NATHAN, D. G. (1976b). Reassessment of the use of desferrioxamine β in iron overload. *New Engl. J. Med.*, **294**, 1421–1423.

RACHMILEWITZ, E. A., SHIFTER, A. & KAHANE, I. (1979). Vitamin E deficiency in β thalassemia major: changes in hematological parameters following therapeutic trial with α-tocopherol. *Amer. J. clin. Nutr.*, **32**, 1850–1858.

RAPAPORT, S. I., REILLY, E. B. & CARPENTER, G. (1957). Clinically "intermediate" thalassemia due to hypersplenism complicating thalassemia minor: a case report illustrating relief of anemia by splenectomy. *Ann. intern. Med.*, **46**, 1199–1207.

REEMTSMA, K. & ELLIOTT, R. H. E. JNR (1956). Splenectomy in Mediterranean anemia: an evaluation of long-term results. *Ann. Surg.*, **144**, 999–1007.

REIMANN, F. & ARKUN, N. S. (1955). Ein Vergleich der osmotischen Resistenz der roten Blutkörperchen bei den eisenempfindlichen chronischen Chloranämien und bei Fällen von Mittelmeeranämie. *Z. klin. Med.*, **153**, 14–34.

REWALD, E. (1964). Substitutive-inhibitory therapy in constitutional non-spherocytic erythrocytic disease. *Acta haemat. (Basel)*, **31**, 303–309.

RISDON, R. A., BARRY, M. & FLYNN, D. M. (1975). Transfusional iron overload: the relationship between tissue iron concentration and hepatic fibrosis in thalassaemia. *J. Path.*, **116**, 83–95.

RODECK, C. H. & CAMPBELL, S. (1978). Sampling pure fetal blood by fetoscopy in second trimester of pregnancy. *Brit. med. J.*, **ii**, 728–730.

RODECK, C. H. & MORSMAN, J. M. (1983). First-trimester chorion biopsy. *Brit. med. Bull.*, **39**, 338–342.

RODECK, C. H. & NICOLAIDES, K. H. (1983). Fetoscopy and fetal tissue sampling. *Brit. med. Bull.*, **34**, 332–337.

ROSATELLI, C., FALCHI, A. M. TUVERI, T., SCALAS, M. T., DI TUCCI, A., MOUNI, G. & CAO, A. (1985). Prenatal diagnosis of beta-thalassaemia with the synthetic-oligomer technique. *Lancet*, **i**, 241–243.

ROSNER, P., PFENNINGER, A. & MARTI, H. R. (1965). Hb H-α-thalassémie. A propos d'un cas. *Schweiz. med. Wschr.*, **95**, 739–742.

ROWLEY, P. T. (1976). The diagnosis of beta-thalassemia trait: a review. *Amer. J. Hemat.*, **1**, 129–137.

RUBIN, E. M. & KAN, Y. W. (1985). A simple sensitive prenatal test for hydrops fetalis caused by α-thalassaemia. *Lancet*, **i**, 75–77.

SCHMAIR, A. H., MAURER, H. M., JOHNSTON, C. L. & SCOTT, R. B. (1973). Alpha thalassemia screening in neonates by mean corpuscular volume and mean corpuscular hemoglobin determination. *J. Pediat.*, **83**, 794–797.

SCHORR, J. B. & RADEL, E. (1964). Transfusion therapy and its complications in patients with Cooley's anemia. *Ann. N.Y. Acad. Sci.*, **119**, 703–708.

SCHRIEVER, H. G. (1973). Differentiation of thalassaemia minor from iron deficiency. *Lancet*, **ii**, 154 (Letter).

SEPHTON SMITH, R. (1962). Iron excretion in thalassaemia major after administration of chelating agents. *Brit. med. J.*, **ii**, 1577–1580.

SEPHTON SMITH, R. (1964). Chelating agents in the diagnosis and treatment of iron loading in thalassaemia. *Ann. N.Y. Acad. Sci.*, **119**, 776–788.

SESHADRI, R., COLEBATCH, J. H. & FISHER, R. (1974). Urinary iron excretion in thalassaemia after desferrioxamine administration. *Arch. Dis. Childh.*, **49**, 195–199.

SESHADRI, R., COLEBATCH, J. H., GORDON, P. & EKERT, H. (1974). Long-term administration of desferrioxamine in thalassaemia major. *Arch. Dis. Childh.*, **49**, 621–626.

SEVEN, M. J., GOTTLIEB, H., ISRAEL, H. L., REINHOLD, J. G. & RUBIN, M. (1954). N-hydroxyethylenediamine triacetic acid, Versenol, in the treatment of hemochromatosis. *Amer. J. med. Sci.*, **228**, 646–651.

SHAHID, M. J. & SAHLI, I. T. (1971). Erythrokinetic studies in thalassaemia. *Brit. J. Haemat.*, **20**, 75–82.

SHAPIRO, I., SCHNECK, H. & ETESS, A. D. (1952). Splenectomy in two Chinese siblings with Mediterranean anemia. *N.Y. St. J. med.*, **52**, 1426–1430.

SHAW, P. J., POYNTON, C. H. & BARRETT, A. J. (1985). Timing of bone-marrow transplantation in thalassaemia major. *Lancet*, **ii**, 153 (Letter).

SHINE, I. & LAL, S. (1977). A strategy to detect β-thalassaemia minor. *Lancet*, **i**, 692–694.

SILVESTRONI, E. & BIANCO, I. (1975). Screening for microcytemia in Italy: analysis of data collected in the last 30 years. *Amer. J. hum. Genet.*, **27**, 198–212.

SILVESTRONI, E., BIANCO, I., GRAZIANI, B., CARBONI, C. & CONSTANTINI, S. (1978). Subcutaneous desferrioxamine in homozygous β-thalassaemia. *Lancet*, **ii**, 1149–1150 (Letter).

SILVESTRONI, B., BIANCO, I., GRAZIANI, B., LERONE, M., VALENTE, M., CONGEDO, P., PONZINI, D. & CONSTANTINI, S. (1982). Intensive iron chelation therapy in beta-thalassaemia major: some effects on iron metabolism and blood transfusion dependence. *Acta haemat. (Basel)*, **68**, 115–123.

SMITH, C. H., ERLANDSON, M. E., SCHULMAN, I. & STERN, G. (1957). Hazard of severe infections in splenectomized infants and children. *Amer. J. Med.*, **22**, 390–404.

SMITH, C. H., ERLANDSON, M. E., STERN, G. & HILGARTNER, M. W. (1962). Postsplenectomy infection in Cooley's anemia: an appraisal of the problem in this and other blood disorders, with a consideration of prophylaxis. *New Engl. J. Med.*, **266**, 737–743.

SMITH, C. H., ERLANDSON, M. E., STERN, G. & HILGARTNER, M. W. (1964). Postsplenectomy infection in Cooley's anemia. *Ann. N.Y. Acad. Sci.*, **119**, 748–757.

SMITH, C. H., ERLANDSON, M. E., STERN, G. & SCHULMAN, I. (1960). The role of splenectomy in the management of thalassemia. *Blood*, **15**, 197–211.

SMITH, C. H., SCHULMAN, I., ANDO, R. E. & STERN, G. (1955a). Studies in Mediterranean (Cooley's) anemia. I. Clinical and hematologic aspects of splenectomy, with special reference to fetal hemoglobin synthesis. *Blood*, **10**, 582–599.

SMITH, C. H., SCHULMAN, I., ANDO, R. E. & STERN, G. (1955b). Studies in Mediterranean (Cooley's) anemia. II. The supression of hematopoiesis by transfusions. *Blood*, **10**, 707–717.

SRIVASTAVA, P. C. (1973). Differentiation of thalassaemia minor from iron deficiency. *Lancet*, ii, 154–155 (Letter).

STEPHENS, A. D. (1985). Abnormal haemoglobins and thalassaemia: methods and control. *Acta haemat. (Basel)*, **74**, 1–5 (Editorial).

STILLMANN, R. G. (1917). A study of von Jaksch's anemia. *Amer. J. med. Sci.*, **153**, 218–231.

STOCKMAN, J. A. III, WEINER, L. S., SIMON, G. E., STUART, M. J. & OSKI, F. A. (1975). The measurement of free erythrocyte porphyrin (FEP) as a simple means of distinguishing iron deficiency from beta-thalassemia trait in subjects with microcytosis. *J. Lab. clin. Med.*, **85**, 113–119.

SUMMERS, M. R., JACOBS, A., TUDWAY, D., PERERA, P. & RICKETTS, C. (1979). Studies in desferrioxamine and ferrioxamine metabolism in normal and iron-loaded subjects. *Brit. J. Haemat.*, **42**, 547–555.

THEIN, S. L., WAINSCOAT, J. S., LYNCH, J. R., WEATHERALL, D. J., SAMPIETRO, M. & FIORELLI, G. (1985a). Direct detection of $\beta^0 39$ thalassaemic mutation with *Mae 1*. *Lancet*, i, 1095 (Letter).

THEIN, S. L., WAINSCOAT, J. S., OLD, J. M., SAMPIETRO, M., FIORELLI, G., WALLACE, R. B. & WEATHERALL, D. J. (1985b). Feasibility of prenatal diagnosis of β-thalassaemia with synthetic DNA probes in two Mediterranean populations. *Lancet*, ii, 345–347.

THOMAS, E. D., BUCKNER, C. D., SANDERS, J. E., PAPAYANNOPOULOU, T., BORGNA-PIGNATTI, C., DE STEFANO, P., SULLIVAN, K. M., CLIFT, R. A. & STORB, R. (1982). Marrow transplantation for thalassaemia. *Lancet*, ii, 227–229.

THOMAS, E. D., SANDERS, J. E., BUCKNER, C. D. PAPAYANNOPOULOU, TH., BORGNA-PIGNATTI, C., DE STEFANO, P., SULLIVAN, K. M., DEEG, H. J., WITHERSPOON, R. P., APPELBAUM, F. R., CLIFT, R. A. & STORB, R. (1985). Marrow transplantation for thalassemia. *Ann. N.Y. Acad. Sci.*, **445**, 417–427.

THOMPSON, R. B., ODOM, J. & BELL, W. N. (1965). Splenomegaly, anemia and thalassemia intermedia. *Amer. J. med. Sci.*, **250**, 298–307.

THORPE, S. J. & HUEHNS, E. R. (1983). A new approach for the antenatal diagnosis of β-thalassaemia: a double labelling immunofluorescence microscopy technique. *Brit. J. Haemat.*, **53**, 103–112.

TORLONTANO, G., TATA, A. & CAMAGNA, A. (1972). A rapid screening test for thalassaemic trait. *Acta haemat. (Basel)*, **48**, 234–238.

TSO, S. C., CHAN, T. K. & TODD, D. (1982). Venous thrombosis in haemoglobin H disease after splenectomy. *Aust. N.Z. J. Med.*, **12**, 635–638.

VATANAVICHARN, S., YENCHITSOMAS, P. & SIDDHIKOL, C. (1985). Vitamin E in β-thalassaemia and α-

thalassaemia (HbH) diseases. *Acta haemat. (Basel)*, **73**, 183.

VIRDIS, S. (1951). Resultati della splenectomia in un caso di ittero-anemia del tipo Rietti-Greppi-Micheli. *Haematologica*, **35**, 1045–1051.

WAHIDIJAT, I., MARKUM, A. H. & ADANG, Z. K. (1972). Early splenectomy in the management of thalassemic children in Djakarta. *Acta haemat. (Basel)*, **48**, 28–33.

WAINSCOAT, J. S., OLD, J. M., THEIN, S. L. & WEATHERALL, D. J. (1984). A new DNA polymorphism for prenatal diagnosis of β-thalassaemia in Mediterranean populations. *Lancet*, ii, 1299–1301.

WALFORD, D. M. (1977). α-thalassaemia in the United Kingdom. *Brit. J. Haemat.*, **35**, 347–350 (Annotation).

WALFORD, D. M. & DEACON, R. (1976). Alpha-thalassaemic trait in various racial groups in the United Kingdom: characterization of a variant of alpha-thalassaemia in Indians. *Brit. J. Haemat.*, **34**, 193–206.

WAPNICK, A. A., LYNCH, S. R., CHARLETON, R. W., SEFTEL, H. C. & BOTHWELL, T. H. (1969). The effect of ascorbic acid deficiency on desferrioxamine-induced urinary iron excretion. *Brit. J. Haemat.*, **17**, 563–568.

WAPNICK, A. A., LYNCH, S. R., KRAWITZ, P., SEFTEL, H. C., CHARLTON, R. W. & BOTHWELL, T. H. (1968). Effects of iron overload on ascorbic acid metabolism. *Brit. med. J.*, iii, 704–707.

WARD, R. H. T., MODELL, B., FAIRWEATHER, D. V. I., SHIRLEY, I. M., RICHARDS, B. A. & HETHERINGTON, C. P. (1981). Obstetric outcome and problems of mid-trimester fetal blood sampling for antenatal diagnosis. *Brit. J. Obstet. Gynaec.*, **88**, 1073–1080.

WASI, P. (1983). Population screening. In: *The Thalassemias (Methods in Hematology*, Vol. 6) (ed. by D. J. Weatherall), pp. 134–143. Churchill Livingstone, Edinburgh.

WASI, P., NA-NAKORN, S. & POOTRAKUL, S. N. (1974). The α thalassaemias. *Clinics Haemat.*, **3**, 383–410.

WASI, P., NA-NAKORN, S., POOTRAKUL, S., SOOKANCK, M., DISTHASONGCHAN, P., PORNPATKUL, M. & PANICH, V. (1969). Alpha- and beta-thalassemia in Thailand. *Ann. N.Y. Acad. Sci.*, **165**, 60–82.

WASI, P., PRAVATMUANG, P. & WINICHAGOON, P. (1979). Immunologic diagnosis of α-thalassemia traits. *Hemoglobin*, **3**, 21–31.

WASI, C., WASI, P. & THONGCHAROEN, P. (1971). Serum-immunoglobulin levels in thalassaemia and the effects of splenectomy. *Lancet*, ii, 237–239.

WAXMAN, H. S. & BROWN, E. B. (1969). Clinical usefulness of chelating agents. In: *Progress in Hematology*, Vol. VI (ed. by E. B. Brown), pp. 338–373. Grune and Stratton, New York.

WEATHERALL, D. J. (1983). The diagnostic features of the different forms of thalassemia. In: *The Thalassemias (Methods in Hematology*, Vol. 6) (ed. by D. J. Weatherall), pp. 1–26. Churchill Livingstone, Edinburgh.

WEATHERALL, D. J. (1985). Prenatal diagnosis of inherited blood diseases. *Clinics Haemat.*, **14**, 747–774.

WEATHERALL, D. J. & CLEGG, J. B. (1981). *The Thalassaemia Syndromes*, 3rd edn. 875 pp. Blackwell Scientific Publications, Oxford.

WEATHERALL, D. J., PIPPARD, M. J. & CALLENDER, S. T. (1977). Iron loading and thalassemia — experimental successes and practical realities. *New Engl. J. Med.*, **297**, 445–446 (Editorial).

WEATHERALL, D. J., PIPPARD, M. J. & CALLENDER, S. T. (1983). Iron loading in thalassemia — five years with the pump. *New Engl. J. Med.*, **308**, 456–458 (Editorial retrospective).

WEINER, M., KARPATKIN, M., HART, D., SEAMAN, C., VORA, S. K., HENRY, W. L. & PIOMELLI, S. (1978). Cooley anemia: high transfusion regimen and chelation therapy, results and perspective. *J. Pediat.*, **92**, 653–658.

WILLIAMS, D. A. & ORKIN, S. H. (1986). Somatic gene therapy. Current status and future prospects. *J. clin. Invest.*, **77**, 1053–1056.

WILLIAMSON, R., ESKDALE, J., COLEMAN, D. V., NIAZI, M., LOEFFLER, F. E. & MODELL, B. M. (1981). Direct gene analysis of chorionic villi. A possible technique for first-trimster antenatal diagnosis of haemoglobinopathies. *Lancet*, **ii**, 1125–1127.

WITZLEBEN, C. L. & WYATT, J. P. (1961). The effect of long survival on the pathology of thalassaemia major. *J. Path. Bact.*, **82**, 1–12.

WÖHLER, F. (1962). Erfahrungen mit Desferrioxamin bei pathologischen Eisenblagerungen. *Schweiz. med. Wschr.*, **92**, 1303–1304 (Gesprach am runden Tisch, Moeschlin, S., Leiter).

WÖHLER, F. (1963) The treatment of haemochromatosis with desferrioxamine. *Acta haemat. (Basel).* **30**, 65–87.

WOLFE, L., OLIVIERI, N., SALLAN, D., COLAN, S., ROSE, V., PROPPER, R., FREEDMAN, M. H. & NATHAN, D. G. (1985). Prevention of cardiac disease by subcutaneous deferoxamine in patients with thalassemia major. *New Engl. J. Med.*, **312**, 1600–1603.

WOLFE, L., SALLAN, D. & NATHAN, D. G. (1985). Current therapy and new approaches to the treatment of thalassemia major. *Ann. N.Y. Acad. Sci.*, **445**, 248–255.

WOLFF, J. A., SITARZ, A. L. & VON HOFE, F. H. (1960). Effect of splenectomy on thalassemia. *Pediatrics*, **26**, 674–678.

WOLFF, J. A., ULTMANN, J. E. & SITARZ, A. (1964). Relationship of erythrocyte survival and reticulocyte levels to splenectomy and need for transfusion in thalassemia major. *Ann. N.Y. Acad. Sci.*, **119**, 686–693.

WOLMAN, I. J. (1964). Transfusion therapy in Cooley's anemia: growth and health as related to long-range hemoglobin levels. A progress report. *Ann. N.Y. Acad. Sci.*, **119**, 736–747.

WOLMAN, I. J. & ORTOLANI, M. (1969). Some clinical features of Cooley's anemia patients as related to transfusion schedules. *Ann. N.Y. Acad. Sci.*, **165**, 407–414.

WOODROW, J. C., NOBLE, R. L. & MARTINDALE, J. H. (1964). Haemoglobin H disease in an English family. *Brit. med. J.*, **i**, 36–38.

WRIGHT, B. M. & CALLAN, K. (1979). Slow drug infusions using a portable syringe driver. *Brit. med. J.*, **ii**, 582.

YANG, T.-Y., YANG, X.-Y., CH'EN, W.-C., QI, S.-L., JIN, Y.-J., GAN, W.-J. & QU, Q. (1985). Thalassemia in China. *Ann. N.Y. Acad. Sci.*, **445**, 92–105.

ZANELLA, A., MILANI, S., FAGNANI, G., MARIANI, M. & SIRCHIA, G. (1983). Diagnostic value of the glycerol lysis test. *J. Lab. clin. Med.*, **102**, 743–750.

ZANNOS-MARIOLEA, L., TZORTZATOU, F., DENDAKI-SVOLAKI, K., KATERELLOS, CH., KAVALLARI, M. & MATSANIOTIS, N. (1974). Serum vitamin E levels with beta-thalassaemia major: preliminary report. *Brit. J. Haemat.*, **26**, 193–199.

ZENG, Y.-T. & HUANG, S.-Z. (1985). α-globin gene organization and prenatal diagnosis of α-thalassaemia in Chinese. *Lancet.*, **i**, 304–307.

Index